MANAGEMENT OF THE
DIFFICULT
AND
FAILED AIRWAY

MANAGEMENT OF THE
DIFFICULT
AND
FAILED AIRWAY

EDITORS

Orlando R. Hung, BSc (Pharmacy), MD, FRCP(C)

Professor, Departments of Anesthesia, Surgery and Pharmacology
Director of Research, Department of Anesthesia
Dalhousie University
Queen Elizabeth II Health Sciences Centre
Halifax, Nova Scotia, Canada

Michael F. Murphy, MD, FRCP(C)

Professor and Chair of Anesthesiology
Professor, Emergency Medicine
Dalhousie University
District Chief Anesthesiology
Capital District Health Authority
Attending Physician Emergency Medicine
Queen Elizabeth II Health Sciences Centre
Halifax, Nova Scotia, Canada

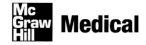

New York   Chicago   San Francisco   Lisbon   London   Madrid
Mexico City   Milan   New Delhi   San Juan   Seoul   Singapore   Sydney   Toronto

Management of the Difficult and Failed Airway

4 5 6 7 8 9 0   CTPS/CTPS   12 11 10

Book: ISBN 978-0-07-150856-8
       MHID   0-07-150856-2
Set: ISBN 978-0-07-144548-1
       MHID   0-07-144548-X
DVD: ISBN 978-0-07-150855-1
       MHID   0-07-150855-4

This book was set in Adobe Garamond by Aptara Inc.
The editor was Joe Rusko.
The production supervisor was Phil Galea.
The cover designer was John Vairo.
The cover photo is by Richard Price/Getty Images.
The interior designer was Alan Barnett.
Production management was handled by Aptara Inc.
China Translation & Printing Services, Ltd., was printer and binder.

This book is printed on acid-free paper.

Library of Congress Cataloging-in-Publication Data

Management of the difficult and failed airway / [edited by] Orlando Hung, Michael F. Murphy.
        p. ; cm.
  Includes bibliographical references and index.
  ISBN 978-0-07-144548-1 (alk. paper)
  1. Airway (Medicine) 2. Respiratory intensive care. 3. Trachea—Intubation. I. Hung, Orlando. II. Murphy, Michael F. (Michael Francis), 1954-
    [DNLM: 1. Airway Obstruction—therapy. 2. Airway Obstruction—prevention & control. 3. Intubation, Intratracheal.
WF 145 M2665 2007]
RC732.M36 2007
616.2—dc22
                                                                                    2007009183

ASSOCIATE EDITORS

Thomas J. Coonan, MD, FRCP(C)
Professor
Departments of Anesthesia and Surgery
Dalhousie University
Queen Elizabeth II Health Sciences Centre
Department of Anesthesia
Halifax, Nova Scotia, Canada

J. Adam Law, BSc, MD, FRCP(C)
Professor
Department of Anesthesia
Dalhousie University
Queen Elizabeth II Health Sciences Centre
Halifax, Nova Scotia, Canada

Ian R. Morris, BEng, MD, FRCP(C), FACEP
Professor
Department of Anesthesia
Dalhousie University
Queen Elizabeth II Health Sciences Centre
Halifax, Nova Scotia, Canada

Ronald D. Stewart, MD, FRCP(C), FACEP, OC
Professor
Departments of Anesthesiology, Emergency Medicine,
    Community Health and Epidemiology and Medical Humanities
Dalhousie University
Queen Elizabeth II Health Sciences Centre
Halifax, Nova Scotia, Canada

CONTENTS

CONTRIBUTORS

David C. Abramson, MBChB, FFA(SA)
North Texas Children's Anesthesia
Dallas, Texas
Airway Management of a 6-Year-Old with a History of Difficult Airway for Bilateral Inguinal Hernia Repair

Steven Abramson, MD
Assistant Professor
Department of Anesthesiology
The University of Texas Medical School at Houston
Houston, Texas
Airway Management of a Patient with History of Difficult Airway Who Refuses To Have Awake Tracheal Intubation

Felice E. Agrò, MD
Professor, Anesthesia and Intensive Care
Chairman, Postgraduate School of Anaesthesia and Intensive Care
Director, Department of Anaesthesiology and Intensive Care
University School of Medicine Campus Bio Medico of Rome, Italy
Medical Director, University Hospital Campus Bio Medico of Rome, Italy
Extraglottic Devices for Ventilation and Oxygenation

Aaron E. Bair, MD
Assistant Professor
Emergency Medicine
U.C. Davis Medical Center
Sacramento, California
Airway Management for Blunt Facial Trauma

Stephen Beed, MD, FRCP(C), DipABA, Cert CCM
Associate Professor Anesthesia and Medicine
Dalhousie University
Attending Anesthesiologist and Critical Care Physician
Departments of Anesthesia and Critical Care Medicine
Queen Elizabeth II Health Sciences Centre
Halifax, Nova Scotia, Canada
Airway Management in the Intensive Care Unit (ICU)

Kerry B. Broderick, MD
Emergency Medicine
Denver Health Medical Center
Denver, Colorado
Patient with Deadly Asthma Requires Intubation; Patient in Cardiogenic Shock

David A. Caro, MD
Associate Residency Director
Assistant Professor
Department of Emergency Medicine
University of Florida Health Science Center – Jacksonville
Jacksonville, Florida
Airway Management with Blunt Anterior Neck Trauma; Airway Management for Blunt Facial Trauma

Idena Carroll, CRNA, MS
Anesthesia Clinical & Educational Services, P.A.
Program Director
Nurse Anesthesia Program
Our Lady of the Lake College
Baton Rouge, Louisiana
Aspiration: Risks and Prevention; Airway Management for a Morbidly Obese Patient Suffering from a Cardiac Arrest

Rita Cataldo, MD
Consultant Anesthesiologist
Department of Anaesthesia
University School of Medicine
Campus Bio Medico of Rome, Italy
Rome, Italy
Extraglottic Devices for Ventilation and Oxygenation

Sabeena K. Chacko, MD
Assistant in Perioperative Anesthesia, Children's Hospital, Boston
Instructor in Anesthesia
Harvard Medical School
Boston, Massachusetts
Airway Management of a Newborn with a Tracheoesophageal Fistula (TEF)

Chris C. Christodoulou, MBChB, FRCP(C)
University of Manitoba
Department of Anesthesia
St. Boniface General Hospital
Winnipeg, Manitoba, Canada
Blind Intubation Techniques

Thomas J. Coonan, MD, FRCP(C)
Professor
Departments of Anesthesia and Surgery
Dalhousie University
Queen Elizabeth II Health Sciences Centre
Department of Anesthesia
Halifax, Nova Scotia, Canada
Extraglottic Devices for Ventilation and Oxygenation

Richard M. Cooper, BSc, MSc, MD, FRCP(C)
Professor
Faculty of Medicine
Department of Anesthesia
University of Toronto
Department of Anesthesia and Pain Management
Toronto General Hospital
Toronto, Ontario, Canada
Rigid and Semirigid Fiberoptic and Video Laryngoscopy and Intubation; Management of Extubation of a Patient Following a Prolonged Period of Mechanical Ventilation

Edward T. Crosby, MD, FRCP(C)
Department of Anesthesiology
Ottawa Hospital B General Campus
Ottawa, Ontario, Canada
The Algorithms; Aspiration: Risks and Prevention; Airway Management of a Patient with Traumatic Brain Injury (TBI)

D. John Doyle, MD, PhD, FRCP(C)
Staff Anesthesiologist
Department of General Anesthesiology
Cleveland Clinic Foundation
Cleveland, Ohio
Airway Evaluation, Extraglottic Devices for Ventilation and Oxygenation; Respiratory Arrest in the Magnetic Resonance Imaging (MRI) Suite

Dennis Drapeau, BSc, MD, FRCP(C)
Dalhousie University
Department of Anesthesia
Queen Elizabeth II Health Sciences Centre
Halifax, Nova Scotia, Canada
Intra-Operative Accidental Dislodgement of the Endotracheal Tube in a Patient in Prone Position

Lorraine J. Foley, MD
Winchester Anesthesia Associates
Clinical Associate Professor of Anesthesia
Tufts School of Medicine
Department of Anesthesia
Winchester Hospital
Winchester, Massachusetts
Airway Management of Patients with a History of Difficult Intubation for a Peripheral Procedure; Documentation of Difficult Airway

Michael Frass, MD
Professor of Medicine
Intensive Care Unit
Department of Internal Medicine
Medical University Vienna
Vienna, Austria
Management of an Accidental Extubation in a Patient in a Halo Jacket

Kyle Friedman, MD
Assistant Professor
Department of Anesthesiology
The University of Texas Medical School at Houston
Houston, Texas
Airway Management of a Patient with History of Difficult Airway Who Refuses To Have Awake Tracheal Intubation

Benedetta Gallì, MD
Staff Anesthesiologist
Department of Anaesthesia
University School of Medicine
Campus Bio Medico of Rome, Italy
Rome, Italy
Extraglottic Devices for Ventilation and Oxygenation

Ronald B. George, MD, FRCPC
Department of Anesthesia
Queen Elizabeth II Health Sciences Centre
Halifax, Nova Scotia, Canada
The Pharmacology of Intubation

Stephen A. Godwin, MD
Residency Director
Assistant Professor
Department of Emergency Medicine
University of Florida Health Science Center
Jacksonville, Florida
Airway Management with Blunt Anterior Neck Trauma; Unique Airway Issues in the Pediatric Population

Angelina Guzzo, MDCM, FRCPC, PhD
Department of Anesthesia
Queen Elizabeth II Health Sciences Centre
Halifax, Nova Scotia, Canada
Performing an Elective Percutaneous Dilational Tracheotomy in a Patient on Mechanical Ventilation

Carin Hagberg, MD
Professor
Department of Anesthesiology
The University of Texas Medical School at Houston
Houston, Texas
Airway Management of a Patient with History of Difficult Airway Who Refuses To Have Awake Tracheal Intubation

John J. Henderson, MB, ChB, FRCA
Consultant Anaesthetist
Gartnavel General Hospital
Glasgow, United Kingdom
Direct Laryngoscopy and Oral Intubation of the Trachea; Airway Management of a Patient with an Unanticipated Difficult Laryngoscopy

Orlando R. Hung, MD, FRCP(C)
Professor, Departments of Anesthesia, Surgery, and Pharmacology
Director of Research, Department of Anesthesia Dalhousie
   University
Queen Elizabeth II Health Sciences Centre
Department of Anesthesia
Halifax, Nova Scotia, Canda
*The Pharmacology of Intubation; Airway Devices and Techniques;
   Blind Intubation Techniques, Extraglottic Devices for Ventilation
   and Oxygenation; Airway Management of an Unconscious
   Patient Who Remains Trapped Inside the Vehicle Following a
   Motor Vehicle Accident; Airway Management of a Motorcyclist
   with a Full Face Helmet Following an Accident; Performing an
   Elective Percutaneous Dilational Tracheotomy in a Patient on
   Mechanical Ventilation; Intra-Operative Accidental
   Dislodgement of the Endotracheal Tube in a Patient in Prone
   Position*

Andy Jagoda, MD, FACEP
Professor and Vice Chair of Emergency Medicine
Mount Sinai School of Medicine
New York, New York
*Airway Management of a Patient with Traumatic Brain Injury
   (TBI)*

Liane B. Johnson, MDCM, FRCS(C)
Department of Otolaryngology
Dalhousie University
Department of Pediatric Otolaryngology
Queen Elizabeth II Health Sciences Centre
Halifax, Nova Scotia, Canada
*Surgical Airway; Performing an Elective Percutaneous Dilational
   Tracheotomy in a Patient on Mechanical Ventilation;
   Management of 12-Year-Old Child with a Foreign Body in the
   Bronchus*

David Kirkpatrick, MD, FRCSC
Professor and Head
Department of Otolaryngology
Dalhousie University
Queen Elizabeth II Health Sciences Centre
Halifax, Nova Scotia, Canada
Airway Management in a Patient with Retropharyngeal Abscess

Niranjan "Tex" Kissoon, MD, FRCP(C), FAAP, FCCM, FACPE
Senior Medical Director
Acute and Critical Care Programs
Associate Head, Department of Pediatrics
Professor, Pediatric and Surgery (EM)
British Columbia Children's Hospital
University of British Columbia
Vancouver, British Columbia, Canada
*Unique Airway Issues in the Pediatric Population; Pediatric Patient
   with a Closed Head Injury*

Babu V. Koka, MD
Division Chief in Perioperative Anesthesia
Senior Associate in Perioperative Anesthesia,
   Children's Hospital, Boston
Assistant Professor in Anesthesia
Harvard Medical School
Boston, Massachusetts
*Airway Management of a Newborn with a Tracheoesophageal
   Fistula (TEF)*

Gordon O. Launcelott, MD, FRCP(C)
Department of Anesthesia
Dalhousie University
Queen Elizabeth II Health Sciences Centre
Halifax, Nova Scotia, Canada
*Surgical Airway, Airway Management of a Patient with Superior
   Vena Cava Obstruction Syndrome*

J. Adam Law, BSc, MD, FRCP(C)
Professor
Department of Anesthesia
Dalhousie University
Queen Elizabeth II Health Sciences Centre
Halifax, Nova Scotia. Canada
*Rigid and Semirigid Fiberoptic and Video Laryngoscopy and
   Intubation Airway Management of a Patient with Traumatic
   Bran Injury (TBI); Management of the Patient with a Neck
   Hematoma Postobstructive Pulmonary Edema (POPE)*

Robert C. Luten, MD
Professor
Pediatrics and Emergency Medicine
College of Medicine
University of Florida
Jacksonville, Florida
*Unique Airway Issues in the Pediatric Population; Pediatric Patient
   with a Closed Head Injury*

Kirk J. MacQuarrie, MD, FRCP(C)
Assistant Professor
Department of Anesthesia
Dalhousie University
Deputy Chief
Department of Anesthesia
Queen Elizabeth II Health Sciences Centre
Halifax, Nova Scotia, Canada
*Airway Management of a Patient with Cardiogenic Pulmonary
   Edema; Airway Management in a Patient with Retropharyngeal
   Abscess*

Neilson J. McLean, MD
Emergency Medicine Resident
Division of Emergency Medicine
University of British Columbia
Vancouver General Hospital
Vancouver, British Columbia, Canada
Airway Management in a Patient with Angioedema

Ian R. Morris, BEng, MD, FRCP(C), FACEP
Professor,
Department of Anesthesia
Dalhousie University
Queen Elizabeth II Health Sciences Centre
Halifax, Nova Scotia, Canada
*Preparation for Awake Intubation; Flexible Fiberoptic Intubation;
Airway Management in the Operating Room of a Patient with a
History of Oral and Cervical Radiation Therapy*

Holly A. Muir, MD, FRCPC
Chief, Division of Women's Anesthesia
Vice Chair Clinical Operations
Director of Perioperative Leaders Group, DN OR
Assistant Professor of Anesthesia
Associate of Obstetrics and Gynecology
Duke University Medical Center
Durham, North Carolina
*Unanticipated Difficult Airway in an Obstetrical Patient Requiring
an Emergency Cesarean Section; Airway Management in the
Pregnant Trauma Victim*

Michael F. Murphy, MD, FRCP(C)
Professor and Chair Anesthesiology
Professor, Emergency Medicine
Dalhousie University
District Chief Anesthesiology
Capital District Health Authority
Attending Physician Emergency Medicine
Queen Elizabeth II Health Sciences, Centre
Halifax, Nova Scotia, Canada
*Airway Evaluation; The Algorithms; Airway Devices and
Techniques; What Is Unique About Airway Management in the
Prehospital Setting?; Airway Management in the Emergency
Department; Airway Management of a Patient with a Stab
Wound to the Neck; Airway Management in a Patient with
Angioedema; Management of an Accidental Extubation in a
Patient in a Halo Jacket; Uncooperative Down Syndrome
Patient; Unique Airway Issues in the Pediatric Population;
Pediatric Patient with a Closed Head Injury; Unique Challenges
of Ectopic Airway Management; Difficult Airway Carts*

Adeyemi J. Olufolabi, MB, BS, DCH, FRCA
Division of Women's Anesthesia
Duke University Medical Center
Durham, North Carolina
*Unanticipated Difficult Airway in an Obstetrical Patient Requiring
an Emergency Cesarean Section; Airway Management in the
Pregnant Trauma Victim*

David Petrie, MD, FRCPC
Attending Emergency Physician
Queen Elizabeth II Health Sciences Centre
Associate Professor, Emergency Medicine
Dalhousie University
Halifax, Nova Scotia, Canada
What Is Unique About Airway Management in the Prehospital Setting?

Tom C. Phu, MD
Department of Anesthesia
Queen Elizabeth II Health Sciences Centre
Halifax, Nova Scotia, Canada
*Airway Management of an Unconscious Patient Who Remains
Trapped Inside the Vehicle Following a Motor Vehicle Accident*

Saul Pytka, MD, FRCP(C)
Associate Professor
Department of Anesthesiology
University of Calgary
Attending Anesthesiologist
Rockyview Hospital
Calgary, Alberta, Canada
*Aspiration: Risks and Prevention; Airway Management of a
Morbidly Obese Patient Suffering from a Cardiac Arrest;
Difficult Airway Carts*

Brian K. Ross, PhD, MD
Professor
Department of Anesthesiology
University of Washington
Seattle, Washington
*What Is Unique about the Obstetrical Airway?, Airway Management
of the Obstetrical Patient with an Anticipated Difficult Airway*

Robert E. Schneider, MD
Emergency Medicine Physician
Consultant: Department of Homeland Security
United States Government
Washington, DC
The Pharmacology of Intubation

Matthew G. Simms, MSc, MD
Resident
Department of Anesthesia, Faculty of Medicine
Dalhousie University
Queen Elizabeth II Health Sciences Centre
Halifax, Nova Scotia, Canada
Postobstructive Pulmonary Edema (POPE)

Christian M. Soder, MD, FRCPC
Chief, Department of Pediatric Critical Care
Associate Professor of Anesthesia and Pediatrics
Dalhousie University
Queen Elizabeth II Health Sciences Centre
Halifax, Nova Scotia, Canada
*Airway Management of a Child with Epiglottitis; Airway
Management in a 1-Year-Old with Pierre Robin Syndrome for
Myringotomy and Tubes*

Ronald D. Stewart, MD, FRCP(C), FACEP, OC
Professor
Departments of Anesthesiology, Emergency Medicine,
    Community Health and Epidemiology and Medical
    Humanities
Queen Elizabeth II Health Sciences Centre
Halifax, Nova Scotia, Canada
*Airway Management of an Unconscious Patient Who Remains
    Trapped Inside the Vehicle Following a Motor Vehicle Accident*

John Tallon, MD, FRCP(C)
Attending Emergency Physician
Queen Elizabeth II Health Sciences Center
Associate Professor, Emergency Medicine
Dalhousie University
Halifax, Nova Scotia, Canada
*What Is Unique About Airway Management in the Prehospital
    Setting?*

Robert J. Vissers, MD, FRCP(C), FACEP
Director
Department of Emergency Medicine
Legacy Emanuel Hospital
Adjunct Associate Professor
Oregon Health Sciences University
Lake Oswego, Oregon
*Airway Management in the Patient with Burns to the Head, Neck,
    Upper Torso and the Airway*

Mark P. Vu, MD, FRCP(C)
Department of Anesthesia
Dalhousie University
Queen Elizabeth II Health Sciences Centre
Department of Anesthesia
Halifax, Nova Scotia, Canada
*Airway Management of a Motorcyclist with a Full Face Helmet
    Following an Accident*

Ron M. Walls, MD
Chairman Department of Emergency Medicine
Brigham and Women's Hospital
Associate Professor of Medicine
Division of Emergency Medicine,
Harvard Medical School
Boston, Massachusetts
Airway Management in the Emergency Department

David T. Wong, MD
Associate Professor
University of Toronto
Department of Anesthesia
Toronto Western Hospital
Toronto, Ontario, Canada
*Management of a SARS Patient Admitted to the ICU with
    Impending Respiratory Failure and a Clinical Suspicion of
    Difficult Airway Airway Management in the Operating Room of
    a Morbidly Obese Patient in a "Can't Intubate, Can't Ventilate"
    (CICV) Situation*

Richard D. Zane, MD
Vice Chair
Department of Emergency Medicine
Brigham and Women's Hospital
Assistant Professor
Harvard Medical School
Boston, Massachusetts
Patient with Deadly Asthma Requires Intubation

FOREWORD

As in all fields of human endeavor, increasing knowledge leads to increasing specialization. No single practitioner of the science and art of anesthesia can be expected to absorb and become skilled in the immense range of procedures which form part of today's practice. The general anesthesiologist, like the general surgeon, is fast becoming an anachronism. We would not wish our child to be anesthetized by anyone other than an experienced pediatric anesthesiologist; nor would we wish to undergo a complex cardiac procedure, were the person responsible for maintaining our bodies in unconscious homeostasis not performing this delicate balancing act on a regular basis. Airway management, often described as the cornerstone of anesthesia practice, is no exception to this general phenomenon. The subject has grown immensely over the last twenty years and, as in other fields, the pace of change is accelerating. But there is a difference. The skills and techniques of airway management are required in all branches of anesthesia and also outside the hospital environment—wherever control of ventilation may be required. Yet because it remains impossible to predict many cases of difficult airways, and because when problems arise disaster may be only minutes away, skill in diagnosis and use of appropriate tools for management of the airway cannot be left to an "airway expert." Whatever branch of anesthesia or emergency care we are involved in, we all need to be able to react appropriately in the face of the airway emergency. Yet how do we become expert at something like managing a truly difficult airway if this situation arises so rarely that we may seldom, if ever, encounter it?

Clearly, there is a problem here and it is a problem which this book goes a long way towards addressing. There is no shortage of airway experts between its covers. They have collaborated to provide a balanced yet very detailed and above all very practical account of the subject, including a careful analysis of what constitutes an acceptable standard of care. Overall, the book offers a very comprehensive survey of the tools of airway management and the situations in which they may be indicated. The use of case histories drawn from actual experience is a particularly valuable approach which adds to the vivid, easy-to-read format. The text is accompanied by abundant high-quality illustrations, particularly valuable in the understanding of the anatomy of the upper airway in relation to regional anesthetic techniques.

It is important to understand what this book does and does not offer, however. It should not be considered as a compendium of rules covering every conceivable airway problem. The case histories represent logical responses to real problems; however, it should not be forgotten that every situation is unique and that there may be more than one valid solution to any given problem. For example, two equally competent practitioners may choose different device options or strategies, depending on their familiarity and skill with a particular device or procedure. Another point to bear in mind is that new studies and techniques are emerging at an ever-increasing rate, so that it is impossible for any textbook of this scope to be fully up-to-date, even at the moment of going to press. The authors have rightly emphasized the importance of tried and tested methods of airway management, but all of us are aware that the pace of change in this field is such that we must keep open minds. The best solutions available today are likely to be challenged sooner or later. Nevertheless, our ability to critically evaluate new possibilities depends on having a clear grasp of the foundations of our practice. Hung et al. have collaborated to offer you just that—whether you are a novice or a seasoned practitioner, the book you hold in your hands is an invaluable compendium of knowledge on the subject of airway management, and deserves a prominent place in your library.

Dr. Archie Brain
December, 2006

PREFACE

Why another textbook addressing "The Airway"? First, this book deals exclusively with the identification and management of *difficult* and *failed* airways which, if not properly managed, are associated with adverse outcomes and increased medical legal liability. Second, difficult and failed airways continue to be a source of great anxiety to practitioners responsible for airway management. Finally, there is no text that presents a consistent approach to the difficult and failed airway in all clinical settings.

Throughout the book, one is reminded that the basic principle of airway management is oxygenation, rather than laryngoscopy and intubation.

Relying to the extent possible on the available evidence, the authors of these chapters provide a conceptual approach and strategies and tactics to manage patients with difficult or failed airways. Sadly, few randomized, double-blind, controlled clinical trials (Level 1 evidence) are available to enable us to evaluate specific airway approaches, techniques, or devices. Most randomized clinical trials examining airway techniques or devices involve small numbers of patients with too few subjects to draw valid conclusions. Most of the existing clinical evidence consists of case reports, case series, and reviews. Although there are limitations in drawing conclusions from these clinical observations, these reports are probably the best evidence we have to guide critical decision making in managing a difficult or failed airway.

There is good clinical evidence that failure to properly evaluate the airway and to predict difficulty is the most important factor leading to a failed airway. For this reason, airway management must be approached with a view that alternative devices or techniques may be necessary should the primary plan fail. Accordingly, the practitioner must evaluate the airway for difficulty relative to each of the alternatives contemplated. For example, Mallampati Classification and thyromental distance may help the practitioner predict difficult laryngoscopy and intubation; but an assessment must also be done for difficulties related to bag-mask-ventilation, ventilation using extraglottic devices, tracheal intubation using other devices (e.g., the Trachlight), and the performance of a surgical airway.

This text adopts a fairly mechanistic approach to the airway, an approach developed by the founders of the "Difficult Airway Course." This approach is reputed by those who have taken these courses to reduce performance anxiety, improve clinical decision-making and performance, and mitigate adverse outcomes. The text, together with the videos, advocate an orderly approach to the evaluation of the airway, the appropriate use of medications to facilitate airway management, and the possession of an array of reliable techniques to rescue the airway in the event it is required. Mnemonics and algorithms are employed as memory aids and management strategies that have proven track records in the evaluation and management of medical emergencies in general, and airway management emergencies in particular. With an organized approach, a competent airway practitioner should be able to reliably predict a difficult airway, to immediately recognize a failed airway, and to be able to secure the airway with adequate gas exchange using alternative airway techniques.

The book is divided into four sections that discuss the principles of difficult and failed airway management; devices and techniques; difficult and failed airways in different patient populations and "practical considerations." The chapters in each section deal with contemporary issues and approaches to difficult and failed airway management in the prehospital arena, in the Emergency Department, operating rooms, intensive care units, and other clinical settings. The "questions" format in each chapter is designed to highlight some issues and concerns for learners and practitioners when faced with patients having a "challenging" airway. The "answers" appear at the end of the book.

It is our hope that this book will provide the reader with a conceptual framework and a practical approach to caring for patients with airway challenges, and that it may, in turn, help result in favorable outcomes for all.

ACKNOWLEDGMENTS

We wish to acknowledge the contributions and collaborations of all the authors. We are grateful for their tireless efforts to be clear, engaging and accurate. We wish to specifically thank Sara Whynot for her editorial assistance, Christopher Hung for scanning and processing all the images, Christopher Hung and David Hung for production of the DVD. We also wish to acknowledge the support of dedicated staff at McGraw-Hill.

Orlando R. Hung, MD
Michael F. Murphy, MD

SECTION 1 — Foundations of Difficult and Failed Airway Management

CHAPTER (1)

Airway Evaluation

Michael F. Murphy and D. John Doyle

1.1 INTRODUCTION

"Airway management" may be defined as the application of therapeutic interventions that are intended to effect gas exchange in patients. "Gas exchange" is the fundamental feature of this definition.[1] A number of devices and techniques are commonly employed in health care settings to achieve this goal, e.g., bag-mask-ventilation (BMV), extraglottic devices (EGDs), oral or nasal endotracheal intubation, and surgical airway management techniques.

The failure to adequately manage the airway has been identified as a major factor leading to poor outcomes in anesthesia, emergency medicine, critical care, and Emergency Medical Services (EMS).[2,3] In fact, adverse respiratory events constituted the largest single cause of injury in the ASA Closed Claims Project.[4] Furthermore, it has been repeatedly shown that the single most important factor leading to a failed airway is the failure to predict the difficult airway.[3–5]

Bedside screening tests designed to predict difficult laryngoscopic intubation in otherwise normal patients have proven to be so unreliable that airway practitioners need to be prepared to manage a failed airway every time they are faced with a patient in need of airway management.[6,7]

This chapter deals with the identification of the difficult and failed airway, particularly in an emergency, in which evaluation and management must be done concurrently in a compressed time frame and cancelling the case or delaying management is not an option. Successful airway management is generally governed by four intertwined factors:

1. A clinical situation of varying urgency, venue, and resources.

2. Patient factors including airway anatomy and vital organ system reserve.

3. Available airway resources.

4. Skills of the airway practitioner.

Because one must choose a method of airway management from an array of techniques, some degree of precision of language is essential. For example, a difficult oral laryngoscopy and intubation may not necessarily constitute a difficult *airway* if BMV is easily performed. In the same way, a failed intubation does not necessarily constitute a failed airway. A failed *intubation,* defined narrowly as the failure to be able to intubate on three attempts,[8] may not constitute a failed *airway* if one is able to effect gas exchange with BMV or with an EGD. However, "intubation failure" ought to conjure a sense of urgency and mandates the airway practitioner to rapidly switch to a failed airway management sequence because such a situation may become life-threatening if gas exchange cannot be provided expeditiously and adequately by other means. Furthermore, the alternative airway technique employed must have the highest degree of success in the practitioner's skill set. It is inappropriate to make random disorganized attempts to manage the airway in the hope that one of the airway techniques might work. Rather, one should have a planned strategy (Chapter 2) including invasive techniques such as cricothyrotomy.[2–5]

Caveat:

Failure to Evaluate the Airway and Predict Difficulty is the Single Most Important Factor Leading to a Failed Airway.

ASA Close Claims Database[4]

1.2   INCIDENCE OF DIFFICULT AND FAILED AIRWAY

1.2.1   How common are the difficult and failed airway?

Bag-mask-ventilation, the use of EGDs, endotracheal intubation, and surgical airway management constitute the four primary avenues by which gas exchange is provided in the event patients are unable to do so adequately for themselves. In each category, difficulty and failure may be encountered. Failure of all four, ordinarily, leads to the demise of the patient.

Until recently, the success or failure of airway management has been defined in terms of BMV and orotracheal intubation. The introduction of EGDs and the heightened profile of cricothyrotomy have broadened such concepts. Fortunately, tracheal intubation is usually straightforward, particularly in the elective setting of the operating room (OR). The same cannot be said for other venues.

Airways that are difficult to manage are fairly common in anesthesia and emergency medicine practice, with some estimates as high as 20% of all emergency intubations.[9–13] However, the incidence of intubation failure is quite uncommon (ranging 0.5–2.5%), and the disastrous situation of being unable to intubate or ventilate rarely occurs (0.1–0.05%).[2,9–18] This translates to a "can't intubate, can't ventilate" failure rate of about 1:1000 to 1:2000 patients in a general surgical population. The incidence is strikingly higher in the parturient undergoing caesarian section (1:280), an almost tenfold increase. In fact, half of the excess mortality (28 times) seen with general anesthesia for caesarian section over regional anesthesia is attributable to airway management failure.[19–21]

1.2.2   How do we avoid airway management failure?

Although circumstances can vary widely, the expectation is the same: timely, flawlessly executed airway management without injury to the patient. In circumstances of multiple trauma, facial or airway swelling, abnormal anatomy, upper-airway hemorrhage, or a myriad of other difficult airway scenarios, intubation may be difficult, or even impossible, and even BMV can fail. Nevertheless, the expectation remains that the patient's airway be promptly secured and oxygenation be maintained.

The American Society of Anesthesiologists (ASA) responding to an identified need to reduce the incidence of airway management failure issued guidelines for management of the difficult airway and an algorithm in 1993, followed by a revision in 2003.[6,22] The guidelines stressed the importance of performing an airway evaluation for difficulty prior to inducing and paralyzing the patient. Planned awake intubation, awakening the patient in the presence of a failed airway, and acquiring skills in alternative airway-management techniques are hallmarks of the 1993 guidelines. The 2003 guidelines reemphasize the importance of the airway evaluation and incorporate the laryngeal mask airway (LMA™) as a discrete step in the algorithm should failure occur. Unfortunately, the guidelines are less useful outside the OR, especially in circumstances in which intubation must be accomplished quickly and awakening the patient is not an option. Even in the OR setting, explicit guidelines for the rapid evaluation of an airway for occult difficulty and the prioritization of rescue maneuvers in the event of a mandated immediate intubation are not well handled by the ASA guidelines and algorithm (see Chapter 2). Furthermore, the ASA guidelines do not take into consideration patients who are uncooperative (e.g., young children or mentally challenged patients) or different patient populations (e.g., parturients).

Further complicating this issue are the many new, effective, and safe airway devices that have been introduced to assist with difficult and failed airway management. Flexible fiberoptic intubating bronchoscopes (FFB) have become more portable and easier to use and have been joined by a collection of rigid fiberoptic scopes (e.g., Shikani Optical Stylet™, Bullard Laryngoscope™, Bonfils™ Stylet, Upsher Laryngoscope™, etc.) and hybrid devices employing cameras or fiberoptics such as video-laryngoscopes (e.g., GlideScope®, Videolaryngoscope™, see Chapter 9). The laryngeal mask airway (LMA™) and intubating laryngeal mask airway (ILMA™ or LMA Fastrach™) have taken on a distinct role in the management of both the difficult and the failed airway. The Combitube™ has often been used as a lifesaving rescue device. Lighted stylet methods (e.g., Trachlight™) may permit light-guided intubation in situations in which the vocal cords cannot be visualized. Certain airways are impossible to manage by any means other than surgical cricothyrotomy—a procedure of increasing importance for all airway practitioners.

The challenge for any airway practitioner is to be able to accurately predict when a difficult airway is present, to *immediately* recognize when an intubation failure has occurred, and to reliably and reproducibly secure continuous gas exchange in both of these unnerving circumstances.

1.3   STANDARD OF CARE

1.3.1   Is there a prevailing standard of care in managing the difficult and failed airway? How is it defined?

The growth in knowledge and evidence related to the practice of airway management is relentless. The challenge for the practitioner is to keep abreast of new information, new techniques, and the changing expectations by our colleagues and patients. Advances in airway management over the past decade have significantly improved patient outcome with a reduction in the incidence of death and disability. Therefore, it is important for practitioners to keep abreast of these advances in airway management in their clinical practice.

Black's Law Dictionary[23] defines the *Standard of Care* as

> The **average** degree of skill, care and diligence exercised by members of the same profession, practicing in the **same or similar locality** in light of the **present state** of medical and surgical science.

This definition incorporates several important features:

- average degree of skill
- same or similar locality
- present state of knowledge

Taking these into consideration, the *Standard of Care* is the conduct and skill of an average and "prudent practitioner" that can be expected by a "reasonable patient." A bad result due to a failure to meet the standard of care is generally considered to be malpractice. There are two main sources of information as to exactly what is the expected standard of care:

- The beliefs and opinions of experts in the field.
- The published scientific evidence, standards of care, practice guidelines, protocols.

Ultimately the standard of care is what a jury says it is!

Driven by the complex nature of this clinical dilemma and the need for successful solutions that are easily learned and maintained (and cost-effective), the standard of care in airway management is exceedingly dynamic. Continuing evolution of new devices and techniques, or ways of thinking, modify the existing standard of care on an ongoing basis. It is incumbent on practitioners to keep abreast of new devices and techniques and remain facile with existing rescue techniques. They can do so by continually perusing the literature and attending educational programs related to airway management.

1.3.2 What is the role of professional organizations in establishing the standard of care?

International, national, regional, and local professional organizations generally address issues relevant to airway management in a variety of ways. Most national societies, such as the American Society of Anesthesiologists (ASA), the Difficult Airway Society (UK), the American Association of Nurse Anesthetists (AANA), the American College of Emergency Physicians (ACEP), the Canadian Anesthesiologists' Society (CAS), and others, engage in crafting standards of care and practice guidelines. [6,22,24,25]

In the event of an untoward outcome, the "reasonable patient" expects the published standards to be observed by the "prudent practitioner." Organizations that craft and publish such practice guidelines are careful to stipulate that such guidelines do not constitute the *Standard of Care*.[6,22] Unfortunately, guidelines are often perceived as the standard of care, particularly in a medical–legal context.

Professional organizations often provide educational initiatives to ensure that their members practice at the prevailing standard. The ASA, ACEP, and the Society for Airway Management (SAM) are good examples. SAM is an organization committed to advancing knowledge and improving the quality of airway care to our patients. This international society blends the expertise of anesthesia, otolaryngology, head and neck surgery, critical care, and emergency medicine to debate issues related to airway management. The SAM serves as a sounding board, not only for new devices and techniques but also for those wishing to challenge traditional dogma and advance new frontiers. Those with a specific interest in airway management are well advised to become involved in this organization.

1.3.3 How can we integrate the *standard of care* into our clinical practice?

Despite all these initiatives, the *Standard of Care* remains elusive, particularly when applied to the management of the difficult and

failed airway. It means different things to different practitioners and is situation dependent. For example,

- to the plaintiff's attorney, it must be precisely defined in the most minute of detail;
- to the practitioner, it is what they do every day;
- to the *defendant* practitioner, it is consistent with their actions.

It is perhaps easier to articulate what it is not:

- It is not so low as to consistently lead to bad outcomes.
- It is neither much better nor much worse care than that delivered on average by one's peers.
- It is not the same as the care provided by "experts" managing difficult and failed airways everyday.
- It is not what ivory tower, academic experts "think" it "ought to be."
- It is not a single study published in a reputable journal last week, or a position advocated by "experts" in an editorial in a similarly reputable journal.

We do know that the *Standard of Care* is dynamic and our patients expect to receive it at a minimum.

Perhaps the best test with respect to difficult and failed airway management is to ask a specific question: "Should the *average, reasonable, and prudent practitioner...*"

- be able to recognize and manage an anticipated difficult airway?
- be able to manage an unanticipated difficult airway?
- be able to use an FFB to intubate the trachea of a patient?
- be able to recognize and manage the failed airway?
- be facile with one or two rescue devices or techniques in the face of a failed airway?
- be able to perform a surgical airway? Or at the least, transtracheal ventilation?

It is reasonable to suspect that most practitioners charged with managing airways would answer *yes* to all of these questions and thereby *define the standard of care.*

1.4 DEVELOPMENT OF LARYNGOSCOPIC INTUBATION

1.4.1 How did the design of laryngoscopes and the basic technique of oral laryngoscopy evolve?

Herholdt and Rafn are generally credited with first describing blind oral intubation in 1796. Subsequently, Desault described blind nasal intubation in 1814. Although Sir William Macewen described direct vision oral intubation in 1880, it is generally accepted that the first description of laryngoscopic-aided oral intubation as we know it today was by Kirsten in 1895. By 1907, Chevalier Jackson, an ENT surgeon of considerable renown, introduced distal lighting to the laryngoscope, and Janeway, in 1913, innovated the insertion of electric batteries into the handle of

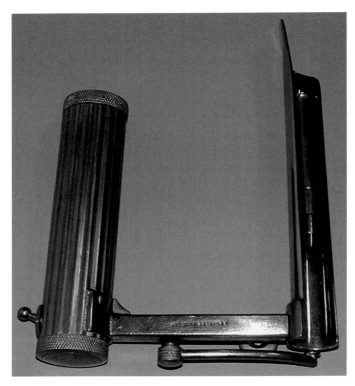

FIGURE 1-1. The Magill's laryngoscope.

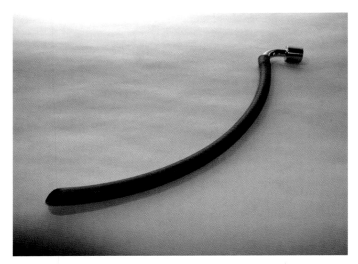

FIGURE 1-2. The Magill bevel on the endotracheal tube.

a laryngoscope to facilitate the procedure. Magill and Rowbotham engineered the straight Magill blade in the 1920s by cutting a wedge out of the side of the blade of the ENT surgeon's anterior commissure laryngoscope to facilitate intubation (Figure 1-1). Across the Atlantic, this design (with minor modifications) became known as the Miller blade in the 1940s. The Macintosh blade was also introduced in the 1940s by Sir Robert Macintosh.[26]

Magill is credited with introducing the "retro-molar" or "para-glossal" approach, reasoning that placing the blade as far to the corner of the mouth as possible when attempting to bring the glottis into view (as opposed to being in the midline) ought to minimize the distance to the glottis and enhance the degree to which it is visible. This technique has recently been resurrected by Henderson.[27]

1.4.2   How did the design of endotracheal tubes evolve?

It was also Sir Ivan Magill (circa 1914) who recommended a left-sided bevel (Magill bevel) be created on the distal tip of an endotracheal tube (ETT) (Figure 1-2). At that time, blind nasal intubation using a nonbeveled, gum-elastic tube was popular. Magill observed that, as the right nostril is usually largest and most anesthesia practitioners are right handed, nasotracheal intubation was usually at first attempted through the right nostril. The natural tendency for a tube introduced through the right nostril was to deviate leftward as it transited the nasopharynx and oropharynx and to deflect off the left glottic structures into the left pyriform recess. Magill reasoned that the left-sided bevel would deflect the ETT into the glottis.[28] Left-side bevel ETTs continue to be the most commonly used tubes to this day.

Curare and succinylcholine were introduced into anesthetic practice during the 1940s. These drugs led to the need for positive pressure ventilation, a tracheal seal being achieved by packing gauze (at times oil soaked) into the glottic opening. A more effective seal could be obtained by incorporating a balloon (initially rubber, thick walled, high pressure, and removable) onto the ETT. However, the possibility that the beveled orifice of the distal tip could rest against the wall of the bronchus in the event of a right mainstem intubation permitting positive pressure inspiration but not passive expiration was noted. This led to the creation of the Murphy eye opposite the bevel orifice.

The bulk of the ETT and balloon hindered its passage through the channel of laryngoscope blades, and this led the Eschmann Corporation to introduce the intubating stylet to facilitate a Seldinger-type intubation over the stylet in 1949.[29]

1.4.3   How has our understanding of how the difficult airway might be predicted developed over the years?

The use of neuromuscular blockade to facilitate oral endotracheal intubation followed the introduction of curare into anesthetic practice in the early 1940s and succinylcholine in the late 1940s. Up until that time, orotracheal intubation was largely performed with the patient ventilating spontaneously under inhalational anesthesia. The consequence of a failed intubation was mitigated by the fact that the patient continued to breathe spontaneously. The threat of failure to intubate in the face of neuromuscular blockade and apnea required anesthesia practitioners to evaluate the airway for difficulty, leading to a landmark publication by Cas;[30] in 1956 this study outlined those anatomical features that might predict difficult laryngoscopic intubation. Thus, the clinical use of neuromuscular blocking agents became inseparable from the ability to perform an airway evaluation and the ability to rescue the airway in the event of failure. Many practitioners continue to fail to recognize a difficult airway when one exists or they overlook the evaluation altogether.[4,6]

The literature regarding the difficult airway was relatively quiet until the mid-1980s when Patil offered the proposition that a thyromental distance of less than 6 cm was associated with

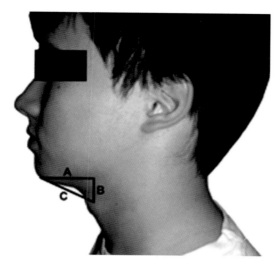

FIGURE 1-3. The Patil's triangle. (**A**) The second "3" of the "3-3-2" evaluation; (**B**) the "2" of the "3-3-2" evaluation; (**C**) the thyromental distance.

orotracheal intubation difficulty. During the 1990s, Savva did the same by using the sternomental distance.[31] The importance of Patil's dimension rests not in the distance described, or in its lack of sensitivity, specificity, or positive predictive value with respect to airway management difficulty, but in the fact that it alludes to the "geometry" of the airway. The thyromental line constitutes the hypotenuse of a right angle triangle (Figure 1-3). The axis is length of the floor of the mouth (a dimension of the mandibular space), and the abscissa locates the larynx in relation to the floor of the mouth. The length of the oral axis affects the ease with which the glottis is exposed during conventional laryngoscopy: too long and the glottis cannot be visualized beyond the horizon of visibility; too short and the larynx is shielded by the base of the tongue ("anterior larynx"). Likewise for the location of the larynx in relation to the base of the tongue: too far down the neck and it is beyond the visible horizon; too high in the neck and it is tucked up under the base of the tongue. Furthermore, the dimensions of the mandibular space (length, width, and depth; or volume) have important implications. The volume of the mandibular space must accommodate the tongue, a fluid-filled noncompressible structure, as it is displaced into this space during laryngoscopy to bring the glottis into view.

Mallampati in 1983 and 1985 created a scoring system,[32,33] modified by Samsoon in 1987,[34] that identified oral and pharyngeal access as an issue of importance in airway management (Figure 1-4). Although the score of and by itself had poor sensitivity, specificity, and positive predictive value, the notion that "access" is important became cemented.

It was during this time that Cormack and Lehane proposed their Laryngeal View Grade scoring system in an effort to provide some structure to the discussion of "difficult laryngoscopy" (Figure 1-5).[35] Although found to be subject to considerable interobserver variability, the scale has been embraced as a valid measure of difficulty; with Grade 3 and 4 views being equated with "difficult laryngoscopy." By the late 1990s, other models with more

reproducible scoring systems, such as Levitan's percentage of glottic opening (POGO) visible, were proposed. However, widespread adoption of these systems over the Cormack/Lehane (C/L) system has yet to occur (Figure 1-6).[36–38]

By the late 1980s, it had become apparent that airway management failure was *the* most important contributor to poor patient outcome in anesthesia practice, lawsuits, and financial settlements.[4] The question facing airway practitioners became: Who should you not paralyze? A variety of investigators pursued univariate and multivariate systems of analysis that attempted to answer this question, but none with much success:

- Wilson, 1988 (*Wilson Risk Sum*): Employed a weighted scoring system 0–2 incorporating body weight, head and neck movement, jaw movement, receding mandible, and prominent (buck) teeth.[39]
- Bellhouse, 1988: Used x-rays to evaluate for difficulty.[40–45]
- Rocke, 1992: Evaluated 1500 parturients using a combination of Mallampati, short neck, receding mandible, and buck teeth.[46]
- Savva, 1994: Identified a sternomental distance <12 cm as a risk for difficulty.[31]
- Tse, 1995: Combined Mallampati, head extension, and thyromental distance.[47]
- El-Ganzouri, 1996: In a large study of 10,507 patients looked at mouth opening, Mallampati, neck movement, mandibular protrusion, body weight, and a positive history of airway management difficulty.[48]
- Karkouti, 2000: Evaluated 461 patients (38 difficult)—correlated mouth opening, chin protrusion, atlanto-occipital extension.[49]

Hot on the heels of the "Who should you not paralyze?" question is the dilemma: How is the airway best rescued in the event that intubation and/or ventilation is impossible, i.e., a failed airway? In the past, BMV was viewed as the most commonly performed fallback technique. This difficult to teach, learn, and perform technique is being supplanted by more user friendly and easily performed EGDs. This has led to a reframing of the way we think about airway

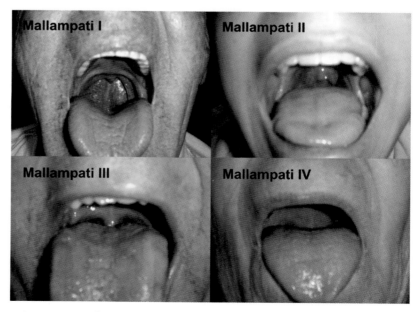

FIGURE 1-4. Mallampati Classes.

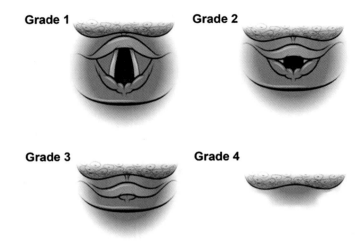

FIGURE 1-5. Cormack/Lehane Laryngeal View Grade score.

management: In the event laryngoscopy and intubation fails, is it likely that gas exchange can be maintained by BMV *or* one of these EGD devices? Furthermore, the recognition that while aspiration is undesirable, it is not usually a deadly occurrence, serves to emphasize the primacy of gas exchange *over* intubation and airway protection.

1.5   DEFINITIONS OF DIFFICULT AND FAILED AIRWAYS

The Difficult Airway is something you anticipate;

the Failed Airway is something you experience.

(Walls, 2002)

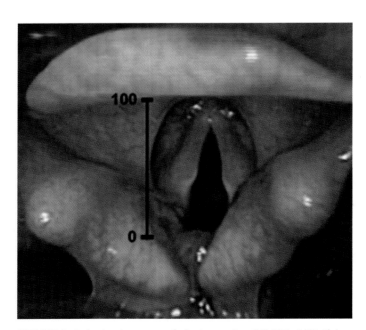

FIGURE 1-6. Levitan's percent of glottic opening (POGO): 100, if the complete glottis can be seen; 0, if no part of the glottis can be seen.

As noted earlier, this chapter explores the concepts of "the difficult" and "the failed" airway. The premise is that the preprocedure recognition and management of the difficult airway should minimize the occurrence of a failed airway. Furthermore, recognizing the failed airway promptly ought to optimize the chances that failing techniques will be abandoned and replaced by techniques reasonably anticipated to succeed.

1.5.1   The difficult airway

When one is presented with a patient that requires intubation, the first decision is whether or not this airway needs to be managed immediately (typically, the "newly dead" or the "nearly dead" "Crash Airway," see Chapter 2) and one simply proceeds to intervene in the airway. If it is not a crash airway, one must ask, "Is this a Difficult Airway?" Asking the question presumes that one has a framework to answer it!

As discussed above, and unlike the failed airway, the difficult airway is not so easily defined. Rather than a definition, in concept, the "Difficult Airway" has five dimensions[8]:

1. difficult BMV
2. difficult laryngoscopy
3. difficult intubation
4. difficult placement of a EGD
5. difficult cricothyrotomy.

These five dimensions can be reduced to four technical operations:

1. difficult BMV
2. difficult laryngoscopy and intubation
3. difficult EGD
4. difficult cricothyrotomy

The evaluation of the airway for difficulty may be leisurely or urgent. In the latter circumstance, it must be done quickly with care taken not to omit anything important. Like well-constructed algorithms, mnemonics are efficient memory-aid strategies that lead to a complete, yet rapid, evaluation. One for each technical operation has been crafted to permit a rapid and complete evaluation, no matter the clinical circumstance.

1.5.2   The failed airway

The *Failed Airway* is easily defined as[8]:

1. three failed attempts at orotracheal intubation by a skilled practitioner and/or
2. failure to maintain acceptable oxygen saturations, typically 90% or above in otherwise normal individuals.

The problem in everyday practice is not so much defining failure; it is *recognizing* failure once it has occurred, and then moving quickly to alternatives. Clinically, the failed airway presents itself in two ways:

1. You have time: "Can't intubate/can ventilate and oxygenate."

2. You have no time: "Can't intubate/can't ventilate or oxygenate" (CICV or CICO).

The intent is to minimize the chance of encountering a failed airway when one might have easily predicted a difficult intubation, difficult BMV, difficult EGD, or a difficult cricothyrotomy.

The adage in anesthesia practice with respect to neuromuscular blockade of a patient who has some effective spontaneous ventilation has always been "Don't take anything away from the patient that you can't replace." While such a rigid principle is not always consistent with the realities of airway management, it is a useful one to remember!

1.6 PREDICTION OF DIFFICULT AND FAILED AIRWAY

The most effective aids work well in all clinical situations, as everyday practice adjuncts. The following mnemonics fall into this category[8]:

1.6.1 Difficult bag-mask-ventilation: MOANS

The importance of BMV in airway management is not taken lightly by airway practitioners, particularly as a rescue maneuver when orotracheal intubation has failed. If the airway practitioner is uncertain that neuromuscular blockade facilitated tracheal intubation will be successful, they must be confident that BMV will be adequate, the use of an EGD be successful, or at the very least, a cricothyrotomy can rapidly be performed.

The bag-mask devices most commonly used in resuscitation settings are capable of generating 50–100 cm of water pressure in the upper airway, provided that they do not have positive pressure relief valves, and an adequate mask seal can be obtained (Figure 1-7).

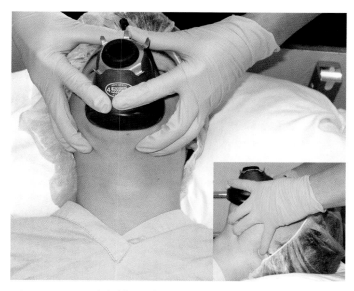

FIGURE 1-7. Mask hold to achieve a mask seal using a two-hand technique.

Pediatric and neonatal devices often incorporate positive pressure relief valves that can be easily defeated if needed. This degree of positive pressure is often sufficient to overcome the moderate degree of upper airway obstruction offered by redundant tissue (e.g., the obese) or edematous tissue (e.g., angioedema, croup, or epiglottitis).

Research[50,51] has validated many of those anatomical features that over the years have been implicated in heralding difficult BMV. The five indicators that have been identified can be easily recalled by using the mnemonic MOANS[8]:

*M*ask seal: Bushy beards, crusted blood on the face, or a disruption of lower facial continuity are the commonest examples of conditions that may make an adequate mask seal difficult. Some recommend smearing a substance such as Vaseline or KY Jelly™ on a beard as a remedy to this problem. However, in the experience of the authors, it simply makes a bad situation worse in that the entire face becomes too slippery to hold the mask in place.

*O*bese: Patients who are obese (defined by Langeron et al.[50] as BMI > 26 kg·m^{-2} as opposed to the conventional definition of obese as 30 kg·m^{-2}) are often difficult to ventilate adequately by bag and mask. BMV can also be difficult in parturients at term and in patients with upper-airway obstruction, angioedema, Ludwig's angina, upper-airway abscesses (e.g., peritonsillar), and epiglottitis. There is a sense among experienced practitioners that edematous lesions (e.g., angioedema, croup, epiglottitis, etc.) are more amenable to bag-mask rescue should sudden obstruction occur or be induced, although the authors would not rely on this opinion. On the other hand, firm, immobile lesions such as hematomas, cancers, and foreign bodies usually cannot be circumvented by BMV. Total airway obstruction must be avoided in these patients, and care must be taken with airway manipulation (positioning, avoidance of bleeding, sedative hypnotic medications, etc.).

*A*ged: Age more than 55 is associated with a higher risk of difficult BMV, perhaps because of a loss of muscle and tissue tone in the upper airway.

*N*o teeth: An adequate mask seal may be difficult in the edentulous patient as the face tends to cave in. An option is to leave dentures in situ (if available) for BMV and remove them for intubation. Alternatively, gauze may be inserted in the cheeks to puff them out in an attempt to improve the seal (vigilance to prevent dislodgement into the airway is required).

*S*nores or *S*tiff: For the former, this mnemonic affords one a reminder to check for sleep apnea, an increasingly important consideration in anesthetic practice today.[52] BMV may be difficult or impossible in the face of substantial increases in airways resistance (e.g., deadly asthma) or decreases in pulmonary compliance (e.g., pulmonary edema).

1.6.2 Difficult laryngoscopy and intubation: LEMON

Difficult laryngoscopy and intubation ordinarily implies that the operator had a poor view of the glottis. Cormack and Lehane[35] provided some clarity to the way we think of the "difficult airway" by parsing the act of intubation into its two subcomponents: laryngoscopy and intubation. They also introduced the most widely utilized system of categorizing the degree to which the glottis can be visualized during laryngoscopy (Figure 1-5).

Cormack/Lehane view Grades 3 (epiglottis only visible) and 4 (no glottic structures at all visible) are often used as surrogates to define a difficult laryngoscopy and predict difficult intubation. View Grades 1 (visualization of the entire laryngeal aperture) and 2 (visualization of the posterior cords and arytenoids) are not typically associated with difficult intubation, though some Grade 2s may be difficult or impossible to intubate. Tough Grade 2s and 3s are "tailor-made" for intubating introducers such as the Eschmann and Frova devices (see Section 10.2.1 and 10.2.2).

As can be gleaned from the descriptions, the Cormack/Lehane grading system is insensitive to the degree to which the laryngeal aperture is visible during laryngoscopy: a little bit of it (Grade 2) or all of it (Grade 1). The question often asked is: How much of the cords must be viewed to assure intubation success? How much is *enough*? In attempting to provide a framework or an approach to answering this question, Levitan et al.[36–38] devised a scoring system to quantify the POGO visible. While attractive in many ways, this scale has yet to gain wide acceptance (Figure 1-6).

The Cormack/Lehane grading system is predicated upon grading during the best attempt at conventional laryngoscopy, and *best attempt in turn requires definition*. Benumof[5] defines best attempt as being composed of six components:

(1) performance by a reasonably experienced practitioner;

(2) no significant muscle tone;

(3) the use of the optimal "sniffing" position;

(4) the use of external laryngeal manipulation (*backward upward rightward pressure* [BURP] or *optimum external laryngeal manipulation* [OELM]);[53]

(5) length of the blade;

(6) type of blade.

Most times an intubation demands that the first attempt *be* the best attempt, particularly in an emergency, although some compromises may be necessary (e.g., residency training). Should an orotracheal intubation attempt fail and an additional attempt be contemplated, it seems reasonable to "change something" on the subsequent attempt to enhance the chances of success. That "something" may be one, some, or all of these factors. Reminding oneself of the components of the *optimum* or *best attempt* provides a framework to address "what to change?"

Optimization of all six components may not be in the patient's best interest in an emergency. For example, if difficulty is anticipated, it may not be advisable to paralyze the patient. Additionally, in the event the cervical spine is immobilized it may not be possible to place them in the "sniffing" position. Most experts on airway management agree that positioning the head and neck is an important step in optimizing conventional laryngoscopy as a prelude to orotracheal intubation.

If it is possible to consistently and precisely predict intubation failure, the initial selection of laryngoscopic oral intubation could be eliminated as a strategy and alternative techniques employed (e.g., fiberoptic intubation, cricothyrotomy). However, they may be technically more challenging, risky, and time consuming. During the last several decades, this has not proven to be possible. Lists of anatomical features, radiologic findings, and complex scoring systems have all been explored without consistent success.

Therefore, we are left to assemble the known risks, match them to the skill, experience, and judgment of the practitioner, and make a decision: Does this airway meet the threshold of being sufficiently difficult to warrant using a Difficult Airway Algorithm, or am I safe to proceed directly to induction, paralysis, and intubation (e.g., rapid sequence intubation or rapid sequence induction known as RSI)?[8]

So, how do we quickly identify as many of the risks as possible? The mnemonic LEMON is a useful guide:

Look externally: If the airway looks difficult, it probably is (Figure 1-8). A litany of physical features has been associated with difficult laryngoscopy and intubation—a small mandible may indicate that the tongue is "retro-fitted" over the larynx; a large mandible elongates the pharyngeal axis serving to extend the distance to the larynx and perhaps move it beyond the horizon of view. Buck teeth block access to the oral cavity and elongate the length of the oral axis. A high, arched palate is often associated with a long, narrow oral cavity making access a problem. A short neck may mean the larynx is positioned higher in the neck relative to the base of the tongue making it more difficult to bring the glottis into view. Lower facial disruption is inconsistent with adequate mask seal and may make the glottis impossible to find. It is often said that when it comes to orotracheal intubation, the 'tongue is your enemy' because it gets in your way and the 'epiglottis is your friend' because once you find it you ought to be able to find the glottic opening. In upper-airway disruption, the

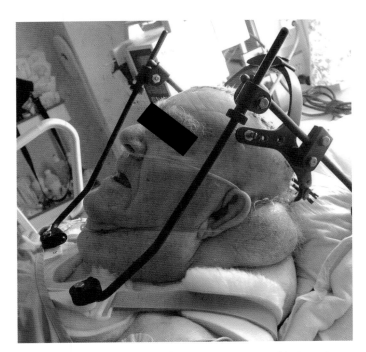

FIGURE 1-8. This patient provides an image recognizable instantly as a difficult airway.

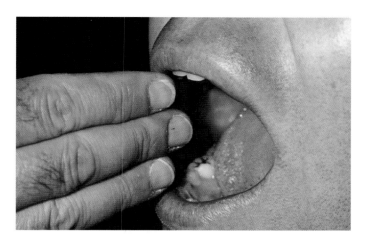

FIGURE 1-9. Airway evaluation: The first 3 of "3-3-2" evaluation indicates the extent of the mouth opening.

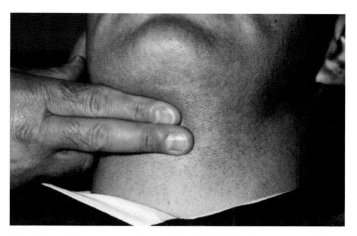

FIGURE 1-11. Airway evaluation: The 2 of "3-3-2" evaluation indicates the position of the larynx relative to the base of the tongue.

tongue may actually be a friend as it leads to the epiglottis and the glottic opening.

*E*valuate 3-3-2: Although there is no scientific basis to support the 3-3-2 rule, it serves to ensure that the relevant geometry of the upper airway is assessed adequately. The first "3" assesses the adequacy of oral access (Figure 1-9). One ought to be able to open one's mouth three of one's own finger breadths (approximately 5 cm). The second "3" and the "2" recognize the interplay of the geometric relationships among the various components of the upper airway as first articulated by Patil in 1983. A thyromental distance of less than 6 cm was associated with difficult intubation (Figure 1-3). As described earlier, the thyromental distance is the hypotenuse of Patil's triangle (Figure 1-3), the base being the length of the mandible (Figure 1-10) and the third leg being the distance between the base of the tongue (neck–mandible junction at the level of the hyoid bone) and the top of the larynx (Figure 1-11). One ought to be able to accommodate three of one's own fingers (approximately 5 cm) between the tip of mentum and the mandible–neck junction (Figure 1-10) and fit two fingers between the mandible–neck junction and

the thyroid notch (Figure 1-11). The second "3" steers one in assessing the capacity of the mandibular space to accommodate the tongue on laryngoscopy. More than, or less than, three fingers are associated with greater degrees of difficulty in visualizing the larynx. The length of the oral axis is elongated if it is longer than three fingers, and the mandibular space may be too small to accommodate the tongue during laryngoscopy if it is shorter than 3 fingers, leaving it to obscure the view of the glottis. The "2" identifies the location of the larynx in relation to the base of the tongue. If more than two fingers are accommodated, meaning the larynx is further below the base of the tongue, it may be difficult to visualize the glottis on laryngoscopy because it is too far down the neck and beyond the visual horizon. Fewer than two fingers may mean that the larynx is tucked up under the base of the tongue and may be difficult to expose. This condition is often called "anterior larynx."

*M*allampati Class:[32,33] Mallampati studied the relationship between the visibility of the posterior oropharyngeal structures and success rate of laryngoscopic intubation. He had patients sit on the side of the bed, open their mouth as widely as possible, and protrude their tongue as far as possible, without phonating. Figure 1-4 depicts how the scale is constructed. Although Class I and II patients are associated with low intubation failure rates, circumspection with respect to the wisdom of utilizing neuromuscular blockade to facilitate intubation rests with those in Classes III and IV, particularly Class IV in which intubation failure rates may exceed 10%. This scale, by itself, is neither sensitive nor specific. However, it is commonly used because it is easily performed, particularly in an emergency, and it may reveal important information about access to the oral cavity and potentially difficult glottic visualization.

*O*bstruction: There are three cardinal signs of upper airway obstruction: muffled voice ("hot potato voice"); difficulty swallowing secretions, either because of pain or obstruction; and stridor. The first two signs do not ordinarily herald imminent total upper-airway obstruction. The presence of stridor generally indicates that the diameter of the airway has been reduced

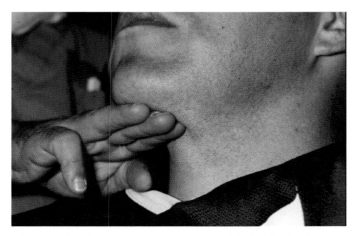

FIGURE 1-10. Airway evaluation: The second 3 of "3-3-2"evaluation indicates the length dimension of the mandibular space.

to 4.0 mm or less.[54] Upper-airway obstruction should always be considered a difficult airway and managed with extreme care. The administration of small doses of opioids and benzodiazepines to manage anxiety may induce total obstruction as the stenting tone of the upper airway musculature relaxes.

*N*eck mobility: The ability to position the head and neck is one of the six components of achieving an optimal view of the larynx on oral laryngoscopy. Though there is some dissention,[55] it has long been taught that the "sniffing the morning air," or "sipping English tea" positioning (neck flexion, head extension) of the head and neck, when possible, is at least the best place to start. While cervical spine immobilization alone may not constitute a difficult laryngoscopy, airway practitioners should be cautious in managing patients with limited cervical spine movement.

1.6.3   Difficult extraglottic device: **RODS**

The insertion of an EGD may be a planned backup maneuver ("Plan B") when faced with a failed conventional orotracheal intubation. It may also serve as a bridging technique to reestablish gas exchange in a CICV setting while one prepares to perform a cricothyrotomy (see Chapter 2). To minimize the wasting of valuable time, airway practitioners should place the EGD concurrently, with setting up to perform a surgical airway.

In the former case, when "Plan B" is an EGD, one ought to have performed an evaluation for difficult EGD placement before it is relied on as a primary or backup plan. RODS is a mnemonic that is intended to identify problem patients when an EGD is contemplated:

*R*estricted mouth opening: Depending on the EGD to be employed, more or less oral access may be needed.

*O*bstruction: Upper-airway obstruction at the level of the larynx or below. An EGD will not bypass this obstruction.

*D*isrupted or distorted airway: At least in as much as the "seat and seal" of the EGD may be compromised.[56]

*S*tiff lungs or cervical spine: Ventilation with an EGD may be difficult or impossible in the face of substantial increases in airways resistance (e.g., deadly asthma) or decreases in pulmonary compliance (e.g., pulmonary edema). Seal may be exceedingly difficult or impossible to achieve in the face of a fixed flexion deformity of the neck.[56] In addition, there are reports of difficult LMA insertion in patients with limited neck movement.[57,58]

1.6.4   Difficult cricothyrotomy: **SHORT**

There are no absolute contraindications to performing an emergency cricothyrotomy. However, some conditions may make it difficult or impossible to perform the procedure, making it imperative to identify those conditions up front, particularly if one is relying on a rapidly performed cricothyrotomy as a rescue technique. The mnemonic SHORT is used to quickly identify features that may indicate a difficult cricothyrotomy:

*S*urgery/disrupted airway: The anatomy of the neck may be furtively or obviously distorted due to previous surgery, making the airway difficult to access.

*H*ematoma or infection: An infective process or hematoma in the pathway of the cricothyrotomy incision may make the procedure technically difficult but should never be considered a contraindication in a life-threatening situation.

*O*bese/access problem: Obesity should be considered a surrogate for any problem that makes percutaneous access to the anterior neck problematic. A fixed flexion deformity of the cervical spine, halo traction, and other situations may also make access to the neck difficult.

*R*adiation: The tissue changes associated with past radiation therapy may distort tissues, making the procedure difficult.

*T*umor: Tumor either in or around the airway may present difficulty, both from an access perspective as well as bleeding.

1.7   SUMMARY

Failure to evaluate the airway and predict difficulty is the single most important factor leading to a failed airway. Despite decades of study, no system of evaluation is able to discern with certainty (100% reliability) those airways that can be managed with conventional laryngoscopic intubation and those where an alternative method is advisable. For this reason, each and every airway management episode must be approached with a view that some other device or technique may be necessary should the primary plan fail. Furthermore, the airway practitioner must evaluate the airway for difficulty relative to each of the alternatives contemplated. Once Plan A has failed, it is too late to suddenly realize that Plan B is also impossible because a factor, which could have been detected, had a prior evaluation for difficulty been conducted.

While not exhaustive in covering all of the features of a difficult airway, the mnemonics MOANS, LEMON, RODS, and SHORT provide guidance in evaluating all airways for difficulty, although they are specifically designed to be employed rapidly in the face of an urgent or emergency clinical circumstance.

Finally, recognizing that one is in the midst of a failed airway is crucial in embarking on maneuvers that may rescue the airway. Persisting with a failing technique is a fundamental contributor to bad outcomes in airway management.

REFERENCES

1. Hung O, Murphy M: Changing practice in airway management: are we there yet? Editorial. *Can J Anaesth.* 2004;51:963–8.
2. Shiga T, Wajima Z, Inoue T, et al.: Predicting difficult intubation in apparently normal patients: a meta-analysis of bedside screening test performance. *Anesthesiology* 2005;103:429–437.
3. Mort TC: Emergency tracheal intubation: complications associated with repeated laryngoscopic attempts. *Anesth Analg* 2004;99:607–613.
4. Cheney FW, Posner KL, Caplan RA: Adverse respiratory events infrequently leading to malpractice suits. A closed claims analysis. *Anesthesiology* 1991;75:932.
5. Benumof JL: The ASA difficult airway algorithm: new thoughts and considerations. 51st Annual Refresher Course Lectures and Clinical Update Program, #235. American Society of Anesthesiologists, 2000.
6. Practice guidelines for management of the difficult airway: an updated report by the American Society of Anesthesiologists Task Force on Management of the Difficult Airway. *Anesthesiology* 2003;98:1269–277.

7. Wilson ME: Predicting difficult intubation. *Br J Anaesth*. 1993;71: 333–334.
8. Murphy M, Walls RM: Identification of the difficult and failed airway. In: *Manual of Emergency Airway Management*. Walls RM, Murphy MF, Luten R, eds. Philadelphia, PA: Lippincott, Williams, Wilkins, 2004:70–81.
9. Sakles JC, Laurin EG, Rantapaa AA, et al.: Airway management in the emergency department: a one-year study of 610 tracheal intubations. *Ann Emerg Med*. 1998;31:325–332.
10. Bair AE, Filbin MR, Kulkarni RG, et al.: The failed intubation attempt in the emergency department: analysis of prevalence, rescue techniques, and personnel. *J Emerg Med*. 2002;23:131–140.
11. Sivilotti MA, Filbin MR, Murray HE, et al.: On behalf of the NEAR investigators. Does the sedative agent facilitate emergency rapid-sequence intubation? *Acad Emerg Med*. 2003;10:612–620.
12. Sagarin MJ, Chiang V, Sakles JC, et al.: on behalf of the NEAR investigators. Rapid sequence intubation for pediatric emergency airway management. *Ped Emerg Care*. 2002;18:417–423.
13. Bair AE, Filbin MR, Kulkarni R, et al.: On behalf of the NEAR investigators. Failed intubation in the emergency department: analysis of prevalence, rescue techniques, and personnel. *J Emerg Med*. 2002;23:131–140.
14. Benumof JL: The unanticipated difficult airway. *Can J Anaesth*. 1999;46: 510–511.
15. Crosby ET: The unanticipated difficult airway-evolving strategies for successful salvage (Editorial). *Can J Anesth*. 2005;52:562–567.
16. Randell T: Thyromental distance-shouldn't we redefine the role in the prediction of difficult laryngoscopy (Letter, reply). *Acta Anaesthesiol Scand*. 1998;42: 136–137.
17. Combes X, Le Roux B, Suen P, et al.: Unanticipated difficult airway in anesthetized patients: prospective validation of a management algorithm. *Anesthesiology*. 2004;100:1146–1150.
18. Rose DK, Cohen MM: The airway: problems and predictions in 18,500 patients. *Can J Anesth*. 1994;41:372.
19. Ezri T, Szmuk P, Evron S, et al.: Difficult airway in obstetric anesthesia: a review. *Obstet Gynecol Surv*. 2001;56:631–641.
20. Ross BK: ASA closed claims in obstetrics: lessons learned. *Anesthesiol Clin North America*. 2003;21:183–197.
21. Levack ID, Masson AH: Difficult tracheal intubation in obstetrics. *Anaesthesia*. 1985;40:384.
22. Practice guidelines for management of the difficult airway. A report by the American Society of Anesthesiologists Task Force on Management of the Difficult Airway. *Anesthesiology*. 1993;78:597–602.
23. Black HC: *Black's Law Dictionary*, 7th edn. Garner BA (ed.). St Paul, MN: West Publishing Co., 1999.
24. Crosby ET, Cooper RM, Douglas MJ, et al.: The unanticipated difficult airway with recommendations for management. *Can J Anaesth*. 1998;45: 757–776.
25. Henderson JJ, Popat MT, Latto IP, Pearce AC: Difficult Airway Society guidelines for management of the unanticipated difficult intubation. *Anaesthesia*. 2004;59:675–594.
26. Stoller JK: The history of intubation, tracheotomy, and airway appliances. *Respir Care*. 1999;44:595–601.
27. Henderson JJ: The use of paraglossal straight blade laryngoscopy in difficult tracheal intubation. *Anaesthesia*. 1997;52:552–560.
28. www.adair.at/eng/museum/equipment/default.htm.
29. Henderson JJ: Development of the gum-elastic bougie'. *Anaesthesia*. 2003;58:103–104.
30. Cass NM, James NR, Lines V: Difficult direct laryngoscopy complicating intubation in anaesthesia. *BMJ*. 1956; 1:488–490.
31. Savva D: Sternomental distance—a useful predictor of difficult intubation in patients with cervical spine disease? *Anaesthesia*. 1996;51:284–285.
32. Mallampati SR: Clinical sign to predict difficult tracheal intubation (hypothesis). *Can Anesth Soc J*. 1983;30:316–317.
33. Mallampati SR, Gatt SP, Gugino LD, et al.: A clinical sign to predict difficult intubation: a prospective study. *Can Anesth Soc J*. 1985;32:429–434.
34. Samsoon GL, Young JR: Difficult tracheal intubation: a retrospective study. *Anaesthesia*. 1987;42:487–490.
35. Cormack RS, Lehane J: Difficult tracheal intubation in obstetrics. *Anaesthesia*. 1984;39:1105.
36. Levitan RM, Ochroch EA, Kush S, et al.: Assessment of airway visualization: validation of the percentage of glottic opening (POGO) scale. *Acad Emerg Med*. 1998;5:919–923.
37. Ochroch EA, Hollander JE, Kush S, et al.: Assessment of laryngeal view: percentage of glottic opening score vs Cormack and Lehane grading. *Can J Anaesth*. 1999;46:987–990.
38. Levitan RM, Hollander JE, Ochroch EA: A grading system for direct laryngoscopy. *Anaesthesia*. 1999;54:1009–1010.
39. Wilson ME, Spiegelhalter D, Robertson JA, et al.: Predicting difficult intubation. *Br J Anaesth*. 1988;61:211–216.
40. Bellhouse CP, Dore C: Criteria for estimating likelihood of difficulty of endotracheal intubation with the MacIntosh laryngoscope. *Anaesth Intensive Care*. 1988;16:329.
41. Bellhouse CP, Dore C: Predicting difficult intubation. *Br J Anaesth*. 1989;62:469.
42. Bellhouse CP: Predicting difficult intubation. *Anaesthesia*. 1992;47:440–441.
43. Bellhouse P: Predicting difficult intubation. *Br J Anaesth*. 1991;67:505.
44. Bellhouse CB: Predicting difficult intubation. *Br J Anaesth*. 1994;72:494.
45. Bellhouse CP: Prediction of difficult tracheal intubation. *Br J Anaesth*. 1995;74:490.
46. Rocke DA, Murray WB, Rout CC, et al.: Relative risk analysis of factors associated with difficult intubation in obstetric anesthesia. *Anesthesiology*. 1992;77:67.
47. Tse JC, Rimm EB, Hussain A: Predicting difficult endotracheal intubation in surgical patients scheduled for general anesthesia: a prospective blind study. *Anesth Analg*. 1995;81:254.
48. El-Ganzouri AR, McCarthy RJ, Turman KJ, et al.: Preoperative airway assessment: predictive value of a multivariate risk index. *Anesth Analg*. 1996;82:1197.
49. Karkouti K, Rose DK, Wigglesworth D, et al.: Predicting difficult intubation: a multivariable analysis. *Can J Anaesth*. 2000;47:730–739.
50. Langeron O, Masso E, Huraux C, et al.: Prediction of difficult mask ventilation. *Anesthesiology*. 2000;92:1229.
51. Adnet F: Difficult mask ventilation: an underestimated aspect of the problem of the difficult airway? *Anesthesiology*. 2000;92:1217–1218.
52. Ezri T, Gewurtz G, Sessler DI, et al.: Prediction of difficult laryngoscopy in obese patients by ultrasound quantification of anterior neck soft tissue. *Anaesthesia*. 2003;58:1111–1114.
53. Benumof JL, Cooper SD: Quantitative improvement in laryngoscopic view by optimal external laryngeal manipulation. *J Clin Anesth*. 1996;8:136–140.
54. Donlon JV: Anesthetic and airway management of laryngoscopy and bronchoscopy. In: *Airway Management: Principles and Practice*. Benumof JL (ed.). St. Louis: Mosby, 1996: 666–685.
55. Adnet F, Baillard C, Borron SW, et al.: Randomized study comparing the "sniffing position" with simple head extension for laryngoscopic view in elective surgery patients. *Anesthesiology*. 2001;95:836–841.
56. Buckham M, Brooker M, Brimacombe J, et al.: A comparison of the reinforced and standard laryngeal mask airway: ease of insertion and the influence of head and neck position on oropharyngeal leak pressure and intracuff pressure. *Anaesth Intensive Care*. 1999;27:628–631.
57. Ishimura H, Minami K, Sata T, et al.: Impossible insertion of the laryngeal mask airway and oropharyngeal axes. *Anesthesiology*. 1995; 83:867–869.
58. Olmez G, Nazaroglu H, Arslan SG, et al.: Difficulties and failure of laryngeal mask insertion in a patient with ankylosing spondylitis. Turk. *J Med Sci*. 2004;34:369–352.

SELF-EVALUATION QUESTIONS

1.1. The most common factor leading to a failed airway is

   A. morbid obesity

   B. distorted airway anatomy

   C. upper airway obstruction

   D. failure to predict a difficult airway

   E. not knowing enough rescue techniques well

1.2. The standard of care in airway management is related to all of the following **EXCEPT**

   A. the skill of an average practitioner

   B. similar localities

   C. procedures that give the best results

   D. the expectations of the reasonable patient

   E. opinions ventured by experts

1.3. The standard of care expects that the average, reasonable practitioner ought to be able to do all of the following **EXCEPT**

A. be able to manage an unanticipated difficult airway

B. be an expert and be able to use a flexible fiberoptic bronchoscope to intubate immediately in the face of a CICV airway

C. be able to recognize and manage a failed airway

D. be facile with one or two rescue devices or techniques in the face of a failed airway

E. be able to perform a surgical airway

CHAPTER (2)

The Algorithms

Michael F. Murphy and Edward T. Crosby

2.1 INTRODUCTION

2.1.1 What is the challenge of difficult and failed airway management?

Airway management is fundamental to the practice of anesthesia, emergency medicine, critical care medicine, and other areas of care. The focus of this chapter is the *management* of the difficult and failed airway in an emergency or urgent situation. Management of the predicted difficult intubation is dealt with in Chapter 3 and in Section II of this book.

The challenge for the airway practitioner is to be able to accurately predict when a difficult airway is more likely to be present, to recognize when an intubation failure has occurred, and to be able to reliably and reproducibly achieve timely and effective oxygenation and ventilation in both of these unnerving circumstances. Appropriate planning, selection of the correct device and technique, and calm execution based on learned methods and experience enhances success even in these most difficult cases. In an airway crisis, there is no question that having a logical and simple approach based on a planned strategy is most likely to be successful.

2.1.2 How reliably can we predict a difficult airway?

In airway management, there are two areas in which difficulty may be encountered: intubation and ventilation. Ventilation most commonly is performed using a bag and a mask, though in more sophisticated settings more advanced devices may be selected (eg, extraglottic devices or EGDs).

In elective situations, difficulty with mask-ventilation is uncommon. Langeron prospectively reviewed the management of 1502 patients undergoing elective surgery under general anesthesia.[1] Difficult mask-ventilation was defined as (1) an inability to maintain $SaO_2 > 92\%$ while using 100% O_2 via the anesthesia circuit bag-mask unit; (2) significant gas leak via the face-mask; (3) a need to increase the fresh gas flow to rates > 15 L·min^{-1} and to use the flush valve more than twice; (4) no perceptible chest wall movement during ventilation; (5) the need to perform a two-handed mask technique; or (6) to change the operator. The anesthesia practitioner was asked to consider ventilation as difficult only if the difficulty was perceived to be clinically relevant, ie, potentially leading to a patient threat. In 5% of the patients ventilation was considered difficult, and in one patient ventilation was impossible. Following multivariate analysis, five criteria were recognized as independent factors for difficult mask-ventilation: age > 55 years; BMI > 26 kg·m^{-2}; lack of teeth; presence of a beard; and a history of snoring (see Section 1.6.1).

In the emergency situation, other scenario-specific factors may become relevant when considering whether difficulty with mask-ventilation is more likely to be encountered. Trauma to the face with resultant edema, bleeding or debris in the airway, and the need to maintain in-line C-spine immobilization where required may increase the degree of difficulty with mask-ventilation. In addition, the use of cricoid pressure, often perceived to be necessary in emergency intubations, spare is recognized to increase the likelihood of difficult mask-ventilation. Petito and Russell evaluated the impact of cricoid pressure on lung ventilation during bag-mask-ventilation (BMV).[2] Fifty patients were randomized to either have or not have cricoid pressure applied during a 3-minute period of standardized mask-ventilation. Patients who had cricoid pressure applied were considered more difficult to ventilate (36% vs. 12%), and these patients tended to have more air in the stomach than those patients considered easy to ventilate with applied cricoid pressure.

The bulk of the literature dealing with assessment of the airway in anticipation of tracheal intubation using a laryngoscope, including Cass' landmark paper in 1956,[3] and the Mallampati classification in the mid 1980s,[4,5] has little applicability to currently available alternative devices (eg, rigid fiberoptic devices, intubating EGDs, video laryngoscopes, etc.). Modification of Mallampati's original schema,[6] as well as alternate strategies to assess the airway (see Section 1.6.2) have been proposed. These have ranged from using simple anatomical descriptors, ranking and summating anatomical scoring systems, and using logistic regression to create predictive scales and to derive performance indices. These different strategies share some common characteristics: they have a high sensitivity but low specificity and low positive predictive value with respect to predicting failure. Additionally, many of the tests have only moderate interobserver reliability.[7] These limitations may help to explain why the tests often fail to predict difficult tracheal intubation, and why perhaps some practitioners question the value of performing preanesthetic airway assessments.[8]

A number of new schemes and techniques used to predict potential airway difficulty have been described; their accuracy and widespread applicability are not yet determined. However, it is likely that they will continue to be characterized by a low positive predictive value, similar to current strategies, because of the low incidence of airway difficulty.[8] Further more, we knew that even with careful evaluation, difficulty will not be predicted in many instances. Therefore strategies to manage the unanticipated difficult airway should be preformulated and practiced to minimize adverse outcomes resulting from false negative predictions.

2.2 AIRWAY EMERGENCIES

2.2.1 How is airway management in an emergency setting different?

Airway management in an emergency setting may be complicated by a multitude of factors. Trauma to the face and neck may distort anatomical features or obscure them with blood and debris. The requirement for in-line stabilization in patients with spinal injury or perceived to be at-risk for a spinal injury may make laryngoscopy more difficult. Unprepared patients are often associated with a full stomach and are at a higher risk of regurgitation and aspiration of gastric contents. The use of cricoid pressure to reduce the risk of regurgitation and aspiration also may make tracheal intubation more difficult. Smith evaluated the ease of rigid fiberoptic (WuScope System™) intubation in anesthetized adults receiving cricoid pressure.[9] Each patient had their trachea intubated under two conditions: with and without cricoid pressure. An easy intubation occurred in 91% of patients without cricoid pressure and in 66% of patients with cricoid pressure applied. Cricoid pressure compressed the vocal cords in 27% of patients and impeded tracheal tube placement in 15%. In three patients (9%), pressure had to be released in order to successfully intubate their tracheas. Hodgson assessed the effect of cricoid pressure on lightwand intubation success in 60 adult female patients presenting for abdominal hysterectomy.[10] All 30 patients allocated to intubation without cricoid

pressure were intubated successfully on the first attempt with a median time of 28 seconds. Lightwand intubation with cricoid pressure was successful in 26 of 30 patients on the first attempt, but the median time to successful intubation was significantly longer at 48.5 seconds. Three patients required two attempts for successful intubation, and one could not be intubated with the lightwand while cricoid pressure was being applied. Shulman compared the Bullard laryngoscope (BL) with the flexible fiberoptic bronchoscope (FFB) in a cervical spine injury model, using in-line stabilization with and without cricoid pressure.[11] The times for laryngoscopy and intubation were longer in the FFB group than in the BL group. Further, there was a significantly lower rate of adequate laryngoscopic view in the FFB group in the presence of cricoid pressure than in either of the BL groups, or in the FFB no cricoid-pressure group. Shulman concluded that the BL is more reliable, quicker, and more resistant to the effect of cricoid pressure than is the FFB when used in the setting of in-line stabilization with cricoid pressure applied.

In summary, cricoid pressure has a limited, though negative, impact on the success rate of airway interventions.

An emergency and hemodynamic instability may mitigate against the use of drugs that are ordinarily employed to facilitate laryngoscopy, resulting in intubation conditions which may be less than ideal. Finally, a chaotic emergency environment may distract the practitioner making it more difficult to concentrate on the task at hand at a time when focus may be essential.

2.3 DIFFICULT AND FAILED AIRWAY

2.3.1 What does experience tell us about rescuing the difficult airway?

Evidence has emerged that having automatic "*default-to*" strategies improves the success of rescue airway interventions and reduces the occurrence of adverse outcomes. Conversely, there are also data demonstrating that persisting with failing techniques rather than defaulting to rescue strategies results in higher rates of morbidity and mortality. Rose and Cohen reported that difficult laryngoscopy in anesthesia practice was most often managed with persistent attempts at direct laryngoscopy, and the use of alternative approaches to tracheal intubation was uncommon.[12] In these patients, there was a higher incidence of desaturation, esophageal intubation, dental damage, and unexpected ICU admissions.[1] Similarly, Mort, in reviewing the airway management of 2833 critically ill patients outside of the operating room, noted that the most common strategy implemented for managing difficult intubations was, again, repeated direct laryngoscopy.[13] There was a significant increase in the rate of airway-related complications as the number of laryngoscopic attempts increased (≤ 2 vs. > 2). These complications included hypoxemia, regurgitation, aspiration, bradycardia, and cardiac arrest.

Contrary to the experiences reported by Rose and Cohen and Mort, Hung noted that immediately choosing an alternate technique (lighted stylet) when direct laryngoscopy had failed was typically rewarded with rapid tracheal intubation.[14] Complications were both rare and minor and generally attributable to the preceding attempts at direct laryngoscopy. Recently, Heidegger reported on a protocol for management of both anticipated and unanticipated difficult intubations that emphasized defaulting to the fiberoptic bronchoscope early when difficult laryngoscopy was anticipated or observed.[15] Applied in 13,248 intubations, the protocol failed in only 6 patients (0.045%); again this strategy was associated with minimal morbidity. Combes reported on the efficacy of an institutional protocol employing the intubating laryngeal mask and Eschmann tracheal introducer.[16] One hundred cases of unanticipated difficulties occurred among 11,257 tracheal intubations. There were three deviations from the protocol and two patients were wakened without further airway management. All patients managed by the protocol were successfully ventilated and intubated. Finally, Mort compared the outcomes of patients undergoing emergency tracheal intubation in his institution before and after the application of the American Society of Anesthesiologists (ASA) guidelines.[17] The rate of cardiac arrest during emergency intubation was reduced by 50%.

It is tempting to conclude from these latter reports that early conversion to adjuncts and alternatives to direct-vision laryngoscopy when direct laryngoscopy proves difficult may result in a high salvage rate with low patient morbidity. The emerging evidence is that the choice of the alternative may be less important than the fact that it is a *practiced alternative* and chosen early in a planned approach when direct laryngoscopy has proven to be difficult or has actually failed.

2.3.2 Is there a pattern to the way airway practitioners behave in the face of a difficult or failed airway?

Tracheal intubation is still predominantly performed orally by direct laryngoscopy. Difficulties related to airway management largely involve failure to achieve tracheal intubation due to difficult direct laryngoscopy. A number of innovative new tools for tracheal intubation have been presented in recent years, which address many of the factors that give rise to difficulties during direct laryngoscopy.[18]

The direct laryngoscope is designed to facilitate tracheal intubation by establishing a line of view from the mouth to the larynx. As has already been noted, there are multiple patient factors, which individually or in combination may conspire to obstruct a laryngeal view. The ability to predict all patients in whom it will be impossible to establish a line of view during laryngoscopy is sufficiently imprecise that sole reliance on the laryngoscope to perform tracheal intubation is a precarious strategy.

It is likely that reliance on limited conventional airway techniques that are less than optimum for the task at hand is a risk-enhancing behavior, which predisposes patients to increased rates of morbidity and mortality. There is evidence that such behavior is common among anesthesiologists. Rosenblatt surveyed a random sample of the active membership of the ASA.[19] The survey presented difficult airway scenarios involving cooperative adult patients who required tracheal intubation. Physicians were asked to identify their preferred management technique. In a scenario described as a patient with a history of previous difficult intubation, 60% of practitioners would induce general anesthesia and 59% would proceed with direct laryngoscopy. Experienced practitioners tended to use higher risk induction techniques and were more likely to use the laryngeal mask airway in situations commonly agreed to be unconventional or contraindicated. Use of alternative devices including the BL, lighted stylet, and other adjuncts was uncommon, occurring in <5% in all scenarios.

Jenkins surveyed 833 Canadian anesthesiologists to assess difficult airway management, training, and access to airway equipment.[20] Respondents were asked to indicate their management choices in 10 difficult airway scenarios. The direct laryngoscopy was the preferred technique overall, with FFB being the second most commonly used device. More experienced, male, and older practitioners were more likely to choose asleep induction for high-risk scenarios, a finding similar to that of Rosenblatt. Respondents were not asked to indicate their degree of comfort in using the alternatives that were chosen to manage the clinical scenarios described in the survey.

Kristensen similarly assessed airway management behavior, experience, and knowledge among Danish anesthesiologists by surveying all members of the Danish Society of Anesthesiologists.[21] Respondents were asked if they had experienced situations during anesthesia in which insufficient oxygenation had caused serious problems that could have been prevented by different airway management. About a quarter of those surveyed answered in the affirmative with 20% of registrars and 26% of specialists agreeing. When asked whether they would perform awake intubation if they expected a difficult intubation, 34% of registrars, 50% of senior registrars, but only 25% of specialists said that they would. Only 48% of registrars and 59% of specialists agreed that a previous difficult intubation was a reliable predictor of difficult intubation in the future. These high-risk attitudes and behaviors are especially concerning. Among the specialists, only 21% use a lighted stylet at least once a year, 11% a BL, and 7% a retrograde technique. Forty percent of specialists had intubated the trachea of an awake, spontaneously breathing patient 10 times or less in their career, and 23% of specialists had never done so using an FFB. Finally, about half the registrars and a third of the specialists reported that they did not routinely have immediate access to an LMA when providing anesthesia.

Ezri's more recent survey of American anesthesiologists suggests that there may be an increasing willingness to use alternatives to the direct laryngoscope in airway scenarios perceived as high risk.[22] However, Ezri also observed that such a willingness persisted even when the anesthesiologists acknowledged that they were neither comfortable nor experienced with the alternate technology that they proposed using in these difficult situations.

2.3.3 What is the medical–legal experience with respect to airway management failure?

The largest series of published medical-legal cases involving airway management is that of the ASA Closed Claims Project. Data from the airway cases reviewed in the ASA Closed Claims Project were originally published in 1990, with a revised publication in 2000.[23] In the 1990 report, Caplan noted that respiratory claims accounted for 34% (522/1541) of all claims. Inadequate ventilation was the most common single event overall, accounting for 12.7% of all claims and more than a third of the respiratory claims. In the original report, esophageal intubation and difficult intubation claims occurred each at about half the rate of those for inadequate ventilation. Caplan speculated that improved monitoring would be the most important intervention needed to reduce the incidence of inadequate ventilation and esophageal intubation. Further, it was stated that enhanced training would be the most important intervention to reduce the occurrence of difficult intubation and its sequelae.

In 2000, a Closed Claims data update was published in the ASA Newsletter.[24] Respiratory claims now accounted for 17.9% of total claims (798/4459), half the original proportion. Inadequate ventilation accounted for 7% of claims and esophageal intubation for 4.5% of claims, both considerably less than in the first report. However, claims for difficult intubation accounted for 6.4% of total claims, 14% higher than in the original report. In 48% of the difficult intubation claims, some difficulty was anticipated preoperatively by the anesthesiologist. Despite this expectation of difficulties, the most common (69% of instances) management strategy employed in these situations was induction of anesthesia followed by persistent attempts at oral laryngoscopic intubation. A similar strategy of multiple attempts orally was employed in scenarios in which difficulty was not anticipated but encountered. Of the cases in which difficulty was anticipated, 69% eventually deteriorated into a "can't intubate, can't ventilate" (CICV) situation.

Airway management was deemed to be below the accepted "standard of care" in 49% of the cases reported in the update. This is significantly higher than that seen for other claims in the database. Claims involving airway management are more likely to be associated with a permanent adverse outcome than others, and it is recognized that such severely adverse outcomes can affect the judgment as to the "appropriateness of care."[25] However, a preoperative airway review was not conducted (or recorded as having been conducted) in 25% of cases, 28% of practitioner's had no explicit plan for dealing with anticipated difficulties, and 25% did not alter their conventional method of airway management despite recognizing the potential for difficulty. Furthermore, when difficulties were encountered, the most common management strategy was persistent nonsurgical attempts at tracheal intubation. In 69% of cases where difficulties were anticipated, a CICV situation arose. Finally, and significantly, no strategy for extubation was outlined in almost half of the cases in which the practitioner encountered difficulties intubating the trachea.

2.4   AIRWAY ALGORITHMS

2.4.1   Why are algorithms useful in airway management?

Fundamental to successfully managing the airway, particularly in an emergency, is the development of a systematic approach ("decision trees" or "algorithms") to clinical situations encountered in day-to-day practice. These algorithms must be evidence based and must be quickly and easily applied. It is fair to say that after years of formal medical education and practice, most of us harbor an aversion to "algorithms." Memorized by rote and seldom used, most algorithms have been forgotten. While it is recognized that rigidity stifles innovation and constrains personal preference, adherence to sensibly constructed decision trees minimizes variation, conserves valuable time, and has been shown to provide the greatest chance for success.

Decision aids such as algorithms are meant to *inform* the practitioner rather than *dictate* to the practitioner. The practitioner is required to correctly identify the clinical problem (ie, a failed airway) before choosing the algorithm. The algorithm should be designed and validated to ensure a high degree of success, provided that it is applied to the correct clinical problem. Many of these situations occur relatively infrequently in a clinical practice, and it is unlikely that practitioners will have an opportunity to generate rules for managing the situations based on experience alone. By providing a limited number of likely-to-be successful options, the algorithm can increase the likelihood of a good outcome.

Reason has defined two basic mechanisms whereby practitioners deal with critical incidents. The first is a rule-based solution, whereby on recognizing the event for what it is, one identifies and applies a solution that experience has shown will likely be useful in solving the problem. Recognizing the event involves a process called "similarity-matching"; based on identifying that the characteristics of the events are similar to those of past events (in a sense, "pattern recognition"). The practitioner then decides upon a particular solution that is likely to be effective in solving the problem and resolving the threat. This presupposes that the practitioner has had sufficient experience with both the situation and the application of the rule to both immediately recognize the problem and to know which rule to apply. This ability constitutes what is called "expertise." Unfortunately, difficult and failed airways are encountered infrequently in practice, and the individual experiences of practitioners may have not been sufficient to earn them "expert" status.

The second mechanism for dealing with critical incidents is to apply a knowledge-based solution. This is a ground-up, first-principle strategy whereby the practitioner, without important past experience with similar situations, attempts to find an appropriate solution. Not surprisingly, such strategies are time consuming, and when made under pressure of time, are more likely to result in failure.

Many airway practitioners will not have sufficient experience with difficult and failed airway scenarios to have, of themselves, created a rule-based, organised approach to these airway dilemmas in which knowledge-based solutions may be inadequate. For this reason, preformulated airway algorithms are helpful in these situations and deserve to be considered by all airway practitioners.

Coincident with the development of the "decision trees" ("strategies") and vital to airway management success is skill in the application of an array of devices and techniques ("tactics") that can optimize clinical outcomes. Techniques and devices advocated in this chapter, as in the case of the decision trees, are anchored by evidence, rather than personal preference.

Algorithms meant to be used in crisis situations must exhibit the following design elements:

- Entry and exit points are easily recognized
- They are based on the best available evidence
- Branch points are binary
- There are a limited number of actions at each step
- They are easy to remember and represent graphically

2.4.2   What are the strengths and weaknesses of the ASA difficult airway algorithm?

The ASA, in an attempt to avert airway management disasters, has produced the "ASA Difficult Airway Algorithm" first in 1993 (Figure 2-1) and a revision in 2003 (Figure 2-2).[26,27] The ASA Difficult Airway

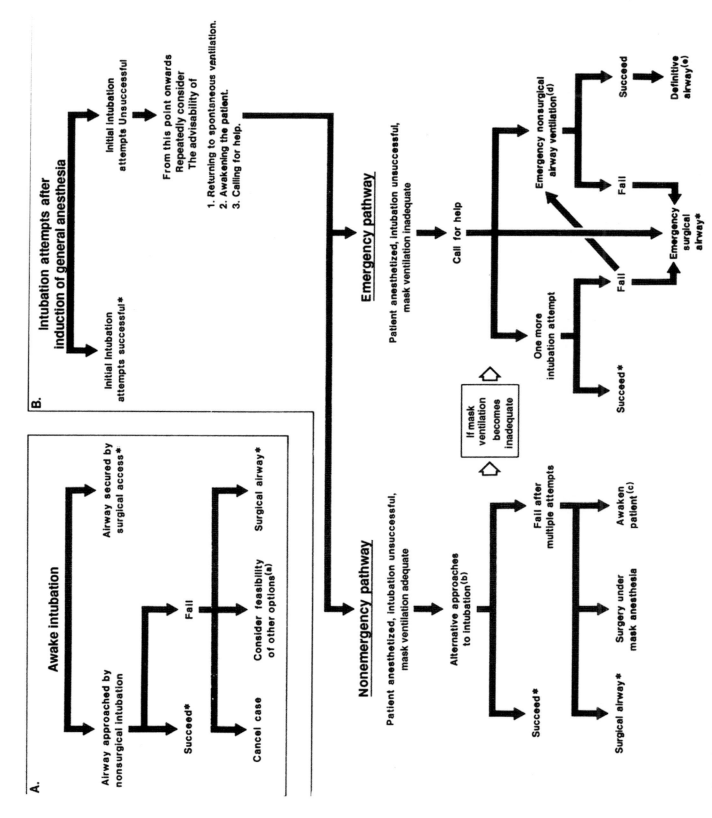

FIGURE 2-1. 1993 ASA Difficult Airway Management Algorithm.

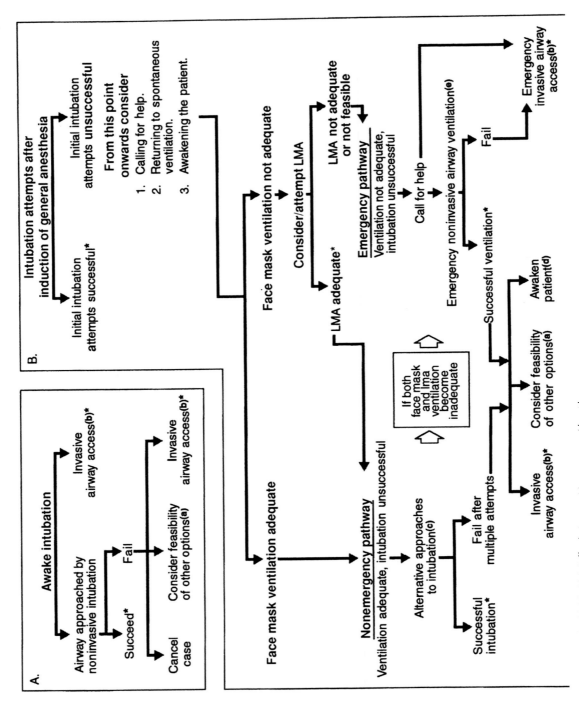

FIGURE 2-2. 2003 ASA Difficult Airway Management Algorithm.

TABLE 2-1

Components of the Preoperative Airway Physical Examination

AIRWAY EXAMINATION COMPONENT	NONREASSURING FINDING
Length or upper incisors	Relatively long
Relation of maxillary and mandibular incisors during normal jaw closure	Prominent overbite (maxillary incisors anterior)
Relation of incisors during protrusion of mandible	Overbite remains present
Interincisor distance	Less than 3 cm
Visibility of uvula (Mallampati class)	Not visible with tongue protruded, patient sitting (>II)
Shape of palate	High arched or narrow
Compliance of mandibular space	Stiff and indurated
Thyromental distance	Less than 5 cm
Length of neck	Short
Thickness of neck	Thick
Range of motion of head on neck	Limited

Adapted from Caplan RA, Benumof JL, Berry FA, et al: Practice guidelines for management of the difficult airway. An updated report by the American Society of Anesthesiologists Task Force on Management of the Difficult Airway. Anesthesiology 2003; 98: 1269–77.

Algorithm is derived from the "Practice Guidelines for the Management of the Difficult Airway," developed by the ASA Task Force on Difficult Airway Management.

In both iterations, Panel A is directed at anticipating the "Difficult Airway" and managing it awake, and Panel B deals with the "Failed Airway." The algorithms guide management strategies when difficulty is predicted and recommend rescue tactics in the event of failure. They emphasize the importance of possessing expertise in more than one airway management technique and that each time an airway is managed the practitioner formulate a variety of backup plans should the primary plan fail ("Plan B and Plan C").

As the ASA guidelines evolved from the first to the second iteration, a number of significant changes were made. Guidance is offered to those anatomic elements that may prove useful in the evaluation of the airway (Table 2-1), although no direction is given as to how to interpret the findings. The concept of a "reassuring" versus "nonreassuring" examination is now included, with the recommendation that a "nonreassuring" examination be a relevant factor in the plan for airway management. The need for the continuous application of oxygen to the patient during management of the difficult airway is emphasized in the second iteration. Finally, the laryngeal mask airway for ventilation has been moved from the emergency pathway of Panel B to an entry point determining whether the emergency pathway is entered. This change is likely due to the worldwide recognition that the laryngeal mask airway is an effective rescue-ventilating device.

A number of other groups have generated evidence-based consensus guidelines for the management of the difficult airway.[18,28] They differ from the ASA guidelines in being relevant only to the unanticipated difficult airway. They are similar to the ASA package in that they recognize the utility of alternatives to both BMV and the direct laryngoscopy for intubation as well as emphasizing the role of salvage plans and physician training with the alternative devices. The essential messages of the ASA "Difficult Airway Algorithms" are:

- If difficulty is anticipated (a nonreassuring airway examination)—secure the airway awake. While recognizing that even with a careful assessment, some airways perceived to be "unlikely to be difficult," in fact may be difficult to manage.

- If difficulty is encountered under anesthesia—awaken the patient. This is an option in an elective situation but clearly may not be an option in an urgent or emergency situation or a case in which airway management is the clinical end point rather than a diagnostic or therapeutic intervention.

- Think ahead—have Plans B and C immediately available or in place. This implies that one has evaluated the airway for difficulty in performing Plans B and C before embarking on Plan A, as stressed in Chapter 1.

Additional essential messages from the ASA Closed Claims Project and the medical–legal experience accumulating in anesthesia include:

- If the airway evaluation is nonreassuring, the plan for airway management should be constructed reflecting this finding.

- When faced with a variety of effective intubation choices, do what you do best!!

- If the technique you do best has not worked, and is not working, after no more than three attempts, use some other technique. Do not persist with a technique already demonstrated to be inadequate for the task at hand.

The ASA Guidelines and Algorithm have served to highlight the importance of predicting and managing the difficult airway and have probably led to a reduction in adverse events related to airway management disasters in the operating room setting. However, several limitations are identified in a detailed study of the algorithm:

- The algorithm actually addresses both difficult and failed airway management, but does not explicitly identify the two pathways. Identifying when a "difficult airway" has progressed to a "failed" one is crucial in selecting management options that will avert a bad outcome.

- The nonbinary nature of the decision matrices and the multiplicity of pathways have limited the clinical usefulness of the algorithm in guiding day-to-day practice, particularly in a crisis posed by an airway management failure (ie, Plans B and C).

- Often, in real life, rescue maneuvers are (and perhaps ought to be) contemplated and executed concurrently (eg, inserting an LMA at the same time preparations are underway to perform a surgical airway). The algorithm is silent in this regard.

- The algorithm does not provide for uncooperative patients (children, mentally challenged, and patients who refuse to cooperate with the planned airway management) and different patient populations (eg, obstetrical and pediatric patients).

- While surgical airway management is the cornerstone of failed airway management, anesthesia practitioners are often reluctant to undertake surgical airway management. Most experts agree that all airway practitioners ought to be able to perform such an intervention. Failure of the practitioner to expeditiously perform a surgical airway is often leveled as a criticism by plaintiff experts in medicolegal actions. It follows then, that when faced with a failed airway, preparations for a surgical airway must begin immediately. Neither the 1993 nor the 2003 ASA algorithm reflects this thinking. Furthermore, the 2003 ASA algorithm inserts an additional LMA step, potentially delaying the performance of a surgical airway.

- The medico-legal context.

  ○ The algorithm is intended to facilitate the management of the difficult airway and to reduce the likelihood of adverse outcomes. Although the determination of whether or not a practitioner met the standard of care will be judged in law, it is likely that reference to existing guidelines will be made in such determination.[29]

  ○ The guidelines and algorithm are silent with respect to whether or not they ought to apply outside the operating room. The performance of a defendant may be expected to comply with the algorithm no matter where the airway management is undertaken.

  ○ The option of "awakening the patient" is often not possible in a failed airway situation, particularly if the intubation is an emergency and the intubation is the actual and necessary clinical end point. This may seem elementary in concept, but the statement may pose a problem in medico-legal proceedings when the simplicity of "awakening the patient" is positioned by the plaintiff as *the* solution in the face of airway management failure, making the failure to do such a simple maneuver inexplicable and arcane. A simple statement by the Task Force that "awakening the patient" is not always feasible would go a long way in legally defending the appropriate actions of a practitioner in emergency airway situations.

  ○ Despite any disclaimer, this document is likely to be referenced by medical experts in establishing the "standard of care" for difficult and failed airway management in anesthesia practice.

2.5   THE EMERGENCY AIRWAY ALGORITHMS[30]

2.5.1   Why do these algorithms work best in emergency situations?

The Emergency Airway Management Algorithms that follow adhere to the design elements of effective algorithms and are specifically intended to be applied in crisis situations in which actions must be intuitive and automatic to increase the changes of a good outcome. They are derived loosely from the ASA algorithm and based on the same evidence. They describe a logical progression of "thinking" and "doing" when faced with the "crash" situation, the difficult airway, and the failed airway. An algorithm dealing with extubation of the difficult airway is also presented.

These algorithms are shown in Figures 2-3 to 2-6. The reader is encouraged to refer to the figures while reading the text descriptions below. The Emergency Airway Algorithms do not address the indications for intubation and do not deal with the decision to intubate. Therefore, the entry point for each one is immediately after the decision to intubate has been made.

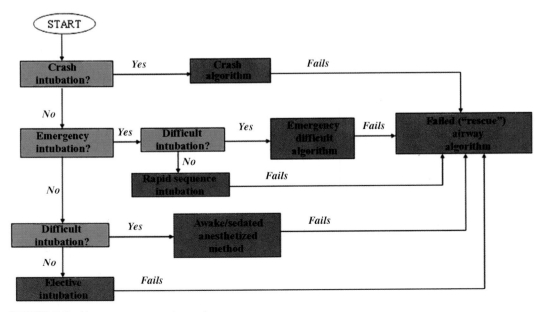

FIGURE 2-3. Airway management overview.

The Crash Airway Algorithm

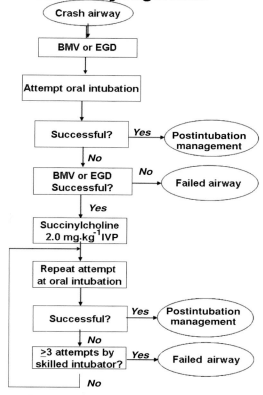

FIGURE 2-4. Crash Airway Algorithm.

The Failed Airway Algorithm

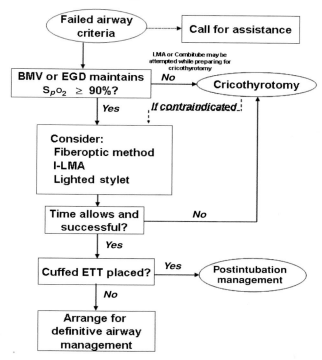

FIGURE 2-6. Failed Airway Algorithm.

The Emergency Difficult Airway Algorithm

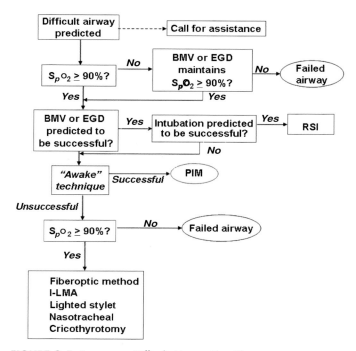

FIGURE 2-5. Emergency Difficult Airway Algorithm.

These algorithms, though consistent with the thinking imbedded in the ASA algorithm, are tailored for urgent and emergency clinical situations and adhere to the principles fundamental to such clinical situations. Importantly, the algorithms presented in this chapter are not meant to be memorized and followed slavishly, as with a recipe. They are the ways of rapidly thinking through urgent clinical situations and helping to make crucial decisions and actions.

The practitioner may fail to appreciate the "failed airway" and subsequently fail to move quickly to a salvage strategy or to secure a surgical airway. It must be emphasized that there ought to be no hesitation in performing a surgical airway or cricothyrotomy in the face of airway management failure.

2.5.2 The overview algorithm

The Overview Algorithm (Figure 2-3) presents the way most practitioners approach the issue of airway management. Most of the time, it is routine, elective, controlled, and deliberate. Most intubations are not "crash" or emergency situations. So the first real question faced in daily practice is "Is this a difficult airway?" If not, it is handled in a routine fashion as preferred by the individual.

If it is deemed to be difficult (based on a nonreassuring airway examination, an awkward environment, poor patient condition, etc.), an awake intubation procedure may be indicated depending on the judgment of the airway practitioner. There are a number of considerations that will inform and influence this decision.

- Is direct laryngoscopy likely to be difficult? If so, is the airway practitioner skilled in an alternative technique that is likely to be effective in the situation or is the skill set limited to direct laryngoscopy? If the latter statement most accurately describes the situation, then awake intubation is likely the most prudent course. If the former statement most accurately describes the case, consideration may be given to induction of anesthesia, with muscle paralysis, followed by tracheal intubation using an alternate strategy, provided that there is no anticipated difficulty in ventilation using BMV or an EGD.

- Is there a need to protect the airway from gastric contents? If so, it should be recognized that the ability to protect the airway with cricoid pressure is limited[31]; and that multiple attempts at direct laryngoscopy over a prolonged period of time are associated with regurgitation and aspiration. The combination of difficult laryngoscopy and a full stomach in a cooperative patient may best be managed with an awake intubation (see Chapters 3 and 5).

In the event the patient is unresponsive or near death, a "crash" intubation is indicated and the "Crash Algorithm" is employed. "Unresponsive" means that the patient does not respond adversely to oral laryngoscopy ("the newly dead or nearly dead").

Failure to meet the criteria for a crash intubation does not mean that the intubation is not an emergency. Intubation is urgently indicated in the event when a patient is unable to:

- maintain reasonable oxygenation,
- protect the airway,
- maintain the airway,
- is faced with intubation to manage some other condition, or is to be paralyzed.

Once the decision is made that this is an urgent or emergency intubation, the next question is "Will this be a difficult intubation?" This decision must be made quickly, and Chapter 1 presents efficient strategies for assessing the airway quickly for difficulty. If the urgent/emergency intubation is not judged to be difficult, a Rapid Sequence Induction/Intubation (RSI) is indicated as the method most likely to rapidly and safely secure the airway.

In the event the airway is judged difficult, the Emergency Difficult Airway Algorithm should be employed. Should any of these approaches fail, the "Failed Airway Algorithm" is used to rapidly and definitively gain control of the airway.

Four algorithms emerge from this conceptual approach to the airway and its management:

- The Crash Airway Algorithm (Figure 2-4)
- The Emergency Difficult Airway Algorithm (Figure 2-5)
- The Failed Airway Algorithm (Figure 2-6)
- The Extubation Algorithm (Figure 2-7)

2.5.3   The crash airway algorithm

Entry at this point requires an unconscious, unresponsive patient with immediate need for airway management. The first step in the crash algorithm is to attempt oral intubation immediately by direct laryngoscopy without pharmacologic assist. If the oral intu-

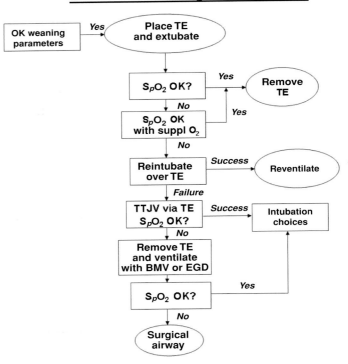

Difficult Airway Extubation

FIGURE 2-7. Difficult Airway Extubation Algorithm.

bation is successful, then the practitioner proceeds with postintubation management. If oral intubation is not initially successful with direct laryngoscopy, then a decision point is reached and several questions must be asked.

2.5.3.1   Is BMV Successful?

If BMV is successful, then one has time and further attempts at oral intubation are possible. If BMV is unsuccessful in the context of a failed oral intubation with a "crash" airway, then a failed airway is present. BMV should be optimized with the use of oral and nasal airways and include maneuvers such as jaw thrust, chin lift, or a head tilt if appropriate. A two-hand mask hold may improve mask seal. Additionally, if cricoid pressure is being applied, consideration should be given to relaxing the force being applied or temporarily discontinuing it and assessing airway patency in its absence. One further attempt at intubation may be indicated, but no more than one, because intubation has failed and the failure of BMV places the patient in serious and immediate jeopardy. This is a CICV situation, and in such circumstances, the "Failed Airway Algorithm" (see Figure 2-6) mandates immediate surgical airway management. If surgical airway management is not *immediately* possible, temporizing methods, such as the placement of an EGD (eg, LMA or Combitube™), should be attempted, but such attempts should not delay preparation for, and the creation of, a surgical airway. The successful use of an EGD in permitting adequate gas exchange may obviate the need for a surgical airway.

2.5.3.2   Is the Patient Completely Relaxed and Flaccid?

During the first attempt at orotracheal intubation in the unconscious, unresponsive patient, the patient is assessed for degree of relaxation to permit intubation. If the impression is one of absolute, complete skeletal muscle relaxation, then further intubation attempts are indicated. If the patient is felt to be exhibiting any resistance whatsoever to intubation, then a single dose of succinylcholine, 2.0 mg·kg^{-1}, should be given and oral intubation attempted again. Usually, only one dose is indicated. It should be noted that this dose of succinylcholine is higher than the 1.0–1.5 mg·kg^{-1} recommended elsewhere in this text. This is an empiric judgment of the authors related to the fact that these patients often have no spontaneous circulation needed to get the medication to the motor endplate. Further, in this situation no induction agent is indicated.

2.5.3.3   Have There Been Three Attempts at Intubation by an Experienced Airway Practitioner?

If the answer to this question is yes, then consistent with the definition above, the situation represents a "failed airway" (Figure 2-5). The futility of further attempts may be evident after the first attempt dictating an immediate move to a different device or technique. If fewer than three attempts have been made by an experienced airway practitioner, and it is the opinion of the practitioner that it is possible to be successful by this route, a repeat attempt at oral intubation is justified. No more than three attempts at direct laryngoscopy can be supported. As detailed above, the evidence suggests that there is a low likelihood of success with persistent use of the direct laryngoscope after three failed attempts and an increased likelihood of patient morbidity and cardiac arrest. Between each intubation attempt, defined by a single laryngoscopy, the patient should receive ventilation and oxygenation through a bag-mask.

2.5.3.4   Is It Appropriate to Repeat Laryngoscopic Intubation Until Three Attempts Have Failed?

As stated above, it is often apparent after a single attempt that further attempts at orotracheal intubation will be futile. In such cases, move to Plan B if oxygenation can be maintained; the "Failed Airway Algorithm" if it cannot be maintained.

2.5.3.5   Were Repeated Efforts Successful?

If intubation is achieved, then proceed to postintubation management; if not, cycle back to make another attempt or to proceed to the failed airway algorithm, depending on the number of attempts which have already been made. The failure of three attempts indicates a very low likelihood of ultimate success with oral intubation. There is a diminishing return with subsequent attempts and an increased risk of hypoxia, aspiration, and cardiac arrest. After three attempts, efforts to ensure oxygenation should be the priority while preparations are being made to perform a surgical airway.

2.5.3.6   Postintubation Management

This is undertaken in the event of a successful intubation.

2.5.4   The emergency difficult airway algorithm

This algorithm (Figure 2-5) is specifically designed to guide airway management in an emergency. Decisions are binary by design. It incorporates the notion of the failed airway. Though a fairly busy-appearing figure with some 13 boxes, in reality it simply poses a series of simple questions:

1. Is the airway difficult (MOANS, LEMON, RODS, and SHORT)? (See Sections 1.6.1–1.6.4.)

2. Do I have time (is the oxygen saturation within a normal range)? Or can I make time (with BMV)?

3. On reconsideration, is an RSI technique reasonable?

4. Failing that, what is my best option?

Bearing in mind that patients presenting in an emergency should almost always considered having a full stomach, some points deserve emphasis.

2.5.4.1   Is a Difficult Airway Predicted?

If, for whatever reason, airway management is predicted to be difficult, nothing should be taken from the patient that the airway practitioner cannot replace. This particularly applies to the administration of paralytic drugs. Furthermore, the ability to protect the airway with cricoid pressure is limited, and multiple attempts at laryngoscopy over a prolonged period of time have been associated with regurgitation and aspiration. Therefore, careful consideration should be given to awake intubation in the setting of dual concerns of difficult airway and full stomach.

2.5.4.2   Is BMV or EGD Ventilation Predicted to Be Successful (MOANS and RODS)? (See Sections 1.6.1 and 1.6.3.)

In other words, if intubation fails, will BMV or rescue with some other device (commonly an EGD) be possible? One must have a high degree of certainty that this question is answered in the affirmative, particularly if one is contemplating the use of paralytic agents. The fact that one is operating within this algorithm presupposes that there is a sense of urgency to the situation *and* the airway practitioner is suspecting difficulty. In this situation, planning for and being prepared to undertake rescue maneuvers (Plans B and C) are crucial, as is the preemptive evaluation for difficulty. As an example, if one is planning to perform a rapid cricothyrotomy (Plan B) should induction and paralysis (Plan A) fail, then an evaluation for difficult cricothyrotomy must be performed (SHORT, see Section 1.6.4) before embarking on Plan A.

2.5.4.3   Is Intubation Deemed Reasonably Likely?

The decision to proceed with an RSI technique in the patient with a predicted difficult airway must be associated with the likelihood that it will be successful. Airway practitioners must be confident in their abilities and must possess a broad array of equipment and skills to rescue the airway in the event that conventional direct vision orotracheal intubation fails.

2.5.4.4   Should an "Awake Look" Employing Topical Anesthesia and Sedation Be Attempted to Assist in Decision Making?

A variety of techniques are available to obtund the airway, the patient, or both, without "burning any bridges." The condition of the patient and the clinical situation will dictate the aggression of this maneuver (ie, how much does one need to see?). It may be that the airway practitioner simply needs to verify that the epiglottis is in the midline to make the decision to back off and move to a rapid-sequence technique. At other times, it may indicate that an awake intubation is appropriate.

The value of the "awake look" as a maneuver to reassure oneself that oral intubation is likely to be possible following the administration of induction and paralytic medications ought to be tempered by the findings of Sivarajan and Fink.[32] These authors measured the position of larynx in lateral radiographs of necks taken in human volunteers when they were awake, and after induction of general anesthesia and muscle paralysis. They found that the hyoid bone and epiglottis were shifted anteriorly and the extraglottic region or the vestibule of the larynx was enlarged with the onset of general anesthesia and muscle paralysis. In addition, the larynx was also stretched longitudinally with wide separation of the vestibular and vocal folds. The authors concluded that consciousness is associated with tonic muscular activity that folds the larynx and partially closes it and that onset of general anesthesia and muscle paralysis opens the larynx wider and shifts it anteriorly, which might make visualization of the larynx difficult during direct laryngoscopy in some patients.

2.5.5   The failed airway algorithm

The failure to intubate is rarely accompanied by the failure to ventilate and oxygenate. This situation has variously been termed CICV or "can't intubate, can't oxygenate" (CICO), the latter being the more precise term. It is a clinical emergency of such magnitude that it leads to neurologic compromise and death if not rectified rapidly. Decisive action in selecting a technique most likely to lead to a secure airway (ie, an emergency surgical airway) is essential to success in such a situation. It cannot be overemphasized that a failing technique (eg, direct laryngoscopy) cannot be considered as an appropriate salvage technique and there is no defence for persistent attempts with a failing technique.

More often the failure to intubate is associated with some degree of success with BMV/oxygenation, giving the airway practitioner time to consider alternative techniques. This CICV/O situation is amenable to nonsurgical rescue techniques. In this scenario, practiced alternatives to the direct laryngoscope such as the lighted stylet, or a rigid or flexible endoscope, may be used or an EGD may be placed to provide a more secure, bridging airway. In the latter case, these EGDs may be used to facilitate intubation (eg, LMA-Fastrach™, Cook ILA™) or provide time to prepare for a more definitive solution (surgical airway).

The Failed Airway Algorithm is presented in Figure 2-6. The essential message from this algorithm is that the decision to move to a surgical airway must be taken early once the failure to maintain oxygenation is recognized. Wasting valuable time attempting a variety of devices or techniques is to be avoided at all costs, unless it is while the practitioner is concurrently preparing to perform a surgical airway. There is little or no value at this time in making attempts with tools or techniques with which the practitioner has no experience.

2.5.5.1   Failed Airway Criteria Have Been Met

This is the entry point to the "Failed Airway Algorithm." The criteria are either three failed attempts at intubation via oral laryngoscopy by an experienced practitioner or a single failed attempt at oral intubation with inability to maintain $SpO_2 \geq 90\%$ using a bag-mask. A mandated intubation in a patient with a difficult or crash airway in whom BMV also fails represents a failed airway. As with the difficult airway, it is advisable to call for assistance when a failed airway has occurred. This is especially true if BMV has also failed and qualified help is immediately available.

2.5.5.2   Is BMV Possible and Adequate?

In the circumstance of a failed airway, if BMV is not adequate, then immediate cricothyrotomy is mandatory. The only exception to this recommendation is the use of a temporizing technique, such as the I-LMA or Combitube™, if cricothyrotomy is not immediately possible. Further attempts at intubation or use of alternate devices will merely prolong the patient's hypoxemic state. If surgical airway management is itself *relatively* contraindicated (in a life and death situation all contraindications to cricothyrotomy are relative), then alternative methods may be tried first. For example, if the patient has known laryngeal pathology in the area of the anticipated surgical intervention, such as a tumor or hematoma, then alternative techniques may be preferred. However, if these methods are not immediately successful, cricothyrotomy should be performed, even in the presence of relative contraindications. SHORT (see Section 1.6.4) identifies conditions that present difficulty and should not be thought of as contraindications.

2.5.5.3   Consider Combitube™, Fiberoptic, I-lma, Lighted Stylet, Trans-Tracheal Jet Ventilation, Retrograde, or Some Other Method

If ventilation and oxygenation by bag-mask can maintain $SpO_2 \geq 90\%$ (or some acceptable number), then a number of different devices and procedures may be attempted to rescue the patient with the failed airway. At all times, the patient must be monitored for adequate oxygenation. If oxygenation becomes inadequate at any time and cannot be restored via BMV, then cricothyrotomy is mandatory. Likewise, if there is failure of each of the techniques considered appropriate, then cricothyrotomy should be undertaken. Videolaryngoscopic (eg, the Glidescope®) and fiberoptic methods, including the FFB, and the rigid fiberoptic laryngoscopes (eg, Shikani, Bonfils, Bullard) have all been shown to be effective and safe rescue techniques. The choice of the tool should be governed primarily by the practitioner's experience and expertise. The application of a tool with which the practitioner has little experience is difficult to defend as a prudent intervention.

2.5.5.4   Time Allows and Successful?

If there is sufficient time to achieve oxygenation and ventilation using one of these devices or techniques, proceed down the main path of the algorithm. If not, cricothyrotomy is mandated.

2.5.5.5   Was an Endotracheal Tube Placed?

If an endotracheal tube is successfully placed at any time, postintubation management may be undertaken. If a Combitube™, King LT Airway, or percutaneous transtracheal ventilation have been employed successfully, then the airway should be considered to be temporary, at best and arrangements for a definitive airway be made. If the airway placed is unable to provide adequate ventilation and oxygenation, then immediate cricothyrotomy is indicated.

2.5.6   The extubation algorithm

The Extubation Algorithm (Figure 2-7) is specifically intended to be employed in those situations in which reintubation, if needed, is judged to be difficult or impossible (eg, patient was initially intubated awake because intubation was judged to be impossible).[33] At the core of the algorithm is a trial of extubation over a 'tube exchanger' (TE) (e.g., Cook Endotracheal Tube Exchange Catheter).

It is important to note that a failure to reintubate should be immediately followed by an assessment of the ability to maintain oxygen saturations. If oxygen saturation can be maintained by jet ventilation through the catheter or by BMV, there is likely some time to use alternative methods of intubation, such as lightwands and fiberscopes. On the other hand, the failure to maintain oxygen saturation should be immediately followed by attempts to employ rescue devices such as Combitube™, Intubating Laryngeal Mask, and Trans-Tracheal Jet Ventilation while preparations are undertaken to perform a surgical airway.

2.6   SUMMARY

The failure to adequately manage the airway is a major contributor to poor outcomes in anesthesia, emergency medicine, critical care, and Emergency Medical Services.[34–36] Adverse respiratory events constitute the largest cause of injury in the ASA Closed Claims Project.[34] The single most important factor leading to a failed airway is failure to predict the difficult airway.[25,35]

Emergency airway management is always stress provoking. Crucial decisions must be made in a timely manner, and the airway practitioner is expected to possess expertise in a variety of primary (Plan A) and backup (Plans B and C) maneuvers.

Well-designed algorithms based on the best available evidence are intended to improve the outcome of difficult and failed airway emergencies. However, it is incumbent on the airway practitioner to identify which algorithm to employ, particularly in the event that a "difficult airway" has progressed to a "failed airway."

REFERENCES

1. Langeron O, Masso E, Huraux C, et al.: Prediction of difficult mask ventilation. *Anesthesiology.* 2000;92:1229–1236.
2. Petito SP, Russell WJ: The prevention of gastric insufflation—a neglected benefit of cricoid pressure. *Anaesth Intens Care.* 1988;16:139.
3. Cass NM, James NR, Lines V: Difficult direct laryngoscopy complicating intubation in anaesthesia. *BMJ.* 1956;1:488–490.
4. Mallampati SR: Clinical sign to predict difficult tracheal intubation (hypothesis). *Can Anesth Soc J.* 1983;30;316–317.
5. Mallampati SR, Gatt SP, Gugino LD, et al.: A clinical sign to predict difficult intubation: a prospective study. *Can Anesth Soc J.* 1985;32:429–434.
6. Samsoon GL, Young JR: Difficult tracheal intubation: a retrospective study. *Anaesthesia.* 1987;42:487–490.
7. Karkouti K, Rose DK, Ferris LE, et al.: Inter-observer reliability of ten tests used for predicting difficult tracheal intubation. *Can J Anaesth.* 1996;43:554–55.
8. Yentis SM: Predicting difficult intubation—worthless exercise or pointless ritual? *Anaesthesia.* 2002;57:105–109.
9. Smith CE, Boyer D: Cricoid pressure decreases ease of tracheal intubation using fibreoptic laryngoscopy. *Can J Anesth.* 2002;49:614–619.
10. Hodgson RE, Gopalan PD, Burrows RC, et al.: Effect of cricoid pressure on the success of endotracheal intubation with a lightwand. *Anesthesiology.* 2001; 94:259–262.
11. Shulman GB, Connelly NR: A comparison of the Bullard Laryngoscope versus the flexible fiberoptic bronchoscope during intubation in patients afforded in-line stabilization. *J Clin Anesth.* 2001;13:182–185.
12. Rose DK, Cohen MM: The airway: problems and predictions in 18,500 patients. *Can J Anaesth.* 1994;41:372–383.
13. Mort TC: Emergency tracheal intubation: complications associated with repeated laryngoscopic attempts. *Anesth Analg.* 2004;99:607–613.
14. Hung OR, Pytka S, Morris I, et al.: Lightwand intubation: II. Clinical trial of a new lightwand for tracheal intubation in patients with difficult airways. *Can J Anaesth.* 1995;42:826–830.
15. Heidegger T, Gerig HJ, Ulrich B, et al.: Validation of a simple algorithm for tracheal intubation: daily practice is the key to success in intubation—an analysis of 13,248 intubations. *Anesth Analg.* 2001;92:517–522.
16. Combes X, Le Roux B, Suen P, et al.: Unanticipated difficult airway in anesthetized patients. Prospective validation of a management algorithm. *Anesthesiology.* 2004;100:1146–1150.
17. Mort TC: The incidence and risk factors for cardiac arrest during emergency tracheal intubation: a justification for incorporating the ASA guidelines in the remote location. *J Clin Anesth.* 2004;16:508–516.
18. Crosby ET, Cooper RM, Douglas MJ, et al.: The unanticipated difficult airway with recommendations for management. *Can J Anaesth.* 1998;45: 757–776.
19. Rosenblatt WH, Wagner PJ, Ovassapian A, et al.: Practice patterns in managing the difficult airway by anesthesiologists in the United States. *Anesth Analg.* 1998;87:153–157.
20. Jenkins K, Wong DT, Correa R: Management choices for the difficult airway by anesthesiologists in Canada. *Can J Anaesth.* 2002;49:850–856.
21. Kristensen MS, Møller J: Airway management behavior, experience and knowledge among Danish anaesthesiologists: room for improvement. *Acta Anaesthesiol Scand.* 2001;45:1181–1185.
22. Ezri TE, Szmuk P, Warters RD, et al.: Difficult airway management practice patterns among anesthesiologists practicing in the United States: have we made any progress. *J Clin Anesth.* 2003;15:418–422.
23. Caplan RA, Posner KL, Ward RJ, et al.: Adverse respiratory events in anesthesia: a closed claims analysis. *Anesthesiology.* 1990;72:828–833.
24. Miller CG: Management of the difficult intubation in closed malpractice claims. ASA Newsletter 200; 64. Available at: www.asahq.org/Newsletters/2000.
25. Caplan RA, Posner KL, Cheney FW: Effect of outcome on physician judgements of appropriateness of care. *J Am Med Assoc.* 1991;265:1957–1960.
26. Caplan RA, Benumof JL, Berry FA, et al.: Practice guidelines for management of the difficult airway. A report by the American Society of Anesthesiologists Task Force on Management of the Difficult Airway. *Anesthesiology.* 1993;78: 597–602.
27. Caplan RA, Benumof JL, Berry FA, et al.: Practice guidelines for management of the difficult airway. An updated report by the American Society of Anesthesiologists Task Force on Management of the Difficult Airway. *Anesthesiology.* 2003;98:1269–1277.
28. Henderson JJ, Popat MT, Latto IP, et al.: Difficult Airway Society guidelines for management of unanticipated difficult intubation. *Anaesthesia.* 2004; 59:675–694.
29. Hyamis AL, Brandenburg JA, Lipsitz SR, et al.: Practice guidelines and malpractice litigation: a two-way street. *Ann Intern Med.* 1995;122:450–455.
30. Walls RM: The emergency airway algorithms. In: *Manual of Emergency Airway Management.* Walls RM, Murphy MF, Luten R, eds. Philadelphia, PA: Lippincott, Williams, and Wilkins, 2004:8–21.
31. Brimacombe J: Cricoid pressure. *Can J Anaesth.* 1997;44:414–425.
32. Sivarajan M, Fink BR: The position and the state of the larynx during general anesthesia and muscle paralysis. *Anesthesiology.* 1990;72:439–442.

33. Miller KA, Harkin CP, Bailey PL: Postoperative tracheal extubation. *Anesth Analg.* 1995;80:149–172.

34. Mort TC: Emergency tracheal intubation: complications associated with repeated laryngoscopic attempts. *Anesth Analg.* 2004;99:607–613.

35. Cheney FW, Posner KL, Caplan RA: Adverse respiratory events infrequently leading to malpractice suits. A closed claims analysis. *Anesthesiology.* 1991; 75:932.

36. Practice guidelines for management of the difficult airway: an updated report by the American Society of Anesthesiologists Task Force on Management of the Difficult Airway. *Anesthesiology.* 2003;98:1269–1277.

SELF-EVALUATION QUESTIONS:

2.1. All of the following are features of well designed, clinically useful algorithms **EXCEPT**

   A. They are designed by reputable organizations

   B. They have clear entry and exit points

   C. Decision points are binary

   D. They are easily remembered in crisis

   E. They are easy to represent graphically

2.2. All of the following are true of the ASA Difficult Airway Algorithm **EXCEPT**

   A. It is evidence based

   B. It has likely helped to reduce the rate of airway management failure in anesthesia practice

   C. It is meant to represent the 'standard of care' in medico-legal proceedings

   D. It has two sections: one for the difficult airway and one for the failed airway

   E. The use of the LMA is a discrete step

2.3. All of the following are identified weaknesses of the ASA Difficult Airway Algorithm **EXCEPT**

   A. The algorithm actually addresses both difficult and failed airway management, but does not explicitly identify the two pathways.

   B. The nonbinary nature of the decision matrices and the multiplicity of pathways have limited the clinical usefulness of the algorithm in guiding day-to-day practice.

   C. The algorithm does not provide for uncooperative patients (children, mentally challenged, and patients who refuse to co-operate with the planned airway management) and different patient populations (e.g. obstetrical and pediatric patients).

   D. The algorithm is silent with respect to whether or not they ought to apply outside the Operating Room.

   E. The algorithm is clear that awakening the patient is not always possible.

CHAPTER (3)

Preparation for Awake Intubation

Ian R. Morris

3.1 INTRODUCTION

3.1.1 What are the fundamentals of an "awake, fiberoptically facilitated" intubation?

If awake fiberoptic intubation is to be achieved rapidly with minimal patient discomfort, an in-depth knowledge of the anatomy and regional anesthesia of the airway is required, as is dexterity with bronchoscopic manipulation. In order to achieve optimal regional anesthesia of the airway and avoid complications, a thorough knowledge of the local anesthetics employed and techniques of administration is necessary. The primary requirement for successful awake intubation is the effective regional anesthesia of the airway.[1]

3.2 AIRWAY ANATOMY

3.2.1 Why is knowledge of upper-airway anatomy beneficial in airway management?

Knowledge of the structure, function, and pathophysiology of the upper airway permits the health care provider to anticipate potential life-threatening problems and better use the full spectrum of airway management techniques.[2] Functionally, the upper airway can be considered to consist of the nasal cavities, pharynx, larynx, and trachea (see Figure 3-1).[3] The oral cavity provides an alternate access route to the pharynx.

3.2.2 The nose

Anatomically, the nose can be divided into an external component and the nasal cavity.[4] The external nose consists of a bony vault posterior superiorly, a cartilaginous vault anteriorly, and the lobule at the inferior-anterior aspect (see Figure 3-2).[3] The cavity of the nose is divided into bilateral compartments by the nasal septum and continues posteriorly from the nostrils (nares), to communicate with the nasopharynx at the posterior aspect of the septum (the choanae) (see Figures 3-3 to 3-5).[3] The nasal vestibule is a small dilatation located immediately inside the nostrils.[3,4] Each nasal cavity is bounded by a floor, a roof, and medial and lateral walls.[3–5] The roof of the nasal cavity extends posteriorly from the bridge of the nose, and it consists of the lateral nasal cartilages, the nasal bones and spine of the frontal bone, the cribriform plate of the ethmoid, and the inferior aspect of the sphenoid.[3,4,6] The nasal septum forms the medial wall, and it is formed by the quadrilateral cartilage, the perpendicular plate of the ethmoid, and the vomer (see Figure 3-5).[3] The lateral wall is formed anterior inferiorly by the frontal process of the maxilla, the nasal bones anterior superiorly, the nasal aspect of the ethmoid superiorly, and the perpendicular plate of the palatine and medial pterygoid plate posteriorly.[3,7] A series of three horizontal scroll-like ridges (conchae or turbinates) project medially from the lateral walls of the nasal cavities, each of which overhangs a corresponding groove or meatus (see Figures 3-2 to 3-4).[3,8] Septal deviation is common, may be associated with compensatory hypertrophy of the turbinates, and can produce nasal obstruction.[3,4] The paranasal sinuses and the nasolacrimal duct empty into the nasal cavity through ostia in the lateral wall.[3] Obstruction of the ostia of the paranasal sinuses can occur with prolonged nasal intubation and can cause sinusitis.[2,3] The floor of each nasal cavity is concave and is formed by the palatine process of the maxilla and the horizontal plate of the palatine

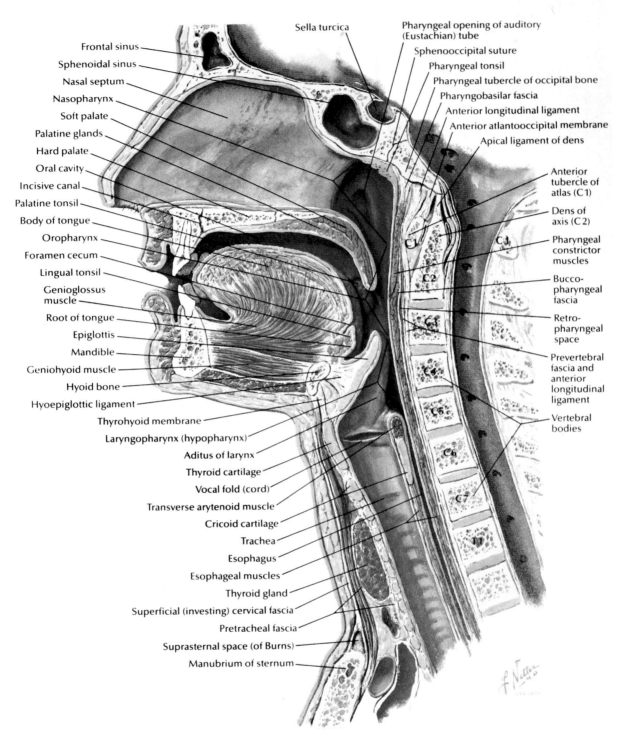

FIGURE 3-1. Sagittal view of the upper airway. *(Reproduced with permission from Netter FH: Atlas of Human Anatomy. Summit. New Jersey: CIBA-GEIGY Corporation, 1989.)*

bone.[3,4] The floor extends posteriorly in a transverse plane from the vestibule.

The major nasal airway is located below the inferior turbinate, declines slightly front to back (~20 degrees), and a nasotracheal tube should be directed backward and slightly inferiorly along the floor of the nose.[2–4] Occasionally, the posterior aspect of the inferior turbinate may be hypertrophied and resistance to the passage

of a nasotracheal tube may be encountered at this location.[4] Alternating counterclockwise/clockwise rotation of the tube changes the orientation of the bevel and may facilitate negotiation of the nasal cavity (see Chapter 10).

The anterior and posterior ethmoidal branches of the internal carotid artery supply the anterior-superior aspect of the nasal cavity and the sphenopalatine branch of the external carotid supplies

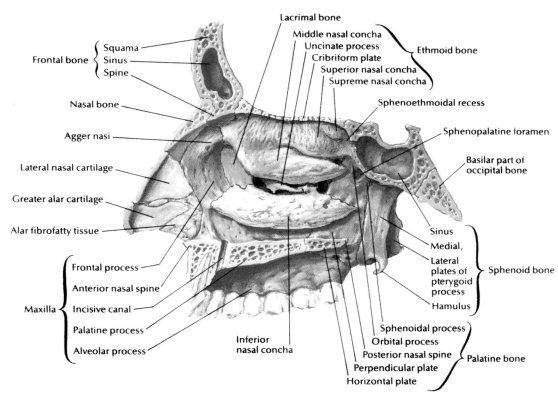

FIGURE 3-2. Bony components of lateral nasal wall. (*Reproduced with permission from Netter FH: Atlas of Human Anatomy. Summit. New Jersey: CIBA-GEIGY Corporation, 1989.*)

the posterior-inferior aspect.[3,9] The vestibule receives blood supply from both the anterior ethmoidal and sphenopalatine arteries as well as from nasal branches of the superior labial branch of the facial artery (see Figure 3-6).[3,9] Anastomoses between vessels from these three different sources occur particularly at the anterior-inferior aspect of the septum (Little's area or Kiesselbach's plexus), and this is a common site of epistaxis.[3,4,9] Tintinalli reported mod-

erate to severe epistaxis in 7% of 71 attempted emergency nasotracheal intubations.[10] The single case of severe epistaxis in this series occurred in a patient with cirrhosis. Minimal epistaxis has been reported in 11–40% of nasal intubations.[10,11] In a series of 99 patients undergoing nasotracheal intubation for oromaxillofacial surgery, epistaxis occurred in 6 patients but was sufficient to result in a visible accumulation of blood in the pharynx in only 1 patient.[12] During nasal intubation passing the tube with the bevel at the tip facing the septum directs the leading edge away from the vascular septum; however the optimum orientation of the tube is controversial (see Section 10.5.3).[13] Perforation into the submucosal space can occur and lead to hematoma and abscess formation in the retropharyngeal space.[2,3] Excessive force must be avoided.[3]

Common sensation to the nasal cavities is supplied by the ophthalmic and maxillary divisions of the trigeminal nerve.[2,3] The posterior aspect of the septum is innervated by the short- and long sphenopalatine branches of the maxillary nerve.[3,4] Anteriorly the septum is supplied by the anterior ethmoidal branch of the ophthalmic nerve (see Figure 3-7). The posterior-superior aspect of the lateral wall is innervated by the short sphenopalatine nerve and the inferior aspect by the posterolateral nasal branches of the sphenopalatine nerve.[3,4,9] Anteriorly, the floor of the nose is supplied by the anterior-superior dental branch of the infraorbital nerve and posteriorly by the greater palatine.[3,4] Rootlets of the olfactory nerve located in the roof of the nose adjacent to the cribriform plate transmit the sense of smell.[3]

In addition to being a respiratory pathway, the nose humidifies and warms inspired air, houses the olfactory receptors, removes bacteria, dust, and other particles from inspired air, and acts as a voice resonator.[3,4,8]

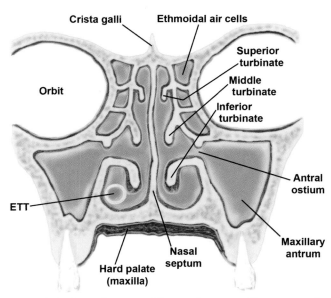

FIGURE 3-3. Coronal section of the maxillary sinus. The position of a nasotracheal tube (ETT) is shown in the right nasal cavity.

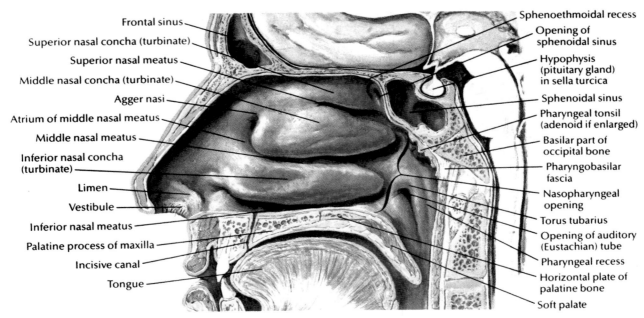

FIGURE 3-4. Lateral nasal wall. (*Reproduced with permission from Netter FH*: Atlas of Human Anatomy. *Summit. New Jersey: CIBA-GEIGY Corporation, 1989.*)

3.2.3   The mouth

Anatomically, the mouth consists of (1) the vestibule which is bounded externally by the lips and cheeks and internally by the gums and teeth and (2) the mouth cavity.[3,4] The mouth cavity is bounded by the alveolar arches and the teeth anteriorly and laterally, the hard palate and the anterior aspect of the soft palate above, and the anterior two-thirds of the tongue and the reflection of its mucosa onto the floor of the mouth and mandible below.[3,4] Posteriorly, the oral cavity opens into the oropharynx at the oropharyngeal isthmus.[3-5] The anterior two-thirds of the palate (hard palate) is composed of the palatine plates of the maxillae and the horizontal plates of the palatine bones (see Figure 3-2).[3,4,14] Posteriorly the hard palate is continuous with the soft palate, which is composed of a tough, fibrous sheath and extends to a free posterior border.[3,4,14] In the midline, the soft palate ends in the uvula[3,4,14]

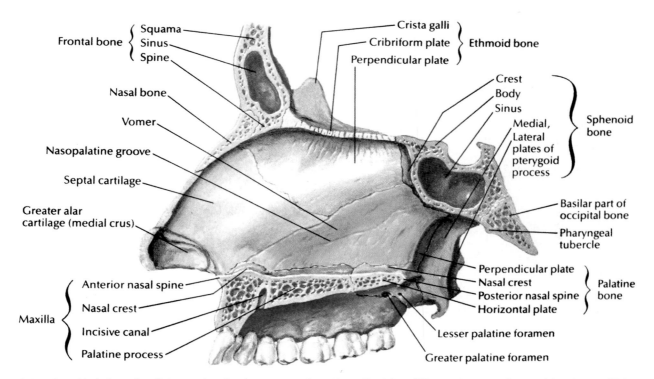

FIGURE 3-5. Medial nasal wall. (*Reproduced with permission from Netter FH*: Atlas of Human Anatomy. *Summit. New Jersey: CIBA-GEIGY Corporation, 1989.*)

Blood supply to lateral wall of nose

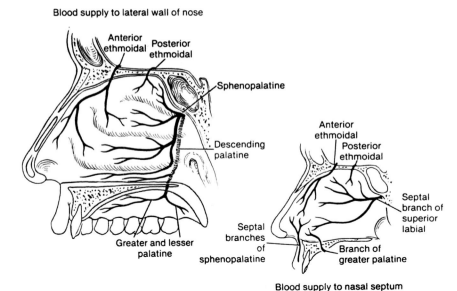

FIGURE 3-6. Blood supply to mucosa of lateral nasal wall and septum. (*Reproduced with permission from Graney DO, Baker SR: Basic science: anatomy. In: Otolaryngology Head and Neck Surgery, 3rd edn. Cummings CW, Fredrickson JM, Herker LA, et al. eds. St. Louis: Mosby, 1998.*)

then curves laterally to blend into the lateral pharyngeal wall at the palatoglossal and palatopharyngeal folds (anterior and posterior tonsillar pillars), respectively.[3,4,14] The anterior aspect of the soft palate faces the mouth cavity and oropharynx, whereas the posterior aspect is part of the nasopharynx.[3,4,14] The uvula is a valuable midline landmark during fiberoptic intubation through the mouth. Movement of the soft palate is controlled by five paired muscles including palatoglossus and palatopharyngeus, which descend in their respective folds to blend with the side of the tongue (palatoglossus) and the side wall of the pharynx (palatopharyngeus) and serve to approximate the folds.[3,4] These folds can be used as

landmarks for transmucosal glossopharyngeal nerve blocks. The palatine muscles help to isolate the nasopharynx from the mouth during swallowing and phonation.[3,4] Paralysis permits regurgitation of food into the nasopharynx and results in nasal speech.[3,4] Sensation to the palate is primarily supplied by the trigeminal nerve; however the glossopharyngeal supplies the most posterior aspect (see Figure 3-8).[3,4]

The anterior two-thirds of the body of the tongue occupies most of the floor of the mouth.[2,3,6] The posterior third of the tongue lies in the oropharynx and is separated from the anterior two-thirds by a V-shaped groove on the dorsal aspect of the tongue, the sulcus terminalis.[3] The pharyngeal third of the tongue has abundant lymphoid nodules, the lingual tonsil,[6] and hypertrophy of this lymphoid tissue can make intubation by direct laryngoscopy difficult or impossible.[15] The tongue is also subdivided by a median vertical fibrous septum represented on the dorsum of the tongue by a shallow midline groove,[14] another useful landmark during fiberoptic intubation (see Figure 3-9). The tongue musculature is divided into intrinsic muscles that alter the shape of the tongue[13] and extrinsic muscles that move the tongue as a whole (see Figure 3-10).[2,3,14] The extrinsic muscles connect the tongue to the symphysis of the mandible (genioglossus), hyoid (hyoglossus), styloid process (styloglossus), and the soft palate (palatoglossus).[14] In the supine unconscious individual, a decrease in genioglossal tone allows the tongue to move posteriorly and airway obstruction can occur. Sensation to the anterior two-thirds of the tongue is supplied by the lingual branch of the mandibular nerve,[3,14] whereas sensation to the posterior third is supplied by the glossopharyngeal and superior laryngeal

Nerve supply of lateral wall of nose

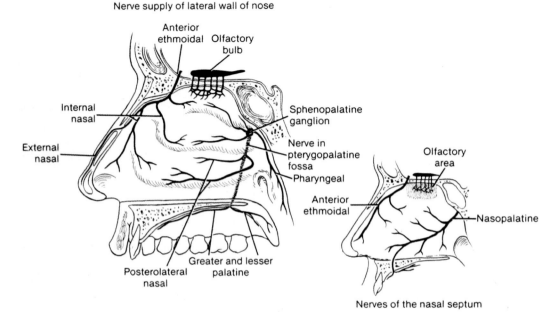

Nerves of the nasal septum

FIGURE 3-7. Nerve supply to mucosa of the lateral nasal wall and nasal septum (*Reproduced with permission from Graney DO, Baker SR: Basic science: anatomy. In: Otolaryngology Head and Neck Surgery, 3rd edn. Cummings CW, et al. eds. St. Louis: Mosby, 1998.*)

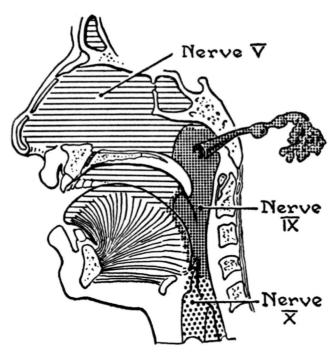

FIGURE 3-8. The sensory distribution of the glossopharyngeal nerve. (*Reproduced with permission from Basmajian JV: Grant's Method of Anatomy, 8th edn. Baltimore: Williams and Wilkins (after Edwards), 1981.*)

nerves.[6,14] Stimulation of the posterior third of the tongue during awake intubation typically provokes the gag reflex and reflex secretions, and can be particularly problematic during fiberoptic intubation. The tongue receives its blood supply from the lingual branch of the external carotid[14] and is a very vascular structure.[2] At the lateral aspect of the tongue, the mucosa is reflected onto the floor of the mouth and extends laterally to reach the gingiva, the "lingual sulcus."[3] Deep to the mucous membrane in the floor of the mouth on either side of the tongue anteriorly lie the sublingual glands, and deep to these structures lies the mylohyoid muscle which forms a sling to support the floor of the mouth (see Figure 3-11).[3,7,14] The submandibular gland straddles the mylohyoid muscle posteriorly.[3] Both the lingual and the hypoglossal nerves travel in the floor of the mouth lateral to the tongue in the lingual sulcus.[3] Lingual branches of the glossopharyngeal nerve lie deep to the mucosa of the palatoglossal arch (anterior tonsillar pillar) at the lateral aspect of the tongue and can be blocked in this location (see Figure 3-12). The mylohyoid muscle divides the floor of the mouth into two potential spaces: the submandibular space below the muscle and the sublingual space above.[2] Hematoma formation or infection in either of these fascial spaces can displace the tongue superiorly and posteriorly to produce airway compromise and can make intubation difficult (e.g., Ludwig's Angina).

The mandible consists of a horseshoe-shaped body anteriorly and two rami posteriorly, which extend superiorly to end in a

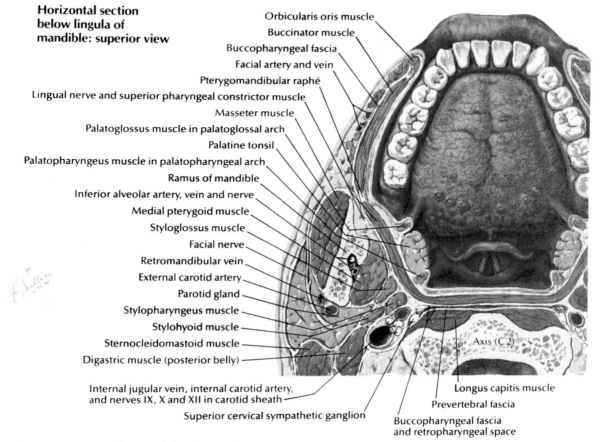

Horizontal section below lingula of mandible: superior view

Orbicularis oris muscle
Buccinator muscle
Buccopharyngeal fascia
Facial artery and vein
Pterygomandibular raphé
Lingual nerve and superior pharyngeal constrictor muscle
Masseter muscle
Palatoglossus muscle in palatoglossal arch
Palatine tonsil
Palatopharyngeus muscle in palatopharyngeal arch
Ramus of mandible
Inferior alveolar artery, vein and nerve
Medial pterygoid muscle
Styloglossus muscle
Facial nerve
Retromandibular vein
External carotid artery
Parotid gland
Stylopharyngeus muscle
Stylohyoid muscle
Sternocleidomastoid muscle
Digastric muscle (posterior belly)

Internal jugular vein, internal carotid artery, and nerves IX, X and XII in carotid sheath
Superior cervical sympathetic ganglion

Axis (C 2)

Longus capitis muscle
Prevertebral fascia
Buccopharyngeal fascia and retropharyngeal space

FIGURE 3-9. Horizontal section below lingua of mandible: superior view. (*Reproduced with permission from Netter FH: Atlas of Human Anatomy. Summit. New Jersey: CIBA-GEIGY Corporation, 1989.*)

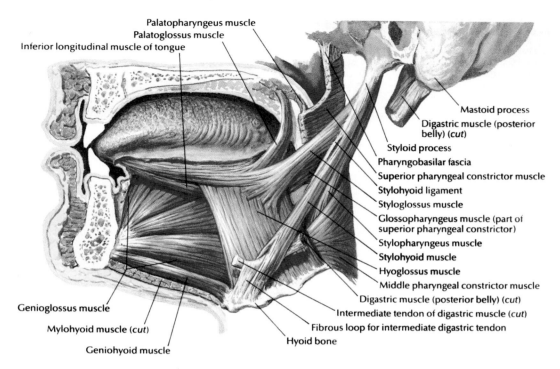

FIGURE 3-10. Extrinsic muscles of the tongue. (*Reproduced with permission from Netter FH: Atlas of Human Anatomy. Summit. New Jersey: CIBA-GEIGY Corporation, 1989.*)

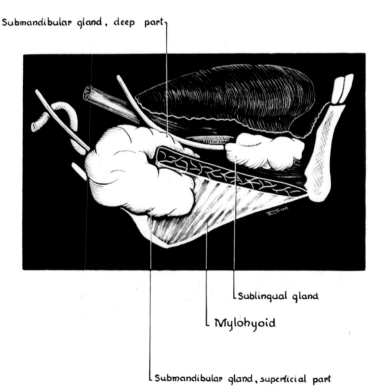

FIGURE 3-11. The floor of the mouth. (*Reproduced with permission from Friedman SM: Visual Anatomy, Vol. 1. Head and Neck. New York: Harper & Row, 1970.*)

condylar head and a coronoid process with an intervening mandibular notch (see Figure 3-13).[3] The condylar head articulates with the mandibular fossa of the temporal bone at the temporomandibular joint (TMJ).[3] Two types of movement occur at the TMJ—rotation and a forward gliding—thereby opening the mouth (see Figure 3-14).[3,6] Normal mandibular opening in the adult is about 4 cm, or at least 2 finger breadths, between the upper and lower incisors.[3,8] Decreased mandibular mobility and anatomic variants, in particular micrognathia, can make intubation by direct laryngoscopy difficult to impossible.

3.2.4 The pharynx

The pharynx is a U-shaped musculofascial tube which extends from the base of the skull to the lower border of the cricoid cartilage where at the level of the sixth cervical vertebrae it is continuous with the esophagus (see Figure 3-1).[2,3,6] Posteriorly, it rests against the prevertebral fascia (see Figures 3-8 and 3-9). Anteriorly, it communicates with the nasal cavity, mouth, and the larynx at the *naso-*, *oro-*, and *laryngo*pharynx, respectively (see Figure 3-15).[3,4] From the internal aspect, outward the pharynx consists of mucosa, submucosa, muscle, and a loose areolar sheath, the buccopharyngeal fascia. This buccopharyngeal fascia is the thin fibrous capsule of the pharynx, contains the plexi of pharyngeal veins and nerves, and is continuous with the areolar sheath of the buccinator muscles and the adventitia of esophagus.[2,3,6] Superiorly, it is attached to the base of the skull.[2] Edema associated with infection in the floor of the mouth, such as Ludwig's angina, is limited by the buccopharyngeal fascia, can spread into the pharynx and larynx, and lead to airway obstruction.[3,4] The muscular layer of the

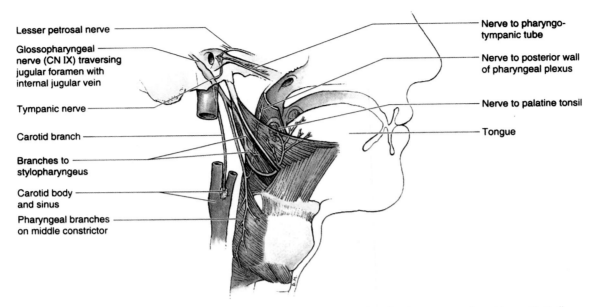

Lesser petrosal nerve

Glossopharyngeal
nerve (CN IX) traversing
jugular foramen with
internal jugular vein

Tympanic nerve

Carotid branch

Branches to
stylopharyngeus

Carotid body
and sinus

Pharyngeal branches
on middle constrictor

Nerve to pharyngo-
tympanic tube

Nerve to posterior wall
of pharyngeal plexus

Nerve to palatine tonsil

Tongue

FIGURE 3-12. Distribution of the glossopharyngeal nerve (CN IX). (*Reproduced with permission from Moore KL, Dalley AF: Clinically Oriented Anatomy, 4th edn. Philadelphia: Lippincott, Williams & Wilkins, 1999.*)

pharynx is made up primarily of three paired constrictor muscles that curve around the pharyngeal lumen and telescope into one another (see Figure 3-16). The inferior constrictor consists of an upper oblique part and a lower transverse part (the cricopharyngeus) that is continuous with the esophagus and functions as an upper esophageal sphincter.[3,6] The junction of the pharynx with the esophagus is the narrowest part of the gastrointestinal tract and is a commonplace for foreign bodies to impact.[3,6]

The *naso*pharynx extends from the posterior choanae to the tip of the uvula[3,9] and forms a backward extension of the nasal cavities (see Figure 3-17).[3,6] It is bounded inferiorly by the soft palate.[3,4,6] It communicates with the oropharynx at the pharyngeal isthmus,

which is closed during swallowing by the soft palate, the palatopharyngeus, and a ridge of the superior pharyngeal constrictor—the ridge of Passavant.[3,4,6] The roof of the nasopharynx is formed by the sphenoid bone[3,9] and curves into the posterior pharyngeal wall at the level of the atlas and axis.[3,6,9] The nasopharyngeal tonsils (adenoids) are located in the roof of the nasopharynx and can extend laterally.[3,6] The Eustachian tube enters the nasopharynx through the lateral wall.[3,4] During nasal intubation, occasionally the passage of the endotracheal tube can impact the mucosa and resist advancement at the ridge of Passavant or at the level of the anterior tubercle of the atlas (Cl). Rotation of the tube will facilitate passage around this prominence; however on occasion digital manipulation through the mouth may be required.

The *oro*pharynx extends from the soft palate to the epiglottis[3,4,9] and lies behind the mouth cavity and posterior third of the tongue. The palatoglossal folds arch downward from the soft palate to the

Head or condyle

Mandibular notch

Coronoid proc.

Antr. border
Oblique line

Alveolar proc.
Incisive fossa

Neck

Angle

For masseter   For facial A.

Mental   Foramen
Tubercle
Protuberance

FIGURE 3-13. Lateral view of mandible. (*Reproduced with permission from Basmajian JV: Grant's Method of Anatomy, 8th edn. Baltimore: Lippincott, Williams & Wilkins, 1981.*)

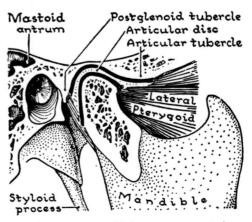

FIGURE 3-14. The temporomandibular joint, on saggital section. (*Reproduced with permission from Basmajian JV: Grant's Method of Anatomy, 8th edn. Baltimore: Lippincott, Williams & Wilkins, 1981.*)

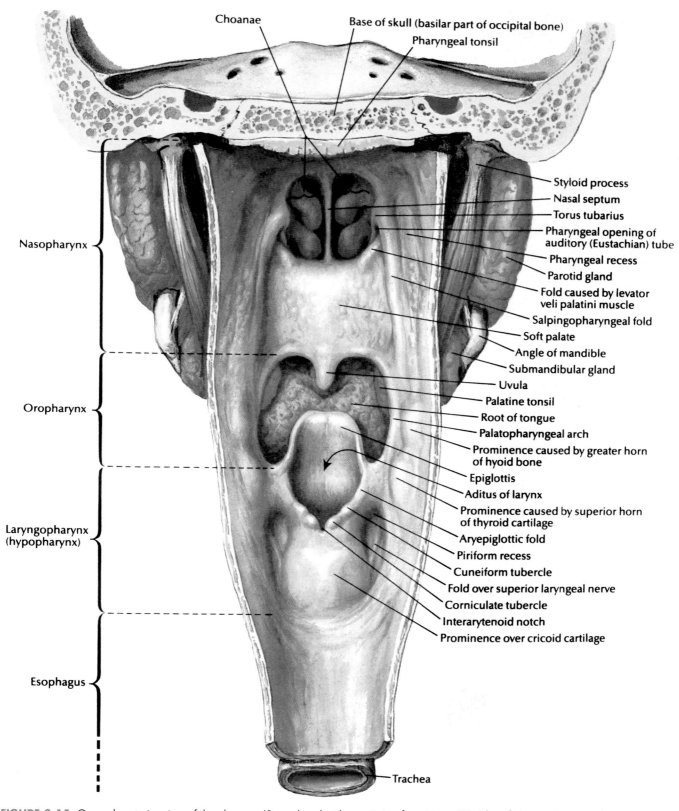

FIGURE 3-15. Opened posterior view of the pharynx. (*Reproduced with permission from Netter FH:* Atlas of Human Anatomy. *Summit. New Jersey: CIBA-GEIGY Corporation, 1989.*)

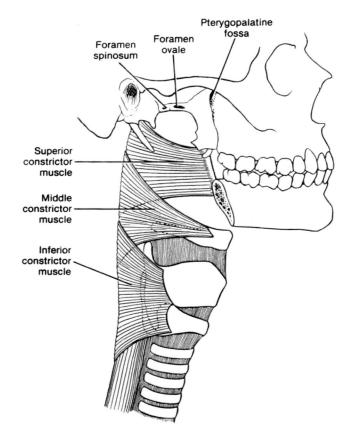

FIGURE 3-16. The lateral view of the pharyngeal muscles. *(Reproduced with permission from Graney DO, Baker SR: Basic science: anatomy. In: Otolaryngology Head and Neck Surgery, 3rd edn. Cummings CW, et al., eds. St. Louis: Mosby 1998.)*

junction of the anterior two-thirds and posterior third of the tongue and provide the dividing line between the mouth and oropharynx (see Figure 3-8).[3,6] This oropharyngeal isthmus is completed by the soft palate and the sulcus terminalis of the tongue.[3] The palatine tonsils lie on either side of the oropharynx in the triangle formed by the tongue and the palatoglossal and palatopharyngeal arches.[3,4,6] The glossopharyngeal nerve can be blocked as it runs deep to the mucosa posterior to the palatopharyngeal fold.

The laryngopharynx extends from the tip of the epiglottis to the lower border of the cricoid cartilage where it is continuous with the esophagus (see Figures 3-15 and 3-17).[3,4,14] The oblique inlet of the larynx bounded by the epiglottis, aryepiglottic folds, arytenoid cartilages, and the posterior commissure lies anteriorly.[3,6] The cylindrical larynx itself bulges posteriorly into the center of the laryngopharynx creating a deep recess, the piriform fossa (or sinus), on either side leading into the esophagus.[3,4] As seen during direct laryngoscopy, the larynx can be conceptualized to be a smaller cylinder eccentrically placed within and at the anterior aspect of the larger cylindrical pharynx. Laterally, the piriform fossae are bounded by the thyroid cartilage and the thyrohyoid membrane.[3,6] Superior to the piriform fossae, the median glossoepiglottic fold connects the epiglottis to the tongue in the midline and the lateral glossoepiglottic folds connect it to the pharyngeal wall.[3,6] The depressions formed between these folds are termed the valleculae[6] and are considered to be within the oropharynx.[9] During direct laryngoscopy, the Macintosh blade is inserted into the base of the

vallecula to engage the hyoepiglottic ligament and thereby move the epiglottis anteriorly to expose the glottis.

Sensation to the nasopharynx and oropharynx is supplied primarily by the glossopharyngeal nerve.[3,6] The glossopharyngeal nerve enters the neck in company with the internal carotid artery and the internal jugular vein.[16] At the level of the styloid process, it leaves this position and winds anteriorly and inferiorly lateral to stylopharyngeus which it supplies (see Figure 3-18).[7] The nerve then passes forward between the superior and middle constrictors and gives off pharyngeal branches as well as lingual branches to the posterior third of the tongue (see Figure 3-12). Glossopharyngeal nerve blocks can be performed posterior to the midpoint of the palatopharyngeal fold or at the base of the palatoglossal fold in the mouth. The maxillary branch of the trigeminal nerve supplies sensation to the roof of the nasopharynx and contributes to the sensory supply of the soft palate and the adjacent part of the tonsil.[3,6] The laryngopharynx receives sensory innervation from the internal branch of the superior laryngeal nerve, which pierces the thyrohyoid membrane and runs in the submucosa of the piriform fossae.[3] This nerve also supplies sensation to the larynx above the level of the false cords[17,18] or true cords.[6,7,19] Cotton pledgets soaked in local anesthetic can be held against the mucosa of the piriform fossa using Kraus or Jackson forceps to produce a block of the internal branch of the superior laryngeal, or the nerve can be approached percutaneously. It has been said that the superior aspect (pharyngeal surface) of the epiglottis is innervated by the glossopharyngeal nerve, whereas the inferior aspect (laryngeal surface) receives sensory innervation from the superior laryngeal nerve.[18,20] Others have stated that both the surfaces of the epiglottis are innervated by the superior laryngeal nerve.[19]

3.2.5 The larynx

The larynx is a complex structure made up of a framework of cartilages and fibroelastic membranes covered by a layer of muscles and lined with mucous membrane.[3,4] It functions as an open valve during respiration, a partially closed valve during phonation, a closed value during swallowing and, when effort is required, to produce increased intrathoracic pressure (Valsalva maneuver).[2,3,9,14] It extends from its oblique entrance or aditus to the lower border of the cricoid cartilage and bulges posteriorly into the laryngopharynx (see Figure 3-15).[3,6] It is suspended from the hyoid bone which is itself attached to the mandible, tongue, and the base of the skull.[14]

The laryngeal cartilages include the thyroid, cricoid, epiglottic and the paired arytenoid, corniculate, and cuneiform cartilages (see Figure 3-19). The quadrilateral laminae of the thyroid cartilage meet in the midline anteriorly to form the thyroid prominence (Adam's apple). Superiorly, the thyroid cartilage is attached to the hyoid by the thyrohyoid membrane.[3] Posteriorly the lower horns of the thyroid cartilage articulate with the posteriorly oriented signet ring shaped cricoid cartilage. Anteriorly the thyroid cartilage is attached to the cricoid by the cricothyroid membrane, a suitable site for emergency surgical airway access in the adult. The cricoid cartilage is the only complete skeletal ring of the airway and can be used to provide cricoid pressure to occlude the esophagus during rapid sequence induction/intubation. The paired arytenoid cartilages articulate with the superior aspect of

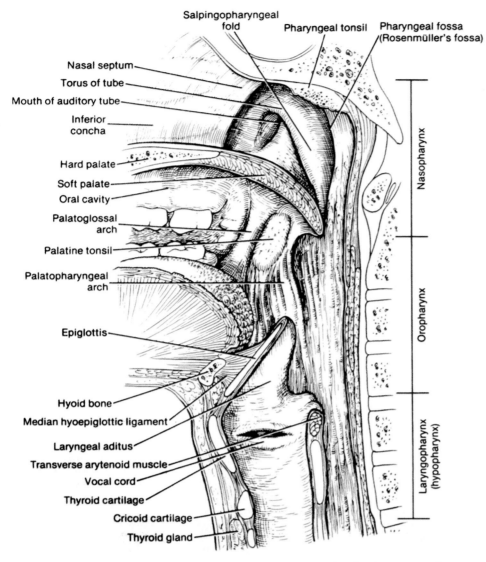

Salpingopharyngeal fold
Pharyngeal tonsil
Pharyngeal fossa (Rosenmüller's fossa)
Nasal septum
Torus of tube
Mouth of auditory tube
Inferior concha
Hard palate
Soft palate
Oral cavity
Palatoglossal arch
Palatine tonsil
Palatopharyngeal arch
Epiglottis
Hyoid bone
Median hyoepiglottic ligament
Laryngeal aditus
Transverse arytenoid muscle
Vocal cord
Thyroid cartilage
Cricoid cartilage
Thyroid gland
Nasopharynx
Oropharynx
Laryngopharynx (hypopharynx)

FIGURE 3-17. The medial view of the pharyngeal mucosa. (*Reproduced with permission from Graney DO, Baker SR: Basic science: anatomy. In: Otolaryngology Head and Neck Surgery, 3rd edn. Cummings CW, et al., eds. St. Louis: Mosby 1998.*).

upper border is free and thickened to form the vocal ligament (true vocal cord).[3,9] In coronal section, the relationship of the true vocal cords to the false vocal cords and the laryngeal ventricle or sinus can be readily appreciated (see Figure 3-21).[3,9] The aryepiglottic, the vestibular, and the vocal folds form a trilevel sphincter mechanism that regulates and protects the airway.[3,9] The folds also divide the larynx into the supraglottic compartment or *vestibule* above the false cords, the *glottic* compartment between the false and true cords, and the *infraglottic* compartment between the true cords and the lower border of the cricoid.[3,6,14] The absence of a submucosal layer at the vocal ligament causes the cords to appear white and limits the collection of edema fluid.[14]

A complex arrangement of intrinsic muscles alters the configuration of the laryngeal folds. The cricothyroid is classified by itself as the only extrinsic muscle of the larynx, and muscles that elevate or depress the larynx as a whole (e.g., during swallowing) are considered to be accessory laryngeal muscles.[3,9]

The larynx receives its nerve supply from the superior and recurrent laryngeal nerves.[3,4] The superior laryngeal nerve arises from the vagus just below the pharyngeal plexus, passes medial to both the internal and external carotids, and then divides into a large sensory internal and a small motor external branch which supplies the cricothyroid muscle (see Figure 3-22).[3,4,7] The internal branch pierces the thyrohyoid membrane to provide sensation to the laryngeal mucosa above the level of the false cords[3,9,17,18] or true cords.[6,7,19]

On the right side, the recurrent laryngeal nerve leaves the vagus as it crosses the subclavian artery, loops posteriorly under the artery, and ascends to the larynx in the groove between the esophagus and trachea. On the left, the nerve leaves the vagus as it crosses the aortic arch and similarly loops posteriorly under the arch and then runs superiorly between the esophagus and the trachea to reach the larynx.[3,4] The recurrent laryngeal nerves supply all the intrinsic muscles of the larynx and provide sensation below the level of the false[3,9,17,18] or true cords.[6,7,19] Hoarseness produced by damage to the superior laryngeal nerve is usually temporary as the contralateral cord exerts a compensatory action.[3,4] Damage to the recurrent laryngeal nerve also produces hoarseness, and if both nerves are affected severe airway obstruction can occur.[3,14]

The cricothyroid membrane or ligament can be identified in the anterior neck as a concavity between the convex inferior border of

the cricoid cartilage posteriorly. The corniculate cartilages in turn articulate with the apices of the pyramidal shaped arytenoids.[3] The shallow depression between the two corniculate cartilages (the posterior commissure) is a useful landmark during laryngoscopy.[3,9] The cuneiform cartilages are located lateral to the corniculate cartilages and lie within the aryepiglottic folds. The leaf-shaped epiglottis is attached to the thyroid cartilage inferiorly and the hyoid bone superiorly.[3] The remaining framework of the larynx consists of two paired fibroelastic folds, the quadrangular and triangular membranes (see Figure 3-20).[3,9] The quadrangular membrane spans the space between the lateral border of the epiglottis and the arytenoid cartilages.[3,9] Its free upper edge forms the aryepiglottic ligament at the laryngeal aditus, and its thickened lower border forms the vestibular ligament (false vocal cord).[3,6] The triangular ligament is attached in the midline anteriorly to the thyroid and cricoid cartilages and extends posteriorly to attach to the arytenoid cartilage. The inferior border of the triangular ligament is attached obliquely to the cricoid cartilage whereas the

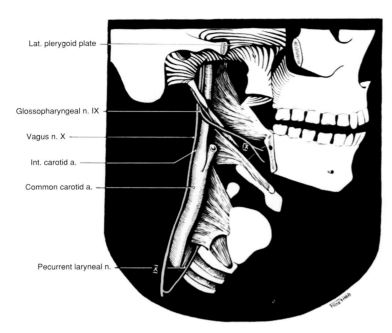

Lat. pterygoid plate

Glossopharyngeal n. IX

Vagus n. X

Int. carotid a.

Common carotid a.

Recurrent laryneal n.

FIGURE 3-18. The glossopharyngeal nerve. (*Reproduced with permission from Friedman SM: Visual Anatomy, Vol. 1. Head and Neck. New York: Harper & Row, 1970.*)

the thyroid cartilage and the superior portion of the cricoid cartilage (see Figures 3-19 and 3-23). The space is trapezoidal in shape with a cross-sectional area of 2.9 cm^2 and a mean height of 9 mm (ranging 5–12 mm).[21,22] The average vertical distance between the true cords and the midpoint of the cricothyroid membrane is 1.3 cm in the adult.[22] The vertical distance from the lower border of the thyroid cartilage to the vocal cords is 5–11 mm.[21,23] The cricothyroid branches of the superior thyroid arteries run transversely across the membrane, usually the upper third,[21,23] and tributaries of the anterior jugular veins occasionally run anterior to the membrane, although considerable variation exists in the vascular pattern.[21] During cricothyrotomy or membrane puncture, the cricothyroid membrane should be traversed at its inferior third to minimize vascular injury.[21,23]

3.2.6 The trachea

The trachea extends inferiorly from its junction with the larynx at the lower border of the cricoid cartilage to the carina (see Figure 3-24).[3,4,24] It is about 10–15 cm in length in the adult and about 9–16 mm in diameter.[3,4,6,17,25] The inferior half of the trachea lies within the superior mediastinum.[6] The cervical trachea is in the midline; however the intrathoracic portion is deviated to the right by the aortic arch.[4] The patency of the trachea is maintained by 16 to 20 U-shaped rings of hyaline cartilage[6] joined by fibroelastic tissue and closed posteriorly by the trachealis muscle.[3,4] Longitudinal mucosal markings can be seen posteriorly when the trachea is viewed through the bronchoscope, and these can be used for spatial orientation. The average distance from the central incisors to the carina is 27 cm in the adult male and 23 cm in the adult female.[26] The distance from the nostrils to the carina is an additional 4 cm.[26] Tracheotomy is usually performed between the second and third or third and fourth tracheal rings.[4,27]

3.2.7 How is the anatomy of the pediatric airway different from that of the adult?

Awake intubation is most often performed in the adult population, and this chapter on preparation for awake intubation is directed to this age group. The reader is directed to the pediatric sections of the text for further information on pediatric airway management. Management of the pediatric airway does require consideration of anatomic differences in this age group, and therefore they are elaborated on here.

The infant head is relatively large and tends to flex the neck on the trunk in the supine position.[2,3,5] The tongue is also large relative to the mouth cavity and the palatine tonsils are prominent.[2,5,25] The nasal passages are relatively narrow and can easily be obstructed by edema, secretions, or the relatively large adenoidal tissues.[2,5] The neonate is an obligate nose breather due to the more cephalad position of the larynx,[24] with the glottis at C3-C4 as compared to C5 in the adult.[2] It also appears to be more anterior on direct laryngoscopy. In children less than 5 years of age, the narrowest part of the upper airway is at the level of the cricoid cartilage and not the glottis, as in the adult.[2] The epiglottis is relatively long, U-shaped, and makes a more acute angle with the vocal cords, which themselves are slanted inferiorly, back to front.[2,3,5] The trachea in the newborn is only 4–5 cm long[28,29] and 3–4 mm in diameter.[26,30] The cricothyroid membrane is small and not readily palpable in children.[31] Due to this fact, cricothyrotomy has been said to be contraindicated in those less than 6 years of age[23] and should be performed with extreme caution in children less than 10 years of age.[21] Usually by 12 years of age, the cricothyroid membrane can be easily palpated and cricothyrotomy may be performed.[28]

3.3 LOCAL ANESTHESIA OF THE AIRWAY

3.3.1 What drugs are useful for airway anesthesia? What are their toxicities and associated complications?

Lidocaine, tetracaine, cocaine, benzocaine, and dyclonine have all been used to achieve topical anesthesia of the airway, and lidocaine is commonly used to perform glossopharyngeal and superior laryngeal nerve blocks.

3.3.2 Lidocaine

Introduced in 1948, lidocaine is the prototypical member of the amide class of local anesthetics and is metabolized in the liver by mixed function oxidases.[32] Lidocaine is probably the local anesthetic most commonly used for regional anesthesia of the airway and has also been used extensively in the past for the treatment of ventricular arrhythmias.[32–34]

Following application to the mucous membranes of the airway, lidocaine produces an anesthetic effect which is limited to the mucous membrane in 1–2 minutes.[25,35] The peak anesthetic effect

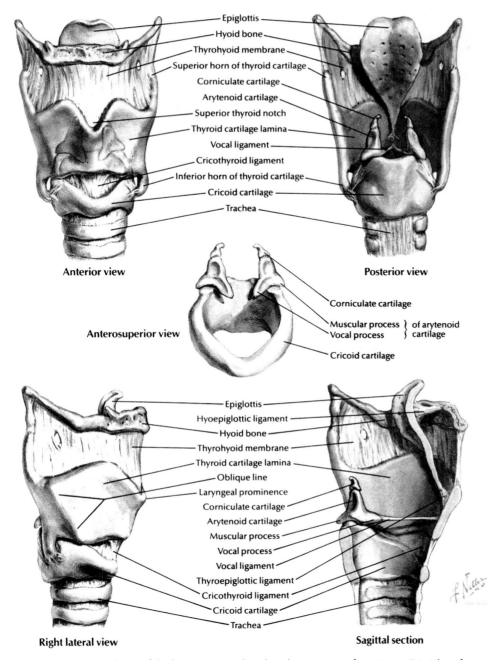

FIGURE 3-19. Cartilages of the larynx. (*Reproduced, with permission, from Netter FH: Atlas of Human Anatomy. Summit. New Jersey: CIBA-GEIGY Corporation, 1989.*)

utes.[35] The latent period has a profound significance when fiberoptic intubation is performed using a "spray as you go" technique and suggests that a significant risk of insufficient anesthesia may exist.[39] Concentrations of lidocaine of 1% (10 mg.mL^{-1}) to 10% (100 mg.mL^{-1}) have been used for topical anesthesia of the airway. Excellent topical anesthesia of the airway in the adult can be produced by 4% lidocaine, but at 2% (20 mg.mL^{-1}) concentration, topical anesthesia may be inadequate and 1% lidocaine has been found to be insufficient for airway instrumentation.[40] Increasing the concentration beyond the optimum level does not affect the latent period or duration of action,[35] and increasing the dose to a given area of mucosa beyond 15 mg of lidocaine per square centimeter does not increase the anesthetic effect.[39] Importantly, topical epinephrine penetrates mucous membranes poorly, has no significant local effect, does not prolong the duration of topical local anesthesia,[32] and will not slow the rate of anesthetic absorption.[41]

Local anesthetics applied to the mucous membranes of the airway are rapidly absorbed into the circulation.[32] The extent of systemic absorption depends on the site and technique of application, tissue vascularity, the total dose administered,[42,43] the state of the mucosa, the concomitant use of drying agents,[38,44] the amount of mucous present, the rate and depth of respiration, the state of the circulation, the patient's disease state,[45,46] and individual variation.[45,46] Slower uptake occurs from the more proximal parts of the respiratory tract.[45,46] Absorption is particularly rapid when local anesthetics are applied to the tracheobronchial tree,[32] whereas decreased rates of absorption occur in the upper airway secondary to decreased vascularity and surface area.[42] Absorption from alveoli may approximate IV administration[47] due to osmotic relationships in the pulmonary vascular bed designed to prevent the collection of fluid in the alveolar spaces.[35,48] The therapeutic serum concentration of lidocaine when the drug is used as an antiarrhythmic is usually considered to be 1.5–4.0 μg.mL^{-1}.[49] As serum lidocaine concentrations increase however, systemic toxicity is produced. At the upper limit of the antiarrhythmic therapeutic range, lightheadedness, tinnitus, and circumoral and tongue numbness can occur.[50] As serum concentrations continue to rise, visual disturbances and muscle twitching occur and can be followed by generalized seizure activity.[50] Seizures are most frequently seen at plasma concentrations greater than 8–10 μg.mL^{-1},[47,51] although they

occurs within 2 to 5 minutes,[32] and the duration of the airway anesthesia is said to be 30–40 minutes,[32] 20–40 minutes,[36] or 15–30 minutes.[37] Watanabe et al. found the duration of anesthesia following the application of lidocaine to the oral mucosa to be 40 minutes with glycopyrrolate pretreatment and 20 minutes without it.[38] Schonemann et al. sprayed 10% (100 mg.mL^{-1}) lidocaine onto the oral mucosa of the lower lip and demonstrated a hypoalgesic effect that lasted 14 mintues.[39] Maximum hypoalgesia was observed after 4–5 minutes.[39] Adriani et al. found that the maximum effective concentration of topical lidocaine applied to the tongue was 4% (40 mg.mL^{-1}) and this concentration had a latent period of 2 minutes and duration of effect of 15.2 min-

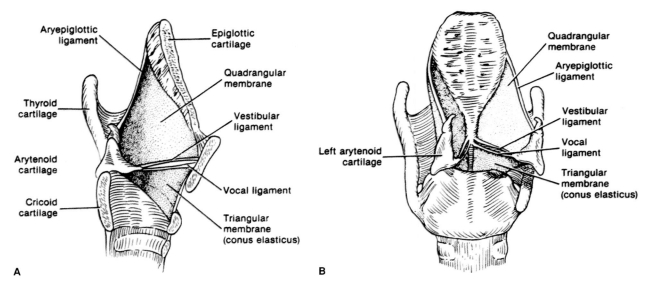

FIGURE 3-20. A. Saggital section of laryngeal membranes. B. Posterior view of laryngeal membranes (right arytenoid cartilage moved laterally). (*Reproduced with permission from Graney DO, Baker SR: Basic science: anatomy. In: Otolaryngology Head and Neck Surgery, 3rd edn. Cummings CW, et al., eds. St. Louis: Mosby, 1998.*)

have occurred at plasma concentrations as low as 6 μg.mL^{-1}.[42] Cardiorespiratory arrest can occur at plasma lidocaine concentrations of 20–25 μg.mL^{-1}.[42,50] Levels in arterial blood have been shown to be 20–30% higher than that in venous samples[44,51,52] and more closely correlate with CNS effects.[53] However, most practitioners consider venous blood levels to be reliable indicators of clinical toxicity.[42] Hypersensitivity reactions to lidocaine, although exceedingly rare, can also occur and be catastrophic.[36] Clinically significant methemoglobinemia has been reported in association with lidocaine administration, although these occurrences have been extremely rare.[54–58] A review of the English literature found only two cases in which no other drug associated with methemoglobinemia had been used.[55,56s]

The maximum safe dose of topical lidocaine has been stated to be 4 mg.kg^{-1},[59–64] 3–4 mg.kg^{-1},[37] and 6.0 mg.kg^{-1}.[26] However, when topically applied to the mucous membranes of the airway, these maximal doses can only be interpreted when the method of

topical administration is known. Lidocaine administered to the airway by nebulization has been reported to produce low-peak plasma concentrations as compared to other techniques.[42,44,53,65] This has been attributed to the loss of up to 50% of the nebulized solution to the environment with continuous nebulization.[53,66] The exact dose of lidocaine delivered to the airway when an inhalational technique is used is difficult to measure,[53] and the dose administered may bear little relation to the dose actually absorbed.[67] Absorption of local anesthetics administered by aerosols is also dependent on droplet size. Typical nebulizers produce droplets that range from 1–20 μm in diameter.[68] The peak deposition of aerosol droplets occurs in the peripheral airway for droplets of about 2 μm, in bronchioles for droplets of about 8 μm, in bronchi for droplets of about 15 μm, and in the upper airway for droplets larger than 40 μm.[69] Higher oxygen flow rates through nebulizers create smaller droplets (less than 30 μm) that travel further distally into the bronchial tree and increase the rate of absorption.[37]

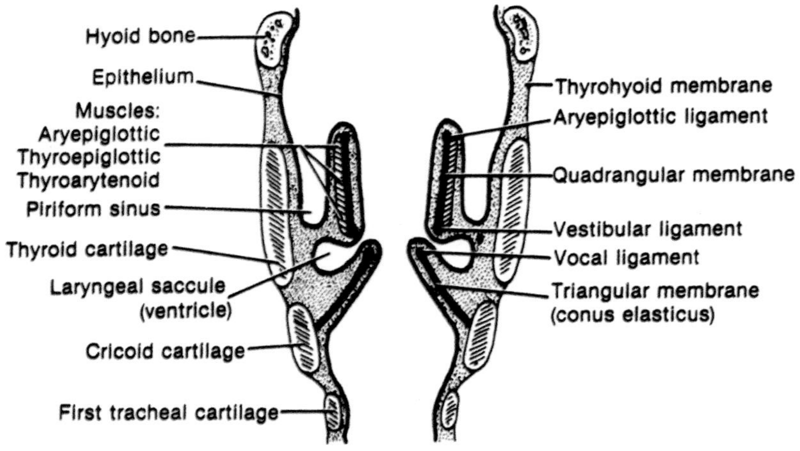

Droplets larger than 60 μm are preferred for airway anesthesia during awake intubation because they "rain out" in the proximal airway where the topical anesthesia is required.[37] The droplet size produced by manually squeezing the bulb of the hand-held DeVilbiss #40 nebulizer tends to be much larger than that produced by conventional aerosol delivery systems and is dependant on the pressure generated in the atomizer.[70] The mean bulb pressure produced by a firm squeeze is 250–340 mmHg (4.86–6.01 psi). The mass median diameter (MMD) of the droplets thus produced was found to be 6.2–12.0 μm with 28–50% of the particles being less than 6.2 μm in diameter, small enough to penetrate the tracheobronchial tree.[70] With increasing firmness of the manual squeeze and increased bulb pressure, these nebulizers increase output and decrease MMD. When an oxygen flow through the RD 15 DeVilbiss atomizer of 5.0 L.min^{-1} was utilized, pressures at the inlet of the device of 3.8–4.0 psi were generated, and at 8 L.min^{-1} oxygen flow this pressure was

FIGURE 3-21. Coronal section of larynx. (*Reproduced with permission from Graney DO, Baker SR: Basic science: anatomy. In: Otolaryngology Head and Neck Surgery, 3rd edn. Cummings CW, et al., ed. St. Louis: Mosby, 1998.*)

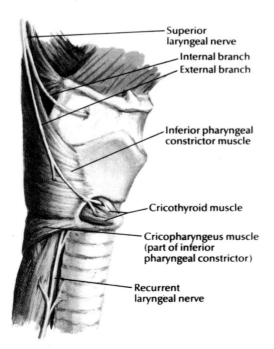

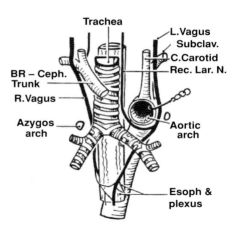

FIGURE 3-24. The trachea and extrapulmonary bronchi, and their relations. (*Reproduced with permission from Basmajian JV: Grant's Method of Anatomy, 8th edn. Baltimore: Lippincott, Williams & Wilkins, 1981.*)

FIGURE 3-22. Nerves innervating the larynx. (*Reproduced with permission from Netter FH: Atlas of Human Anatomy. Summit. New Jersey: CIBA-GEIGY Corporation, 1989.*)

11.2–11.4 psi. This technique may produce smaller droplets leading to increased systemic absorption, although it has been shown that only about 7–12% of the nebulized dose of a drug actually reaches the lung.[71,72] Furthermore the anesthetic expectorated after gargle and atomizer administration must be subtracted from the total dose administered.

Many investigators have endeavored to link route of administration and dosage of lidocaine used for airway anesthesia to plasma levels and toxicity:

- In a study performed by Melby et al., 1.5 mg.kg^{-1} of 4% lidocaine was injected into the endotracheal tube of six patients under general anesthesia. Peak serum lidocaine concentrations of 1.4–3.3 μg.mL^{-1} occurred at 11.7 ± 5.2 minutes following administration. Three of the six patients experienced almost instantaneous absorption.[49]

- Chu et al. measured plasma lidocaine concentrations produced by tracheal spraying using 3.3 mg.kg^{-1} of 4% lidocaine and IV injection of 1 mg.kg^{-1} of 2% lidocaine. After tracheal spraying, maximum plasma lidocaine levels of 2.0–5.6 μg.mL^{-1} were recorded at 15–20 minutes. Following IV administration, peak concentrations of 5.0–6.85 μg.mL^{-1} were reached within 12 minutes.[69]

  - Curran et al. measured the concentration of lidocaine in venous blood following tracheal as compared to laryngeal spraying in 10 patients under general anesthesia. Each group received 3 mL of 10% lidocaine. The peak lidocaine concentration in the tracheal group ranged from 1.9 to 8.2 μg.mL,$^{-1}$ whereas in the laryngeal group the range was 0.4–2.5 μg.mL^{-1}. Lidocaine levels in the tracheal group tended to rise more rapidly and reach a peak earlier than in the laryngeal group.[73]

  - Eyres et al. administered 4 mg.kg^{-1} of 4% lidocaine into the larynx and immediate subglottic area of 96 children under general anesthesia and measured plasma lidocaine levels at 2, 4, 6, 10, 15, 20, and 30 minutes after administration. Mean peak lidocaine levels measured were 4.3 ± 1.9 μg.mL^{-1} for those less than 1 year of age, 5.7 ± 2.0 for those 1–3 years of age, 5.3 ± 1.4 for those 3–5 years of age, and 5.3 ± 2.0 for those more than 5 years of age. Plasma lidocaine levels exceeded 8.0 μg.mL^{-1} in 13 patients. The time to peak concentration varied from 8.5 ± 2.5 minutes in those less than 1 year of age to 11.7 ± 4.3 minutes in those more than 5 years of age.[74]

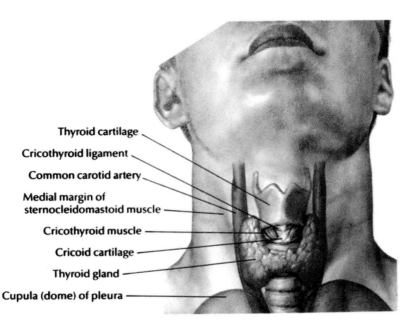

FIGURE 3-23. Anterior view of cricothyroid membrane (ligament). (*Reproduced with permission from Netter FH: Atlas of Human Anatomy. Summit. New Jersey: CIBA-GEIGY Corporation, 1989.*)

- Patterson et al. reported the administration of up to 380 mg of lidocaine almost entirely delivered as a 1% solution through the bronchoscope to 21 adult patients. With the exception of one patient, the maximum blood levels of lidocaine recorded were <2.48 μg.mL^{-1}. The peak concentration occurred between 5 and 75 minutes following lidocaine administration, usually between 5 and 30 minutes. Again, considerable individual variation in the maximum concentration measured was noted. One patient with abnormal liver function was found to have a plasma concentration of 18.2 μg.mL^{-1} but developed no signs of toxicity.[75]

- Parks et al. administered 6 mg.kg^{-1} of 10% lidocaine to 10 ASA I volunteers via a nebulizer connected to a facemask powered by an oxygen flow of 6 L.min^{-1}. The mean peak serum concentration of lidocaine produced was 0.29 μg.mL^{-1}, and the highest measurement was 0.45 μg.mL^{-1}. The peak concentration occurred 30 minutes after nebulization was commenced.[44]

- Mostafa et al. similarly administered 6 mg.kg^{-1} of 10% lidocaine to 14 ASA I and II patients scheduled for head and neck surgery using a nebulizer system with a mouthpiece and an oxygen flow of 7 L.min^{-1}. The mean plasma lidocaine level 10 minutes after nebulization was 0.95 $\pm$ 0.62 μg.mL,$^{-1}$ and at 20 minutes it was 0.68 $\pm$ 0.32 μg.mL^{-1}.[72]

- Sutherland and Williams administered 5 mL of 4% lidocaine to 20 adult patients using a standard nebulizer connected to a mouthpiece and an oxygen flow of 8 L.min^{-1}. The mouthpiece was connected to an oral airway intubator that was advanced into the oropharynx during the latter part of the nebulization process. The subjects also gargled 5 mL of 2% lidocaine gel for 1 minute, and 2 mL of 2% lidocaine was injected through the bronchoscope onto the vocal cords, as well as 2 mL into the trachea. The dosage range was 2.5–11 mg.kg^{-1} (mean dose, 5.3 $\pm$ 2.1 mg.kg^{-1}). The mean peak plasma concentration was 0.7 $\pm$ 0.4 μg.mL^{-1}, and the highest plasma concentration was 1.6 μg.mL^{-1}. The mean peak concentration occurred 23 minutes following airway intubator insertion.[76]

- Efthimiou et al. measured plasma concentrations of lidocaine in a group of 41 patients who underwent topical airway anesthesia before fiberoptic bronchoscopy. In 32 patients, 14 sprays of 10% lidocaine were administered to the nose and oropharynx followed by 8 mL of 4% lidocaine solution administered via the bronchoscope to the pharynx and vocal cords, and 14 mL of 1% lidocaine to the bronchial tree. In nine patients, 8 mL of 2% lidocaine gel was applied to the nose and the use of the 10% spray was omitted. The average dose of lidocaine administered was 9.3 $\pm$ 0.5 mg.kg^{-1}. The average peak plasma concentration was 2.9 $\pm$ 0.5 μg.mL^{-1} and correlated with dose per unit body weight. Two patients had plasma levels above 5 μg.mL^{-1} but demonstrated no clinical evidence of toxicity. The average time to peak concentration was 42.6 minutes in the aerosol group and 48.4 minutes in the gel group. In a second study of 10 volunteers, plasma concentrations following 4% lidocaine gargle and swallow was compared with 10% oropharyngeal spray. The dose in each group was 6.8 mg.kg^{-1}. The gargle produced a peak concentration of 2.4 μg.mL^{-1}, whereas the spray produced a peak concentration of 1.9 μg.mL^{-1} at 50 minutes.[43]

- Reasoner et al. randomized 40 adult patients undergoing awake fiberoptic intubation and surgery for cervical spine instability into topical and nerve block groups. Up to 20 mL of 4% lidocaine was administered to the topical group via a nebulizer attached to a facemask using a flow rate of 10 L.min^{-1}. Nebulization required about 10 minutes and was followed by cricothyroid puncture and injection of an additional 3 mL of 4% lidocaine. In the nerve block group, airway anesthesia was achieved with 50 mg of 10% lidocaine spray applied to the tongue, bilateral glossopharyngeal nerve block at the palatoglossal fold using 0.5–1.0 mL 2% lidocaine, superior laryngeal nerve block using 1–2 mL 2% lidocaine, and 3 mL 4% lidocaine injected through the cricothyroid membrane. Arterial blood was sampled for the plasma lidocaine level following administration of local anesthesia, 2 minutes prior to intubation (time zero), and again 10 minutes later. The topical group received 815 $\pm$ 208 mg of lidocaine whereas the nerve block group received 349 $\pm$ 44 mg. Mean plasma lidocaine levels at time zero were 2.16 $\pm$ 1.48 μg.mL^{-1} in the topical group, and 4.23 $\pm$ 1.12 μg.mL^{-1} in the nerve block group. Ten minutes later, the levels were 3.34 $\pm$ 1.87 μg.mL^{-1} and 4.02 $\pm$ 1.02 μg.mL^{-1}, respectively. No plasma sampling was performed after the 10-minute recording. The quality of anesthesia achieved was similar with both the techniques, and intubation was achieved in 3.2 minutes on average. No complications were identified.[77]

- Ameer et al. administered topical lidocaine for bronchoscopy to 19 adults using a combination of lidocaine gargle, atomized lidocaine, lidocaine jelly, and lidocaine solution injected through the bronchoscope. The time over which lidocaine was administered was 0.79 $\pm$ 0.31 hours in 5 young patients and 0.69 $\pm$ 0.22 hours in 14 elderly subjects. The total dosage administered was 19.01 $\pm$ 1.67 mg.kg^{-1} in the young adults, and 17.15 $\pm$ 2.28 mg.kg^{-1} in the elderly. The mean maximum plasma concentration achieved was 3.04 $\pm$ 1.27 μg.mL^{-1} in the young and 2.40 $\pm$ 0.92 μg.mL^{-1} in the elderly. The times required to reach peak levels were 0.77 $\pm$ 0.28 hours in the young and 1.21 $\pm$ 0.55 hours in the elderly. No serious drug toxicity occurred.[78]

Toxicity associated with lidocaine topically applied to the airway can however occur.

- Wu et al. reported a grand mal seizure which occurred following the topical application of 300–320 mg of lidocaine applied as a 4% spray to the larynx and 10–12 mL of 1% viscous lidocaine to the oropharynx and trachea of a 30-year-old, 48-kg female with renal failure, congestive heart failure, cardiomyopathy, and abnormal liver function tests. The plasma lidocaine level shortly after the seizure was 12 μg.mL^{-1}. They also reviewed seven cases of seizure after the administration of topical lidocaine to mucous membranes of the airway. In each of these seven cases, the topical lidocaine was administered as 2% viscous or 2–4% solution.[42]

- Kotaki et al. in 1996 reported a seizure following the application of up to 800 mg of lidocaine as a 2% viscous preparation and 4% solution to the oropharynx. The serum lidocaine concentrations were found to be 11.6 μg.mL^{-1} and 9.0 μg.mL^{-1} after 30 and 150 minutes postseizure, respectively. The authors reviewed three cases of seizure in addition to those reviewed by Wu et al. associated with topical application of lidocaine to the mucous membranes of the oral cavity and pharynx. In each of these three cases, the lidocaine had been administered as a 4% solution or 2% viscous preparation.[51]

In summary, determination of the maximum safe dose of lidocaine that can be topically applied to the mucous membrane of the airway is difficult and must take into account the method of topicalization employed as well as the time course of administration. Traditional dosage guidelines may be excessively conservative when some or the entire dose is administered by aerosol based on the available evidence with respect to serum levels and toxicity occurrences. Caution must be exercised however and a precalculated dose should not be exceeded. As always, clinical judgment is required and meticulous attention to detail should be employed when lidocaine is applied to the airway such that effective anesthesia is achieved without producing toxicity.

3.3.3 Can topical anesthesia of the upper airway cause airway obstruction?

Several studies have looked at this issue:

- In a study of seven normal subjects, Gal administered 4% lidocaine by ultrasonic aerosol and measured airway responses. After the inhalation of lidocaine, the subjects noted an impaired ability to swallow, and a husky voice suggesting vocal cord paresis. Three of the seven subjects described a sensation of obstruction during deep inspiration, although this was not reflected by significant changes in peak inspiratory flow as recorded in maximum effort flow volume loops. Peak expiratory flow rates were also unchanged. However, statistically significant increases in maximum inspiratory flow were observed at 60%, 50%, and 40% of forced vital capacity (FVC) following the lidocaine aerosol. The author concluded that administration of 4% lidocaine by ultrasonic nebulization produced mild bronchodilation and did not adversely affect airway function in normal subjects.[79]

- Gove et al. administered 10 mL of 4% lidocaine by means of an ultrasonic nebulizer attached to a mouthpiece to 33 patients prior to bronchoscopy. Five of the 33 patients required additional boluses of lidocaine to the bronchial tree during the procedure. Spirometry was recorded in 32 patients. A wide variation in individual response to the nebulized lidocaine was observed. Forced expiratory volume in 1 second (FEV1) varied between −18% and +45%, FVC between −27% and +18%, and peak expiratory flow rate (PEFR) between −41% and +34%. However, no overall effect on airflow was demonstrated. The bronchoconstriction that did occur was not clinically significant and bronchodilator therapy was not required.[80]

- Kuna et al. performed pulmonary function tests (PFTs) on 11 normal subjects before and after topical anesthesia of the airway. The topical anesthesia was achieved using 4% lidocaine spray to the soft palate and posterior oropharynx, internal approach superior laryngeal nerve block using cotton pledgets soaked in 4% lidocaine, and 1.5 mL of 10% cocaine applied by means of a cannula to the epiglottis and vocal cords by direct laryngoscopy. The PFTs consisted of flow volume loops, body box determinations of functional residual capacity (FRC), and airway resistance. The area under the inspiratory curve, peak inspiratory flow, and forced inspiratory flow at 25%, 50%, and 75% of FRC were decreased after airway anesthesia, as was peak expiratory flow. However the area under the expiratory curve and forced expiratory flow at 25, 50, and 75% FVC were unchanged. The authors noted that the configuration of the flow volume envelope following anesthesia in most subjects demonstrated a plateau or sudden reversible reduction in airflow on inspiration but a relative preservation of gas flow on expiration, and concluded that laryngeal anesthesia can compromise upper airway patency.[81]

- Listro et al. measured specific airway conductance and maximum inspiratory and expiratory flow rates before and 15, 35, and 45 minutes after topical anesthesia of the upper airway. Anesthesia was achieved using four 10% lidocaine sprays to the oropharynx and hypopharynx, and 2 mL of 4% lidocaine solution instilled twice onto the vocal cords using a laryngeal syringe. Average values of maximum inspiratory flow rate (MIFR) decreased 15 minutes after upper-airway anesthesia, but returned to control levels or nearly so at 45 minutes. Transient decreases in flow rates reaching zero flow on some occasions were observed in 13 of 16 subjects during forced inspiratory vital capacity (FIVC) and in 7 of 16 during forced expiratory vital capacity (FEVC) maneuvers. The site of obstruction to air flow was determined in 13 patients using simultaneous measurements of supraglottic pressure, flow rates, and lung volume. In 12 of this 13 patients, the site of obstruction was localized to the glottis, and in one, both supraglottic and glottic obstruction occurred. However, upper-airway anesthesia in the absence of maximum forced respiratory maneuvers did not result in a decrease in flow rates. The authors concluded that topical anesthesia of the upper airway induces a glottic obstruction that produces a profound but transient decrease in maximum inspiratory and expiratory gas flow consistent with reflex regulation of upper airway caliber.[82]

- Weiss and Patwardhan administered lidocaine aerosols to 22 patients with stable asthma and demonstrated an initial decrease of expiratory gas flow of approximately 20% within 5 minutes of aerosol administration. Following this initial response, 12 of 22 patients continued to demonstrate a reduction in measured expiratory gas flow that persisted up to 60 minutes, whereas the remaining 10 patients revealed a significant improvement in expiratory gas flow above baseline.[83]

- MacAlpine and Thomson similarly measured FEV1 in 20 asthmatic patients following the administration of 6 mL of 4% nebulized lidocaine. The maximum percentage change in FEV1 following lidocaine inhalation varied from −42.1% to +28.2%, with a mean of −8.2%. Five of the 20 patients experienced a decrease in FEV1 greater than 15%.[84]

- Groben et al. measured changes in FEV1 in 10 volunteers with mild asthma after topical airway anesthesia with either lidocaine or dyclonine and awake fiberoptic intubation. The local anesthetic was initially administered by nebulizer and supplemented with a gargle and administration of the anesthetic solution onto the epiglottis via the bronchoscope. Following baseline measurements, FEV1 was measured after saline or salbutamol inhalation, local anesthetic inhalation, intubation, and extubation. No significant difference was found in FEV1 following lidocaine or dyclonine inhalation. Salbutamol inhalation significantly increased FEV1. Following awake fiberoptic intubation under lidocaine anesthesia, FEV1 decreased 35%, and 51% after dyclonine. This decrease in FEV1 was significantly attenuated by salbutamol pretreatment in both groups. After 2–5 minutes of extubation, FEV1 returned to values close to those obtained following saline or salbutamol administration. No significant difference was found between FEV1 values after extubation as compared to the respective FEV1 baseline.[85]

- Thomson also reported a fall in specific conductance of the airway following bupivacaine aerosol administration to asthmatics.[86]

- Shaw et al. reported a case of respiratory distress following the administration of 10% lidocaine spray to the tongue and oropharynx in the presence of a compromised airway associated with goiter. Air entry could not be maintained despite repositioning the patient onto her left side, jaw thrust, chin lift, and placement of an oral airway. The authors felt that a combination of laryngospasm due to irritation caused by the lidocaine spray, and loss of muscle tone as a result of the local anesthetic action, contributed to the airway obstruction.[87]

- McGuire and El-Beheiry reported complete airway obstruction during attempted awake fiberoptic intubation under local anesthesia in two patients with unstable cervical spine fractures. Both required surgical airways. Both patients also received sedative agents. One patient developed stridor then complete airway obstruction following introduction of the flexible fiberoptic bronchoscope (FFB) after topicalization using 1% lidocaine spray and cricothyroid puncture. The second patient was topicalized using swabs soaked in 4% lidocaine. Insertion of the fiberscope was associated with gagging and coughing followed by complete airway obstruction.[88]

- Ho et al. reported a case of complete airway obstruction which occurred following the topical administration of 2% lidocaine onto the tongue and pharynx and suctioning in a patient with recurrent neck carcinoma following radiotherapy, who had hoarseness and stridor preoperatively.[89]

Extensive clinical experience with lidocaine has shown it to be an effective topical agent for airway anesthesia and to have a wide margin of safety.[72,75] However, in the presence of preexisting airway compromise, topical anesthesia and instrumentation of the airway can be associated with complete airway obstruction and in this setting, due consideration must be given to the performance of an awake tracheotomy under local anesthesia.[89–91]

3.3.4 Tetracaine

Introduced in 1932, tetracaine (pontocaine) is a long-acting amino ester derivative of para-aminobenzoic acid[32,41] and is still used extensively for spinal anesthesia and topical anesthesia of the eye.[41] Although once widely used for topical anesthesia of the airway,[92] its use for this indication fell into disfavor after reports of toxic reactions including fatalities were published in the 1950s.[48,92] Of the local anesthetics possessing topical action, dibucaine and tetracaine are the most potent as well as the most toxic.[48] The maximal effective concentration of topical tetracaine is 1%. This concentration has a latent period of 0.6–1.1 minutes and a duration of 50.2–55.5 minutes.[35] When applied to the tongue, 0.5% tetracaine has a latent period of 1.6 minutes and a duration of action of 18.1 minutes.[35] The latent period for 0.4% tetracaine is 3.8 minutes and the duration of action is 35.8 minutes, while for 2% tetracaine, these are 11 and 48.6 minutes, respectively.[35] The duration of action on the conjunctiva is approximately twice than that at the tip of the tongue, whereas the duration of action on the lip and palate is intermediate. Tetracaine appears to be superior

to other topical anesthetics and this may be due to its ability to anesthetize structures deep to the mucous membrane.[48,93]

Tetracaine applied to the mucous membranes of the pharynx and trachea is rapidly absorbed into the circulation such that blood levels are almost comparable to those obtained after IV injection.[93,94] Epinephrine added to the tetracaine does not retard its absorption.[93] In 1951, Weisel and Tella reported a series of 1000 bronchoscopies performed with topical tetracaine.[92] There were 12 minor and 7 severe toxic reactions including 6 seizures and 1 severe bronchospasm. Loss of consciousness preceded convulsions in two of the cases. Cotton pledgets were dipped into a solution of 2% tetracaine and placed successively between the faucial pillars and in each piriform fossa for about 1 minute at each location. Then 1 mL of 2% tetracaine was injected into the trachea using a syringe and a laryngeal cannula.[92] The dose administered was estimated to be ≤40 mg in most cases although measurement was inexact. The toxic reaction occurred following application of the fourth pledget in two patients, and tracheal instillation in five patients, and was heralded by syncope or presyncope.[92] Adriani and Campbell noted 10 fatalities at their institution over a 15-year period caused by topical tetracaine.[48] The maximum safe dosage of tetracaine has never been clearly defined.[93] However, maximum safe doses cited in the literature are said to be 50 mg,[32] 80 mg,[25] or 100 mg[95,96] in the adult. Again, when maximum safe doses are considered, the method of administration must also be taken into account. In a 1995 review, topical tetracaine was said to be no longer recommended for topical airway anesthesia because of its narrow margin of safety[64]; however, topical tetracaine continues to be widely used for awake intubation. Tetracaine (0.45%) administered by atomizer produces excellent intubating conditions; however, the potential for toxicity must be appreciated. Allergic reaction, although rare, is more likely with the ester group of local anesthetics as compared to the amides.

3.3.5 Does cocaine have a role in providing topical airway anesthesia in current anesthesia practice?

Cocaine, an ester of benzoic acid and a nitrogen base was first isolated in 1860 and serendipitously discovered to have anesthetic properties.[32,41] It is the only local anesthetic that inhibits reuptake of norepinephrine and thereby produces vasoconstriction, hence its continued popularity for nasal procedures.[33,34,97] The maximum effective concentration of topical cocaine is 20%, and this solution produces an anesthetic effect within 0.3 minutes and has a duration of action of 54.5 minutes.[35] Topical anesthesia is produced with 4% cocaine after a latent period of 4 minutes and has a duration of action of 10.2 minutes,[35] whereas 10% cocaine has a latent period of 2 minutes and duration of action of 31.5 minutes.[35] The same degree of blockade is produced with 20% cocaine as with 1% tetracaine.[35] Typically 1–10% cocaine is used clinically.[32,63] The vasoconstriction produced by cocaine occurs after a latent period of 5–10 minutes.[59] The maximum recommended dose for topical nasal application has been said to be from 1.5 mg.kg^{-1} (Ref. 98) to 3.0 mg.kg^{-1} (Ref. 37) and 1–3 mg.kg^{-1} (Ref. 99); however, toxic reactions have occurred after nasal administration of as little as 20–30 mg.[99,100] The use of cocaine has been associated with coronary artery vasoconstriction, increased myocardial demand,[64] and hypertension.[98] Doses as small as 0.4 mg.kg^{-1} may cause ventricular fibrillation,[98] and fatalities have been reported.[41] Cocaine should be avoided or used cautiously in the presence of hypertension, hyperthyroidism, angina, or in patients taking monoamineoxidase inhibitors (MAOIs).[37] Blood levels of cocaine after topical application to the piriform fossae were similar to levels produced after IV injection.[41,94] Oxymetazoline has been shown to be as effective as cocaine in the prevention of epistaxis caused by nasotracheal intubation[101,102] as has normal saline,[102] phenylephrine/lidocaine,[12,100] and phenylephrine alone.[100]

From the available evidence, the disadvantages associated with the use of cocaine to produce nasal anesthesia for awake intubation appear to outweigh the advantages.

3.3.6   How safe and effective is benzocaine?

Benzocaine, an ethyl ester of para-aminobenzoic acid,[103] is a water soluble ester type local anesthetic that is widely used for topicalization of the airway.[96] It is available as a 20% spray which can deliver 60 mg[95] to 200–295 mg per 1 second spray.[103] Benzocaine is also a component of cetacaine which consists of 14% benzocaine, 2% tetracaine, and 2% butyl aminobenzoate (butamben).[104] The maximum effective concentration of topical benzocaine is 20%, has a latent period of 0.17 minutes, and a duration of action of 4.3 minutes.[35] An onset time of 15–30 seconds and a duration of action of 5–10 minutes have also been cited.[64] The maximum dose recommended for upper-airway anesthesia has been quoted to be 1.5 mg.kg^{-1} (Ref. 37), although a dose of 100 mg in the adult has also been cited to be toxic.[96] Benzocaine can produce methemoglobinemia following the administration of as little as 150–300 mg in the adult.[105] As of 1999, 58 cases of benzocaine-induced methemoglobinemia had been reported in the literature.[104] Additional cases have occurred since that time[37,105–107] leading to a letter of warning from the Federal Drug Administration (FDA) in the USA. Methemoglobinemia is potentially fatal[104] and treatment with a 1% solution of methylene blue 1–2 mg.kg^{-1} is recommended for methemoglobin levels greater than or equal to 30% or at lower levels if symptoms of hypoxia are present.[108] Benzocaine is metabolized by plasma cholinesterase[103] to para-aminobenzoic acid, a highly allergenic molecule[64] and allergic reactions to benzocaine can occur. Given its short duration of action, and its potential for toxicity, the use of benzocaine as a topical anesthetic for airway management seems difficult to justify.

3.3.7   Dyclonine hydrochloride

Dyclonine, a ketone, is a unique local anesthetic agent that was introduced in 1952 and is structurally distinct from the aminoesters and aminoamides.[109] It can be used as a 0.5–1% solution for topical anesthesia.[32,109] When applied to mucous membranes, the onset time is 2–10 minutes and the duration of action is 20–30 minutes. Adriani et al. noted that dyclonine had limited systemic toxicity but a saturated solution may cause residual numbness that persists for many hours suggesting local injury.[35] One percent dyclonine administered by aerosol has been shown to produce topical airway anesthesia as effective as, and longer lasting than, 4% lidocaine.[85] In a study of 10 volunteers with mild asthma, 4 of the 10 subjects reported much more intense topical anesthesia following 1% dyclonine inhalation as compared to 4% lidocaine.[85] However, FEV1 decreased to a greater extent in the dyclonine group and the authors

concluded that dyclonine must be considered relatively contraindicated in the setting of bronchial hyperreactivity.

Bacon et al. reported the use of dyclonine for awake fiberoptic intubation in a patient with apparent allergy to local anesthetics.[109] The patient gargled and then swallowed 25 mL of 1% dyclonine solution, and 5 mL of 1% dyclonine was then administered by nebulizer. Adequate anesthesia was achieved.[109] Dyclonine has not been widely used, however, for airway anesthesia and is no longer marketed for this purpose in the USA or Canada.

3.4   AIRWAY ANESTHESIA TECHNIQUES

3.4.1   What techniques are available for upper-airway anesthesia?

Regional anesthesia of the airway can be achieved using a wide variety of techniques. Each technique requires a meticulous approach, attention to detail, and knowledge of relevant anatomy, as well as the pharmacology of the agents employed, if an adequate block is to be achieved. The most important prerequisite for a successful awake intubation is adequate regional anesthesia of the airway.

3.4.2   Spray/ointment/gel/EMLA/cream

The posterior third of the tongue, the soft palate, the tonsillar pillars, and the adjacent pharynx can be sequentially anesthetized using commercially available 10% lidocaine spray,[33,34,97] simply by directing the spray onto the relevant structures. A tongue depressor can be used to gently retract the tongue. The commercially available 10% lidocaine aerosol is fitted with a metered valve that delivers 10 mg of lidocaine with each depression of the release button.[47] The aerosol is generated by a simple pump mechanism using manually compressed air as the driving force. Adequate regional anesthesia for awake intubation by direct laryngoscopy can readily be achieved in this manner, and in the emergency setting, time may not permit additional regional techniques. The 10% lidocaine aerosol is marketed in Canada by Odan Laboratories Limited but is not currently marketed in the USA (see Figure 3–25). Alternatively, 4% lidocaine administered using a

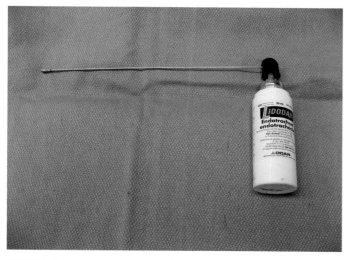

FIGURE 3-25. Lidocaine aerosol fitted with a malleable stainless steel nozzle (*Reproduced with permission from Odan Laboratories Ltd., Montreal, Canada*).

mucosal atomization device can be used (Wolf Tory Medical Incorporated, Salt Lake City, Utah). A curved metal cannula can also be used to inject lidocaine solution into the laryngopharynx and larynx as time and circumstances permit; however this is not necessary for awake intubation by direct laryngoscopy, and blood levels of lidocaine produced with this technique will probably be higher than those produced by aerosol techniques.[44] Cooperative patients can also gargle 2–4% lidocaine in order to achieve topical anesthesia of the posterior tongue and adjacent oropharynx. Residual anesthetic should be expectorated to avoid excessive drug exposure and potential nausea and vomiting.[33,97,110] Lidocaine ointment (5%) can be very useful to anesthetize the posterior third of the tongue especially when patients are unable to gargle. Lidocaine gel 2% can also be used. With any of these techniques, time (at least 1 minute[25] to 2 minutes[35] and perhaps as long as 5 minutes[32]) must be allowed for the anesthetic effect to occur.

Benzocaine spray has no apparent advantage over lidocaine and can produce allergic reactions as well as methemoglobinemia.

EMLA cream, a 1:1 eutectic mixture of 2.5% lidocaine and 2.5% prilocaine, has also been used to produce airway anesthesia. Larijani et al. applied up to 4 g of EMLA cream to the tongue and pharynx in a series of 20 patients who underwent awake fiberoptic intubation.[111] The intubation was performed via a Williams airway. The mean time from the application of the EMLA cream to placement of the oral airway was 11 ± 6 minutes. All patients were successfully intubated but all coughed when the scope was passed into the trachea. No toxic plasma levels of lidocaine or prilocaine occurred. A statistically significant increase in methemoglobin levels occurred within 6 hours; however these levels did not exceed normal values (1.5%).[111] Sohmer et al. used 4 mL of EMLA cream applied to the tongue and gargled before performing awake bronchoscopy in 57 patients.[112] In addition, 79.05 ± 14.39 mg of lidocaine was administered through the FFB for laryngeal anesthesia. Fifty-six of the cases did not require supplemental anesthesia. Bronchoscopic conditions were excellent in 55 cases and good in the remaining 2 cases.[112] The mean time from EMLA application to insertion of the bronchoscope was 5.10 ± 0.45 minutes. EMLA cream applied to the nostril prior to the passage of an FFB provoked rhinorrhea and sneezing that persisted for several hours in 21 of 31 individuals, although the fiberoscopy was well tolerated.[113] EMLA cream may be an alternative for oropharyngeal topical anesthesia although experience is limited.

3.4.3 Aerosols

Excellent anesthesia of the airway can be produced by the administration of aerosolized local anesthetic delivered by an atomizer such as the DeVilbiss RD 15 (see Figure 3-26). The device consists of a glass reservoir, which holds the anesthetic solution, and a nozzle assembly, which can be connected to a high-pressure oxygen source by means of standard oxygen tubing. A small bleed hole is cut in the oxygen tubing at a convenient location near its connection to the atomizer. When oxygen flow is delivered into the tubing at about 6–8 L.min^{-1} occlusion of the bleed hole with a fingertip produces a fine spray of local anesthetic from the atomizer nozzle. When held at the nostril, and coordinated with deep breaths on command, the device can produce profound anesthesia of the airway from the nose to the trachea and beyond in about 5 minutes.[33,97] The atomized

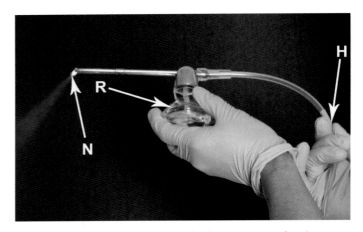

FIGURE 3-26. DeVilbiss Atomizer: The device consists of a glass reservoir (R), which holds the anesthetic solution, and a nozzle assembly, which can be connected to standard oxygen tubing. A small bleed hole (H) is cut in the oxygen tubing. When oxygen flow is delivered into the tubing at about 6.0–8.0 L.min^{-1}, occlusion of the bleed hole with a finger produces a fine spray of local anesthetic from the atomizer nozzle (N).

local anesthetic can also be administered through the mouth, although superior gas flow characteristics through the nose may deliver the anesthetic more efficiently to the pharynx, larynx, and trachea.[33,97] Obstruction of the nasal cavity of course precludes nasal administration. At the author's institution, the DeVilbiss atomizer has been used routinely for awake intubation for more than two decades with excellent results and no toxic reactions. Preferred local anesthetic by most clinicians has been 10–20 mL of 0.45% tetracaine, although an excellent block can also be achieved with 10–12 mL of 3% lidocaine. Others have recommended up to 20 mL of 0.5% tetracaine or 10 mL of 4% lidocaine with this technique.[96]

Aerosolized local anesthetic can also be administered through the mouth using a standard nebulizer attached to a mouthpiece.[114] An oral airway intubation device can be attached to the nebulizer and advanced into the oropharynx as tolerated to deliver the anesthetic to the more distal airway (see Figure 3-27).[114] The authors

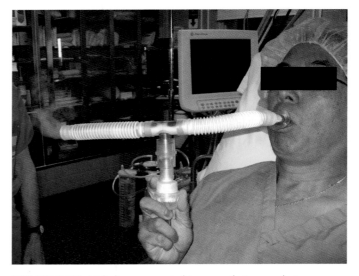

FIGURE 3-27. Nebulizer connected to a mouthpiece and airway intubator.

of the noted report used 4 mL of 4% lidocaine at 8 L.min⁻¹ oxygen flow with this technique and the nebulization required 8 minutes.[114] Additionally, 4 mL of 2% lidocaine was administered through the FFB during intubation.[114]

Nebulized local anesthetic has also been administered by facemask using 4–20 mL of 4% lidocaine[53,65,68,77] or 6 mg.kg⁻¹ of 10% lidocaine.[44] Nebulization by this technique required 10–22 minutes.[44,53,65,68,77] In a study reported by Kundra, 7 of 24 patients required supplemental lidocaine through the FFB after nebulization by mask,[65] and two of three other reports of awake intubation or bronchoscopy using nebulization by mask also used supplemental anesthesia.[53,65,68,77]

3.4.4   Local anesthetic aspiration

Local anesthesia of the airway can also be achieved using an aspiration technique.[115] In this technique, lidocaine solution is simply dripped onto the dorsum of the tongue of a supine patient during tongue traction.[115] The swallowing reflex is initially stimulated but lidocaine subsequently pools in the posterior pharynx and is aspirated into the trachea.[115] Gargling with two consecutive 5 mL aliquots of 2% lidocaine can decrease the intensity of this swallowing reflex.[115] Chung et al. instilled the lesser of 0.2 mL.kg⁻¹ or 20 mL of 1.5% lidocaine following the gargle as described above and reported satisfactory fiberoptic intubating conditions in 39 patients although mild coughing or gagging did occur with the scope in the trachea in 10 patients, and with the tube in the trachea in another 21 patients. Supplemental local anesthesia was not required. Eighteen patients were intubated orally, using a Williams airway, whereas 21 were intubated nasally. Gauze packing soaked in 1.5 mL of 5% lidocaine was used for nasal anesthesia. The time required for intubation varied from 1 to 10 minutes (median time 3.25 minutes).[115] By comparison, intubation after a DeVilbiss technique can usually be accomplished in about 30 seconds.

During fiberoptic intubation, lidocaine is commonly sprayed onto the mucosa of the airway through the suction channel of the bronchoscope, the so-called "spray as you go" technique. However, since the time course to maximum analgesia for topical lidocaine may be as long as 5 minutes after application, this approach seems illogical and may provoke unnecessary reflex glottic closure and cough. Furthermore, extending the duration of the procedure can adversely affect patient comfort.

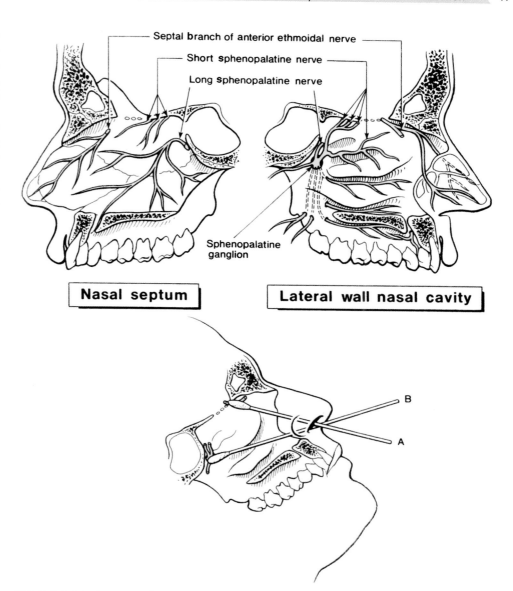

FIGURE 3-28. Placement of cotton-tipped applicators to contact the anterior ethmoidal nerve (A) and the sphenopalatine ganglion and nerves (B). (*Reproduced with permission from Murphy TM: Somatic blockade of the head and neck. In: Neural Blockade in Clinical Anesthesia and Management of Pain, 3rd ed. Cousins MJ, Bridenbaugh PO, eds. Philadelphia: Lippincott-Raven Publishers, 1998:489–574.*)

3.4.5   Nasal anesthesia

Local anesthesia of the nasal cavity can be achieved by a variety of methods. Nebulized lidocaine can be administered by facemask and the patient instructed to breathe through the nose.[65,68] Lidocaine or tetracaine administered with a DeVilbiss atomizer can also be very effective in achieving topical anesthesia of the nasal cavity. Alternatively, long cotton tipped applicators or pledgets, held in bayonet forceps and soaked in 4% lidocaine or 4% cocaine, can be introduced into the selected nostril.[96] One applicator can be inserted parallel to the anterior border of the nasal cavity along the septum until it reaches the anterior end of the cribriform plate at a depth of about 5 cm (see Figure 3-28).[116] The local anesthetic soaked applicator can then be left in place for 5–15 minutes to produce a transmucosal block of the anterior ethmoidal nerve.[96,116] A second applicator can be inserted at an angle of about

20–45 degrees to the floor of the nose until bony resistance is felt at a depth of about 6–7 cm.[116] In this location, the tip of the applicator is adjacent to the sphenopalatine ganglion located deep to the nasal mucosa and similarly can be left in contact with the mucosa for 5–15 minutes to produce a transmucosal block of the sphenopalatine nerves.[96,116] Nasal anesthesia has also been produced using sprays from a multiorificed cannula,[100] a 20-gauge angiocatheter,[96] an epidural catheter,[117] 10% lidocaine aerosol, and lidocaine gel.

A vasoconstrictor is frequently applied topically to the nasal mucosa in an effort to prevent the epistaxis that can occur with nasotracheal intubation.[101] In a prospective, randomized, double-blind study of 36 patients, Rector et al found no difference in the incidence of epistaxis associated with nasotracheal intubation following nasal spraying with 0.05% oxymetazoline, 10% cocaine, or normal saline.[102] Similarly, Gross et al. found no significant difference among groups pretreated with 4% cocaine, 3% lidocaine with 0.25% phenylephrine or 0.25% phenylephrine.[100] Mitchell et al. compared 5% cocaine, 4% lidocaine/0.5% phenylephrine, and normal saline and again found no significant difference in the prevention of epistaxis,[118] and Latorre et al. compared 10% cocaine with 3% lidocaine/0.25% phenylephrine and found no difference.[12] Katz et al. found lidocaine 4% with epinephrine 1:100000 to be less effective than 0.05% oxymetazoline but no difference between 10% cocaine and oxymetazoline, or cocaine and lidocaine with epinephrine.[101]

Thus, the efficacy of the practice of administering vasoconstrictors to prevent epistaxis associated with nasotracheal intubation is doubtful and cocaine would appear to offer no significant advantage over oxymetazoline or phenylephrine.

3.4.6 Translaryngeal anesthesia

Injection of local anesthetic through the cricothyroid membrane was described in the 1920s, and use of this technique to facilitate endotracheal intubation was described in 1949.[22,119] A 21–23-gauge needle can be passed posteriorly in the midline immediately cephalad to the cricoid cartilage to enter the larynx (see Figure 3-29).[22,33,120] Alternatively, a 20-gauge angiocatheter can be used.[96] Directing the needle caudally will direct it away from the

vocal cords which are located 1.3 cm cephalad from the transverse plane at the midpoint of the cricothyroid membrane.[22] The correct intraluminal position of the needle can be confirmed by the aspiration of air.[22,96] Then, 1.5–2.0 mL of 4% lidocaine,[120,121] 3 mL of 4% lidocaine,[77] 4 mL of 2–4% lidocaine,[96] or 2–3 mL of 2% lidocaine[122] can be injected either at end exhalation[123] or inspiration.[96] The cough precipitated by the injection facilitates the spread of the anesthetic which has been shown to reach the superior aspect of the true cords in 95% of cases.[124] If the goal is to spread anesthetic into the larynx and pharynx then injection at end inspiration seems most logical. Also, 4 mL of 2.5% cocaine[125] or 3 mL of 4% cocaine[121] have been used for translaryngeal anesthesia. Tetracaine has also been used in the past[22]; however, severe reactions have been reported with the injection of tetracaine solution into the larynx.[92] Serum lidocaine levels following injection of 5 mg.kg^{-1} of a 10% solution into the larynx via a cricothyroid puncture have been found to be in the antiarrhythmic therapeutic range at a mean time of 5.1 ± 3.2 minutes.[126]

Contraindications to cricothyroid puncture include coagulopathy, local pathology, and an inability to clearly identify the cricothyroid membrane due to obscured landmarks as in the morbidly obese.[22,121] Relative contraindications include those circumstances in which vigorous cough could be deleterious, such as raised intracranial pressure or intraocular pressure, open eye injury, or unstable cervical spine injuries.[96] The use of translaryngeal anesthesia in the presence of a full stomach is controversial.[64] Complications of laryngeal anesthesia including laryngospasm and soft tissue infection have been rarely reported.[22,120] Potential complications include bleeding, subcutaneous emphysema, pneumomediastinum, pneumothorax, vocal cord damage, and esophageal perforation.[96] A review of 17,500 cricothyroid punctures revealed only 8 complications: 2 laryngospasms, 2 broken needles, and 4 soft tissues infections of the neck.[22] In a series of 286 emergency department nasal intubations using translaryngeal anesthesia, Danzl and Thomas reported only 1 complication due to the cricothyroid membrane puncture, a case of superficial cellulitis.[120]

3.4.7 Glossopharyngeal nerve block

In the majority of individuals, the application of topical anesthesia to the mucosa of the oropharynx is sufficient to abolish the gag reflex. However, in the presence of a very pronounced gag reflex or excess secretions, glossopharyngeal nerve block may be a reasonable alternative approach. Submucosal pressure receptors in the posterior third of the tongue may also be involved in the gag reflex[62,96,127–130] and are not felt to be susceptible to topically applied local anesthetics.[96,130]

The glossopharyngeal nerve can be blocked using a posterior approach as it runs about 1 cm deep to the mucosa behind the midpoint of the posterior tonsillar pillar (see Figure 3-30).[34,96,97,127,129–131] A 23-gauge angled tonsillar needle with 1 cm exposed shaft at the tip can be inserted 0.5 cm behind the midpoint of the palatopharyngeal fold, directed laterally and slightly posteriorly to a depth of about 1 cm.[127,131] Following a negative aspiration test, 2 mL of 2% lidocaine[127] or 3–5 mL of 1% lidocaine[129,131] can be injected. Mouth opening must be sufficient to permit visualization of the palatopharyngeal fold (posterior tonsillar pillar),[62] and adequate

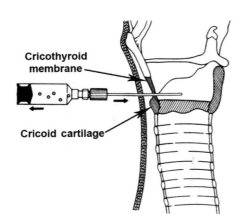

FIGURE 3-29. Anatomical relationships in translaryngeal anesthesia (lateral view). The needle punctures the cricothyroid membrane immediately cephalad to the cricoid cartilage to enter the larynx. (*Reproduced with permission from of Cook® Incorporated, Bloomington, IN*).

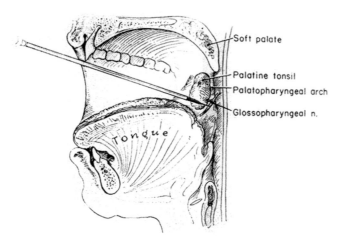

FIGURE 3-30. Glossopharyngeal nerve block. Posterior to palatopharyngeal fold (*Reproduced, with permission, from Barton S, Williams JD: Glossopharyngeal nerve block. Arch Otolaryng. 1971;93:186–188.*)

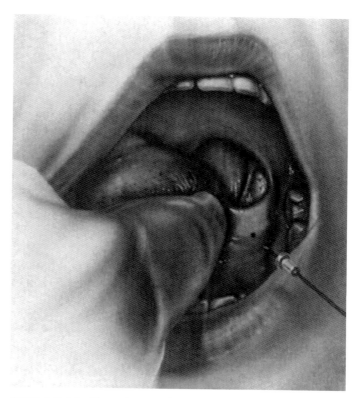

FIGURE 3-31. Glossopharyngeal nerve block at the palatoglossal fold. (*Reproduced with permission from Bogdonoff DL, Stone DJ: Emergency management of the airway outside the operating room. Can J Anaesth. 1992;39(10):1069–1089*).

topical anesthesia of the tongue and adjacent pharyngeal mucosa is necessary to permit exposure of the tonsillar pillar with a tongue blade or laryngoscope.[62,96] Barton and Williams reported a series of 130 patients who underwent glossopharyngeal nerve block for endoscopic procedures or tonsillectomy with no complications, and elimination of the gag reflex in all but 3 patients.[127] Cooper and Watson similarly reported a series of 893 patients who underwent bronchoscopy or tonsillectomy using glossopharyngeal block.[131] Again no complications were reported. Onset time of the block has been noted to be about 1 minute[131] and the duration of the block to be 45–60 minutes.[129] DeMeester and Skinner performed glossopharyngeal nerve block on 500 patients who underwent endoscopic procedures.[129] Superior laryngeal nerve blocks were also performed and supplemental anesthetic was administered through the bronchoscope. An inadequate block occurred in 10 patients. Blood was aspirated in six patients requiring needle repositioning and four additional patients complained of headache thought to have been due to partial intra-arterial injection of the local anesthetic. Two patients had a seizure during the endoscopy and five developed an arrhythmia following the block. The overall complication rate secondary to the glossopharyngeal nerve block was reported to be 2%.[129] Complications in addition to those noted above include local infection and hematoma formation.[96] Contraindications include coagulopathy and local pathology. This posterior approach, glossopharyngeal nerve block, is not widely used and may be impractical in the setting of difficult intubation.

Alternatively, the lingual branch of the glossopharyngeal nerve can be blocked as it runs deep to the mucosa of the palatoglossal fold (anterior tonsillar pillar) (see Figure 3-31).[96,128,130,132] Although the lingual branch of the nerve supplying the posterior third of the tongue is blocked primarily, in some cases retrograde submucosal tracking of the local anesthetic has been shown to occur, with blockade of the pharyngeal and tonsillar branches.[96,133] A 22–27-gauge needle is inserted in the floor of the mouth, 0.5 cm lateral, to the lateral aspect of the base of the tongue at the palatoglossal fold (see Figure 3-31).[96,130,132] The needle is inserted to a depth of about 0.5 cm,[130,132] and following a negative aspiration test, 2 mL of 2% lidocaine[128,130] or 2–5 mL

of 1% lidocaine[96,132] can be injected. If blood is aspirated, the needle should be redirected medially.[96] If air is aspirated, the needle has passed through the palatoglossal fold to enter the oropharynx and should be withdrawn until no air is aspirated.[96] Woods and Landers reported 34 anterior approach glossopharyngeal nerve blocks and noted a duration of action of 15–20 minutes with plain lidocaine and 60 minutes with lidocaine and epinephrine.[130] The blocks were performed with a minimum of patient discomfort.[130] The gag reflex was not completely obliterated in "a number of patients."[130] Sitzman et al. reported a prospective randomized single blinded crossover study of airway anesthesia for direct laryngoscopy on 11 anesthesiologist volunteers which compared 2% viscous lidocaine swish and gargle (S&G), S&G combined with 10% lidocaine spray, and S&G combined with bilateral anterior glossopharyngeal nerve blocks.[132] There was no significant difference between the S&G/spray and S&G/block groups with respect to discomfort during direct laryngoscopy; however the S&G group did experience significantly more discomfort than the other two groups. A trend toward less coughing and gagging with S&G/spray compared with S&G/block was noted although the difference was not significant. Oropharyngeal discomfort lasting 24 hours or more occurred in 91% of the participants in the block group, and four participants had discomfort lasting more than 3 days. The study was stopped due to this oropharyngeal discomfort. The study used 5 mL of 1% plain lidocaine bilaterally, and the authors suggest that the discomfort may have been related to the volume of solution injected.[132]

Contraindications include coagulopathy and local pathology. Potential complications include intra-arterial injection, patient discomfort, hematoma formation, and anatomic distortion. In addition, local anesthetic injected into the floor of the mouth *anterior* to the palatoglossal fold may produce bilateral hypoglossal nerve block and impair the ability to swallow.[130] The block is considered to be acceptable in the presence of a full stomach.[120]

3.4.8 Superior laryngeal nerve block

The internal branch of the superior laryngeal nerve can be blocked as it runs just deep to the mucosa of the piriform fossa using Kraus or Jackson forceps to hold a cotton pledget soaked in 4% lidocaine against the mucosa for about 1 minute (see Figure 3-32).[17,33,60,63,97] Keeping the lidocaine-soaked pledget in contact with the mucosa of the piriform fossa for 5 minutes has also been recommended[63,64,96] but in the author's experience, this is not necessary.

Alternatively, this block can be performed using an external approach to the superior laryngeal nerve as it penetrates the thyrohyoid membrane just below the greater cornu of the hyoid bone.[17,33,63,64,96,97,123,134] With the patient supine and the head extended, the hyoid can be palpated as a freely mobile bony structure cephalad from the thyroid cartilage (see Figures 3-33 and 3.34).[123,134] The hyoid can be fixed between the operator's index finger and thumb[120] and displaced manually toward the side to be

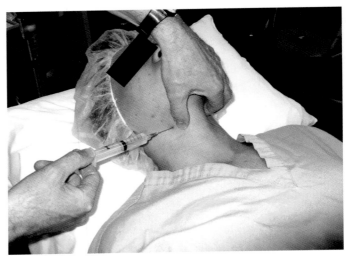

FIGURE 3-33. Percutaneous superior laryngeal nerve block: The hyoid can be fixed between the operator's index finger and thumb and displaced manually toward the side to be blocked. A 22-gauge needle is passed medially in the frontal plane through the skin to contact the hyoid at or near the greater cornu.

blocked.[62] A 21–25-gauge needle[62,63,123] can be passed medially in the frontal plane through the skin to contact the hyoid at or near the greater cornu[123,134] and then walked caudad until it slips off the bone.[123] The needle is then advanced 2–3 mm.[62,96] In this location, the needle tip has entered a closed space bounded by the thyrohyoid membrane laterally and the mucosa of the piriform fossa medially. A slight resistance may be appreciated as the needle is advanced

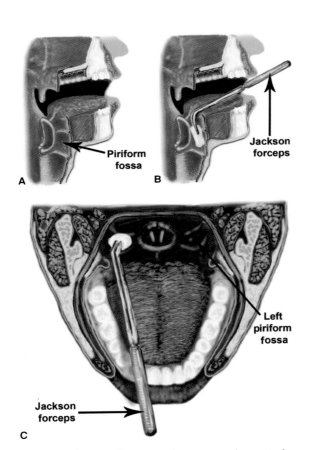

FIGURE 3-32. Schematic illustration of transmucosal superior laryngeal nerve block using Jackson forceps and a cotton pledget soaked in 4% lidocaine. A and B show the lateral view of the block and C shows the superior view of the block.

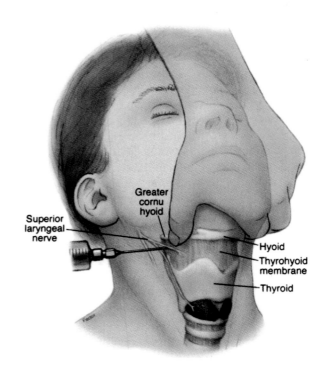

FIGURE 3-34. Schematic illustration of superior laryngeal nerve block (*Reproduced with permission from Brown D, ed. Atlas of Regional Anesthesia, 2nd edn. Philadelphia: Saunders, 1999:205–208.*)

through the ligament,[96] and a definite give as the needle passes through the deep aspect of the membrane.[122] Following a negative aspiration, 2–3 mL of 2% lidocaine[63,64,123] can then be injected. If blood is aspirated, the needle may have entered the superior laryngeal artery or vein or the carotid artery, and in this circumstance it should be withdrawn and redirected anteriorly.[96] If air is aspirated, the pharyngeal lumen has been entered and the needle must be withdrawn until no air is aspirated prior to injection.[96] Entry into the laryngopharynx has been used as an integral part of the technique,[129,135] although this is not necessary. If the hyoid bone cannot be identified by palpation or if palpation produces undue patient discomfort, the thyroid cartilage can be used as a landmark.[33,34,62–64,96,97,123,135] The thyroid cartilage can be displaced toward the side to be blocked and the needle passed medially in the frontal plane to contact the cartilage at a point at or near the greater cornu[64,96,97] or at a point 1/3 of the distance from the midline to the superior cornu.[86] The needle is then walked cephalad to reach and perforate the thyrohyoid membrane.[32,62–64,123,134] Alternatively, the thyrohyoid membrane itself can be identified by palpation with the index finger immediately cephalad to the lateral aspect of the thyroid cartilage.[62,129,135] The carotid pulse can be felt posteriorly (see Figure 3-35).[129] The needle can then be passed medially anterior to the fingertip.[129,135] The feeling of resistance changes as the needle punctures the membrane and is relied on to indicate proper depth.[62] The needle may also be advanced to contact the thyroid cartilage as a depth guide and then walked cephalad.[135]

The onset time for the block is 5–10 minutes[37,63,64] and the duration of action is at least 90 minutes[133] and may be as long as 4–6 hours when 2% lidocaine is used.[64,134] Complications include intra-arterial injection, hematoma (reported incidence 1.4%),[9] unintended pharyngeal perforation,[37,64,123,129] hypotension, and bradycardia.[96] Contraindications include local pathology, coagulopathy, and poor anatomic landmarks.[37,64,123,129] The block has also been said to be contraindicated in patients at risk of aspiration.[17,96,123,133]

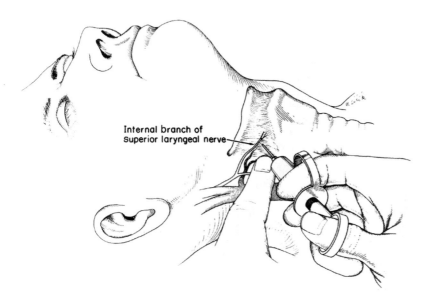

FIGURE 3-35. Alternative technique of superior laryngeal nerve block. (*Reproduced with permission from DeMeester TR, Skinner DB, Evans RH, et al.: Local nerve block anesthesia for peroral endoscopy. Ann Thoracic Surg. 1977; 24(3): 278–282.*)[129]

3.5 OTHER CONSIDERATIONS

3.5.1 Is regional anesthesia of the airway contraindicated in the presence of a full stomach?

Local anesthesia of the larynx and trachea obtunds protective airway reflexes and may predispose to aspiration.[33,34,121,136] However, local anesthesia of the airway has been used in circumstances associated with an increased risk of aspiration without aspiration actually occurring.[22,120–122,136–139] Thomas reported a series of 25 patients who were intubated awake, 21 of whom had a full stomach.[122] Topical anesthesia was administered to all 25 and bilateral superior laryngeal nerve blocks were performed on 21 patients. Nine patients were given translaryngeal injections. No incident of aspiration occurred.[122] Duncan reported 12 patients who underwent awake intubation for emergency surgery under regional anesthesia of the airway including transtracheal injection and recorded no incident of aspiration.[121] Kopman et al. reported 55 awake intubations in patients with full stomachs under topical anesthesia to the nose, mouth, pharynx, and larynx. There was no evidence of aspiration in any of the patients.[137] Danzl and Thomas performed 286 emergency nasotracheal intubations under transtracheal anesthesia and reported no aspirations.[120] Meschino et al. reported a series of 165 patients with cervical spine fracture who underwent awake intubation.[138] Sixty-four patients required emergency endotracheal intubation, and "a regional block or local anesthesia of the larynx" was administered in 137 patients. No evidence of aspiration of gastric contents was documented during intubation.[138] Ovassapian et al. performed 114 awake fiberoptic intubations on patients with a full stomach risk under regional anesthesia of the airway including translaryngeal injection or injection into the larynx and trachea through the flexible bronchoscope.[139] Again no aspirations occurred.[139,137] Gold and Buechel reviewed 17,500 cases of translaryngeal anesthesia reported in the literature.[22] They recorded eight complications, but no aspirations.[22]

The risk of aspiration during awake intubation under regional anesthesia of the airway must be weighed against the risks associated with other airway management modalities.[33,34] As always, good clinical judgment and a common sense approach are mandatory.[33,34]

3.5.2 Are antisialagogues helpful or even essential in awake fiberoptic intubation?

Secretions in the airway interpose a mechanical barrier between the mucosa and topically applied local anesthetics, dilute the anesthetic solution, and wash it away from the intended site of action.[33,34,36,63,64,97,140,141] The view through the bronchoscope can also be impaired by the presence of secretions.[37] Antisialagogues are therefore invaluable adjuncts to facilitate awake fiberoptic intubation.[33,34,47,97] Atropine and glycopyrrolate are both effective, although glycopyrrolate is the more potent drying agent.[33,97,142] Scopolamine has also been used as an antisialagogue; however it produces sedation as well as amnesia and can produce delirium.[63]

These antimuscarinic drugs dry the airway by decreasing the *production* of secretions.[37,63,64] They must therefore be administered far enough in advance of planned airway manipulation to allow eradication of secretions that have already accumulated, as well as to permit the drug to exert its antisialagogic effect.[37,63] Following IV administration of glycopyrrolate to volunteers, dryness of the mouth was noted 7 minutes after injection and a significant drying effect was observed after 15 minutes.[38] Following IM administration, glycopyrrolate has an onset of action of 20–40 minutes[63,143] and the peak effect occurs at 30–45 minutes.[143] Inhibition of salivary secretions persists for up to 7 hours after parenteral administration of glycopyrrolate[144] and is dose related.[142] The appropriate dose of IM glycopyrrolate when used as a drying agent is 0.2–0.4 mg in the adult.[142] The corresponding dose in children is about 10 $\mu g.kg^{-1}$ (Ref. 142). Glycopyrrolate can also be given subcutaneously.[63,64,144] After IM administration, doses of glycopyrrolate sufficient to produce a 75% inhibition of salivation produced only minimal heart rate changes,[142] although an increase in heart rate can occur after IV administration.[142] Glycopyrrolate is a quaternary ammonium compound and does not cross the normal blood–brain barrier.[37,96]

Following the IM administration of atropine, inhibition of salivation is seen within 30 minutes,[143] the peak effect is seen at 1.0–1.6 hours,[143] and the duration of action is 4 hours.[63] The heart rate increases 5–40 minutes after the IM administration of atropine and peaks within 20–60 minutes.[143] At doses necessary to produce a 75% inhibition of salivation, atropine increases the heart rate by more than 15%.[142] When used as an antisialagogue, 0.2–0.8 mg of atropine can be given IM or subcutaneously 30–60 minutes before airway manipulation.[63,143] Rarely at low doses, atropine can exert a parasympathomimetic effect and produce a bradycardia.[143] Atropine readily crosses the blood–brain barrier and can produce a CNS effect.[145]

In a prospective randomized double-blind study of 37 surgical patients, the drying effect of glycopyrrolate 0.2 mg IM administered 90 minutes preoperatively was compared to 0.2 mg IV given 10 minutes preoperatively,[146] to 2 mg given by mouth 90 minutes preoperatively, and to placebo. No significant difference was found in the patient's sensation of mouth dryness 10 minutes after IV injection of glycopyrrolate or placebo, and no difference between groups in the anesthetist's perception of dryness of the airway following intubation by direct laryngoscopy. Ten minutes may not be sufficient time to permit significant drying to occur after IV injection as the effect has been shown to increase for up to 15 minutes.[38] The peak effect of IM glycopyrrolate occurs at 30–45 minutes following injection[143] and 90 minutes following injection may not have been the optimal time for observation. Furthermore, the inhibition of salivation is dose related and 0.2 mg is at the low end of the dose range recommended in the adult.[142] Direct laryngoscopy is also a different stimulus as compared to awake fiberoptic intubation under local anesthesia. Cowl et al. reported a double-blind placebo-controlled study of 217 patients who underwent bronchoscopy and intubation under local anesthesia and sedation.[147] Patients were randomly allocated to receive atropine 0.01 mg.kg^{-1} IM, glycopyrrolate 0.005 mg.kg^{-1} IM, or saline placebo 2 mL IM, 15–45 minutes preoperatively. The time of administration in each patient was not recorded however, and the number of patients who received glycopyrrolate 15 minutes before the procedure is unknown. The operators noted no significant difference in antisialagogic effect or cough suppression for either atropine or glycopyrrolate as compared to placebo. However the patients reported significantly higher visual analog scores for secretion control with glycopyrrolate.[147] Roffe et al. randomly allocated 190 consecutive patients undergoing bronchoscopy employing local anesthesia and sedation to receive either IM atropine 0.6 mg, IM glycopyrrolate 0.3 mg, or no antisialagogue 30 minutes preoperatively.[148] Troublesome coughing was less frequent in the glycopyrrolate group as was patient movement. Mouth dryness was most common with glycopyrrolate but overall assessment of discomfort was similar in all three groups. Brookman et al. randomized 80 adult patients undergoing elective dental extraction to receive 0.4 mg hyoscine hydrobromide PO, 0.4 mg hyoscine hydrobromide IM, 0.4 mg glycopyrrolate IM, or placebo 60 minutes preoperatively.[149] All patients underwent nasal fiberoptic intubation. The clarity of the visual field was noted to be significantly improved in all three anticholinergic groups.[149]

The results of these studies are somewhat difficult to extrapolate to the awake fiberoptic intubation setting. In the author's experience, drying agents are immensely helpful in facilitating awake fiberoptic intubation. Glycopyrrolate 0.4 mg IM given to the adult 30 minutes before airway manipulation will provide optimum conditions for topical anesthesia of the airway in the vast majority of patients. Inflammatory conditions of the airway can be associated with excess secretion production and antisialagogues may be less effective in this setting. In the absence of pathology at the site of injection, superior laryngeal nerve block or glossopharyngeal nerve block may be more effective in this circumstance; however intubation under topical anesthesia alone can usually be achieved. The nasal approach requires less suppression of the gag reflex and may be the more appropriate route in the presence of excess secretions.

3.5.3 Is sedation useful in facilitating awake intubation?

If adequate local anesthesia of the airway can be achieved, awake intubation can be rapidly and easily accomplished, and the use of sedation is not necessary. Regional anesthesia of the airway can in itself be achieved with minimal patient discomfort, although stimulation of the gag and cough reflexes can be unpleasant.[112] The emphasis should however be placed on the development of regional anesthesia skills, rather than on the use of sedation in an attempt to compensate for poor airway anesthesia.[34] As time and circumstances permit however, sedation can be used to further minimize discomfort, produce anxiolysis, and attenuate recall,[34] although the need for anxiolysis or amnesia is reduced or eliminated if airway anesthesia can be rapidly and skillfully achieved. In the presence of airway compromise or respiratory distress, any additional impairment of the level of consciousness can lead to deterioration in the clinical situation. The goal of sedation during awake intubation is to produce a calm and cooperative patient who remains crisply responsive to command.[33,34] During awake fiberoptic intubation, the ability of the patient to breathe deeply on command improves visualization of the airway structures, moves the epiglottis anteriorly out of the path of the advancing bronchoscope and endotracheal tube, and by producing maximum abduction of the vocal cords facilitates glottic cannulation. Sedation can therefore make fiberoptic intubation more difficult.

Sedation to facilitate awake intubation can be achieved using a variety of drugs. In general, the minimum amount of sedation required for anxiolysis should be used and the dose carefully titrated to effect.[96]

Midazolam administered in increments of 0.25–0.5 mg to the adult produces anxiolysis and amnesia,[150] and titration to a suitable end point without losing patient cooperation is usually achievable.[34] The onset time is 1–3 minutes and the duration of action is about 2 hours.[34,64] Fentanyl can provide sedation, analgesia, and euphoria, can attenuate laryngeal reflexes, and has an antitussive effective.[34,37,64] Respiratory depression can also occur,[34] as can bradycardia.[150] When used in combination, a synergism between fentanyl and midazolam occurs which potentiates the effects of both drugs.[34,64] Hypotension and apnea can occur. However, when administered in low doses and titrated carefully to affect, midazolam and fentanyl in combination can be used to produce excellent sedation, and side effects can be avoided.[34] Diazepam, lorazepam, and long-acting opioids do not appear to provide any advantage during awake intubation and may be more difficult to titrate. Overdose with benzodiazepines or opioids can be reversed with flumazenil and naloxone, respectively.

Droperidol, a butyrophenone that produces a state of quiescence with reduced motor activity and indifference to one's surroundings,[150] also has been used to facilitate awake intubation. However, about 10% of individuals exposed to droperidol experience a feeling of mental restlessness and agitation, so-called dysphoria,[25,37] and prolongation of the QT interval can occur even at low doses.[151] Ketamine can produce excessive secretions, hallucinations, and mild respiratory depression and is not commonly used to facilitate awake intubation.[64]

In the emergency situation, when judicious chemical restraint is required to permit airway management of combative and intoxicated patients, haloperidol, also a butyrophenone, can be immensely helpful.[33] Intravenous doses of 2–10 mg in the adult can be carefully titrated to effect.[33]

Recently, the use of remifentanil for awake fiberoptic intubation as a single agent and in combination with propofol or midazolam has been reported.[152–157]

- Reusche and Egan reported a case of Ludwig's angina in which awake nasotracheal intubation was performed using a remifentanil infusion at 0.05–0.175 μg.kg^{-1}.min^{-1} (Refs. 156, 157). The patient was also given glycopyrrolate 0.2 mg, droperidol 0.625 mg, and midazolam 2.0 mg IV. After 4 mL of 4% lidocaine was administered by nebulizer, the right naris was swabbed with 4% cocaine, and 2 mL of 4% lidocaine was sprayed on the vocal cords through the FFB. The patient was intubated without gagging, bucking, or coughing.[156,157]

- Johnson et al. reported the use of a remifentanil bolus of 3.2 μg.kg^{-1} in addition to 26 μg.kg^{-1} of midazolam to perform direct laryngoscopy on a patient who was predicted to be a difficult intubation on physical examination.[153] The patient remained conscious and followed commands throughout the direct laryngoscopy and subsequent intubation, appeared to tolerate the pro-

cedure well, and had no recall of the event. No local anesthetic was used.

- Puchner et al. reported the use of a remifentanil infusion to facilitate awake nasotracheal intubation of a patient with odontogenic facial and cervical infection.[156] The nose was anesthetized with 4% lidocaine spray, and 2 mL of 4% lidocaine was sprayed through the FFB onto the vocal cords and subglottic area. The patient remained conscious, calm, and cooperative. No reflex glottic closure was observed.[156] Remifentanil infusion was subsequently compared to a combination of fentanyl and midazolam during awake fiberoptic intubation in 74 patients.[155] Remifentanil was administered in dosages of 0.1–0.5 μg.kg^{-1}.min^{-1}. Both groups received PO midazolam 1 hour preoperatively. Four percent lidocaine spray was administered to the nose, and 4 mL of 4% lidocaine was sprayed through the FFB onto supraglottic and subglottic areas. Patients in the remifentanil group had a significantly reduced response to the nasal passage of the tube and less cough as the larynx was intubated. The investigators felt that remifentanil suppressed laryngeal reflexes significantly better than fentanyl and midazolam and improved intubating conditions.[155]

- Machata et al. compared a remifentanil 0.75 μg.kg^{-1} bolus, followed by 0.075 μg.kg^{-1}.min^{-1} with a 1.5 μg.kg^{-1} bolus followed by 0.15 μg.kg.min^{-1} for awake intubation in 24 patients.[154] All patients were premedicated with midazolam 0.05 mg.kg^{-1} and glycopyrrolate 0.2 mg IV. The nostril was anesthetized using 2% lidocaine gel coating on nasopharyngeal tubes. The supraglottic region was sprayed with 5 mL of 2% lidocaine and 2 mL were administered onto the vocal cords through the working channel of the FFB. No respiratory rate less than eight breaths per minute occurred, no patient recalled pain, and all patients remained cooperative. Intubating conditions were adequate in all patients and comparable between the groups.[154] Both regimens blunted airway reflexes sufficiently.

The ester structure of remifentanil is unique among fentanyl congeners and results in very rapid metabolism. The peak effect–site concentration of remifentanil occurs within 1 to 2 minutes of bolus injection,[153] and the offset is also rapid. The time necessary to reach a 50% decrease in concentration after stopping a continuous infusion at steady state is 4 minutes.[156] The median dose of remifentanil administered over 2 minutes required to produce loss of consciousness has been found to be 12 μg.kg^{-1}, and at doses $\leq$5 μg.kg^{-1} no subjects lost consciousness.[153,158] It has been recommended that dosing should be calculated on lean body mass and reduced by as much as 50–70% in the elderly.[153] Remifentanil therefore appears to be very easily titrated. Jhaveri et al. noted mild muscle rigidity in 40% and moderate rigidity in an additional 40% of a group of elective surgical patients following the administration of 2 μg.kg^{-1} of remifentanil over 2 minutes.[158] No severe muscle rigidity was observed at doses less than 4 μg.kg^{-1}. Wilhelm et al. administered remifentanil by infusion to a group of patients undergoing oocyte removal and did not observe muscle rigidity at doses up to 0.4 μg.kg^{-1}.min^{-1} (Ref. 159).

Anecdotally, remifentanil infusion appears to attenuate the gag reflex as well as laryngeal reflexes and can facilitate airway anesthesia. It may be particularly useful in patients with hyperactive gag reflexes, and in the presence of excess secretions, remifentanil may be an invaluable adjunct in awake intubation. Remifentanil may prove to be an exception to the general rule that sedatives cannot or should not be used to compensate for poor regional anesthesia of the airway. Remifentanil has also been administered by infusion in combination with low-dose propofol during awake intubation.[152]

Dexmedetomidine is an alpha 2-adrenoceptor agonist, which produces sedation, analgesia, some degree of amnesia, and commonly xerostomia. Dexmedetomidine infusion in combination with ketamine infusion has been used for awake fiberoptic intubation.[160] Scher and Gitlin administered a bolus of 1 μg.kg^{-1} of dexmedetomidine over 10 minutes and followed this with an infusion of 0.7 μg.kg^{-1}.h^{-1} (Ref. 160). Upon completion of the dexmedetomidine bolus, 15 mg of ketamine was administered as a bolus, and then followed by an infusion of 20 mg.h^{-1}. The patient remained responsive to command and calm. Regional anesthesia of the airway was then performed "in the usual manner," and fiberoptic intubation via an intubating airway was performed.[160] Intubating conditions were reported to be excellent and included a secretion-free airway. The patient had no recall of the procedure. Dexmedetomidine may be a desirable drug for use with fiberoptic intubation but experience is limited.

3.5.4 How should a patient be prepared psychologically to undergo awake intubation?

Undergoing any medical procedure can be intimidating, anxiety provoking, even frightening, and the physician must make every effort to minimize patient anxiety. As time permits in the emergency setting, and routinely in the elective situation, a full explanation of the circumstances requiring awake intubation should be given to the patient.[34] This explanation of the procedure and its necessity should be provided in as controlled a manner as possible, again as time and circumstances permit. The explanation should be delivered in a calm, unhurried, sincere, methodical manner[36,63] and should emphasize the margin of safety maintained as well as the dangers associated with intubation under general anesthesia in the presence of a difficult airway.[34,64] The explanation should be frank and straightforward, yet sufficiently detailed that the patient understands the necessity for the procedure as well as what to expect during the procedure itself.[37,63] Possible adverse consequences can be discussed as appropriate.[63] The patient must be able to develop a sense of trust in the operator's judgment and expertise if cooperation is to be established.[64] Perhaps in no other procedure is a good bedside manner more important than in awake fiberoptic intubation.

Following the preoperative interview, the patient should be brought into the procedure room (e. g., operating room) only after all the equipment has been made ready. The room should be calm and quiet. Only those who are working in the room should be present. One learner is appropriate, but spectators should be minimized or disallowed. The practitioner and an assistant should perform the awake intubation in a controlled methodical manner, and the practitioner should calmly explain each step of the procedure to further allay anxiety. Nervous behavior by individuals in the room should be avoided. Local anesthesia of the airway should be achieved in 15 minutes or less and the intubation itself in about 30 seconds.

3.5.5 What technique works well for the average patient?

In the emergency setting, regional anesthesia of the airway for awake intubation by direct laryngoscopy can be readily achieved using 10% lidocaine spray. The spray can be directed onto the posterior third of the tongue, the uvula, and the tonsillar pillars using the malleable, stainless steel nozzle, and a tongue depressor to retract the tongue. Sprays can also be delivered into the piriform fossae; however spraying into the larynx should be avoided as laryngospasm, cough, and a loss of patient cooperation may be precipitated. An explanation of the procedure should be provided to the patient as time and circumstances permit. In general, the use of sedation should be avoided in the emergency awake intubation and the time required for antisialagogues to provide mucosal drying is not available. If neck movement is permissible, then awake intubation by direct laryngoscopy is most easily performed with the patient in the sitting position.

In the setting of an anticipated difficult intubation in which awake fiberoptic intubation is planned, profound regional anesthesia of the airway can be achieved using the following technique:

- A full explanation of the procedure should be provided to the patient.

- An antisialagogue should be administered about 20–30 minutes prior to planned airway manipulation.

- If neck movement is allowed, the patient should be in the sitting or semisitting position.

- The patient can then be asked to gargle 40–50 mL of 4% lidocaine solution and expectorate the residual. If the patient is unable to gargle or if an attempt to gargle produces gagging, then the posterior third of the tongue can be anesthetized using 5% lidocaine ointment gently applied with a tongue depressor, or 10% lidocaine spray can be directed onto the posterior third of the tongue, uvula and fauces.

- About 12 mL of aerosolized 3% lidocaine can then be administered optimally via the nose using a DeVilbiss atomizer attached to a high-pressure oxygen source. The spray delivered by the atomizer should be coordinated with respiration, with inhalation through the nose and exhalation through the mouth. Alternatively, the aerosol can be administered via the mouth.

- Cotton pledgets soaked in 4% lidocaine can then be gently advanced over the tongue into the piriform fossa on each side using Jackson forceps to confirm the block or supplement it as necessary. As the pledget is removed, the mucosa of the oropharynx can be swabbed to confirm the absence of the gag reflex.

Fiberoptic intubation can then be rapidly achieved as described in Chapter 8.

3.6 SUMMARY

Awake intubation can be achieved rapidly and with minimal patient discomfort. Knowledge of airway anatomy, the medications that can be employed and techniques of regional anesthesia of the airway are necessary. Manual dexterity, gentleness, and an appropriate bedside manner are also essential.

REFERENCES

1. Mongan PD, Culling RD: Rapid oral anesthesia for awake intubation. *J Clin Anesth.* 1992;4:101–105.
2. Redden RJ: Anatomic airway considerations in anesthesia. In: *Handbook of Difficult Airway Management*, 1st edn. Hagberg CA, ed. Philadelphia: Churchill Livingstone, 2000:1–13.
3. Morris IR: Functional anatomy of the upper airway. *Emerg Med Clin North Am.* 1988;6:639–669.
4. Ellis H, Feldman S: *Anatomy for Anesthetists*, 4th edn. Oxford: Blackwell Scientific Publications, 1983.
5. Morris IR: Airway management. In: *Emergency Medicine: Concepts and Clinical Practice.* Rosen P, et al., eds. St. Louis, Mosby Yearbook, 1992:79–105.
6. Basmajian JV: *Grant's Method of Anatomy*, 8th edn. Baltimore, Williams & Wilkins, 1981.
7. Friedman SM: *Visual Anatomy. Volume 1 Head and Neck.* New York, Harper & Harper, 1970.
8. Hall IS: *Diseases of the Nose, Throat and Ear: A Handbook for Students and Practitioners*, 11th edn. Edinburgh, Churchill Livingstone, 1985.
9. Graney DO: Basic science: anatomy. In: *Otolaryngology Head and Neck surgery.* Cummings CW, et al., St. Louis, Mosby, 1986.
10. Tintinalli JE, Claffey J: Complications of nasotracheal intubation. *Ann Emerg Med.* 1981;10:142–144.
11. Iserson KV: Blind nasotracheal intubation. *Ann Emerg Med.* 1981;10: 468–471.
12. Latorre F, Otter W, Kleemann PP, Dick W, Jage J: Cocaine or phenylephrine/lignocaine for nasal fibreoptic intubation? *Eur J Anaesthesiol.* 1996;13:577–581.
13. Smith JE, Reid AP: Identifying the more patent nostril before nasotracheal intubation. *Anaesthesia.* 2001;56:258–262.
14. Ellis H: *Clinical Anatomy: A Revision and Applied Anatomy for Clinical Students*, 6th edn. Oxford, Blackwell Scientific Publications, 1977.
15. Ovassapian A, Glassenberg R, Randel GI, et al.: The unexpected difficult airway and lingual tonsil hyperplasia: a case series and a review of the literature. *Anesthesiology.* 2002;97:124–132.
16. Snell RS: *Clinical Neuroanatomy for Medical Students*, 5th edn. Philadelphia, Lippincott, Williams & Wilkins, 2001.
17. Stone DJ, Gal TJ: Airway Management In: *Anesthesia*, 5th edn. Miller RD (ed.). Philadelphia, Churchill Livingstone, 2000:1414–1451.
18. Donlon JV Jr: Anesthetic and airway management of laryngoscopy and bronchoscopy. In: *Airway Management Principles and Practice.* Benumof JL, ed. St. Louis, Mosby, Inc., 1996:666–685.
19. *Gray's Anatomy*, 37th edn. Williams PL, Warwick R, Dyson L, et al., (eds.) New York, Churchill Livingstone, 1989.
20. Stoelting RK: Endotracheal intubation. In: *Anesthesia.* Miller RD. ed. New York, Churchill Livingstone, 1981:233–255.
21. Melker RJ, Florete OG Jr: Percutaneous dilatational cricothyrotomy and tracheostomy. In: *Airway Management Principles and Practice.* Benumof JL ed. St. Louis, Mosby, Inc., 1996:448–572.
22. Gold MI, Buechel DR: Translaryngeal anesthesia: a review. *Anesthesiology.* 1959;20:181–185.
23. Wong MEK, Bradick JP: Surgical approaches to airway management fo anesthesia practitioners. In: *Handbook of Difficult Airway Management*, 1st edn. Hagberg CA (ed.) Philadelphia, Churchill Livingstone, 2000:185–218.
24. Kastendiek JG: Airway management. In: *Emergency Medicine Concepts and Clinical Practice*, 2nd edn. Rosen P, et al., (eds.) St. Louis, Mosby, Inc., 1988:26–53.
25. Dripps RD, Eckenhoff JE, VanDam LD: Introduction to anesthesia. In: *The Principles of Safe Practice*, 6th edn. Philadelphia, WB Saunders Co., 1982.
26. Atkinson RS, Rushman GB, Lee JA: *A Synopsis of Anaesthesia*, 8th edn. Bristol, John Wright & Sons, 1977.
27. Davidson TM, Mogit AE: Surgical airway. In: *Airway Management Principles and Practice.* Benumof JL, ed. St. Louis, Mosby, Inc., 1996:513–530.
28. Meredith JW, et al.: ATLS Advanced Trauma Life Support Program for Doctors. Course Manual, 7th edn Chicago, American College of Surgeons Committee on Trauma, 2004.
29. Steward DJ: *Manual of Pediatric Anesthesia.* New York, Churchill Livingstone, 1979.
30. Levin RM: *Pediatric Anesthesia Handbook*, 2nd edn. Garden City, Medical Examination Publishing, 1980.
31. Kress TD, Balasubramaniam S: Cricothyroidotomy. *Ann Emerg Med.* 1982;11:197–201.
32. Catterall W, Mackie K: Local anesthetics. In: *Goodman and Gilman's The Pharmacological Basis of Therapeutics*, 10th edn. Hardman JG, Limbird LE, Gilman AG (eds.). New York, McGraw-Hill, 2001:367–384.
33. Morris IR: Fibreoptic intubation. *Can J Anaesth.* 1994;41:996–1007;discussion 1007–1008.
34. Morris IR: Airway Anesthesia, Sedation and Awake Intubation In: *The Difficult Airway Course: Anesthesia Airway, Course Manual*, 64–81.
35. Adriani J, Zepernick R, Arens J, Authement E: The comparative potency and effectiveness of topical anesthetics in man. *Clin Pharmacol Ther.* 1964;45:49–62.
36. Kirkpatrick MB: Lidocaine topical anesthesia for flexible bronchoscopy. *Chest.* 1989;96:965–967.
37. Walsh ME, Shorten GD: Preparing to perform an awake fiberoptic intubation. *Yale J Biol Med.* 1998;71:537–549.
38. Watanabe H, Lindgren L, Rosenberg P, Randell T: Glycopyrronium prolongs topical anaesthesia of oral mucosa and enhances absorption of lignocaine. *Br J Anaesth.* 1993;70:94–95.
39. Schonemann NK, van der Burght M, Arendt-Nielsen L, Bjerring P: Onset and duration of hypoalgesia of lidocaine spray applied to oral mucosa–a dose response study. *Acta Anaesthesiol Scand.* 1992;36:733–735.
40. Ovassapian A: The flexible bronchoscope. A tool for anesthesiologists. *Clin Chest Med.* 2001;22:281–299.
41. Schenck NL: Local anesthesia in otolaryngology. A re-evaluation. *Ann Otol Rhinol Laryngol.* 1975;84:65–72.
42. Wu FL, Razzaghi A, Souney PF: Seizure after lidocaine for bronchoscopy: case report and review of the use of lidocaine in airway anesthesia. *Pharmacotherapy.* 1993; 13: 72–8
43. Efthimiou J, Higenbottam T, Holt D, Cochrane GM: Plasma concentrations of lignocaine during fibreoptic bronchoscopy. *Thorax.* 1982;37:68–71.
44. Parkes SB, Butler CS, Muller R: Plasma lignocaine concentration following nebulization for awake intubation. *Anaesth Intensive Care.* 1997;25:369–371.
45. Pelton DA, Daly M, Cooper PD, Conn AW: Plasma lidocaine concentrations following topical aerosol application to the trachea and bronchi. *Can Anaesth Soc J.* 1970;17:250–255.
46. Rosenberg PH, Heinonen J, Takasaki M: Lidocaine concentration in blood after topical anaesthesia of the upper respiratory tract. *Acta Anaesthesiol Scand.* 1980;24:125–128.
47. Scott DB, Littlewood DG, Covino BG, Drummond GB: Plasma lignocaine concentrations following endotracheal spraying with an aerosol. *Br J Anaesth.* 1976;48:899–902.
48. Adriani J, Campbell D: Fatalities following topical administration of local anesthetics to musous membranes. *JAMA* 1956;162:1527–1530.
49. Melby MJ, Raehl CL, Kruel JK: Pharmacokinetic evaluation of endotracheally administered lidocaine. *Clin Pharm.* 1986;5:228–231.
50. Berde CB, Strichartz GR: Local Anesthetics. In: *Anesthesia*, 5th edn. Miller RD (ed.). Philadelphia, Churchill Livingstone, 2000:494–521.
51. Kotaki H, Tayama N, Ito K, et al.: Safe and effective topical application dose of lidocaine for surgery with laryngomicroscopy. *Clin Pharmacol Ther.* 1996;60:229–235.
52. Karvonen S, Jokinen K, Karvonen P, Hollmen A: Arterial and venous blood lidocaine concentrations after local anaesthesia of the respiratory tract using an ultrasonic nebulizer. *Acta Anaesthesiol Scand.* 1976;20:156–159.
53. Korttila K, Tarkkanen J, Tarkkanen L: Comparison of laryngotracheal and ultrasonic nebulizer administration of lidocaine in local anaesthesia for bronchoscopy. *Acta Anaesthesiol Scand.* 1981;25:161–165.
54. Rothrock SG, Green SM: Methemoglobinemia resulting from an unusual treatment for costochondritis. *J Emerg Med.* 1992;10:494–495.
55. Karim A, Ahmed S, Siddiqui R, Mattana J: Methemoglobinemia complicating topical lidocaine used during endoscopic procedures. *Am J Med.* 2001; 111:150–153.
56. Deas TC: Severe methemoglobinemia following dental extractions under lidocaine anesthesia. *Anesthesiology.* 1956;17:204.
57. O'Donohue WJ, Jr., Moss LM, Angelillo VA: Acute methemoglobinemia induced by topical benzocaine and lidocaine. *Arch Intern Med.* 1980;140: 1508–1509.
58. Burne D, Doughty A: Methaemoglobinaemia Following Lignocaine. *Lancet.* 1964;67:971.
59. Donlon JV Jr: Anesthetic for eye, ear, nose and throat surgery. In: *Anesthesia.* Miller RD, ed. New York, Churchill Livingstone, 1981:1265–1321.
60. Donlon JV Jr: Anesthetic management of patients with compromised airways. *Anesth Rev.* 1980;7:22–31.
61. Donlon Jr: Anesthetic for eye, ear, nose and throat surgery. In: *Anesthesia.* Miller RD, ed. New York, Churchill Livingstone, 1986:1897–1894.
62. Simmons ST, Schleich AR: Airway regional anesthesia for awake fiberoptic intubation. *Reg Anesth Pain Med.* 2002;27:180–192.
63. Reed AP, Han DG: Preparation of the patient for awake fiberoptic intubation. *Anesth Clin North Amer.* 1991;9:69–81.

64. Reed AP: Preparation for intubation of the awake patient. *Mt Sinai J Med.* 1995;62:10–20.

65. Kundra P, Kutralam S, Ravishankar M: Local anaesthesia for awake fibreoptic nasotracheal intubation. *Acta Anaesthesiol Scand.* 2000;44:511–516.

66. Chinn WM, Zavala DC, Ambre J: Plasma levels of lidocaine following nebulized aerosol administration. *Chest.* 1977;71:346–348.

67. Jenkins SA, Marshall CF: Awake intubation made easy and acceptable. *Anaesth Intensive Care.* 2000;28:556–561.

68. Bourke DL, Katz J, Tonneson A: Nebulized anesthesia for awake endotracheal intubation. *Anesthesiology.* 1985;63:690–692.

69. Chu SS, Rah KH, Brannan MD, Cohen JL: Plasma concentration of lidocaine after endotracheal spray. *Anesth Analg.* 1975;54:438–441.

70. Chan KN, Clay MM, Silverman M: Output characteristics of DeVilbiss No. 40 hand-held jet nebulizers. *Eur Respir J.* 1990;3:1197–1201.

71. Clay MM, Clarke SW: Wastage of drug from nebulizers: a review. *J R Soc Med.* 1987;80:38–39.

72. Mostafa SM, Murthy BV, Hodgson CA, Beese E: Nebulized 10% lignocaine for awake fibreoptic intubation. *Anaesth Intensive Care.* 1998;26: 222–223.

73. Curran J, Hamilton C, Taylor T: Topical analgesia before tracheal intubation. *Anaesthesia.* 1975;30:765–768.

74. Eyres RL, Bishop W, Oppenheim RC, Brown TC: Plasma lignocaine concentrations following topical laryngeal application. *Anaesth Intensive Care.* 1983;11:23–26.

75. Patterson JR, Blaschke TF, Hunt KK, Meffin PJ: Lidocaine blood concentrations during fiberoptic bronchoscopy. *Am Rev Respir Dis.* 1975;112:53–57.

76. Sutherland AD, Williams RT: Cardiovascular responses and lidocaine absorption in fiberoptic-assisted awake intubation. *Anesth Analg.* 1986;65: 389–391.

77. Reasoner DK, Warner DS, Todd MM, Hunt SW, Kirchner J: A comparison of anesthetic techniques for awake intubation in neurosurgical patients. *J Neurosurg Anesthesiol.* 1995;7:94–99.

78. Ameer B, Burlingame MB, Harman EM: Systemic absorption of topical lidocaine in elderly and young adults undergoing bronchoscopy. *Pharmacotherapy* 1989;9:74–81.

79. Gal TJ: Airway responses in normal subjects following topical anesthesia with ultrasonic aerosols of 4% lidocaine. *Anesth Analg.* 1980;59:123–129.

80. Grove RI, Wiggins J, Stableforth DE: A study of the use of ultrasonically nebulized lignocaine for local anaesthesia during fibreoptic bronchoscopy. *Br J Dis Chest.* 1985;79:49–59.

81. Kuna ST, Woodson GE, Sant'Ambrogio G: Effect of laryngeal anesthesia on pulmonary function testing in normal subjects. *Am Rev Respir Dis.* 1988; 137:656–661.

82. Liistro G, Stanescu DC, Veriter C, Rodenstein DO, D'Odemont JP: Upper airway anesthesia induces airflow limitation in awake humans. *Am Rev Respir Dis.* 1992;146:581–585.

83. Weiss EB, Patwardhan AV: The response to lidocaine in bronchial asthma. *Chest.* 1977; 72: 429–38.

84. McAlpine LG, Thomson NC: Lidocaine-induced bronchoconstriction in asthmatic patients. Relation to histamine airway responsiveness and effect of preservative. *Chest.* 1989;96:1012–1015.

85. Groeben H, Schlicht M, Stieglitz S, Pavlakovic G, Peters J: Both local anesthetics and salbutamol pretreatment affect reflex bronchoconstriction in volunteers with asthma undergoing awake fiberoptic intubation. *Anesthesiology.* 2002;97:1445–1450.

86. Thomson NC: The effect of different pharmacological agents on respiratory reflexes in normal and asthmatic subjects. *Clin Sci (Lond).* 1979;56:235–241.

87. Shaw IC, Welchew EA, Harrison BJ, Michael S: Complete airway obstruction during awake fibreoptic intubation. *Anaesthesia.* 1997;52:582–585.

88. McGuire G, EL-Beheiry H: Complete upper airway obstruction during awake fibreoptic intubation in patients with unstable cervical spine fractures. *Can J Anaesth.* 1999;46:176–178.

89. Ho AM, Chung DC, To EW, Karmakar MK: Total airway obstruction during local anesthesia in a non-sedated patient with a compromised airway. *Can J Anaesth.* 2004;51:838–841.

90. Wong DT, McGuire GP: Management choices for the difficult airway. *Can J Anaesth.* 2003; 50: 624.

91. Mason RA, Fielder CP: The obstructed airway in head and neck surgery. *Anaesthesia.* 1999;54:625–628.

92. Weisel W, Tella RA: Reaction to tetracaine (pontocaine) used as topical anesthetic in bronchoscopy; study of 1000 cases. *J Am Med Assoc.* 1951;147:218–222.

93. Noorily AD, Noorily SH, Otto RA: Cocaine, lidocaine, tetracaine: which is best for topical nasal anesthesia? *Anesth Analg.* 1995;81:724–727.

94. Campbell D, Adriani J: Absorption of local anesthetics. *J Am Med Assoc.* 1958;168:873–877.

95. Benumof JL: *Anesthesia for Thoracic Surgery.* Philadelphia, WB Saunders Company, 1995.

96. Sanchez AF, Morrison DE: Preparation of the patient for awake intubation. In: *Handbook of Difficult Airway Management*, 1st edn. Hagberg CA (ed.). Philadelphia, Churchill Livingstone, 2000.

97. Morris IR: Pharmacologic aids to intubation and the rapid sequence induction. *Emerg Med Clin North Am.* 1988;6:753–768.

98. Donlon JV Jr: Anesthesia for eye, ear, nose and throat surgery. In: *Anesthesia*, 5th edn. Miller RD (ed.). Philadelphia, Churchill Livingstone, 2000, pp 2173–2198.

99. Lewin NA, Goldfrank LR, Hoffman RS: Cocaine. In: *Toxicologic Emergencies*, 5th edn. Goldfrank LR, Weisman RS, Flomenbaum NE, et al., (eds.). Norwalk, Appleton and Lange, 1994:847–862.

100. Gross JB, Hartigan ML, Schaffer DW: A suitable substitute for 4% cocaine before blind nasotracheal intubation: 3% lidocaine-0.25% phenylephrine nasal spray. *Anesth Analg.* 1984;63:915–918.

101. Katz RI, Hovagim AR, Finkelstein HS, et al.: A comparison of cocaine, lidocaine with epinephrine, and oxymetazoline for prevention of epistaxis on nasotracheal intubation. *J Clin Anesth.* 1990;2:16–20.

102. Rector FT, DeNuccio DJ, Alden MA: A comparison of cocaine, oxymetazoline, and saline for nasotracheal intubation. *AANA J.* 1987;55:49–54.

103. Drugdex System, Thompson Micromedex. Edited by Klesco RK. Greenwood Village, Colorado Healthcare Services. Expires 9/2001; Volume 109. (on-line reference by subscription)

104. Nguyen ST, Cabrales RE, Bashour CA, et al.: Benzocaine-induced methemoglobinemia. *Anesth Analg.* 2000;90:369–371.

105. Rinehart RS, Norman D: Suspected methemoglobinemia following awake intubation: one possible effect of benzocaine topical anesthesia–a case report. *AANA J.* 2003;71:117–118.

106. Kern K, Langevin PB, Dunn BM: Methemoglobinemia after topical anesthesia with lidocaine and benzocaine for a difficult intubation. *J Clin Anesth.* 2000;12:167–172.

107. Haynes JM: Acquired methemoglobinemia following benzocaine anesthesia of the pharynx. *Am J Crit Care.* 2000;9:199–201.

108. White CD, Weiss LD: Varying presentations of methemoglobinemia: two cases. *J Emerg Med.* 1991;9(Suppl 1):45–49.

109. Bacon GS, Lyons TR, Wood SH: Dyclonine hydrochloride for airway anesthesia: awake endotracheal intubation in a patient with suspected local anesthetic allergy. *Anesthesiology.* 1997;86:1206–1207.

110. Benumof JL: Upper airway obstruction. *Can J Anaesth.* 1999;46:906–907.

111. Larijani GE, Cypel D, Gratz I, et al.: The efficacy and safety of EMLA cream for awake fiberoptic endotracheal intubation. *Anesth Analg.* 2000;91: 1024–1026.

112. Sohmer B, Bryson GL, Bencze S, Scharf MM: EMLA cream is an effective topical anesthetic for bronchoscopy. *Can Respir J.* 2004;11:587–588.

113. Randell T, Yli-Hankala A, Valli H, Lindgren L: Topical anaesthesia of the nasal mucosa for fibreoptic airway endoscopy. *Br J Anaesth.* 1992;68: 164–167.

114. Sutherland AD, Sale JP: Fibreoptic awake intubation–a method of topical anaesthesia and orotracheal intubation. *Can Anaesth Soc J.* 1986;33:502–504.

115. Chung DC, Mainland PA, Kong AS: Anesthesia of the airway by aspiration of lidocaine. *Can J Anaesth.* 1999;46:215–219.

116. Murphy TM: Somatic blockade of the head and neck. In: *Nerual Blockade in Clinical Anesthesia and Management of Pain*, 3rd edn. Cousins MJ, Bridenbaugh P (eds.). Philadelphia, Lippincott Raven, 1998:489–574.

117. Hannenberg AA: An atraumatic method for topical application of local anesthetics to the nasal mucosa. *Anesthesiology.* 1983;59:596–597.

118. Mitchell RL, DeNuccio DJ, Alden MA: A comparison of nasal spray with cocaine, lidocaine/phenylephrine and saline for nasal intubation. *Anesthesiology.* 1984;61:A217.

119. Bonica JJ: Transtracheal anesthesia for endotracheal intubation. *Anesthesiology.* 1949;10:736–738.

120. Danzl DF, Thomas DM: Nasotracheal intubations in the emergency department. *Crit Care Med.* 1980;8:677–682.

121. Duncan JA: Intubation of the trachea in the conscious patient. *Br J Anaesth.* 1977;49:619–623.

122. Thomas JL: Awake intubation. Indications, techniques and a review of 25 patients. *Anaesthesia.* 1969;24:28–35.

123. Gotta AW, Sullivan CA: Superior laryngeal nerve block: an aid to intubating the patient with fractured mandible. *J Trauma.* 1984;24:83–85.

124. Walts LF, Kassity KJ: Spread of local anesthesia after upper airway block. *Arch Otolaryngol.* 1965;81:77–79.

125. Graham DR, Hay JG, Clague J, Nisar M, Earis JE: Comparison of three different methods used to achieve local anesthesia for fiberoptic bronchoscopy. *Chest.* 1992;102:704–707.
126. Boster SR, Danzl DF, Madden RJ, Jarboe CH: Translaryngeal absorption of lidocaine. *Ann Emerg Med.* 1982;11:461–465.
127. Barton S, Williams JD: Glossopharyngeal nerve block. *Arch Otolaryngol.* 1971;93:186–188.
128. Bogdonoff DL, Stone DJ: Emergency management of the airway outside the operating room. *Can J Anaesth.* 1992;39:1069–1089.
129. DeMeester TR, Skinner DB, Evans RH, Benson DW: Local nerve block anesthesia for peroral endoscopy. *Ann Thorac Surg.* 1977;24:278–283.
130. Woods AM, Lander CJ: Abolition of gagging and the hemodynamic response to laryngoscopy. *Anesthesiology.* 1987;67:A220.
131. Cooper M, Watson RL: An improved regional anesthetic technique for peroral endoscopy. *Anesthesiology.* 1975;43:372–374.
132. Sitzman BT, Rich GF, Rockwell JJ, et al.: Local anesthetic administration for awake direct laryngoscopy. Are glossopharyngeal nerve blocks superior? *Anesthesiology.* 1997;86:34–40.
133. Benumof JL: Management of the difficult adult airway. With special emphasis on awake tracheal intubation. *Anesthesiology.* 1991;75:1087–1110.
134. Gotta AW, Sullivan CA: Anaesthesia of the upper airway using topical anaesthetic and superior laryngeal nerve block. *Br J Anaesth.* 1981;53:1055–1058.
135. Gaskill JR, Gillies DR: Local anesthesia for peroral endoscopy. Using superior laryngeal nerve block with topical application. *Arch Otolaryngol.* 1966;84:654–657.
136. Walts LF: Anesthesia Of The Larynx In The Patient With A Full Stomach. *JAMA* 1965;192:705–706.
137. Kopman AF, Wollman SB, Ross K, Surks SN: Awake endotracheal intubation: a review of 267 cases. *Anesth Analg.* 1975;54:323–327.
138. Meschino A, Devitt JH, Koch JP, Szalai JP, Schwartz ML: The safety of awake tracheal intubation in cervical spine injury. *Can J Anaesth.* 1992;39:114–117.
139. Ovassapian A, Krejcie TC, Yelich SJ, Dykes MH: Awake fibreoptic intubation in the patient at high risk of aspiration. *Br J Anaesth.* 1989;62:13–16.
140. Derbyshire DR, Smith G, Achola KJ: Effect of topical lignocaine on the sympathoadrenal responses to tracheal intubation. *Br J Anaesth.* 1987;59:300–304.
141. Telford RJ, Liban JB: Awake fibreoptic intubation. *Br J Hosp Med.* 1991;46:182–184.
142. Mirakhur RK, Dundee JW: Glycopyrrolate: pharmacology and clinical use. *Anaesthesia.* 1983;38:1195–1204.
143. Compendium of Pharmaceuticals and Specialties. *The Canadian Drug Reference for Health Professionals.* Repchinsky C (editor-in-chief). Ottawa: Canadian Pharmacist's Association, 2004:868–869.
144. McEvoy GK: Glycopyrrolate. In: *AHFS Drug Information.* Bethesda: American Society of Health System Pharmacists Inc., 2005:1243–1244.
145. Stoelting RK: *Pharmacology and Physiology in Anesthetic Practice.* Philadelphia, JB Lippincott Company, 1991.
146. Bernstein CA, Waters JH, Torjman MC, Ritter D: Preoperative glycopyrrolate: oral, intramuscular, or intravenous administration. *J Clin Anesth.* 1996;8:515–518.
147. Cowl CT, Prakash UB, Kruger BR: The role of anticholinergics in bronchoscopy. A randomized clinical trial. *Chest.* 2000;118:188–192.
148. Roffe C, Smith MJ, Basran GS: Anticholinergic premedication for fibreoptic bronchoscopy. *Monaldi Arch Chest Dis.* 1994;49:101–106.
149. Brookman CA, Teh HP, Morrison LM: Anticholinergics improve fibreoptic intubating conditions during general anaesthesia. *Can J Anaesth.* 1997;44:165–167.
150. Marshall BE, Wollman H: General anesthetics. In: *Goodman and Gillman's The Pharmacological Basis of Therapeutics,* 6th edn. New York, MacMillan Publishing Company, 1980.
151. Merchant RN: Droperidol. *Canadian Anesthesiologists' Society Newsletter.* 2002;4.
152. Donaldson AB, Meyer-Witting M, Roux A: Awake fibreoptic intubation under remifentanil and propofol target-controlled infusion. *Anaesth Intensive Care.* 2002;30:93–95.
153. Johnson KB, Swenson JD, Egan TD, Jarrett R, Johnson M: Midazolam and remifentanil by bolus injection for intensely stimulating procedures of brief duration: experience with awake laryngoscopy. *Anesth Analg.* 2002;94:1241–1243.
154. Machata AM, Gonano C, Holzer A, et al.: Awake nasotracheal fiberoptic intubation: patient comfort, intubating conditions, and hemodynamic stability during conscious sedation with remifentanil. *Anesth Analg.* 2003;97:904–908.
155. Puchner W, Egger P, Puhringer F, et al.: Evaluation of remifentanil as single drug for awake fiberoptic intubation. *Acta Anaesthesiol Scand.* 2002;46:350–354.
156. Puchner W, Obwegeser J, Puhringer FK: Use of remifentanil for awake fiberoptic intubation in a morbidly obese patient with severe inflammation of the neck. *Acta Anaesthesiol Scand.* 2002;46:473–476.
157. Reusche MD, Egan TD: Remifentanil for conscious sedation and analgesia during awake fiberoptic tracheal intubation: a case report with pharmacokinetic simulations. *J Clin Anesth.* 1999;11:64–68.
158. Jhaveri R, Joshi P, Batenhorst R, Baughman V, Glass PS: Dose comparison of remifentanil and alfentanil for loss of consciousness. *Anesthesiology.* 1997;87:253–259.
159. Wilhelm W, Biedler A, Hammadeh ME, Fleser R, Gruness V: [Remifentanil for oocyte retrieval: A new single-agent monitored anaesthesia care technique]. *Anaesthesist.* 1999;48:698–704.
160. Scher CS, Gitlin MC: Dexmedetomidine and low-dose ketamine provide adequate sedation for awake fibreoptic intubation. *Can J Anaesth.* 2003;50:607–610.

SELF-EVALUATION QUESTIONS

3.1. The lower border of the quadrangular ligament forms

A. the true vocal cord

B. the false vocal cord

C. the aryepiglottic ligament

D. the triangular ligament

E. the hyoepiglottic ligament

3.2. The maximum effective concentration of topical lidocaine applied to the tongue is

A. 1%

B. 2%

C. 4%

D. 10%

E. 15%

3.3. Benzocaine

A. is an ester

B. is metabolized to para-aminobenzoic acid

C. can produce methemoglobinemia

D. is an effective topical anesthetic

E. all of the above

CHAPTER (4)

Pharmacology of Intubation

*Ronald B. George, Orlando R. Hung, and
Robert E. Schneider*

4.1 PHYSIOLOGY OF TRACHEAL INTUBATION

4.1.1 What are the physiological responses to tracheal intubation?

The goal of intubation is to provide a secure, definitive airway. Unfortunately, laryngoscopy and intubation can result in a cascade of physiological and pathophysiological reflex responses. These responses are initiated by stimulation of afferent receptors in the posterior pharynx from the glossopharyngeal and vagus nerves. The central nervous system (CNS), cardiovascular system, and respiratory system all respond predictably to these afferent stimuli, and in selected patients the resultant physiologic manifestations may adversely affect the patients' outcome. Though no outcome data exist to suggest that patient outcomes are altered by attenuating the increases in intracranial pressure (ICP), stimulation of the autonomic nervous system with increases in the heart rate and blood pressure, and stimulation of the upper and lower respiratory tract resulting in increases in airway resistance. In light of the possible adverse effects in a compromised patient, it seems both reasonable and logical to attenuate these responses.

The CNS responds to airway manipulation by increasing cerebral metabolic oxygen demand ($CMRO_2$) and cerebral blood flow (CBF). If the intracranial compliance is decreased, the increase in CBF will further increase the ICP. This response is important in situations in which there is a loss of autoregulation such that blood flow to the brain or regions of the brain is pressure-passive (i.e., increases in blood pressure result in increases in ICP).

The act of laryngoscopy stimulates the patients' protective reflexes and predictably leads to alteration of the cardiovascular and respiratory systems via the sympathetic nervous system. In children, this process is considered to be primarily a monosynaptic reflex promoting vagal stimulation of the sinoatrial node that results in bradycardia. In adults, a polysynaptic event predominates whereby impulses travel afferently via the ninth and tenth cranial nerves to the brain stem and spinal cord. They then return efferently through the cardioaccelerator nerves and sympathetic ganglia. This event results in norepinephrine release from the adrenergic nerve terminals, epinephrine release from the adrenal glands, and activation of the renin–angiotensin system, which leads to further increases in the blood pressure. This increase in heart rate and blood pressure may be detrimental in those patients with myocardial ischemia, with known intracerebral or aortic aneurysms, major vessel dissection, or those with a penetrating trauma in whom increases in pressure may exacerbate hemorrhage. In similar fashion, increases in blood pressure may result in significant increases in ICP if autoregulation has been lost (e.g., acute severe head injury or intracranial hemorrhage).

The respiratory system responds in two important ways to airway manipulation. There is activation of the upper-airway reflexes leading to laryngospasm and coughing, both of which may compromise the patient. Laryngospasm, a forceful involuntary spasm of the laryngeal musculature, may produce difficulty with intubation as well as ventilation. Persistent and life-threatening laryngospasm is treated with a gentle continuous positive airway pressure with 100% oxygen, intravenous lidocaine ($1.5 \ mg.kg^{-1}$), or if persistent, neuromuscular blockade (e.g., succinylcholine at 10% of the intubating dose). Negative intrathoracic pressure created by inspiration attempts against a closed glottis (laryngospasm) may result in pulmonary edema (see Chapter 55).

Coughing may produce significant adverse effects in patients with increased ICP, unstable cervical spine injury, or penetrating eye injuries. Activation of the lower airway reflexes leads to an increase in airway resistance. This reaction is most often manifested by bronchospasm brought about by reflexes, irritants, or antigens.

Whether mitigation of these reflexes improves patient outcome is not known, but the current data argue for the use of specific pre-laryngoscopy therapy capable of mitigating these potentially harmful physiologic effects. The useful agents are most easily remembered by the mnemonic *LOAD,* which stands for *L*idocaine, *O*pioid, *A*tropine, and *D*efasciculating agent. This chapter provides a general discussion of the appropriate pharmacological agents and their relevant properties. It should be emphasized that the goal of this chapter is not to discuss the rationale of using a specific sedative or muscle relaxant in an anticipated difficult airway. Rather, this discussion will center on the drugs used to facilitate tracheal intubation and mitigate adverse physiological consequences.

4.2   PRETREATMENT AGENTS USING THE *LOAD* APPROACH

4.2.1   What is the LOAD approach and why do we use it?

Pre-laryngoscopy agents are used to attenuate the adverse physiologic responses to laryngoscopy and intubation. LOAD is the mnemonic used to enhance recall of lidocaine, opioids, atropine, and defasciculating agents when the use of pretreatment agents may be indicated. Ideally, all pretreatment agents should be administered shortly before (typically about 3 minutes) induction to synchronize the peak drug effects of all drugs administered in the airway management sequence.

While short-acting beta blockers, such as esmolol, have been shown to be beneficial in attenuating the sympathetic response to laryngoscopy,[1] they are not effective in attenuating to any extent a rise in ICP. They potentially increase airway resistance, especially in patients with reactive airways disease. Furthermore, beta-blockers are also negative inotropes and in some clinical situations, particularly emergencies in which maximum cardiac reserve should be preserved, the combination of beta-blockers and the negative cardiovascular effects of most induction agents could be catastrophic.

4.2.2   What is the rationale of using lidocaine for tracheal intubation?

Local anesthetics bind to sodium channels in the closed-inactivated form and prevent subsequent channel activation. Sodium channels in the closed-inactivated state are not permeable to sodium and therefore action potentials cannot be generated. Local anesthetics are a combination of a lipophilic benzene ring and a hydrophilic amine either linked by an amide or an ester. Lidocaine is a low-potency, rapid-onset, and intermediate-acting amide local anesthetic. The literature is replete with articles that offer varying conclusions as to the efficacy of lidocaine in the pretreatment phase of tracheal intubation.

Attenuation of the elevation of ICP related to airway manipulation is ascribed to lidocaine's ability to increase the depth of anesthesia, decrease $CMRO_2$ demand globally, decrease CBF, and increase cerebrovascular resistance. Patients with intracranial pathology may have an abnormal intracranial pressure–volume relationship which can predispose them to abrupt and extreme elevations of ICP. Such increases can contribute to secondary injury of the brain, herniation of the brain, impaired perfusion, and subsequent ischemia. Although direct evidence is lacking, indirect evidence exists that lidocaine can attenuate the intracranial hypertensive response to laryngoscopy and intubation. Intracranial hypertension associated with suctioning of the endotracheal tube has been suppressed with intravenous lidocaine.[2–5] Intratracheal lidocaine is equally as effective.[4] Lidocaine (1.5 $mg.kg^{-1}$) administered 3 minutes before intubation suppresses the cough reflex and attenuates the increase in airway resistance resulting from irritation of the airway by the endotracheal tube.

Lidocaine's effect on antigenic bronchospasm is more controversial. Lidocaine and other local anesthetics are suspected of causing bronchoconstriction in patients with reactive airway disease when given via the inhalational route.[6] In normal individuals, lidocaine does not alter global airflow resistance, though it has been shown to produce mild bronchodilation.[7] Groeben et al.[8–10] in three similar trials showed that intravenous lidocaine attenuates the response to an inhalational histamine challenge in patients with mild asthma. The inhalational administration of lidocaine to such patients, however, was met with short-lived initial increases in airway resistance.[10] Intravenous lidocaine but not inhalational lidocaine seems appropriate for the attenuation of the bronchorestrictive response to tracheal manipulation. Lidocaine (1.5 $mg.kg^{-1}$) 3 minutes before induction is advocated for patients with reactive airway disease (i.e., "tight lungs") or elevated ICP (i.e., "tight brains"). Lidocaine has a wide safety margin, particularly at a dose of 1.5 $mg.kg^{-1}$. The primary toxic effect is the development of seizures, which usually occurs with much greater doses.

4.2.3   Why do we use opioids prior to tracheal intubation?

Opium, derived from poppy seeds (*Papaver somniferum*), has more than 20 alkaloids that serve as the foundation of modern opioids. A German pharmacist isolated the first alkaloid from opium in 1806 and named it morphine after the Greek god of dreams, Morpheus.[11] A broad definition of the term *opioid* includes all drugs, synthetic and natural, with morphine-like behavior, covering agonists, antagonists, and endogenous substances. Opioids are a routine part of an anesthetic induction and with the advent of newer, more rapid acting agents like remifentanil, opioids will continue to have a role in airway management.

The list of opioid receptors continues to expand. Mu (μ), kappa (κ), and delta (δ) receptor classes have been firmly established.[12] Most clinically useful opioids are highly selective μ agonists, which are responsible for the bulk of supraspinal and spinal analgesia. Although highly selective, opioid effects typically involve complex interactions among the various receptor sites. Opioids act throughout the nervous system, including the dorsal horn of the spinal cord (substantia gelatinosa), periaqueductal gray matter, and in the periphery. They inhibit presynaptic release and postsynaptic response to excitatory neurotransmitters such as acetylcholine (ACh) and substance P by altering the potassium and calcium conductance.[11]

TABLE 4-1

Pharmacokinetics of Opioids in Clinical Use[11]

	MORPHINE	FENTANYL	SUFENTANIL	REMIFENTANIL
pK$_a$	7.9	8.4	8	7.2
% Ionization	23	8.5	20	58
% Protein bound	35	84	90	66
Rapid Redistribution- $t_{1/2\pi}$ (min)		1.2–1.9	1.4	0.4–0.5
Redistribution- $t_{1/2\alpha}$ (min)	1.5–4.4	9.2–19	17	2–3.7
Elimination- $t_{1/2\beta}$ (h)	1.7–3.3	3.6–6.6	2.2–4.1	0.17–0.33

Opioids are typically of low molecular weight but vary widely in their lipid solubility, percent of ionization, and degree of binding to proteins (Table 4-1). Commonly used opioids for induction (fentanyl, sufentanil, and remifentanil) are more lipid soluble, which accounts for their speed of onset of action. Redistribution is responsible for the termination of their CNS drug action. Metabolism of most opioids occurs through a two-stage hepatic process that generally results in an inactive metabolite. The exception is remifentanil, which contains an ester linkage and is rapidly hydrolyzed by nonspecific esterases in the blood and tissue.

Physiologically, opioids exert their effect on all organ systems. Venodilation and depressed sympathetic reflexes typically result in a decrease in heart rate and blood pressure. Neither fentanyl, sufentanil, nor remifentanil releases histamine. This is part of the reason why they cause less hypotension than morphine. All opioids depress ventilation by blunting the carbon dioxide response at the respiratory center, essentially raising the apneic threshold and depressing the slope of the CO_2 response curve.

The primary reason to include an opioid in the intubation sequence is their ability to significantly attenuate the sympathetic response that occurs with manipulation of the airway. Unfortunately, the rapid administration of fentanyl and its derivatives has been associated with brief episodes of coughing and chest wall rigidity.[13–15] Large induction doses of an opioid can decrease pulmonary compliance in 50–86% of patients and potentially induce glottic closure interfering with ventilation of the patient.[13–16] Doses of this magnitude are seldom if ever employed in emergency airway management, in or out of the operating room (OR).

4.2.4 What types of opioids are commonly used for tracheal intubation?

The hemodynamic and intracranial responses to tracheal intubation are usually short lived. Therefore, the "ideal" choice of an opioid for tracheal intubation should be based on its pharmacokinetic and pharmacodynamic characteristics, namely, a rapid onset and a brief duration of drug effect. While there are currently many opioids available, the following discussion will be restricted to only those opioids with a rapid onset and short duration of drug effect.

4.2.4.1 Fentanyl

Fentanyl is a phenylpiperidine-derived synthetic opioid agonist. It is roughly 100 times more potent than morphine. Fentanyl in large doses (10–30 μg.kg^{-1}) causes chest wall rigidity in 35–85% of patients.[13,15,17] This side effect is present in all age groups.[18] Rigidity is a unique and idiosyncratic response to opioids and is probably related to the dose and speed of administration. Tagaito et al.[19] characterized respiratory and laryngeal responses to laryngeal irritation during increasing doses of fentanyl under propofol anesthesia. Increasing doses of fentanyl reduced the incidences of all these responses.

For the purpose of airway management, fentanyl is a short-acting opioid, though with repeated dosing accumulation can limit its use. Peak onset of the drug effect occurs in 3–5 minutes following intravenous administration and an equilibration time between the plasma and brain of 5 minutes.[20] Doses recommended for attenuating the adverse effects of airway manipulation range from 1 to 4 μg.kg^{-1}. One must be prepared to treat dose-related hypotension and respiratory depression that may occur with fentanyl administration.

4.2.4.2 Sufentanil

A thienyl derivative of fentanyl, sufentanil is 10–15 times more potent than fentanyl. Sufentanil is a highly specific μ agonist with similar pharmacokinetic properties as fentanyl. It is extremely lipophilic; therefore, its high tissue affinity permits rapid penetration of the blood–brain barrier and onset of CNS effects. Sufentanil 0.3–1 μg.kg^{-1}, 1–3 minutes prior to intubation, will blunt the response to laryngoscopy. Rigidity has been reported with larger doses.[17] The difficult ventilation associated with opioid rigidity may be due in part to vocal cord closure.[14,16]

4.2.4.3 Remifentanil

Remifentanil is a structurally unique opioid: it is a piperdine analog with a methyl ester side chain. The ester linkage renders it susceptible to cleavage by nonspecific plasma and tissue esterases.[21] The rapid metabolism of remifentanil is responsible for its ultrashort duration of action and with no redistribution there is no accumulation. It is rapidly cleared from the plasma (3 L.min^{-1}).[17] Remifentanil is not, however, a substrate for pseudocholinesterase and therefore it is unaffected by pseudocholinesterase deficiency.

Remifentanil is a potent μ receptor agonist with a similar potency to fentanyl. Doses of 0.25–3 μg.kg^{-1} have successfully attenuated the response to laryngoscopy.[22–27] At higher doses, centrally mediated depression of sympathetic tone and vagally induced bradycardias may occur. Remifentanil-induced bradycardia can be attenuated with prior administration of glycopyrrolate or other antimuscarinics.[11] Peak respiratory depression occurs 5 minutes after bolus dosing, lasting 10 minutes with 1.5 μg.kg^{-1}

and 20 minutes with 2 $\mu g.kg^{-1}$ (Ref. 28). Remifentanil, like other opioids, may cause chest wall rigidity dependent on the dose and speed of administration.[29]

The clinical usefulness of remifentanil is reflected in its distinctive pharmacokinetic characteristics. Its rapid onset, brief duration, and easily titratable nature have sparked an interest with respect to airway management, particularly in emergency settings or for short surgical procedures. A small dose of remifentanil (0.25 $\mu g.kg^{-1}$) can provide excellent conditions for laryngeal mask airway insertion with minimal hemodynamic disturbance.[30] The trachea may be successfully intubated without muscle relaxants with the combination of remifentanil and an induction agent. Remifentanil, 2–4 $\mu g.kg^{-1}$, provides good to excellent intubating conditions.[23,31–33] Suppression of airway reflexes while maintaining patient comfort without compromising spontaneous ventilation for awake tracheal intubation is possible with remifentanil via continuous infusion (0.07–0.25 $\mu g.kg^{-1}.min^{-1}$).[34–36] Puchner et al.[37] successfully used remifentanil, 0.07 $\mu g.kg^{-1}.min^{-1}$, for procedural sedation in a case of severe neck swelling in a morbidly obese patient with no alternative to awake fiberoptic intubation.

4.2.5 What is the role of atropine (or other antimuscarinic) administration prior to tracheal intubation?

Succinylcholine-induced bradycardia may be seen in children because of their sensitivity to vagal stimulation. Bradycardia can be attenuated or abolished by administering atropine 0.02 $mg.kg^{-1}$ or glycopyrrolate 0.01 $mg.kg^{-1}$ (Ref. 38) as pretreatment before administering succinylcholine. The age after which atropine need not be given is unknown. Regardless of the age, repeated doses of succinylcholine may produce vagotonic effects and the administration of atropine may be necessary.

Unlike the natural derivatives of *Atropa belladonna*, atropine and scopolamine, glycopyrrolate is a synthetic, quaternary ammonium antimuscarinic agent. Because of its polar nature, glycopyrrolate is unable to cross the blood–brain barrier, and so is devoid of CNS activity. It is a potent antisialagogue with minimal sedative properties, which makes glycopyrrolate a useful pretreatment medication. Glycopyrrolate increases the heart rate in a manner similar to atropine with an onset of effect in 2 minutes, lasting 30–60 minutes.[39] Typically, increases in the heart rate following glycopyrrolate administration are more gradual than those with atropine, thereby avoiding a rapid tachycardia of particular concern in patients with cardiovascular disease.

4.2.6 Why do we use defasciculating agents for tracheal intubation?

Fasciculations are involuntary muscle contractions. Practically all patients who receive succinylcholine will experience fasciculations. Fasciculations have been associated with an increase in catecholamine release and elevations of ICP. Small doses of nondepolarizing muscle relaxants (NDMRs), such as vecuronium, rocuronium, and pancuronium, when administered prior to succinylcholine have been clearly shown to decrease the incidence of succinylcholine-induced fasciculations.[40–45]

Arguably their greatest benefit is in mitigating the increase in ICP caused by succinylcholine. The appropriate defasciculating dose for any of the NDMRs is 10% of their ED_{95}. Typically, the suggested intubating dose is twice the ED_{95}. Therefore, the defasciculating dose would be approximately 5% of the intubating dose of the NDMRs. The use of higher doses will increase the incidence of muscle weakness and apnea prior to the induction of anesthesia. When used as a defasciculating agent, rocuronium 0.03 $mg.kg^{-1}$ should be administered 1.5–3 minutes prior to succinylcholine.[46]

4.3 INDUCTION AGENTS

The ideal induction agent would quickly render the patient unconscious, unresponsive, and amnestic in one arm/heart/brain circulation time. Such an agent would also provide analgesia, maintain stable cerebral perfusion pressure (CPP) and cardiovascular hemodynamics, be immediately reversible, and have few, if any, adverse side effects. Unfortunately, such an induction agent does not exist.

Most induction agents are highly lipophilic, and therefore have a rapid onset of effect within 30 to 45 seconds of intravenous administration. Their clinical effect is likewise terminated quickly as the drug rapidly redistributes from the CNS to less well-perfused tissues. All induction agents have the potential to cause myocardial depression and subsequent hypotension. These effects depend on the particular drug and the patient's underlying physiologic condition. The faster the drug is administered, the larger the amount of the drug that will be delivered to those organs with the greatest blood flow (such as the brain and heart) and the more pronounced the effect. The choice of drug and the dose must be individualized to each patient to capitalize on desired effects, while minimizing those that might adversely affect the patient.

Anesthetic induction is intended to rapidly render the patient unable to appreciate, respond to, or recall noxious stimuli, and is therefore at the end of a spectrum spanning mild sedation on one end and deep plane anesthesia (and death) on the other. The induction agents include short-acting barbiturates: thiopental and methohexital; benzodiazepines: principally midazolam; and miscellaneous agents: etomidate, ketamine, and propofol. Opioids can function as anesthetic induction agents when used in very large doses (e.g., fentanyl 30 $\mu g.kg^{-1}$) but are rarely, if ever, used for that purpose during emergency intubation, so will not be discussed in this chapter.

All of the induction agents discussed in this chapter share similar pharmacokinetic characteristics. As mentioned previously, they are highly lipophilic, and therefore a standard induction dose of an induction agent administered to a euvolemic, normotensive patient will take effect within 30 seconds. The duration of observed clinical effect of each drug is measured in minutes and is due to the redistribution of the drug from the central circulation (brain) to larger, but less well-perfused tissues, for example, fat and muscle. The elimination half-life ($t_{1/2\beta}$, usually measured in hours) is characterized by each drug's reentry from fat and lean muscle into plasma down a concentration gradient followed by hepatic metabolism which precedes renal excretion. Generally it requires four to five elimination half-lives to clear the drug completely from the body.

Because the target organ is the brain, and the desired effect is produced rapidly following bolus injection of the drug, dosing of induction agents in normal-sized and obese adults should be based on ideal body weight in kilograms. Hypovolemia results in the patient having a contracted central compartment; therefore, lower doses of induction agents are necessary to achieve adequate levels at the target organ (brain). Aging affects the pharmacokinetics of induction agents. In older adults, lean body mass and total body water decrease while total body fat increases, resulting in an increased volume of distribution, an increase in $t_{1/2\beta}$, and an increased duration of drug effect. Older adults are also much more sensitive to the hemodynamic and respiratory depressant effects of these agents, and consequently, most induction doses should be reduced.

4.3.1   Barbiturates

4.3.1.1   Discuss the Different Types of Barbiturate Induction Agents

Barbiturates are derived from barbituric acid, a cyclic compound obtained by the combination of urea and malonic acid. They are prepared as water soluble, alkaline (2.5% solution $\Rightarrow$ pH $>$ 10) sodium salts that are dissolved in isotonic saline or water. These agents act at the barbiturate receptor, which forms part of the GABA-receptor complex to enhance and mimic the action of GABA. Thiopental decreases GABA dissociation from its receptor, which enhances GABA's neuroinhibitory activity, directly opens the chloride channel, and, at higher drug concentrations, causes hyperpolarization of this chloride channel resulting in global depression of neuronal excitation and subsequent unconsciousness. The most commonly used barbiturates are thiopental and methohexital.

Thiopental is the prototypical barbiturate. It is highly lipid soluble and protein bound. Thiopental undergoes hepatic oxidation to hydroxythiopental and carboxylic acid derivatives, which are water soluble and excreted via the kidney. Methohexital shares similar clinical pharmacologic properties with thiopental although it is significantly less lipid soluble and is two to three times more potent than thiopental. The elimination of methohexital is three to four times faster than thiopental.[47]

4.3.1.2   What Are the Indications and Contraindications of Barbiturate Induction Agents?

Barbiturates are primarily used as an induction agent for patients suspected of having increased ICP. Their ability to decrease ICP stems from the cerebral vasoconstriction and subsequent decreased CBF. The decreased systemic vascular resistance is not matched by the decreased CBF and so CPP is maintained and possibly increased.[48] Barbiturates remain a mainstay of intravenous cerebroprotective measures despite limited outcome data.[49–52]

Barbiturates have significant anticonvulsant activities in addition to their cerebroprotective properties.[53] Methohexital is often used in those patients undergoing electroconvulsive therapy where its rapid onset of amnesia and short duration of action are desirable. Thiopental and other barbiturates are absolutely contraindicated in patients with acute intermittent porphyria, or variegate porphyria, as they can activate the enzyme responsible for precipitating an acute attack, which can be life-threatening.

4.3.1.3   What Are the Clinical Doses of Barbiturate Induction Agents?

The dosing of thiopental depends on the hemodynamic status of the patient and the concomitant use of other agents. Apart from stimulating the release of histamine from mast cells, thiopental is a potent venodilator and myocardial depressant.[54,55] Consequently, the dose must be decreased in patients with decreased intravascular volume, those with compromised myocardial function, older adults, and whenever thiopental is used with other drugs that affect sympathetic tone or cardiovascular function. In euvolemic, normotensive adults, a recommended induction dose of thiopental is 3–5 mg.kg^{-1}. For most emergency intubations, the lower dose of this range (3 mg.kg^{-1}) achieves excellent sedation and intubating conditions with fewer tendencies to cause hypotension that often occurs with the 5 mg.kg^{-1} dose. Thiopental should be avoided entirely in severely hypotensive patients for whom other drugs, especially etomidate or ketamine, may preserve greater hemodynamic stability. The onset of methohexital is more rapid and the duration of action shorter than it is with thiopental. The recommended induction dose of methohexital in the euvolemic, normotensive patient is 1.5 mg.kg^{-1}.

4.3.1.4   What Are the Common Side Effects of Barbiturates?

The chief side effects of thiopental include central respiratory depression, venodilation, and myocardial depression. These last two may produce hypotension that tends to be greater in treated, and untreated, hypertensive patients compared with normotensive patients. Both of these effects may be detrimental in patients where optimal preload is required to maintain cardiac output and prevent organ ischemia. Thiopental causes a dose-related release of histamine (anaphylactoid response) which in most situations is not clinically significant, but may exacerbate hypotension or bronchospasm in patients with reactive airways disease.[54] Although barbiturates produce dose-dependent depression of ventilation centers, they do not completely blunt airway reflexes.[56]

There is a 10–20% incidence of nausea and vomiting that occurs during recovery from a barbiturate induction. Two to five percent of patients will experience pain on injection of thiopental or methohexital, especially if small veins on the dorsum of the hand are used. Inadvertent intra-arterial injection or subcutaneous extravasation of thiopental can result in chemical endarteritis and distal thrombosis, ischemia, and tissue necrosis. Methohexital has a greater incidence than thiopental of twitching and hiccups (excitatory phenomena) that may be misdiagnosed as seizures.[57]

4.3.2   Benzodiazepines

4.3.2.1   Discuss the Clinical Pharmacology of Benzodiazepines

Although chemically distinct from the barbiturates, the benzodiazepines also exert their effects via the GABA-receptor complex. Benzodiazepines specifically facilitate the binding of GABA to the benzodiazepine receptor, which in turn modulates chloride conduction inhibiting neuronal function. The benzodiazepines provide amnesia, anxiolysis, sedation, anticonvulsant effects, and hypnosis. This potent, dose-related amnestic property is perhaps their greatest asset.

Benzodiazepines generally contain a benzene and diazepine ring. All have similar pharmacologic profiles, though various substitutions in the ring structures make each agent pharmacologically unique and their clinical usefulness variable. The lipophilicity of the benzodiazepines varies widely. Greater lipid solubility confers a more rapid onset of action because of the brain's high lipid content. The two benzodiazepines most clinically used during airway manipulation are midazolam and diazepam. Of the two, midazolam is the most lipid soluble. Although, prepared as a water-soluble agent, the imdazole ring structure closes at physiological pH greatly increasing the lipid solubility. Many studies have shown that the onset of effect is slower for midazolam compared to diazepam.[58] Regardless, the time to clinical effectiveness of benzodiazepines is longer than any of the other induction agents, which mitigates their role in airway management. The termination of action of these drugs is due to initial redistribution and subsequent hepatic metabolism via cytochrome P450–3A4 microsomal oxidation for midazolam and diazepam. The innate structure of each parent compound will determine the precise mechanism of hepatic degradation and the production of active or inactive metabolites, both of which will dictate the eventual elimination half-life of each drug. Midazolam has one insignificant active metabolite and a $t_{1/2}$ of 2–4 hours. Diazepam has two active metabolites, both of which can prolong its sedative effect but more importantly are metabolized and excreted more slowly than diazepam and account for its prolonged $t_{1/2}$ of 20–40 hours. The benzodiazepines do not release histamine, and allergic reactions are very rare.

4.3.2.2 What Are the Clinical Uses and Adverse Effects of Benzodiazepines?

The primary indications for benzodiazepines are to promote antianxiety, amnesia, and sedation. In this regard, the benzodiazepines are unparalleled. Midazolam is primarily used for procedural sedation, anxiolysis, and seizure management. Because of their dose-related reduction in systemic vascular resistance and direct myocardial depression, dosage must be adjusted in volume-depleted or hemodynamically compromised patients. Unlike the other induction agents, including those that cause hypotension, midazolam is generally significantly under-dosed during emergency induction. It is postulated that this is due to the clinicians' familiarity with sedating doses of midazolam employed during procedural sedation and lack of familiarity with the dosing and pharmacokinetics of midazolam as an induction agent.

The dose of midazolam for induction of anesthesia is 0.1–0.3 mg.kg^{-1}. Bergrin and Erikson[59] prospectively demonstrated that midazolam 0.4 mg.kg^{-1} provided anesthetic depth similar to that of thiopental 6 mg.kg^{-1}, in 60 female patients undergoing induction for elective abortion. Driessen et al.[60] found that 0.2 mg.kg^{-1} midazolam and 5 mg.kg^{-1} thiopental provided similar depth of anesthesia in 40 women undergoing outpatient anesthesia. Jensen et al.[61] found similar results using 0.2 mg.kg^{-1} midazolam versus 3 mg.kg^{-1} of thiopental for 40 orthopedic surgeries and Izuora et al.[62] found 0.15–0.2 mg.kg^{-1} midazolam comparable to thiopental 4–6 mg.kg^{-1} in 145 patients undergoing surgical procedures. Interestingly, Sagarin et al.[63] recently demonstrated that most emergency intubations are per-

formed using midazolam doses in the range of 0.03–0.04 mg.kg^{-1}. The lower dosing appears to be due to the inexperience with the larger doses of midazolam used for induction or the concern that hypotension may ensue. Other induction agents, including thiopental and etomidate, were used in recommended doses.[63]

Except for midazolam, the benzodiazepines are insoluble in water and are usually supplied in solution in propylene glycol. Unless injected into a large vein, pain and venous irritation on injection can be significant.

4.3.3 Etomidate

4.3.3.1 Discuss the Clinical Pharmacology of Etomidate

Etomidate is a carboxylated imdazole derivative that is primarily an intravenous hypnotic agent used for the rapid induction of anesthesia. It is available in a 0.2% solution dissolved in 35% propylene glycol. It inhibits the reticular activating system, mimicking GABA at the GABA-receptor complex. Etomidate owes its rapid onset to its high lipid solubility and large nonionized portion at physiological pH (pK = 4.2).[17] Its rapid redistribution leads to prompt awaking following administration. The elimination half-life of etomidate is 2–5 hours. It is rapidly hydrolyzed by hepatic metabolism and plasma esterases to water-soluble inactive metabolites excreted primarily by the kidneys.

Etomidate is a potent direct cerebral vasoconstrictor.[64] It attenuates underlying elevated ICP by decreasing CBF and CMRO$_2$. Its hemodynamic stability preserves CPP. The use of etomidate in patients with seizure disorders ought to be limited to the induction of anesthesia and not its maintenance. Etomidate has been shown to increase electroencephalographic activity in certain leads[65] and is less effective than other agents in attenuating the motor activity associated with seizures.[66]

The respiratory system may be centrally stimulated by etomidate, so administration is not usually associated with apnea unless opioids are coadministered.[17,67] Etomidate lacks any direct bronchodilatory properties. Eames et al.[56] prospectively demonstrated that 2.5 mg.kg^{-1} of propofol was superior to either 0.4 mg.kg^{-1} etomidate or 5 mg.kg^{-1} pentothal in decreasing mean airway pressure during bronchoscopy in 75 patients.

Etomidate is touted as the most hemodynamically stable induction agent.[68–70] It mildly decreases the systemic vascular resistance but appears to have no direct effect on cardiac output or contractility. Gauss et al.[71] conducted an echocardiogenic assessment of the hemodynamics of various induction agents. Etomidate showed no changes in the hemodynamic variables measured.

4.3.3.2 What Is the Role of Etomidate as an Induction Agent for Tracheal Intubation?

Etomidate is becoming the induction agent of choice for most emergency rapid sequence inductions because of its rapid onset, its profound hemodynamic stability, its positive CNS profile, and its rapid recovery. As with any induction agent, dosage must be adjusted in hemodynamically compromised patients. The use of etomidate to facilitate airway management in the patient with status epilepticus is not contraindicated, as it does depress the level of consciousness, and long-term medication with benzodiazepines or propofol ordinarily follows the intubation.

In euvolemic and hemodynamically stable patients, the normal induction dose of etomidate is 0.2–0.4 $mg.kg^{-1}$. In compromised patients, the induction dose should be reduced commensurate with the patient's clinical status. Etomidate has no analgesic properties.

4.3.3.3 What Are the Adverse Effects of Etomidate?

Etomidate is associated with nausea and vomiting during recovery in 30–40% of patients undergoing general anesthesia. Pain on injection is common because of the propylene glycol solvent. The incidence can be as high as 80%.[72] Myoclonic movements due to an imbalance of inhibition and excitation in the thalamocortical tract are common and have been confused with seizure activity.[65] It is of no clinical consequence and generally terminates promptly. The occurrence of hiccups, usually during awakening, is highly variable, 0–70%.[73]

The most significant and controversial side effect of etomidate is its reversible blockade of 11-beta-hydroxylase. Etomidate causes reversible adrenocortical suppression by interfering with 11-beta-hydroxylation of 11-deoxycortisol, which prevents its conversion to cortisol. It decreases both serum cortisol and aldosterone levels. Single bolus induction doses of etomidate have transiently inhibited cortisol and aldosterone synthesis.[74–76] The possible long-term adrenocortical suppression has limited the growth of etomidate as a sedative for intensive care management and total intravenous anesthesia.

4.3.4 Ketamine

4.3.4.1 Discuss the Clinical Pharmacology of Ketamine

Ketamine, an arylcyclohexylamine, is a structural analog of phencyclidine, which may account for the psychomimetic side effects such as hallucinations and nightmares. The compound has a chiral center producing stereoisomers and is commercially available as a racemic mixture. It is fairly lipid soluble and minimally protein bound accounting for its rapid onset (45–60 second). Ketamine is extensively taken up by the liver and metabolized by the cytochrome P-450 biotransformation system. The primary metabolite, norketamine, has roughly 1/5 the potency of the parent molecule. Its high lipid solubility and large volume of distribution are responsible for a short duration of effect secondary to redistribution, while the rapid hepatic uptake is responsible for the short elimination half-life of 2–3 hours. Ketamine has been touted as a "complete" anesthetic by many, as it provides analgesia, amnesia, and hypnosis (unconsciousness). Besides blocking polysynaptic spinal cord reflexes, ketamine is a noncompetitive antagonist of N-methyl-D-aspartate (NMDA) receptors at the GABA-receptor complex, promoting the inhibition of excitatory neurotransmitters in selected areas of the brain. An interaction between ketamine and a number of the opioid receptors may be partially responsible for its analgesic properties. Ketamine produces dissociative anesthesia by electrophysiologically separating the thalamus from the limbic system. Patients may appear conscious but are unable to respond to stimuli. Ketamine centrally stimulates the sympathetic nervous

system, which in turn releases catecholamines, augmenting the heart rate and blood pressure in those patients who are not catecholamine depleted secondary to the demands of their underlying disease. Similar to most other anesthetics, however, ketamine in the face of catecholamine depletion causes dose-dependent myocardial depression.

Traditionally, ketamine's direct stimulation of the CNS is thought to increase cerebral metabolism, $CMRO_2$, and CBF, thus potentially increasing ICP in patients with CNS injury. These generalizations may not be valid. Pfenninger et al.[77] investigated the effect of 2 $mg.kg^{-1}$ of ketamine on the ICP and CPP of ventilated pigs. There was no increase in ICP in normal pigs with induced intracranial hypertension. Likewise, in ventilated goats, ketamine significantly decreased the $CMRO_2$, while the ICP did not increase.[78] Albanese et al.[79] studied the effects of ketamine (5 $mg.kg^{-1}$) in eight patients with traumatic brain injury who were ventilated and sedated with propofol. There was a significant decrease in the ICP, while the CPP and middle cerebral artery blood flow velocity were unchanged. Mayberg et al.[80] found similar results with a cohort of patients presenting for a craniotomy anesthetized with isoflurane and nitrous oxide who received 1 $mg.kg^{-1}$ of ketamine. The mean arterial blood pressure, CPP, and arterial carbon dioxide did not change, while the ICP significantly decreased. There is emerging evidence that the antagonist behavior of ketamine at NMDA receptors may have a neuroprotective benefit.[81] Unfortunately, the evidence with respect to the use of ketamine for induction of anesthesia specifically in the patient with intracranial hypertension is lacking. However, it can be said that ketamine may be used in the sedated, mechanically ventilated patient with little concern for worsening intracranial hypertension. Ketamine's long-term exclusion from the induction of patients with decreased intracranial compliance may be an overgeneralization.

A key feature of ketamine is its effects on the respiratory system. Despite inducing a profound anesthesia, upper airway reflexes and central respiratory drive are preserved to a degree following ketamine administration, though with extremes of dosing, hypoventilation and apnea will occur. In addition, ketamine directly relaxes bronchial smooth muscle, producing bronchodilation. Ketamine has been successfully used to treat status asthmaticus and less severe bronchospasm.[82–86] Hemmingsen et al.[83] in a placebo-controlled trial showed that ketamine (1 $mg.kg^{-1}$) successfully relieved bronchospasm in ventilated subjects.

4.3.4.2 With Its Unique Characteristics, What Is the Role of Ketamine as an Induction Agent in Management of the Airway?

Ketamine is the traditional induction agent for patients with reactive airways disease who require tracheal intubation. Because of its unique pharmacologic profile, ketamine may also be considered for induction in patients who are hypovolemic and for patients with hemodynamic instability due to cardiac tamponade or distributive shock. In normotensive or hypertensive patients with ischemic heart disease, catecholamine release may adversely increase myocardial oxygen demand, but it is not known whether this effect is clinically significant. Ketamine's preservation of central respiratory drive makes it appealing for awake upper airway evaluation in the difficult airway patient. On the basis of the previous discussion, the use of ketamine in patients with elevated ICP remains controversial.

Traditional teaching would have us avoid ketamine despite there being little to no evidence to support such a practice.

4.3.4.3   Discuss the Clinical Use and Adverse Effects of Ketamine

The induction dose of ketamine is 1–2 mg.kg^{-1}. This dose needs to be adjusted for hypovolemic and/or hypotensive patients. Ketamine is commonly mixed with propofol as a 50:50 mixture (5 mg.mL^{-1} of each), "ketofol," a combination that produces less hypotension and respiratory depression than propofol alone. Because of its stimulating effects, ketamine enhances laryngeal reflexes and increases pharyngeal and bronchial secretions. These secretions may precipitate laryngospasm and be bothersome during upper airway examination in the difficult airway patient or during procedural sedation. An antimuscarinic agent such as glycopyrrolate may be administered in conjunction with ketamine to promote a drying effect. The maintenance of airway reflexes does not negate the need for intubation and airway protection when faced with patients at risk for aspiration.

Five to thirty percent of patients will experience hallucinations or dreams on emergence from ketamine. They are more common in the adult than in the child and can be eliminated by the concomitant or subsequent administration of a benzodiazepine.[87] This is less of an issue in emergency airway management, in which often the patient is sedated with benzodiazepines for prolonged periods.

4.3.5   Propofol

4.3.5.1   Discuss the Clinical Pharmacology of Propofol

Propofol (2,6-diisopropylphenol) is an alkylphenol derivative with hypnotic properties. Propofol is supplied in an emulsion of 10% soybean oil, 2.25% glycerol, and 1.2% egg lecithin.[88] It is highly lipid soluble and hence rapidly acting. The initial redistribution half-life is 2–8 minutes. It is rapidly metabolized to inactive, water-soluble metabolites.

Propofol enhances GABA activity at the GABA-receptor complex. It decreases CMRO$_2$ and ICP.[89–91] Propofol causes a direct reduction in blood pressure through vasodilation and direct myocardial depression, resulting in a decrease in CPP, which may be detrimental in a compromised patient.[92] Propofol has profound anticonvulsant properties.[93] It is a potent depressor of ventilation inhibiting hypoxic and hypercarbic ventilatory drive.

4.3.5.2   What Is the Role of Propofol as an Induction Agent for Tracheal Intubation?

Propofol is an excellent induction agent in hemodynamically stable patients. Its potential for hypotension and reduction in CPP may reduce its role as an induction agent for rapid sequence intubation/induction (RSI). However, it remains a commonly used agent in this setting as the adverse hemodynamic changes and other pharmacological effects of propofol are very predictable. Altered dosing for the unstable patients or using it in conjunction with ketamine, "ketofol," helps to attenuate the undesirable hemodynamic effects. Apart from avoiding the use of propofol in patients with known egg allergy (egg lecithin emulsion), there are no absolute contraindications to the use of propofol.

The induction dose of propofol is 1–2 mg.kg^{-1} in a euvolemic, normotensive patient. Because of its predictable tendency to reduce mean arterial blood pressure, smaller doses are generally used when propofol is given as an induction agent for emergency induction. Young adults and children may require 2–3 mg.kg^{-1}.

The pain associated with the injection of propofol is comparable to that of methohexital, less than etomidate, and more than thiopental.[11] This effect can be attenuated by injecting the medication through a rapidly running intravenous infusion in a large vein. Alternatively, pretreatment with a small dose of 1% lidocaine (4 mL)[94] or mixing the propofol with a small amount of 1% lidocaine (2–4 mL) prior to injection[95] have both been shown to minimize the discomfort. Propofol can cause mild clonus but to a lesser degree than thiopental, etomidate, or methohexital.[65]

4.3.6   Inhalational agents

4.3.6.1   What Is the Role of Inhalational Anesthetics as Sedating/Induction Agents in Management of the Airway?

From the beginnings of anesthesia, volatile anesthetics have been an integral part of anesthesia induction. This technique is more commonly used in pediatrics than in adults. In the early days of ether anesthesia, inductions were stormy affairs. With the advent of newer volatile agents that are potent, less pungent, and poorly soluble/rapid onset, a smooth inhalational induction can be easily accomplished.[96]

The major advantage of an inhalational induction is that spontaneous ventilation can be preserved and patients can regulate their own depth of anesthesia. This technique of inhalational induction in pediatric epiglottitis is well established. The safety of extending this practice to other causes of upper airway obstruction, and in adults with upper airway obstruction of any cause, has yet to be conclusively established. However, some have reported that tracheal intubation can be successfully carried out using this technique while maintaining spontaneous ventilation in an uncooperative patient with a difficult airway.[97–99] While halothane mask induction had played a major role in inducing pediatric patients in the past, most practitioners currently favor sevoflurane. Theoretically, the addition of nitrous oxide may speed the onset of anesthesia. However, unconsciousness can be accomplished in less than 60 seconds with sevoflurane and oxygen when using a primed circuit with 8% sevoflurane and fresh gas flow of 8 L.min^{-1}.[98,100]

4.4   NEUROMUSCULAR BLOCKING AGENTS

Neuromuscular blocking agents are the cornerstone of emergency airway management and are used to obtain total control of the patient to facilitate rapid endotracheal intubation while minimizing the risks of aspiration or other adverse physiologic events. Neuromuscular blocking agents do not provide analgesia, sedation, or amnesia, and an induction or sedative agent must be used during RSI in patients who are not completely unresponsive. Similarly, appropriate sedation is essential when neuromuscular blockade is maintained for controlled mechanical ventilation following intubation.

4.4.1 Discuss the clinical pharmacology of neuromuscular blocking agents

In order to understand the pharmacology of neuromuscular blocking agents, it is important to understand their effects at the postjunctional, cholinergic, nicotinic receptors at the neuromuscular junction. Under normal circumstances, the neuron synthesizes ACh from choline and acetate and packages it in vesicles. Each vesicle contains 5000–10,000 ACh molecules. Calcium enters the nerve through channels that open in response to the action potential propagating the length of the nerve. Calcium permits the binding of specific proteins to the vesicles necessary for them to bind to the nerve end membrane. Binding produces fusion and the release of ACh. The ACh migrates across the synaptic cleft and attaches to nicotinic ACh receptors, promoting muscle fiber depolarization producing muscle contraction. ACh then detaches from the receptor to be eligible for reuptake into the nerve terminal or hydrolysis by acetylcholinesterase, which also resides in the cleft.

Neuromuscular blocking agents are either ACh agonists (depolarizers of the motor end plate) or antagonists (nondepolarizers of the motor end plate). The antagonists attach to the receptors and competitively block ACh from accessing ACh receptors. Because they are in competition with ACh for the motor end plate, they can be displaced from the end plate by increasing concentrations of ACh, the end result of reversal agents (the cholinesterase inhibitors), such as neostigmine and edrophonium, that inhibit acetylcholinesterase and allow ACh accumulation and the return of neuromuscular function.

In clinical practice, there are two classes of neuromuscular blocking agents: the noncompetitive or depolarizing neuromuscular blocking agents, of which succinylcholine is the prototype and the only one in common clinical use. The competitive or nondepolarizing agents are divided into two main classes: the benzylisoquinolinium compounds and the aminosteroid compounds. The benzylisoquinolines, *d*-tubocurarine, metocurine, atracurium, cisatracurium, and mivacurium share common properties. The aminosteroids, vecuronium, pancuronium, rapacuronium, and rocuronium also share common attributes that are distinct from those of the benzylisoquinolines.

The ideal muscle relaxant to facilitate tracheal intubation would have a rapid onset, a short duration of action, no significant adverse side effects, and metabolism and excretion independent of liver and kidney function. Unfortunately, such an agent does not exist. Succinylcholine comes closest to meeting all these desirable goals. Despite the historic and well-known adverse effects of succinylcholine and the continuous advent of new competitive neuromuscular blocking agents, succinylcholine remains an essential drug in facilitating tracheal intubation.

4.4.2 Depolarizing neuromuscular blocking agent

4.4.2.1 What Are the Clinical Pharmacological Characteristics of Succinylcholine That Make It a Unique Neuromuscular Blocking Agent?

Succinylcholine is chemically similar to ACh. It consists of two molecules of ACh linked by an ester bridge and, as does ACh, succinylcholine stimulates the nicotinic and muscarinic cholinergic receptors of the sympathetic and parasympathetic nervous systems. Once succinylcholine reaches the neuromuscular junction, it binds tightly to the ACh receptors. ACh receptors related to neuromuscular transmission are located in three areas:

- The presynaptic receptors, responsible for regulation of ACh vesicles release, generate an action potential along the neuron.

- The postsynaptic receptors: the principle paralyzing component of succinylcholine occurs at the postsynaptic receptor. The resultant depolarization and subsequent desensitization to further stimulation produced by succinylcholine occurs because unlike ACh, succinylcholine is not rapidly hydrolyzed by acetylcholinesterase. Succinylcholine is resistant to degradation by cleft acetylcholinesterase and is susceptible to rapid hydrolysis by pseudocholinesterase, an enzyme of the liver and plasma not present at the neuromuscular junction. Therefore, diffusion away from the neuromuscular junction motor end plate and back into the vascular compartment is ultimately responsible for succinylcholine metabolism. This also explains why only a fraction of the initial intravenous dose of succinylcholine ever reaches the motor end plate to promote paralysis.

- Extrajunctional receptors, although numerous, are generally not of clinical significance. In pathological states such as denervation injuries or severe muscle crush injury, these receptors become unregulated and proliferate. The depolarization of the extrajunctional receptors in large numbers can result in clinically significant hyperkalemia.

Succinylmonocholine, the initial metabolite of succinylcholine, sensitizes the cardiac muscarinic receptors in the sinus node to repeat doses of succinylcholine, which may then cause bradycardia that will respond to atropine.

4.4.2.2 What Are the Indications and Contraindications for Succinylcholine?

Succinylcholine remains the neuromuscular blocking agent of choice for emergency RSI because of its rapid onset and relatively brief duration of action. A personal or family history of malignant hyperthermia (MH) is an absolute contraindication to the use of succinylcholine. Patients judged to be at risk for succinylcholine-related hyperkalemia represent absolute contraindications to its use. Under these circumstances, to facilitate tracheal intubation rapidly, a large dose of a competitive, nondepolarizing neuromuscular blocking agent should be used.[101] Relative contraindications to the use of succinylcholine are dependent on the skill and proficiency of the intubator and individual patient's clinical circumstance. A patient who is felt to represent a difficult intubation, and in whom ventilation with a bag and mask is also felt to be difficult or impossible, should not receive any neuromuscular blocking agents except as part of a planned approach to the difficult airway.

4.4.2.3   How Can Succinylcholine Be Used Safely?

In the normal-sized adult patient, the recommended dose of succinylcholine for intubation is 1–2 $mg.kg^{-1}$. In a rare, life-threatening circumstance when succinylcholine must be given IM because of inability to secure venous access, a dose of 3–4 $mg.kg^{-1}$ IM may be used.

The intubating dose is typically felt to be two to three times the dose that produces on average 95% decrease in twitch height of the adductor pollicis muscle (effective dose or ED_{95}). The ED_{95} of succinylcholine is 0.3–0.6 $mg.kg^{-1}$ in adults,[102,103] 0.5 $mg.kg^{-1}$ in children, and 0.7 $mg.kg^{-1}$ in infants and neonates.[104] Therefore, an appropriate intubating dose of succinylcholine for a normal-sized adult is 1 $mg.kg^{-1}$. The average onset time is 1–1.5 minutes. Defasciculation with a nondepolarizing muscle relaxant will decrease the potency of succinylcholine by half. Therefore, if one intends to pretreat the fasciculations with a nondepolarizing agent, a succinylcholine dose of 1.5–2 $mg.kg^{-1}$ is required for intubation.[103]

Succinylcholine is a rapidly cleared drug dependent on pseudocholinesterase for its metabolism. Pseudocholinesterase is an enzyme, manufactured in the liver, found primarily in the plasma. Once succinylcholine diffuses out of the synaptic cleft it is hydrolyzed to succinylmonocholine and then to succinic acid. The mean elimination half-life of succinylcholine is 43 seconds.[105] The rate of metabolism determines the duration of action. A normal adult has a theoretical 8-minute apneic reserve of oxygen. The mean time to return of spontaneous ventilation after an intubating dose of succinylcholine (1 $mg.kg^{-1}$) is approximately 5–8 minutes.[106] Hayes et al.[106] did however have 10% of their patients desaturate before the return of spontaneous ventilation. The airway practitioner still has to provide mechanical ventilation until the function of the respiratory muscles returns. Doses less than 1 $mg.kg^{-1}$ may not compromise the intubation nor do they shorten the apneic period.[107]

4.4.2.4   What Are the Adverse Effects of Succinylcholine and How Can We Minimize These Side Effects?

The recognized side effects of succinylcholine include fasciculations, hyperkalemia, bradycardia, prolonged neuromuscular blockade, MH, and masseter muscle spasm. Each of these will be discussed separately.

Fasciculations. Fasciculations are involuntary, unsynchronized muscle contractions caused by depolarization of ACh receptors, which initiates an action potential that propagates to all of the muscles supplied by this nerve. Fasciculations cause muscle damage that manifests itself as myalgias, increased creatinine kinase, myoglobinemia, and an increase in catecholamines leading to increases in heart rate and blood pressure. These uncontrolled muscle contractions increase oxygen consumption, and carbon dioxide production can lead to increased cardiac output and potentially CBF and ICP. In an animal study, the increase in ICP was found to be secondary to the increase in muscle spindle activation caused by succinylcholine-induced spindle depolarization.[108]

Lastly, fasciculations tend to increase intragastric pressure, though this is not clinically significant as it is offset by an increase in lower esophageal sphincter tone.

Virtually all patients receiving succinylcholine will experience fasciculations. The same cannot be said for postoperative myalgias which occur following the administration of succinylcholine at a rate 1.5–89%.[109] However, 15–20% subjects undergoing surgery without being exposed to succinylcholine will suffer from postoperative myalgias.[110] Not only is the link between fasciculations and myalgias controversial, there is no evidence that the severity of fasciculations corresponds with more severe myalgias,[109] nor does it appear to be a dose-related side effect. McLoughlin et al.[111] suggest that actually increasing the dose may decrease the incidence of myalgias, suggesting that the larger dose leads to a more synchronous contraction and less shearing forces.

Small doses of NDMRs have clearly been shown to decrease the incidence of fasciculations,[40–45] but their ability to effectively relieve postoperative myalgias is not quite as clear.[41–43] A meta-analysis did determine that atracurium, *d*-tubocurarine, galamine, and pancuronium can decrease the frequency of fasciculations and myalgias.[40] Traditionally, 10% of the intubating dose of a NDMR has been given to pretreat for fasciculations. However, at this dose, a significant number of patients experience weakness. While a dose of 0.06 $mg.kg^{-1}$ of rocuronium has been shown to decrease the incidence of fasciculations, it does not decrease the incidence of myalgias.[42–44,112] Harvey et al.[41] showed that rocuronium at doses 0.03 and 0.05 $mg.kg^{-1}$ was equally effective and decreasing the incidence of fasciculations. The timing of rocuronium administration (3 vs. 1.5 minutes) prior to the succinylcholine does not seem to affect it effectiveness.[44]

Lidocaine is an alternative to nondepolarizing muscle relaxants for defasciculation. At doses of 1.5 $mg.kg^{-1}$, lidocaine effectively decreases the incidence of fasciculation and myalgias following the administration of succinylcholine.[40,109] Lidocaine appears to work by preventing ionic exchange across the sodium channels.

Hyperkalemia. Under normal circumstances, serum potassium increases minimally when succinylcholine is administered (0–0.5 $mEq.L^{-1}$) due to depolarization of the myocytes. A pathological response to succinylcholine can occur, however, resulting in rapid and dramatic increases in serum potassium. These pathologic hyperkalemia responses occur by two distinct mechanisms: receptor upregulation and rhabdomyolysis. In either situation, potassium increase may approach 4 times the normal efflux of potassium, resulting in hyperkalemic, dysrhythmias, or cardiac arrest.[113] Two forms of postjunctional ACh receptors exist, mature (junctional) and immature (extrajunctional). Each ACh receptor is composed of five proteins arranged in circular fashion around a common channel. Both types of receptors contain two alpha subunits. ACh must attach to both alpha subunits to open the channel and affect depolarization and muscle contraction. When receptor upregulation occurs, the mature receptors at and around the motor end plate are gradually converted over a 4–5-day period to immature receptors that propagate throughout the entire muscle membrane. Upregulated receptors are characterized by low conductance and prolonged channel opening times, resulting in increasing levels of potassium, clinically significant dysrhythmias, and cardiac arrest.[112] Most of the entities associated with hyperkalemia during emergency

RSI are the result of receptor upregulation. Interestingly, these same extrajunctional nicotinic receptors are relatively refractory to nondepolarizing agents, so larger doses of vecuronium, pancuronium, or rocuronium will be required to produce paralysis. (One would not expect hyperkalemia with nondepolarizing agents as there would not be any fasciculation or depolarization.)

Rhabdomyolysis is the other mechanism by which hyperkalemia may occur. It is most often associated with myopathies. In cardiac arrest situations related to rhabdomyolysis and continued loss of potassium, resuscitation seems to be less successful than in receptor upregulation. Gronert[113] reviewed 129 cases of cardiac arrest from hyperkalemia; 57 were due to rhabdomyolysis and 78 due to upregulation. The mortality was higher in those cases of rhabdomyolysis (30%) compared to cases of upregulation (11%). Succinylcholine is a toxin to unstable membranes in any patient with a myopathy and should be avoided.

Receptor upregulation occurs in the following circumstances: In burn victims, extrajunctional receptor sensitization becomes clinically significant at 4–5 days postburn. It lasts an indefinite period of time or at least until healing of the burned area is complete. It is prudent not to administer succinylcholine to burned patients if any question exists regarding the status of their burn. The percent of body surface area burned does not determine the magnitude of hyperkalemia; significant hyperkalemia has been reported in patients with as little as 8% total body surface area burn.[114] Most emergency intubations for burns are performed well within the safe 4-day window after the burn occurs. There have been no reports of hyperkalemia in the first 24 hours postburn. It seems rational to avoid the administration of succinylcholine until the burn has completely healed.

The patient who suffers a denervation event secondary to a lower motor neuron or upper motor neuron injury is at risk for hyperkalemia. Following lower motor neuron denervation injuries, patients exhibit a sensitivity to succinylcholine, which begins 3–4 days postinjury[112] and patients suffering from severe polyneuropathies display increased potassium release following the administration of succinylcholine.[115,116] Upper motor neuron lesions, such as stroke and traumatic closed head injuries, display a similar sensitivity to succinylcholine, usually 3–5 days after the event.[112] As long as any neuromuscular disease is dynamic, one ought to expect that there will be augmentation of the extrajunctional receptors and the risk for hyperkalemia with the use of succinylcholine. Congenital upper motor neuron and lower motor neuron lesions, such as cerebral palsy and myelomeningocele, do not exhibit an altered response to succinylcholine.[117,118] The duration of the upregulation and altered response to succinylcholine in neuromuscular disorders is not clear. Upregulation has been observed 3 years following an injury and may last even longer in progressive disease types.[112] Unlike fasciculations, the hyperkalemic response cannot be attenuated by administering defasciculating doses of NDMRs, and therefore, these specific clinical situations should be considered absolute contraindications to succinylcholine during the designated time periods.

Infection or inflammation can alter the neuromuscular junction response to muscle relaxants.[112] This situation is complicated by the intensive care unit environment where total body disuse atrophy and chemical denervation of the ACh receptors can occur if muscle relaxants are chronically infused. Exaggerated hyperkalemic responses to succinylcholine have been observed in patients with life-threatening infections.[119,120] The at-risk time period appears to be 5 days after the illness has begun and continues indefinitely as long as the disease process is present.

Succinylcholine is absolutely contraindicated in patients with inherited myopathies such as Duschene and Becker's muscular dystrophies. The combination of the succinylcholine-induced contractures and the fragile muscle membrane of the myopathic patients predisposes them to rhabdomyolysis.[46] In children up to 10 years of age, an elevated creatine kinase is a highly sensitive indicator of muscular dystrophy.[121] Myopathic rhabdomyolysis and hyperkalemia-induced cardiac arrest is associated with a significant degree of mortality. The hyperkalemic efflux can be four times the expected normal response. Any inappropriate response by young males following the use of succinylcholine should alert the practitioner to the possibility of undiagnosed Duschene muscular dystrophy.[122]

There is a paucity of evidence supporting the notion that chronic renal failure patients with normal levels of serum potassium present a risk of an exaggerated hyperkalemic response with the administration of succinylcholine. Indeed, the majority of renal failure patients are successfully intubated using succinylcholine without adverse cardiovascular complications. A review of the literature by Thapa et al.[123] concluded that there was insufficient evidence to support avoiding succinylcholine in patients with renal failure.

Patients with hyperkalemia may be different. Despite succinylcholine being used successfully in patients with hyperkalemia[124] without any adverse events, succinylcholine still cannot be recommended to such patients. Even the normal 0.5 mEq.L^{-1} efflux of potassium could be lethal in a patient with preexisting significant hyperkalemia and acidosis.

Bradycardia. Bradycardia following the administration of succinylcholine is seen most commonly in children because of their heightened vagotonic state. This is especially so as the sympathetic nervous system does not mature until 4–6 months of age. Bradycardia is attenuated or abolished by administering atropine 0.02 mg.kg^{-1} or glycopyrrolate 0.01 mg.kg^{-1} (Ref. 38) as pretreatment before administering succinylcholine. The age above which prophylactic atropine is no longer needed is unknown. But McAuliffe et al.[125] suggest that the incidence of bradycardia following succinylcholine in children 1–12 years of age is lower than expected and that atropine may not be necessary. Regardless of the age, repeated doses of succinylcholine may produce the same vagotonic effects in adults and the administration of atropine may be necessary.

Prolonged Neuromuscular Blockade. Prolonged neuromuscular blockade may result from either an acquired reduction in pseudocholinesterase concentration, a congenital absence of pseudocholinesterase, or the presence of an atypical form of pseudocholinesterase, all three of which will delay the degradation of succinylcholine and prolong paralysis. Reduced concentrations of pseudocholinesterase may be a result of liver disease, pregnancy, burns, oral contraceptives, uremia, or plasmapheresis. This quantitative loss of pseudocholinesterase is rarely clinically significant. Atypical or abnormal genetic variants of pseudocholinesterase can be uncovered by testing. The patient who is a homozygous for atypical pseudocholinesterase (1:1500) may have paralysis for 3–6 hours after a single dose of succinylcholine.

Increase in Intraocular Pressure. Elevated intraocular pressure results from muscle contractures of the orbital muscles that occur following stimulation of the postsynaptic ACh receptors. Though succinylcholine can increase the intraocular pressure by 6–8 mmHg,[126] there have been no cases of vitreous extrusion in the presence of an opened globe eye injury related to the administration of succinylcholine or the act of intubation. The use of succinylcholine has been advocated in patients for whom the prompt securing of the airway is indicated in the face of open globe injuries.[127] The more pressing concern should be protection and the prevention of the deleterious side effects of intubation, such as hypoxia and coughing.

Malignant Hyperthermia. A personal or family history of MH is an absolute contraindication to the use of succinylcholine. MH is an acute hypermetabolic disorder of skeletal muscle. The incidence of MH ranges from 1:50000 to 1:4000.[128] It is an inherited syndrome typified by alteration of the Ry1 ryanodine receptor which modulates calcium release from the sarcoplasmic reticulum. It can be triggered by halogenated anesthetics and succinylcholine. Following the initiating event, its onset can be acute and progressive or delayed for hours. Generalized awareness of MH, earlier diagnosis, and the availability of dantrolene have decreased the mortality to approximately 10%.[129]

MH is characterized by an acute loss of intracellular calcium control. This results in a cascade of rapidly progressive events manifested primarily by increased metabolism (increased oxygen consumption and carbon dioxide production) as well as muscular rigidity, autonomic instability, hypoxia, hypotension, severe lactic acidosis, hyperkalemia, and myoglobinemia. An elevation in temperature is a highly variable manifestation. The treatment for MH consists of discontinuing the known or suspected precipitant and the immediate administration of dantrolene. Dantrolene is essential to successful resuscitation and should be given as soon as the diagnosis is seriously entertained. Dantrolene is a hydantoin derivative that acts directly on skeletal muscle to prevent calcium release from the sarcoplasmic reticulum without affecting calcium reuptake. The initial dose is 2.5 mg.kg^{-1} and is repeated every 5 minutes until muscle relaxation occurs or the maximum dose of 10 mg.kg^{-1} is administered. Dantrolene is free of any serious side effects. Additionally, measures to control body temperature, manage hyperkalemia, maintain acid–base balance, and enhance urinary output to preserve renal function must be instituted as soon as possible.

All cases of MH require constant monitoring of pH, arterial blood gases, and serum potassium. Immediate and aggressive management of hyperkalemia with the administration of calcium gluconate, glucose, insulin, and sodium bicarbonate may be necessary. Following an acute MH crisis, intensive care monitoring is recommended for 24–36 hours. Arterial pH, myoglobinemia, and creatine kinase should be serially monitored. Recrudescence occurs in 25% of MH cases.[128] Patients should be maintained on dantrolene (1 mg.kg^{-1} every 6–8 hours) for the first 24 hours after a crisis.

Masseter Muscle Rigidity. Masseter muscle rigidity (MMR) is defined as the transient inability to distract the mandible from the maxilla such that the mouth cannot be opened or opened only with force.[130] The incidence of MMR following succinylcholine is 0.3–1%.[131] Pretreatment with defasciculating doses of nondepolarizing NMBAs will not prevent masseter rigidity. MMR typically subsides in 2–3 minutes. More than 50% of patients with MMR are susceptible to MH based on caffeine–halothane contracture studies.[132] In the setting of the OR where an operation is contemplated, continuance of a nontriggering anesthetic following tracheal intubation is reasonable if proper monitoring is available (end-tidal carbon dioxide, temperature, creatine kinase, and myoglobin) and the anesthesia provider is comfortable treating MH,[131] otherwise the anesthetic should be discontinued and patient monitored for signs of MH.

4.4.3 Nondepolarizing (competitive) neuromuscular blocking agents

4.4.3.1 Discuss the Clinical Pharmacology of Nondepolarizing Neuromuscular Blocking Agents

Nondepolarizing muscle relaxants (NDMRs) competitively antagonize the action of ACh transmission at the postjunctional, cholinergic, nicotinic receptors at the neuromuscular junction. They are incapable of inducing the conformational change necessary to initiate the depolarization of the neuromuscular junction. NDMRs prevent ACh access to both alpha subunits of the nicotinic receptor, which is required for muscle contraction. This competitive blockade is characterized by the absence of fasciculations and the reversal of paralysis by acetylcholinesterase inhibitors that prevent metabolism of ACh to allow its reaccumulation and retransmission at the motor end plate, promoting a muscle contraction. Metabolism and elimination of NDMRs occurs through a variety of biochemical pathways involving the liver, kidney, and Hoffman degradation. Hoffman degradation, a nonenzymatic degradation, is largely responsible for the metabolism of cisatracurium.

Mivacurium is a benzylisoquinoline derivative that unlike the rest of the NDMRs is metabolized by pseudocholinesterase. Intubating doses range from 0.15 to 0.2 mg.kg^{-1} with a short onset time and brief duration. Mivacurium duration will be prolonged in patients with atypical pseudocholinesterase. As well, mivacurium releases histamine that can induce hypotension.

Cisatracurium, as previously mentioned, undergoes Hoffman degradation and elimination, rendering it virtually independent of liver and renal function. It is devoid of autonomic side effects. Cisatracurium has a relatively long onset time and intermediate duration.

Rocuronium, an aminosteroid, is eliminated primarily by the liver. It has an ED$_{95}$ at a dose of 0.3 mg.kg^{-1}. A dose of 0.6 mg.kg^{-1} can provide good intubating conditions in 90 seconds. In order to provide good intubating conditions in 60 seconds, similar to that of succinylcholine, a larger dose (1–1.2 mg.kg^{-1}) is commonly required for an RSI.[101] However, it has an intermediate duration of action. Rapacuronium, a newer rapid onset aminosteroid NDMR, provides good intubating conditions in doses of 1.5 mg.kg^{-1} and has a short duration of action (17 minutes).[133] Unfortunately, rapacuronium has caused life-threatening bronchospasm and as a result its sale has been suspended.[134]

4.4.3.2 What Are the Indications and Contraindications of NDMRs?

The NDMRs serve a multipurpose role in emergency airway management. They can be used as pretreatment agents to attenuate the

TABLE 4-2

Commonly Used NDMRs, Their Therapeutic Intubating Doses, Pretreatment Doses for Preventing Fasciculation and Myalgias, and Their Basic Pharmacokinetics[11]

	INTUBATING DOSE (mg·kg^{-1})	PRETREATMENT (mg·kg^{-1})	ONSET (sec)	DURATION (min)
Rocuronium	0.6–1.2	0.03	60–90	45
Vecuronium	0.15	0.005	300	45
Cisatracurium	0.15	0.005	300	45
Mivacurium	0.2	0.01	120–180	30
Rapacuronium	1.5	0.07	60	15

many undesirable side effects associated with muscle fasciculations (e.g., myalgia, and the increase in ICP, IOP, etc.) following the use of succinylcholine. They can also serve as the muscle relaxant of choice if succinylcholine is contraindicated or unavailable, or to maintain postintubation paralysis. NDMRs are contraindicated in the face of difficult ventilation/intubation and an inexperienced airway practitioner.

4.4.3.3   How Can We Use NDMRs Effectively?

Defasciculation prior to the administration of succinylcholine is used in patients to minimize myalgias and the elevation of ICP secondary to the increased CBF associated with the increase of carbon dioxide production from the fasciculations and muscle spindle activation. The appropriate dose is 10% of the ED$_{95}$ of any of the nondepolarizing agents. Presently, rocuronium appears to be the most commonly used NDMR to abate fasciculations[46] and it can be given 1.5 to 3 minutes prior to the induction of anesthesia.[44]

NDMRs are the only option for rapid sequence induction when succinylcholine is contraindicated or not available. In these situations, NDMRs can be used for emergency RSI. The drug of choice is rocuronium 1–1.2 mg·kg^{-1} based on its time to onset. If rocuronium is not available, vecuronium 0.15 mg·kg^{-1} is a reasonable alternative (Table 4-2).

4.4.4   How do we decide when to use a nondepolarizing muscle relaxant versus succinylcholine for tracheal intubation?

The use of neuromuscular blocking agents to facilitate endotracheal intubation results in an increased success rate and fewer complications.[101,135–137] Whether succinylcholine or an NDMR is used to accomplish the task is a hotly debated topic. Succinylcholine is superior to the slower onset NDMRs such as pancuronium, atracurium, and vecuronium.[138] The most commonly used muscle relaxants in a rapid sequence induction/intubation are succinylcholine and rocuronium based on their pharmacokinetic and pharmacodynamic profiles. For each drug, the dosage is critical to their success of intubation. The most appropriate dose of succinylcholine is 1–2 mg·kg^{-1} (Refs. 102, 103, 107). Doses of 1–1.2 mg·kg^{-1} of

rocuronium provide better intubating conditions within 60–90 seconds than the lower dose of 0.6 mg·kg^{-1} (Refs. 101, 139, 140). In the emergency department and the OR, succinylcholine (1–2 mg·kg^{-1}) and rocuronium (1–1.2 mg·kg^{-1}) in the appropriate doses have been used safely and efficaciously with paralleled success.[136,137,140,141] However, one must always be weary of the potentially difficult intubation, and in those cases the selection of rocuronium would be unwise.

4.4.5   Are there any new muscle relaxants with a better pharmacodynamic profile?

The next generation of neuromuscular blocking drugs aims for a rapid onset with a short duration of action, mimicking succinylcholine, but with minimal side effects. The ideal NDMR was thought to be rapacuronium, a newer rapid onset aminosteroid NDMR. It provided good intubating conditions with a short duration of action.[133] After widespread usage of rapacuronium, it became evident that it can cause severe bronchospasm associated with arterial desaturation and difficult ventilation.[133,134,139] As a result of its life-threatening bronchospasm, rapacuronium was withdrawn from the market in 2001.

The most promising of this new generation is an asymmetrical mixed-tetrahydroisoquinolinium chlorofumarate, GW280430A. It is an NDMR with an ultrashort duration of action. Belmont[142] has estimated the ED$_{95}$ to be 0.19 mg·kg^{-1}. The onset of action of doses 2.5 to 3 times the ED$_{95}$ was within 90 seconds. Clinical duration was less than 10 minutes.[142] GW280430A's metabolism is said to be "degradation by chemical mechanisms in vitro."[134] The early studies indicate no adverse cardiovascular or respiratory side effects in humans.[134]

4.5   SUMMARY

Tracheal intubation and manipulation of the airway are associated with significant physiological changes. Although it is unknown if pharmacological attenuation of these responses will improve the outcome, it seems both reasonable and logical to minimize these responses, particularly in compromised patients. This chapter provides a general discussion of the appropriate pharmacological agents and their relevant properties. Successful and safe use of these drugs requires a clear understanding of patient's physiology, the pharmacokinetic and pharmacodynamic properties of the drugs, as well as the associated side effects.

REFERENCES

1. Figueredo E, Garcia-Fuentes EM: Assessment of the efficacy of esmolol on the haemodynamic changes induced by laryngoscopy and tracheal intubation: a meta-analysis. *Acta Anaesthesiol Scand.* 2001;45:1011–1022.

2. Donegan MF, Bedford RF: Intravenously administered lidocaine prevents intracranial hypertension during endotracheal suctioning. *Anesthesiology.* 1980;52:516–518.

3. Yano M, Nishiyama H, Yokota H, et al.: Effect of lidocaine on ICP response to endotracheal suctioning. *Anesthesiology.* 1986;64:651–653.

4. White PF, Schlobohm RM, Pitts LH, Lindauer JM: A randomized study of drugs for preventing increases in intracranial pressure during endotracheal suctioning. *Anesthesiology.* 1982;57:242–244.

5. Robinson N, Clancy M: In patients with head injury undergoing rapid sequence intubation, does pretreatment with intravenous lignocaine/lidocaine lead to an improved neurological outcome? A review of the literature. *Emerg Med J.* 2001;18:453–457.

6. McAlpine LG, Thomson NC: Lidocaine-induced bronchoconstriction in asthmatic patients. Relation to histamine airway responsiveness and effect of preservative. *Chest.* 1989;96:1012–1015.

7. Kirkpatrick MB, Sanders RV, Bass JB Jr: Physiologic effects and serum lidocaine concentrations after inhalation of lidocaine from a compressed gas-powered jet nebulizer. *Am Rev Respir Dis.* 1987;136:447–449.

8. Groeben H, Foster WM, Brown RH: Intravenous lidocaine and oral mexiletine block reflex bronchoconstriction in asthmatic subjects. *Am J Respir Crit Care Med.* 1996;154:885–888.

9. Groeben H, Silvanus MT, Beste M, Peters J: Combined intravenous lidocaine and inhaled salbutamol protect against bronchial hyperreactivity more effectively than lidocaine or salbutamol alone. *Anesthesiology.* 1998;89:862–868.

10. Groeben H, Silvanus MT, Beste M, Peters J: Both intravenous and inhaled lidocaine attenuate reflex bronchoconstriction but at different plasma concentrations. *Am J Respir Crit Care Med.* 1999;159:530–535.

11. Barash PG, Cullen BF, Stoelting RK: *Clinical Anesthesia*, 4th edn. Philadelphia: Lippincott Williams & Wilkins, 2001.

12. Atcheson R, Lambert DG: Update on opioid receptors. *Br J Anaesth.* 1994;73:132–134.

13. Bailey PL, Wilbrink J, Zwanikken P, Pace NL, Stanley TH: Anesthetic induction with fentanyl. *Anesth Analg.* 1985;64:48–53.

14. Bennett JA, Abrams JT, Van Riper DF, Horrow JC: Difficult or impossible ventilation after sufentanil-induced anesthesia is caused primarily by vocal cord closure. *Anesthesiology.* 1997;87:1070–1074.

15. Streisand JB, Bailey PL, LeMaire L, et al.: Fentanyl-induced rigidity and unconsciousness in human volunteers. Incidence, duration, and plasma concentrations. *Anesthesiology.* 1993;78:629–634.

16. Abrams JT, Horrow JC, Bennett JA, Van Riper DF, Storella RJ: Upper airway closure: a primary source of difficult ventilation with sufentanil induction of anesthesia. *Anesth Analg.* 1996;83:629–632.

17. Stoelting RK: *Pharmacology and Physiology in Anesthetic Practice*, 3rd edn. Philadelphia: Lippincott-Raven, 1999.

18. Muller P, Vogtmann C: Three cases with different presentation of fentanyl-induced muscle rigidity—a rare problem in intensive care of neonates. *Am J Perinatol.* 2000;17:23–26.

19. Tagaito Y, Isono S, Nishino T: Upper airway reflexes during a combination of propofol and fentanyl anesthesia. *Anesthesiology.* 1998;88:1459–1466.

20. Shafer SL, Varvel JR: Pharmacokinetics, pharmacodynamics, and rational opioid selection. *Anesthesiology.* 1991;74:53–63.

21. Egan TD, Lemmens HJ, Fiset P, et al.: The pharmacokinetics of the new short-acting opioid remifentanil (GI87084B) in healthy adult male volunteers. *Anesthesiology.* 1993;79:881–892.

22. McAtamney D, O'Hare R, Hughes D, Carabine U, Mirakhur R: Evaluation of remifentanil for control of haemodynamic response to tracheal intubation. *Anaesthesia.* 1998;53:1223–1227.

23. Grant S, Noble S, Woods A, Murdoch J, Davidson A: Assessment of intubating conditions in adults after induction with propofol and varying doses of remifentanil. *Br J Anaesth.* 1998;81:540–543.

24. Batra YK, Al Qattan AR, Ali SS, et al.: Assessment of tracheal intubating conditions in children using remifentanil and propofol without muscle relaxant. *Paediatr Anaesth.* 2004;14:452–456.

25. Blair JM, Hill DA, Wilson CM, Fee JP: Assessment of tracheal intubation in children after induction with propofol and different doses of remifentanil. *Anaesthesia.* 2004;59:27–33.

26. Habib AS, Parker JL, Maguire AM, Rowbotham DJ, Thompson JP: Effects of remifentanil and alfentanil on the cardiovascular responses to induction of anaesthesia and tracheal intubation in the elderly. *Br J Anaesth.* 2002;88:430–433.

27. Maguire AM, Kumar N, Parker JL, Rowbotham DJ, Thompson JP: Comparison of effects of remifentanil and alfentanil on cardiovascular response to tracheal intubation in hypertensive patients. *Br J Anaesth.* 2001;86:90–93.

28. Glass PS, Hardman D, Kamiyama Y, et al.: Preliminary pharmacokinetics and pharmacodynamics of an ultra-short-acting opioid: remifentanil (GI87084B). *Anesth Analg.* 1993;77:1031–1040.

29. Joshi GP, Warner DS, Twersky RS, Fleisher LA: A comparison of the remifentanil and fentanyl adverse effect profile in a multicenter phase IV study. *J Clin Anesth.* 2002;14:494–499.

30. Lee MP, Kua JS, Chiu WK: The use of remifentanil to facilitate the insertion of the laryngeal mask airway. *Anesth Analg.* 2001;93:359–362.

31. Erhan E, Ugur G, Alper I, Gunusen I, Ozyar B: Tracheal intubation without muscle relaxants: remifentanil or alfentanil in combination with propofol. *Eur J Anaesthesiol.* 2003;20:37–43.

32. Alexander R, Olufolabi AJ, Booth J, El-Moalem HE, Glass PS: Dosing study of remifentanil and propofol for tracheal intubation without the use of muscle relaxants. *Anaesthesia.* 1999;54:1037–1040.

33. Klemola UM, Mennander S, Saarnivaara L: Tracheal intubation without the use of muscle relaxants: remifentanil or alfentanil in combination with propofol. *Acta Anaesthesiol Scand.* 2000;44:465–469.

34. Puchner W, Egger P, Puhringer F, et al.: Evaluation of remifentanil as single drug for awake fiberoptic intubation. *Acta Anaesthesiol Scand.* 2002;46:350–354.

35. Donaldson AB, Meyer-Witting M, Roux A: Awake fibreoptic intubation under remifentanil and propofol target-controlled infusion. *Anaesth Intensive Care.* 2002;30:93–95.

36. Machata AM, Gonano C, Holzer A, et al.: Awake nasotracheal fiberoptic intubation: patient comfort, intubating conditions, and hemodynamic stability during conscious sedation with remifentanil. *Anesth Analg.* 2003;97:904–908.

37. Puchner W, Obwegeser J, Puhringer FK: Use of remifentanil for awake fiberoptic intubation in a morbidly obese patient with severe inflammation of the neck. *Acta Anaesthesiol Scand.* 2002;46:473–476.

38. Lerman J, Chinyanga HM: The heart rate response to succinylcholine in children: a comparison of atropine and glycopyrrolate. *Can Anaesth Soc J.* 1983;30:377–381.

39. Bevan DR, Donati F, Kopman AF: Reversal of neuromuscular blockade. *Anesthesiology.* 1992;77:785–805.

40. Pace NL: Prevention of succinylcholine myalgias: a meta-analysis. *Anesth Analg.* 1990;70:477–483.

41. Harvey SC, Roland P, Bailey MK, Tomlin MK, Williams A: A randomized, double-blind comparison of rocuronium, d-tubocurarine, and "mini-dose" succinylcholine for preventing succinylcholine-induced muscle fasciculations. *Anesth Analg.* 1998;87:719–722.

42. Mencke T, Schreiber JU, Becker C, Bolte M, Fuchs-Buder T: Pretreatment before succinylcholine for outpatient anesthesia? *Anesth Analg.* 2002;94:573–576.

43. Martin R, Carrier J, Pirlet M, Claprood Y, Tetrault JP: Rocuronium is the best non-depolarizing relaxant to prevent succinylcholine fasciculations and myalgia. *Can J Anaesth.* 1998;45:521–525.

44. Motamed C, Choquette R, Donati F: Rocuronium prevents succinylcholine-induced fasciculations. *Can J Anaesth.* 1997;44:1262–1268.

45. D'Honneur G, Gall O, Gerard A, et al.: Priming doses of atracurium and vecuronium depress swallowing in humans. *Anesthesiology.* 1992;77:1070–1073.

46. Donati F: Succinylcholine in modern anesthesia. *Anesthesiology Rounds* 2002;1:1–6.

47. Beskow A, Werner O, Westrin P: Faster recovery after anesthesia in infants after intravenous induction with methohexital instead of thiopental. *Anesthesiology.* 1995;83:976–979.

48. Bedford RF, Persing JA, Pobereskin L, Butler A: Lidocaine or thiopental for rapid control of intracranial hypertension? *Anesth Analg.* 1980;59:435–437.

49. Randomized clinical study of thiopental loading in comatose survivors of cardiac arrest. Brain Resuscitation Clinical Trial I Study Group. *N Engl J Med.* 1986;314:397–403.

50. Ward JD, Becker DP, Miller JD, et al.: Failure of prophylactic barbiturate coma in the treatment of severe head injury. *J Neurosurg.* 1985;62:383–388.

51. Gunaydin B, Babacan A: Cerebral hypoperfusion after cardiac surgery and anesthetic strategies: a comparative study with high dose fentanyl and barbiturate anesthesia. *Ann Thorac Cardiovasc Surg.* 1998;4:12–17.

52. Nussmeier NA, Arlund C, Slogoff S: Neuropsychiatric complications after cardiopulmonary bypass: cerebral protection by a barbiturate. *Anesthesiology.* 1986;64:165–170.

53. Modica PA, Tempelhoff R, White PF: Pro- and anticonvulsant effects of anesthetics (Part II). *Anesth Analg.* 1990;70:433–444.

54. Hirshman CA, Edelstein RA, Ebertz JM, Hanifin JM: Thiobarbiturate-induced histamine release in human skin mast cells. *Anesthesiology.* 1985;63:353–356.

55. Filner BE, Karliner JS: Alterations of normal left ventricular performance by general anesthesia. *Anesthesiology.* 1976;45:610–621.

56. Eames WO, Rooke GA, Wu RS, Bishop MJ: Comparison of the effects of etomidate, propofol, and thiopental on respiratory resistance after tracheal intubation. *Anesthesiology.* 1996;84:1307–1311.

57. Todd MM, Drummond JC, U HS: The hemodynamic consequences of high-dose methohexital anesthesia in humans. *Anesthesiology.* 1984;61:495–501.

58. Mould DR, DeFeo TM, Reele S, et al.: Simultaneous modeling of the pharmacokinetics and pharmacodynamics of midazolam and diazepam. *Clin Pharmacol Ther.* 1995;58:35–43.

59. Berggren L, Eriksson I: Midazolam for induction of anaesthesia in outpatients: a comparison with thiopentone. *Acta Anaesthesiol Scand.* 1981;25: 492–496.

60. Driessen JJ, Booij LH, Crul JF, Vree TB: Comparative study of thiopental and midazolam for induction of anesthesia. *Anaesthesist.* 1983;32:478–482.

61. Jensen S, Schou-Olesen A, Huttel MS: Use of midazolam as an induction agent: comparison with thiopentone. *Br J Anaesth.* 1982;54:605–607.

62. Izuora KL, Ffoulkes-Crabbe DJ, Kushimo OT, et al.: Open comparative study of the efficacy, safety and tolerability of midazolam versus thiopental in induction and maintenance of anaesthesia. *West Afr J Med.* 1994;13:73–80.

63. Sagarin MJ, Barton ED, Sakles JC, et al.: Underdosing of midazolam in emergency endotracheal intubation. *Acad Emerg Med.* 2003;10:329–338.

64. Milde LN, Milde JH, Michenfelder JD: Cerebral functional, metabolic, and hemodynamic effects of etomidate in dogs. *Anesthesiology.* 1985;63:371–377.

65. Reddy RV, Moorthy SS, Dierdorf SF, Deitch RD Jr, Link L: Excitatory effects and electroencephalographic correlation of etomidate, thiopental, methohexital, and propofol. *Anesth Analg.* 1993;77:1008–1011.

66. Avramov MN, Husain MM, White PF: The comparative effects of methohexital, propofol, and etomidate for electroconvulsive therapy. *Anesth Analg.* 1995;81:596–602.

67. Choi SD, Spaulding BC, Gross JB, Apfelbaum JL: Comparison of the ventilatory effects of etomidate and methohexital. *Anesthesiology.* 1985;62: 442–447.

68. Choi YF, Wong TW, Lau CC: Midazolam is more likely to cause hypotension than etomidate in emergency department rapid sequence intubation. *Emerg Med J.* 2004;21:700–702.

69. Jellish WS, Riche H, Salord F, Ravussin P, Tempelhoff R: Etomidate and thiopental-based anesthetic induction: comparisons between different titrated levels of electrophysiologic cortical depression and response to laryngoscopy. *J Clin Anesth.* 1997;9:36–41.

70. Guldner G, Schultz J, Sexton P, Fortner C, Richmond M: Etomidate for rapid-sequence intubation in young children: hemodynamic effects and adverse events. *Acad Emerg Med.* 2003;10:134–139.

71. Gauss A, Heinrich H, Wilder-Smith OH: Echocardiographic assessment of the haemodynamic effects of propofol: a comparison with etomidate and thiopentone. *Anaesthesia.* 1991;46:99–105.

72. Holdcroft A, Morgan M, Whitwam JG, Lumley J: Effect of dose and premedication on induction complications with etomidate. *Br J Anaesth.* 1976;48:199–205.

73. Ghoneim MM, Yamada T: Etomidate: a clinical and electroencephalographic comparison with thiopental. *Anesth Analg.* 1977;56:479–485.

74. Wagner RL, White PF: Etomidate inhibits adrenocortical function in surgical patients. *Anesthesiology.* 1984;61:647–651.

75. Duthie DJ, Fraser R, Nimmo WS: Effect of induction of anaesthesia with etomidate on corticosteroid synthesis in man. *Br J Anaesth.* 1985;57:156–159.

76. Wagner RL, White PF, Kan PB, Rosenthal MH, Feldman D: Inhibition of adrenal steroidogenesis by the anesthetic etomidate. *N Engl J Med.* 1984;310:1415–1421.

77. Pfenninger E, Dick W, Ahnefeld FW: The influence of ketamine on both normal and raised intracranial pressure of artificially ventilated animals. *Eur J Anaesthesiol.* 1985;2:297–307.

78. Schwedler M, Miletich DJ, Albrecht RF: Cerebral blood flow and metabolism following ketamine administration. *Can Anaesth Soc J.* 1982;29:222–226.

79. Albanese J, Arnaud S, Rey M, et al.: Ketamine decreases intracranial pressure and electroencephalographic activity in traumatic brain injury patients during propofol sedation. *Anesthesiology.* 1997;87:1328–1334.

80. Mayberg TS, Lam AM, Matta BF, Domino KB, Winn HR: Ketamine does not increase cerebral blood flow velocity or intracranial pressure during isoflurane/nitrous oxide anesthesia in patients undergoing craniotomy. *Anesth Analg.* 1995;81:84–89.

81. Hirota K, Lambert DG: Ketamine: its mechanism(s) of action and unusual clinical uses. *Br J Anaesth.* 1996;77:441–444.

82. Hemming A, MacKenzie I, Finfer S: Response to ketamine in status asthmaticus resistant to maximal medical treatment. *Thorax.* 1994;49:90–91.

83. Hemmingsen C, Nielsen PK, Odorico J: Ketamine in the treatment of bronchospasm during mechanical ventilation. *Am J Emerg Med.* 1994;12:417–420.

84. Hirshman CA, Downes H, Farbood A, Bergman NA: Ketamine block of bronchospasm in experimental canine asthma. *Br J Anaesth.* 1979;51:713–718.

85. Sarma VJ: Use of ketamine in acute severe asthma. *Acta Anaesthesiol Scand.* 1992;36:106–107.

86. L'Hommedieu CS, Arens JJ: The use of ketamine for the emergency intubation of patients with status asthmaticus. *Ann Emerg Med.* 1987;16:568–571.

87. Cartwright PD, Pingel SM: Midazolam and diazepam in ketamine anaesthesia. *Anaesthesia.* 1984;39:439–442.

88. Bryson HM, Fulton BR, Faulds D: Propofol. An update of its use in anaesthesia and conscious sedation. *Drugs.* 1995;50:513–559.

89. Cavazzuti M, Porro CA, Barbieri A, Galetti A: Brain and spinal cord metabolic activity during propofol anaesthesia. *Br J Anaesth.* 1991;66:490–495.

90. Pinaud M, Lelausque JN, Chetanneau A, et al.: Effects of propofol on cerebral hemodynamics and metabolism in patients with brain trauma. *Anesthesiology.* 1990;73:404–409.

91. Lagerkranser M, Stange K, Sollevi A: Effects of propofol on cerebral blood flow, metabolism, and cerebral autoregulation in the anesthetized pig. *J Neurosurg Anesthesiol.* 1997;9:188–193.

92. Searle NR, Sahab P: Propofol in patients with cardiac disease. *Can J Anaesth.* 1993;40:730–747.

93. Ebrahim ZY, Schubert A, Van Ness P, Wolgamuth B, Awad I: The effect of propofol on the electroencephalogram of patients with epilepsy. *Anesth Analg.* 1994;78:275–279.

94. King SY, Davis FM, Wells JE, Murchison DJ, Pryor PJ: Lidocaine for the prevention of pain due to injection of propofol. *Anesth Analg.* 1992;74:246–249.

95. Johnson RA, Harper NJ, Chadwick S, Vohra A: Pain on injection of propofol. Methods of alleviation. *Anaesthesia.* 1990;45:439–442.

96. Doi M, Ikeda K: Airway irritation produced by volatile anaesthetics during brief inhalation: comparison of halothane, enflurane, isoflurane and sevoflurane. *Can J Anaesth.* 1993;40:122–126.

97. Mostafa SM, Atherton AM: Sevoflurane for difficult tracheal intubation. *Br J Anaesth.* 1997;79:392–393.

98. Thwaites A, Edmends S, Smith I: Inhalation induction with sevoflurane: a double-blind comparison with propofol. *Br J Anaesth.* 1997;78:356–361.

99. Muzi M, Robinson BJ, Ebert TJ, O'Brien TJ: Induction of anesthesia and tracheal intubation with sevoflurane in adults. *Anesthesiology.* 1996;85:536–543.

100. Yogendran S, Prabhu A, Hendy A, et al.: Vital capacity and patient controlled sevoflurane inhalation result in similar induction characteristics. *Can J Anaesth.* 2005;52:45–49.

101. Andrews JI, Kumar N, van den Brom RH, et al.: A large simple randomized trial of rocuronium versus succinylcholine in rapid-sequence induction of anaesthesia along with propofol. *Acta Anaesthesiol Scand.* 1999;43:4–8.

102. Kopman AF, Klewicka MM, Neuman GG: An alternate method for estimating the dose-response relationships of neuromuscular blocking drugs. *Anesth Analg.* 2000;90:1191–1197.

103. Szalados JE, Donati F, Bevan DR: Effect of d-tubocurarine pretreatment on succinylcholine twitch augmentation and neuromuscular blockade. *Anesth Analg.* 1990;71:55–59.

104. Meakin G, McKiernan EP, Morris P, Baker RD: Dose-response curves for suxamethonium in neonates, infants and children. *Br J Anaesth.* 1989;62:655–658.

105. Roy JJ, Donati F, Boismenu D, Varin F: Concentration-effect relation of succinylcholine chloride during propofol anesthesia. *Anesthesiology.* 2002;97: 1082–1092.

106. Hayes AH, Breslin DS, Mirakhur RK, Reid JE, O'Hare RA: Frequency of haemoglobin desaturation with the use of succinylcholine during rapid sequence induction of anaesthesia. *Acta Anaesthesiol Scand.* 2001;45:746–749.

107. Donati F: The right dose of succinylcholine. *Anesthesiology.* 2003;99: 1037–1038.

108. Lanier WL, Milde JH, Michenfelder JD: Cerebral stimulation following succinylcholine in dogs. *Anesthesiology.* 1986;64:551–559.

109. Wong SF, Chung F: Succinylcholine-associated postoperative myalgia. *Anaesthesia.* 2000;55:144–152.

110. Mikat-Stevens M, Sukhani R, Pappas AL, et al.: Is succinylcholine after pretreatment with d-tubocurarine and lidocaine contraindicated for outpatient anesthesia? *Anesth Analg.* 2000;91:312–316.

111. McLoughlin C, Leslie K, Caldwell JE: Influence of dose on suxamethonium-induced muscle damage. *Br J Anaesth.* 1994;73:194–198.

112. Martyn JA, White DA, Gronert GA, Jaffe RS, Ward JM: Up-and-down regulation of skeletal muscle acetylcholine receptors. Effects on neuromuscular blockers. *Anesthesiology.* 1992;76:822–843.

113. Gronert GA: Cardiac arrest after succinylcholine: mortality greater with rhabdomyolysis than receptor upregulation. *Anesthesiology.* 2001;94:523–529.

114. Viby-Mogensen J, Hanel HK, Hansen E, Graae J: Serum cholinesterase activity in burned patients. II: anaesthesia, suxamethonium and hyperkalaemia. *Acta Anaesthesiol Scand.* 1975;19:169–179.

115. Feldman JM: Cardiac arrest after succinylcholine administration in a pregnant patient recovered from Guillain-Barre syndrome. *Anesthesiology.* 1990;72:942–944.

116. Fergusson RJ, Wright DJ, Willey RF, Crompton GK, Grant IW: Suxamethonium is dangerous in polyneuropathy. *Br Med J (Clin Res Ed)* 1981;282:298–299.

117. Dierdorf SF, McNiece WL, Rao CC, et al.: Effect of succinylcholine on plasma potassium in children with cerebral palsy. *Anesthesiology.* 1985;62:88–90.

118. Dierdorf SF, McNiece WL, Rao CC, Wolfe TM, Means LJ: Failure of succinylcholine to alter plasma potassium in children with myelomeningocoele. *Anesthesiology.* 1986;64:272–273.

119. Kohlschutter B, Baur H, Roth F: Suxamethonium-induced hyperkalaemia in patients with severe intra-abdominal infections. *Br J Anaesth.* 1976;48:557–562.

120. Khan TZ, Khan RM: Changes in serum potassium following succinylcholine in patients with infections. *Anesth Analg.* 1983;62:327–331.

121. Larach MG, Rosenberg H, Gronert GA, Allen GC: Hyperkalemic cardiac arrest during anesthesia in infants and children with occult myopathies. *Clin Pediatr (Phila)* 1997;36:9–16.

122. Smith CL, Bush GH: Anaesthesia and progressive muscular dystrophy. *Br J Anaesth.* 1985;57:1113–1118.

123. Thapa S, Brull SJ: Succinylcholine-induced hyperkalemia in patients with renal failure: an old question revisited. *Anesth Analg.* 2000;91:237–241.

124. Schow AJ, Lubarsky DA, Olson RP, Gan TJ: Can succinylcholine be used safely in hyperkalemic patients? *Anesth Analg.* 2002;95:119–122.

125. McAuliffe G, Bissonnette B, Boutin C: Should the routine use of atropine before succinylcholine in children be reconsidered? *Can J Anaesth.* 1995;42:724–729.

126. Cunningham AJ, Barry P: Intraocular pressure—physiology and implications for anaesthetic management. *Can Anaesth Soc J.* 1986;33:195–208.

127. Vachon CA, Warner DO, Bacon DR: Succinylcholine and the open globe. Tracing the teaching. *Anesthesiology.* 2003;99:220–223.

128. Rosenbaum HK, Miller JD: Malignant hyperthermia and myotonic disorders. *Anesthesiol Clin North America* 2002;20:623–664.

129. Rosenberg H FJ, Brandom BW: Malignant hyperthermia and other pharmacogenetic disorders. In: *Clinical Anesthesia,* 4 edn. Barash PG, Cullen BF, Stoelting RK, eds.. Philadelphia: Lippincott Williams & Wilkins, 2001: 521–549.

130. Rosenberg H: Trismus is not trivial. *Anesthesiology.* 1987;67:453–455.

131. Littleford JA, Patel LR, Bose D, Cameron CB, McKillop C: Masseter muscle spasm in children: implications of continuing the triggering anesthetic. *Anesth Analg.* 1991;72:151–160.

132. O'Flynn RP, Shutack JG, Rosenberg H, Fletcher JE: Masseter muscle rigidity and malignant hyperthermia susceptibility in pediatric patients. An update on management and diagnosis. *Anesthesiology.* 1994;80:1228–1233.

133. Sparr HJ, Mellinghoff H, Blobner M, Noldge-Schomburg G: Comparison of intubating conditions after rapacuronium (Org 9487) and succinylcholine following rapid sequence induction in adult patients. *Br J Anaesth.* 1999;82:537–541.

134. Moore EW, Hunter JM: The new neuromuscular blocking agents: do they offer any advantages? *Br J Anaesth.* 2001;87:912–925.

135. Kovacs G, Law JA, Ross J, et al.: Acute airway management in the emergency department by non-anesthesiologists. *Can J Anaesth.* 2004;51:174–180.

136. Laurin EG, Sakles JC, Panacek EA, Rantapaa AA, Redd J: A comparison of succinylcholine and rocuronium for rapid-sequence intubation of emergency department patients. *Acad Emerg Med.* 2000;7:1362–1369.

137. Mazurek AJ, Rae B, Hann S, et al.: Rocuronium versus succinylcholine: are they equally effective during rapid-sequence induction of anesthesia? *Anesth Analg.* 1998;87:1259–1262.

138. Mehta MP, Sokoll MD, Gergis SD: Accelerated onset of non-depolarizing neuromuscular blocking drugs: pancuronium, atracurium and vecuronium. A comparison with succinylcholine. *Eur J Anaesthesiol.* 1988;5:15–21.

139. McCourt KC, Salmela L, Mirakhur RK, et al.: Comparison of rocuronium and suxamethonium for use during rapid sequence induction of anaesthesia. *Anaesthesia.* 1998;53:867–871.

140. Perry JJ, Lee J, Wells G: Are intubation conditions using rocuronium equivalent to those using succinylcholine? *Acad Emerg Med.* 2002;9: 813–823.

141. Cheng CA, Aun CS, Gin T: Comparison of rocuronium and suxamethonium for rapid tracheal intubation in children. *Paediatr Anaesth.* 2002;12: 140–145.

142. Belmont MR, Lien CA, Tjan J, et al.: Clinical pharmacology of GW280430 A in humans. *Anesthesiology.* 2004;100:768–773.

SELF-EVALUATION QUESTIONS

4.1. Which of the following is a true statement about the elimination of remifentanil?

A. It is metabolized by hepatic enzymes.

B. It is primarily removed from the body unchanged by the kidneys.

C. It is metabolized primarily by plasma and tissue esterases.

D. It is primarily removed from the body by Hoffman elimination.

4.2. To avoid serious hyperkalemia, which of the following is **NOT** considered a safe period to administer succinylcholine to a burned patient?

A. immediately after the burn

B. more than 1 day after the burn

C. more than 2 days after the burn

D. more than 3 days after the burn

E. more than 4 days after the burn

4.3. Which of the following statements is **NOT** true about propofol?

A. It is highly lipid soluble.

B. It is contraindicated for patients with a history of egg allergy.

C. Mixing the propofol with a small dose of lidocaine (2–4 mL) has not been shown to minimize the discomfort associated with injection.

D. It is rapidly metabolized by the liver into inactive water-soluble metabolites.

E. It decreases ICP.

CHAPTER (5)

Aspiration: Risks and Prevention

Saul Pytka, Idena Carroll, and Edward Crosby

5.1 INTRODUCTION

Pulmonary aspiration, although an uncommon occurrence associated with anesthesia, may lead to a spectrum of sequelae, from no discernable effects to significant morbidity and mortality. In this chapter, we will outline the known factors that increase the risks of aspiration and how anesthetic management may be optimized to reduce the risks to the patient.

Although reported in the literature as a relatively uncommon complication of anesthesia, the majority of anesthesia practitioners will acknowledge that the risk of aspiration is a major concern to them in daily practice. Most would acknowledge that if they have not had an episode of aspiration in one of their patients, they know a colleague who has had to deal with the complication. Kluger[1] reported in 1998 that over 71% of all responders to a national mail-in survey in New Zealand had had at least one case of aspiration in their careers.

5.2 HISTORICAL PERSPECTIVE

5.2.1 When was gastric aspiration first described?

Mendelson was the first to describe the occurrence of aspiration in conjunction with the delivery of anesthesia.[2] Since that time, a plethora of publications have followed, outlining the risks and ways of preventing the problem. Unfortunately, much of the information is conflicting, and conclusions have been derived from studies with surrogate endpoints that may have very little to do with actual clinical risks. For example, the often-quoted study by

Roberts and Shirley[3] suggested a gastric volume of greater than 25 mL and pH of less than 2.5, as a specific risk factor for aspiration. This postulation was accepted by subsequent investigators who directed their efforts for prevention of aspiration to the assumption that these specific values were critical factors in predicting the outcome of aspiration.

5.2.2 What was Sellick's approach to minimize the risk of gastric aspiration?

In the discussion of his 1961 paper advocating the use of cricoid pressure during induction of anesthesia to prevent gastric regurgitation, Sellick examined alternatives available at the time.[4] He identified inhalational induction in the supine or lateral position (with head-down tilt) and rapid IV induction of anesthesia in the sitting position. He commented that, with inhalational induction, vomiting usually occurred in lighter stages of anesthesia when protective reflexes were hopefully still present and noted that any difficulty during induction predisposed to regurgitation and anoxia. Rapid IV induction in the sitting position often led to cardiovascular collapse in critically ill patients, and pulmonary aspiration was made more likely by the sitting position, if gastric reflux occurred. Sellick advocated the use of cricoid pressure during induction of anesthesia as a third option.

Sellick suggested that the stomach should be emptied before induction and the nasogastric tube then be removed. He was of the opinion that the nasogastric tube would prevent esophageal occlusion with cricoid pressure. The patient was positioned with the head and neck fully extended and, following denitrogenation, induction ideally occurred with an IV barbiturate muscle relaxant combination. Cricoid pressure was instituted before induction, moderate pressure was applied during induction, and this was increased to firm pressure once consciousness was lost. Sellick suggested that the lungs may be ventilated without risk of gastric regurgitation. Once intubation was completed and the cuff inflated, cricoid pressure could be safely released.

In his description of cricoid pressure, Sellick reported its application in 23 high-risk cases. He noted no instance of pulmonary aspiration in any patient but did report that, in three cases, release of cricoid pressure after intubation was followed immediately by reflux into the pharynx of gastric or esophageal contents, suggesting that cricoid pressure had indeed been effective.

5.3   INCIDENCE AND RISK

5.3.1   What is the incidence of aspiration?

The difficulty in determining the actual incidence of aspiration relates to a number of factors. Firstly, it is a rare occurrence, and as such, large studies need to be undertaken. Most, if not all, of the investigations to date have been studies from large computerized databases. Secondly, aspiration is not always easy to recognize and, as will be illustrated below, rarely leads to clinical findings, let alone serious sequelae. Hence, it is an event likely to be missed and therefore underreported.

The recognition of gastric material in the pharynx is not a diagnosis of aspiration in itself. Despite the evident regurgitation, pulmonary aspiration may not have occurred. If material has been seen below the level of the true vocal cords, there may again be a wide spectrum of clinical presentations. Silent aspiration may occur, wherein the patient exhibits no signs, or symptoms, of aspiration and there are no disruptions of physiological parameters. Indeed, it has been reported that asymptomatic aspiration may occur in up to 45% of normal subjects during sleep, and as many as 70% of people who have a blunted level of consciousness and responsiveness.[5]

Aspiration may become symptomatic, with cough and audible wheeze. Acute lung injury may induce tachypnea, increase in alveolar-arterial (A-a) gradient, hypoxemia, and radiological evidence of lung injury—with infiltrates and/or atelectasis. Frank respiratory failure may ensue, with the development of acute respiratory distress syndrome (ARDS), the need for ventilatory support, and (rarely) death.

Although many papers have reviewed the topic of aspiration, there has been a notable absence of consistent end point. In 1993, Warner[6] published a retrospective review of 215,488 general anesthetics during a period of 6 years. Aspiration was defined as:

> either the presence of bilious secretions, or particulate matter, in the tracheobronchial tree; or, in patients who did not have their tracheobronchial airways directly examined after regurgitation, the presence of an infiltrate on postoperative chest roentgenogram that was not identified by preoperative roentgenogram, or physical examination.

Of the anesthetics included, 202,061 were elective and the remaining 13,427 were emergency cases. There were 52 and 15 aspirations in these two groups, respectively. The overall incidence of aspiration was 1:3,216. Aspiration occurred in 1:3,886 of elective surgeries and 1:895 of emergency procedures. Sixty-seven cases of aspiration were recognized; one patient died from surgical causes intraoperatively. Of the remaining 66 patients, 42 (64%) experienced no obvious sequelae from the aspiration. Of the remaining 24 patients, 13 required mechanical ventilation with 6 needing prolonged (>24 hours) mechanical support. Half of these (three) died of complications from their aspiration, giving a death rate of 1:71,829.

Mellin-Olsen,[7] in 1996, reported a prospective review of 85,594 cases over a 5-year period. They defined aspiration as "what the anesthetist has interpreted as such during, or immediately after the anesthetic procedures, based on clinical signs like gastric content, in the pharynx/larynx/trachea and a drop in O_2 saturation." In their study, a total 25 cases of aspiration were recorded; 52,650 patients had received a general anesthetic, with the remainder undergoing either regional or IV sedation. All cases of aspiration occurred in the general anesthetic population, giving an incidence of 1:2,106. The incidence of aspiration was 1:3,303 in elective procedures under general anesthetic and 1:809 for emergency procedures, both rates similar in magnitude to those reported by Warner. In the patients who had aspirated, there were similar complications to those described by Warner.[6] No deaths occurred and 22/25 patients had either no or minimal sequelae; three experienced more serious consequences. One patient required ventilation for 7 days, but made a complete recovery from his lung injury.

Ollson et al.[8] reported a similar retrospective review, with an incidence of aspiration of 1:2,131 and a mortality rate of 1:46,000. All these studies reaffirm that aspiration is a relatively uncommon occurrence and the mortality due to aspiration in the perioperative period is rare.

Kluger and Short[9] reported, in 1999, the analysis of data from the Australian Anaesthetic Incident Monitoring Study (AIMS). AIMS is a voluntary, anonymous reporting system of anesthesia-related incidents, collected in a central database. Unfortunately, the nature of this type of study does not allow for a denominator (i.e., the total number of anesthetics performed by all reporting clinicians) and the incidence is unavailable. Of the 5,000 reported events, 133 dealt with aspiration. Aspiration was deemed to have occurred if *any obvious nonrespiratory secretions were suctioned via a tracheal tube, there was chest X-ray evidence of new pathology after an incident, and/or there were signs of new wheeze or crackles after an episode of regurgitation or vomiting.* In this group of 133 aspirations, 5 deaths were recorded. Of interest, aspiration did occur in a number of patients undergoing regional anesthesia in the AIMS study (7 out of the 133), whereas none were reported to have occurred in almost 31,000 regional and sedation cases in the paper by Mellin-Olsen et al.[7]

The American Society of Anesthesiologists (ASA) Closed Claims Database reviewed the incidence of aspiration as a cause of liability to anesthesiologists. In 2000, Cheney[10] reported that aspiration represented 3.5% of all claims as a primary or secondary event, and in half of those it was the offending event leading to a claim. Seven percent of the aspiration claims were during regional anesthesia.

In conclusion, the incidence of aspiration in a population is consistently estimated at between 1:2,000 and 1:4,000, depending on the population studied, and when the data had been reported.

Emergency surgery increases the risk of aspiration fourfold, or more, yet overall mortality remains low.

5.3.2 What are the risk factors that contribute to aspiration?

In published studies measuring the incidence of aspiration, the most common association was with emergency surgery.[6–10] Ollson[8] reported that the timing of surgery also correlated with an increased incidence of aspiration, with a sixfold increase in the rate of aspiration between 18:00 and 06:00 hours. The causative factors that relate to the increased risk of aspiration with emergency surgery are not outlined in the studies, but numerous issues such as lack of fasting, stress, depression of GI motility, less staff availability, higher dependence upon less-experienced anesthesia staff, and fatigue may all play contributing roles. A preponderance of the cases of aspiration reported by Ollson[8] occurred in patients who had abdominal surgery performed, with esophageal and upper abdominal procedures predominating. The incidence of aspiration in cesarean section was 1:661. Interestingly, Warner,[6] roughly 10 years later, had no cases of aspiration during cesarean section. In another paper reviewing the incidence of aspiration in children, Warner[11] reviewed 63,180 anesthetics in children under the age of 18 and also found the incidence of aspiration in the emergency patient (1:373) to be significantly higher than that in the elective situation (1:4,544).

There is a paucity of well-controlled, clinical trials that examine the incidence of aspiration in the prehospital and emergency department (ED) settings. In the prehospital setting, the rates of occurrence of aspiration vary from 6% to 90%, depending on the study populations and facilities, and whether the study considered survivors, nonsurvivors, or postmortem examinations.[12,13] Often, aspiration had already occurred prior to attempted intervention and provision of care. In some papers, the incidence of failure to intubate the airway is as high as 47%.[14,15] In the study by Gausche,[14] patients were randomized into intubation group versus transport by bag-valve-mask. There was an intubation success rate by the paramedics of only 57% and the only aspirations occurred in the intubation group. The outcomes between the two groups, in terms of survival, were similar. In the prehospital literature, the source of aspirate in trauma patients differs from that of the emergency surgical population. In the study by Lockey,[12] 34%, or a total of 18 of the trauma patients, had evidence suggestive of aspiration. Of these, 15 had blood contaminating their airway, while only 3 had evidence of gastric contents. All had significant head injuries, with a Glasgow Coma Scale of 8 or less.[12]

Taryle reviewed 43 consecutive intubations in the ED in a major teaching institution and reported a total of 38 complications in half of the patients (22/43). Aspiration occuring prior to airway manipulation was not included as an aspiration. There was a total eight aspirations, the second most common complication after prolonged intubating time.[16] Sakles[17] reported a 1-year review of all intubations in an ED that had a census of 60,000 patients per year. In 610 consecutive intubations, 49 patients had a total of 57 immediate complications. Although there were 10 cases of vomiting, they did not report any occurrences of aspiration. Mort,[18] reporting on airway complications during emergency intubation occurring outside of the operating room, noted that fewer aspirations occurred in

the ED than on the wards or the medical ICU. The obstetrical population will be discussed later in this chapter.

5.3.3 What happens during an aspiration that determines its severity?

The consequences of aspiration can occur as a result of a chemical injury to the airway mucosa from either acid or bile. Injury may occur from particulate material in the aspirate causing either airway obstruction, or an inflammatory response. Finally, there may be pneumonia secondary to contamination from bacteria in the stomach or upper airway.

Injury resulting from aspiration is often that of an acute burn and is a function of both volume and pH of the aspirate. Subsequent release of inflammatory substances, such as cytokines and interleukins from injured tissue, provokes neutrophil migration to the affected areas and further airway reaction. Airway edema, as well as capillary leak in the alveoli, can increase airway resistance and worsen lung compliance. The end result is ventilation–perfusion mismatching and hypoxemia, as well as inflammatory infiltration and/or atelectasis.

The initial chemical burn effect occurs within seconds, followed by neutralization of the acid within 15 seconds. A sudden onset of bronchospasm and laryngospasm may occur. Full evolution of injury can take several days. Repair of the injury is of the order of 3–7 days. Particulate materials can induce a local reaction themselves and lead to a pneumonia. Indeed, attempts to neutralize the gastric pH with particulate antacids may aggravate reaction in the lung due to the particles rather than from the acid itself. Particulate materials of sufficient size or number can produce substantive airway obstruction in their own right.

Pneumonia may follow, related to organisms from the upper airway, esophagus and stomach. This is usually of a mixed flora, with anaerobes and aerobes present. Depending on the organism and the premorbid condition of the patient, this may progress to lung abscess. This is unlikely in the healthy patient. Differentiating between inflammatory pneumonitis and pneumonia may be difficult. The clinical and radiological picture may be similar. Pneumonitis is usually acute, resolving in hours to a day. If the presentation is one of progression without resolution, lasting days, with fever and purulent sputum, a diagnosis of pneumonia is more likely.[19–23]

5.4 PATIENT POPULATIONS AT RISK

5.4.1 What is the relevance of the issues of gastric volume, pH, and constituency of the gastric contents?

Roberts and Shirley[3] concluded that a pH of >2.5 and a gastric volume of 25 mL (or 0.4 mL·kg^{-1}) correlate with aspiration and resultant pneumonitis. In their study, an acid solution was injected directly into the bronchus of a monkey and extrapolations were made in regard to the volume and pH that would place humans at risk. These conclusions have been challenged by numerous investigators.[24,25] Schreiner[25] in 1998 pointed out that over 30–60% of patients have a gastric fluid volume of greater than 0.4 mL·kg^{-1} (median 0.3, as high as 4.5 mL·kg^{-1}), yet the incidence of aspiration is quite rare. Indeed, it has been demonstrated that gastroesophageal reflux (GER) is not associated with residual gastric volume (RGV).[26] On the other hand, it has been shown that GER during anesthesia is related to episodes of straining on an endotracheal tube when inadequate anesthesia has been provided.[27]

Maltby[24] argues that the risk of aspiration is due to loss of the barrier pressure at the gastroesophageal sphincter (GES). Normally, stomach contents are prevented from refluxing into the esophagus by the pressure exerted by the lower esophageal sphincter (LES). The difference between LES pressure and intragastric pressure is the barrier pressure. The stomach is a very compliant structure and intragastric pressure can remain stable until volumes greater than 1,000 mL are present.[28] Indeed, as intragastric pressure rises, so does LES pressure, maintaining the barrier pressure. In one study, measurements of the intragastric pressure and LES pressure during laparoscopy demonstrated that a rise in mean gastric pressure from 5.2 to 15.7 was matched by a rise in LES tone from 31.2 to 47.0 cm H$_2$O.[29]

There is a clear association between aspiration and vomiting or gagging.[1,6–9] With active vomiting, or gagging, the sudden onset of high intragastric pressure is associated with relaxation of both the lower and upper esophageal sphincter mechanisms. This combination enhances the risk of pulmonary aspiration.

The higher the baseline intragastric pressure, the greater the tendency for GER and pulmonary aspiration. With an intestinal obstruction, for example, the intragastric pressure is high in association with the large RGV. This accounts for the high incidence of aspiration in this patient population and the finding that it is one of the commonest factors associated with aspiration in most publications. By the same reasoning, patients with a documented hiatal hernia, or a history of GER disease (GERD), are also exposed to a higher risk of regurgitation and aspiration.

Active vomiting, in association with an unprotected airway, is most likely to occur during induction of anesthesia, with airway manipulation prior to placement of the endotracheal tube, and at the end of a procedure as the patient is awakening and the airway is no longer protected. Inadequate levels of anesthesia at these times, as well as difficulty securing an airway, provide the circumstances most favorable for aspiration to occur. Two-thirds of aspirations are reported during induction and extubation, equally divided between the two periods.[6]

5.4.2 How important is a history of heartburn? acid taste or burping? A history of GERD? How much reflux is significant?

Reflux occurs prevent when the barrier pressure fails to prevent gastric contents from moving from the stomach into the esophagus. Intuitively, those with a clear history of reflux should be at greater risk of aspiration. Kluger[9] found that a history of reflux and hiatal hernia were the ninth and tenth most common predisposing factors for aspiration, representing 7 and 6 cases, respectively, in the database of 133 total cases of aspiration. The patient with a history of acid reflux, with complaints of acid taste or choking at night, represents a more significant risk than one with only complaints of heartburn. The latter may suggest gastric mucosa pathology only. However, no specific data are available indicating that one symptom is more helpful than the other in delineating who is at greater risk. Again the larger the volume of reflux, the more significant is the risk of aspiration.

5.4.3 What clinical situations and characteristics predispose to aspiration?

5.4.3.1 Emergency Surgery

Emergency surgery is the most significant risk factor associated with aspiration in the studies outlined earlier, increasing the incidence of aspiration by four- to sixfold.[6]

5.4.3.2 ASA Physical Status

When Warner[6] compared the ASA status to the risk of aspiration in elective situations, the risk or aspiration increased by almost sevenfold as ASA status rose from I to IV or V. In emergency situations, the occurrence of aspiration increased from 1:2,949 for ASA I patients to 1:343 for ASA IV and V patients, or almost a ninefold increment (Table 5-1). Ollson[8] also reported an increased risk of aspiration and increased morbidity with increasing ASA status. Most, if not all, of the reported aspiration-associated deaths occur in ASA IV and V patients.

5.4.3.3 Airway and Intubation Difficulties

Difficult intubation is associated with an increased risk of aspiration. Vomiting during airway interventions is frequently associated with aspiration, far more so than passive regurgitation. In Ollson's paper,[8] out of 15 cases of aspiration in elective patients where no risk factors predisposing to aspiration could be identified from the chart review, 10 of these (67%) had difficulty with intubation preceding the vomiting and aspiration. In total, 58 out of the 87 patients who aspirated did so due to difficulty with intubation or,

TABLE 5-1

Risk of Pulmonary Aspiration in Elective and Emergency General Anesthetics by ASA Physical Status Classification[6]

ASA PHYSICAL STATUS	ELECTIVE	EMERGENCY	P
I	4/36,916 (1:9,229)	1/2,949 (1:2,949)	.319
II	11/82,436 (1:7,494)	3/5,036 (1:1,679)	.043
III	31/74,301 (1:2,397)	8/4,413 (1:552)	<.001
IV and V	6/8,409 (1:1,401)	3/1,029 (1:343)	.066
Total	52/202,061 (1:3,886)	15/13,427 (1:895)	<.001

with airway manipulation. Warner[6] described aspiration in 69% of his patients in whom active vomiting or gagging occurred during intubation or extubation. Mort demonstrated that when the number of intubation attempts went from ≤2 to >2, a significant increase in complications occurred. The incidence of regurgitation rose from 1.9% to 22% and aspiration went from 0.8% to 13%, directly correlated with an increase in the number of intubation attempts.[18]

In summary, there are multiple studies describing morbidity and mortality associated with airway difficulties.[18,30–32]

5.4.3.4   Obesity

There was no correlation between obesity and aspiration in the studies by Warner et al.[6] or Mellin-Olson et al.[7] Ollson,[8] however, did find obesity to be a contributing factor to the risk of aspiration. Obesity is frequently listed as an aspiration-associated factor in many other references. The association of obesity with a higher risk of aspiration may relate to a high incidence of pertinent comorbidities. For example, delayed gastric emptying is known to be associated with diabetes, which is a more frequent finding in the obese. Other factors related to the obese include GER, difficult intubation, and inadequate anesthesia at the time of induction. This may account for the larger number of obese patients included in some reported aspiration populations.[9]

Obese patients have the same gastric emptying rate as nonobese patients for liquids. Depending on the meal content, the gastric emptying of obese patients for solids may be faster, slower, or the same as in the nonobese.[24,33–36] Maltby[24] reported that obesity did not slow gastric emptying in the absence of other predisposing comorbid conditions and suggested that fasting guidelines should be applied to obese patients using the same criterion as for the nonobese. In their paper, obese patients, with no comorbid conditions, were randomized into fasting and nonfasting groups. The later received a 300-mL clear fluid challenge preoperatively, with no difference demonstrated in the two groups with respect to the RGV postintubation. In a paper reviewing anesthesia for electroconvulsive therapy in 50 obese patients, no incidences of aspiration occurred during 660 procedures.[37]

5.4.3.5   Pregnancy

It has been well accepted that the obstetrical population is at increased risk of aspiration. This has been felt to be secondary to a number of factors. Hormones particularly progesterone, cause relaxation of the GES and impaired gastric emptying. Mechanical effects of the gravid uterus alter the position of the stomach and, as term approaches, create a gastric 'pinchcock' partially obstructing the gastroduodenal junction. The gravid uterus also increases intra-abdominal pressure, which then increases intragastric pressure. It has been demonstrated that the intragastric pressure in pregnancy is increased to 17.2 cm H_2O from the nonpregnant level of 7.3 cm H_2O. Women experiencing heartburn in pregnancy have a drop in the LES tone from the normal in pregnancy of 44 cm H_2O to 24 cm H_2O. Heartburn in pregnancy is reported in some series to be between 45% and 70%, with 27% of these patients having hiatal hernias. The onset of labor with pain and stress, coupled with the presence of opioid analgesics, are independent factors associated

with a reduction in gastric emptying. Increased difficulty with intubation occurs in the parturient related to hormonally induced mucosal edema and increased breast mass. For many reasons, the parturient is at an increased risk for aspiration.[3,38–40]

Interestingly, however, this risk has significantly decreased since Mendelson reported a maternal death rate from aspiration during C-section of 1:667.[2,5] This may well be due to the increased use of regional anesthesia, as well as the application of rapid sequence induction (RSI) techniques, with cricoid pressure and cuffed endotracheal tubes. The use of pharmacologic interventions, although not proven to alter the incidence, may also be a contributing factor. The adoption of difficult airway practices that discourage persistence in failed attempts at intubation may be an important factor, as is the increased use of regional anesthesia.

5.4.3.6   Age

According to Warner,[6] age was not found to be an independent risk factor for aspiration. Ollson,[8] however, did find that extremes of age increased the risk of aspiration. Warner[11] reviewed 63,180 anesthetics in children under the age of 18. The incidence of aspiration in that population was not dissimilar to adults, except that there was an increased incidence of aspiration in patients less than 3 years of age. Over 91% of the aspirations in this population had either a bowel obstruction or ileus perhaps skewing the incidence in young children, although there is some uncertainty as to the effectiveness of the LES in this population. Distended stomachs from both fluids and air entrained during crying or using a pacifier predisposes to gastric reflux when these infants cry or gag. The efficacy and method of application of cricoid pressure during RSI in small children has not been defined.

Borland found that the incidence of aspiration in the pediatric population was 10.2:10,000, higher than Warner's reported 3.8:10,000.[11,41]

5.4.3.7   Decreased Levels of Consciousness and Neurological Disease

It is recognized that the incidence of aspiration of extraglottic (e.g., blood) and lower GI tract (e.g., stomach contents) contaminants is increased in patients with a reduced level of consciousness.[8,12] In these patient populations, loss of function of the LES and upper esophageal sphincter and delayed gastric emptying combine with a reduction of upper airway protective reflexes to promote both regurgitation and aspiration.[42,43] This has relevance for the postanesthetic period as well, as it has been shown that patients left in the supine position with a reduced level of consciousness have an increased incidence of aspiration.

Patients with other underlying neurological diseases, such as Parkinson's disease and multiple sclerosis, are also at increased risk of aspiration due to impairment of their protective airway reflexes.[44] The diabetic with autonomic neuropathy has been demonstrated to have delayed gastric emptying, sometimes manifested by early postprandial satiety but usually asymptomatic. Diabetics also have a theoretically increased incidence of difficult laryngoscopy and intubation due to glycosylation of collagen in the cervical vertebrae. In spite of this speculation of increased risk of regurgitation and aspiration,[45,46] no studies have found diabetes to be an independent risk factor for aspiration.[1,6–11,41]

5.4.3.8   Bowel Obstruction or Other Gastrointestinal Pathology

As discussed in Section 5.3.1 in this chapter, increased gastric volume predisposes patients to an increased risk of aspiration. Gastric obstruction, and or ileus, is one of the commonest associations with aspiration.[8,9,11] The incidence of aspiration in esophageal endoscopy is 1:188, and appendectomy 1:751.

5.4.3.9   Full Stomach

Even in the absence of bowel pathology, recent ingestion of a meal has been documented to be a risk factor for aspiration.[6,11] Guidelines for fasting have been developed for the elective population. However, fasting does not guarantee an empty stomach and RGVs can be quite variable.

5.4.4   Is there a difference in gastric emptying in emergency patients or those who have received opioids?

Trauma patients, have been shown to have delayed gastric emptying up to a week after injury. Patients who are critically ill, in ICU, also have significantly delayed gastric emptying.[47] Neurological injury, either head or spinal cord, is associated with significant delays in gastric emptying related, in part, to catecholamine surge.[48]

Opioids, irrespective of the manner of administration, have been shown to decrease gastric emptying significantly.[49–51]

5.5   STRATEGIES AIMED AT MINIMIZING ASPIRATION RISK

5.5.1   What are the current fasting guidelines? What evidence supports their use?

The American Society of Anesthesiologists has published a set of fasting guidelines, generated from a review of the available literature and input of expert opinion.[52] These guidelines were developed with the healthy patient in mind, booked for elective surgery. They are not intended to be applied to patients with comorbidities that would increase the risk of aspiration. There is a striking paucity of evidence around the relationships between fasting times, gastric volume, pH, and the risk of pulmonary aspiration. The consensus guidelines recommended the following:

For clear fluids, the Task Force recommended a minimum 2-hour period of preoperative abstinence. Clear fluids consist of water, black tea or coffee, pulp free juices, fat and protein free drinks, and carbonated drinks. There is controversy as to the benefits of ingestion of carbohydrate containing beverages. Some investigators feel that they may reduce gastric volume and raise pH, although this difference is not of clinical significance. There is some evidence to suggest that fasting itself may have detrimental effects, particularly in the pediatric population, resulting in greater anxiety and hunger.

For breast milk, the Task Force recommended a fasting period, for both infants and neonates, of 4 hours. Commercial milk and infant formula have a recommended fasting period of 6 hours.

A minimum period of 6 hours is recommended from the last ingestion of solids until the provision of anesthesia for elective surgery following a light meal. Indeed, some studies have noted that solids, particularly fats, can be found in the stomach for periods of over 8 hours after a meal. The Task Force recommended that consideration should be taken into account of the amount and type of food prior to the provision of anesthetic care after consumption of meals other that what is considered "light" (i.e., clear liquids and toast).

There is growing controversy as to the application of these guidelines in the parturient,[53] a complex group, as there is always a potential need for emergency surgery. It would seem reasonable to allow the moderate intake of clear fluids or ice chips for the low-risk parturient. However, the high-risk parturient, either due to comorbidities or at increased risk of requiring an operative delivery, should be fasted.[54] For elective cesarean sections, a fast of 8 hours following solids is recommended.

5.5.2   What role do pharmacological agents play at minimizing aspiration risk?

Although evidence exists to support the contention that pharmacological agents reduce gastric acid production, gastric volume, or both, no evidence exists to support their use in preventing or reducing the incidence of aspiration or improving outcome if aspiration was to occur. Furthermore, the administration of many of the pharmacological agents could not be justified on the basis of cost-benefit analysis. Subsequently, the ASA Task Force has not recommended the routine use of any pharmacological interventions for the prophylaxis of aspiration.

Similarly, there are no recommendations regarding the "at risk" patient, other than the use of nonparticulate antacids in the obstetrical population. The majority of studies looking at the efficacy of these drugs have been carried out in the healthy, low-risk populations.

H-2 antagonists, such as ranitidine, famotidine, and nazatidine, act by binding competitively to the histamine receptors on the gastric parietal cell. They are effective in increasing gastric pH and reducing gastric volume within 2–3 hours of administration. Unfortunately, the effect of the drug diminishes after a few days as tolerance develops.[55]

Proton pump inhibitors interfere with the H^+/K^+ ATPase pump on the parietal cells. They are less effective than H-2 antagonists if the intent is to use them for a single dose as they require at least two doses to be effective, both the night before and the morning of surgery. Tachyphylaxis does not develop with these agents.

Although reductions in gastric acid and volume have been shown with these agents, they do not reduce the harm from bile reflux or particulate matter aspiration. Evidence from the animal literature suggests that pulmonary injury from bile is as significant, if not more so, as acid alone.[56] Bile, with a pH of 7.19, caused severe chemical pneumonitis and edema in one animal study.[56]

Prokinetic agents are used to accelerate emptying of the stomach, thereby reducing RGV. The most commonly used of these is metoclopramide. It has multiple effects, including prokinetic properties, antiemetic properties, and finally, an effect on increasing the tone of the LES. It acts by antagonizing dopamine and serotonin receptors. Depending on the receptor subtype, it may also act as an agonist. Its antiemetic effects are largely due to the 5HT3 antagonism and the prokinetic effects from the 5HT4 agonism. Its prokinetic properties, however, are quickly inhibited by the presence of opioids and anticholinergic agents.

Of interest, the antibiotic erythromycin has been shown to be an effective agent in stimulating gastric motility, thereby increasing the rate of gastric emptying. It exerts its effect via the motilin receptor. Unlike metoclopramide, it has no extrapyramidal side effects and its prokinetic properties are not inhibited by opioids or anticholinergics. Doses of $1-2$ mg.kg^{-1} have been reported to be effective in reducing gastric fluid volume.[57,58]

The use of antacids has been demonstrated to reduce the pH of gastric contents for variable lengths of time. As discussed earlier in this chapter, the administration of particulate antacids can be problematic. The use of clear nonparticulate antacids has been in wide use for the past two decades, primarily in the obstetrical population. Sodium citrate is in routine use, prior to elective or emergency obstetrical procedures. Bicitra is a commercially available form of sodium citrate. The mechanism of action is by conversion to sodium bicarbonate. Rebound acidity will occur with prolonged use, increasing the volume of acid production.[59]

5.5.3 What is the role of rapid sequence induction?

Rapid sequence induction with cricoid pressure has been described as the standard of care in anesthesia for patients at risk for gastric regurgitation.[60] As well, it is cited to be the most common method of airway management by emergency physicians for critically ill and injured emergency patients. It is characterized by a high success rate and a low rate of serious complications.[17,61,62] RSI is also the principal salvage technique when other oral or nasal intubation methods fail in the emergency room.[8]

The use of a rapid sequence technique results in fewer attempts, more rapid intubations, and higher success rates when compared to intubation with no sedation or sedation alone, both in hospital and in the prehospital setting.[63–65] Concerns about the role of rapid sequence techniques in the prehospital setting for the care of severely head-injured patients relate to the potential for hypoxemia under some circumstances. The major issues seem to be the occurrence of severe hypoxia during induction in patients who were not hypoxic before induction and the excess morbidity and mortality, which results in these patients. An effective strategy for maintenance of oxygenation is needed before it can be concluded that rapid sequence intubation is of value in the out-of-hospital care of patients with serious closed head injury.[66,67]

5.5.4 Describe the technique of RSI

The patient should be placed at a height that is most convenient for the airway practitioner performing laryngoscopy. The head should be placed in the "sniffing" position with a firm pillow under the occiput. Although the benefit of the "sniffing" position compared to simple extension was recently challenged by Adnet, it did provide an advantage in patients who were obese or in whom there was at least one factor predictive of difficult intubation.[68]

5.5.4.1 Denitrogenation

The usual method for denitrogenating patients involves having the patient breathe 100% oxygen normally (tidal-volume breathing) through a snug-fitting facemask for 3–5 minutes. An alternative strategy is to have patients take four vital capacity breaths, but there is evidence that the former methodology is preferable.[69] For this reason, whenever possible, it is recommended that the tidal-volume breathing technique be employed.

5.5.4.2 Cricoid Pressure

The cricoid cartilage should be identified by the assistant during denitrogenation, before induction of anesthesia, and the accuracy of the landmark should be confirmed by the airway practitioner. Cricoid pressure may be gently applied at the start of the induction sequence and the pressure increased to that required concurrent with induction of anesthesia. The pressure should not be released until the cuff is inflated and the intratracheal position of the tube has been confirmed.

5.5.4.3 Nasogastric Tubes and Gastric Evacuation

Sellick recommended evacuating the stomach with a gastric tube and then removing the tube before induction of anesthesia.[4] Stept[70] argued that there was little evidence to support an effect of the tube on esophageal sphincter competence and suggested that the risk would be outweighed by the advantage of continuous gastric decompression when the tube was left in situ. Satiani et al.[71] demonstrated no difference in the incidence of regurgitation with or without a nasogastric tube. Salem and colleagues demonstrated the effectiveness of cricoid pressure in preventing reflux in both infant and adult cadavers with nasogastric tubes in place.[72] It is recommended that a nasogastric tube be used to empty the stomach and then be left open to atmosphere to limit increases in intragastric pressure during induction of anesthesia.

5.5.4.4 The Choice of Sedatives/Hypnosis During RSI

Despite wide acceptance and use of RSI, no single agent has emerged as the drug of choice for sedation and hypnosis during RSI. A deeper plane of anesthesia may improve intubating conditions in emergency patients undergoing RSI by complementing incomplete muscle paralysis.[73]

The use of etomidate, ketamine, a benzodiazepine, or no sedative agent prior to neuromuscular blockade is associated with a lower likelihood of successful intubation on the first attempt, as compared with thiopental, methohexital, or propofol.[73] The use of the benzodiazepine midazolam alone is associated with a prolonged delay to time of laryngoscopy and doses >0.1 mg·kg^{-1} are associated with a dose-related incidence of hypotension.[73–76]

Etomidate, thiopental, and propofol have a favorable effect on intraocular pressure (IOP) and intracranial pressure (ICP).[77–79] Barbiturates have cerebral protective qualities against ischemia caused by elevated ICP. However, barbiturates may significantly lower mean arterial blood pressure and thereby lower cerebral perfusion pressure, potentially compromising collateral blood flow to ischemic regions of the brain.[79] Although propofol also reduces ICP, it reduces mean arterial pressure (MAP) more than barbiturates and thus can cause a significant reduction of cerebral perfusion pressure.[80] Etomidate, in contrast to barbiturates and propofol, reduces ICP to a similar degree while maintaining or increasing MAP and thus cerebral perfusion pressure, but there is evidence of neurotoxicity in experimental models.[81,82] Ketamine is contraindicated in the patient with a head or ocular injury because it elevates ICP, IOP, and cerebral metabolic demands. It is also associated with neurotoxicity in experimental models.

Ketamine, when used in the presence of hypovolemic shock, can be unpredictable in its effect on the hemodynamic profile. It possesses both indirect sympathomimetic stimulation and direct myocardial depressant properties, which support or raise systemic blood pressure in the acutely injured and hypovolemic patient. However, a patient who has been physiologically stressed for an extended period may be depleted of endogenous catecholamines, thereby rendering indirect autonomic stimulation ineffective and allowing the direct myocardial depressant effects to dominate.

Although it clearly has some advantages in a compromised patient, a significant disadvantage of etomidate is that it does not blunt the sympathetic response to endotracheal intubation.[83] This may result in hypertension and tachycardia during endotracheal intubation secondary to sympathetic stimulation. This response may raise ICP and increase myocardial work. Mitigation of this effect is achieved with the use of 1.5–5 μg·kg^{-1} of fentanyl in conjunction with etomidate.[84]

Lidocaine is widely used as an adjunct with induction for its reputed ability to decrease the magnitude of increases in ICP in patients with closed head injury (with or without increased ICP). In fact, there is limited evidence that IV lidocaine reduces the magnitude of the increase in ICP with elective tracheal intubation or suctioning in patients with increased ICP, and there is no evidence that a similar effect occurs in head-injured patients undergoing RSI.[85]

5.5.4.5 The Choice of Muscle Relaxant During Rapid Sequence Techniques

Succinylcholine is widely used in anesthesia and emergency medicine during rapid sequence techniques. Doses approximating 1 mg·kg^{-1} have been conventionally used for intubation; the average time to return to 50% of twitch height following this dose is 8–9 minutes, and to return to 90% twitch height 10–11 minutes are required. A number of authors have explored the use of smaller doses to decrease the time to recovery and to limit the dose-dependent sequelae. El-Orbany[86] assessed onset times and time to twitch recovery for succinylcholine in doses of 0.3, 0.4, 0.5, 0.6, and 1 mg·kg^{-1} after anesthesia was induced with fentanyl and propofol. Onset times ranged between 82 and 52 seconds, decreasing with

increasing doses of succinylcholine but not differing between 0.6 and 1 mg·kg^{-1}. Intubation conditions were often unacceptable after 0.3 and 0.4 mg·kg^{-1} doses, but acceptable conditions were achieved in all patients receiving more than 0.5 mg·kg^{-1}; intubation conditions in patients receiving 0.6 and 1.0 mg·kg^{-1} were identical. The times to twitch recovery and to regular spontaneous reservoir bag movements were significantly shorter in the 0.6 mg·kg^{-1} dose group compared with patients receiving 1 mg·kg^{-1}. Naguib[87] carried out a similar study administering succinylcholine 0.3–1.0 mg·kg^{-1} after anesthesia was induced with fentanyl and propofol. Intubating conditions were acceptable (excellent plus good grade combined) in 30%, 92%, 94%, and 98% of patients after 0.0, 0.3, 0.5, and 1.0 mg·kg^{-1} succinylcholine, respectively. The calculated doses of succinylcholine that were required to achieve acceptable intubating conditions in 90% and 95% of patients at 60 seconds were 0.24 mg·kg^{-1} and 0.56 mg·kg^{-1}, respectively.

While these results may have significant clinical implications, more studies are needed to examine the effectiveness of these smaller doses of succinylcholine in different patient populations, including obese, pregnant, pediatric, trauma, and critically ill patients. It must also be emphasized that the ideal is 100% acceptable intubating conditions, particularly in an emergency.

There is considerable enthusiasm in anesthesia practice to replace succinylcholine with a nondepolarizing muscle relaxant. At this time, rocuronium has emerged as the most likely nondepolarizer to fill this role. Rocuronium 1 mg·kg^{-1} given after induction in a rapid sequence technique is clinically equivalent to succinylcholine 1 mg·kg^{-1}.[88] The incidences of clinically acceptable intubating conditions with rocuronium and succinylcholine were 93.2% and 97.1%, respectively. Clinically acceptable conditions occurred less frequently when rocuronium 0.6 mg·kg^{-1} was used. The use of propofol 2.5 mg·kg^{-1} combined with rocuronium 0.6 mg·kg^{-1} results in satisfactory intubating conditions in 90% of patients within 61 seconds (range 50–81 seconds).[89] The use of either thiopental (5.0 mg·kg^{-1}) or etomidate (0.3 mg·kg^{-1}) combined with rocuronium 0.6 mg·kg^{-1} results in a longer time to achieve as well as a lower incidence of satisfactory intubating conditions than that achieved with propofol/rocuronium combinations.[90,91] The addition of alfentanil 10 μg·kg^{-1} to these doses of etomidate and thiopental results in an increased likelihood of acceptable intubation conditions at 60 seconds following rocuronium administration.[92]

Rocuronium 1 mg·kg^{-1} is a suitable alternative to succinylcholine during RSI. The time to full twitch recovery of doses of rocuronium studied may be in excess of 1 hour, which may again exceed the comfort level of some practitioners.

5.5.4.6 Positive Pressure Ventilation During RSI

In the eighteenth century, application of pressure in the cricoid area was advocated to allow for ventilation of the lungs without causing gastric distention.[89] Sellick,[4] in his description of cricoid pressure, also recommended ventilating the lungs while awaiting onset of muscle paralysis. On the other hand, Stept et al. recommended against the use of ventilation after application of cricoid pressure[70] and conventional practice has favored this recommendation. However, there is now evidence that not only is there a benefit to ventilating the patient's lungs during the period of apnea but also that it can be done safely.

The average time to return to 90% of twitch height following an intubating dose of succinylcholine is considerably longer than it will take most patients to desaturate, even under ideal circumstances.[93] Using a simulator model, Hardman et al. have identified the factors that shorten the time to desaturate with apnea.[94] The factors that have a moderate effect are a reduced ventilatory minute volume preceding apnea and a reduced duration of denitrogenation. Those that have a large effect are increased oxygen consumption and reduced functional residual capacity. All of those factors are likely to be relevant in many instances of RSI.

There is a relationship between airway pressure and gastric inflation.[95,96] In subjects ventilated by bag-mask without cricoid pressure, airway pressures below 15 cm H_2O rarely cause stomach inflation. Pressures between 15 and 25 cm H_2O will result in gastric insufflation in some patients, and pressures greater than 25 cm H_2O do so in most patients.[95] Application of cricoid pressure during BMV increases the maximum pressure that may be generated during mask-ventilation, without air entering the stomach, to about 45 cm H_2O.[96]

Petito and Russell measured the ability of cricoid pressure to prevent gastric inflation during BMV of the lungs.[97] Fifty patients were randomized to either have or not have cricoid pressure applied during a 3-minute period of standardized mask-ventilation. Patients who had cricoid pressure applied had less gas in the stomach after mask-ventilation. However, more patients who had cricoid pressure applied (36% vs. 12%) were considered more difficult to ventilate and these patients tended to have more air in the stomach than those patients considered easy to ventilate with applied cricoid pressure.

In summary, the application of cricoid pressure significantly reduces the volume of air entering the stomach at low to moderate ventilation pressures. It allows for continued ventilation of the lungs even in situations where past convention would have discouraged it, such as in RSI. Ventilating the lungs while awaiting the onset of muscle block would clearly be a useful maneuver to prevent oxygen desaturation, and there is an evidence base that supports this intervention. In order to prevent gastric insufflation, every effort should be made to ventilate the lungs at the lowest pressure possible.

5.6   CRICOID PRESSURE

5.6.1   Discuss the applied anatomy of cricoid pressure

The cricoid cartilage is shaped like a signet ring with the narrow part of the ring being oriented anteriorly. The anterior arch of the cricoid cartilage is attached to the thyroid cartilage by the cricothyroid membrane. Laterally the cricothyroid muscles are situated in the cricothyroid gap (see Figure 3-23). The inferior horns of the thyroid cartilage articulate with the lateral surfaces of the cricoid cartilage. The cricoid cartilage is attached to the first tracheal ring by the cricotracheal ligament. The esophagus begins at the lower border of the posterior aspect of the cricoid cartilage. Sellick proposed the application of cricoid pressure during induction of anesthesia, to prevent regurgitation of gastric or esophageal contents by compressing the esophagus between the cricoid and the cervical spine, obliterating the esophageal lumen.[4] To perform the maneuver, the neck was extended, increasing the anterior convexity of the cervical spine and stretching the esophagus. Sellick hypothesized that this prevented lateral displacement of the esophagus when cricoid pressure was applied. However, Vanner[98] reported that contrast CT scanning in one patient revealed that when cricoid pressure was applied, although the cricoid cartilage and cervical vertebrae were approximated, only part of the esophageal lumen was obliterated. There was also slight lateral movement of the cricoid cartilage, which allowed the nonobliterated lumen to be pressed against the body of the longus colli muscle adjacent to the vertebral body. Smith[99] reviewed 51 cervical CT scans of normal patients to assess the anatomic relationships between the cricoid cartilage and the esophagus. Lateral esophageal displacement relative to the cricoid cartilage was evident in half (25 of 51) of the patients; 64% of those with lateral displacement had esophageal displacement beyond the lateral border of the cricoid cartilage. Smith subsequently reported on MRI taken of 22 volunteers with and without cricoid pressure applied. The esophagus was again seen to be displaced laterally relative to the cricoid cartilage in 52.6% of the subjects; this increased to 90.5% with the application of cricoid pressure. Lateral laryngeal displacement and airway compression were observed in 66.7% and 81% of the necks, respectively, with the application of cricoid pressure.[100] In neither study by Smith were the patients placed in the tonsillectomy position as recommended by Sellick. However, there is no evidence that doing so would have resulted in different findings than those reported.

The potential for lateral positioning and displacement of the esophagus relative to the cricoid cartilage possibly explains a number of case reports where, despite seemingly appropriate application of cricoid pressure during RSI, regurgitation and aspiration occurred.

5.6.2   What is the Sellick technique?

Sellick[101] outlined a number of steps in his original description of cricoid pressure applied concurrent with anesthetic induction. The patient was placed in the tonsillectomy position with the cervical spine in extension. Before induction of anesthesia, the cricoid was palpated and lightly held between the thumb and index finger; as induction commenced, pressure was exerted on the cricoid cartilage mainly by the index finger. As the patient lost consciousness, Sellick recommended firm pressure sufficient to seal the esophagus. Cricoid pressure was initially felt to be contraindicated by Sellick in the setting of active vomiting, in the belief that the esophagus may be damaged by vomit under high pressure. He later modified this stand, stating that he felt the risk of rupture to be almost nonexistent.[101] Since his original description, the technique has been exposed to much study and critique. Data have now accumulated to provide evidence to support many of Sellick's recommendations.

5.6.3   Does cricoid pressure reliably protect against regurgitation and aspiration?

There are no outcome studies confirming the clinical benefit of cricoid pressure when used either in anesthesia or resuscitation.

Brimacombe cites numerous case reports documenting the occurrence of aspiration despite the application of cricoid pressure.[60] There are also multiple studies documenting a negative impact of cricoid pressure on patient interventions, usually relating to airway management. There is also a single case report in the literature attributing rupture of the esophagus to cricoid pressure.[102] It involved an elderly female subjected to laparotomy after repeated episodes of hematemesis. The patient, who vomited on induction, was positioned laterally, cricoid pressure was released, and the trachea was intubated after pharyngeal suctioning. At surgery, a longitudinal split was found in the lower esophagus. It was concluded, by the reporting authors, that the esophageal rupture represented an esophageal injury attributable to the cricoid pressure. However, the diagnosis of rupture of the esophagus as a result of the repeated episodes of hematemesis represents as likely a diagnosis, as the stomach adjacent to the area of esophageal injury was noted to be bruised and swollen during the surgery, suggesting a temporally more remote injury.

There are a number of factors that would explain why cricoid pressure cannot provide absolute protection against aspiration, in addition to the anatomic factors already outlined. The landmarks on the patient's neck may not be identified properly and, as a result, pressure not exerted on the cricoid cartilage itself. Cricoid pressure may not have been commenced prior to induction, allowing for an interval between loss of consciousness and application of pressure, during which the patient is at risk for aspiration. Personnel may be inadequately trained. Cricoid pressure may be released inadvertently before the trachea is intubated and the cuff inflated. Finally, it may be difficult to maintain occlusive pressures for prolonged periods and the maneuver may become less effective in preventing aspiration during instances of difficult intubation.

Despite the lack of conclusive evidence supporting the role of cricoid pressure in the emergency management of the airway in the setting of a full stomach, it is likely to continue to be encouraged as a pattern of practice.

5.6.4   How much cricoid pressure is needed to prevent gastric regurgitation?

Twenty newtons of applied cricoid pressure are probably adequate in many instances and 30 N is more than enough to prevent regurgitation into the pharynx in most patients. Pressures of greater than 30 N (approximately 3 kg, or 7 lb) are unlikely to be necessary.[103–106] The originally described forces (40 N) would rarely be necessary to prevent gastric regurgitation.

5.6.5   How do you measure the performance of cricoid pressure?

Meek investigated the cricoid pressure technique of anesthetic assistants.[107] A large variation in the force applied (from <10 N to >90 N) was observed. Performance was improved markedly by providing simple instruction and further improved by practical training in the application of target force on a simulator. Meek also studied six operating room assistants performing simulated cricoid pressure (on a model of the larynx) to determine how long and under what conditions cricoid pressure could be sustained.[108] Subjects were asked to maintain forces of 20, 30, and 40 N for a target time of 20 minutes, with the arm either extended or flexed; most could not do so. Mean times to release of cricoid pressure varied from 3.7 minutes (flexed) to 7.6 minutes (extended) at 40N, to 6.4–10.2 minutes at 30 N, and 13.2–14.6 minutes at 20 N, respectively. These findings suggest that the ability to generate forces sufficient to provide esophageal occlusion and airway protection is limited.

5.6.6   Is bimanual cricoid pressure better than a one-handed technique?

Flexion of the head on the neck may occur as a result of cricoid pressure and this may impede laryngoscopy. Bimanual (two-handed) cricoid pressure with the free hand of the assistant placed behind and supporting the neck or alternatively, with the use of a small support placed behind the patient's neck, has been recommended to overcome the tendency to neck flexion.[109] However, Vanner found no benefit for laryngoscopy when a cushion was placed behind the neck to prevent neck flexion during the application of cricoid pressure.[110] Cook compared the view of the larynx at laryngoscopy in 121 patients with one- or two-handed cricoid pressure applied.[111] In 28 cases the laryngeal view was better with one-handed cricoid pressure, and in 11 cases the laryngeal view was better with two-handed cricoid pressure. In 81 cases, the view was unaffected by the type of cricoid pressure applied. Two-handed cricoid pressure was not demonstrated to routinely provide an advantage over the one-handed technique.

Yentis[112] also studied the effect of the two different methods of cricoid pressure on laryngoscopic view in 94 patients and reached contrary conclusions to those of Cook. In 21 cases, a better laryngoscopic view was obtained with the bimanual technique; in 8 cases it was better with the single-handed technique; and in 65 cases the method of cricoid pressure made no difference. The force applied may have some impact on both the amount of neck flexion and the balancing potential of a bimanual technique. In the study by Yentis, considerably larger forces were applied (50–55 N) than in either Vanner's (30 N) or Cook's (40 N) studies. It is possible that more neck flexion occurred with the larger applied force and more benefit was thus realized when a bimanual technique was employed.

In summary, the technique of cricoid pressure which produces the best laryngoscopic view in an individual patient cannot be predicted. However, an alternative technique should be considered if it is suspected that the technique of cricoid pressure application is having a deleterious effect on direct laryngoscopy.

5.6.7   Does it matter which hand is used to apply cricoid pressure?

Cook assessed the cricoid force applied by trained anesthesia assistants, as well as the ability to maintain the applied force, and compared the two hands.[113] Overall, the assistants applied a lower force than is classically taught but were able to maintain the force with either hand for a sustained period. The use of the left hand resulted in slightly lower applied forces but the differences were not felt to be clinically relevant. Thus, no recommendation can be made regarding position of the assistants as it relates to the handedness of the cricoid pressure.

5.6.8 How does cricoid pressure affect ventilation and airway interventions?

A concern about cricoid pressure in general, and at higher applied pressures in particular, has been the potential for compromise of either the quality of the airway or the effectiveness of airway interventions.[114–116] In a recent report of 23 failed intubations over a 17-year period in one maternity unit, cricoid pressure was maintained during the failed intubation drill.[117] In 14 patients (60%), ventilation via a facemask was not difficult, indicating that cricoid pressure was at least not harmful in these patients. In the remaining nine patients, ventilation was difficult in seven patients (30%) and impossible in two (9%). Although some patients had laryngeal edema, it is possible that cricoid pressure contributed to the difficult ventilation in these patients.[114]

Vanner[116] reported that difficulty breathing occurred in about half of awake patients with 40 N forces applied, and Lawes[118] reported that airway obstruction occurred in about 10%. Hartsilver and Vanner investigated whether airway obstruction is related strictly to the force applied or whether the technique of application was also relevant.[119] They recorded expired tidal volumes and inflation pressures during mask-ventilation in anesthetized patients. Airway obstruction occurred in 2% of patients with pressure applied at 30 N, and in 35% with 44 N. If the force is applied in an upward and backward direction, obstruction at 30 N occurs in 56%.

Aoyama assessed the effect of cricoid pressure (prior to insertion) on the positioning of and ventilation through the laryngeal mask airway (LMA).[120] Ventilation was considered adequate in all patients in the group with no cricoid pressure applied but in only 25% of those with pressure applied. The glottis was visible fiberoptically below the mask aperture in all patients when no pressure was applied, suggesting correct placement. Correct placement was evident in only 15% of patients who had the LMA placed with cricoid pressure applied. Fiberoptic evaluation showed that the mask was not inserted far enough in the remaining 85% of patients. Radiographs taken showed that the tip of the mask in the no-cricoid-pressure group was located below the level of the cricoid cartilage (C6 or C7 vertebra), whereas the mask tip in the cricoid pressure group was above this level (C4 or C5).

Asai[121] studied 50 patients to assess if the cricoid pressure applied after placement of the laryngeal mask prevented gastric insufflation, without affecting ventilation. Cricoid pressure significantly decreased mean expiratory volume delivered through an LMA. This inhibitory effect was greater when the pressure was applied without support of the neck. Cricoid pressure also reduced the incidence of gastric insufflation. In no patient was the mask dislodged. The inhibitory effect of cricoid pressure on ventilation without support of the neck was greater than cricoid pressure with support of the neck.

MacG Palmer and Ball[122] studied the effect of cricoid pressure on airway anatomy in 30 anesthetized patients examined fiberoptically through an LMA. They assessed the effect of 20, 30, and 44 N on the internal appearance of the cricoid and vocal cords. At 44 N, cricoid deformation occurred in 90% of patients and 50% had cricoid occlusion; 43% had cricoid occlusion at 30 N and 23% at 20N. Associated difficulty in ventilation was present in 50% of

patients and 60% had vocal cord closure with associated difficult ventilation, at forces up to 44 N.

Smith and Boyer evaluated the ease of rigid fiberoptic (WuScope System™) intubation in anesthetized adults receiving cricoid pressure.[123] Each patient had their trachea intubated under two conditions: with and without cricoid pressure. An easy intubation occurred in 91% of patients without cricoid pressure and in 66% of patients with cricoid pressure applied. Cricoid pressure compressed the vocal cords in 27% of patients and impeded tracheal tube placement in 15%. In three patients (9%), pressure had to be released in order to successfully intubate their tracheas.

Hodgson[124] assessed the effect of application of cricoid pressure on the success of lightwand intubation in 60 adult female patients presenting for abdominal hysterectomy. All 30 patients allocated to intubation without cricoid pressure were intubated successfully, at the first attempt, within a median time of 28 seconds. Lightwand intubation with cricoid pressure was successful in 26 of 30 patients at the first attempt, but the median time to successful intubation was significantly longer at 48.5 seconds. Three patients required two attempts for successful intubation and one could not be intubated with the lightwand, while cricoid pressure was applied.

Shulman compared the Bullard laryngoscope (BL) with the flexible fiberoptic bronchoscope (FFB) in a cervical spine injury model. Using in-line stabilization with or without cricoid pressure, he concluded that BL is more reliable when used in the setting of in-line stabilization with cricoid pressure applied. He determined as well that BL is also quicker and more resistant to the effect of cricoid pressure than is FFB.[125]

In summary, properly applied cricoid pressure has a limited impact on the ability to ventilate the lungs, the quality of the airway realized, and the effectiveness of airway interventions. However, as applied pressures are increased, the potential for compromise of both the airway and airway interventions is also increased.

5.6.9 What is the impact of cricoid pressure on cervical spine movement?

In the setting of potential or actual cervical injury, concerns have been expressed that the application of cricoid pressure may result in cervical spine displacement, causing or worsening cord injury. Although cricoid pressure is widely used during airway management in trauma settings, there are no data either affirming its safety or implying that it actually poses a risk. Gabbott[126] assessed the impact of single-handed cricoid pressure applied concurrent with manual in-line stabilization of the neck in a neutral position in 30 healthy patients undergoing general anesthesia with neuromuscular paralysis. Vertical displacement was measured from the midpoint of the neck (directly below the cricoid cartilage), and mean neck displacement (vertebral) was 4.6 mm with a range of 0–8 mm.

Gabbott then measured the effect of single-handed cricoid pressure on cervical spine movement after applying manual in-line stabilization in cadavers.[127] The median vertical displacement measured from the body of C5 was 0.5 mm (range 0–1.5 mm). There was no disruption of the lines formed by the anterior or posterior borders of the cervical bodies. In this second study, Gabbott was unable to demonstrate that single-handed cricoid pressure caused clinically significant displacement of the cervical spine in a cadaver model.

Wood[128] studied the effect of cricoid pressure on the view obtained at laryngoscopy with concurrent cervical stabilization maneuvers. Laryngoscopic view was best in the unrestrained position, with 77.4% of these views being Grade 1. More frequently, Grade 3 views were obtained in the presence of cervical stabilization with or without cricoid pressure. When in the stabilized position, application of cricoid pressure improved the view in 26% of patients. Wood concluded that cricoid pressure may actually improve the view of the larynx when the neck is stabilized even though it is often detrimental to the view in the absence of stabilization.

In summary, there is no evidence which would either encourage or discourage the use of cricoid pressure in the setting of real or potential cervical injury. However, its use in this setting is common and there is no evidence of harm caused. Cricoid pressure may actually facilitate laryngoscopy when cervical immobilization is employed, in much the same fashion that anterior laryngeal pressure does.

5.7   OTHER CONSIDERATIONS

5.7.1   What is the aspiration risk associated with the use of extraglottic devices?

When discussing extraglottic devices, the focus is generally on the LMA and its various forms. Other devices are available such as the Cuffed Oro-Pharyngeal Airway. However, the vast majority of the literature relates to the LMA.

The LMA has enjoyed over a decade of widespread use in anesthesia worldwide and has been hailed for its ease of use, efficacy, and low incidence of complications. As its use expanded, so did the nature of its application and it began to be employed for positive pressure ventilation, prolonged anesthesia (more than 2 hours duration), laparoscopic and nonlaparoscopic abdominopelvic surgery, and for surgery in the prone position. These applications have been labeled nonconventional applications and as these patterns of practice have become more common, increasing concerns about aspiration are being expressed.

Authors have addressed these concerns in three ways:

(1) Esophageal pH probes have been employed to determine the incidence and extent of GER during anesthesia with LMAs in place;

(2) Deliberate pharyngeal soiling has been used to measure the protection afforded to the respiratory tract by the LMA. Clinical studies have compared the incidence of reflux when the LMA was employed relative to endotracheal tubes or alternate airways;

(3) Finally, retrospective series and case reports have been presented to both estimate the incidence of aspiration associated with LMA and detail the clinical events and sequelae when aspiration occurred. The bulk of the published literature refers to the LMA Classic™ but more recently, literature relating to

the newer iterations of the LMA, including the LMA ProSeal™ (PLMA) and the intubating LMA, has appeared.

Roux et al.[129] studied esophageal reflux, using esophageal pH probes, in 60 patients administered anesthesia with either a facemask or an LMA. They concluded that the use of the LMA was associated with an increased incidence of gastric reflux in the lower esophagus, but not mid-esophagus, and that reflux was not influenced by either volume of air or pressure inside the LMA cuff. Joshi et al.[130] found no evidence of hypopharyngeal aspiration using pH probes in a study that compared the LMA with the endotracheal tube in spontaneously breathing patients. Ho et al.[131] reported that the use of positive pressure ventilation in a similar setting did not increase the risk of reflux. Hagberg et al.[132] studied both reflux and tracheal aspiration using pH electrodes measuring in both the proximal and distal esophagus, as well as the trachea. The patients were managed with either an LMA or a Combitube™. No changes in esophageal or pharyngeal pH were observed, but 12% of the LMA group and 4% of the Combitube' group had pH changes at the tracheal level. No patient demonstrated clinical signs or symptoms of aspiration.

Using pH probes, McCrory and McShane[133] determined the incidence and level of reflux during spontaneous respiration with the LMA and compared the supine and lithotomy positions. The pH was measured in both the esophagus and the bowl of the LMA. Esophageal reflux occurred in 38% of the patients in the supine position and 100% of the patients in the lithotomy position. A change in pH was also measured in the bowl of the LMA in 57% of patients in the lithotomy position, but was not seen in the supine position.

Cheong et al.[134] compared the incidence of reflux and regurgitation in adults associated with LMA removal and compared the incidence when two strategies were employed for removal. In one group, the LMA was removed when signs of rejection were observed (swallowing, struggling, restlessness) and in the second, when the patients could open their mouth to command. A pH probe was used to assess reflux and a gelatin capsule containing methylene blue, swallowed before anesthesia induction, was employed to identify regurgitation. Instances of reflux measured with the pH probe were more common in the late-removal group. There were no regurgitation events observed in either group.

Evans et al.[135] assessed the ability of the PLMA to isolate the respiratory tract from the digestive tract. Methylene blue-dyed saline was instilled into the hypopharynx via the drainage tube once the mask was in place in 102 patients. A fiberoptic bronchoscope was used to view the bowl of the mask to assess for evidence of methylene blue. Although an effective barrier was observed in all patients initially, mask displacement occurred in two patients (2%) and dye leaked into the bowl of the mask.

Verghese and Brimacombe[136] surveyed the use of the LMA in 11,910 patients, with special emphasis on nonconventional use of the LMA, and the occurrence of airway-related complications. Of the 11,910 uses recorded, 2,222 were considered to be nonconventional. Eighteen of the 44 documented critical incidents related to the airway including laryngospasm (8), regurgitation (4), bronchospasm (3), vomiting (2), and aspiration (1). There was no difference between the rates of occurrence of critical incidents in conventional (0.16%) versus nonconventional (0.14%) use of the LMA. Brimacombe and Berry[137] performed a meta-analysis of the published literature relevant to the association of LMA use and aspiration. In the reviewed papers, there were three cases of aspiration in 12,901 patients, with no death or permanent disabilities recorded.

Keller et al.[138] described 3 cases of aspiration: the first death and the first case of severe permanent neurological injury associated with aspiration and the use of the LMA. All three patients were considered by the authors to be at increased risk of aspiration; two had previous gastric surgery and the third had a hiatus hernia. Keller also reported a literature review designed to assess risk factors for LMA-associated aspiration. Twenty case reports were identified in the literature. In 14 cases, there were factors that could increase the risk of aspiration, including inadequate depth of anesthesia (7), intra-abdominal surgery (3), upper GI tract disease (2), lithotomy position (2), exchanging the LMA (2), a full stomach (1), multiple trauma (1), multiple insertion attempts (1), obesity (1), opioid use (1), and cuff deflation (1).

In summary, there is evidence that gastric reflux into the lower esophagus occurs with some frequency during anesthesia provided with an LMA even in healthy patients without obvious risk factors. Reflux to higher levels of the esophagus or into the pharynx appears to be less common but does occur. It may be increased by patient positioning, such as the lithotomy and lateral decubitus positions. Although the LMA cuff may provide somewhat a protective barrier to refluxing materials, the barrier is not absolute and aspiration may occur even with a PLMA in place. The incidence of aspiration associated with LMA use seems low and not significantly altered when the LMA is used in an unconventional manner. However, it is likely that many cases of LMA-associated aspirations have occurred and gone unreported. When aspirations are reported, it is common that factors traditionally associated with a higher risk of aspiration are present.

In the opinion of the authors, in situations suggesting that the patient is at an increased or high risk of aspiration, it would seem prudent to employ alternate methods to the LMA when managing the airway.

5.7.2 Is it safe to use a lightwand intubation technique (e.g., Trachlight™) in patients at risk of aspiration?

The Trachlight™ represents an alternate airway device that has proven its efficacy in many clinical situations. Studies have shown that it is both safe and effective, with minimal trauma and its ability to secure the airway in clinical situations where anatomical features make the use of the laryngoscope less likely to be successful. Indeed, features that predict difficult laryngoscopy have little or no correlation with the ease or difficulty of Trachlight™ intubation.[139]

The question of the safety of the Trachlight™ in the patient at risk of aspiration is one not well addressed in the literature. Only one paper[125] exists which reviews the use of the Trachlight™ in the presence of cricoid pressure and RSI in a randomized trial and it suggests that the use of the Trachlight is hampered by the presence of cricoid pressure. Sixty healthy patients were randomized into a cricoid pressure group and a noncricoid pressure group. Of the noncricoid pressure group, there was a 100% success rate on the

first attempt. In the cricoid pressure group of 30 patients, only 26 were intubated on the first attempt, three on the second, and one failed with the Trachlight™. The conclusion was that the Trachlight™ should not be used as a first-line choice for RSI.

As discussed earlier, a failed or difficult intubation increases the risk of aspiration. Under circumstances where a difficult laryngoscopic intubation is predicted, one could argue that the use of the Trachlight™ might represent a safer choice. Hung et al.[139] documented that the success of the Trachlight™ was at least as good, if not better than, as the laryngoscope in a series of 950 patients randomized into Trachlight™ and laryngoscope intubation. In another study, Hung et al.[140] studied 265 patients deemed to be difficult laryngoscopic intubations. Of these, 206 were felt to be difficult either because of previously documented problems or anatomical factors predicting difficulty, such as cervical fusion, small mandibles, and impaired mouth opening. The remaining 59 were unanticipated failed laryngoscopic intubations whose airways were secured with the Trachlight™. A total of two failures occurred, both of which could have predicted due to anatomical abnormalities that made the transillumination difficult.

Clearly, clinical judgment is required. The patient with the full stomach from a recent meal does not have the same risk of aspirating as the patient with an acute bowel obstruction. In addition, coughing and gagging in relation to prolonged attempts at laryngoscopy are as likely, if not more so, to expose the patient to the potential of aspirating than if the assistant releases cricoid pressure momentarily to facilitate insertion of a Trachlight™.

Unfortunately, apart from the solitary paper cited above, there is not enough evidence to draw a firm conclusion.

5.7.3 Is awake intubation with an anesthetized airway associated with a lower risk of aspiration than under anesthesia?

Airway anesthesia is routinely used for awake intubation. Many sources caution against these airway anesthesia techniques in the patient with a "full stomach," fearing that anesthetizing the upper airway impairs the cough reflex, leaving the patient at risk should regurgitation occur.[141–144] The question then arises how should one proceed in a patient who has an anticipated difficult airway in the presence of elevated risk of regurgitation? Only one relevant study[142] has been published, in 1989. The tracheas of 123 patients at high risk for aspiration were intubated awake, but sedated, with a FFB. In 114 cases, the vocal cords were anesthetized by either injection of 4% lidocaine through the working channel of the bronchoscope or by transtracheal injection of lidocaine. No local anesthetics were used on 15 occasions. Topical anesthesia was applied to the oropharynx by benzocaine–amethocaine (Cetacaine) spray and benzocaine ointment for oral intubations. Patients having nasal intubations received topical 4% cocaine to the nasal mucosa. No incidences of aspiration were identified in this study.

While many use propofol boluses for awake intubation, this technique must be used with great caution. Propofol and other sedatives decrease LES tone, predisposing to aspiration. In addition, the patient with airway compromise may depend on voluntary muscle tone for airway patency.[144]

Clearly, each situation is unique. An anesthetized airway in an awake patient can prevent gagging, retching, and coughing during intubation. In addition, the awake, cooperative patient maintains the LES tone and can anticipate vomiting and assist in maneuvers to prevent aspiration—turning their head to the side, opening their mouth for suctioning, etc.[142] On the other hand, sedation can produce an uncooperative patient with depressed airway reflexes.

In the patient at high risk for aspiration, one must weigh each technique carefully in securing an airway while minimizing the risks of aspiration.

5.7.4 What is the appropriate management for aspiration?

When aspiration is suspected prompt measures should be taken to prevent further aspiration. The head of the bed should immediately be adjusted to a 30-degree head down position and the patient's head turned to the left side to facilitate drainage of secretions. The upper airway should be suctioned thoroughly. If the patient aspirates on induction, intubation should follow immediately with aggressive tracheal suctioning before ventilation, if possible. If intubation was not intended (as in procedural sedation) and the patient is spontaneously breathing, then supplemental oxygen by face mask should be applied after suctioning as one prepares for further assessment.[5,145,146]

As was mentioned earlier, damage to the lungs after the aspiration of gastric contents occurs within seconds, with subsequent neutralization of acid in 15 seconds. Consequently, bronchoscopy is not indicated except to remove large particulate matter. The decision to proceed with or cancel the surgery should depend on the severity of the aspiration, the patient's clinical status, and the urgency of the procedure. The patient should be notified that aspiration has occurred, when it is appropriate to do so and observed for signs of pneumonitis initially and pneumonia over the ensuing days.

Since gastric acid normally prevents the growth of bacteria, antibiotics are not indicated following aspiration alone. The incidence of progression to bacterial pneumonia following chemical lung injury is unknown. Symptoms of pneumonitis include wheezing, coughing, dyspnea, and cyanosis. Further complications may include pulmonary edema, hypotension, hypoxemia, and severe ARDS.[22] Treatment of pneumonitis largely consists of supportive therapy, varying from simple oxygen supplementation to full ventilatory support.

5.7.5 Should corticosteroids be administered following the aspiration of gastric contents?

The use of steroids in aspiration has been historically based on theoretical considerations, which remain unproven. These relate to anti-inflammatory properties, stabilizing effects on lysosomal membranes, ability to reduce platelet aggregation, and improvement of peripheral release of oxygen from erythrocytes.[147] Studies conducted in the 1960s, 1970s, and 1980s consistently failed to prove a benefit of high- dose steroids after aspiration.[148–150] Nevertheless, the practice continues[22] despite a significantly higher death rate from secondary infections in the group receiving steroids.[151]

The use of high-dose steroids has not been proven effective and can adversely affect mortality in the critically ill population.[5,151] Therefore, its use in episodes of aspiration is not recommended.

5.7.6 Should antibiotics be administered to prevent pneumonia following the aspiration of gastric contents?

The majority of literature on the treatment of aspiration pneumonia is related to aspiration of colonized oropharyngeal secretions,[22] not gastric contents. Treatment should focus on supportive care to maintain oxygenation followed by organism-specific antibiotic therapy should bacterial pneumonia develop. The incidence of post aspiration pneumonia is more common in debilitated patients with comorbid conditions, and patients who have been on ventilatory support, due to leakage around the tracheal tube cuff that occurs in these patients.

The prophylactic use of antibiotics after aspiration has not been demonstrated to prevent infectious pneumonia and is not recommended.[152] Some exceptions may include patients with bowel obstruction[22] and elderly or debilitated patients.[152] The choice of antibiotics varies according to the syndrome and the clinical situation. For example, institutionalized elderly patients with aspiration pneumonia more commonly have anaerobic microorganisms cultured[153] than other population.

The recommendations for antibiotic selection change frequently and current guidelines for antibiotic therapy should be consulted. Such guidelines have been published by the following medical societies: American Thoracic Society,[154] Infectious Diseases Society of America,[155] Canadian Infectious Disease Society,[156] and the Canadian Thoracic Society.[156] Most commonly, it is recommended that antibiotic selection be guided by culture and sensitivity determinations.[22]

5.7.7 How long should the patient be observed following the aspiration of gastric contents?

In a retrospective study of the perioperative course of 172,334 patients receiving general anesthesia, Warner et al.[6] reviewed 67 cases of aspiration. Forty-two of these patients, who were asymptomatic at 2 hours postaspiration or procedure, never manifested any symptoms, acute or delayed. Eighteen of these were day surgeries, and 12 were discharged home on the day of surgery. Twenty-four developed symptoms within 2 hours including cough or wheeze (17), decrease in arterial oxygen saturation of $> 10\%$ on room air (10), an increase in the A-a gradient >300 (1), or radiographic changes (12). Of the 24 with symptoms, 18 required respiratory support or ICU admission, with 6 being ventilated for more than 24 hours because of the development of ARDS. Only one patient developed pneumonia and required antibiotics.

Patients who have been discharged home after suspected episodes of aspiration should be informed of the symptoms of pulmonary complications and instructed to report them promptly.

5.8 SUMMARY

The prevention of aspiration is a significant focus of the airway practitioner. Certain factors markedly increase the risk of this event occurring. Some are inherent to the patients themselves, primarily premorbid conditions known to predispose to aspiration, some related to the patients' pathology and planned intervention, such as emergency surgery, bowel pathology, high ASA risk scores, pregnancy, difficult airway, and decreased level of consciousness. Airway management in the semiconscious patient may lead to coughing and gagging during attempts to secure the airway, accounting for over ⅔ of the perioperative aspirations.

Recognition of high-risk patients is important. Maneuvers to reduce gastric acid and volume, both pharmacologically and with drainage, may have their role but need to be targeted to specific situations. Bile and particulate materials are potentially as harmful to the lung as is the acid that tends to be the primary focus. Thus use of particulate antacids has been abandoned in the perioperative setting should their be aspirated.

Although the efficacy of the Sellick maneuver has come under recent criticism, it is still a standard of care in the protection of the airway at risk. A well-trained assistant is crucial. Under certain conditions when it hampers intubation or ventilation, the reduction or even release of cricoid pressure momentarily may be appropriate. The wisdom of the use of extraglottic devices in the high aspiration-risk patient, when other options are available, should be critically analyzed.

Finally, in the unlikely event that aspiration does occur, guidelines that are evidence based should used in the assessment and management of these patients.

REFERENCES

1. Kluger MT, Willemsen G: Anti-aspiration prophylaxis in New Zealand: a national survey. *Anaesth Intensive care.* 1998;26:70–77.
2. Mendelson C: The aspiration of stomach contents into the lungs during obstetric anesthesia. *Am J Obstet Gynecol.* 1946;52:191–205.
3. Roberts RB, Shirley MA: Reducing the risk of acid aspiration during cesarean section. *Anesth Analg.* 1974;53:859–868.
4. Sellick BA: Cricoid pressure to control regurgitation of stomach contents during induction of anesthesia. *Lancet.* 1961;2:404–406.
5. Engelhardt T, Webster NR: Pulmonary Aspiration of gastric contents in anaesthesia. *Br J Anaesth.* 1999;83:453–460.
6. Warner MA, Warner ME, Weber JG: Clinical significance of pulmonary aspiration during the perioperative period. *Anesthesiology.* 1993;78:56–62.
7. Mellin-Olsen J, Fasting S, Gisvold SE: Routine preoperative gastric emptying is seldom indicated. A study of 85,594 anaesthetics with special focus on aspiration pneumonia. *Acta Anaesthesiol Scand.* 1996;40:1184–1188.
8. Ollson GL, Hallen B, Hambreaus-Jonzon K: Aspiration during anaesthesia: a computer aided study of 185,358 anaesthetics. *Acta Anaesthesiol Scand.* 1986;30:84–92.
9. Kluger MT, Short TG: Aspiration during anaesthesia: a review of 133 cases from the Australian Anaesthetic Incident Monitoring Study (AIMS). *Anaesthesia.* 1999;54:19–26.
10. Cheney FW, Aspiration: A Liability Hazard for the Anesthesiologist? ASA Newsl June 2000;64:N6.
11. Warner MA, Warner ME, Warner DO, Warner LO, Warner EJ: Perioperative Pulmonary Aspiration in Infants and Children. *Anesthesiology.* 1999;90:66–71.
12. Lockey DJ, Coates T, Parr MJ: Aspiration in severe trauma: a prospective study. *Anaesthesia.* 1999;54:1097–1098.
13. McNicholl BP: The golden hour and prehospital care. *Injury.* 1994;25:251–254.
14. Gausche M, Lewis RJ, Stratton SJ, et al.: Effect of out-of-hospital pediatric endotracheal intubation on survival and neurologic outcome. A controlled clinical trial. *JAMA.* 2000;283:783–790.
15. Nolan JD: Prehospital and resuscitative airway care: should the gold standard be reassessed? *Curr Opin Crit Care.* 2001;7:413–421.
16. Tayrle DA, Chandler JE, Good JT Jr., Potts DE, Sahn SA: Emergency room intubations-complications and survival. *Chest.* 1979;75:541–543.
17. Sakles JC, Laurin EG, Rantapaa AA, Panacek EA: Airway management in the emergency department: a one-year study of 610 tracheal intubations. *Ann Emerg Med.* 1998;31:325–332.
18. Mort TC: Emergency tracheal intubation: complications associated with repeated laryngoscopic attempts. *Anesth Analg.* 2004;99:607–613.
19. Coriat P, Labrouse J, Vilde F, Tenaillon A, Lissac J: Diffuse interstitial pneumonitis due to aspiration of gastric contents. *Anaesthesia.* 1984;39:703–705.
20. Knight PR, Druskovich G, Tait AR, Johnson KJ: The role of neutrophils, oxidants, and proteases in the pathogenesis of acid pulmonary injury. *Anesthesiology.* 1992;77:772–778.
21. Knight PR, Tutter AR, Coleman E, Johnson KJ: Pathogenesis of gastric particulate lung injury: a comparison and interaction with acidic pneumonitis. *Anesth Analg.* 1993;77:754–760.
22. Marik PE: Aspiration pneumonitis and aspiration pneumonia. *N Engl J Med.* 2001;344:665–671.
23. Smith G, Ng A: Gastric reflux and pulmonary aspiration in anaesthesia. *Minerva Anestesiol.* 2003;69:402–406.
24. Maltby JR, Pytka S, Watson NC, et al.: Drinking 300 mL of clear fluid two hours before surgery has no effect on gastric fluid volume and pH in fasting and non-fasting obese patients. *Can J Anaesth.* 2004;51:111–115.
25. Schreiner MS: Gastric fluid volume: is it really a risk factor for pulmonary aspiration? *Anesth Analg.* 1998;87:754–756.
26. Hardy JF, Lepage Y, Bonneville-Chouinard N: Occurrence of gastroesophageal reflux does not correlate with gastric contents. *Can J Anaesth.* 1990;37:502–508.
27. Illing L, Duncan PG, Yip R: Gastroesophageal reflux during anaesthesia. *Can J Anaesth.* 1992;39:466–470.
28. Guyton AD, Hall JE: *Textbook of Medical Physiology*, 10th edn. Philadelphia: WB Saunders, 2000:728–733.
29. Jones MJ, Mitchell RW, Hindocha N: Effect of increased intra-abdominal pressure during laparoscopy on the lower esophageal sphincter. *Anesth Analg.* 1989;68:63–65.
30. Mort TC: The incidence and risk factors for cardiac arrest during emergency tracheal intubation: a justification for incorporating the ASA guidelines in the remote location. *J Clin Anesth.* 2004;16:508–516.
31. Rose DK, Cohen MM: The airway: problems and predictions in 18500 patients. *Can J Anaesth.* 1994;39:1105–1111.
32. Schwartz DE, Mathay MA, Cohen NH: Death and other complications of emergency airway management in critically ill patients: A prospective investigation of 297 tracheal intubations. *Anesthesiology.* 1995;82:367–376.
33. Dubois A: Obesity and gastric emptying. Editorial. *Gastroenterology.* 1983;84:875–876.
34. Horowitz M, Collins PJ, Harding PE, Shearman DI: Abnormalities of gastric emptying in obese patients. *Int J Obes.* 1983;7:415–421.
35. Maddox A, Horowitz M, Wishart J, Collins P: Gastric and esophageal emptying in obesity. *Scan J Gastroenterol.* 1989;24:593–598.
36. Wright RA, Krinsky S, Fleeman C, Trujillo J, Teague E: Gastric emptying and obesity. *Gastroenterology.* 1983;84:747–751.
37. Kadar AG, Ing CH, White PF, et al.: Anesthesia for electroconvulsive therapy in obese patients. *Anesth Analg.* 2002;94:360–361.
38. Ewah B,Yau K, King M: Effect of epidural opioids on gastric emptying in labour. *Int J Obstet Anaesth.* 1993;2:125–128.
39. MacFie AG, Magides AD, Richmond MN, Reilly CS: Gastric emptying in pregnancy. *Br J Anaesth.* 1991;67:54–57.
40. Shinder SM, Levinson G: *Anesthesia for Obstetrics*, 2nd edn. Philadelphia: Lippincott Williams & Wilkins, 1987:300–315.
41. Borland LM, Sereika SM, Woelfel SK: Pulmonary aspiration in pediatric patients during general anaesthesia. *J Clin Anesth.* 1998;10:95–102.
42. Kao CH, Chang Lai SP, Chieng PU: Gastric emptying in head-injured patients. *Am J Gastroenterol.* 1998;93:1108–1112.
43. Saxe JM, Ledgerwood AM, Lucas CE, Lucas WF: Lower esophageal sphincter dysfunction precludes safe gastric feeding after head injury. *J Trauma.* 1994;37:581–584.
44. Hardoff R, Sula M, Tamir A, et al.: Gastric emptying time and gastric motility in patients with Parkinson's disease. *Mov Disord.* 2001;16:1041–1047.
45. Kalinowski CPH, Kirsch JR: Strategies for prophylaxis and treatment for aspiration. *Best Pract Res Clin Anaesthesiol.* 2004;18:719–737.
46. McAnulty GR, Robertshaw HJ, Hall GM: Anaesthetic management of patients with diabetes mellitus. *Br J Anaesth.* 2000;85:80–90.
47. Heyland DK, Tougas G, King D, Cook DJ: Impaired gastric emptying in mechanically ventilated, critically ill patients. *Intensive Care Med.* 1996;22:1339–1344.
48. Kao CH, Ho YJ, Changlai SP, Ding HJ: Gastric emptying in spinal cord injury patients. *Dig Dis Sci.* 1999;44:1512–1515.

49. Kelly MC, Carabine UA, Hill DA, Mirakhur RK: A comparison of the effect of intrathecal and extradural fentanyl on gastric emptying in labouring women. *Anesth Analg.* 1997;85:834–838.

50. Murphy DB, Sutton JA, Prescott LF, Murphy MB: Opioid-induced delay in gastric emptying: a peripheral mechanism in humans. *Anesthesiology.* 1997;87:765–770.

51. Porter JS, Bonello E, Reynolds F: The influence of epidural administration of fentanyl infusion on gastric emptying in labour. *Anaesthesia.* 1997;52:1151–1156.

52. American Society Task Force on Preoperative Fasting: Practice guidelines for preoperative fasting and the use of pharmacologic agents to reduce the risk of pulmonary aspiration: application to healthy patients undergoing elective procedures. *Anesthesiology.* 1999;79:482–485.

53. O'Sullivan G, Scrutton M: NPO during labour. Is there any scientific validation? Anesthesiology. *Clin N Am.* 2003;21:87–98.

54. Practice guidelines for obstetric anesthesia: A report by the American Society of Anesthesiologists Task Force on Obstetric Anesthesia. *Anesthesiology.* 1999;90:600–611.

55. Hatlebakk JG, Berstad A: Pharmacokinetic optimisation in the treatment of gastroesophageal reflux disease. *Clin Pharmacokinet.* 1996;31:386–406.

56. Porembka DT, Kier A, Sehlhorst S, et al.: The pathophysiologic changes following bile aspiration in a porcine lung model. *Chest.* 1993;104:919–924.

57. Sturm A, Holtmann G, Goebell H, Gerken G: Prokinetics in patients with gastroparesis: a systemic analysis. *Digestion.* 1999;60:422–427.

58. Zatman TF, Hall JE, Harmer M: Gastric residual volume in children: A study comparing efficiency of erythromycin and metoclopramide as prokinetic agents. *Br J Anaesth.* 2001;86:869–871.

59. Gibbs CP, Schwartz DJ, Wynne JW, Hood CI, Ruck EJ: Antacid pulmonary aspiration in the dog. *Anesthesiology.* 1979;51:380–385.

60. Brimacombe JR, Berry AM: Cricoid pressure. *Can J Anaesth.* 1997;44:414–425.

61. Bair AE, Filbin MR, Kulkarni RG, Walls RM: The failed intubation attempt in the emergency department: analysis of prevalence, rescue techniques, and personnel. *J Emerg Med.* 2002;23:131–140.

62. Sloane C, Vilke GM, Chan TC, et al.: Rapid sequence intubation in the field versus trauma patients. *J Emerg Med.* 2000;19:259–264.

63. Pearson S: Comparison of intubation attempts and completion times before and after the initiation of a rapid sequence intubation protocol in an air medical transport program. *Air Med J.* 2003;22:28–33.

64. Ricard-Hibon A, Chollet C, Leroy C, Marty J: Succinylcholine improves the time of performance of a tracheal intubation in prehospital critical care medicine. *Eur J Anaesthesiol.* 2002;19:361–367.

65. Rocca B, Crosby E, Maloney J, Bryson G: An assessment of paramedic performance during invasive airway management. *Prehosp Emerg Care.* 2000;4:164–167.

66. Davis DP, Dunford JV, Poste JC, et al.: The impact of hypoxia and hyperventilation on outcome after paramedic rapid sequence intubation of severely head-injured patients. *J Trauma.* 2004;57:1–8.

67. Dunford JV, Davis DP, Ochs M, Doney M, Hoyt OB: Incidence of transient hypoxia and pulse rate reactivity during paramedic rapid sequence intubation. *Ann Emerg Med.* 2003;42:721–728.

68. Adnet F, Baillard C, Borron SW, et al.: Randomized study comparing the "sniffing position"@ with simple head extension for laryngoscopic view in elective surgery patients. *Anesthesiology.* 2001;95:836–841.

69. Gambee AM, Hertzka RE, Fisher DM: Preoxygenation techniques: comparison of three minutes and four breaths. *Anesth Analg.* 1987;66:468–470.

70. Stept WJ, Safar P: Rapid induction/intubation for prevention of gastric content aspiration. *Anesth Analg.* 1970;49:633–635.

71. Satiani B, Bonner JT, Stone H: Factors influencing intraoperative gastric regurgitation. A prospective random study of nasogastric tube drainage. *Arch Surg.* 1978;113:721–723.

72. Salem MR, Wong AY, Fizzotti GF: Efficacy of cricoid presure in preventing aspiration of gastric contents in paediatric patients. *Br J Anaesth.* 1972;44:401–404.

73. Sivilotti ML, Filbin MR, Murray HE, Slasor P, Walls RM: NEAR Investigators. Does the sedative agent facilitate emergency rapid sequence intubation? *Acad Emerg Med.* 2003;10:612–620.

74. Sivilotti ML, Ducharme J: Randomized, double-blind study on sedatives and hemodynamics during rapid-sequence intubation in the emergency department: The SHRED Study. *Ann Emerg Med.* 1998;31:313–324.

75. Davis DP, Kimbro TA, Vilke GM: The use of midazolam for prehospital rapid-sequence intubation may be associated with a dose-related increase in hypotension. *Prehosp Emerg Care.* 2001;5:163–168.

76. Adams P, Gelman S, Reves JG, et al.: Midazolam—pharmacodynamics and pharmacokinetics during acute hypovolemia. *Anesthesiology.* 1985;63:140–146.

77. Thomson MF, Brock-Utne JG, Bean P, et al.: Anesthesia and intraocular pressure; a comparison of total anaesthesia using etomidate with conventional inhalation anaesthesia. *Anaesthesia.* 1982;37:758–761.

78. Mirakhur RK, Elliot P, Sheperd WFI, et al.: Intra-ocular pressure changes during induction of anaesthesia and tracheal intubation: a comparison of thiopentone and propofol followed by vecuronium. *Anesthesia.* 1988;43:54–57.

79. Michenfelder JD, Milde JH, Sundi TM Jr: Cerebral protection by barbiturate anesthesia. *Arch Neurol.* 1976;33:345–350.

80. Hartung HJ: Intracranial pressure after propofol and thiopental administration in patients with severe head trauma. *Anaesthesist.* 1987;36:285–287.

81. Moss E, Powell D, Gibson RM, et al.: Effect of etomidate on intracranial pressure and cerebral perfusion pressure. *Br J Anaesth.* 1979;51:347–351.

82. McCollum JSC, Dundee JW: Comparison of induction characteristics of four intravenous anaesthetic agents. *Anaesthesia.* 1986;41:995–1000.

83. Giese JL, Stockham RJ, Stanley TH, Pace NL, Nelissen RH: Etomidate versus thiopental for induction of anesthesia. *Anesth Analg.* 1985;64:871–876.

84. Weiss-Bloom LJ, Reich DL: Haemodynamic responses to tracheal intubation following etomidate and fentanyl for anaesthetic induction. *Can J Anesth.* 1992;39:780–785.

85. Robinson N, Clancy M: In patients with head injury undergoing rapid sequence intubation, does pretreatment with intravenous lignocaine/lidocaine lead to an improved neurological outcome? A review of the literature. *Emerg Med J.* 2001;18:453–457.

86. El-Orbany MI, Joseph NJ, Salem MR, Kiowden AJ: The neuromuscular effects and tracheal intubation conditions after small doses of succinylcholine. *Anesth Analg.* 2004;98:1680–1685.

87. Naguib M, Samarkandi A, Riad W, Alharby SW: Optimal dose of succinylcholine revisited. *Anesthesiology.* 2003;99:1045–1049.

88. Andrews JI, Kumar N, van den Brom RH, et al.: A large simple randomized trial of rocuronium versus succinylcholine in rapid-sequence induction of anaesthesia along with propofol. *Acta Anaesthesiol Scand.* 1999;43:4–8.

89. Dobson AP, McCluskey A, Meakin G, Baker RD: Effective time to satisfactory intubation conditions after administration of rocuronium in adults. Comparison of propofol and thiopentone for rapid sequence induction of anaesthesia. *Anaesthesia.* 1999;54:172–176.

90. Skinner HJ, Biswas A, Mahajan RP: Evaluation of intubating conditions with rocuronium and either propofol or etomidate for rapid sequence induction. *Anaesthesia.* 1998;53:702–706.

91. Fuchs-Buder T, Sparr HJ, Ziegenfuss T: Thiopental or etomidate for rapid sequence induction with rocuronium. *Br J Anaesth.* 1998;80:504–506.

92. Salem MR, Sellick BA, Elam JO: The historical background of cricoid pressure in anesthesia and resuscitation. *Anesth Analg.* 1974;53:230–232.

93. Fammery AD, Roe PG: A model to describe the rate of oxyhemoglobin desaturation during apnoea. *Br J Anaesth.* 1996;76:284.

94. Hardman JG, Wills JS, Aitkenhead AR: Factors determining the onset and course of hypoxemia during apnea: an investigation using physiological modeling. *Anesth Analg.* 2000;90:619–624.

95. Lawes EG, Campbell I, Mercer D: Inflation pressure, gastric insufflation and rapid sequence induction. *Br J Anaesth.* 1987;59:315.

96. Ruben H, Krudsen EJ, Carngati G: Gastric inflation in relation to airway pressure. *Acta Anaesth Scand.* 1961;5:107.

97. Petito SP, Russell WJ: The prevention of gastric insufflation—a neglected benefit of cricoid pressure. *Anaesth Intensive care.* 1988;16:139–143.

98. Vanner RG, Pryle BJ: Nasogastric tubes and cricoid pressure. *Anaesthesia.* 1993;48:112–113.

99. Smith KJ, Ladak S, Choi PTL, Dobranowski J: The cricoid cartilage and the esophagus are not aligned in close to half of adult patients. *Can J Anesth.* 2002;49:503–507.

100. Smith KJ, Dobranowski J, Yip G, Dauphin A, Choi PT: Cricoid pressure displaces the esophagus: an observational study using magnetic resonance imaging. *Anesthesiology.* 2003;99:60–64.

101. Sellick BA: Rupture of the oesophagus following cricoid pressure? *Anaesthesia.* 1982;37:213–214.

102. Ralph SJ, Wareham CA: Rupture of the oesophagus during cricoid pressure. *Anaesthesia.* 1991;46:40–41.

103. Hein C, Owen H: The effective application of cricoid pressure. *J Emerg Prim Health Care.* 2005; 3(Issue 1–2).

104. Vanner RG, O'Dwyer JP, Pryle BJ, Reynolds F: Upper oesophageal sphincter pressure and the effect of cricoid pressure. *Anaesthesia.* 1992;47:95–100.

105. Wraight WJ, Chamney AR, Howells TH: The determination of an effective cricoid pressure. *Anaesthesia.* 1983;38:461–466.

106. Vanner RG, Pryle BJ: Regurgitation and oesophageal rupture with cricoid pressure: a cadaver study. *Anaesthesia.* 1992;47:732–735.

107. Meek T, Gitins N, Duggan JE: Cricoid pressure: knowledge and performance amongst anaesthetic assistants. *Anaesthesia.* 1999;54:59–62.

108. Meek T, Vincent A, Duggan JE: Cricoid pressure: can protective force be sustained? *Br J Anaesth.* 1998;80:672–674.

109. Crowley DS, Giesecke AH: Bimanual cricoid pressure. *Anaesthesia.* 1990;45:588–589.

110. Vanner RG, Clarke P, Moore WJ, Raftery S: The effect of cricoid pressure and neck support on the view at laryngoscopy. *Anaesthesia.* 1997;52:896–900.

111. Cook TM: Cricoid pressure: are two hands better than one? *Anaesthesia.* 1996;51:365–368.

112. Yentis SM: The effects of single-handed and bimanual cricoid pressure on the view at laryngoscopy. *Anaesthesia.* 1997;52:332–335.

113. Cook TM, Godfrey I, Rockett M, Vanner RG: Cricoid pressure: which hand? *Anaesthesia.* 2000;55:648–653.

114. Allman KG: The effect of cricoid pressure on airway patency. *J Clin Anesth.* 1995;7:197–199.

115. Moynihan RJ, Brock-Utne JG, Archer JH, Feld LH, Krietzman TR: The effect of cricoid pressure on preventing gastric insufflation in infants and children. *Anesthesiology.* 1993;78:652–656.

116. Vanner RG: Tolerance of cricoid pressure by conscious volunteers. *Int J Obstet Anesth.* 1992;1:195–198.

117. Hawthorne L, Wilson R, Lyons G, Dresener M: Failed intubation revisited: 17-yr experience in a teaching maternity unit. *Br J Anaesth.* 1996;76:680–684.

118. Lawes EG, Duncan PW, Bland B, Gemmel L, Downing JW: The cricoid yoke—a device for providing consistent and reproducible cricoid pressure. *Br J Anaesth.* 1986;58:925–931.

119. Hartsilver EL, Vanner RG: Airway obstruction with cricoid pressure. *Anaesthesia.* 2000;55:208–211.

120. Aoyama K, Takenaka I, Sata T, Shigematsu A: Cricoid pressure impedes positioning and ventilation through the laryngeal mask airway. *Can J Anaesth.* 1996;43:1035–1040.

121. Asai T, Barcaly K, McBeth C, Vaughan RS: Cricoid pressure applied after placement of the laryngeal mask prevents gastric insufflation but inhibits ventilation. *Br J Anaesth.* 1996;76:772–776.

122. MacG Palmer JH, Ball DR: The effect of cricoid pressure on the cricoid cartilage and vocal cords: an endoscopic study in anaesthetised patients. *Anaesthesia.* 2000;55:263–268.

123. Smith CE, Boyer D: Cricoid pressure decreases ease of tracheal intubation using fibreoptic laryngoscopy. *Can J Anesth.* 2002;49:614–619.

124. Hodgson RE, Gopalan PD, Burrows RC, Zuma K: Effect of cricoid pressure on the success of endotracheal intubation with a lightwand. *Anesthesiology.* 2001;94:259–262.

125. Shulman GB, Connelly NR: A comparison of the Bullard Laryngoscope versus the flexible fiberoptic bronchoscope during intubation in patients afforded in-line stabilization. *J Clin Anesth.* 2001;13:182–185.

126. Gabbott DA: The effect of single-handed cricoid pressure on neck movement after applying manual in-line stabilisation. *Anaesthesia.* 1997;52:586–588.

127. Helliwell V, Gabbott DA: The effect of single-handed cricoid pressure on cervical spine movement after applying manual in-line stabilisation—a cadaver study. *Resuscitation.* 2001;49:53–57.

128. Wood PR: Direct laryngoscopy and cervical spine stabilization. *Anaesthesia.* 1994;49:77–78.

129. Roux M, Drolet P, Girard M, Grenier Y, Petit B: Effect of the laryngeal mask airway on oesophageal pH: influence of the volume and pressure inside the cuff. *Br J Anaesth.* 1999;82:566–569.

130. Joshi GP, Morrison SG, Okonwo NA, White PF: Continuous hypopharyngeal pH measurements in spontaneously breathing anesthetized outpatients: laryngeal mask airway versus tracheal intubation. *Anesth Analg.* 1996;82:254–257.

131. Ho BY, Skinner HJ, Mahajan RP: Gastro-esophageal reflux during day case gynaecological laparoscopy under positive pressure ventilation: laryngeal mask vs. tracheal intubation. *Anaesthesia.* 1998;53:921–924.

132. Hagberg CA, Vartazarian TN, Chelly JE, Ovassapian A: The incidence of gastroesophageal reflux and tracheal aspiration detected with pH electrodes is similar with the Laryngeal Mask Airway and Esophageal Tracheal Combitube—a pilot study. *Can J Anaesth.* 2004;51:243–249.

133. McCrory CR, McShane AJ: Gastroesophageal reflux during spontaneous respiration with the laryngeal mask airway. *Can J Anaesth.* 1999;46:268–270.

134. Cheong YP, Park SK, Son Y, et al.: Comparison of incidence of gastroesophageal reflux and regurgitation associated with timing of removal of the laryngeal mask airway: on appearance of signs of rejection versus after recovery of consciousness. *J Clin Anesth.* 1999;11:657–662.

135. Evans NR, Gardner SV, James MF: ProSeal laryngeal mask protects against aspiration of fluid in the pharynx. *Br J Anaesth.* 2002;88:584–587.

136. Verghese C, Brimacombe JR: Survey of laryngeal mask airway usage in 11910 patients: safety and efficacy for conventional and non-conventional usage. *Anesth Analg.* 1996;82:129–133.

137. Brimacombe JR, Berry A: The incidence of aspiration associated with the laryngeal mask airway: a meta-analysis of published literature. *J Clin Anesth.* 1995;7:297–305.

138. Keller C, Brimacombe J, Bittershol J, Lirk P, von Goedecke A: Aspiration and the laryngeal mask airway: three cases and a review of the literature. *Br J Anaesth.* 2004;93:579–582.

139. Hung OR, Pytka S, Morris I, et al.: Clinical Trial of a New Lightwand Device (Trachlight) to Intubate the Trachea. *Anesthesiology.* 1995;83:509–514.

140. Hung OR, Pytka S, Morris I, Murphy M, Stewart RD. Lightwand intubation: II-Clinical trial of a new lightwand for tracheal intubation in patients with difficult airways. *Can J Anaesth.* 1995;42:826–830.

141. Bourke DL, Katz J, Tonneson A: Nebulized anesthesia for awake endotracheal intubation. *Anesthesiology.* 1985;63:690–692.

142. Ovassapian A, Krejcie TC, Yelich SJ, Dykes MH: Awake fiberoptic intubation in the patient at high risk of aspiration. *Br J Anaesth.* 1989;62:13–16.

143. Simmons ST, Schleich AR: Airway regional anesthesia for awake fiberoptic intubation. *Reg Anesth Pain Med.* 2002;27: 180–192.

144. Walsh ME, Shorten GD: Preparing to perform an awake fiberoptic intubation. *Yale J Biol Med.* 1998;71:537–549.

145. Benumof JL: Management of the difficult adult airway. *Anesthesiology.* 1991;75:1087–1107.

146. McCormick PW: Immediate care after aspiration of vomit. *Anaesthesia.* 1975;30:658–665.

147. Wynne JW, Modell JH: Respiratory aspiration of stomach contents. *Ann Intern Med.* 1977;87:466–474.

148. Lee M, Sukumaran M, Berger HW, Reilly TA: Influence of corticosteroid treatment on pulmonary function after recovery from aspiration of gastric contents. *Mt Sinai J Med.* 1980;47:341–346.

149. Sukumaran M, Granada MJ, Berger HW, Lee M, Reilly TA: Evaluation of corticosteroid treatment in aspiration of gastric contents: a controlled clinical trial. *Mt Sinai J Med.* 1980;47:335–340.

150. Wolfe JE, Bone RC, Ruth WE: Effects of corticosteroids in the treatment to patients with gastric aspiration. *Am J Med.* 1977;63:719–722.

151. Bone RC, Fisher CJ Jr., Clemmer TP, et al.: A controlled clinical trial of high-dose methylprednisolone in the treatment of severe sepsis and shock. *N Eng J Med.* 1987;317:653–658.

152. Johnson JL, Hirsch CS. Aspiration pneumonia. *Postgrad Med.* 2003; 113:99–102, 105–106, 111–112.

153. El-Solh AA, Pietrantoni C, Bhat A, et al.: Microbiology of severe aspiration pneumonia in institutionalized elderly. *Am J Respir Crit Care Med.* 2003;167:1650–1654.

154. Niederman MS, Bass JB Jr., Campbell GD, et al.: Guidelines for the initial management of adults with community-acquired pneumonia: diagnosis, assessment of severity, and initial antimicrobial therapy. American Thoracic Society. Medical Section of the American Lung Association. *Am Rev Respir Dis.* 1993;148:1418–1426.

155. Bernstein JM: Treatment of community-acquired pneumonia—IDSA Guidelines. *Chest.* 1999;115:98–138.

156. Mandell LA, Marrie TJ, Grossman RF, Chow AW, Hyland RH: Canadian guidelines for the initial management of community-acquired pneumonia: an evidence-based update by the Canadian Infectious Diseases Society and the Canadian Thoracic Society. The Canadian Community-Acquired Pneumonia Working Group. *Clin Infect Dis.* 2000;31:383–421.

SELF-EVALUATION QUESTIONS

5.1. How much cricoid pressure has been shown to prevent gastric regurgitation?

A. 10 N

B. 20 N

C. 30 N

D. 40 N

E. 50 N

5.2. Which of the following is **NOT** true about cricoid pressure and airway techniques?

A. The difficulty in ventilation using the LMA is dependent on the amount of pressure applied.

B. Cricoid pressure reduces the incidence of gastric insufflation when using a LMA.

C. Improper LMA placement can occur when cricoid pressure is applied.

D. Ventilation via a facemask has not been shown to be affected by cricoid pressure.

E. Tracheal intubation using a rigid fiberoptic laryngoscope (e.g., WuScope System™) is more difficult to perform when cricoid pressure is applied.

5.3. Which of the following is **NOT** a known factor that increases the risk of aspiration?

A. Emergency surgery

B. Timing of surgery

C. Lack of fasting

D. Pregnant patients

E. Children

SECTION 2

Devices and Techniques for Difficult and Failed Airway Management

CHAPTER (6)

Airway Devices and Techniques

Michael F. Murphy and Orlando R. Hung

6.1 INTRODUCTION

Fundamental to airway management is the maintenance of adequate oxygenation and ventilation, and protection of the airway from the aspiration of foreign substances. Though this may be achieved in a variety of ways, the primary method is by orotracheal intubation employing a conventional laryngoscope.

6.1.1 Why is there such continuing emphasis on the difficult and failed airway?

The answer to this question is easy: death, disability, liability, and money.

Practitioners consistently fail to recognize a "difficult airway." Simple evaluation maneuvers can identify a difficult airway and prevent intubation failure. Previously, if three attempts at direct laryngoscopy were unsuccessful, a "failed airway" existed. The definition of a "failed airway" now, however, includes the inability to maintain acceptable oxygenation. In other words, if at any time during the airway management sequence oxygen saturations cannot be maintained with whatever device one chooses, regardless of the number of attempts at tracheal intubation, a failed airway has occurred. The airway practitioner is then obliged to switch from a "difficult airway" management pathway to a "failed airway" management pathway. The finding that extraglottic devices (EGDs) are often effective in permitting ventilation and oxygenation in "can't intubate, can't ventilate" (CICV) situations has re-emphasized the fundamental goals of airway management: gas exchange and in particular, oxygenation.[1–4]

6.1.2 I have always been told that if I failed on the first attempt at orotracheal intubation, I should change something before the next attempt. What "something" can I change?

Achieving the best view of the glottis employing conventional laryngoscopy results from the interplay of *six* factors[3,5]:

- The skill set of the individual performing the intubation. All authorities recommend that at the moment one recognizes that difficulty or failure is encountered help should be summoned.[6–8]
- Position of the head and neck. The "sniffing the morning air" or "sipping English tea" position has been enshrined as the best position for visualization of the glottic opening using a conventional straight or curve blade laryngoscope, though there has been some controversy in this regard.[9–12] Regardless of the controversy, most would agree that the "sniffing position" is the best position for direct-vision laryngoscopic intubation.[13–15] There is also evidence to suggest that an exaggerated sniffing position with the use of a ramp is particularly useful in obese patients (see Chapter 17).[16]
- Degree of induced neuromuscular block. It is well known that inadequate muscle relaxation can lead to difficult laryngoscopic visualization of the larynx. This serves to crystallize the dilemma as to whether or not neuromuscular blockade should be employed in the face of a potentially difficult airway.
- Optimum laryngeal manipulation. Often called "optimal external laryngeal manipulation" (OELM) or "backward upward rightward pressure" (BURP), this maneuver is distinct from Sellick's maneuver.[14,17,18]

- Length of laryngoscope blade.
- Design of the laryngoscope blade.

6.1.3 How many ways are there to steer an endotracheal tube into the trachea and to get some idea immediately that I am in the right spot?

Visualizing the endotracheal tube passing through the glottis into the trachea is not the only way to verify intratracheal placement (e.g., confirmation by end tidal carbon dioxide detection), but it is the one most commonly used. There are four broad categories of methods that are used to "steer" an endotracheal tube into the trachea:

1. Direct vision of the glottic opening using a conventional laryngoscope,

2. Indirect vision using fiberoptic or video techniques as with rigid and flexible fiberoptic scopes, and video laryngoscopes employing camera technology,

3. Inferential methods
   a. visually identified transillumination as with a lighted stylet (e.g., Trachlight™) or a fiberoptic device
   b. hearing and feeling the movement of air as the tube enters the trachea such as with "blind" nasotracheal intubation in spontaneously breathing patients
   c. feeling for upper-airway structures with the fingers and guiding the endotracheal tube into the trachea (tactile digital intubation)

4. Blind intubation—simply inserting an endotracheal tube through the mouth, an intubating EGD, or the nose, in the hope that it will find its way into the trachea.

6.2 INNOVATION AND SKILL

Innovation over the past 15 years in the field of airway management has led to the proliferation of new and improved techniques and devices, particularly EGDs and fiberoptic/camera technologies. These innovations are driven by several forces:

- the inherent technical difficulty associated with bag-mask-ventilation (BMV)
- the opportunity and the convenience of being able to free hands from holding a mask on a spontaneously breathing, nonintubated, anesthetized patient in and out of the operating room, such as in the MRI unit or during transport
- the need for options to solve the problems posed by the difficult airway
- the need for options to manage the failed airway

Over this same period of time,

- aspiration has become less feared,
- substantial clinical evidence demonstrating the efficacy and safety of these EGDs has become available,

- EGDs and endotracheal intubation are supplanting BMV by basic and advanced emergency health care providers,
- growing familiarity of airway practitioners in general with the use of these devices, particularly practitioners in anesthesia.

6.2.1 With all of these new devices and techniques, what is happening to the old standbys: BMV and orotracheal intubation?

The introduction of these new techniques has had a measurable and predictable effect on perishable, difficult to master skills such as BMV and orotracheal intubation, from both a teaching perspective and in one's ability to maintain facility with conventional techniques.[19–21] Student practitioners of airway management, whether EMTs, first responders, or anesthesia providers, appear to have increasing difficulty in achieving proficiency in mask sealing and maintaining an open airway, both of which are essential for adequate BMV.[22] Completing their training programs with, at best, marginal skills, they now have difficulty maintaining them.[23–25]

The increasing use of an EGD in place of endotracheal intubation in elective surgical patients has led to practitioners being less able to achieve and retain the skill of endotracheal intubation, as described above for BVM.

6.2.2 What other technological advances have provided new tools for managing airways?

Technological advances over the past two decades have dramatically improved the clinical utility of many airway devices, including

1. Enhanced light intensity of some airway instruments. For example, the transillumination or light-guided technique is substantially improved with the introduction of high-intensity bulbs in lightwands such as the Trachlight™. Adequate transillumination is usually possible under ambient indoor lighting conditions obviating the need to dim the light or darken the environment during the procedure. In fact, a large clinical study involving 950 patients showed that nearly 88% of intubations using the Trachlight™ could be effectively performed under ambient light with or without shading of the neck.[26]

2. Recent advances in the technology of video resolution and color fidelity, coupled with improved video display, have permitted the development of improved video camera and fiberoptic instruments. These include the Video Macintosh Intubating Laryngoscope System (VMS, K. Storz Endoscopy Co., Culver City, CA), the Glidescope®, and the LMA CTrach™. There is some evidence that devices with small diameters and when coupled with improved optics result in a substantial improvement over the last decade, particularly in pediatrics.[27]

3. Portability factors. Technological advances have made it possible to make airway devices more portable, lightweight, and robust in construction. For example, lightweight battery powered fiberoptic bronchoscopes, making it possible to carry this equipment to the bedside without additional equipment such as an external power source.

6.3   DEVICES AND TECHNIQUES

6.3.1   How many airway management devices or techniques should I be proficient in using?

While it is impossible, and perhaps impractical, to be proficient in using all of the available airway devices or techniques, individuals called upon to manage airways need to be proficient in at least BMV, the use of an EGD, oral and nasal intubation, and cricothyrotomy. In certain instances, particularly in children below the age of 8 to 10 where the cricothyroid space is small or nonexistent and cricothyrotomy is relatively contraindicated, one ought to be able to perform some form of transtracheal ventilation.

Increasingly, at least in a hospital setting, practitioners are expected to be proficient in using more technically sophisticated airway equipment, such as fiberoptic and camera-based devices. Though this is particularly so for anesthesia practitioners,[28,29] there is a growing body of literature suggesting that nonanesthesia airway practitioners may need to acquire these skills as well.[30–34]

6.3.2   Are intubating stylets rescue devices?

No. The Eschmann Introducer (EI, also known as the "gum elastic bougie"), the Frova Catheter (Cook Critical Care), and other related intubation aids are as routine to airway management as a laryngoscope. Specifically designed to facilitate intubation for the Cormack/Lehane (C/L) Grade 3 view, these devices have been shown to facilitate laryngoscopic intubation when conventional methods have failed.[35–37]

6.3.3   What EGDs should I incorporate into my practice?

The existing literature supports the use of the laryngeal mask airway (LMA) and the Combitube™ in providing effective ventilation and oxygenation.[6,7,38–43] The intubating LMA (Fastrach™, reusable and disposable varieties) are particularly useful in the failed airway. Although a myriad of other EGDs have been introduced over the last several years, it remains unclear whether their success rates approach those of the LMA and the Combitube™.

Although the role of EGDs in routine airway management has been well established, these devices cannot replace an endotracheal tube in some situations, particularly in those patients at high risk for aspiration or those requiring high ventilation pressures. During the last several years, the Intubating LMA (LMA Fastrach™) has emerged as a particularly useful rescue device conferring the ability to ventilate coupled with the ability to serve as a conduit for tracheal intubation either blindly or with the assistance of a lightwand or fiberoptic bronchoscope.[44,45]

The Cook ILA (Mercury Medical) also permits intubation, though the lack of a "handle" as with the LMA Fastrach™ may limit its effectiveness in the "failed airway" situation. Employing similar logic and design as the Combitube™ is the King LT Airway (King Systems). Personal experience with this device suggests that it has an advantage over the Combitube™ in that it is easier to insert and appears to be equally effective.

Finally, among the disposable, nonintubating laryngeal mask/EGDs currently on the market, the Ambu LMA (Ambu USA) demonstrates superior insertion and seal characteristics that may make it superior to other similar devices.

6.3.4   What is the best way to confirm placement of an endotracheal tube in the trachea?

Flexible fiberoptic bronchoscopy remains the "gold standard" of verifying correct endotracheal tube placement by permitting indirect visualization of tracheal rings.[46] Visualization of the endotracheal tube entering the larynx also provides a highly reliable method of verifying intratracheal placement.

Detection of exhaled carbon dioxide provides reliable evidence of tracheal rather than esophageal intubation and represents the current standard of care.[47,48] In patients with intact circulation, carbon dioxide detection is a highly reliable indicator of correct placement 99%–100% of the time.[49–51] Soft drinks in the stomach containing carbon dioxide may mimic the exhaled carbon dioxide from the lungs for several breaths, the so-called "Cola-complication," though this confounding result ought not to persist beyond six breaths.[52]

The migration of an endotracheal tube from the trachea to the esophagus is an ever-present hazard during the tosses and turns of transport. It has been demonstrated that the continuous monitoring of exhaled carbon dioxide during the prehospital phase of care minimizes the risk of such displacement going unrecognized.[53,54]

As might be expected in patients with circulatory arrest, carbon dioxide detection techniques tend to be less accurate in identifying correct placement of the endotracheal tube, with reported false negative rates (carbon dioxide not detected, tube in the trachea) as high as 30%–35%.[51] In this circumstance, the endotracheal placement of the tube can be evaluated by an "esophageal detector device" that consists of a self-inflating suction bulb or syringe armed with an adapter to fit a standard endotracheal tube connector (see Figure 13–1). The collapsed bulb or syringe rapidly fills with air if the endotracheal tube is in the trachea; it does not inflate if the tube is in the esophagus. It has a specificity rate of about 99%.[55] Use of this device *instead of* carbon dioxide detection is not recommended due to its failure to detect esophageal intubation as often as 20% of the time.[56]

Physical examination techniques used to confirm intratracheal placement of an endotracheal tube, while neither sensitive nor specific, remain important adjuncts to more elaborate techniques, particularly in the patient suffering a cardiopulmonary arrest. Auscultation of the chest for breath sounds and of the epigastrium for absence of air entry into the stomach, and observation of chest motion during ventilation and condensation inside the endotracheal tube during extubation are common but notoriously unreliable methods of ascertaining proper endotracheal tube placement.[54]

In summary, although carbon dioxide detection remains the most reliable method of confirming correct tracheal placement, the combination of several methods of confirmation is superior to any single method.

6.4   TRAINING AND EDUCATION

6.4.1   How do I become proficient with these devices and techniques?

Effective airway management demands that the practitioner be proficient not just in "Plan A" but "Plans B, C, and D" as well. In other words, one must approach every airway management situation armed with several options for establishing and maintaining ventilation and oxygenation, and must become comfortable with and adept at several techniques.

Airway management workshops that present an array of devices and techniques are conducted worldwide. Most have well defined learning objectives that focus on varying clinical approaches, devices, and techniques and use both manikin and animal models to enhance technical and cognitive learning. It is incumbent on the learner to identify those alternative techniques (Plan "B," "C," etc.), which they will employ in the event Plan "A" fails and integrate these techniques into their daily practice to maintain skill levels.

Mulcaster et al. reported that, after training on a manikin, considerable experience in intubating the trachea of live patients is required before a trainee becomes proficient in laryngoscopic intubation.[57] Their model demonstrated that 47 patient intubations were necessary to achieve proficiency in laryngoscopic intubation. These findings serve to counter the notion that airway management training using standard manikins alone is adequate.

6.4.2   What is the role of airway simulators in teaching airway management?

In an ideal world, all airway practitioners would be adequately trained in the expert use of an array of airway devices. For many practitioners, the cost-effectiveness of "adequate" training is an important consideration. If training takes too long and is too expensive, few may opt for it. This is particularly true in training airway practitioners to deal with relatively uncommon events, such as the "difficult" and "failed" airway.

However, there is hope on the horizon. The use of high-fidelity human patient simulators, coupled with the evolution of simulation experts, has been shown to be effective in teaching some aspects of airway management.[58-60]

6.5   SUMMARY

Airway management is a constant challenge for the practitioner. BMV and endotracheal intubation skills are difficult to master let alone maintain. The increase in awareness of *difficult airway* and its associated adverse events has led to the search for alternative solutions to management of this clinical problem, such as EGDs and enhanced indirect vision techniques. Cricothyrotomy is an essential airway management skill that all airway practitioners must be able to perform and be willing to carry out in the setting of a CICV failed airway.

All practitioners need to approach every airway management episode with a Plan "A" and at least two backup plans should cascading failure ensue. This suggests that all airway practitioners ought to have facility with BMV, laryngoscopy and intubation, cricothyrotomy, a CICV alternative device (e.g., Trachlight™, rigid or flexible fiberoptic scopes, etc.), and a CICV device (e.g., Fastrach™, Combitube™, King LT) that can be employed while setting up for a cricothyrotomy.

REFERENCES

1. Benumof JL: Laryngeal mask airway and the ASA difficult airway algorithm. *Anesthesiology*. 1996;84:686–699.
2. Ezri T, Szmuk P, Warters RD, Katz J, Hagberg CA: Difficult airway management practice patterns among anesthesiologists practicing in the United States: have we made any progress? *J Clin Anesth*. 2003;15:418–422.
3. Benumof J: The ASA difficult airway algorithm: new thoughts and considerations. Fifty-first Annual Refresher Course Lectures and Clinical Update Program, #235. American Society of Anesthesiologists, 2000.
4. Parmet JL, Colonna-Romano P, Horrow JC, et al.: The laryngeal mask airway reliably provides rescue ventilation in cases of unanticipated difficult tracheal intubation along with difficult mask ventilation. *Anesth Analg*. 1998;87: 661–665.
5. Benumof JL: Difficult laryngoscopy: obtaining the best view. *Can J Anaesth*. 1994;41:361–365.
6. Walls R: The emergency airway algorithms. In: *Manual of Emergency Airway Management*. Walls R, Murphy M, Luten R, et al., eds. Philadelphia, PA: Lippincott Williams and Wilkins, 2004:8–21.
7. Practice guidelines for management of the difficult airway: an updated report by the American Society of Anesthesiologists Task Force on Management of the Difficult Airway. *Anesthesiology*. 2003;98:1269–1277.
8. Practice guidelines for management of the difficult airway. A report by the American Society of Anesthesiologists Task Force on Management of the Difficult Airway. *Anesthesiology*. 1993;78:597–602.
9. Adnet F, Baillard C, Borron SW, et al.: Randomized study comparing the "sniffing position" with simple head extension for laryngoscopic view in elective surgery patients. *Anesthesiology*. 2001;95:836–841.
10. Adnet F, Borron SW, Dumas JL, et al.: Study of the "sniffing position" by magnetic resonance imaging. *Anesthesiology*. 2001;94:83–86.
11. Adnet F, Borron SW, Lapostolle F, Lapandry C: The three axis alignment theory and the "sniffing position": perpetuation of an anatomic myth? *Anesthesiology*. 1999;91:1964–1965.
12. Adnet F, Lapostolle F, Borron SW, et al.: Optimization of glottic exposure during intubation of a patient lying supine on the ground. *Am J Emerg Med*. 1997; 15:555–557.
13. Levitan RM, Mechem CC, Ochroch EA, Shofer FS, Hollander JE: Head-elevated laryngoscopy position: improving laryngeal exposure during laryngoscopy by increasing head elevation. *Ann Emerg Med*. 2003;41:322–330.
14. Schneider R, Murphy M: Bag mask ventilation and endotracheal intubation. In: *Manual of Emergency Airway Management*. Walls R, Murphy M, Luten R, et al., eds. Philadelphia, PA: Lippincott Williams and Wilkins, 2004:43–69.
15. Murphy MF: Bringing the larynx into view: a piece of the puzzle. *Ann Emerg Med*. 2003;41:338–341.
16. Collins JS, Lemmens HJ, Brodsky JB, Brock-Utne JG, Levitan RM: Laryngoscopy and morbid obesity: a comparison of the "sniff" and "ramped" positions. *Obes Surg*. 2004;14:1171–1175.
17. Knill RL: Difficult laryngoscopy made easy with a "BURP". *Can J Anaesth*. 1993;40:279–282.
18. Benumof JL, Cooper SD: Quantitative improvement in laryngoscopic view by optimal external laryngeal manipulation. *J Clin Anesth*. 1996;8:136–140.
19. Chamberlain D, Smith A, Woollard M, et al.: Trials of teaching methods in basic life support (3): comparison of simulated CPR performance after first training and at 6 months, with a note on the value of re-training. *Resuscitation*. 2002;53:179–187.
20. Kovacs G, Bullock G, Ackroyd-Stolarz S, Cain E, Petrie D: A randomized controlled trial on the effect of educational interventions in promoting airway management skill maintenance. *Ann Emerg Med*. 2000;36:301–309.
21. Zautcke JL, Lee RW, Ethington NA: Paramedic skill decay. *J Emerg Med*. 1987;5:505–512.

22. Alexander R, Hodgson P, Lomax D, Bullen C: A comparison of the laryngeal mask airway and Guedel airway, bag and facemask for manual ventilation following formal training. *Anaesthesia.* 1993;48:231–234.

23. Burton JH, Baumann MR, Maoz T, Bradshaw JR, Lebrun JE: Endotracheal intubation in a rural EMS state: procedure utilization and impact of skills maintenance guidelines. *Prehosp Emerg Care.* 2003;7:352–356.

24. Nelson MS: Medical student retention of intubation skills. *Ann Emerg Med.* 1989;18:1059–1061.

25. Jez W, Rutkowski B, Cieslawski J: Training phantoms for endotracheal intubation. *Pol Tyg Lek.* 1966;21:593–594.

26. Hung OR, Pytka S, Morris I, et al.: Clinical trial of a new lightwand device (Trachlight) to intubate the trachea. *Anesthesiology.* 1995;83:509–514.

27. Schellhase DE: Pediatric flexible airway endoscopy. *Curr Opin Pediatr.* 2002; 14:327–333.

28. Rosenblatt WH, Wagner PJ, Ovassapian A, Kain ZN: Practice patterns in managing the difficult airway by anesthesiologists in the United States. *Anesth Analg.* 1998;87:153–157.

29. Ovassapian A: The flexible bronchoscope. A tool for anesthesiologists. *Clin Chest Med.* 2001;22:281–299.

30. Afilalo M, Guttman A, Stern E, et al.: Fiberoptic intubation in the emergency department: a case series. *J Emerg Med.* 1993;11:387–391.

31. Ovassapian A, Randel GI: The role of the fiberscope in the critically ill patient. *Crit Care Clin.* 1995;11:29–51.

32. Levitan RM, Kush S, Hollander JE: Devices for difficult airway management in academic emergency departments: results of a national survey. *Ann Emerg Med.* 1999;33:694–698.

33. Delaney KA, Hessler R: Emergency flexible fiberoptic nasotracheal intubation: a report of 60 cases. *Ann Emerg Med.* 1988;17:919–926.

34. Bauer PC, Heye M, Kottmann R: Importance of fiberoptic bronchoscopy in emergency medicine. *Internist (Berl).* 1983;24:89–94.

35. Phelan MP, Moscati R, D'Aprix T, Miller G: Paramedic use of the endotracheal tube introducer in a difficult airway model. *Prehosp Emerg Care.* 2003;7:244–246.

36. Murphy MF, Walls RM: Endotracheal tube introducer. *Ann Emerg Med.* 2001; 37:361–362.

37. Frova G: Role of the long stylet in difficult intubations. *Rev Med Suisse Romande.* 1999;119:903–906.

38. Ferson DZ, Rosenblatt WH, Johansen MJ, Osborn I, Ovassapian A: Use of the intubating LMA-Fastrach in 254 patients with difficult-to-manage airways. *Anesthesiology.* 2001;95:1175–1181.

39. Crosby ET, Cooper RM, Douglas MJ, et al.: The unanticipated difficult airway with recommendations for management. *Can J Anaesth.* 1998;45: 757–776.

40. Rumball CJ, MacDonald D: The PTL, Combitube, laryngeal mask, and oral airway: a randomized prehospital comparative study of ventilatory device effectiveness and cost-effectiveness in 470 cases of cardiorespiratory arrest. *Prehosp Emerg Care.* 1997;1:1–10.

41. Levitan RM, Frass M: The Combitube as rescue device: recommended use of the small adult size for all patients six feet tall or shorter. *Ann Emerg Med.* 2004;44:92–93.

42. Agro F, Frass M, Benumof J, et al.: The esophageal tracheal combitube as a non-invasive alternative to endotracheal intubation. A review. *Minerva Anestesiol.* 2001;67:863–874.

43. Agro F, Frass M, Benumof JL, Krafft P: Current status of the Combitube: a review of the literature. *J Clin Anesth.* 2002;14:307–314.

44. Fan KH, Hung OR, Agro F: A comparative study of tracheal intubation using an intubating laryngeal mask (Fastrach) alone or together with a lightwand (Trachlight). *J Clin Anesth.* 2000;12:581–585.

45. Henderson JJ, Popat MT, Latto IP, Pearce AC: Difficult Airway Society guidelines for management of the unanticipated difficult intubation. *Anaesthesia.* 2004;59:675–694.

46. Grmec S: Comparison of three different methods to confirm tracheal tube placement in emergency intubation. *Intensive Care Med.* 2002;28: 701–704.

47. Li J: Capnography alone is imperfect for endotracheal tube placement confirmation during emergency intubation. *J Emerg Med.* 2001;20:223–229.

48. Dykes MH, Ovassapian A: Dissemination of fibreoptic airway endoscopy skills by means of a workshop utilizing models. *Br J Anaesth.* 1989;63:595–597.

49. Erasmus PD: The use of end-tidal carbon dioxide monitoring to confirm endotracheal tube placement in adult and paediatric intensive care units in Australia and New Zealand. *Anaesth Intensive Care.* 2004;32:672–675.

50. Goldberg JS, Rawle PR, Zehnder JL, Sladen RN: Colorimetric end-tidal carbon dioxide monitoring for tracheal intubation. *Anesth Analg.* 1990;70: 191–194.

51. MacLeod BA, Heller MB, Gerard J, Yealy DM, Menegazzi JJ: Verification of endotracheal tube placement with colorimetric end-tidal CO2 detection. *Ann Emerg Med.* 1991;20:267–270.

52. Zbinden S, Schupfer G: Detection of oesophageal intubation: the cola complication. *Anaesthesia.* 1989; 44: 81.

53. Bledsoe BE, Eckstein M, Gandy WE, Katz SH, Silvestri S: The misplaced endotracheal tube? *JEMS* 2004;29:36–38; discussion 38–50.

54. Katz SH, Falk JL: Misplaced endotracheal tubes by paramedics in an urban emergency medical services system. *Ann Emerg Med.* 2001;37:32–37.

55. Wee MY: The oesophageal detector device. Assessment of a new method to distinguish oesophageal from tracheal intubation. *Anaesthesia.* 1988;43: 27–29.

56. Hendey GW, Shubert GS, Shalit M, Hogue B: The esophageal detector bulb in the aeromedical setting. *J Emerg Med.* 2002;23:51–55.

57. Mulcaster JT, Mills J, Hung OR, et al.: Laryngoscopic intubation: learning and performance. *Anesthesiology.* 2003;98:23–27.

58. Owen H, Plummer JL: Improving learning of a clinical skill: the first year's experience of teaching endotracheal intubation in a clinical simulation facility. *Med Educ.* 2002;36:635–642.

59. Parry K, Owen H: Small simulators for teaching procedural skills in a difficult airway algorithm. *Anaesth Intensive Care.* 2004;32:401–409.

60. Rosenthal E, Owen H: An assessment of small simulators used to teach basic airway management. *Anaesth Intensive Care.* 2004;32:87–92.

SELF-EVALUATION QUESTIONS

6.1. Based on the information available, how many tracheal intubations in patients one ought to perform before one can achieve the proficiency in laryngoscopic intubation?

A. 10

B. 20

C. 30

D. 40

E. 50

6.2. Which of the following methods is the **LEAST** reliable to confirm the placement of an endotracheal tube in the trachea?

A. exhaled carbon dioxide

B. esophageal detector device

C. observation of chest motion during ventilation

D. visualization of the endotracheal tube passing through the vocal cords

E. flexible fiberoptic bronchoscopy

6.3. Which of the following factors is **NOT** known to improve the view of the glottis during conventional direct laryngoscopy?

A. the skill set of the individual performing the intubation

B. sniffing position of the head and neck

C. the Sellick maneuver

D. length of laryngoscope blade

E. optimum laryngeal manipulation

CHAPTER (7)

Direct Laryngoscopy and Oral Intubation of the Trachea

John J. Henderson

7.1 HISTORY

7.1.1 When was tracheal intubation first used to provide an airway in anesthesia and what technique was used? What pharmacological technique was used?

The first use of tracheal intubation as a dedicated airway in anesthesia was by William Macewen (Glasgow) in 1878,[1] on a patient with cancer of the base of the tongue. The standard airway management for oral surgery at that time was tracheotomy with a cuffed tube. Macewen's intubation predated the first report of the local anesthetic properties of cocaine in 1884.[2] Macewen gained experience on cadavers and then practiced tracheal intubation, on awake subjects, on several occasions before the day of surgery. He used his fingers to guide a metal tube into the trachea, and then packed the pharynx. It is impossible nowadays to comprehend the fortitude of both the patient and the surgeon.

On the day of the surgery, chloroform anesthesia was administered after tracheal intubation had been achieved. Anesthesia and surgery went well, with a good outcome. A secure airway had been achieved and tracheotomy avoided.

7.1.2 Who first performed tracheal intubation under vision, and what equipment was used?

The first direct laryngoscopy, described by Kirstein[3] in 1895, used a straight blade. The original technique of laryngoscopy involved passing the tip of the laryngoscope posterior to the epiglottis, which was then elevated directly to expose the vocal cords. Diagnostic and therapeutic laryngoscopy developed rapidly with leading figures, including Killian in Germany and Jackson in the United States. Elsberg (New York) had been using tracheal intubation for anesthesia but had found the digital technique of Macewen impossible in large patients. In 1910,[4] he described the use of the Killian and Jackson straight laryngoscopes to perform tracheal intubation under vision in patients undergoing thoracic and general surgery. Tracheal intubation under vision was now practical and many centers soon reported large series.[5]

7.1.3 How did the technique of direct laryngoscopy for tracheal intubation develop in subsequent decades?

Jackson[6] stated that the head must be placed on a pillow, but in full extension, and that the tip of the laryngoscope should be placed sufficiently beyond the tip of the epiglottis such that the latter would not slip into the field of vision. He postulated that the epiglottis must be identified for successful intubation, cautioned against using the teeth as a fulcrum, and emphasized that the force applied to the laryngoscope was designed to lift the hyoid and epiglottis.[7] He recommended inserting the laryngoscope from the right side of the tongue, i.e., passage along the paraglossal gutter, when a tracheal tube was passed.

Magill[8] also recommended passage of the laryngoscope along the paraglossal gutter. He further suggested that, when laryngoscopy proved difficult, the proximal end of the laryngoscope should be positioned as lateral as possible in the mouth.[9] Bonfils later described this technique as "retromolar",[10] but this term is misleading as the laryngoscope is almost never passed posterior to the molar teeth. The key feature of the techniques suggested by Magill, and Bonfils, is the passage of the laryngoscope along the paraglossal gutter, a position which facilitates optimum lateral displacement of the entire tongue. "Paraglossal" is a more accurate description for this technique.[11]

7.1.4 When did Macintosh describe his curved laryngoscope and what differentiated it from previous designs?

The Macintosh curved laryngoscope was described in 1943.[12] The laryngoscope design was radically different from existing straight laryngoscopes in many respects. In particular, the long axis of the blade is curved, the cross section is a right-angled "Z" section, the web and flange are bulky, the tip is atraumatic, and the light bulb is shielded by the web. The latter two features offered significant advances over the straight laryngoscopes used at that time. However, Macintosh's key innovation was not the design of the laryngoscope but his novel technique of indirect elevation of the epiglottis, achieved by tensioning the hyoepiglottic ligament after the laryngoscope tip has been positioned in the vallecula. The importance of the technique is often overlooked but it is the key to understanding the success of the Macintosh laryngoscope and its limitation.

7.2 LARYNGOSCOPE FUNCTION

The structure and function of a laryngoscope are linked to the technique of laryngoscopy.

7.2.1 What is the purpose of direct laryngoscopy for tracheal intubation?

The purpose of direct laryngoscopy is to achieve sight of the vocal cords so that tracheal intubation can be performed under vision. Although it is desirable to see the entire length of the vocal cords, including the anterior commissure, tracheal intubation under vision can be achieved when only a portion of the vocal cords can be seen. This author agrees with Levitan[13] that visualization of the interarytenoid notch is generally sufficient to permit tracheal intubation under direct vision.

7.2.2 How is the efficacy of direct laryngoscopy measured?

The efficacy of direct laryngoscopy is measured in terms of the best view of the vocal cords which can be achieved. The need for an

objective scale to describe the view at laryngoscopy was met by Cormack and Lehane[14] (Figure 1-5). The definitions they used are as follows:

Grade 1—most of the glottis is visible.

Grade 2—only the posterior extremity of the glottis is visible.

Grade 3—no part of the glottis, but only the epiglottis, is visible.

Grade 4—not even the epiglottis can be seen.

Many modifications of this classification have been suggested. A particularly useful modification is the subclassification of Cormack/Lehane (C/L) Grade 3[15] into 3a, in which the epiglottis can be lifted from the posterior pharyngeal wall, and 3b, in which it cannot be lifted (Figure 7-1). This modification of C/L Grade 3 should be used routinely as the introducer technique does not[15] work well in C/L Grade 3b situation, where no further attempts at blind intubation with the Macintosh laryngoscope can be justified.

7.2.3 What is meant by difficult tracheal intubation?

Many definitions[16] of difficult intubation have been proposed and challenges in reaching a useful definition have been reviewed.[17] In practice, laryngoscopy which fails to provide a view of the glottis (C/L Grade 3 or Grade 4 view) is synonymous with difficult intubation in most patients.[18]

The complexity of the tracheal intubation may be quantified with the Intubation Difficulty Scale[19] (IDS), a numerical score based on seven parameters (number of attempts, number of operators, number of alternative techniques, laryngeal view, lifting force required, application of laryngeal pressure, and vocal cord mobility) associated with difficult intubation. The IDS alone does not specify the cause of difficulty; thus, it is important to communicate the scores of the individual elements of the IDS.[20]

7.2.4 What is the incidence of failure to see the vocal cords with a Macintosh laryngoscope?

Although incidences of 1–2% were found in early studies, the incidence of C/L Grade 3 or 4 views has been higher in recent detailed prospective studies. Many factors, including an increasing proportion of elderly patients, and a decreasing incidence of edentulous patients, may contribute to this increase. Recently reported incidences of patients with C/L Grade 3 or 4 view are 10% in patients undergoing coronary artery surgery,[21] 20% in

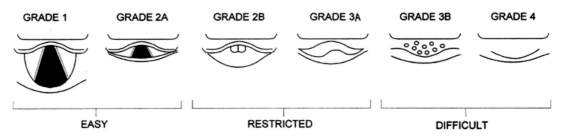

FIGURE 7-1. Modified Cormack/Lehane Classification of laryngeal grade as suggested by Cook. (*Reproduced with permission, Cook TM: A new practical classification of laryngeal view. Anaesthesia. 2000;55:274–91.*)

patients with cervical spine disease,[22] and 10–18%[16,15,23] in patients presenting for surgery.

7.2.5 What is the theory of optimum patient position for direct laryngoscopy for tracheal intubation?

The optimum position for direct laryngoscopy has long been controversial.[24] Jackson emphasized full head extension.[6] The concept of the "sniff" position was introduced by Magill[25] who stated, "The head itself is slightly extended on the atlas, so that the mandible is approximately at right angles to the table. When he wishes to sniff the air, a man in the normal erect posture instinctively and unconsciously takes this attitude." The triple axis alignment was first proposed by Bannister (an anesthetist) and MacBeth (an ENT surgeon) in 1944.[24] They suggested that positioning with neck flexion and head extension aligned the axes of the mouth, pharynx, and larynx.

Subsequently, in a study of awake patients in either simple head extension or the sniff position, Adnet has shown that it is not possible to achieve alignment of the axes of the mouth, pharynx, and larynx[26] in either position. In counterpoint, Candido et al.[27] argue that it is not position alone but a combination of position and use of the laryngoscope that is necessary to create the line of sight (LOS) of the larynx.

The three axis alignment theory is much less important to the understanding of laryngoscopy than is the influence of the tongue and epiglottis on the LOS.[14,28] This does not imply that the sniff position is not the best initial position for direct laryngoscopy for most patients, though neck flexion is probably less important than other maneuvers.

7.2.6 What is the clinical evidence regarding head position on the view achieved at laryngoscopy?

There is clinical evidence of the value of the sniff position.[29] Head extension facilitates insertion of the laryngoscope, reduces contact between the laryngoscope and the maxillary teeth, improves the view of the larynx, and is essential for full mouth opening.[30] Adnet et al.[23] compared the view achieved during laryngoscopy in patients in the sniff position (neck flexion) with simple head extension. They concluded that the sniff position was particularly beneficial in patients who are obese or have limited head extension. The sniff position improved glottic visualization in 18% of patients and worsened it in 11%. In those patients in whom the sniff position improved the view, the grade was improved from C/L Grade 4 to Grade 3 in two patients, from Grade 3 to Grade 2 in 16 patients, and from Grade 2 to Grade 1 in 66 patients. These improvements are clinically important. Furthermore, the sniff position improves pharyngeal airway patency in patients with obstructive sleep apnea.[31]

7.2.7 What are the anatomical objectives of direct laryngoscopy?

The purpose of direct laryngoscopy is to facilitate tracheal intubation under vision. Successful direct laryngoscopy depends on achieving a LOS from the maxillary teeth to the larynx. Cormack

and Lehane[14] and others[28] have highlighted the importance of the base of the tongue and the epiglottis as the anatomical structures that intrude into the LOS. Management of the tongue and epiglottis is therefore central to successful direct laryngoscopy. Before the laryngoscope is inserted, the patient is positioned in the "sniff" position by placing a pillow (or similar bolster) under the head to flex the lower neck, and by extension of the head on the neck. Probably the more important feature of this position is maximum head extension, as it rotates the maxillary teeth out of the LOS. The laryngoscope blade is then used to displace the tongue and epiglottis out of the LOS.

The tongue is displaced horizontally (normally to the left) from the LOS, the hyoid bone and epiglottis are moved anteriorly, and the epiglottis is elevated. Forward movements of the hyoid bone and epiglottis are achieved by the general forward movement of the laryngoscope tip, and elevation of the epiglottis is achieved by stretching the hyoepiglottic ligament. A significant lifting force, causing considerable tissue distortion, may be required in direct laryngoscopy.

7.2.8 What factors influence anterior lifting force applied to the laryngoscope during direct laryngoscopy?

There is considerable difference in the lifting force applied during laryngoscopy; the weight of the patient is a significant factor.[32] The required lifting force is lower with the McCoy laryngoscope[33] and is 30% less with a straight blade than with the Macintosh laryngoscope.[34] The importance of applying adequate lifting force to the laryngoscope handle in difficult laryngoscopy patients has long been recognized[35] as a key factor in successful direct laryngoscopy. Increased (described as "abnormal") lifting force was secondary only to the use of external laryngeal pressure in a prospective study of factors influencing successful tracheal intubation.[36] Recognition of the appropriate force which achieves an optimum view of the larynx with a minimal risk of trauma is gained with experience.

7.2.9 What is the theoretical basis of the Macintosh technique of laryngoscopy?

The key differences between the Macintosh and the straight laryngoscope techniques are that the anatomical basis of tongue displacement is different and that, in the former, the epiglottis is elevated indirectly by stretching the hyoepiglottic ligament. The epiglottis lies behind and along the posterior surface of the Macintosh laryngoscope blade. The hyoepiglottic ligament can only be stretched when the tip of the Macintosh laryngoscope is positioned deep in the vallecula and the vector of the force applied to the laryngoscope is optimal. For a variety of anatomical reasons, it is not possible to correctly position the Macintosh laryngoscope in a significant proportion of patients.

7.2.10 What is the mechanism of failure to achieve a line-of-site with the Macintosh laryngoscope?

Many factors may cause difficulty with direct laryngoscopy. Charters and colleagues suggest that there might be a final common pathway in many cases. Laryngoscopy, with lateral radiographic monitoring, was performed under topical anesthesia[37] in a volunteer group that included subjects in whom direct laryngoscopy had failed. In the four most difficult of eight patients, the tongue was compressed into a "peardrop" shape by the laryngoscope, forcing the tip of the laryngoscope blade posteriorly to deflect the epiglottis against the posterior pharyngeal wall. In these subjects, and in patients with a "partial pear drop" effect,[38] the tip of the blade was displaced some distance posterior to the hyoid bone. This prevented tongue displacement to the left of the laryngoscope.

Failure to displace some of the tongue to the left of the blade occurs most obviously when there is increased tongue size or reduced mouth space. However, reduced mouth opening can also result in posterior displacement of the blade so that some of the tongue is trapped between the blade and the hyoid. Trapping of the tongue between the Macintosh blade and the hyoid makes it impossible for the tip of the laryngoscope to pass into the vallecula. Consequently, it is not possible to stretch the hyoepiglottic ligament and elevate the epiglottis. This is probably the final common pathway of many causes of failure to see the vocal cords with the Macintosh laryngoscope.

7.2.11   What are the strengths and weaknesses of the Macintosh technique?

The Macintosh laryngoscope works well in most patients and competence with the technique in these patients is gained relatively quickly. Insertion is usually easy as the curved blade follows the natural curve from the mouth to the laryngopharynx. Although the laryngoscope is inserted to the right of the tongue, it is moved into the midline as it is advanced and this helps to locate the epiglottis, and larynx, in the majority of patients. However, there are the inherent limitations, as described, and it is necessary to be skilled in alternative techniques.[39]

7.2.12   What is the theoretical basis regarding ability of the straight laryngoscope to facilitate visualization of the larynx in most patients in whom this proves impossible with the Macintosh laryngoscope?

Some authors[40,41] have suggested that the mechanism of the greater efficacy of the straight laryngoscope is an improved LOS, as there is no laryngoscope curve to intrude into the LOS.[40,41] In addition, the paraglossal technique allows a further slight improvement in the LOS, as the proximal end of the laryngoscope is moved laterally, and hence posteriorly, in relation to the maxillary incisors which limit the proximal LOS with the Macintosh laryngoscope. However, the improvement of the view with the straight laryngoscope is often so dramatic,[42] that other mechanisms must be contributory.[39] These mechanisms are probably both more effective displacement of the tongue and more reliable elevation of the epiglottis. These differences are particularly important in the situation where the larynx cannot be seen with the Macintosh laryngoscope. In this situation, placement of a narrow straight laryngoscope in the paraglossal gutter may avoid the adverse

effects[37] of the Macintosh laryngoscope on the tongue and epiglottis and allow effective displacement of the tongue to the left of the laryngoscope.[39] This is consistent with the reduced force and head extension needed with a straight laryngoscope.[34]

7.2.13   What evidence of the value is seen using a straight laryngoscope in patients in whom unanticipated difficult laryngoscopy occurs with the Macintosh laryngoscope?

The first series that defined the efficacy of the straight laryngoscope in patients in whom the larynx could not be visualized with the Macintosh laryngoscope was published in 1983.[10] Six further series were reviewed, in 1997,[11] in a paper which also cited corroborative evidence of the value in this situation of the same technique with either the ENT straight laryngoscope or the rigid bronchoscope. A subsequent series has confirmed the much greater value of the Belscope (Bellhouse angulated straight laryngoscope), relative to the McCoy[42] laryngoscope, in patients in whom the larynx could not be seen with the Macintosh laryngoscope. There is further supporting evidence in recent reports of the successful use of the straight ENT laryngoscope,[43–47] and rigid bronchoscope,[48] in patients in whom tracheal intubation with the Macintosh laryngoscope has proved impossible. These reports raise the question why most anesthesia practitioners prefer to use a curved laryngoscope[49]? Arino et al. confirmed[50] the more reliable visualization of the larynx with straight than with curved laryngoscopes, but found tracheal intubation with the Miller laryngoscope difficult. This has been challenged by others[51,52] who believe that Arino's group might have come to different conclusions if they had used a visual introducer technique with the Miller laryngoscope, or used alternative straight laryngoscopes, which are designed to facilitate passage of the tracheal tube.

7.3   LARYNGOSCOPE DESIGN

A laryngoscope should have some mechanism for displacing and controlling the tongue so that it does not intrude into the LOS and should have a mechanism for elevating the epiglottis. Some laryngoscopes have additional design features which facilitate passage of the tracheal tube.

7.3.1   What standard terminology is used to describe the components of a laryngoscope?

The terms used to describe the parts of a laryngoscope have been well described (see Figure 7-2).[53] Most laryngoscopes employed primarily to place endotracheal tubes have two parts, a handle and a blade, which connect with a hook-on fitting. Until recently, the handle contained a battery connected to a terminal in the blade. This conducted current through wires to a tungsten bulb in the blade. The system now most widely used contains the bulb in the handle and light is conducted through a fiberlight bundle to the distal end of the blade. The blade of the laryngoscope is that part which

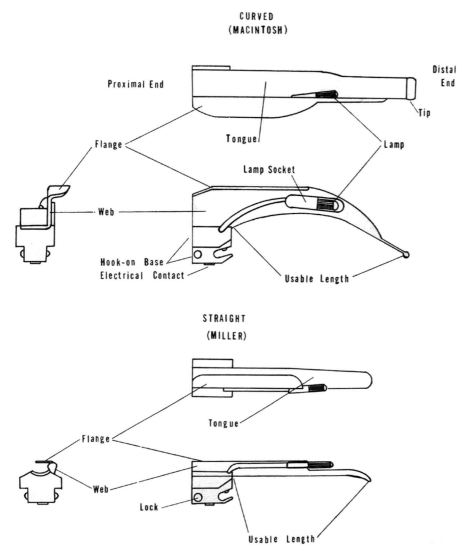

CURVED (MACINTOSH)

STRAIGHT (MILLER)

FIGURE 7-2. Characteristics of a curved blade (Macintosh) and a straight blade (Miller). *(Reproduced with permission from Dorsch JA, Dorsch SE: Laryngoscopes. In: Understanding Anesthesia Equipment, 2nd edn. Dorsch JA, Dorsch SE, eds. Baltimore: Williams & Wilkins, 1984.)*

not relevant. These laryngoscopes should be described in terms of their tip and cross section.

7.3.3 What light sources are used for laryngoscopes?

The first light source used was a tungsten light bulb. The output of these bulbs increased by about 30–40% when xenon, rather than halogen, was used to surround the tungsten filament (Jan Häring, Karl Storz Endoscopy). Early laryngoscopes using this type of light source were prone to problems including reliability, burns,[55] and the loss of bulbs.[56,57] They were difficult to clean, the bulbs and the surrounding part of the blade, and corrosion occurred readily.

The term "fiberlight" has been used to describe laryngoscopes in which light is transmitted from the handle to the tip through optical fibers. Light sources include a sealed bulb in the blade and external light connected through a cable. The "Green" system is designed to allow interchangeability of handles and blades from different manufacturers. Early fiberlight laryngoscopes provided poorer illumination than did conventional tungsten bulb models.[58–60] Light transmission of fiberlight laryngoscope blades deteriorates with repeated steam autoclaving at 134°C[61] and there is a substantial difference among the products of different manufacturers. The fiberlight system has the following advantages: thorough cleaning is easier and there is no risk of detachment of the bulb, or of tissue burns from the heat of the bulb.

is inserted into the mouth. The parts of the blade are the base, tongue (or spatula), flange, web, tip, and the light mechanism. The base of the blade makes physical and electrical, or optical, connection with the handle. The tongue is the main shaft of the blade and is designed to manipulate soft tissues. The flange and web are important structures in the curved laryngoscope. They are designed to facilitate displacement and control of the tongue. The tip is designed to work in the tissues close to the epiglottis, which may be elevated directly or indirectly.

7.3.2 How is this terminology relevant in the description of straight laryngoscopes?

The terms flange and web are appropriate for straight laryngoscopes (see Figure 7-2), such as the Soper,[54] which have a cross section similar to the Macintosh laryngoscope. However, most straight laryngoscopes have a semitubular cross section and these terms are

7.3.4 What modifications have been made to the Macintosh laryngoscope?

Many variations have been described, most without significant data about their efficacy, and few have stood the test of time. Blades vary greatly in curvature.[62] The versions of the Macintosh laryngoscope based on the original "English" design differs[63] from the US ("standard") version in several respects, particularly in the curve and the flange. An important difference is that the flange in the US version is much deeper proximally than that in the English version, so that the contact with incisor teeth is more likely. In a prospective study of 300 patients, the performance of the "English" model was better in most patients.[63]

The Callander modification in which the proximal, but not the central, part of the flange is removed reduces contact with the upper teeth and improves the view of the glottis.[64] A size four Macintosh laryngoscope[65] may be successful in cases in which the size three has failed to achieve a view of the glottis, although it is not clear

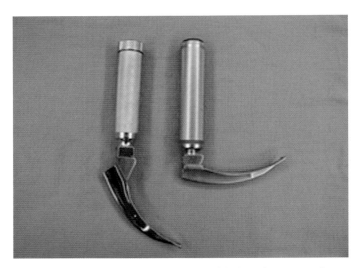

FIGURE 7-3. Characteristics of the "polio" blade and a Macintosh curved blade.

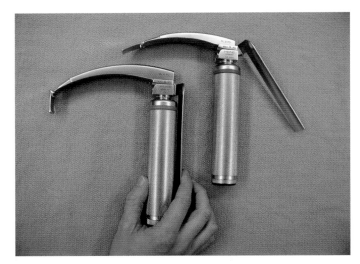

FIGURE 7-4. The McCoy laryngoscope is a modified Macintosh-type laryngoscope with a hinged tip which flexes when a lever on the handle is depressed.

whether this applies to both the English and US versions of the blade. The Polio version of the Macintosh laryngoscope, in which the handle forms an obtuse angle with the blade, was introduced in 1954[66] for use in patients in iron lung respirators (Figure 7-3). Its use in surgical patients who have been prepped and draped has been advocated because of these unique design features.[66] However, it is probable that the Polio blade gives a poor mechanical advantage[67] in relation to the standard blade and its use in a difficult situation by those without prior experience cannot be recommended.

Left-entry[68,69] (often called "left-handed") laryngoscopes are designed for insertion to the left of the tongue, which is then displaced to the right of the midline. They may be particularly useful in the presence of lesions or awkward dentition in the right side of the mouth.[69–71] This is an important version of the Macintosh laryngoscope and should be widely available. In the "Improved Vision"[72] version, the central part of the blade is concave, creating a groove, which may slightly improve the view of the larynx.

7.3.5 What is the role of the flex-tip Macintosh laryngoscope (also known as the levering or McCoy laryngoscope)?

A modern Macintosh-type laryngoscope with a hinged tip, which flexes when a lever on the handle is depressed, was introduced by McCoy in 1993 (Figure 7-4).[73] The mechanism of tongue displacement and elevation of the epiglottis is similar to the Macintosh laryngoscope; in that, the tip of the laryngoscope is inserted into the vallecula and the epiglottis is elevated indirectly by stretching the hyoepiglottic ligament. There have been many reports of conversion of C/L Grade 3 views to Grade 1 or 2.[74–77] However, there have been reports of failures.[76,78–80] In prospective studies, it was found that in patients with C/L Grade 3 Macintosh laryngoscopy the view improved with the McCoy laryngoscope in 50%[81] and 83%[82] of patients. Levitan has sought to explain the variable effectiveness of the McCoy laryngoscope.[83] Prospective studies in patients with simulated cervical spine injuries, in whom manual in-line stabilization was used, showed an improved view

with the McCoy in comparison with the Macintosh[84,85] laryngoscope. However, the Belscope (angulated straight laryngoscope) performed much better than the McCoy[42] in a comparison with patients in whom unanticipated difficult intubation occurred with the Macintosh laryngoscope. Despite its many advocates, the McCoy laryngoscope does not allow tracheal intubation under vision in a sufficient proportion of patients with a failed Macintosh laryngoscopy for it to be considered the *only* alternative laryngoscopy technique one may need.

7.3.6 What is the role of prisms and mirrors in direct laryngoscopy?

The Huffman prism[86] was designed for use with the Macintosh laryngoscope (Figure 7-5) and a dedicated prism was designed for use with the Belscope[41] angulated straight laryngoscope. There is evidence[50] that the laryngeal view can be improved, although Bellhouse did not find its use necessary.[41] Mirror laryngoscopes[87,88]

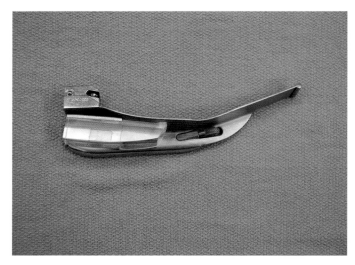

FIGURE 7-5. Huffman prism attached to the web of a curved blade.

have been described. Use of a laryngeal mirror has been helpful in adult[89] and pediatric[90] patients. However, there are practical problems with the use of prisms and mirrors. Passage of the tracheal tube while maintaining an LOS through a prism, or mirror, can be difficult. Mist from condensation may form on both prisms[91] and mirrors. In addition, mirror laryngoscopes cause reversal of image. Prisms and mirrors have been superseded by alternative devices that give better views and are easier to use.

7.3.7 What modifications of the straight laryngoscope have been made?

Two early straight laryngoscope blades were designed by Jackson[6] and Magill.[8] The reader is referred to textbooks[53] on anesthesia equipment for detailed descriptions of the Flagg, Guedel, Wisconsin, Wisconsin-Forreger, and other straight laryngoscopes. Straight blades have been made with reduced proximal cross sections,[92–95] angulation,[41,95] or other modifications[96] designed to reduce contact with maxillary teeth.

The Miller laryngoscope[97] has probably been the most popular straight laryngoscope for many years. It has a lower cross section as compared to other straight laryngoscopes, and this feature, which facilitates insertion and positioning, is responsible for its popularity. However, illumination is a problem with many Miller laryngoscopes as it has been positioned in such a way that it can be readily obscured by tissues or secretions.[98] This problem has been resolved in some[99] of the most recent fiberlight models.

There are other problems with Miller blades. The tip curves forward in the longitudinal and transverse axes and, as a consequence, the point of contact with the posterior surface of the epiglottis is small. This increases the risk of trauma and unstable elevation of the epiglottis. In addition, as it is not possible to see the tip of the blade, precise positioning is difficult. Finally, the greatest problem with the Miller laryngoscope is that the small cross section impedes passage of the tracheal tube.

7.3.8 What straight laryngoscopes have been designed specifically for use with the paraglossal technique?

The Belscope[41] is an angulated straight laryngoscope manufactured in three sizes. It is narrow and has a low profile and an atraumatic tip. It is designed to be used with the paraglossal technique as described by Bellhouse.[41] The efficacy of the Belscope in improving the view of the larynx and preventing contact with the maxillary incisors has been confirmed[100] despite the use of a suboptimal, central technique. Its efficacy in patients in whom the larynx cannot be seen with the Macintosh laryngoscope has been confirmed in three series.[41,42,101]

The Phillips laryngoscope has a semitubular cross section[102] which tapers, the wider diameter being proximal. The tip is similar to the tip of the Miller laryngoscope. The Piquet–Crinquette–Vilette (PCV) laryngoscope[103] has a gentle curve but allows a straight LOS. It has a semitubular cross section and an external light source.

The Henderson[A] laryngoscope[13,49,104] was designed to overcome the drawbacks of the Miller laryngoscope. It has been shown[105] that the passage of tracheal tubes in straight laryngoscopes is facilitated by a C-shaped cross section. The uniform semitubular cross section of the Henderson laryngoscope is slightly wider than that of the Miller and is designed to facilitate both visualization of the larynx and passage of an 8.0 mm ID inner diameter (ID) tracheal tube down the lumen of the laryngoscope (larger tubes, including double-lumen tubes, can be passed lateral to the lumen of the laryngoscope). The cross section of the laryngoscope allows steering of the tip of the tracheal tube during passage, so that the tip emerges at the larynx. The illumination site from the fiberlight lies within the lumen of the laryngoscope, so that it cannot be easily obscured by soft tissue, or secretions. The laryngoscope has an atraumatic tip which remains in vision during passage and positioning of the laryngoscope. It has been well reviewed.[13]

7.4 DIRECT LARYNGOSCOPY PREPARATION

7.4.1 What are the fundamental priorities during tracheal intubation?

The purpose of tracheal intubation is to achieve protection of the airway and facilitate mechanical ventilation by correct positioning of the tube in the trachea. The risk of complications should be minimized by using best practice. Four principles are central to prevention of complications:

1. Maintenance of oxygenation must take priority over all other issues. Regular use of mask-ventilation between attempts at tracheal intubation is essential.[106]

2. Soft tissue trauma must be prevented. The number of attempts with blind techniques should ideally be zero and certainly not more than three or four.[106,107]

3. The practitioner should always have back-up plans before starting the primary technique.[106]

4. The airway practitioner should seek the best help available ("call for help") as soon as difficulty with laryngoscopy is experienced.[106]

7.4.2 What assessments should be used as a guide to whether tracheal intubation should be performed in the conscious or anesthetized patient?

Before proceeding to tracheal intubation under general anesthesia, it is essential to assess the probability of difficult direct laryngoscopy. A history of previous anesthesia and/or intubations should be sought. An examination should be made to detect signs of anatomical factors that could make laryngoscopy difficult. Detection of such signs does not imply that direct laryngoscopy will be difficult, and the airway practitioner must assess the risk based on the degree of abnormality, the number of abnormal factors, and personal experience. Scoring systems[108,109] have been

---

[A]***Statement of Interest***: Dr. John Henderson has leased his patents for the Henderson laryngoscope and receives royalties on their sales.

developed to assist with that decision, but they are not completely reliable. The most important factors include reduced head extension, mouth opening, and reduced space for displacement of the tongue. These are often associated with conditions such as micrognathia, or submandibular lesions.[110] Some dental patterns can impede insertion, or manipulation, of the laryngoscope.

The author prefers the examination (mouth opening, ability to prognath, head extension, thyromental distance, and Mallampati class) described by El-Ganzouri[109] and used by Ovassapian.[111] Even such a detailed assessment may miss serious problems. These include asymptomatic lesions[111] in the vicinity of the larynx and skeletal factors.[112,113] Airway assessment overestimates the risk of difficulty and fails to detect some patients in whom tracheal intubation proves to be very difficult and its very value has been questioned.[114] However, the fallacy of these arguments has been shown[115] and routine airway assessment is recommended in all guidelines.

If no difficulties are anticipated, preparations are made for tracheal intubation under general anesthesia. However, if difficulties with mask-ventilation are anticipated, spontaneous ventilation must be maintained by avoiding the use of muscle relaxants or any other drug combination which may cause apnea. The safest course in such situations is to perform tracheal intubation under topical anesthesia in the awake patient.

7.4.3 What factors are important during direct laryngoscopy preparation for tracheal intubation?

Adequate personnel, drugs, and equipment must be available. A minimum list of equipment is described in the ASA guidelines[107] and the Difficult Airway Society Web site (www.das.uk.com). The first attempt at direct laryngoscopy should always be performed under optimal conditions.[18,106] The airway practitioner should always be prepared for unanticipated difficulty, so that adequate expertise, equipment, and assistance are available. It should not be necessary to make major adjustments to the patient position or the shape of the tracheal tube. Time spent making these adjustments after induction may delay successful tracheal intubation and increase the risk of hypoxemia or airway trauma. Wherever possible, the patient should be positioned at a height comfortable for the airway practitioner. Intravenous access is secured (in a few patients this may not be possible and access may be achieved by a colleague during inhalational induction of anesthesia if an anesthetic is the goal).

Monitoring[116] is established, the minimum being electrocardiogram, noninvasive blood pressure and pulse oximeter – with audible signals activated. Denitrogenation should precede laryngoscopy and intubation. The vocal cords should be abducted and made nonreactive before passage of the tracheal tube is attempted.

7.4.4 What pharmacological techniques are used to facilitate direct laryngoscopy for tracheal intubation? What are their advantages and disadvantages?

The purpose of pharmacological adjuvants is to permit optimal use of direct laryngoscopy while ensuring maximum safety, minimal

patient discomfort, as well as attenuating the patient's memory of the event. In the routine practice, the most frequent choice is the combination of an intravenous anesthetic with a nondepolarizing muscle relaxant, while in an emergency a depolarizing relaxant is often the choice. The onset of effect is rapid and excellent conditions for intubation are usually assured. However, this pharmacological approach can be dangerous. Neuromuscular blocking drugs produce apnea, and oxygenation following their use can be maintained only by effective ventilation with a face-mask or extraglottic airway device. Thus, safety is predicated upon ones capacity to continually provide effective ventilation. It has been suggested that succinylcholine might be a safer choice, as its shorter duration of action allows earlier return of spontaneous ventilation.

Although the duration of succinylcholine is shorter than that of nondepolarizing drugs, time to desaturation after denitrogenation varies greatly.[117] The return of normal neuromuscular function may not occur until after hypoxemic tissue damage. Administration of neuromuscular blockers in the face of doubt about ability to maintain oxygenation and ventilation is extremely problematic. Substitution of short-acting opiates and hypnotics for neuromuscular blocking drugs with the intention of preserving spontaneous ventilation has been advocated and, also, disputed.[118,119] Conditions for direct laryngoscopy and tracheal intubation are inferior to those when neuromuscular blockers are used[120–123] and there is a higher risk of failed intubation and of airway trauma.[124,125] Judicious use of intravenous adjuvants, in conjunction with good topical analgesia, would be a preferable option.[126,22] A slow infusion of propofol,[127] with topical anesthesia,[127] has been used successfully.

Use of inhalational induction has been advocated when difficulty with airway management is anticipated.[128–131] Deep anesthesia is necessary for direct laryngoscopy and tracheal intubation, but prior administration of topical anesthesia[128] can facilitate passage of the tracheal tube under lighter anesthesia. Although its use has been advocated in the presence of stridor,[132,133] it can be a dangerous technique.[134] Patients with stridor depend both on muscle tone, to maintain the shape of the thorax, and on powerful contraction of the diaphragm. During inhalational induction, respiratory drive and muscle tone are reduced and hypoventilation, airway obstruction, and arterial hypotension occur frequently.[135] In addition, conditions for laryngoscopy are often suboptimal and the time available is limited. When the airway is lost during inhalational induction, emergency cricothyrotomy is indicated, though likely to be more difficult and dangerous as a response to an airway emergency iatrogenically created than if selected as a primary airway technique.

7.5 MACINTOSH LARYNGOSCOPY TECHNIQUE

7.5.1 What are the standard technique components of direct laryngoscopy with the Macintosh laryngoscope?

It is usually possible to achieve tracheal intubation with a rapid sequence of movements in which all components of a complex technique merge into one another. An ideal technique might emerge from analysis of underlying components. Direct laryngoscopy for tracheal intubation can be divided into four overlapping steps: insertion of the laryngoscope, optimization of the position of the laryngoscope (and the view of the larynx), passage of the tracheal tube, and confirmation of intubation.

7.5.2 What is the insertion technique of the Macintosh laryngoscope?

The value of head extension has been discussed.[30] If mouth opening remains limited, despite optimal head positioning, the scissor technique (Benumof's intraoral technique[136]) can be a very useful means of achieving maximum mouth opening. When the right hand is used in this technique, the thumb pushes caudally and anteriorly on the mandibular teeth as the first or middle finger push upward on the maxillary teeth. This action can help to achieve maximum sliding as well as rotation of the temporomandibular joint before the laryngoscope is inserted and it may help in the presence of intermittent temporomandibular joint malfunction.

The laryngoscope handle is normally held in the left hand. The laryngoscope is inserted from the right side of the mouth and to the right of the tongue. Care is taken in that the lips are not trapped between the laryngoscope blade and the teeth. The laryngoscope is advanced and simultaneously moved medially into the midline to displace the entire tongue to the left of the midline. Visualization of anatomical structures is essential to minimize the risk of trauma. The first key anatomical landmark is the epiglottis. As the laryngoscope is advanced, a moderate lifting force is applied to the laryngoscope handle to maintain displacement of the tongue, to achieve maximum mouth opening, and to reduce contact between the laryngoscope and the maxillary teeth. As the epiglottis comes into view, the tip of the laryngoscope is advanced into the vallecula and the epiglottis is elevated indirectly by tensioning the hyoepiglottic ligament to reveal the vocal cords.

7.5.3 What is the basic exposure technique of the larynx and creation of an optimum view with the Macintosh laryngoscope?

When a good view of the larynx is achieved, the vocal cords, the aryepiglottic folds, posterior cartilages, and interarytenoid notch can be identified. A frequent error is to accept a partial view of the vocal cords when a better view can be achieved. Precise positioning (depth of insertion of the laryngoscope) and application of the laryngoscope lifting force are necessary and these should be adjusted to achieve the best view of the larynx.[136] The airway practitioner must be ready to use a further range of maneuvers and there is little predictability as to which maneuver may be most effective in any particular patient. Once the best view has been achieved, the airway practitioner should not take his eye off the vocal cords until the tube is seen pass between them.

7.5.4 What maneuvers are of proven value at improving the view with the Macintosh laryngoscope?

First, it is necessary to check that maximum head extension has been used, that the entire tongue is displaced to the left of the laryngo-

scope, and that mouth opening is maximum. Small adjustments to the depth of insertion of the laryngoscope should be made to determine whether these improve elevation of the epiglottis and hence the view. The lifting force applied to the laryngoscope should be adjusted in direction and magnitude to optimize the view. It is important not to lever on the maxillary teeth, as this may cause dental damage and reduce the view of the larynx.[137] These first checks of the basic technique should be made before using other maneuvers.

The most important additional maneuver is external laryngeal manipulation, which should be an integral part of direct laryngoscopy. This technique has long been used by ENT surgeons to improve the view in patients undergoing diagnostic laryngoscopy.[138,139] Wilson[108] was the first to quantify the value of laryngeal pressure when he used it to reduce the incidence of C/L Grade 3 and 4 views from 9.3% to 5.9%. Benumof[140] found that the technique, which he called optimal external laryngeal manipulation (OELM), could consistently improve the laryngeal view by one grade. He stressed the importance of the manipulation being performed with the right hand of the airway practitioner, who then guides an assistant to provide identical manipulation. BURP[141] (Backward Upward Right Pressure) applied to the larynx is of proven value, but OELM describes the technique better as the force and direction are adjusted by the airway practitioner. The best term is probably "bimanual laryngoscopy"[142] as it emphasizes the coordinated internal movement of the laryngoscope with the external manipulation of the laryngeal cartilages. Bimanual laryngoscopy should be an integral part of direct laryngoscopy and should be the first maneuver employed to improve the view of the larynx.

Some other maneuvers may help. Increased neck flexion, achieved by head elevation, can make intubation under vision possible in some patients who are initially C/L Grade 3.[143] Laryngeal lift by an assistant may help to improve the view.[144] Manual forward displacement of the mandible by an assistant can improve the view of the vocal cords.[45] If the larynx still cannot be seen, alternative techniques will be necessary and adequacy of ventilation becomes a paramount consideration. Maintenance of oxygenation and prevention of trauma take precedence over all other considerations in the elective surgery patient in this situation.

7.5.5 What is the technique used to pass the tracheal tube after the vocal cords are seen with the Macintosh laryngoscope?

The view of the vocal cords is maintained while the airway practitioner takes the tracheal tube (close to the 15 mm connector) in the right hand and guides the tube between the vocal cords under vision. The tube is passed from the right side of the mouth so that the progress of the tracheal tube toward and between the vocal cords can be observed. In order to keep the vocal cords in sight, the tube should be placed in the right hand by an assistant. Passage of the tube is greatly facilitated if an assistant pulls the side of the mouth open and the tube has an optimal shape.[145] A tube in the shape of an ice-hockey stick[146–149] facilitates steering of the tip of the tube. This shape is most readily created by the use of a stylet, "a metallic rod, usually coated with plastic, inserted into the lumen of a flexible tracheal tube to stiffen it and give it the desired shape during its passage."[145] The stylet should be well lubricated and should not protrude beyond the tip of the tracheal tube. Its ease of withdrawal should be checked before starting laryngoscopy.[150] When the tip of the tube has passed 1.0–2.0 cm beyond the vocal cords, the stylet should be withdrawn by an assistant, who uses counter-pressure on the tracheal tube connector to ensure that the tracheal tube is not pulled out of the larynx. The tracheal tube is then advanced until the cuff is about 2.0 cm distal to the vocal cords. The cuff is inflated to slightly higher than the "just-seal" pressure, which should then be maintained,[151] as excessive cuff pressure can cause postoperative laryngeal dysfunction.[152,153] Finally, the correct position of the tube is confirmed. The stylet should always be inspected after use to check that it is intact.[154,155] If the larynx cannot be seen with the Macintosh laryngoscope, blind techniques (usually an introducer) will be required unless the airway practitioner is skilled in alternative techniques of laryngoscopy under vision. Oxygenation should be maintained with mask-ventilation between intubation attempts.

7.5.6   What are tracheal tube introducers and how were they developed?

Tracheal tube introducers (e.g., Eschmann Introducer or commonly known as "gum-elastic bougie") are devices which are passed (introduced) into the trachea and then used as a guide over which the tracheal tube is passed ("railroaded") into the trachea (see Section 10.2.1).[145] Although introducers have a role when the larynx can be seen (particularly with the straight and video laryngoscopy techniques), they are most frequently used with the Macintosh laryngoscope when the larynx cannot be seen. In this application, the technique can be legitimately described as a blind introducer technique.

The material used to manufacture the original Eschmann Introducer probably contributed to its success.[156] It gives moderate stiffness, yet holds a new shape reasonably well at body temperature. It is flexible enough to follow a tortuous course and yet yields if pressed gently against soft tissues. Its length (60 cm) also contributed to its success. Early introducers were relatively short and were passed within the tracheal tube as a single unit, the tip of the introducer protruding several centimeters beyond the tip of the tracheal tube. The greater length of the Eschmann Introducer allowed initial positioning of the introducer in the trachea and subsequent "railroading" of the tracheal tube over the introducer into the trachea. Initial passage of the introducer allows tactile verification[157,158] of blind placement in the trachea and the angled tip[159–161] and narrow, flexible nature of the introducer contribute to successful entry into the trachea. Other introducers have been manufactured but have not been used as frequently. The single-use Eschmann Introducer seems less effective[162–164] than the multiple-use device but introduction of new versions is imminent. Other single-use introducers have been manufactured and the Frova hollow introducer is of proven value[165,166] (see Section 10.2.1).

7.5.7   How should the blind introducer technique be used most effectively?

The technique is described in detail elsewhere (see Section 10.2.1).[106,145] The technique can be divided into three parts:

passage of the introducer, confirmation of tracheal position, and passage ("railroading") of the tube over the introducer into the trachea. As with other equipment, the integrity of the device should be checked before use.[167,168] Creation of a curve in the introducer[161] greatly increases the success rate. The laryngoscope is kept in the midline and the airway practitioner tries to visualize the likely location of the larynx distal to the epiglottis. The tip of the introducer is passed from the side of the mouth, posterior to the epiglottis and blindly into the larynx. A gentle technique should always be used in order to minimize trauma and facilitate verification of passage into the trachea. A sensation of clicks, due to the introducer hitting the tracheal cartilages, is detected in 90% of correct intratracheal placements as the introducer passes down the lumen of the trachea.[158] If clicks are not elicited, the introducer has either passed down the center of the trachea or is in the esophagus. The second sign of tracheal positioning is distal holdup, sensed as slight resistance to further advancement. Holdup at 24–40 cm was detected in 100% of instances of tracheal placement.[158] In the case of hollow introducers, intratracheal position may be confirmed with a self-inflating bulb.[165] If none of these signs are detected, the introducer is almost certainly in the esophagus. The introducer should be removed and, if another attempt with the blind introducer can be justified, the laryngoscopy technique should be optimized and another attempt made to pass the introducer into the trachea. Successful positioning of the introducer in the trachea must be followed by passage ("railroading") of the tracheal tube over the introducer and into the trachea.[106]

Railroading sometimes proves difficult or impossible.[169,170] Dogra confirmed the value of 90 degree anticlockwise rotation of the tube[171] and demonstrated the importance of keeping the laryngoscope in place during railroading. Small tracheal tubes facilitate railroading[172,173] and their use is the most important aid to effective railroading. Many reports support the use of wire-reinforced tracheal tubes to increase success with railroading during fiberoptic intubation.[174,175] It can be difficult to pass a preformed tube (e.g., an oral RAE tube) over an introducer.[145]

7.5.8   What are the success rates and limitations of the introducer technique?

There are many reports[169,176–179] of failure of the introducer technique, but it does have a high success rate. The success rate in the Australian Incident Monitoring Study was 75%.[180] A success rate of 96.5% by the second attempt[181] was found in a prospective survey, and another prospective study[182] recorded a 90% success rate in two attempts. The technique works well when the epiglottis can be elevated from the posterior pharyngeal wall[15] but not when the best view is C/L Grade 3b (see Figure 7-1). These findings are in keeping with the comment by Cormack and Lehane that the technique does not work well when only the tip of the epiglottis can be seen.[14] The great merit of the introducer technique is that it combines simplicity of the technique with a high success rate. The introducer technique was developed before alternative techniques of tracheal intubation under vision. Now that such techniques are available,[183] the role of the blind use of introducers should be reevaluated.[184–186]

Unpublished cases of death from mediastinitis after use of the introducer technique are present in the files of the medical defense societies. Closed claims analysis of anesthetic cases[187] and review of emergency medicine cases[188] confirm the association of persistent attempts at intubation with death. Persistent attempts at tracheal intubation can lead to increasing difficulty with mask-ventilation[189] and to pharyngeal or esophageal perforation which results in mediastinitis.[190] Other adverse effects of repeated attempts at intubation include a risk of awareness if the depth of anesthesia is not maintained, a risk of pulmonary aspiration as security of the airway is not achieved, and the risk of hypertension and tachycardia.[187] Although this author believes that the introducer technique still has a place in management of C/L Grade 3a patients, there can be no justification for the use of more than three or four blind attempts at intubation,[106,107] and the limit of two attempts is recommended.[182] The one exception is a single additional attempt by a more experienced airway practitioner, which may be successful.[35,191] The airway practitioner should have sought help whenever difficulty was experienced and should move to plan B early if the blind introducer technique proves unsuccessful.[192]

7.5.9   What makes insertion of the Macintosh laryngoscope difficult in the presence of mammomegaly and what are the solutions?

The angle between the blade of the Macintosh laryngoscope and the handle can make insertion of the laryngoscope difficult, as the handle can make contact with the anterior chest wall. Conditions[193] that lead to contact between the chest wall and the handle of the Macintosh laryngoscope include mammomegaly (e.g., morbid obesity and parturients at term), kyphosis, short neck, and fixed flexion of the head and neck (conditions often managed more safely with awake flexible fiberoptic intubation). Excessive neck flexion caused by placing several pillows under the head makes it more likely that the handle will make contact with the anterior chest wall. In a morbidly obese patient, optimal position often requires building a ramp of sheets or towels under the shoulders, neck, and head of the patient (see Section 17.4.3 and Figure 17-2). The assistant's hand which applies cricoid pressure can also impede the handle of the laryngoscope and this can be corrected by ensuring that the hand which applies cricoid pressure is kept parallel to the neck. Use of a short handle[194] (although light intensity may be reduced[58]), a pediatric laryngoscope handle,[195] and a Polio blade (Figure 7-3)[193,196] have been recommended. Adaptors have been designed with the aim of increasing the angle between the blade and the handle[197–200] or of allowing lateral swivelling[201] between the blade and the handle. It has been claimed that insertion of the blade alone, followed by connection to the handle, is usually simple.[67] However, there is little evidence of the efficacy of these techniques. Alternatively, mastery in the use of the straight laryngoscope technique ensures that the handle never impinges on the chest because of the angle between the handle and the blade.

7.5.10   What is the importance of confirmation of tracheal intubation?

Confirmation of tube position is *mandatory* since avoidable deaths from hypoxemia, as a consequence of unrecognized esophageal intubation, although less frequent than formerly, continue to occur.[187] The two fail-safe signs of tracheal intubation are visualization of the

tracheal tube between the vocal cords and use of a flexible fiberoptic bronchoscope within the tracheal tube to visualize the cartilaginous rings of the trachea and the tracheal carina.[136] If visual confirmation is not possible, a high degree of suspicion that the tube may be misplaced should be maintained and other methods to confirm proper tube position should be used. Although a characteristic pattern on the capnograph confirms tracheal intubation, capnography is not completely reliable. Malfunction of the capnograph may lead to removal of a properly positioned tracheal tube. Low or zero CO_2 concentrations may be detected in very low cardiac output states or severe respiratory disease. A low and decreasing pattern of CO_2 excretion may be detected when the tube is in the esophagus. The negative-pressure (esophageal detector) device works on the principle that air can be aspirated from the trachea but not the esophagus.[202] It is simple and inexpensive, but not completely reliable.

Signs suggestive of esophageal intubation include distension of the left upper abdomen with no chest movement and auscultation of air entry into the stomach.[203] Early hypoxemia (2-20 min) after tracheal intubation should be regarded as esophageal intubation until proved otherwise. If there is any suspicion of esophageal intubation, the only safe maxim is *"If in doubt, take it out."*[203] If the practitioner thinks the tube is probably in the trachea, an introducer, or airway exchange catheter, may be passed before removing the tracheal tube. Mask-ventilation with 100% oxygen is used to restore oxygenation. Further management will depend on factors such as the degree of muscle relaxation, urgency of surgery, difficulty of tracheal intubation, and the help available.[106]

When esophageal intubation has been excluded, it is necessary to confirm that the tip of the tube lies in the trachea and not the right main bronchus. Auscultation for equal breath sounds over both axillae is performed. Hypoxemia or an increase in airway pressure should trigger a check for correct position of the tracheal tube, as tubes can migrate into the right main bronchus during surgery or position changes of the patient following intubation. Once satisfactory tracheal tube position is confirmed, it is secured with tape,[204] a secure knot,[205] or both in order to prevent accidental extubation, or accidental endobronchial intubation. The depth marking on the tube at the patient's teeth or lips should be documented. A bite-block should be inserted in order to prevent occlusion of the airway (by biting the tracheal tube) during emergence from anesthesia. Such occlusion can lead to hypoxemia and negative-pressure pulmonary edema[206,207] (see Chapter 55). For surgical procedures shorter than a few hours, this author prefers to insert an oropharyngeal airway after tracheal intubation.

7.5.11   What are the limitations of the Macintosh laryngoscope?

There has been no significant reduction in the number of reports in the ASA Closed Claims Study[187] of adverse outcome associated with tracheal intubation. This failure to make tracheal intubation safer is one of the most important challenges facing anesthesia in particular, and all airway practitioners generally. It would seem that the problem lies in the significant incidence of failure to see the vocal cords with conventional laryngoscopy leading to blind techniques that produce airway trauma. This in turn is related to the fact that many anesthesia practitioners have failed to master alternative airway management techniques. Use of extraglottic devices for elective surgery in patients in whom tracheal intubation was planned is not recommended in airway guidelines.[106,107] All airway practitioners should be skilled in at least one alternative technique of tracheal intubation under vision, and the rigid fiberoptic laryngoscope or straight laryngoscope have been recommended.[39]

7.6   STRAIGHT LARYNGOSCOPE: PARAGLOSSAL TECHNIQUE AND ROLE IN ANESTHETIC PRACTICE

7.6.1   What is the role of the straight laryngoscope for tracheal intubation in the adult patient?

It is now appreciated that the straight laryngoscopy technique is more effective than the Macintosh technique, implying that all airway practitioners ought to employ this technique with some degree of regularity to develop and maintain skill in the technique.[183] As discussed, it can facilitate tracheal intubation under vision in most patients in whom this proves impossible with the Macintosh laryngoscope. Factors that contribute to the better view achieved with the straight laryngoscope are more effective displacement of the tongue from the LOS and more reliable elevation of the epiglottis. The straight laryngoscope may have particular niche roles in patients with mandibular hypoplasia; patients with lesions in the region of the vallecula, epiglottis, or larynx; and in patients with some awkward dentition patterns. The technique is completely different from the Macintosh technique and effort and commitment are required for its mastery. Differences from the Macintosh technique will be highlighted.

7.6.2   Is there an optimum technique with the straight laryngoscope?

More than one technique has been described and all techniques have advantages and disadvantages. The techniques described are based on the paraglossal technique described by Magill,[9] Wiggin,[208] Philips and Duerksen,[102] Arai,[40] Bellhouse,[41] and Crinquette et al.[103] Others[24,209,210] have supported these approaches. They have been developed by the author during more than 2,000 tracheal intubations with the Henderson laryngoscope. Two variations are described:

1. The standard epiglottic visualization technique. This technique depends on progressive visualization of anatomical structures, using the tip of the epiglottis as the principal landmark, as recommended by Chevalier Jackson.[6]
2. The alternative technique of direct passage to the larynx. This technique depends on external observation of movement of the laryngeal cartilages in the anterior neck by the laryngoscope blade, followed by the adjustment of the laryngoscopic view using bimanual laryngoscopy.

As with the Macintosh laryngoscope, the techniques can be divided into four steps (insertion of laryngoscope and passage along the paraglossal gutter, optimization of the position of the laryngo-scope and the view of the larynx, passage of the tracheal tube, and confirmation of intubation) and all components of the technique are important. The steps in the standard technique will be discussed in detail, followed by the differences in the alternative technique.

7.6.3   What is the technique of insertion of the straight laryngoscope and passage along the paraglossal gutter in the standard epiglottic visualization technique?

Before laryngoscopy, the patient's head and neck should be placed in maximum extension. Maximum extension facilitates mouth opening[30] and insertion of the laryngoscope, reduces contact between the maxillary teeth and the laryngoscope, and improves the view of the larynx. Maximum mouth opening requires use of the sliding and rotational functions of the temporomandibular joint, and it is important to the displacement of the entire tongue to the left of the laryngoscope. The laryngoscope is inserted lateral to the tongue on the right and advanced carefully along the paraglossal gutter between the tongue and the tonsil. Care is taken that the lips are not trapped between the laryngoscope blade and the teeth. Continued application of a moderate lifting force with the laryngoscope during its passage helps to maintain anterior displacement of the mandible, control of the tongue, and reduce contact between the laryngoscope and the maxillary teeth. As the laryngoscope is advanced, the epiglottis comes into view and the tip of the laryngoscope is passed posterior to it.

7.6.4   What further maneuvers may be used to optimize passage of the straight laryngoscope?

Two further maneuvers can minimize contact between the laryngoscope and the incisor teeth: (1) passage of the laryngoscope as far *right* in the mouth as possible (Magill's paraglossal technique,[9] rediscovered by Bonfils and erroneously called the "retromolar" technique[10]) and (2) rotation of the head to the left. The lateral teeth are less vulnerable than the incisors to damage. Furthermore, these maneuvers can improve the view of the larynx.[10]

7.6.5   What is the optimum position of the straight laryngoscope for passage of the tracheal tube?

When the straight laryngoscope has been positioned optimally, the tip of the laryngoscope lies in the midline of the posterior surface of the epiglottis, close to the anterior commissure of the vocal cords.[6] This position reduces the risk that slight withdrawal of the laryngoscope may allow the epiglottis to flip posteriorly and obstruct the view of the larynx. It also facilitates passage of the tracheal tube.

7.6.6   What maneuvers can be used to optimize the position of the laryngoscope and the view of the larynx?

The laryngoscope should be maneuvered into a position as close to the optimal as possible. If a partial view of the vocal cords is achieved, an attempt should always be made to achieve the best view possible, as this facilitates passage of the tracheal tube. If the vocal cords cannot be seen, the first step is to identify the location of the tip of the laryngoscope. Both the view and the tactile clues experienced during bimanual laryngoscopy are important.

If the larynx is not visible, it is probable that the tip of the laryngoscope is located in the vallecula, pyriform fossa (usually the right), posterior pharyngeal wall, or the esophagus. The view when the tip is in the vallecula is of the flat pale cartilage of the anterior surface of the epiglottis. The pyriform fossa is asymmetrical, with the aryepiglottic fold at one side. The pharynx and esophagus are featureless and symmetrical (sometimes part, or the entire featureless circular orifice, of the esophagus is seen).

The tactile sensations produced during bimanual laryngoscopy[142] can be a very useful guide. When the tip of the laryngoscope is positioned in the esophagus, it lies behind the cricoid cartilage. External movement of the larynx, when the tip of the laryngoscope lies in the esophagus, creates a distinctive sensation of rolling of the larynx on the blade, similar to that described[211] with esophageal placement of a tracheal tube. When the laryngoscope is withdrawn slowly from this position, there is a characteristic backward movement of the larynx, as the laryngoscope tip moves from posterior to the cricoid to its new position posterior to the epiglottis. The view will now depend on whether the tip is centered behind the epiglottis or lies laterally in the pyriform fossa. External lateral movement of the larynx and internal lateral movement of the tip of the laryngoscope during bimanual laryngoscopy should now reveal the vocal cords.

When the vocal cords are visualized, the view should next be optimized, with the aim of producing a view of the entire length of the vocal cords. If the view is poor, the basic maneuvers should be checked: the head is maximally extended; the tongue is displaced entirely to the left of the laryngoscope; the mouth is fully open; the mandible is maximally advanced using the sliding, as well as the rotational components of temporomandibular joint function; the laryngoscope has been inserted to the optimum depth; optimum lifting force has been applied to the laryngoscope in the correct direction; and bimanual laryngoscopy (OELM) has been optimized. The direction of the force applied to the handle of the straight laryngoscope is different from that applied to the Macintosh laryngoscope, because of the different angle between the handle and the tip of the laryngoscope. The direction of this force is at right angles to the line of the straight laryngoscope blade (and LOS of the larynx) and is produced by lifting in the line of the laryngoscope handle. Under *no* circumstances should a levering action be applied to the teeth. Not only does this *risk* dental damage, but it worsens the view.

If an adequate view is impossible, with the recommended maneuvers, a different technique of laryngoscopy, or of tracheal intubation, is indicated. Neck flexion, achieved by head elevation, can improve the view,[212,139] but the appropriate degree of head flexion has been questioned.[212] Manual forward displacement of the mandible by an assistant may improve the view of the vocal cords, with both the straight and curved laryngoscopes,[213] but these variations on head position are probably less important than maintaining head extension and optimizing the lifting force.

7.6.7 What are the features of the alternative (direct passage to larynx) technique of straight laryngoscopy?

In this technique, external landmarks are used to indicate the position of the larynx, to which the laryngoscope is passed directly without visualizing the tip of the epiglottis. The mandible is held anteriorly as the tip of the laryngoscope is passed posterior to the epiglottis along the paraglossal gutter and into the hypopharynx. An increased lifting force is applied to the laryngoscope while movement of the laryngeal cartilages in the anterior of the neck is observed. The position of the laryngoscope is adjusted so that maximum movement is apparent in the midline of the neck. When midline advancement of the laryngeal cartilages in the neck has been confirmed, the view down the laryngoscope is checked. As with the standard technique (visualization of the tip of the epiglottis), it is important to be able to recognize the features of the vallecula, pyriform fossa, pharynx, and esophagus. Bimanual laryngoscopy is now used to optimize the view. If any resistance is experienced with this technique, it is abandoned and the technique of visual identification of the epiglottis is used.

7.6.8 What techniques of passage of the tracheal tube are used with the straight laryngoscope?

Three techniques of passage of the tracheal tube may be used with the Henderson (and other "C channel" designs, e.g., the Phillips blade) laryngoscope[104] (see 7.6.12 for other straight blade techniques). The technique chosen depends on the experience of the practitioner and on the best view achieved.

1. Direct passage of the tracheal tube down the lumen of the laryngoscope. This technique is rapid, but sight of the larynx may be lost during passage of the tracheal tube. However, visual confirmation is nearly always possible. The advantages of the direct passage technique are as follows:

   • Problems (need for extra hand, extra time, problems with railroading) associated with the use of an introducer are avoided;

   • tracheal intubation is achieved rapidly;

   • routine use of an optimum laryngoscopy technique is encouraged.

2. Visual introducer technique (the blind introducer technique is *not* recommended with the paraglossal straight laryngoscopy technique). Passage ("railroading") of the tracheal tube (usually down the lumen of the laryngoscope) over an introducer placed in the trachea, under vision, is reliable, but requires an extra step.

3. Passage lateral to the lumen of the laryngoscope. This technique is used when larger tracheal tubes, such as double lumen tubes, are required.

7.6.9 How is the technique of direct passage of the tracheal tube used?

The tip of the tracheal tube is steered while it is passed *directly* down the lumen of the Henderson laryngoscope. Optimum steering and exit of the tube at the tip of the laryngoscope are achieved when the concavity of the tracheal tube curve faces a position between 300 and 330 degrees inside the lumen of the laryngoscope. It is possible to visualize passage of the tip down the laryngoscope, and between the vocal cords, if the bulk of the tracheal tube is kept just to the right of the lumen of the laryngoscope. It is important to maintain the optimum position of the laryngoscope during passage of the tracheal tube. If resistance is felt, the tube should be withdrawn and the view of the larynx optimized. If the vocal cords are not seen, it is likely that the tube has passed between the cords. A view of the tube lying between the vocal cords can usually be achieved by using the index finger of the right hand to displace the proximal part of tube rightward out of the lumen of the laryngoscope.

If the first attempt at this technique fails, the visual introducer (e.g., the Eschmann Introducer) technique should be used.

7.6.10   When should the visual introducer technique be used?

This technique is recommended during early experience with the Henderson laryngoscope and always when the Miller laryngoscope is used. It is sometimes easier to guide the straight rather than the angled end of the introducer between the vocal cords. The technique is useful whenever it proves difficult to guide the tube to the larynx.[214,215] This technique should *always* be used with straight blades in general and the Henderson laryngoscope in particular if:

- less than 50% of vocal cords is visualized (*not* best *view*);
- the tip of the laryngoscope is not close to the anterior commissure (*not* best *depth of insertion*);
- right aryepiglottic fold overlies right vocal cord (larynx *not* optimally *centered*);
- a tooth intrudes into the lumen of the laryngoscope and it proves difficult to pass the tracheal tube down the lumen of the laryngoscope. Either the introducer and tube are passed from the right side of the tooth or the introducer is passed down the lumen of the laryngoscope, and the laryngoscope is then repositioned before passage of the tracheal tube.

After the introducer has been positioned in the trachea under vision, passage ("railroading") of the tracheal tube is similar to the technique to that with the Macintosh laryngoscope. In particular, *the laryngoscope should be kept in its optimum position, until passage of the tracheal tube is complete.*

7.6.11   When and how is the lateral passage of tracheal tube technique used with the straight laryngoscope?

This technique is required when tracheal tubes larger than 8-mm ID, such as double lumen tubes, are used. The tracheal tube is passed lateral to the lumen of the laryngoscope, so that it is observed to pass between the vocal cords. Use of a straight stylet (with slight tip flexion) within the tracheal tube is recommended if more than 50% of the vocal cords is visible. The visual introducer technique should be used if less than 50% of the vocal cords are visible. Lateral traction on the corner of the mouth by an assistant will help passage of the tracheal tube into the mouth.

7.6.12   What technique is used with the Miller laryngoscope?

The technique is similar to that used with the Henderson laryngoscope. However, the view is more restricted and passage of the tracheal tube is more awkward. The tube must be passed initially to the right of the laryngoscope and it must then travel medially to reach the vocal cords. Although the tracheal tube may be passed directly (preferably with minimal angulation of the tip with a stylet), the visual introducer technique is more reliable.[52] An assistant should retract the corner of the mouth laterally.

7.6.13   Are there any disadvantages to deliberate passage of the straight laryngoscope into the esophagus?

Deliberate passage of the laryngoscope into the esophagus with subsequent withdrawal is recommended by some[216] and is widely used in pediatric practice. This author believes that there is a risk of dislocation of the arytenoid cartilages when the laryngoscope moves from behind the cricoid cartilage to behind the epiglottis. This technique should not be used deliberately, as dislocation of the arytenoids cartilages can cause serious morbidity. Furthermore, this technique impedes development of a more precise technique.

7.6.14   Are there any niche roles for the straight laryngoscope?

The straight laryngoscope may be particularly useful in patients with mandibular hypoplasia.[10,44,217-220] There is much evidence of the value of the straight laryngoscope in management of patients with lesions of the vallecula,[221] such as lingual tonsil hyperplasia.[47] The ENT tubular straight laryngoscopes are of proven value[47,222] for intubation of patients with friable laryngeal tumors and it is probable that semitubular straight laryngoscopes are particularly useful in this clinical situation. The straight laryngoscope can be extremely useful in patients with awkward dentition. Maxillary incisors can interfere with the placement of the Macintosh laryngoscope and particular problems may arise with the prominent teeth and a gap between the incisors into which the laryngoscope slots. In the latter case, the laryngoscope is often directed away from the midline and any attempt to correct this deviation can result in dental damage. These problems can be circumvented by using the straight laryngoscope from the side of the mouth. This is particularly useful in patients who have a gap in their right upper dentition, although considerable expertise with the technique may be required.

7.6.15   Are there limitations to the use of the straight laryngoscope?

A significant commitment is required to master the technique. The number of uses required to achieve moderate competence has not been studied, but there is considerable individual variation in the speed of achieving a satisfactory success rate. Optimum results, when direct laryngoscopy proves difficult, can only be achieved if the straight laryngoscope is used regularly.

There are patients in whom direct laryngoscopy cannot provide a view of the vocal cords, for example, in patients with limited mouth opening. If such difficulty is anticipated, alternative techniques, such as indirect rigid laryngoscopes (Bullard laryngoscope or other video-laryngoscopy systems[39]) may be necessary and awake flexible fiberoptic intubation may be the technique of choice. There will always be patients in whom difficulty is not anticipated or is greater than anticipated. Plan B in the DAS guidelines is flexible fiberoptic intubation through the ILMA.[106] Alternative indirect techniques may also be useful.

7.7   PROCEDURES AFTER TRACHEAL INTUBATION

7.7.1   What are the responsibilities of the airway practitioner following tracheal intubation?

The airway practitioner has a continuing responsibility for relevant management of the patient,[107] including a responsibility to minimize the risk of complications of tracheal intubation. Temporomandibular joint function should be checked immediately after any procedure that involves maximum mouth opening, paying particular attention to ensure that dislocation has not occurred. Serious soft tissue injuries after direct laryngoscopy and tracheal intubation have long been reported in the ENT literature, but have only recently received much attention in the anesthesia literature.[190] In particular, pharyngeal or esophageal damage may cause mediastinitis. Death is less likely if the diagnosis is made promptly and treatment started immediately. Domino et al.[190] state, "Patients in whom tracheal intubation has been difficult should be observed for, and told to watch for, the development of symptoms and signs of retropharyngeal abscess, mediastinitis, or both."

Although most laryngeal injuries caused by tracheal intubation are relatively mild and resolve without intervention,[223,224] expert management of more serious complications is required.[225] Potential complications of difficult airway management should be evaluated and their care optimized.[190] Follow-up care when airway management has proved difficult is strongly supported by expert opinion in the ASA guidelines.[107]

7.7.2   What record of laryngoscopy should be made in the patients' notes? What other communication may be necessary?

The communication of details of problems with tracheal management is very important. The best view of the larynx achieved during laryngoscopy should be recorded in the patient care record. Documentation should include description of the airway difficulties and the management used. It is summarized well in the ASA guidelines.[107] Notification systems to be considered include a written report or letter to the patient, a written report in the medical chart, communication with the patient's surgeon or primary caregiver, and a notification bracelet or equivalent device (see Chapter 57 for details). All of these should be used. Since only a bracelet may be available if the patient is admitted unconscious to hospital, use of a system such as Medic Alert® (www.medicalert.com) is recommended[226,227] for all C/L Grade 3b or Grade 4 patients.

7.8   INDICATIONS AND CONTRAINDICATIONS TO DIRECT LARYNGOSCOPY FOR TRACHEAL INTUBATION

7.8.1   What are the indications for direct laryngoscopy for tracheal intubation?

Tracheal intubation may be required for one or more of the following purposes[228]: need for reliable patency of the upper airway, need for protection of the lungs from pulmonary aspiration, conduit for positive pressure ventilation, and conduit for aspiration of pulmonary secretions. These indications occur most frequently in patients undergoing major surgery, or other surgery close to the airway, and in patients who are critically ill. Tracheal intubation is also indicated in other situations in which other airway techniques prove ineffective. In all these situations, the presence of a cuffed tracheal tube in the trachea provides the most reliable method of securing the airway.

7.8.2   Are there some absolute contraindications to direct laryngoscopy?

There are no absolute contraindications to tracheal intubation. However, there are contraindications to the use of muscle relaxants, anesthesia, or direct laryngoscopy. It has long been recognized that muscle relaxants should not be given if there is doubt about the ability to ventilate the patient with a mask, should tracheal intubation prove difficult. Awake intubation has long been advocated if there is serious doubt about the possibility of achieving tracheal intubation with direct or indirect laryngoscopy.[229] Awake intubation with a flexible fiberoptic laryngoscope (or bronchoscope) was first used in 1972[230] and this has become the method of choice for awake intubation.[209,231–237] It is not possible to make a comprehensive list of all the clinical situations in which awake fiberoptic intubation is the technique of choice, but an index situation is the patient with a dental abscess (e.g., Ludwig's Angina)[238] and difficulty with mouth opening. In some patients with severe airway obstruction, tracheotomy under local anesthesia is the safest technique, although not without risks. Whenever there is significant doubt about the ability to maintain oxygenation, to manage bag-mask-ventilation, or to achieve tracheal intubation, awake fiberoptic intubation or tracheotomy under local anesthesia should be considered the technique of choice. We do not have the right to take risks with the safety of our patients.

7.9   SUMMARY

Placement of a tracheal tube under direct vision, using a laryngoscope, remains one of the most important skills to master for all airway practitioners. Many types of laryngoscopes with curve and straight blades have been developed over the years with the objectives to improve visualization of the vocal cords and easy passage of the tracheal tube. While these devices are highly effective and safe, they all have limitations. To minimize the risk of complications and improve outcome, basic principles must be applied when performing a laryngoscopic intubation. These are as follows: (1) Maintenance of oxygenation must take priority over all other issues, (2) must have backup plans (Plan "A," "B," and "C"); (3) keep the number of intubation attempts to a minimum (not more than three or four); and (4) call for help early.

REFERENCES

1. Macewen W: Clinical observations on the introduction of tracheal tubes by the mouth instead of performing tracheotomy or laryngotomy. *Br Med J.* 1880;1:163–165.
2. Wawersik J: History of anesthesia in Germany. *J Clin Anesth.* 1991;3: 235–244.
3. Kirstein A: *Autoskopie des larynx und der trachea.* Berlin: Klinische Wochenschrift 1895;32:476–478.
4. Elsberg CA: Clinical experiences with intratracheal insufflation (Meltzer), with remarks upon the value of the method for thoracic surgery. *Ann Surg.* 1910;52:23–29.
5. Kelly RE: Intratracheal anaesthesia. *Proc Roy Soc Med.* 1914;7:25–28.
6. Jackson C: The technique of insertion of intratracheal insufflation tubes. *Surg Gynecol Obstet.* 1913;17:507–509.
7. Jackson C: Bronchoscopy and esophagoscopy. Gleanings from experience. *JAMA.* 1909;13:1009–1013.
8. Magill IW: An improved laryngoscope for anaesthetists. *Lancet.* 1926;1:500.
9. Magill IW: Technique in endotracheal anaesthesia. *Br Med J.* 1930;2: 817–820.
10. Bonfils P: Difficult intubation in Pierre-Robin children, a new method: the retromolar route. *Anaesthesist.* 1983;32:363–367.
11. Henderson JJ: The use of paraglossal straight blade laryngoscopy in difficult tracheal intubation. *Anaesthesia.* 1997;52:552–560.
12. Macintosh RR: A new laryngoscope. *Lancet.* 1943;1:205.
13. Levitan RM: *The AirwayCam™ guide to intubation and practical emergency airway management.* Wayne: AirwayCam Technologies Inc, 2004.
14. Cormack RS, Lehane J: Difficult tracheal intubation in obstetrics. *Anaesthesia.* 1984;39:1105–1111.
15. Cook TM: A new practical classification of laryngeal view. *Anaesthesia.* 2000;55:274–279.
16. Rose DK, Cohen MM: The incidence of airway problems depends on the definition used. *Can J Anaesth.* 1996;43:30–34.
17. Crosby ET, Cooper RM, Douglas MJ, et al.: The unanticipated difficult airway with recommendations for management. *Can J Anaesth.* 1998;45: 757–776.
18. Benumof JL: Difficult laryngoscopy: obtaining the best view. *Can J Anaesth.* 1994;41:361–365.
19. Adnet F, Borron SW, Racine SX, et al.: The intubation difficulty scale (IDS): proposal and evaluation of a new score characterizing the complexity of endotracheal intubation. *Anesthesiology.* 1997;87:1290–1297.
20. Benumof JL: Intubation difficulty scale: anticipated best use. *Anesthesiology.* 1997;87:1273–1274.
21. Ezri T, Weisenberg M, Khazin V, et al.: Difficult laryngoscopy: incidence and predictors in patients undergoing coronary artery bypass surgery versus general surgery patients. *J Cardiothorac Vasc Anesth.* 2003;17:321–324.
23. Adnet F, Baillard C, Borron SW, et al.: Randomized study comparing the "sniffing position" with simple head extension for laryngoscopic view in elective surgery patients. *Anesthesiology.* 2001;95:836–841.
22. Calder I, Calder J, Crockard HA: Difficult direct laryngoscopy in patients with cervical spine disease. *Anaesthesia.* 1995;50:756–763.
24. Bannister FB, MacBeth RG: Direct laryngoscopy and tracheal intubation. *Lancet.* 1944;2:651–654.
25. Magill IW: Endotracheal anaesthesia. *Am J Surg.* 1936;34:450–455.
26. Adnet F, Borron SW, Dumas JL, et al.: Study of the "sniffing position" by magnetic resonance imaging. *Anesthesiology.* 2001;94:83–86.
27. Candido KD, Ghaleb AH, Saatee S, Khorasani A: Reevaluating the "cornerstone of training in anesthesiology." *Anesthesiology.* 2001;95:1043–1044.
28. Isono S: Common practice and concepts in anesthesia: time for reassessment. Is the sniffing position a "gold standard" for laryngoscopy? *Anesthesiology.* 2001;95:825–827.
29. Horton WA, Fahy L, Charters P: Defining a standard intubating position using "angle finder." *Br J Anaesth.* 1989;62:6–12.
30. Calder I, Picard J, Chapman M, O'Sullivan C, Crockard HA: Mouth opening: a new angle. *Anesthesiology.* 2003;99:799–801.
31. Isono S, Tanaka A, Ishikawa T, Tagaito Y, Nishino T: Sniffing position improves pharyngeal airway patency in anesthetized patients with obstructive sleep apnea. *Anesthesiology.* 2005;103:489–494.
32. Bishop MJ, Harrington RM, Tencer AF: Force applied during tracheal intubation. *Anesth Analg.* 1992;74:411–414.
33. McCoy EP, Mirakhur RK, Rafferty C, Bunting H, Austin BA: A comparison of the forces exerted during laryngoscopy. The Macintosh versus the McCoy blade. *Anaesthesia.* 1996;51:912–915.
34. Hastings RH, Hon ED, Nghiem C, Wahrenbrock EA: Force and torque vary between laryngoscopists and laryngoscope blades. *Anesth Analg.* 1996;82:462–468.
35. Williams KN, Carli F, Cormack RS: Unexpected difficult laryngoscopy: a prospective survey in routine general surgery. *Br J Anaesth.* 1991;66:38–44.
36. Adnet F, Racine SX, Borron SW, et al.: A survey of tracheal intubation difficulty in the operating room: a prospective observational study. *Acta Anaesthesiol Scand.* 2001;45:327–332.
37. Horton WA, Fahy L, Charters P: Factor analysis in difficult tracheal intubation: laryngoscopy-induced airway obstruction. *Br J Anaesth.* 1990;65:801–805.
38. Fahy L, Horton WA, Charters P: Factor analysis in patients with a history of failed tracheal intubation during pregnancy. *Br J Anaesth.* 1990;65:813–815.
39. Henderson JJ: Tracheal intubation of the adult patient. In: *Core Topics in Airway Management.* Calder IA, Pearce AC, eds. Cambridge: Cambridge University Press, 2004:69–79.
40. Arai T, Nagaro T, Nitta K: Management of the difficult endotracheal intubation; advantages of the Miller blade and a facilitated nasotracheal intubation with a fiberoptic bronchoscope. *Masui* 1987;36:1112–1116.
41. Bellhouse CP: An angulated laryngoscope for routine and difficult tracheal intubations. *Anesthesiology.* 1988;69:126–129.
42. Henderson JJ, Frerk CM: Remember the straight laryngoscope. *Br J Anaesth.* 2002;88:151–152.
43. Sofferman RA, Johnson DL, Spencer RF: Lost airway during anesthesia induction: alternatives for management. *Laryngoscope.* 1997;107:1476–1482.
44. Chen PP, Cheng CK, Abdullah V, Chu CPW: Tracheal intubation using suspension laryngoscopy in an infant with Goldenhar's syndrome. *Anaesth Intensive Care.* 2001;29:548–551.
45. Davies R, Balachandran S: Anterior commisure laryngoscope. *Anaesthesia.* 2003;58:721–722.
46. Dering A, Corbridge R, Kitching A: The Negus slotted laryngoscope. *Anaesthesia.* 2003;58:1242.
47. Davies S, Ananthanarayan C, Castro C: Asymptomatic lingual tonsillar hypertrophy and difficult airway management: a report of three cases. *Can J Anaesth.* 2001;48:1020–1024.
48. Hulme GJ, Blues CM: Acromegaly and papillomatosis: difficult intubation and use of the airway exchange catheter. *Anaesthesia.* 1999;54:787–789.
49. Henderson JJ: ENT vs. anaesthesia "straight" laryngoscopes. *Anaesth Intensive Care.* 2002;30:250–251.
50. Arino JJ, Velasco JM, Gasco C, Lopez-Timoneda F: Straight blades improve visualization of the larynx while curved blades increase ease of intubation: a comparison of the Macintosh, Miller, McCoy, Belscope and Lee-Fiberview blades. *Can J Anaesth.* 2003;50:5016.
51. Lim M, Demspey C, Pead M: Choosing a laryngoscope blade: straight vs curved. *Can J Anaesth.* 2003;50:1078–1079.
52. Miller L: Choosing a laryngoscope blade: straight vs curved. *Can J Anaesth.* 2003;50:1079–1080.
53. Dorsch JA, Dorsch SE: Laryngoscopes. In: *Understanding Anesthesia Equipment,* 2nd edn. Dorsch JA, Dorsch SE, eds. Baltimore: Williams & Wilkins, 1984:338–352.
54. Soper RL: A new laryngoscope for anaesthetists. *Br Med J.* 1947;1:265.
55. Toung TJK, Donham RT, Shipley R: Thermal burn caused by a laryngoscope. *Anesthesiology.* 1981;55:184–185.
56. Perel A, Katz E, Davidson JT: Fiberbronchoscopic retrieval of an aspirated laryngoscope bulb. *Intensive Care Med.* 1981;7:143–144.
57. Ince Z, Tugcu D, Coban A: An unusual complication of endotracheal intubation: ingestion of a laryngoscope bulb. *Pediatr Emerg Care.* 1998;14: 275–276.
58. Tousignant G, Tessler MJ: Light intensity and area of illumination provided by various laryngoscope blades. *Can J Anaesth.* 1994;41:865–869.
59. Skilton RW, Parry D, Arthurs GJ, Hiles P: A study of the brightness of laryngoscope light. *Anaesthesia.* 1996;51:667–672.
60. Crosby E, Cleland M: An assessment of the luminance and light field characteristics of used direct laryngoscopes. *Can J Anaesth.* 1999;46:792–796.

61. Bucx MJ, De Gast HM, Veldhuis J, et al.: The effect of mechanical cleaning and thermal disinfection on light intensity provided by fibrelight Macintosh laryngoscopes. *Anaesthesia.* 2003;58:461–465.

62. Daley MD, Norman PH: The sniffing position. *Anesthesiology.* 2002;97:751–752.

63. Asai T, Matsumoto S, Fujise K, Johmura S, Shingu K: Comparison of two Macintosh laryngoscope blades in 300 patients. *Br J Anaesth.* 2003;90:457–460.

64. Lee J, Choi JH, Lee YK, et al.: The Callander laryngoscope blade modification is associated with a decreased risk of dental contact. *Can J Anaesth.* 2004;51:181–184.

65. Eldor J, Gozal Y: The length of the blade is more important than its design in difficult tracheal intubation. *Can J Anaesth.* 1990;37:268.

66. Weeks DB: A new use for an old blade. *Anesthesiology.* 1974;40:200–201.

67. Bourke DL, Lawrence J: Another way to insert a Macintosh blade. *Anesthesiology.* 1983;59:80.

68. Cartwright FF: Devices for anaesthesia in throat surgery. *Anaesthesia.* 1953;8:119.

69. Pope ES: Left-handed laryngoscope. *Anaesthesia.* 1960;15:326–328.

70. Lagade MR, Poppers PJ: Use of the left-entry laryngoscope blade in patients with right-sided oro-facial lesions. *Anesthesiology.* 1983;58:300.

71. Buckland RW: The left-handed laryngoscope. *Anaesthesia.* 1999;54:602–603.

72. Racz GB: Improved vision modification of the Macintosh laryngoscope. *Anaesthesia.* 1984;39:1249–1250.

73. McCoy EP, Mirakhur RK: The levering laryngoscope. *Anaesthesia.* 1993;48:516–519.

74. Farling PA: The McCoy levering laryngoscope blade. *Anaesthesia.* 1994;49:358.

75. Johnston HML, Rao U: The McCoy levering laryngoscope blade. *Anaesthesia.* 1994;49:358.

76. Ward M: The McCoy levering laryngoscope blade. *Anaesthesia.* 1994;49:357–358.

77. Chadwick IS, McCluskey A: Another trachea intubated with the McCoy laryngoscope. *Anaesthesia.* 1995;50:571.

78. Haridas RP: The McCoy levering laryngoscope blade. *Anaesthesia.* 1996;51:91.

79. Wakeling HG, Ody A, Ball A: Large goitre causing difficult intubation and failure to intubate using the intubating laryngeal mask airway: lessons for next time. *Br J Anaesth.* 1998;81:979–981.

80. Asai T, Hirose T, Shingu K: Failed tracheal intubation using a laryngoscope and intubating laryngeal mask. *Can J Anaesth.* 2000;47:325–328.

81. Chisholm DG, Calder I: Experience with the McCoy laryngoscope in difficult laryngoscopy. *Anaesthesia.* 1997;52:906–908.

82. Uchida T, Hikawa Y, Saito Y, Yasuda K: The McCoy levering laryngoscope in patients with limited neck extension. *Can J Anaesth.* 1997;44:674–676.

83. Levitan RM, Ochroch EA: Explaining the variable effect on laryngeal view obtained with the McCoy laryngoscope. *Anaesthesia.* 1999;54:599–601.

84. Gabbott DA: Laryngoscopy using the McCoy laryngoscope after application of a cervical collar. *Anaesthesia.* 1996;51:812–814.

85. Laurent SC, de Melo AE, Alexander-Williams JM: The use of the McCoy laryngoscope in patients with simulated cervical spine injuries. *Anaesthesia.* 1996;51:74–75.

86. Huffman JP, Elam JO: Prisms and fiber optics for laryngoscopy. *Anesth Analg.* 1971;50:64–67.

87. Siker ES: A mirror laryngoscope. *Anesthesiology.* 1956;17:38–42.

88. Biro P: A modified Macintosh blade for difficult intubation. The mirror blade. *Anaesthesist.* 1993;42:105–110.

89. Weisenberg M, Warters RD, Medalion B, et al.: Endotracheal intubation with a gum-elastic bougie in unanticipated difficult direct laryngoscopy: comparison of a blind technique versus indirect laryngoscopy with a laryngeal mirror. *Anesth Analg.* 2002;95:1090–1093.

90. Patil VU, Sopchak AM, Thomas PS: Use of a dental mirror as an aid to tracheal intubation in an infant. *Anesthesiology.* 1993;78:619–620.

91. Bucx MJ, Droogers W, Mallios C: A method to prevent clouding of the Belscope prism. *Anesth Intensive Care.* 1994;22:320.

92. Gould RB: Modified layngoscope blade. *Anaesthesia.* 1954;9:125.

93. Portzer M, Wasmuth CE: Endotracheal anesthesia using a modified Wis-Foregger laryngoscope blade. *Cleve Clin Q.* 1959;26:140–143.

94. Schapira M: A modified straight laryngoscope blade designed to facilitate endotracheal intubation. *Anesth Analg.* 1973;52:553–554.

95. Choi JJ: A new double-angle blade for direct laryngoscopy. *Anesthesiology.* 1990;72:576.

96. Orr RB: A new laryngoscope blade designed to facilitate difficult endotracheal intubation. *Anesthesiology.* 1969;31:377–378.

97. Miller RA: A new laryngoscope. *Anesthesiology.* 1941;2:317–320.

98. Bruin G: The Miller blade and the disappearing light source. *Anesth Analg.* 1996;83:888.

99. Raw D, Skinner A: Miller laryngoscope blades. *Anaesthesia.* 1999;54:500.

100. Watanabe S, Suga A, Asakura N, et al.: Determination of the distance between the laryngoscope blade and the upper incisors during direct laryngoscopy: comparisons of a curved, an angulated straight, and two straight blades. *Anesth Analg.* 1994;79:638–641.

101. Mayall RM: The Belscope for management of the difficult airway. *Anesthesiology.* 1992;76:1059–1060.

102. Phillips OC, Duerksen RL: Endotracheal intubation: a new blade for direct laryngoscopy. *Anesth Analg.* 1973;52:691–698.

103. Crinquette V, Vilette B, Solanet C, et al.: Appraisal of the PCV, a laryngoscope for difficult endotracheal intubation. *Ann Fr Anesth Réanim.* 1991;10:589–594.

104. Henderson JJ: Solutions to the problem of difficult tracheal tube passage associated with the paraglossal straight laryngoscopy technique. *Anaesthesia.* 1999;54:601–602.

105. Whittaker JD, Moulton C: Emergency intubation of infants: does laryngoscope blade design make any difference? *J Accid Emerg Med.* 1998;15:308–311.

106. Henderson JJ, Popat MT, Latto IP, Pearce AC, Difficult Airway Society: Difficult Airway Society guidelines for management of the unanticipated difficult intubation. *Anaesthesia.* 2004;59:675–694.

107. American Society of Anesthesiologists Task Force on Management of the Difficult Airway: Practice guidelines for management of the difficult airway. An updated report by the American Society of Anesthesiologists Task Force on Management of the Difficult Airway. *Anesthesiology.* 2003;98:1269–1277.

108. Wilson ME, Spiegelhalter D, Robertson JA, Lesser P: Predicting difficult intubation. *Br J Anaesth.* 1988;61:211–216.

109. El-Ganzouri AR, McCarthy RJ, Tuman KJ, Tanck EN, Ivankovich AD: Preoperative airway assessment: predictive value of a multivariate risk index. *Anesth Analg.* 1996;82:1197–1204.

110. Lee L: You can smell the difference. *Anesthesiology.* 2001;95:1045.

111. Ovassapian A, Glassenberg R, Randel GI, et al.: The unexpected difficult airway and lingual tonsil hyperplasia: a case series and a review of the literature. *Anesthesiology.* 2002;97:124–132.

112. White A, Kander PL: Anatomical factors in difficult direct laryngoscopy. *Br J Anaesth.* 1975;47:468–474.

113. Chou HC, Wu TL: Mandibulohyoid distance in difficult laryngoscopy. *Br J Anaesth.* 1993;71:335–339.

114. Yentis SM: Predicting difficult intubation—worthwhile exercise or pointless ritual. *Anaesthesia.* 2002;57:105–109.

115. Kristensen M: Predicting difficult intubation 2. *Anaesthesia.* 2002;57:612–613.

116. Eichhorn JH, Cooper JB, Cullen DJ: Standards for patient monitoring during anesthesia at Harvard Medical Schools. *JAMA.* 1986;256:1017–1020.

117. Benumof JL, Dagg R, Benumof R: Critical hemoglobin desaturation will occur before return to an unparalyzed state following 1 mg/kg intravenous succinylcholine. *Anesthesiology.* 1997;87:979–982.

118. Woods AW, Grant S, Harten J, Noble JS, Davidson JA: Tracheal intubating conditions after induction with propofol, remifentanil and lignocaine. *Eur J Anaesthesiol.* 1998;15:714–718.

119. Ng KP, Wang CY: Alfentanil for intubation under halothane anaesthesia in children. *Paediatr Anaesth.* 1999;9:491–494.

120. Wong AK, Teoh GS: Intubation without muscle relaxant: an alternative technique for rapid tracheal intubation. *Anaesth Intensive Care.* 1996;24:224–230.

121. Harsten A, Gillberg L: Intubating conditions provided by propofol and alfentanil—acceptable, but not ideal. *Acta Anaesthesiol Scand.* 1997;41:985–987.

122. Schlaich N, Mertzlufft F, Soltesz S, Fuchs-Buder T: Remifentanil and propofol without muscle relaxants or with different doses of rocuronium for tracheal intubation in outpatient anaesthesia. *Acta Anaesthesiol Scand.* 2000;44:720–726.

123. Kopman AF, Klewicka MM, Neuman GG: Re-examined: the recommended endotracheal intubating dose for nondepolarizing neuromuscular blockers of rapid onset. *Anesth Analg.* 2001;93:954–959.

124. Mencke T, Echternach M, Kleinschmidt S, et al.: Laryngeal morbidity and quality of tracheal intubation: a randomized controlled trial. *Anesthesiology.* 2003;98:1049–1056.

125. Donati F: Tracheal intubation: unconsciousness, analgesia and muscle relaxation. *Can J Anaesth.* 2003;50:99–103.

126. Bulow K, Nielsen TG, Lund J: The effect of topical lignocaine on intubating conditions after propofol-alfentanil induction. *Acta Anaesthesiol Scand.* 1996;40:752–756.

127. Ludbrook GL, Hitchcock M, Upton RN: The difficult airway: Propofol infusion as an alternative to gaseous induction. *Anaesth Intensive Care.* 1997;25:71–73.

128. Edwards RM: Adult inhalational induction. *Anaesth Intensive Care.* 1997;25:198–199.

129. Sjogren P, Pedersen T, Steinmetz H: Mucopolysaccharidoses and anaesthetic risks. *Acta Anaesthesiol Scand.* 1987;31:214–218.

130. Mehta Y, Schou H: The anaesthetic management of an infant with frontometaphyseal dysplasia (Gorlin-Cohen syndrome). *Acta Anaesthesiol Scand.* 1988;32:505–507.

131. Mostafa SM, Atherton AM: Sevoflurane for difficult tracheal intubation. *Br J Anaesth.* 1997;79:392–393.

132. Watters MP, McKenzie JM: Inhalational induction with sevoflurane in an adult with severe complex central airways obstruction. *Anaesth Intensive Care.* 1997;25:704–706.

133. Mason RA, Fielder CP: The obstructed airway in head and neck surgery. *Anaesthesia.* 1999;54:625–628.

134. Burtner DD, Goodman M: Anesthetic and operative management of potential upper airway obstruction. *Arch Otolaryngol.* 1978;104:657–661.

135. Smith M, Calder I, Crockard A, Isert P, Nicol ME: Oxygen saturation and cardiovascular changes during fibreoptic intubation under general anaesthesia. *Anaesthesia.* 1992;47:158–161.

136. Benumof JL: Conventional (laryngoscopic) orotracheal and nasotracheal intubation (single-lumen tube). In: *Airway Management.* Benumof JL, ed. St. Louis: Mosby-Year Book; 1996:261–276.

137. Riddell PL: Reshaping the Macintosh blade. *Anaesthesia.* 1997;52: 1017–1018.

138. Zeitels SM, Vaughan CW: "External counterpressure" and "internal distention" for optimal laryngoscopic exposure of the anterior glottal commissure. *Ann Otol Rhinol Laryngol.* 1994;103:669–675.

139. Hochman II, Zeitels SM, Heaton JT: Analysis of the forces and position required for direct laryngoscopic exposure of the anterior vocal folds. *Ann Otol Rhinol Laryngol.* 1999;108:715–724.

140. Benumof JL, Cooper SD: Quantitative improvement in laryngoscopic view by optimal external laryngeal manipulation. *J Clin Anesth.* 1996;8: 136–140.

141. Knill RL: Difficult laryngoscopy made easy with a "BURP." *Can J Anaesth.* 1993;40:279–282.

142. Levitan RM, Mickler T, Hollander JE: Bimanual laryngoscopy: a videographic study of external laryngeal manipulation by novice intubators. *Ann Emerg Med.* 2002;40:30–37.

143. Schmitt HJ, Mang H: Head and neck elevation beyond the sniffing position improves laryngeal view in cases of difficult direct laryngoscopy. *J Clin Anesth.* 2002;14:335–338.

144. Krantz MA, Poulos JG, Chaouki K, Adamek P: The laryngeal lift: a method to facilitate endotracheal intubation. *J Clin Anesth.* 1993;5:297–301.

213. Tamura M, Ishikawa T, Kato R, Isono S, Nishino T: Mandibular advancement improves the laryngeal view during direct laryngoscopy performed by inexperienced physicians. *Anesthesiology.* 2004;100:598–601.

145. Henderson JJ: Intubation techniques for unanticipated difficult intubation: Stylets and introducers. In: *Der schwerige Atemweg.* Dörges V, Paschen H-R, eds. Berlin: Springer-Verlag; 2004.

146. Deutsch EV: A stilet for endotracheal intubation. *Anesthesiology.* 1951;15: 667–670.

147. Linder GS: New polyolefin-coated endotracheal tube stylet. *Anesth Analg.* 1974;53:341–342.

148. Kubota Y, Toyoda Y, Kubota H, Ueda Y: Shaping tracheal tubes. *Anaesthesia.* 1987;42:896.

149. Smith M, Buist RJ, Mansour NY: A simple method to facilitate difficult intubation. *Can J Anaesth.* 1990;37:144–145.

150. Black AE, Tratman AJ: Stylets for small tracheal tubes. *Anaesthesia.* 1994;49:549.

151. Mehta S: Safer endotracheal intubation. *Lancet.* 1986;1:1148.

152. Ellis PDM, Pallister WK: Recurrent laryngeal nerve palsy and endotracheal intubation. *J Laryngol Otol.* 1975;89:823–826.

153. Cavo JW, Jr.: True vocal cord paralysis following intubation. *Laryngoscope* 1985;95:1352–1359.

154. Bhargava M, Pothula SN, Joshi S: The obstruction of an endotracheal tube by the plastic coating sheared from a stylet: a revisit. *Anesthesiology.* 1998;88:548–549.

155. Sinha PK, Dubey PK: Shearing of plastic coating of stylet with double lumen tube: another incident. *Anesthesiology.* 1999;90:326–327.

156. Henderson JJ: Development of the "gum-elastic bougie." *Anaesthesia.* 2003;58:103–104.

157. Sellers WFS, Jones GW: Difficult tracheal intubation. *Anaesthesia.* 1986;41:93.

158. Kidd JF, Dyson A, Latto IP: Successful difficult intubation. Use of the gum elastic bougie. *Anaesthesia.* 1988;43:437–438.

159. Mushambi MC, Iyer GA: Gum elastic bougies. *Anaesthesia.* 2002;57:727.

160. Sellers WFS: Gum elastic bougies. *Anaesthesia.* 2002;57:289.

161. Hodzovic I, Wilkes AR, Latto IP: To shape or not to shape ... simulated bougie-assisted difficult intubation in a manikin. *Anaesthesia.* 2003;58: 792–797.

162. Annamaneni R, Hodzovic I, Wilkes AR, Latto IP: A comparison of simulated difficult intubation with multiple-use and single-use bougies in a manikin. *Anaesthesia.* 2003;58:45–49.

163. Marfin AG, Pandit JJ, Hames KC, Popat MT, Yentis SM: Use of the bougie in simulated difficult intubation. 2: Comparison of single-use bougie with multiple-use bougie. *Anaesthesia.* 2003;58:852–855.

164. Rucklidge MW, Patel A: Failure of the single-use bougie in acute epiglottitis. *Anaesthesia.* 2004;59:925–926.

165. Tuzzo DM, Frova G: Application of the self-inflating bulb to a hollow intubating introducer. *Minerva Anestesiol.* 2001;67:127–132.

166. Frova G: Comparison of tracheal introducers. *Anaesthesia.* 2005;60:516–517.

167. Latto IP: Fracture of the outer varnish layer of a gum elastic bougie. *Anaesthesia.* 1999;54:497–498.

168. Kumar DS, Jones G: Is your bougie helping or hindering you? *Anaesthesia.* 2001;56:1121.

169. Boys JE: Failed intubation in obstetric anaesthesia. A case report. *Br J Anaesth.* 1983;55:187–188.

170. Alexander R, Moore C: The laryngeal mask airway and training in nasotracheal intubation. *Anaesthesia.* 1993;48:350–351.

171. Dogra S, Falconer R, Latto IP: Successful difficult intubation. Tracheal tube placement over a gum-elastic bougie. *Anaesthesia.* 1990;45:774–776.

172. Viswanathan S, Campbell C, Wood DG, Riopelle JM, Naraghi M: The Eschmann Tracheal Tube Introducer. (Gum elastic bougie). *Anesthesiol Rev.* 1992;19:29–34.

173. Koh KF, Hare JD, Calder I: Small tubes revisited. *Anaesthesia.* 1998;53:46–50.

174. Brull SJ, Wiklund R, Ferris C, et al.: Facilitation of fiberoptic orotracheal intubation with a flexible tracheal tube. *Anesth Analg.* 1994;78:746–748.

175. Calder I: When the endotracheal tube will not pass over the flexible fiberoptic bronchoscope. *Anesthesiology.* 1992;77:398.

176. Christian AS: Failed obstetric intubation. *Anaesthesia.* 1990;45:995.

177. Gordon PC, Carr AS: Difficult intubation prior to coronary artery surgery. *J Cardiothorac Vasc Anesth.* 1994;8:485.

178. McClune S, Regan M, Moore J: Laryngeal mask airway for caesarean section. *Anaesthesia.* 1990;45:227–228.

179. Russell SH, Hirsch NP: Simultaneous use of two laryngoscopes. *Anaesthesia.* 1993;48:918.

180. Williamson JA, Webb RK, Szekely S, Gillies ER, Dreosti AV: The Australian Incident Monitoring Study. Difficult intubation: an analysis of 2000 incident reports. *Anaesth Intensive Care.* 1993;21:602–607.

181. Latto IP, Stacey M, Mecklenburgh J, Vaughan RS: Survey of the use of the gum elastic bougie in clinical practice. *Anaesthesia.* 2002;57:379–384.

182. Combes X, Le Roux B, Suen P, et al.: Unanticipated difficult airway in anesthetized patients: prospective validation of a management algorithm. *Anesthesiology.* 2004;100:1146–1150.

183. Henderson JJ: Questions about the Macintosh laryngoscope and technique of laryngoscopy. *Eur J Anaesthesiol.* 2000;17:2–5.

184. Williamson R: Endotracheal intubation in temporo-mandibular ankylosis. *Anesth Analg.* 1988;67:602–603.

185. Bryan AG, Jones A: Skier's neck: an unusual cause of difficult intubation. *Anaesthesia.* 1991;46:802.

186. Gilbert SM: *Wrongful Death.* New York: Norton; 1997.

187. Peterson GN, Domino KB, Caplan RA, et al.: Management of the difficult airway: a closed claims analysis. *Anesthesiology.* 2005;103:33–39.

188. Mort TC: Emergency tracheal intubation: complications associated with repeated laryngoscopic attempts. *Anesth Analg.* 2004;99:607–613.

189. Caplan RA, Posner KL, Ward RJ, Cheney FW: Adverse respiratory events in anesthesia: a closed claims analysis. *Anesthesiology.* 1990;72:828–833.

190. Domino KB, Posner KL, Caplan RA, Cheney FW: Airway injury during anesthesia: a closed claims analysis. *Anesthesiology.* 1999;91:1703–1711.

191. Fear DW: Failed intubation in the parturient. *Can J Anaesth.* 1989;36:614–616.

192. Henderson JJ, Popat MT, Latto IP, Pearce AC: Difficult Airway Society guidelines for management of the unanticipated difficult intubation. *Anaesthesia.* 2004;59:675–694.

193. Lagade MRG, Poppers PJ: Revival of the polio laryngoscope blade. *Anesthesiology.* 1982;57:545.
194. Datta S, Briwa J: Modified laryngoscope for endotracheal intubation of obese patients. *Anesth Analg.* 1981;60:120–121.
195. Kay NH: Mammomegaly and intubation. *Anaesthesia.* 1982;37:221.
196. Jephcott A: Mammomegaly and intubation: the polio blade. *Anaesthesia.* 1982;37:780.
197. Jellicoe JA, Harris NR: A modification of a standard laryngoscope for difficult tracheal intubation in obstetric cases. *Anaesthesia.*1984;39:800–802.
198. Patil VU, Stehling LC, Zauder HL: An adjustable laryngoscope handle for difficult intubations. *Anesthesiology.* 1984;60:609.
199. Nunn G: A new laryngoscope. A modified laryngoscope to facilitate intubation in cases of restricted access. *Anaesthesia.* 1987;42:877–878.
200. Dhara SS, Cheong TW: An adjustable multiple angle laryngoscope adaptor. *Anaesth Intensive Care.* 1991;19:243–245.
201. Yentis SM: A laryngoscope adaptor for difficult intubation. *Anaesthesia.* 1987;42:764–766.
202. Sanehi O: Confirmation of tracheal intubation. In: *Core Topics in Airway Management.* Calder I, Pearce A, eds. Cambridge: Cambridge University Press; 2005:81–85.
203. Clyburn P, Rosen M: Accidental oesophageal intubation. *Br J Anaesth.* 1994;73:55–63.
204. Patel N, Smith CE, Pinchak AC, Hancock DE: Taping methods and tape types for securing oral endotracheal tubes. *Can J Anaesth.* 1997;44:330–336.
205. Rodenberg H, Edwards K, Hayes T: The modified clove hitch: a technique to maintain endotracheal tube position in the intubated patient. *J Emerg Med.* 1992;10:185–188.
206. Lang SA, Duncan PG, Shephard DA, Ha HC: Pulmonary oedema associated with airway obstruction. *Can J Anaesth.* 1990;37:210–218.
207. Liu EH, Yih PS: Negative pressure pulmonary oedema caused by biting and endotracheal tube occlusion-a case for oropharyngeal airways. *Singapore Med J.* 1999;40:174–175.
208. Wiggin SC: A new modification of the conventional laryngoscope and technic for laryngoscopy. *Anesthesiology.* 1944;5:61–68.
209. Brown ACD, Sataloff RT: Special anesthetic techniques in head and neck surgery. *Otolaryngol Clin North Am.* 1981;14:587–514.
210. Brown A, Norton ML: Instrumentation and equipment for management of the difficult airway. In: *Atlas of the Difficult Airway.* Norton ML, Brown ACD, eds. St. Louis: Mosby-Year Book; 1991: 24–32.
211. Dean VS, Jurai SA: The "roll" sign for oesophageal intubation. *Anaesthesia.* 1996;51:803.
212. Levitan RM, Mechem CC, Ochroch EA, Shofer FS, Hollander JE: Head-elevated laryngoscopy position: improving laryngeal exposure during laryngoscopy by increasing head elevation. *Ann Emerg Med.* 2003;41:322–330.
214. Dutta A, Batra YK, Mohari AR, Chari P: An unusual solution to unsuspected difficult airway: the esophageal dilator guide. *Can J Anaesth.* 2001;48:1048–1049.
215. Al Shamaa M, Jefferson P, Ball DR: Lingual tonsil hypertrophy: airway management. *Anaesthesia.* 2003;58:1134–1135.
216. Schneider RE, Murphy MF: Bag/mask ventilation and endotracheal intubation. In: *Manual of Emergency Airway Management,* 2nd edn. Walls RM, Murphy MF, Luten RC, Schneider RE, eds. Philadelphia, PA: Lippincott Williams & Wilkins, 2004: 43–69.
217. Handler SD, Keon TP: Difficult laryngoscopy/intubation: the child with mandibular hypoplasia. *Ann Otol Rhinol Laryngol.* 1983;92:401–404.
218. Benjamin B, Walker P: Management of airway obstruction in the Pierre Robin sequence. *Int J Pediatr Otorhinolaryngol.* 1991;22:29–37.
219. Stevenson GW, Hall SC, Bauer BS, Vicari FA, Seleny FL: Anaesthetic management of Miller's syndrome. *Can J Anaesth.* 1991;38:1046–1049.
220. Diaz JH, Guarisco JL, LeJeune FE, Jr.: Perioperative management of paediatric microstomia. *Can J Anaesth.* 1991;38:217–221.
221. Kamble VA, Lilly RB, Gross JB: Unanticipated difficult intubation as a result of an asymptomatic vallecular cyst. *Anesthesiology.* 1999;91:872–873.
222. Wolf C, LeJeune FE, Jr., Douglas JR, Jr.: A technique for intubation of the difficult airway. *Otolaryngol Head Neck Surg.* 1987;96:278–281.
223. Peppard SB, Dickens JH: Laryngeal injury following short-term intubation. *Ann Otol Rhinol Laryngol.* 1983;92:327–330.
224. Avrahami E, Frishman E, Spierer I, Englender M, Katz R: CT of minor intubation trauma with clinical correlations. *Eur J Radiol.* 1995;20:68–71.
225. Tolley NS, Cheesman TD, Morgan D, Brookes GB: Dislocated arytenoid: an intubation-induced injury. *Ann R Coll Surg Engl.* 1990;72:353–356.
226. Davies JM, Weeks S, Crone LA, Pavlin E: Difficult intubation in the parturient. *Can J Anaesth.* 1989;36:668–674.
227. Buckland RW, Pedley J: Lingual thyroid—a threat to the airway. *Anaesthesia.* 2000;55:1103–1105.
228. Benumof JL: Indications for tracheal intubation. In: *Airway Management. Principles and Practice.* Benumof JL, ed. St. Louis: Mosby, 1996: 255–260.
229. Giuffrida JG, Bizzari DV, Latteri FF, et al.: Prevention of major airway complications during anesthesia by intubation of the conscious patient. *Anesth Analg.* 1960;39:201.
230. Conyers AB, Wallace DH, Mulder DS: Use of the fiberoptic bronchoscope for nasotracheal intubation: case report. *Can Anaesth Soc J.* 1972;19:654–656.
231. Ovassapian A, Doka JC, Rosma DE: Acromegaly—use of fiberoptic laryngoscopy to avoid tracheostomy. *Anesthesiology.* 1981;54:429–430.
232. Ovassapian A, Randel GI: The role of the fiberscope in the critically ill patient. *Crit Care Clin.* 1995;11:29–51.
233. Hains JD, Gibbin KP: Fiberoptic laryngoscopy in ankylosing spondylitis. *J Laryngol Otol.* 1973;87:699–703.
234. Schwartz HC, Bauer RA, Davis NJ: Ludwig's angina: use of fiberoptic laryngoscopy to avoid tracheostomy. *J Oral Surg.* 1974;32:608–611.
235. Mulder DS, Wallace DH, Woolhouse FM: The use of the fiberoptic bronchoscope to facilitate endotracheal intubation following head and neck trauma. *J Trauma.* 1975;15:638–640.
236. Venus B: Acromegalic patient—indications for fiberoptic bronchoscopy but not tracheostomy. *Anesthesiology.* 1980;52:100.
237. Vaughan RS: Airways revisited. *Br J Anaesth.* 1989;62:1–3.
238. Ovassapian A, Tuncbilek M, Weitzel EK, Joshi CW: Airway management in adult patients with deep neck infections: a case series and review of the literature. *Anesth Analg.* 2005;100:585–589.

SELF-EVALUATION QUESTIONS

7.1. All of the following maneuvers are of proven value at improving the glottic view with the macintosh laryngoscope **EXCEPT**
   A. maximum head extension
   B. the entire tongue is displaced to the left of the laryngoscope
   C. optimal external laryngeal manipulation
   D. place the laryngoscope as far right in the mouth as possible
   E. increase neck flexion

7.2. All of the following are useful maneuvers to optimize visualization of the glottis using the straight laryngoscope **EXCEPT**
   A. place the laryngoscope as far right in the mouth as possible
   B. maintain the head in a midline position
   C. rotation of the head to the left
   D. maximum head extension
   E. displace the entire tongue to the left of the laryngoscope

7.3. Which of the following is not a true statement about the straight laryngoscope for tracheal intubation of the adult patient?
   A. Straight laryngoscopy technique is generally more effective than the Macintosh technique.
   B. More effective displacement of the tongue from the **LOS**.
   C. It is not particularly useful in patients with mandibular hypoplasia.
   D. More reliable elevation of the epiglottis.
   E. It may be particularly useful or patients with awkward dentition patterns.

CHAPTER (8)

Flexible Fiberoptic Intubation

Ian R. Morris

8.1 INTRODUCTION

8.1.1 How did fiberoptic intubation develop?

The first recorded fiberoptic tracheal intubation was reported by Murphy in 1967.[1] In that case report, the trachea of a patient with Still's disease was successfully intubated through the nose using a flexible choledochoscope.[1] The flexible fiberoptic bronchoscope (FFB) was introduced into clinical practice in 1964, and although it was not developed for the purpose of airway management, its value as a device to facilitate endotracheal intubation was soon appreciated.[2,3] A series of 100 fiberoptic endotracheal intubations using the FFB was reported in 1972, with a success rate of 96%.[4] However, utilization of flexible fiberoptic technology for endotracheal intubation remained limited among health care providers throughout the 1970s and 1980s.[5] Seventy-five percent of those who completed questionnaires at a series of fiberoptic workshops between 1984 and 1989 had either no or minimal experience with the technique.[5] Following the publication of the ASA Guidelines on Difficult Airway Management in 1993,[6] the use of flexible fiberoptic intubation among anesthesia practitioners greatly increased[7] and the technique has come to play a pivotal role in the management of the difficult airway.[8]

Although it has been advocated as the technique of choice in the management of the difficult intubation,[9–12] this view is not universally accepted and a reluctance to perform awake fiberoptic intubation continues to occur.[13,14] However, surveys from the United States, France, and Denmark published between 1998–2001 confirm the widespread use of FFB particularly for management of the anticipated difficult airway.[15–18]

8.2 INDICATIONS AND CONTRAINDICATIONS

8.2.1 When is fiberoptic intubation indicated?

The primary indication for fiberoptic intubation is in the elective (or at least nonemergency) management of the anticipated difficult airway.

When endotracheal intubation is required and there has been a history of previous difficult intubation, or if difficult direct laryngoscopy is predicted on airway assessment, and in particular, when mask-ventilation is predicted to be difficult, fiberoptic intubation can be an invaluable alternative intubation technique. Although fiberoptic intubation in this setting can be achieved under general anesthesia (GA), awake intubation maintains a wide margin of safety.[19–21] In general, if airway compromise or respiratory distress exists, awake intubation similarly maintains a wide margin of safety.[20] However, in this circumstance, the urgency with which airway control must be achieved and the extent of the airway compromise may limit the choice of technique and fiberoptic intubation may not be feasible or appropriate. In addition, incomplete local anesthesia of the upper airway makes fiberoptic intubation more difficult as does the presence of blood and secretions in the airway. Complete airway obstruction has been reported following the administration of local anesthesia to the airway and suctioning in preparation for awake intubation in a stridorous patient with recurrent neck carcinoma and radiation therapy.[22] Complete airway obstruction after application of topical local anesthesia to the upper airway was also reported by Shaw et al. in a patient with a compromised airway secondary to goiter.[23] Listro et al. demonstrated a transitory but profound obstruction at the level of the glottis or supraglottis during forced inspiratory and expiratory vital capacity maneuvers that was produced in normal subjects with local anesthesia of the upper airway.[24] Kuna et al. also found a decrease in upper-airway caliber following local anesthesia of the airway in normal subjects.[25] Patients with severe airway obstruction due to edema or tumor must be approached with extreme caution if completion airway obstruction is to be avoided (see Chapter 3).[3]

In the presence of potential cervical spine instability, no intubation technique has been shown to be clearly superior.[19,20,26–29] However, movement of the cervical spine must be minimized during intubation if neurologic injury is to be avoided. Fiberoptic intubation can be a valuable alternative in this setting and has been extensively used.[29,30] Complete airway obstruction has however been reported during attempted awake fiberoptic intubation in this patient population.[30]

Fiberoptic intubation can also be used as an alternative to direct laryngoscopy in any patient for whom intubation is indicated, and in particular when a high risk of dental injury exists.[3] In the setting of failed intubation by direct laryngoscopy or other techniques, fiberoptic intubation can be an invaluable option.

8.2.2 When is fiberoptic intubation best avoided?

Contraindications to fiberoptic intubation must be considered relative and weighed against the risks associated with alternative airway management techniques.[20] Some measure of patient cooperation is required for awake fiberoptic intubation, and the total absence of cooperation may preclude this technique, as can bleeding in the airway and massive tissue disruption.[3,20] Fixed laryngeal obstruction with stridor at rest implies a reduction in the caliber of the airway to about 4.0 mm or less in diameter.[31] Fiberoptic intubation is unlikely to be successful in this setting and at best will produce a higher grade of obstruction when the scope is passed through the involved area. In this setting, a surgical airway (e.g., awake tracheotomy) performed under local anesthesia is a better alternative.[32] Fiberoptic intubation is contraindicated when immediate airway control is necessary and the time required to complete the procedure is not available.[7]

Patient refusal in the adult population without psychiatric disease is exceedingly rare if an appropriate explanation of the procedure has been provided.

8.3 EQUIPMENT

8.3.1 How do fiberoptic bronchoscopes work? What is the best instrument for fiberoptic intubation?

The standard "adult" bronchoscope remains unsurpassed as an instrument for flexible fiberoptic intubation in the vast majority of circumstances in the adult population. These bronchoscopes have a sufficient length (about 60 cm) to accommodate an endotracheal tube ensleeved proximally while leaving an adequate distal segment for maneuverability. Shorter fiberscopes tend to make fiberoptic

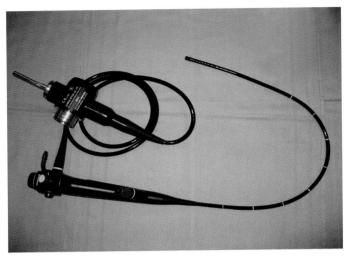

FIGURE 8-1. The adult flexible fiberoptic bronchoscope. An Olympus BF-XT160 is shown here with an insertion cord diameter of 6.3 mm and a length of 600 mm.

intubation more difficult. A bronchoscope with an outside diameter of 5.9–6.0 mm will readily accommodate a 7-mm inner diameter (ID) endotracheal tube and has adequate stiffness to function well as a stylet over which to advance the endotracheal tube (see Figure 8-1).[20,33] Bronchoscopes with thinner insertion cords tend to be more flexible and form a floppy stylet that is easily buckled away from the glottis as the ensleeved endotracheal tube is advanced into the airway (see Figure 8-2).[19]

The flexible bronchoscope consists of a proximal handle and a distal insertion cord or shaft. An umbilical or universal cord is attached to the side of the handle and connects the bronchoscope to an external light source (see Figure 8-3). Modern flexible bronchoscopes include fiberoptic bronchoscopes, video bronchoscopes, and hybrid designs. Flexible fiberoptic bronchoscopes are also available with a battery-operated light source, which greatly improves portability. The handle of the bronchoscope is fitted with

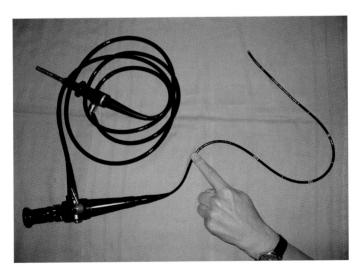

FIGURE 8-2. The "pediatric" flexible fiberoptic bronchoscope. An Olympus LF2 is shown here with an insertion cord diameter of 4 mm and a length of 600 mm. Note the increased flexibility of the thinner insertion cord.

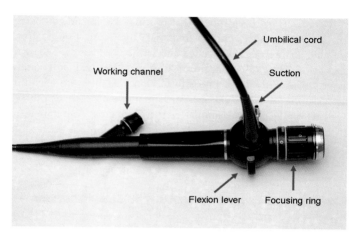

FIGURE 8-3. Features of the flexible fiberoptic bronchoscope: it consists of a proximal handle and a distal insertion cord or shaft. An umbilical or universal cord is attached to the side of the handle and connects the bronchoscope to an external light source. The handle also contains the proximal port of the working channel, a suction port, and the flexion lever.

a lever which controls flexion of the tip of the scope (the bending section)[9,34] in a single plane; the movement of the tip being produced by two wires which connect the control lever to the tip of the scope (see Figure 8-3).[9] The handle also contains the proximal port of the working channel which extends distally to the tip of the scope. This channel can be used to pass various instruments into the airway and can be used for irrigation, administration of medications, and suction. Oxygen insufflation has been used via the working channel; however gastric rupture has been reported with this technique.[35] Light is transmitted from the external light source to the tip of the insertion cord via a fiberoptic bundle made up of thin glass rods (see Figure 8-4).[9,34,36] In the flexible fiberoptic scope

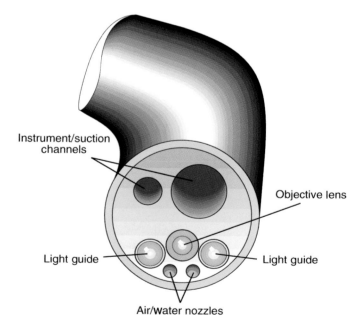

FIGURE 8-4. Schematic diagram of the cross section of the insertion cord of a flexible fiberoptic bronchoscope. (*Reproduced with permission from ECRI. Bronchoscopes. In: Healthcare Product Comparison System, Hospital edn. Plymouth Meeting, PA: ECRI, 2004.*)

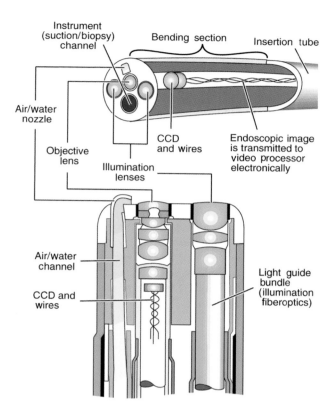

FIGURE 8-5. Schematic diagram of the insertion cord of a flexible videobronchoscope. (*Reproduced with permission from ECRI. Bronchoscopes. In: Healthcare Product Comparison System, Hospital edn. Plymouth Meeting, PA: ECRI, 2004.*)

light reflected from the object being viewed is focused by a lens located at the tip of the insertion cord onto the distal end of a second fiberoptic bundle which then transmits the image to a second lens located in the eye piece.[9,34] The glass fibers in this image transmission bundle remain in the same relative location along the length of the bundle (coherent bundle) such that a mosaic image is accurately reconstructed at the eye piece.[9,34] The image seen through the scope is focused by means of a control located in the handle. In the video bronchoscope, a charged coupled device or silicone chip is located at the distal tip of the insertion cord and is used to sense and transmit the image (see Figure 8-5).[34] The image data are then transmitted electronically through the bronchoscope to an external video processing unit.[34] The image is then displayed on a screen and can be printed, stored electronically, or transmitted to a remote location.[34] A video camera can be coupled to the eye piece of a conventional fiberoptic bronchoscope. However, the image obtained is inferior to that provided by the video bronchoscope.[34]

Bronchoscopes are produced by a number of different manufacturers and are available with insertion cord diameters ranging from 2.2 to 6.3 mm.[34] In general, minimizing the discrepancy between the outside diameter of the bronchoscope and the internal diameter (ID) of the ensleeved endotracheal tube facilitates passage of the tube through the larynx over the scope.[2,3,19,37–43] Bronchoscopes with smaller diameter insertion cords have allowed fiberoptic intubation to be performed in the pediatric population, and very thin scopes such as the Olympus BF-N$_2$O with a shaft diameter of 2.2 mm can be used in infants. However, use of "pediatric" bronchoscopes to perform fiberoptic intubation of the adult in general makes the procedure more difficult.[19] The use of a pediatric bronchoscope to perform awake intubation in the adult with severe upper-airway obstruction may be complicated by complete obstruction and must be approached with great caution.[3,22,32,44]

Bronchoscopes are delicate instruments and must be handled with care if damage to the instrument is to be avoided. Damage to the bronchoscope is not only costly to repair but it also means that the scope is unavailable for clinical use for a period of time.[9] Striking the distal tip of the insertion cord against a hard surface or excessive bending or twisting of the shaft of the scope can damage the lens and fiberoptic bundles, respectively.[34] If the external shaft of the insertion cord or the working channel wall is punctured, fluids can enter the inside of the scope and lead to a degradation or loss of the image transmitted.[34]

Flexible bronchoscopes with shaft diameters of 3.5–4.0 mm can readily be passed through the lumen of a #35-Fr or larger double lumen tube and are invaluable for the precise tube placement required for lung isolation.

8.3.2   How are fiberoptic bronchoscopes disinfected?

In general, the issue of sterilization of bronchoscopes is addressed by infection control and risk management personnel in each health-care facility.[34] Specific recommendations for sterilization are also provided by each manufacturer.[9,34] A typical sterilization process is as follows. Immediately following a bronchoscopic procedure, a premixed enzymatic solution is suctioned through the working channel(s) of the bronchoscope and the instrument is wiped down with a lint-free cloth saturated with the premixed enzymatic solution. This is considered to be a "preclean setup" in the sterilization process and is performed at the bedside. The scope is then transferred to the sterile processing department where a leak tester is connected to the umbilical cord or handle and the inside of the scope is then pressurized with air. The scope is then immersed in a water bath for 30 seconds and observed for escaping bubbles. The scope is removed from the water bath, the leak tester disconnected from the pressure source, and the scope allowed to vent at atmospheric pressure before the tester is disconnected from the self-sealing port. The scope is then placed in a predetermined concentration of an enzymatic solution and the working channels and external controls manually cleaned with appropriate brushes. The working channels are also flushed with the enzymatic solution followed by water and air. The scope is then immersed in a solution of peracetic acid using specially designed equipment that ensures flow through the working channels. These channels are subsequently irrigated with air and alcohol before the scope is dried manually and with an air flush. The sterilization process requires about 50–60 minutes to complete. If the scope is not reused within 1 week of the sterilization process, the sterilization is repeated. Glutaraldehyde, hydrogen peroxide, and orthophthaldehyde (Cidex OPA) can also be used for disinfection of bronchoscopes.[34] Ethylene oxide (ETO) sterilization is also an effective agent for sterilization of bronchoscopes although the process requires about 18 hours to complete. When the scope is "gassed," an ETO cap must be attached to the leak tester port to permit the gas to enter the scope and thereby equalize internal and external pressures.[9]

Recently, it has been shown that routine cleaning and autoclaving do not remove protein material, including prions, from reusable airway devices,[45] and concern has been expressed with respect to the possible transmission of infection with subsequent usage.[46] Currently there is no information available with regard to the cleaning of bronchoscopes such that the absence of protein deposits can be ensured. Similarly, the risk of cross-contamination of patients following a standard cleaning procedure for the flexible fiberoptic bronchoscope is unknown.

8.4   TECHNIQUE

8.4.1   How is the bronchoscope maneuvered? What are the key aspects of technique for fast, successful fiberoptic intubation?

The bronchoscope is most easily maneuvered by holding the handle of the scope in the palm of the dominant (usually right) hand with the thumb placed on the flexion lever (see Figure 8-6). The fingers should comfortably encircle the handle of the scope and the index finger can be used to activate the suction mechanism, although if antisialogogues are used, suction is rarely required during fiberoptic intubation. When the scope is held such that the flexion lever is in the 6 o'clock position, moving the lever downward (toward the shaft of the scope) flexes the tip of the scope upward toward the 12 o'clock position. Conversely, moving the lever up toward the proximal aspect of the handle flexes the tip downward toward the 6 o'clock position (see Figure 8-7). Movement of the flexion lever then flexes the tip of the scope in a single plane. To flex the tip in any other plane, the entire instrument must be rotated clockwise or counterclockwise using the wrist connected to the hand holding the handle of the scope. This wrist rotation is the second important and perhaps not intuitively obvious movement required when manipulating the bronchoscope

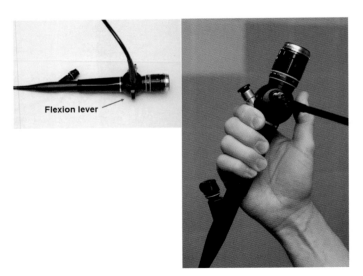

Flexion lever

FIGURE 8-6. Holding the bronchoscope. The fingers comfortably encircle the handle. The thumb is placed on the flexion lever.

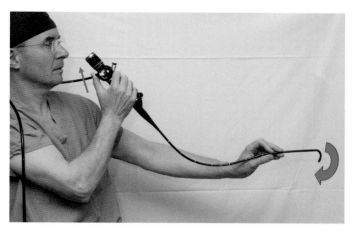

FIGURE 8-7. Movement of the flexion lever flexes the tip of the insertion cord in a single plane.

during fiberoptic intubation (see Figures 8-8 A and B). The tip of the bronchoscope can then be manipulated to view objects in any plane within the scope's field of vision by a combination of wrist rotation and thumb flexion. Many bronchoscopes have a triangular marker or divot[7,47] located at the 12 o'clock position at the periphery of the scope's field of vision (see Figure 8-9). This

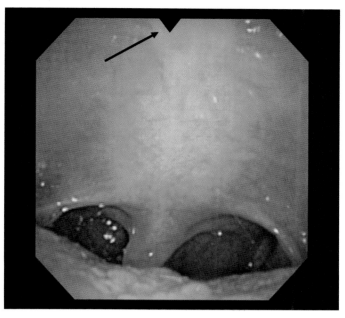

FIGURE 8-9. The marker located at 12 o'clock (arrow) in the scope's field of vision.

marker helps the practitioner maintain spatial orientation as the tip of the scope always flexes in the diametrical plane of the marker. When a video camera is coupled to a fiberoptic bronchoscope, the divot must be adjusted to the 12 o'clock position (opposite the flexion lever on the handle) to maintain correct orientation.[47] The practitioner's nondominant (usually left) hand holds the shaft or insertion cord of the bronchoscope a few centimeters proximal to the tip with the forearm pronated (see Figure 8-10). The shaft should be held between the thumb and index finger and stabilized between the ring and middle finger or some other combination of digits. The hand that holds the distal shaft of the scope must feed the scope forward into the airway in a controlled manner without excessive (shaky) movement that can make visualization difficult.

Generally it is easier to rotate the bronchoscope using the dominant (usually right) hand positioned at the handle. The nondominant

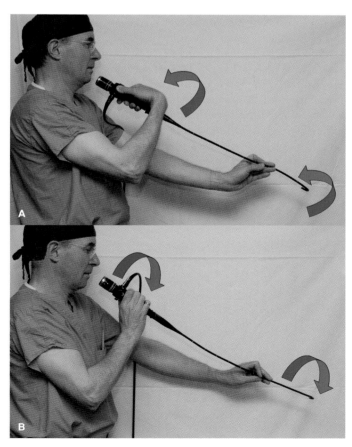

FIGURE 8-8. (A) Rotation of the bronchoscope counterclockwise. (B) Rotation of the bronchoscope clockwise. The entire instrument is rotated using the wrist at the handle of the scope. The hand holding the shaft allows the instrument to rotate.

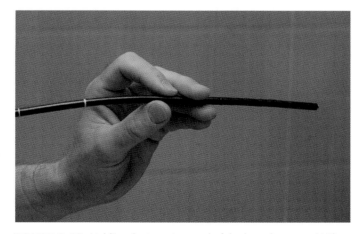

FIGURE 8-10. Holding the insertion cord of the bronchoscope. With the forearm pronated, the nondominant hand holds the insertion cord a few centimeters proximal to the tip of the bronchoscope.

hand holding the distal aspect of the shaft must however allow the shaft to rotate, and therefore the shaft cannot be gripped tightly. If the distal aspect of the shaft is held tightly, rotation at the handle twists the insertion cord, the scope fails to go in the desired direction, and the components in the shaft can be damaged. Although rotation of the scope is usually more easily controlled by the hand positioned at the handle, the nondominant hand holding the distal shaft can also be used to rotate the instrument. In that maneuver, the hand at the handle must follow the movement and allow the entire instrument to rotate, or again, twisting of the shaft will occur and the scope fails to go in the desired direction (see Figures 8-8 A and B). As experience is gained in manipulation of the scope, the shaft does not need to be held taut to maneuver the tip. However, holding the shaft of the scope relatively straight can be useful to maintain orientation and control movement. The most important concepts to master are thumb flexion and wrist rotation. In addition, during fiberoptic intubation, movement of the scope (flexion, rotation, and forward feeding) should be small, slow, and deliberate. Oversteering of the scope is a common error.

The endotracheal tube can be precut to a desired length to maximize the length of the insertion cord beyond the tube and thereby optimize maneuverability.[20] The inside of the tube can be lubricated using lidocaine spray and the tube ensleeved proximally and fixed to the handle with a single piece of easily removable tape (sometimes called a "jacketed scope" with the endotracheal tube being the "jacket") (see Figure 8-11).[20] A lubricant jelly placed on the cuff of the tube may facilitate glottic entry. Lubricating the shaft of the scope is unnecessary and makes it difficult to handle.

8.4.2   Is fiberoptic intubation more easily performed from the head of the bed or from the patient's right side? What instructions should be given to the patient during the procedure?

Awake fiberoptic intubation can be performed with the practitioner standing at the head of the bed, and for those who are most

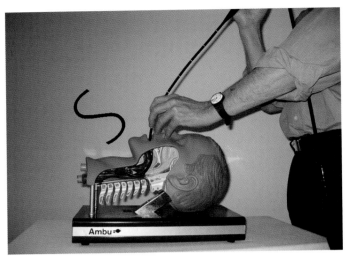

FIGURE 8-12. Fiberoptic intubation performed from the head of the bed requires the insertion cord to negotiate an S-shaped curve and the patient must be supine or nearly supine.

familiar with visualization of the airway by direct laryngoscopy, this position preserves the spatial orientation of the airway structures as they are viewed through the scope.[19,20] However, this position requires the practitioner to negotiate an S-shaped curve to the trachea (see Figure 8-12) and the patient to be supine or nearly supine. Standing at the patient's right side facing cephalad facilitates negotiation of the natural C-shaped curve of the airway, permits easy visualization of patient monitors, and as eye contact can be readily maintained this position may be less intimidating for the patient (see Figure 8-13).[19,20] The patient may be supine or in the semi-sitting position.[19] The semi-seated position may also be less intimidating for the awake patient and may better maintain the patency of the pharyngeal lumen.[19,48] Extension at the atlanto-occipital joint moves the epiglottis anteriorly away from the posterior pharyngeal wall and facilitates passage of the bronchoscope through the pharynx.[3,19,36,49,50] Neck flexion, however, tends to produce pharyngeal obstruction and can make fiberoptic intubation more difficult.[19,49–51]

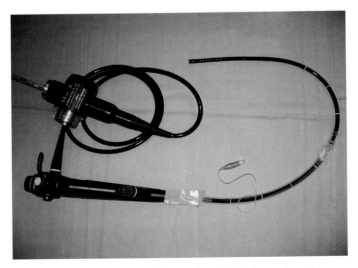

FIGURE 8-11. A #7.5 mm ID PVC endotracheal tube ensleeved over the adult bronchoscope and fixed to the handle with a single piece of tape.

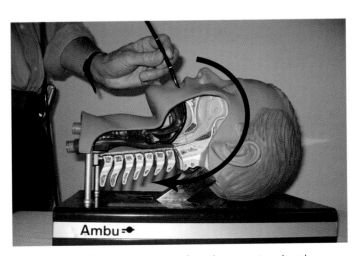

FIGURE 8-13. Fiberoptic intubation from the patient's right side requires the scope to negotiate a C-shaped curve.

For awake oral fiberoptic intubation, the author prefers to be positioned at the semi seated patient's right side (see Figure 8-13). The light source is to the practitioner's left, and the video screen is located in front and to the left of the practitioner. Oxygen can be administered by nasal prongs. An assistant is positioned at the patient's left side and provides gentle tongue traction using a piece of gauze.[19] The bronchoscope can be focused on printed material prior to insertion. Use of a bite block tends to push the tongue posteriorly and cephalad into the oropharyngeal isthmus, can make passage of the scope more difficult, and if adequate local anesthesia has been achieved, is not necessary.[19] The lens can be defogged using silicone solution or simply by holding the tip of the scope in warm water or against the buccal mucosa for a few seconds to warm it and thereby prevent condensation.[19,20] The scope should be inserted into the oral cavity to the level of the dental arches in the midline, and then advanced a few centimeters posteriorly over the dorsum of the tongue following the midline groove toward the first midline landmark, the uvula, seen in the superior aspect of the scope's field of vision (see Figure 8-9).[19] Gently resting the hand holding the shaft of the scope on the patient's chin may help keep the scope in the midline.[19,38] If the uvula is in contact with the dorsal aspect of the tongue, the patient can be instructed to take a deep breath, thereby elevating the uvula and opening the oropharyngeal isthmus.[19,20] The scope is then advanced slowly forward just past the uvula and flexed caudally to visualize the second midline landmark, the epiglottis, seen inferiorly in the scope's field of vision (see Figure 8-14).[19,20] If the epiglottis is oriented posteriorly or is in contact with the posterior pharyngeal wall, the awake patient can again be instructed to take a deep breath and thereby move the epiglottis anteriorly to create an air space through which to pass the scope.[19,20] The scope is then passed, posterior to the epiglottis to visualize the third midline landmark, the vocal cords (see Figure 8-15).[19,20] If the bronchoscope

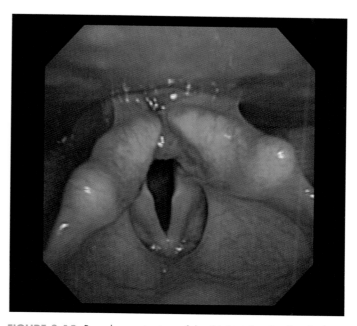

FIGURE 8-15. Bronchoscopic view of the third midline landmark (the vocal cords) during fiberoptic intubation with the practitioner on the patient's right side facing the patient.

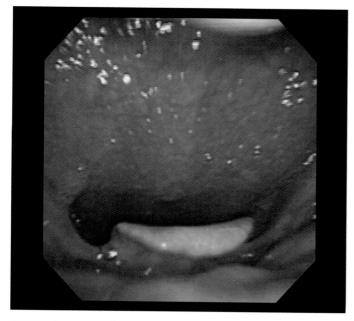

FIGURE 8-14. Bronchoscopic view of the second midline landmark (the epiglottis) during fiberoptic intubation with the practitioner on the patient's right side facing the patient.

is passed behind the epiglottis in the midline, then it is naturally lined up for the approach to the larynx. Conversely, if the bronchoscope is off midline at the level of the epiglottis, the approach to the larynx can be much more difficult. The scope is then advanced in the midline through the glottis and positioned proximal to the carina.[19,20] As the scope is advanced through the larynx, the patient is again instructed to take a deep breath to maximally abduct the vocal cords and thereby facilitate passage of the scope. As the bronchoscope is passed from the level of the dental arches to the trachea, flexion and rotation movements should be small and deliberate such that the scope can be kept in the midline and advanced along the C-shaped curve analogous to staying in a given lane during highway driving using small movements of the steering wheel. Unnecessary touching of the mucosa by the bronchoscope should be avoided. Having positioned the tip of the bronchoscope in the trachea, the practitioner should then look directly at the patient and advance the endotracheal tube over the scope being careful to aim for the midline and to follow the natural curve of the airway (see Figure 8-16).[19,20] The bronchoscope must be kept stationary as the tube is advanced[9] in order to avoid inadvertent contact with the carina or cannulation of a mainstem bronchus or premature removal of the scope from the trachea. Again, as the tube is advanced, the patient should be instructed to take a deep breath to move the epiglottis anteriorly away from the advancing tube and to maximally abduct the vocal cords.[19,20] The correct intratracheal position of the endotracheal tube can be confirmed endoscopically before the scope is removed.[19,20] However the presence of both the bronchoscope and tube in the trachea produces a degree of airway obstruction that can be distressing for the awake patient, and the bronchoscope should be removed expeditiously once the tube is in proper position. Correct position can be further confirmed by listening to and feeling gas exhaled via the tube and by capnography.

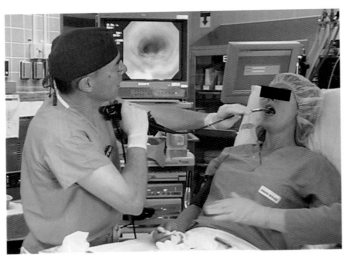

FIGURE 8-16. Advancing the endotracheal tube in the midline during a deep inspiration while looking directly at the patient and following the natural C-shaped curve of the airway.

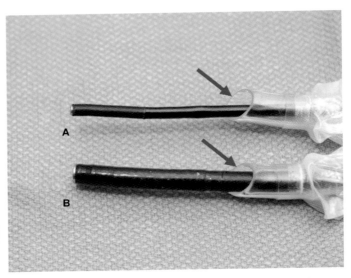

FIGURE 8-18. A #7.5-mm ID PVC endotracheal tube ensleeved over (A) a standard adult bronchoscope and (B) a pediatric bronchoscope. Note the discrepancy between the external diameters of the scopes and the IDs of the endotracheal tubes (arrows).

8.4.3   How can difficulty in passing the ensleeved endotracheal tube into the trachea over the fiberoptic bronchoscope be minimized?

Difficulty in passing the ensleeved endotracheal tube through the larynx has been variously reported to occur in 5–90% of fiberoptic intubations,[40,52–56] and has occurred in awake patients, as well as those under GA and with both the nasal and oral routes of tracheal intubation. During oral fiberoptic intubation, as the tube is advanced with the concave aspect of the tube facing anteriorly and the bevel facing toward the patient's left, the leading edge of the tube may meet resistance at the right arytenoid or aryepiglottic fold (see Figure 8-17).[55,57,58] Rotation of the tube 90 degrees counterclockwise orients the bevel posteriorly and the leading edge anteriorly and has been advocated to improve passage of the endotracheal tube through the larynx.[57,59–61] Rotation of the tube coun-

terclockwise may also keep the leading edge in closer contact with the bronchoscope and provide less of a gap between the two with which to catch a laryngeal structure.[62] During nasal fiberoptic intubation, it has been postulated that the tube tends to impinge on the epiglottis.[55,57] However the usual point of obstruction during nasal tracheal intubation may also be the right arytenoid.[63] Improved success rates have been reported for glottic cannulation during nasal fiberoptic intubation, using a 90-degree counterclockwise rotation of the tube.[55] Conversely, nasal fiberoptic intubation performed with the bevel up has also been advocated such that impingement on the epiglottis may be avoided.[59] In addition to the right arytenoid and epiglottis, impingement can occur at the posterior pharyngeal wall or other laryngeal structures.[56] The larger the discrepancy between the outside diameter of the bronchoscopic stylet and the ID of the ensleeved endotracheal tube, the greater is the chance that the tube may impinge on laryngeal structures and resist entry into the trachea (see Figure 8-18).[2,3,19,40,43,58] Therefore this discrepancy should be minimized by choosing the largest bronchoscope which will easily fit into the endotracheal tube to be used.[19,38,39] In the adult, a bronchoscope with an outside diameter of 5.9–6.0 mm works well when used with a 7.5–8.5 mm ID endotracheal tube. When the combination of a relatively large bronchoscope and an endotracheal tube are both present in the trachea, the practitioner must be aware that a degree of airway obstruction has been produced[37] and the bronchoscope should be removed without delay following tube placement and confirmation. If the bronchoscope must remain inside the tube positioned in the trachea for a relatively long period as during diagnostic or therapeutic bronchoscopy, then the concentric airway remaining must be adequate to permit ventilation to occur.[19,37,64] Wire reinforced spiral tubes are more flexible than polyvinyl chloride (PVC) tubes and may more easily follow the curve of the bronchoscopic stylet as it passes through the larynx.[19,58,64–67] Although flexible wire reinforced tubes were reported to be associated with a lower rate of impingement in the larynx than a standard tube,[67] subsequent studies reported

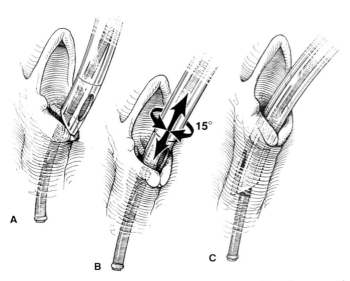

FIGURE 8-17. Impingement of endotracheal tube at the right arytenoid or right epiglottic fold. (*Reproduced with permission from, Crit Care Med. 1990;18(8):883*).

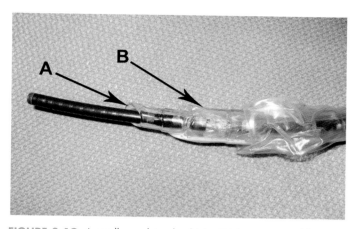

FIGURE 8-19. A smaller endotracheal tube (A) interpositioned between the bronchoscopic insertion cord and a larger endotracheal tube (B).

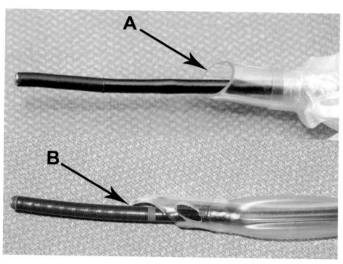

FIGURE 8-21. The Parker Flex-Tip™ tube: a #7-mm ID PVC endotracheal tube ensleeved over a standard pediatric bronchoscope (A) and a #7-mm ID Parker Flex-Tip™ tube ensleeved over a pediatric bronchoscope (B). Note the discrepancy between the leading edge of the two different types of endotracheal tubes (arrows).

frequent laryngeal impaction with spiral tubes.[52,53] Various methods to minimize the discrepancy between the outside diameter of the bronchoscope and the ID of the endotracheal tube have been proposed. These include the interposition of a smaller endotracheal tube between the scope and the larger endotracheal tube to be positioned in the trachea (see Figure 8-19),[41,66] or the use of a sleeve such as an airway exchange catheter,[66] split nasogastric tube,[68] or a custom-designed conical-shaped PVC sleeve.[69] The use of a Cook airway exchange catheter passed alongside the bronchoscope through the endotracheal tube into the trachea to "centralize" the tube and facilitate glottic cannulation has also been reported.[70] Preformed PVC endotracheal tubes can also be warmed to increase flexibility.[9,19,20] Laryngeal cannulation with the ensleeved endotracheal tube may also be facilitated by using a tube with a modified tip design.[19,20,58,61] The intubating laryngeal mask airway (ILMA) tube is reusable and has a soft hemispherical bevel that has a leading edge in the midline (see Figure 8-20).[58] Greer et al. found that the incidence of difficulty in passage of the endotracheal tube was significantly less using the IMLA tube as compared to the flexometallic tube during *oral* fiberoptic intubation under GA.[58] Barker et al. found the Intravent Orthofix ILMA tube

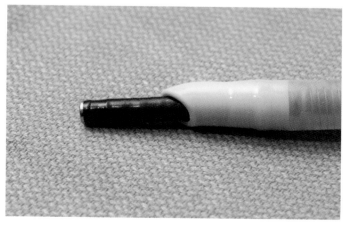

FIGURE 8-20. The ILMA reusable silicone endotracheal tube ensleeved over a standard adult bronchoscope; note the hemispherical bevel with a leading edge in the midline of the tube.

to be superior to both the reinforced and standard tubes during *naso*tracheal intubation under GA.[53] All 15 Intravent tubes were easily passed through the larynx on the first attempt, whereas difficulty in passing the ensleeved tube was encountered in 8/15 in the standard-tube group, and 6/15 in the flexible-tube group.[53] The Parker Flex-Tip™ tube shown in Figure 8-21 has a flexible tip that points toward the center of the distal lumen and the convex side of the tube.[40] Kristensen has reported a greater incidence of initial success with passage of the tube through the larynx as compared to a standard endotracheal tube in a series of 76 patients who underwent oral fiberoptic intubation under GA.[40] A higher cuff pressure was required with this Parker Flex-Tip™ tube to establish a seal. However, in a recent randomized prospective study involving 111 patients with difficult airways or unstable cervical spines, Joo et al. did not find any significant difference in the success rate between the Parker Flex-Tip™ tube and the PVC tube for awake oral fiberoptic intubation.[71] Difficulty in advancing the endotracheal tube through the larynx may be encountered as well in the awake patient without obtunded laryngeal reflexes.[3]

Difficulty with passage of the endotracheal tube through the larynx is exceedingly rare in the awake cooperative patient in the sitting position with adequate topical anesthesia of the airway, when an optimally sized bronchoscope is used relative to the endotracheal tube, and the tube is advanced during a deep inspiration.

8.5 OTHER TECHNIQUES AND ADJUNCTS TO FACILITATE FIBEROPTIC INTUBATION

8.5.1 Are oral intubating airways useful or necessary?

Various oral intubating airways are available and can be used during fiberoptic intubation. The purpose of these airways is to keep

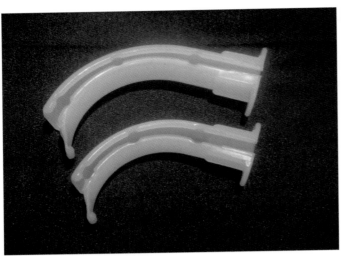

FIGURE 8-22. The Berman Intubating Pharyngeal Airway: the Berman Intubating Pharyngeal Airway is cylindrical and has a longitudinal opening along its side which permits its disengagement from the endotracheal tube following intubation (*Reproduced with permission from Ovassapian A, Wheeler M: Fiberoptic endoscopy-aided techniques. In: Airway Management Principles and Practice. Benumof JL, ed. St. Louis: Mosby, Inc., 1996:289*).

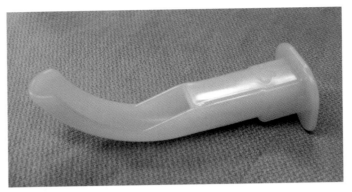

FIGURE 8-23. The Williams Airway Intubator: the Williams Airway Intubator has a cylindrical proximal half whereas the distal half of the device has an open lingual surface.

the bronchoscope in the midline and align it with the glottic opening, displace the tongue anteriorly, and the soft palate superiorly thus opening the pharyngeal space, and to protect the scope from bite damage.[47,72]

The Berman Intubating Pharyngeal Airway, also known as the Berman Breakaway Airway (see Figure 8-22), is cylindrical and has a longitudinal opening along its side which permits its disengagement ("breakaway") from the endotracheal tube.[9] The maneuverability of the bronchoscope is limited when inside the airway, and if the airway is not in line with the glottis, visualization requires manipulation of the device.[9]

The Patel-Syracuse Intubating Airway is made of aluminum and is available in only one size. A central groove is located on the lingual surface for the bronchoscope, but manipulation of the bronchoscope is restricted.[45] An endotracheal tube will not pass through the airway.[9]

The Williams Airway Intubator has a cylindrical proximal half, whereas the distal half of the device has an open lingual surface (see Figure 8-23).[9,47] The airway is available in two sizes (90 and 100 mm ID) which admit 8.0 and 8.5 endotracheal tubes, respectively.[9,47] Manipulation of the bronchoscope inside the airway is limited.[9] If the distal aspect of the airway is not aligned with the glottis, visualization of the vocal cords can be difficult.[9,47]

The Ovassapian Fiberoptic Intubating Airway has a flat lingual surface at the proximal half of the device which minimizes its movement (see Figure 8-24).[9,47] The distal half of the airway has a wide curve designed to prevent the tissues of the anterior pharyngeal wall from moving posteriorly. The posterior distal aspect of the airway is open.

A split Guedel airway has also been used for fiberoptic intubation.[10]

Randall et al. found that the Berman airway was superior to the Ovassapian fiberoptic intubating airway during fiberoptic

intubation.[73] However, only 1 of 63 bronchoscopies failed using the Ovassapian airway. Greenland et al. compared the Williams airway intubator and the Ovassapian fiberoptic intubating airway in 60 Asian patients who underwent oral fiberoptic intubation under GA.[72] They reported that the Williams airway provided an unobstructed view of the glottis in 68.3% of cases, whereas the Ovassapian airway provided an unobstructed view in 25%. Four bronchoscopies failed using the Williams airway and 26 using the Ovassapian airway. Intubating conditions with either airway were similar when the glottis was visible.[72] Asai and Shingu suggest that it may be better to remove an airway intubator after the bronchoscope has been positioned in the trachea as it may interfere with the endotracheal tube.[42]

Airway intubators can be used to facilitate fiberoptic intubation. However, fiberoptic intubation can be rapidly achieved without the use of these devices and the emphasis should be on the development of skill with bronchoscopic manipulation, positioning, and regional anesthesia of the airway.

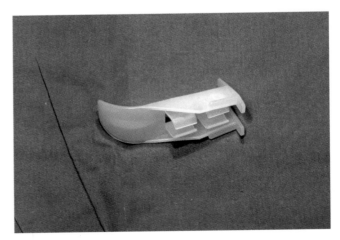

FIGURE 8-24. The Ovassapian intubating airway: the Ovassapian Fiberoptic Intubating Airway has a flat lingual surface at the proximal half of the device which minimizes its movement (*Reproduced with permission from Ovassapian A, Wheeler M: Fiberoptic endoscopy-aided techniques. In: Airway Management Principles and Practice. Benumof JL, ed. St. Louis: Mosby, Inc., 1996:289*).

8.5.2 Is nasal fiberoptic intubation easier? Which nostril is the more appropriate for intubation?

If the nasal route is chosen for fiberoptic intubation, an attempt to identify the more patent nostril can be made by asking the patient to assess airflow through each nasal cavity in turn during exhalation, and by palpating airflow from the nostril.[74] However, these simple diagnostic tests have been shown to have a failure rate of about 45%.[74] Some degree of nasal obstruction can be present in the absence of a history of nasal trauma, surgery, or obstruction and can interfere with the attempted passage of a nasal tube. The mucosa over the turbinates is easily traumatized.[74] Fiberoptic examination of the nasal cavity may be helpful in identifying the more appropriate nostril for intubation.[74] Administration of a nasal vasoconstrictor may also increase the caliber of the nasal airway. In the absence of a history of nasal obstruction, it is controversial whether the left or right nostril should be used for nasal intubation as it is not known whether the bevel or the tip of the tube is more responsible for potential damage to the nasal mucosa (see also Section 10.6.3).

During nasal fiberoptic intubation, either the endotracheal tube or the bronchoscope can be passed initially through the nasal cavity.[2,19,20,36] If the tube is passed first, it can be advanced along the floor of the nose using a gentle alternating clockwise–counterclockwise motion to facilitate its passage until the tip of the tube exits the choana to enter the nasopharynx.[2,19] The scope can then be passed through the lubricated tube and as it exits the distal aspect of the tube, the glottis is usually in view (see Figure 8-25). If on exiting the tip of the endotracheal tube the view is obstructed, the tube may be in contact with the pharyngeal mucosa or the tip of the scope may be covered with blood or debris. The scope can be removed, the tip cleaned and warmed, and then replaced into the tube. If on exiting the distal aspect of the tube still no recognizable structures are visualized, then the scope and tube should be slowly retracted together until pharyngeal or laryngeal landmarks (the uvula, epiglottis or larynx) are

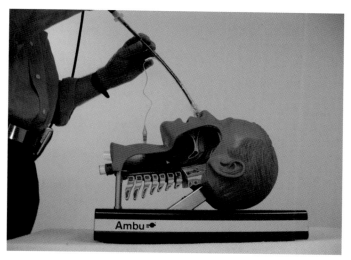

FIGURE 8-26. Nasal intubation using a flexible fiberoptic bronchoscope: the bronchoscope can be passed first into pharynx and trachea. The endotracheal tube is then advanced over the bronchoscope.

identified.[20] If the epiglottis is oriented posteriorly against the posterior pharyngeal wall, the patient can be instructed to take a deep breath and thereby move the epiglottis anteriorly and create an adequate airspace for the scope to pass behind it without touching mucosa and losing the visual field.[19] The fiberoptic bronchoscope is then advanced into the trachea and the endotracheal tube advanced over the scope as for oral intubation during a deep inspiration, optimally with the patient in the semi-sitting or sitting position.[19,20] Alternatively, the fiberoptic bronchoscope can be passed through the nasal cavity initially under fiberoptic control and then on into the trachea and the ensleeved endotracheal tube passed over the scope (see Figure 8-26). On advancing the endotracheal tube over the fiberoptic bronchoscope, the leading edge of the tube may impact on the laryngeal structures and resist further advancement.[55] The most likely site of impingement during nasotracheal fiberoptic intubation is controversial.[57,63] Rotating the tube such that the bevel faces anteriorly,[59] or posteriorly,[55] or advancing with a twisting motion[19,37,57] may facilitate glottic entry. A lubricated nasopharyngeal airway can be inserted temporarily into the nose before subsequent insertion of the endotracheal tube to explore the nasal cavity such that an appropriately sized endotracheal tube can be chosen.[19] Further decompression of the nasal mucosa may also be thereby achieved[75] and trauma due to the more rigid endotracheal tube may be reduced. Alternatively, a nasopharyngeal airway split longitudinally can be inserted into the nasopharynx and used as a guide through which to pass the bronchoscope.[19,75] The guide can then be removed before subsequent passage of the endotracheal tube. On occasion, the caliber of the nasal cavity may be such that it will permit passage of the endotracheal tube but not the bronchoscope through the tube due to external compression of the tube.[19,20] Conversely, the nasal cavity may permit initial passage of the scope but not the tube over the scope.[19,20] In this circumstance, it may be necessary to use a smaller scope, a smaller tube, the other nostril, oral intubation, or another means of airway management.

Nasotracheal intubation produces less stimulation of the gag reflex[3,7,54] and requires less patient cooperation, but is generally

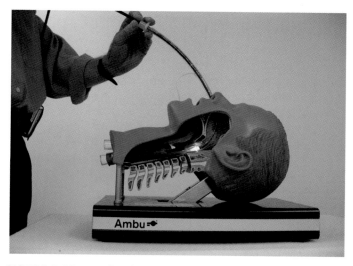

FIGURE 8-25. Nasal intubation using a flexible fiberoptic bronchoscope: the bronchoscope is passed through the endotracheal tube which was initially positioned in the pharynx.

more uncomfortable for the awake patient. If the nasal cavity can be readily cannulated, it is technically somewhat easier than oral fiberoptic intubation.

Nasotracheal intubation has been considered to be contraindicated in the presence of a coagulopathy, intranasal abnormalities, paranasal sinusitis, extensive facial fractures, and basal skull fracture.[76–79] Conversely, basal skull fracture has been said not to be a contraindication to nasotracheal intubation.[76] Complications peculiar to nasotracheal intubation include epistaxis,[26,78–82] damage to the nasal or nasopharyngeal mucosa with creation of a false passage[3,80] and potential abscess formation,[78] bacteremia,[3,26,79] damage to nasal polyps or adenoidal tissue with possible dislodgement and aspiration,[26,79] nasal necrosis,[3,26,78,79] sinusitis,[26,78,79] and otitis.[3,26,79] Minimal epistaxis has been reported in 11–40% of emergency nasotracheal intubations[80,81] and moderate to severe bleeding in 7%.[81] In a series of 99 patients undergoing maxillofacial surgery, nasotracheal intubation was associated with mild epistaxis in 5 patients and bleeding sufficient to produce a visible accumulation of blood in the pharynx in 1 patient.[82]

8.5.3 When is fiberoptic intubation under GA indicated? What are the problems with this technique?

Fiberoptic intubation under GA can be performed as easily as intubation by direct laryngoscopy in patients with normal airway anatomy.[3] Orotracheal fiberoptic intubation has also been successfully performed following simulated rapid sequence induction (RSI),[83] and fiberoptic intubation under GA has been used for training purposes.[84] Fiberoptic intubation of the anticipated and unanticipated difficult intubation under GA has also been reported although some intubation failures did occur.[10,85]

As consciousness is lost, loss of tone in the submandibular muscles allows the tongue and epiglottis to move posteriorly and potentially obstruct the airway at the level of the pharynx and larynx, respectively.[86,87] The soft palate also approximates the posterior pharyngeal wall.[86] The degree of airway obstruction produced is influenced by variations in airway anatomy, body habitus, and depth of coma.[19,50] In the unconscious individual, this reduction in the caliber of the pharyngeal lumen can make fiberoptic visualization more difficult.[3,19,88] Contact of the bronchoscope lens with the mucosa results in loss of the visual field, and the practitioner's ability to maneuver past an epiglottis in contact with the posterior pharyngeal wall is limited.[19,33,38,88] In the supine individual under GA, lingual traction with Duval's forceps has been shown to move the tongue away from the uvula and soft palate better than the jaw thrust maneuver, whereas jaw thrust moved the epiglottis away from the posterior pharyngeal wall more effectively than tongue traction.[87] Jaw thrust and tongue traction applied simultaneously opened the airway at the soft palate and epiglottic level in all patients studied.[87] These combined maneuvers require two assistants.[87] Intubating airways such as the Berman or Ovassapian airway can also be used to keep the pharyngeal airway open as well as to direct the fiberoptic bronchoscope toward the larynx; however multiple manipulations may be required, the intubation may be prolonged, and failure can occur.[87] Anterior displacement of the tongue base using the rigid laryngoscope may also improve visualization,[2,3,19,33] as can placing the patient in the semi-left lateral position with the head turned to the left.[89] If resistance is encoun-

tered in passing the endotracheal tube over the bronchoscope despite rotation of the tube, digital manipulation may be useful to facilitate glottic entry.[38] An endoscopy mask fitted with a diaphragm permits endoscopy during positive pressure mask-ventilation[90] and can be used in conjunction with an intubating airway.[3,7,9,90] The nasotracheal route can also be used in the unconscious individual.[2,88] In the presence of apnea or suboptimal ventilation, arterial desaturation imposes a time limit on fiberoptic techniques.[3,19,20] Fiberoptic intubation of a patient under GA can be difficult and arterial desaturation can occur,[91] although the technique has been used with high levels of success.[83,85]

8.6 UTILIZATION OF FIBEROPTIC INTUBATION IN DIFFERENT SETTINGS

8.6.1 How useful is fiberoptic intubation in the emergency setting?

Immediate airway control in the emergency setting can be difficult using fiberoptic techniques due to the presence of blood, emesis, or secretions in the airway.[19,91–93] Poor preparation of the patient and lack of patient cooperation can also be problematic.[3,19,91,94] Fiberoptic intubation can nevertheless be a valuable option in selected patients such as those with confirmed or suspected cervical spine injury,[93] those with anticipated difficult direct laryngoscopic intubation due to variant anatomy,[93] and in the presence of airway pathology such as Ludwig's angina,[95] burn injury,[96] or angioedema.[92] Complete airway obstruction has however been reported during attempted fiberoptic intubation in the presence of upper-airway compromise.[22,30]

The optimal initial airway management approach in the patient with penetrating neck injury remains controversial.[97,98] Mandavia et al. reported a series of 58 patients with penetrating neck trauma who required emergency airway control.[97] Out of 58 patients, 39 underwent rapid sequence orotracheal intubation with a 100% success rate, 5 unconscious patients underwent orotracheal intubation by direct laryngoscopy without paralysis, and 2 underwent successful emergency tracheotomy.[97] Fiberoptic intubation was attempted in 12 patients. Three of these intubations failed, but all three were subsequently successfully orotracheally intubated by direct laryngoscopy following RSI.[97] Of 107 patients with penetrating neck trauma reported by Shearer and Giesecke, 8 patients underwent orotracheal fiberoptic intubation with a 100% success rate.[98] Eighty-nine patients underwent orotracheal intubation by direct laryngoscopy after RSI, six had a primary surgical airway, and four had blind nasotracheal intubation. Ninety-eight percent of the direct laryngoscopy RSI group was successfully intubated. The authors concluded that the technical and time constraints of fiberoptic intubation led them to prefer RSI and direct laryngoscopy or a primary surgical airway when an emergency airway was required.[98]

Fiberoptic intubation has also been advocated for the emergency management of blunt injury to the airway, although reported experience is limited.[99] Awake nasotracheal fiberoptic intubation of a patient with unstable bilateral mandibular fractures in the semi-prone position has been reported.[100] The patient was unable to tolerate the supine or sitting position due to airway obstruction.[100] Successful awake fiberoptic orotracheal intubation has also been performed via an LMA in a patient with massive oropharyngeal bleeding following blunt trauma.[101] An attempt at fiberoptic intubation had failed due to blood in the airway, and an LMA was inserted to maintain gas exchange during a planned awake tracheotomy. Cuff inflation produced an unobstructed airway, resolution of respiratory distress, and permitted fiberoptic intubation through the LMA.[101] Emergency fiberoptic intubation has also been performed successfully in patients with respiratory failure, congestive heart failure, altered consciousness due to stroke, overdose, head trauma, status asthmaticus, hematemesis, and partial upper-airway obstruction.[91,93,94]

Success rates of emergency fiberoptic intubation have been reported by various authors to be 72%,[91] 87%,[94] 83%,[93] and 75%.[102] Visualization can be improved by pharyngeal suctioning.[19,94] Insufflation of oxygen via the working channel of the fiberoptic bronchoscope has been used to disperse secretions or vomitus and improve visualization.[94] However, gastric rupture has occurred with this technique,[35] and the potential for other barotrauma exists.[3,20]

In 1999, Levitan et al. published a survey of devices used for difficult airway management in academic emergency departments in the United States.[103] Of 95 programs who responded, only 64% had a fiberoptic bronchoscope, and although the most commonly used alternative to intubation by direct laryngoscopy was the flexible fiberoptic bronchoscope, it was in fact rarely used.[103] Only a small minority of patients requiring emergency endotracheal intubation need fiberoptic techniques,[93] and as a result skills' maintenance is problematic.

8.6.2 Can the fiberoptic bronchoscope be combined with other intubation techniques?

Fiberoptic intubation via the LMA has been described by a number of authors.[2,3,9,104–110] A 7.0 mm ID endotracheal tube can be passed through a #5 LMA and a 6-mm tube through a #4 LMA.[36] The appropriately sized bronchoscope can then be passed through the endotracheal tube into the trachea and the tube advanced over the scope. The length of a #4 LMA is 20 cm from the proximal edge of the LMA adapter to the grille,[109] and the distance from the grill to the cords is about 3.5–4.0 cm.[9,111] A standard #6 endotracheal tube will therefore only be able to extend about 5 cm below the cords and will not provide an adequate length of endotracheal tube for satisfactory endotracheal placement.[9] However, a #6 microlaryngoscopy tube with a length of 40 cm can be used to overcome this problem.[112] A #6 or #7 nasal Ring-Adair-Elwyn (RAE) tube can also be used, although the nasal RAE may need to be shortened by 2 cm to permit an adequate depth of intratracheal intubation by the fiberoptic bronchoscope.[111] The LMA can be removed over the endotracheal tube using a second tube to exert counterpressure on the endotracheal tube in the trachea to prevent its inadvertent dislodgement during removal of the LMA.[113] The airway tube of the ILMA has a minimal ID of 13 mm and can accommodate any cuffed endotracheal tube size up to an 8-mm ID.[104] Fiberoptic intubation through the LMA and ILMA has been performed with the patient awake or anesthetized.[3,9,114]

The cuffed oropharyngeal airway (COPA) has also been used to facilitate fiberoptic intubation.[2,115–117] The COPA is a modified Guedel-type oropharyngeal airway fitted with an inflatable cuff which separates the tongue from the posterior pharyngeal wall. The device is fitted with a standard proximal 15-mm adaptor that can be connected to a bag-mask device or an anesthesia breathing circuit.[2,116] The device may be inserted under regional anesthesia of the airway followed by spontaneous ventilation inhalation induction,[115] or after induction of GA.[116,117] Fiberoptic intubation can be performed through the nose[2,115,116] or through the mouth alongside the COPA.[2] During nasotracheal fiberoptic intubation, the fiberoptic bronchoscope having passed the cuff of the airway may encounter the larynx at the 9 o'clock position of the visual field, and rotation and flexion of the scope is then required to enter the larynx.[116] After the bronchoscope has entered the trachea, the cuff of the COPA should be deflated to permit the advancement of the endotracheal tube over the scope.[2,116] During fiberoptic orotracheal intubation, the bronchoscope can be advanced alongside the COPA into the trachea.[2] The cuff is then deflated and the device removed before passing the tube into the trachea.[2] Alternatively, a fiberoptic scope with an ensleeved Aintree Intubation Catheter® (AIC) can be passed through the lumen of the COPA into the trachea, the AIC then passed over the bronchoscope into the trachea, and the scope and oropharyngeal airway removed.[117] An endotracheal tube can then be passed over the AIC and the AIC removed. Jaw thrust or forward tilting of the COPA may be required to improve visualization of the vocal cords.[117] Cervical extension may be required to achieve optimal airway patency and therefore the device may not be suitable in the presence of potential or confirmed C-spine instability.[116] Ventilation during fiberoptic intubation using the COPA can be controlled or spontaneous.[2,115–117]

The fiberoptic bronchoscope can also be used to facilitate retrograde intubation.[2,3,118] During retrograde intubation, the tip of the endotracheal tube being advanced into the trachea over the wire may impinge on laryngeal structures and resist further advancement.[2,3] The flexible bronchoscope can be passed through the tube alongside the wire to visualize the glottis and then passed on into the trachea.[2,3] The wire can then be removed and the endotracheal tube advanced over the bronchoscope.[2,3] Alternatively, the wire can be passed in a retrograde direction through the working channel of the bronchoscope loaded with an ensleeved endotracheal tube.[2,118] The bronchoscope is then advanced over the wire into the trachea and the guidewire removed.[2,3] The endotracheal tube is then passed over the bronchoscope into the trachea.[2,3,118]

Blind nasotracheal intubation can also be assisted by the fiberoptic bronchoscope.[2,3] The bronchoscope can be passed through the contralateral nostril to visualize and thereby facilitate manipulation of the endotracheal tube into the trachea.[2,3]

8.7 OTHER CONSIDERATIONS

8.7.1 What are the limitations and complications of fiberoptic intubation?

Fiberoptic intubation in the presence of secretions, emesis, or blood in the airway is difficult and the applicability of the technique in the emergency situation is limited. Some measure of patient cooperation is also necessary. When both the bronchoscope and the ensleeved endotracheal tube are in the larynx or trachea, significant airway obstruction can be produced[8,37] and can cause respiratory distress. Bronchoscopes are delicate expensive instruments and require careful use if damage is to be avoided. The sterilization process is complex and requires time and resources.

Although they are rare, complications associated with fiberoptic intubation can occur. These include laryngospasm,[2,3] complete airway obstruction,[22,23,30] local anesthetic toxicity,[119] respiratory depression secondary to sedative overdose,[3] loss of the endoscopy mask diaphragm into the airway,[2,3] and laryngeal trauma.[120] The endotracheal tube is advanced blindly over the bronchoscope and may impinge on laryngeal or pharyngeal structures. Supraglottic swelling, pharyngeal hematoma, and vocal cord immobility and bruising have been reported after fiberoptic intubation.[120] The endotracheal tube should be advanced gently over the bronchoscope, the gap between the endotracheal tube and scope diameters minimized, and the use of tubes with modified bevels may be considered. Additional studies are required to determine the mechanism of pharyngeal or laryngeal injury during fiberoptic intubation as well as their incidence and severity.[120] In a series of 2,031 fiberoptic intubations, complications were limited to laryngospasm in 51, pain or hematoma secondary to cricothyroid injection in 33, gagging or vomiting in 8, and mild epistaxis in 70 who were nasally intubated.[3] None of the cases of epistaxis required packing.

8.7.2   How much training is required to develop proficiency in fiberoptic intubation? How can the training be acquired?

Fiberoptic intubation is not a difficult skill to master; however it requires familiarity with the anatomy of the upper airway, and dexterity in bronchoscopic manipulation. Awake fiberoptic intubation requires skill in regional anesthesia of the airway and gentleness on the part of the practitioner. Each step of the procedure must be planned in advance and methodically carried out. The ability to quickly and reliably maneuver the bronchoscope in a given direction is an absolute requirement for fast, successful, and safe fiberoptic intubation. Readily available intubation mannequins can be used to develop manual dexterity with the bronchoscope and threading the endotracheal tube over the scope. Fiberoptic intubation workshops can also be effective in improving skills.[121] Ideally, fiberoptic intubation should be demonstrated by a knowledgeable and skilled instructor.[5] The learner should then be supervised until the principles of bronchoscopic manipulation are mastered. The availability of video bronchoscopes permit the instructor to easily coach the learner in the flexion and rotation movements required to properly steer the bronchoscope and appears to facilitate fiberoptic skill acquisition.[122] Independent practice is then required to further develop and improve psychomotor skills. A reasonable level of dexterity in manipulating the bronchoscope can be achieved within 3 to 4 hours of independent mannequin practice.[5]

Fiberoptic intubation has been advocated as an alternate technique that may be used whenever tracheal intubation is indicated,[3] and this fiberoptic intubation of normal airways under GA may be beneficial in learning to manipulate the bronchoscope and to advance the endotracheal tube over the scope.[3,84,123] However, the use of "nonroutine" techniques may require discussion with the patient beforehand.[124] Furthermore, the fiberoptic intubation of patients with normal airways under GA may not extrapolate well to the intubation of the difficult airway in the awake patient.[123,125]

An acceptable level of technical expertise may be achievable after 10 fiberoptic intubations in anesthetized patients[126] and 15–20 awake fiberoptic intubations in patients with normal anatomy.[5] Smith and Jackson reported that trainees were "becoming reasonably proficient" after performing 20 fiberoptic intubations in anesthetized patients in whom intubation was predicted to be difficult.[127] It has also been suggested that 30 fiberoptic intubations in conscious and anesthetized patients be performed before a practitioner is ready to handle the difficult intubation.[128] The amount of experience and training required for safe and effective use of the fiberoptic bronchoscope in the difficult airway is unknown[9,19]; however an experience of 100 or more fiberoptic procedures may be necessary to acquire expertise in this setting.[5,9,19]

8.8   SUMMARY

Fiberoptic intubation is widely accepted as an invaluable alternate technique in the management of the difficult airway. It should be mastered by all anesthesia practitioners and other practitioners responsible for airway management.

REFERENCES

1. Murphy P: A fibre-optic endoscope used for nasal intubation. *Anaesthesia.* 1967;22:489–491.
2. Ovassapian A: The flexible bronchoscope. A tool for anesthesiologists. *Clin Chest Med.* 2001;22:281–299.
3. Ovassapian A, Wheeler M: Flexible fiberoptic tracheal intubation. In: *Handbook of Difficult Airway Management.* Hagberg CA, ed. Philadelphia, PA: Churchill Livingstone, 2000: 83–114.
4. Stiles CM, Stiles QR, Denson JS: A flexible fiber optic laryngoscope. *JAMA.* 1972;221:1246–1247.
5. Ovassapian A, Yelich SJ: Learning Fiberoptic Intubation. *Anesthesiol Clin North America.* 1991;9:175–186.
6. Practice guidelines for management of the difficult airway. A report by the American Society of Anesthesiologists Task Force on Management of the Difficult Airway. *Anesthesiology.* 1993;78:597–602.
7. Stackhouse RA: Fiberoptic airway management. *Anesthesiol Clin North America.* 2002;20:933–951.
8. Weiss YG, Deutschman CS: The role of fiberoptic bronchoscopy in airway management of the critically ill patient. *Crit Care Clin.* 2000;16:445–451.
9. Ovassapian A, Wheeler M: Fiberoptic Endoscopy-Aided Techniques. In: *Airway Management Principles and Practice.* Benumof JL, ed. St. Louis: Mosby, Inc., 1996: 282–319.
10. Heidegger T, Gerig HJ, Ulrich B, Kreienbuhl G: Validation of a simple algorithm for tracheal intubation: daily practice is the key to success in emergencies–an analysis of 13248 intubations. *Anesth Analg.* 2001;92:517–522.
11. Sidhu VS, Whitehead EM, Ainsworth QP, Smith M, Calder I: A technique of awake fiberoptic intubation. Experience in patients with cervical spine disease. *Anaesthesia.* 1993;48:910–913.
12. Benumof JL: Management of the difficult adult airway. With special emphasis on awake tracheal intubation. *Anesthesiology.* 1991;75:1087–1110.
13. Allan AG: Reluctance of anaesthetists to perform awake intubation. *Anaesthesia.* 2004;59:413.
14. Basi SK, Cooper M, Ahmed FB, Clarke SG, Mitchell V: Reluctance of anaesthetists to perform awake intubation. *Anaesthesia.* 2004;59:918.
15. Heidegger T, Gerig H: Anticipated difficult airway: the role of fiberoptics. *Anesth Analg.* 2002;95:1124.
16. Rosenblatt WH, Wagner PJ, Ovassapian A, Kain ZN: Practice patterns in managing the difficult airway by anesthesiologists in the United States. *Anesth Analg.* 1998;87:153–157.
17. Avargues P, Cros AM, Daucourt V, Michel P, Maurette P: Procedures use by French anesthetists in cases of difficult intubation and the impact of a conference of experts. *Ann Fr Anesth Reanim.* 1999;18:719–724.
18. Kristensen MS, Moller J: Airway management behaviour, experience and knowledge among Danish anaesthesiologists—room for improvement. *Acta Anaesthesiol Scand.* 2001;45:1181–1185.

19. Morris IR: Fibreoptic intubation. *Can J Anaesth*. 1994;41:996–1008.
20. Morris IR: Airway anesthesia, sedation and awake intubation. In: *The Difficult Airway Course: Anesthesia*. Course Manual, 2001:64–81.
21. Reed AP: Preparation for intubation of the awake patient. *Mt Sinai J Med*. 1995;62:10–20.
22. Ho AM, Chung DC, To EW, Karmakar MK: Total airway obstruction during local anesthesia in a non-sedated patient with a compromised airway. *Can J Anaesth*. 2004;51:838–841.
23. Shaw IC, Welchew EA, Harrison BJ, Michael S: Complete airway obstruction during awake fibreoptic intubation. *Anaesthesia*. 1997;52:582–585.
24. Liistro G, Stanescu DC, Veriter C, Rodenstein DO, D'Odemont JP: Upper airway anesthesia induces airflow limitation in awake humans. *Am Rev Respir Dis*. 1992;146:581–585.
25. Kuna ST, Woodson GE, Sant'Ambrogio G: Effect of laryngeal anesthesia on pulmonary function testing in normal subjects. *Am Rev Respir Dis*. 1988;137:656–651.
26. Morris IR: Airway management. In: *Emergency Medicine: Concepts and Clinical Practice*, 3rd edn. Rosen P et al. eds. St. Louis: Mosby Inc., 1992.
27. Walls RM: Airway management. In: *Emergency Medicine: Concepts and Clinical Practice*. 9th ed. Rosen P, et al. eds. St. Louis: Mosby Inc., 1998:2–24.
28. Suderman VS, Crosby ET, Lui A: Elective oral tracheal intubation in cervical spine-injured adults. *Can J Anaesth*. 1991;38:785–789.
29. Meschino A, Devitt JH, Koch JP, Szalai JP, Schwartz ML: The safety of awake tracheal intubation in cervical spine injury. *Can J Anaesth*. 1992;39:114–117.
30. McGuire G, el-Beheiry H: Complete upper airway obstruction during awake fibreoptic intubation in patients with unstable cervical spine fractures. *Can J Anaesth*. 1999;46:176–178.
31. Donlon JV, Jr: Anesthetic management of patients with compromised airways. *Anesth Rev*. 1980;7:22–31.
32. Wong DT, McGuire GP: Management choices for the difficult airway. *Can J Anaesth*. 2003;50:624.
33. Edens ET, Sia RL: Flexible fiberoptic endoscopy in difficult intubations. *Ann Otol Rhinol Laryngol*. 1981;90:307–309.
34. ECRI. Bronchoscopes. In: *Healthcare Product Comparison System*, Hospital edn. Plymouth Meeting, PA: ECRI, 2004.
35. Hershey MD, Hannenberg AA: Gastric distention and rupture from oxygen insufflation during fiberoptic intubation. *Anesthesiology*. 1996;85:1479–1480.
36. Fulling PD, Roberts JT: Fiberoptic intubation. *Int Anesthesiol Clin*. 2000;38:189–217.
37. Dellinger RP: Fiberoptic bronchoscopy in adult airway management. *Crit Care Med*. 1990;18:882–887.
38. Witton TH: An introduction to the fiberoptic laryngoscope. *Can Anaesth Soc. J*. 1981;28:475–478.
39. Sutherland AD, Williams RT: Cardiovascular responses and lidocaine absorption in fiberoptic-assisted awake intubation. *Anesth Analg*. 1986;65:389–391.
40. Kristensen MS: The Parker Flex-Tip tube versus a standard tube for fiberoptic orotracheal intubation: a randomized double-blind study. *Anesthesiology*. 2003;98:354–358.
41. Marsh NJ: Easier fiberoptic intubations. *Anesthesiology*. 1992;76:860–861.
42. Asai T, Shingu K: Difficulty in advancing a tracheal tube over a fibreoptic bronchoscope: incidence, causes and solutions. *Br J Anaesth*. 2004;92:870–881.
43. El-Orbany MI, Salem MR, Joseph NJ: Tracheal tube advancement over the fiberoptic bronchoscope: size does matter. *Anesth Analg*. 2003;97:301.
44. Deam R, McCutcheon C: Management choices for the difficult airway. *Can J Anaesth*. 2003;50:623–624.
45. Taylor DM, Brimacomb J, Stone T: Inactivation of prions by physical and chemical means. *J Hosp Infect*. 1999;43(Suppl):S69–S76.
46. Walsh EM: Reducing the risk of prion transmission in anaesthesia. *Anaesthesia*. 2006;61:64–65.
47. Walsh ME, Shorten GD: Preparing to perform an awake fiberoptic intubation. *Yale J Biol Med*. 1998;71:537–549.
48. Telford RJ, Liban JB: Awake fibreoptic intubation. *Br J Hosp Med*. 1991;46:182–184.
49. Morikawa S, Safar P, Decarlo J: Influence of the headjaw position upon upper airway patency. *Anesthesiology*. 1961;22:265–270.
50. Safar P: Ventilatory efficacy of mouth-to-mouth artificial respiration; airway obstruction during manual and mouth-to-mouth artificial respiration. *J Am Med Assoc*. 1958;167:335–341.
51. Boyson PG: Fiberoptic instrumentation for airway management. *ASA Refresher Course Lectures*. 1993;266:1–5.
52. Hakala P, Randall T, Valli H: Comparison between tracheal tubes for orotracheal fibreoptic intubation. *Br J Anaesth*. 1999;82:135–136
53. Barker KF, Bolton P, Cole S, Coe PA: Ease of laryngeal passage during fibreoptic intubation: a comparison of three endotracheal tubes. *Acta Anaesthesiol Scand*. 2001;45:624–626.
54. Ovassapian A: Flexible bronchoscopic intubation of awake patients. *J Bronchology*. 1994;1:240–245.
55. Hughes S, Smith JE: Nasotracheal tube placement over the fibreoptic laryngoscope. *Anaesthesia*. 1996;51:1026–1028.
56. Randell T: Fibreoptic orotracheal intubation. *Br J Anaesth*. 1999;83:683–684.
57. Katsnelson T, Frost EA, Farcon E, Goldiner PL: When the endotracheal tube will not pass over the flexible fiberoptic bronchoscope. *Anesthesiology*. 1992;76:151–152.
58. Greer JR, Smith SP, Strang T: A comparison of tracheal tube tip designs on the passage of an endotracheal tube during oral fiberoptic intubation. *Anesthesiology*. 2001;94:729–731.
59. Wheeler M, Dsida RM: Fiberoptic intubation: troubles with the "Tube"? *Anesthesiology*. 2003;99:1236–1237.
60. Schwartz D, Johnson C, Roberts J: A maneuver to facilitate flexible fiberoptic intubation. *Anesthesiology*. 1989;71:470–471.
61. Jones HE, Pearce AC, Moore P: Fiberoptic intubatin: influence of tracheal tube tip design. *Anaesthesia*. 1993;48:672–674.
62. Cossham PS: Fibreoptic orotracheal intubation. *Br J Anaesth*. 1999;83: 683–684.
63. Nakayama M, Kataoka N, Usui Y, et al: Techniques of nasotracheal intubation with the fiberoptic bronchoscope. *J Emerg Med*. 1992;10:729–734.
64. Raj PP, Forestner J, Watson TD, Morris RE, Jenkins MT: Techniques for fiberoptic laryngoscopy in anesthesia. *Anesth Analg*. 1974;53:708–714.
65. Calder I: When the endotracheal tube will not pass over the flexible fiberoptic bronchoscope. *Anesthesiology*. 1992;77:398.
66. Tan I: Easier fiberoptic intubation. *Anaesthesia*. 1994;49:830–831.
67. Brull SJ, Wiklund R, Ferris C, et al.: Facilitation of fiberoptic orotracheal intubation with a flexible tracheal tube. *Anesth Analg*. 1994;78:746–748.
68. Aoyama K, Yasunaga E, Takenaka I: Another sleeve for fiberoptic tracheal intubation. *Anesth Analg*. 2003;97:1205.
69. Ayoub CM, Rizk MS, Yaacoub CI, Baraka AS, Lteif AM: Advancing the tracheal tube over a flexible fiberoptic bronchoscope by a sleeve mounted on the insertion cord. *Anesth Analg*. 2003;96:290–292.
70. Ayoub CM, Lteif AM, Rizk MS, et al.: Facilitation of passing the endotracheal tube over the flexible fiberoptic bronchoscope using a Cook airway exchange catheter. *Anesthesiology*. 2002;96:1517–1518.
71. Joo HS, Naik VN, Savoldelli GL: Parker Flex-Tip are not superior to polyvinylchloride tracheal tubes for awake fibreoptic intubations. *Can J Anaesth*. 2005;52:297–301.
72. Greenland KB, Lam MC, Irwin MG: Comparison of the Williams Airway Intubator and Ovassapian Fiberoptic Intubating Airway for fibreoptic orotracheal intubation. *Anaesthesia*. 2004;59:173–176.
73. Randell T, Valli H, Hakala P: Comparison between the Ovassapian intubating airway and the Berman intubating airway in fibreoptic intubation. *Eur J Anaesthesiol*. 1997;14:380–384.
74. Smith JE, Reid AP: Identifying the more patent nostril before nasotracheal intubation. *Anaesthesia*. 2001;56:258–262.
75. Lee AC, Wu CL, Feins RH, Ward DS: The use of fiberoptic endoscopy in anesthesia. *Chest Surg Clin N Am*. 1996;6:329–347.
76. Arrowsmith JE, Robertshaw HJ, Boyd JD: Nasotracheal intubation in the presence of frontobasal skull fracture. *Can J Anaesth*. 1998;45:71–75.
77. Dauphinee K: Nasotracheal intubation. *Emerg Med Clin North Am*. 1988;6:715–723.
78. Bainton CR: Complications of Managing the Airway. In: *Airway Management Principles and Practice*. Benumof JL, ed. St. Louis: Mosby, Inc., 1996: 886–899.
79. Stone DJ, Gal TJ: Airway Management. In: *Anesthesia*, 5th edn. Miller RD, ed. Philadelphia, PA: Churchill Livingstone, 2000.
80. Iserson KV: Blind nasotracheal intubation. *Ann Emerg Med*. 1981;10: 468–471.
81. Tintinalli JE, Claffey J: Complications of nasotracheal intubation. *Ann Emerg Med*. 1981;10:142–144.
82. Latorre F, Otter W, Kleemann PP, Dick W, Jage J: Cocaine or phenylephrine/lignocaine for nasal fibreoptic intubation? *Eur J Anaesthesiol*. 1996;13:577–581.
83. Pandit JJ, Dravid RM, Iyer R, Popat MT: Orotracheal fibreoptic intubation for rapid sequence induction of anaesthesia. *Anaesthesia*. 2002;57:123–127.
84. Hartley M, Morris S, Vaughan RS: Teaching fibreoptic intubation. Effect of alfentanil on the haemodynamic response. *Anaesthesia*. 1994;49:335–337.
85. Heidegger T, Gerig HJ, Ulrich B, Schnider TW: Structure and process quality illustrated by fibreoptic intubation: analysis of 1612 cases. *Anaesthesia*. 2003;58:734–739.
86. Albanon-Sofelo R, Atkins JM, Broom RS, et al.: *Textbook of Advanced Cardiac Life Support*. American Heart Association, 1987.

87. Durga VK, Millns JP, Smith JE: Manoeuvres used to clear the airway during fibreoptic intubation. *Br J Anaesth.* 2001;87:207–211.

88. Coe PA, King TA, Towey RM: Teaching guided fibreoptic nasotracheal intubation. An assessment of an anaesthetic technique to aid training. *Anaesthesia.* 1988;43:410–413.

89. Yushi A, Satomoto M, Hiquchi H, et al.: Fiberoptic orotracheal intubation in the left semi lateral position. *Anesth Analg.* 2002;94:477–478.

90. Patil V, Stehling LC, Zauder HL, Koch JP: Mechanical aids for fiberoptic endoscopy. *Anesthesiology.* 1982;57:69–70.

91. Afilalo M, Guttman A, Stern E, et al.: Fiberoptic intubation in the emergency department: a case series. *J Emerg Med.* 1993;11:387–391.

92. Hamilton PH, Kang JJ: Emergency airway management. *Mt Sinai J Med.* 1997;64:292–301.

93. Mlinek EJ, Jr, Clinton JE, Plummer D, Ruiz E: Fiberoptic intubation in the emergency department. *Ann Emerg Med.* 1990;19:359–362.

94. Delaney KA, Hessler R: Emergency flexible fiberoptic nasotracheal intubation: a report of 60 cases. *Ann Emerg Med.* 1988;17:919–926.

95. Doyle DJ, Arellano R: Medical conditions affecting the airway: A synopsis. In: *Handbook of Difficult Airway Management.* Hagberg CA, ed. Philadelphia, PA: Churchill Livingstone, 2000:227–256.

96. Doyle DJ, Arellano R: The Airway and clinical postoperative conditions. In: *Handbook of Difficult Airway Management.* Hagberg CA, ed. Philadelphia, PA: Churchill Livingstone, 2000:219–225.

97. Mandavia DP, Qualls S, Rokos I: Emergency airway management in penetrating neck injury. *Ann Emerg Med.* 2000;35:221–225.

98. Shearer VE, Giesecke AH: Airway management for patients with penetrating neck trauma: a retrospective study. *Anesth Analg.* 1993;77:1135–1138.

99. Morris IR: *Anaesthesia and Airway Management of Laryngoscopy and Bronchoscopy, Benumof's Airway management Principles and Practice,* 2nd edn. Hagberg CA, ed. Philadelphia, PA Mosby Elsevier, 2007:859–888).

100. Neal MR, Groves J, Gell IR: Awake fiberoptic intubation in the semi-prone position following facial trauma. *Anaesthesia.* 1996;51:1053–1054.

101. Preis CA, Hartmann T, Zimpfer M: Laryngeal mask airway facilitates awake fiberoptic intubation in a patient with severe oropharyngeal bleeding. *Anesth Analg.* 1998;87:728–729.

102. Schafermeyer RW: Fiberoptic laryngoscopy in the emergency department. *Am J Emerg Med.* 1984;2:160–163.

103. Levitan RM, Kush S, Hollander JE: Devices for difficult airway management in academic emergency departments: results of a national survey. *Ann Emerg Med.* 1999;33:694–698.

104. Brain AI, Verghese C, Addy EV, Kapila A: The intubating laryngeal mask. I: Development of a new device for intubation of the trachea. *Br J Anaesth.* 1997;79:699–703.

105. Benumof JL: Use of the laryngeal mask airway to facilitate fiberscope-aided tracheal intubation. *Anesth Analg.* 1992;74:313–315.

106. Choi JE, Leal YR, Johnson MD: Fiberoptic intubation through the laryngeal mask airway. *J Clin Anesth.* 1996;8:687–688.

107. Breen PH: In Response (Letter). *Anesth Analg.* 1997;84:470.

108. Preis CA, Preis IS: Oversize endotracheal tubes and intubation via laryngeal mask airway. *Anesthesiology.* 1997;87:187.

109. Benumof JL: Laryngeal mask airway and the ASA difficult airway algorithm. *Anesthesiology.* 1996;84:686–699.

110. Pennant JH, White PF: The laryngeal mask airway. *Anesthesiology.* 1993; 79:144–163.

111. Benumof JL: A new technique of fiberoptic intubation through a standard LMA. *Anesthesiology.* 2001;95:1541.

112. Preis C, Preis I: Concept for easy fiberoptic intubation via a laryngeal airway mask. *Anesth Analg.* 1999;89:803–804.

113. Watson NC, Hokanson M, Maltby JR, Todesco JM: The intubating laryngeal mask airway in failed fibreoptic intubation. *Can J Anaesth.* 1999;46:376–378.

114. Joo HS, Kapoor S, Rose DK, Naik VN: The intubating laryngeal mask airway after induction of general anesthesia versus awake fiberoptic intubation in patients with difficult airways. *Anesth Analg.* 2001;92:1342–1346.

115. Asai T, Matsumoto H, Shingu K: Awake insertion of the cuffed oropharyngeal airway for nasotracheal intubation. *Anaesthesia.* 1999;54:492–493.

116. Uezono S, Goto T, Nakata Y, et al.: The cuffed oropharyngeal airway, a novel adjunct to the management of difficult airways. *Anesthesiology.* 1998;88:1677–1679.

117. Hawkins M, O'Sullivan E, Charters P: Fibreoptic intubation using the cuffed oropharyngeal airway and Aintree intubation catheter. *Anaesthesia.* 1998;53:891–894.

118. Sanchez AF, Morrison DE: Preparation of the patient for awake intubation. In: *Handbook of Difficult Airway Management,* 1st edn. Hagberg CA, ed. Philadelphia, PA: Churchill Livingstone, 2000:49–82.

119. Wu FL, Razzaghi A, Souney PF: Seizure after lidocaine for bronchoscopy: case report and review of the use of lidocaine in airway anesthesia. *Pharmacotherapy* 1993;13:72–78.

120. Maktabi MA, Hoffman H, Funk G, From RP: Laryngeal trauma during awake fiberoptic intubation. *Anesth Analg.* 2002;95:1112–1114.

121. Dykes MH, Ovassapian A: Dissemination of fibreoptic airway endoscopy skills by means of a workshop utilizing models. *Br J Anaesth.* 1989; 63: 595–597.

122. Smith JE, Fenner SG, King MJ: Teaching fibreoptic nasotracheal intubation with and without closed circuit television. *Br J Anaesth.* 1993;71:206–211.

123. Ball DR: Awake versus asleep fibreoptic intubation. *Anaesthesia.* 1994; 49:921.

124. Bray JK, Yentis SM: Attitudes of patients and anaesthetists to informed consent for specialist airway techniques. *Anaesthesia.* 2002;57:1012–1015.

125. Mason RA: Learning fiberoptic intubation: fundamental problems. *Anaesthesia.* 1992;47:729–731.

126. Johnson C, Roberts JT: Clinical competence in the performance of fiberoptic laryngoscopy and endotracheal intubation: a study of resident instruction. *J Clin Anesth.* 1989;1:344–349.

127. Smith JE, Jackson AP: Learning fiberoptic endoscopy. Nasotracheal or orotracheal intubations first? *Anaesthesia.* 2000;55:1072–1075.

128. Sia RL, Edens ET: How to avoid problems when using the fibre-optic bronchoscope for difficult intubation. *Anaesthesia.* 1981;36:74–75.

SELF-EVALUATION QUESTIONS

8.1. Complications associated with fiberoptic intubation include

A. laryngospasm

B. complete airway obstruction

C. local anesthesia toxicity

D. laryngeal trauma

E. all of the above

8.2. Which of the following is a reliable method of removing prions from the flexible fiberoptic bronchoscope following its use in a patient with Creutzfeldt-Jakob disease?

A. immersed in a solution of peracetic acid

B. disinfection of bronchoscopes using orthophthaldehyde (Cidex)

C. disinfection of bronchoscopes using ethylene oxide

D. disinfection of bronchoscopes using an autoclave

E. none of the above

8.3. During fiberoptic intubation, which of the following can facilitate advancement of the ensleeved endotracheal tube into the trachea over the fiberoptic bronchoscope?

A. Profound regional anesthesia of the airway.

B. Rotation of the tube 90 degree counterclockwise may be necessary to orient the bevel posteriorly.

C. Minimize the discrepancy between the outside diameter of the bronchoscope and the internal diameter of the endotracheal tube.

D. The use of the ILMA tube which has a soft hemispherical bevel and a leading edge in the midline.

E. All of the above.

CHAPTER (9)

Rigid and Semirigid Fiberoptic and Video Laryngoscopy and Intubation

Richard M. Cooper and J. Adam Law

9.1 INTRODUCTION

9.1.1 Why were rigid and semirigid fiberoptic and video laryngoscopes developed?

Direct laryngoscopy (DL) depends upon achieving a line-of-sight from the practitioner to the larynx. While positioning of the head and neck of the patient is critical to optimize alignment of the oral, pharyngeal, and laryngeal axes, this concept has recently been challenged.[1-4] In addition to positioning, the tongue must be displaced and compressed, the mandible and epiglottis elevated, and frequently the larynx manually depressed. Despite these maneuvers, the larynx cannot be visualized by DL in up to 8.5% of cases.[5] The inability to see the larynx does not preclude successful intubation but it increases the likelihood of prolonged or multiple attempts, hypertension, inadequate ventilation, arterial desaturation, and esophageal intubation.[5] Instruments that are more or less anatomically shaped can overcome restrictions in patient anatomy that may make DL difficult or impossible. Fiberoptic and video laryngoscopes are designed specifically for this purpose.

Another significant limitation of DL is that the experience is difficult to share.[6] Only the laryngoscopist is able to visualize the procedure and this complicates the teaching and recording of laryngoscopy and conduct of airway research. Video laryngoscopy circumvents many of these limitations but generally relies upon alternative devices. Visualizing the anatomy and the procedure of intubation can be achieved using a conventional laryngoscope. The Airway Cam®, developed by Dr. Richard Levitan, is a head-mounted camera which captures the laryngoscopist's view through an eye-level pentaprism and conveys the image to a video monitor and/or a recording device.[7,8] This device enables a student and mentor to simultaneously view the same object, capturing the image and playing it back at a pace suitable for teaching, clinical documentation, and research. While these achievements are clearly worthwhile, this technology does not improve laryngeal exposure.

Flexible fiberoptic bronchoscopes* (FFBs) have greatly expanded our ability to diagnose and manage problems in previously inaccessible body parts. These devices are versatile but complex. For tracheal intubation, FFBs demand a different skill set than does DL. Nonetheless, practitioners must master these devices, since they are the best choice for some airway challenges. Their complexity and versatility also add to their cost and fragility. Although occasionally flexible bronchoscopes are essential to solve an airway problem, in many situations other devices can do the job more easily. Using fiberoptic and video technology, semirigid or rigid devices have been designed specifically for intubation and share the attributes of providing illumination and viewing around "anatomical corners." They may be stylet-like (e.g., the Shikani Optical Stylet), flat (e.g., the Bullard laryngoscope), hollow (e.g., WuScope System™ [WS]), or resemble a conventional laryngoscope (Storz Video Macintosh or GlideScope®). As this is an evolving field, this chapter is not an exhaustive review of all the currently available devices.

---

* In discussing the features, costs, and cleaning of these devices, every effort has been made to obtain information from the manufacturer, current at the time of the writing. Prices and device configurations change and the authors strongly advise prospective users to consult further with the manufacturer and national and institutional authorities regarding acceptable methods of disinfection. All prices are in US dollars unless otherwise stated. All prices were accurate at the time of publication but may be subject to change.

9.2   FIBEROPTIC STYLETS

9.2.1   What are fiberoptic stylets?

Liem and coworkers have recently reviewed the development and proposed a classification of flexible fiberoptic stylets.[9] Since 1972, many such devices have been introduced but only a few have survived commercially. Fiberoptic stylets are inserted within the endotracheal tube (ETT) and, through an eyepiece or on a video monitor, allow the practitioner to view ETT advancement. The instruments vary with respect to diameter, image resolution, the source of illumination, and flexibility. At this point, the commercially available optical stylets with reasonable accompanying narrative in the literature include the Bonfils Retromolar Intubation Fiberscope (Bonfils, Karl Storz Endoscopy, Culver City, CA), the Shikani Optical Stylet (SOS, Clarus Medical LLC, Minneapolis, MN), the fiberoptic StyletScope (FSS, Nihon Kohden Corp., Tokyo, Japan), and the Video-Optical Intubation Stylet (VOIS, Acutronic Medical Systems AG, Baar, Switzerland). The Levitan FPS Scope (Clarus Medical LLC, Minneapolis, MN) is a recently introduced fiberoptic stylet that shows promise as a low-cost version of this class of instruments.

9.2.2   What Are the unique characteristics of fiberoptic stylets?

Common to all optical stylets is a rigid or semirigid shaft, with a proximal tube holder compatible with the 15-mm connector an ETT. Most tube holders can be positioned at variable locations on the stylet shaft, enabling reliable positioning of the tip of the endoscope just proximal to the distal end of the ETT. All optical stylets transmit light distally and the image proximally to an eyepiece or camera through glass or plastic fibers, with variable resolution. The distal viewing angle varies from 50 to 90 degrees. Light is supplied via a cable from a remote light source and/or from an attached battery handle to enhance portability. Few of these devices have a hollow working channel of the type present in other classes of fiberoptic device.

9.2.3   Individual fiberoptic stylet description

9.2.3.1   What Are the Characteristics of the Bonfils Retromolar Intubation Fiberscope?

The Bonfils is the only scope in this class of instrument that is nonmalleable. The shaft is 40-cm long and has an anterior bend of 40 degrees at the distal end. It is available in versions with and without a 1.2-mm working channel; both editions are 5.0 mm in diameter, so the instrument will accommodate ETTs down to a 6.0-mm internal diameter (ID) (Figure 9-1). A movable adapter allows for ETT fixation on the stylet as well as oxygen insufflation down the ETT. Light is provided via a cable from a standard remote light source or through a portable battery-powered xenon light source. The distal viewing angle is 90 degrees. The image is transferred by glass fiber (12,000 pixels) to a movable proximal eyepiece with an adjustable diopter correction or an available

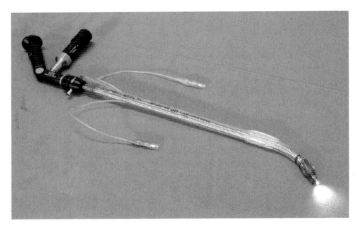

FIGURE 9-1. The Bonfils Retromolar Intubation Fiberscope, shown here with the micro video module camera unit, enabling image display on an accompanying monitor (*Reproduced with permission from Karl Storz*).

attached microvideo module, compatible with standard Storz camera control units.

9.2.3.2   What Are the Characteristics of the Shikani Optical Stylet?

The Shikani Optical Stylet (SOS) incorporates a semirigid, distally malleable stylet (Figure 9-2). It is supplied with a bending tool and can accommodate an arc of up to 120 degrees. The stylet shaft is 27-cm long, has a diameter of 5.0 mm, and is capable of accepting an ETT ≥ 5.5-mm ID. A pediatric version is compatible with ETTs in the 2.5–5.5-mm ID range. ETT fixation is achieved by a movable tube stop device, incorporating a nipple through which O_2 can be delivered down the ETT. The distal viewing angle of the adult scope is 70 degrees. Glass fiberoptic bundles of 30,000 pixels are used to deliver the image to a fixed-focus, proximal eyepiece (the SITEcoupler™). The coupler can be removed to enable complete submersion of the stylet for disinfection, although this feature will be absent in future versions of the device. Lighting is supplied from one of three sources: via fiberoptic cable from a remote light source; a battery 'SITElight™' handle, containing a 6-V halogen bulb; or using an adapter, via a Green specification fiberoptic laryngoscope handle. The eyepiece is compatible with proximally attached camera adapters, if desired. A passively flexible version of this stylet is available, compatible with the company's

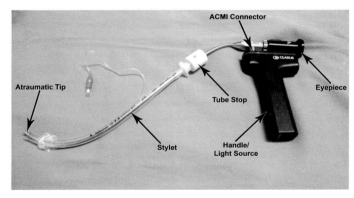

FIGURE 9-2. The Shikani Optical Stylet, adult version (*Reproduced with permission from Clarus Medical*).

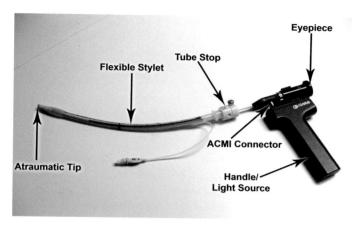

FIGURE 9-3. The Foley Airway Stylet (FAST) (*Reproduced with permission from Clarus Medical*).

handles: the Foley Airway Stylet (FAST, Figure 9-3) can be used to help confirm ETT placement or patency as well as aiding with LMA Fastrach™ intubation.

9.2.3.3 What Are the Characteristics of the Levitan FPS scope?

The Levitan FPS Scope, developed by Dr. Richard Levitan, has recently been introduced as a low-cost fiberoptic stylet (Figure 9-4). The light source is supplied via an adapter from a standard Greenline handle or a dedicated attached portable light-emitting diode. The shaft of the instrument is malleable through 90 degrees. Unlike other fiberoptic stylets, the 15.0-mm connector adapter is fixed on the handle, so that in order to have the distal stylet tip appropriately placed, the ETT will have to be cut to 27 cm prior to use with the scope. A proximal nipple permits O_2 insufflation down the ETT once attached. The proximal eyepiece has a fixed focus. The developer suggests shaping the Levitan FPS Scope "straight to cuff" (i.e., with an otherwise straight shaft bent anteriorly at an angle of no more than 25–35 degrees just proximal to the ETT cuff) (R. Levitan, personal communication, June 2005) and using it in conjunction with DL.

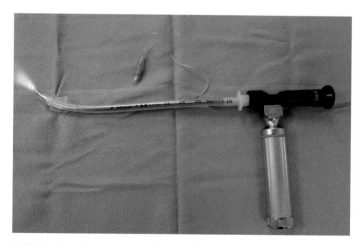

FIGURE 9-4. The Levitan FPS Scope, shown with a Greenline-compatible laryngoscope handle. (*Reproduced with permission from Clarus Medical*).

9.2.3.4 What Are the Characteristics of the StyletScope?

The fiberoptic StyletScope (FSS) is unique among the optical stylets in incorporating a lever adjacent to the proximal handle enabling manipulation of the distal stylet angle during the tracheal tube placement. When depressed, the distal stylet tip, with loaded ETT, will flex anteriorly up to 75 degrees (Figure 9-5). A proximal ETT 15-mm adapter stabilizes the ETT, whereupon stylet length can be adjusted appropriately. Light supply is built in to the proximal battery handle, powered by two 1.5-V alkaline batteries.[10] Fiberoptic imaging is through plastic bundles (3500 pixels) and the obtainable field of view is 50 degrees. At 6.0 mm, the FSS is one of the largest-diameter stylets, compatible with an ETT minimum ID of 7.0 mm. The scope can be sterilized in ethylene oxide (ETO).

9.2.3.5 What Are the Characteristics of the Video-Optical Intubating System (VOIS)?

The VOIS is a semirigid stylet malleable along its distal 40 cm (Figure 9-6). With an OD of 5.0 mm, glass fiberoptic bundles of 10,000 pixels transfer the image to a proximal ocular, which in turn is compatible with various CCD camera systems. With light supplied from a remote source via a fiberoptic cable, a 50-degree angle of view can be obtained.

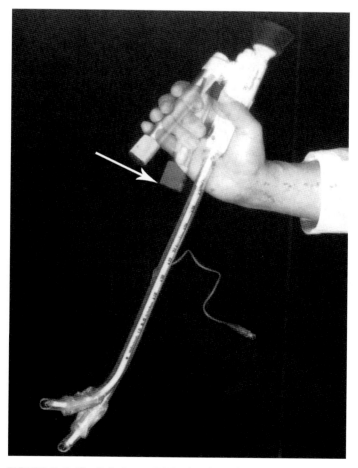

FIGURE 9-5. The StyletScope (FSS). The photo shows the neutral and activated positions: as the proximal lever is depressed toward the device handle (arrow), the distal stylet and ensleeved tube flex anteriorly. (*Reproduced with permission from Kimura et al.,[29]*)

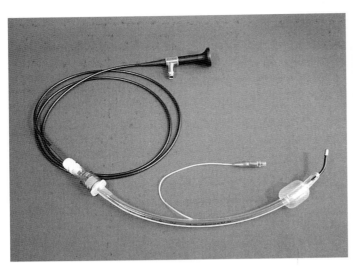

FIGURE 9-6. Video-Optical Intubating Stylet (VOIS) *(Reproduced with permission from Dr. Marcus Weiss).*

9.2.4   Fiberoptic stylet use

Most of the fiberoptic stylets described above are similar in their structure, from which it follows that their function will also be similar. The following narrative describing the use of fiberoptic stylets, in general, can be applied to all.

9.2.4.1   How Are Fiberoptic Stylets Prepared for Tracheal Intubation?

As with all fiberoptic instruments, insertion of a cold instrument in a patient will result in an obscured view. To prevent fogging, the device can be warmed by immersing the stylet shaft in a container of warm water, or a commercial antifog solution can be applied. As the presence of blood and secretions can interfere with viewing, the patient's hypopharynx should be suctioned prior to insertion of a fiberoptic stylet or any fiberoptic device. For semirigid devices, the desired degree of distal angulation will depend on the technique of use: stand-alone use requires more angulation (e.g., 40–90 degrees), while fiberoptic stylet use as adjunct to DL requires a distal curvature of no more than 25–35 degrees.

9.2.4.2   How Are Fiberoptic Stylets Used to Perform Tracheal Intubation?

Optical stylets can be used alone or in conjunction with DL, although most practitioners opt for stand-alone use. A number of different techniques have been described. A jaw lift or thrust should be performed to enlarge the hypopharyngeal space[11] by elevating the tongue and epiglottis away from the posterior pharyngeal wall; indeed, a combination of jaw and tongue pull has been described.[12] The jaw thrust may also be beneficial by expanding the laryngeal aperture.[13] Following suctioning, the stylet/tube assembly can then be inserted from the side of the mouth (i.e., advanced over or behind the molars) and slowly rotated upright and toward the midline during advancement,[12] or alternatively, it can be primarily inserted in a midline location. With a midline approach, the uvula and epiglottis should be identified through the eyepiece or on the video monitor to help orientation to the

location of the tip of the device. Once at the laryngeal aperture, the tube can be advanced off the stylet through the cords.

Description has also been made of optical stylet use in conjunction with DL. Faced, for example, with a persistent Cormack/Lehane (C/L) Grade 3 (epiglottis only) view at DL, a fiberoptic stylet loaded with an ETT can be carefully placed beneath the epiglottis under direct vision. With the ETT tip under but no more than 0.5 cm beyond the tip of the epiglottis, the vocal cords should be immediately visible through the eyepiece, facilitating advancement of the ETT up to and through the cords. If stand-alone use has failed, some practitioners elect to use the direct laryngoscope to help control the tongue.[12,14,15] Most (but not all) authors agree that ETT tube advancement should occur with the fiberoptic stylet remaining outside the cords.

9.2.5   Clinical experience

9.2.5.1   What Is the Learning Curve for Fiberoptic Stylet Use?

Fiberoptic stylets are generally easier to use in manikins than in anesthetized humans. Unlike manikins, patients under anesthesia must have the oro- and hypopharynx opened to permit endoscopic navigation to the laryngeal opening. As previously indicated, this can be done with a jaw lift/thrust, tongue pull, or use of a direct laryngoscope.[12] In addition, meticulous attention to scope and patient preparation (by antifogging and suctioning, respectively) will help to avoid disappointment, as will a good appreciation of upper airway anatomy—in the pharynx, the tip of the fiberoptic stylet should be kept anterior, at the level of the laryngeal inlet, and not allowed to sink posteriorly toward the esophagus. One study using the Bonfils suggests that proficiency is attained after 20–25 intubations.[16] Other published reports of experience with fiberoptic stylets detail most of the failures at the beginning of their respective series (i.e., within the first 10 uses).[12,14]

9.2.5.2   How Effective Are Fiberoptic Stylets for Intubation of the Patient with a Difficult Airway?

Pfitzner and colleagues[17] reported on the successful use of the SOS in a series of seven children with anticipated difficult laryngoscopic intubations. Six of seven patients had confirmed C/L Grade 3 views at DL. Tracheal intubation was successful in all six patients at the first attempt using the SOS, in most cases by practitioners using the scope for the first time. Single case reports have documented successful tracheal intubation with an FSS of a patient with mouth opening limited to 1.5 cm[18] and another in whom neck movement was contraindicated.[19]

In addition to these clinical reports, other prospective studies have evaluated the efficacy and safety of these devices. Using the Bonfils stylet, Rudolph in 1996 reported on a series of 107 patients, of whom 18 presented C/L Grade 3 or 4 views at DL. Tracheal intubation was successful in 16 of 18 cases with the Bonfils, including all four C/L Grade 4 cases. Twenty-one percent of the total series required concomitant use of DL.[15] Shikani, in his initial study of the SOS,[14] looked at 120 patients, 74 of them children, including 7 patients with C/L Grade 3 or 4 views (although graded through the scope, not at DL). The Trachea of all patients in the series, including 5 awake patients, were successfully intubated with the scope, 88% on the first attempt. Five of the 7 C/L Grade 3 and 4 patients required concomitant use of DL. Bein et al.[20] studied the use of the Bonfils in 80 patients with predictors of difficult DL, comparing it to LMA Fastrach™ use. Thirty-nine of 40 patients randomized to Bonfils use were intubated on the first attempt, in a median time of 40 seconds, in contrast to a 70% first attempt success rate for the LMA Fastrach™. A second study looked at Bonfils use after failed DL. In 25 patients recruited following two failed DL attempts, 88% were successfully intubated with the Bonfils at the first attempt, and all but one (96%) by the second attempt, in a median time of 47.5 seconds.[11]

9.2.5.3 How Effective Are Fiberoptic Stylets for Tracheal Intubation in the Simulated Difficult Airway?

Humphries et al. compared use of the SOS to DL with Macintosh or Miller blades in a manikin study. Even with various difficult airway features activated, no difference was appreciated in early acquired skills with the SOS.[21] Evans and coworkers compared the SOS to the bougie in a manikin study with a fixed C/L Grade 3 view. In this model, the SOS permitted significantly faster intubation times than did the bougie and significantly fewer esophageal intubations.[22]

Two studies have been reported using the VOIS in a manikin with a fixed C/L Grade 3 laryngoscopic view. The first study, comparing VOIS use to DL with a conventionally styletted ETT, found that VOIS intubation took twice as long, but resulted in fewer esophageal or endobronchial intubations, and was rated easier.[23] The second study, also with fixed C/L Grade 3 views, compared the VOIS with the Bullard laryngoscope (BL) in the hands of inexperienced users.[24] The VOIS was associated with fewer failed intubations than the BL (8 vs. 41 of 800 intubations), with fewer esophageal intubations (1 vs. 21) and was also rated less difficult to use. The VOIS has also been evaluated in 50 pediatric patients in whom a C/L Grade 3 view had been simulated by suboptimal DL: tracheal intubation was successful in 92% (46/50) of patients within 60 seconds.[25]

9.2.5.4 What Is the Role of the Fiberoptic Stylet for Intubation of the Patient with Known or Possible Cervical Spine Instability?

Kihara and colleagues[26] compared the FSS to DL with a conventionally styletted tube in 193 elective surgical patients with applied manual in-line neck stabilization. Of the 65% of patients thus rendered Grade 3, intubation using the FSS was successful more frequently (98.5 vs. 87%) and with fewer attempts than that using DL. Kitamura and colleagues,[10] studying a series of 32 patients with head and neck in the neutral position and electively revealing only a C/L Grade 3 view with gentle laryngoscopy, achieved a 94% first attempt success rate using the FSS, in a mean time of 29 seconds. A third study compared the use of Macintosh blade DL with Bonfils stylet, BL, or Fastrach™ (ILMA) aided intubations in a series of elective surgical patients. Each of the Bonfils, Bullard, and LMA Fastrach™ resulted in significantly less cervical-spine (C-spine) movement than Macintosh blade facilitated intubation, although Bonfils and LMA Fastrach™ intubations took significantly longer than those using the Macintosh and Bullard blades.[27] Finally, Rudolph et al. studied upper C-spine movement with fluoroscopy

during laryngoscopy using the Bonfils and the Macintosh laryngoscope. Again, significantly less extension of the upper C-spine was found during Bonfils use.[28]

9.2.6 Fiberoptic stylets—other considerations

9.2.6.1 What Are the Potential Complications Associated with the Use of Fiberoptic Stylets?

To date, complications reported in the literature have been limited to failures to intubate; there have been no reports of airway trauma with any of the devices under discussion. In many cases, failure to intubate has resulted from a view being obscured by fog or secretions, a preventable complication. Fiberoptic stylets have been associated with a lower incidence of adverse hemodynamic response than DL.[29,30]

9.2.6.2 What Are the Potential Advantages of Fiberoptic Stylets?

As a class, fiberoptic stylets are portable and, relative to their flexible counterparts, less expensive and possibly more durable. Their rigidity may make them easier to navigate to the laryngeal inlet than flexible devices. Particularly if used in conjunction with DL, they may permit visualization of the glottic opening in situations in which DL permits only a C/L Grade 3 or 4 views. As outlined above, published studies and case series suggest a high rate of success in difficult situations. With the substantial reduction in price of newer fiberoptic stylets, and more future studies confirming a steep learning curve, fiberoptic capability may well be extended to out-of-OR locations such as emergency departments and intensive care units.

9.2.6.3 What Are the Disadvantages of Fiberoptic Stylets?

As indicated above, meticulous scope preparation is needed by performing an antifogging maneuver and ensuring the oropharynx has been suctioned prior to tracheal intubation. Some fiberoptic stylets require cutting of the ETT to a slightly shorter length. During tracheal intubation, orientation within the upper airway can be difficult, particularly when the fiberoptic stylet is used alone with a jaw lift. It is possible that the use of these fiberoptic stylets may be more successful in the hands of operators already experienced in the use of FFBs. However, to the practitioner inexperienced in fiberoptic device use, fiberoptic stylets still hold promise used as an adjunct to DL.

Fiberoptic stylets can be quite expensive, although the cost varies substantially. At the time of writing, the Bonfils costs $5500 without the camera control unit, the SOS (each of the adult and pediatric versions) costs $2495, and the Levitan FPS Scope costs $1295.

9.2.6.4 How Are Fiberoptic Stylets Disinfected?[†]

Most of the fiberoptic stylets can be cleaned in similar fashion to FFBs (see Section 8.3.2), although individual recommendations should be sought from the manufacturer. After use, the stylet shaft

---

[†] Please consult with the manufacturer for detailed cleaning instructions.

should be washed with a detergent solution, while those stylets with a hollow working channel should have it cleaned with a brush supplied for the purpose. Most can be sterilized with ETO, Steris® or Sterrad® systems, or have high-level disinfection applied by cold-soak solutions (e.g., Cidex).

9.3 RIGID FIBEROPTIC LARYNGOSCOPES

9.3.1 What are rigid fiberoptic laryngoscopes?

These devices have in common a fiberoptic bundle and viewing channel within a rigid exoskeleton. The fibers are thereby protected from damage, making these devices more robust. Eliminating the angulation controller found on flexible scopes decreases their complexity, making rigid devices less expensive, but also rendering them less versatile. Rigid fiberoptic laryngoscopes are designed only to view the larynx and observe the insertion and advancement (or removal and exchange) of an ETT; they are not intended for positioning of the tip of endobronchial tubes, performing endoscopy through the nose or a tracheotomy or viewing the trachea or the bronchi.

During DL using a laryngoscope, the view of the glottis is frequently obscured by the ETT. This is particularly true with the straight blade laryngoscope. During intubation using an FFB, typically the scope is advanced into the distal trachea under indirect vision, after which the ETT is advanced blindly over the scope into the trachea. The flexible scope essentially functions in this setting as a tracheal introducer (e.g., Eschmann Introducer). In contrast, the viewing element of the rigid fiberoptic laryngoscope is placed distally on the blade and to the side, providing an unobstructed view of the ETT as it advances through the larynx. This offers a superior degree of control, potentially reducing the danger of laryngeal injury caused by blind tube advancement.

The BL, UpsherScope (UL) and WS have been available for at least a decade. Although clearly these devices have their champions, and despite their apparent utility in a wide variety of challenging settings, they do not enjoy widespread popularity.[31–33]

9.3.2 Specific devices

9.3.2.1 Bullard and Bullard Elite (Circon) Laryngoscopes (BL)

9.3.2.1.1 What Are the Characteristics of the BL?

The BL is an indirect rigid fiberoptic laryngoscope, developed by Roger Bullard and manufactured by ACMI Corporation of Norwalk, Ohio. It is available in adult, pediatric, and neonatal sizes (Figure 9-7). The blade is anatomically shaped and has three channels: a 3.7-mm working channel, a light bundle, and an image bundle all close to the distal tip. The image bundle has 9500 pixels, producing an adequate though lower image resolution than other devices in its class. The unit is reasonably compact when field illumination is provided by an incandescent bulb powered by a battery handle. An external halogen light source and a fiberoptic bundle provide more intense illumination and is better suited if a video camera is utilized. The work-

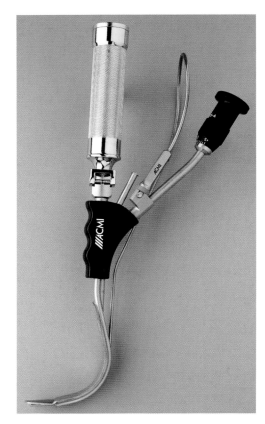

FIGURE 9-7. The Adult Bullard Elite™ Laryngoscope is shown with the dedicated stylet and battery handle. Note how the stylet is tucked tightly beneath the 6-mm spatula-like blade. An external fiberoptic light source is advised when a video camera is attached to the eyepiece. The working channel can be seen between the battery handle and the stylet. This can accommodate a suction catheter, oxygen or an epidural catheter to apply topical anesthesia. (*Reproduced with permission from ACMI.*)

ing channel can be used for oxygen insufflation, suction, or the application of topical anesthesia using an epidural catheter. The eyepiece on the BL Elite has an integrated knob for diopter adjustment. The eyepiece on both the BL and BL Elite can be connected to a standard 35-mm video attachment allowing the image to be displayed on a large video monitor. This facilitates teaching and permits the airway images to be digitally stored.

The blade design resembles a spatula having a thickness of only 6.0 mm, allowing excellent glottic visualization even when mouth opening is very limited and cervical movement is restricted. The ETT can be introduced freehanded with a malleable stylet or with one of two types of dedicated stylets:

1. *Bullard intubating stylet.* This stylet anchors directly to the BL and fits snugly against the posterior and inferior aspect of the BL blade. It is recommended that its tip be passed through the Murphy eye. Alternatively, the ETT can be rotated 180 degrees to reduce contact with the right arytenoids during tube passage.

2. *Straight-tipped "multi-functional stylet."* This stylet also attaches to the BL and fits against its inferior aspect. In contrast to the intubating stylet, it is longer, straight at its distal end, and tubular in order to accommodate an intubation catheter over which the ETT is advanced.

A plastic blade extender can be attached to the distal tip of the laryngoscope for additional length. One of the authors uses the blade extender only when the patient's size would require a larger size conventional laryngoscope blade (e.g., Macintosh #4).

9.3.2.1.2   How Is the BL Used?

To facilitate tracheal intubation using the BL, we suggest the following steps:

- Minimize secretions of the upper airway by using an antisialagogue prior to intubation.

- Prepare the device with an antifogging spray or warm water immersion.

- Prepare freehanded, dedicated Bullard intubating stylet or multifunctional stylet with lubricant and appropriately sized ETT.

- Place the head and neck of the patient in neutral position.

- Topical airway anesthesia should be used if laryngoscopy is to be done awake. This can be achieved by applying topical anesthesia to the tongue to suppress the gag reflex, lidocaine or EMLA ointment to the BL and advancing an epidural catheter through the working channel. The epidural catheter is attached to a syringe containing local anesthetic. This allows topical airway anesthesia to be applied under visual control.

- The blade is inserted by rotation behind and around the tongue. With the scope handle now vertical, the blade is allowed to gently drop against the posterior pharyngeal wall, and then advanced in a caudad direction before lifting it vertically so that the viewing channel is directly pointing at the glottic opening. A jaw lift will often elevate the epiglottis and create additional working space between the epiglottis and the posterior pharyngeal wall.

- When using either of the attached stylets, it is essential to grasp the stylet/ETT together with the handle such that they remain closely applied to the inferior aspect of the blade. This in turn will keep the tip of the stylet visible through the eyepiece.

- A clear view of the larynx should be obtained prior to advancing the ETT. If the dedicated wire stylet is used, it should be pointed toward the left arytenoid cartilage. As the practitioner begins to advance the ETT, subtle adjustments of the scope are still possible, but if the tube fails to enter the glottis, it is often necessary to withdraw the scope and reload the ETT.

- If the multifunctional stylet is used, ETT advancement can be preceded by passage of an intubation catheter through the hollow lumen of the stylet.

- Use of a "freehand" technique involves advancing an ETT off a well-lubricated stylet bent at an acute angle corresponding to that of the BL blade (90 degrees). To reduce the risk of "hang up" against the anterior tracheal wall, Hung et al. have suggested reverse loading of the tracheal tube onto the stylet.[34]

- After intubation, the BL should be removed from the patient by forward rotation of the scope out of the patient's mouth.

9.3.2.1.3   How Effective Is the BL for Tracheal Intubation in Patients with a History of Difficult Laryngoscopy?

MacQuarrie and coworkers compared the BL using a freehanded stylet and the dedicated multifunctional stylet in 80 adult patients lacking anatomical features predictive of a difficult laryngoscopy. A cervical collar was applied to simulate a difficult airway.[35] This resulted in a C/L Grade 3 view in 65% of their patients when DL was performed using a Macintosh #3 blade. BL intubation however was unsuccessful in 12/80 patients (15%). Fogging or secretions were responsible for half of these failures. The cervical collar reduced mouth opening to 2.3 and 2.6 cm in the two groups making it difficult to manipulate the ETT. There was no significant difference between the two different stylets with respect to the number of attempts required, success rate, trauma, or time to tracheal intubation (TTI). Nasal tube insertion might have overcome the problems encountered in the patients in whom mouth opening did not permit manipulation of the ETT.

Use of the BL has been advocated in a wide variety of conditions associated with difficult or failed DL including microstomia, micrognathism, Pierre Robin syndrome, and morbid obesity. These and other case reports have suggested that the BL may be useful in a variety of difficult airway situations.[36–38]

Comparing the BL with the FFB in awake patients with cervical spine disease, the BL provided a better laryngeal view in less time.[39] Hastings and coworkers compared head and C-spine movement and the laryngeal views obtained with the BL, Macintosh, and Miller laryngoscopes in 35 unrestrained adult patients with normal C-spine anatomy. Each patient underwent three laryngoscopies. Compared with DL, the BL resulted in a comparable or superior glottic view, with DL failing to visualize the larynx in 10% of cases. Less head and cervical extension was required for BL.[40] On the other hand, Watts et al. found that simulating emergency conditions by applying in-line stabilization and cricoid pressure resulted in longer intubation times using the BL compared with Macintosh DL.[41]

Insertion of a double lumen tube in a patient with a difficult airway may be difficult since the tube is both larger requiring more pharyngeal space and longer with a complex preformed shape, which makes manipulation more difficult. The reduced inner diameter may not be compatible with available flexible fiberoptic scopes. Shulman and Connelly used the BL in 29 consecutive adult patients requiring lung separation.[42] This resulted in a C/L Grade 1 view in all patients and tracheal intubation was successful in 28 with a time to intubation of 28 ± 10 (14–55) seconds. Tracheal intubation was unsuccessful in the remaining patients who also had a failed intubation under DL owing to the selection of too large a double-lumen tube (DLT). (Two other patients had a failed DL but their tracheas were successfully intubated by BL.) Seven patients, however, had to have their DLTs exchanged because of a torn cuff (one patient) or inadequate size (six patients). This study was conducted using the standard dedicated stylet rather than the multifunctional stylet. The latter has greater length and will permit the use of a larger sized DLT.

9.3.2.1.4   What Is the Role of the BL for Unanticipated Difficult Laryngoscopy for Patients with Lingual Tonsillar Hypertrophy?

Though its prevalence is unknown, lingual tonsillar hypertrophy (LTH) may be responsible for some situations in which despite a careful preoperative airway evaluation, a patient proves to be difficult or impossible to ventilate by mask or intubate by DL.[43] These patients may truly challenge our airway management skills. Even in the most expert hands, an LMA is not always successful in achieving adequate ventilation. Intubation by FFB may also be difficult.[43] Crosby and Skene described a patient who on a previous occasion had been found to have LTH following an unexpected failed DL.

On subsequent presentation to the operating room, Bullard laryngoscopy was performed and intubation was achieved using glycopyrrolate, topical anesthesia, and sedation.[44] When using a BL in the patient with LTH, the practitioner may have difficulty elevating the epiglottis, particularly if the tonsillar tissue is markedly enlarged or when using the dedicated stylet.

9.3.2.1.5   What Is the Learning Curve of the BL?

Shulman and colleagues tested their impression that BL trainees acquire skill faster if their initial instruction is done with a video system rather than direct viewing through the eyepiece. They found that the use of a video system did in fact reduce the laryngoscopy time and improved success; however, the benefits were not discernible after 15 intubations.[45] They demonstrated significant skill acquisition after 5 laryngoscopies in the video group and after 10 in the standard (eyepiece) group.

9.3.2.1.6   What Are the Advantages of the BL?

As indicated above, all of the rigid fiberoptic and video laryngoscopes allow visually controlled ETT insertion and advancement. Compared with the blind approach employed with the FFB, this may be less stimulating and could avoid arytenoid or vocal fold injury.[46]

One distinctive advantage of the BL is its flat spatula-like blade, permitting insertion and laryngoscopy even when mouth opening is very limited. Even with an inter-incisor distance of 6.0 mm, it may be possible to perform laryngoscopy, although in this instance there would likely be insufficient space to allow oral insertion of an ET tube. Nasal intubation could, however, still be achieved.

Although none of the abovementioned stylets are appropriate when intubating nasally, some directional control can be achieved using an Endotrol® ETT (Mallinckrodt, Pleasanton, CA) or a Parker Flex-It™ stylet (Parker Medical, Englewood, CO). An alternative approach is to elevate the head or depress the larynx to influence the position of the ETT relative to the larynx in the anterior–posterior position and to apply torque to rotate the ETT from side to side. The relatively flat spatula-like blade also makes it relatively easy to pass the BL beneath the epiglottis, thereby exposing the glottic aperture. When this is difficult, pulling the mandible (or tongue) forward may elevate the epiglottis and facilitate passage of the BL.

The width and depth of the visual field enables the practitioner to easily discern anatomical landmarks. This is helpful, particularly in settings in which the structures may be altered by disease. Establishing reference landmarks, remaining in the midline, and advancing the BL toward a patent lumen will increase the likelihood of success. The working channel of the BL is a useful conduit for oxygen, suction or topical anesthesia, all under visual control. The latter is best accomplished by advancing an epidural catheter through the working channel.

9.3.2.1.7   What Are the Disadvantages of the BL?

Like many of the rigid fiberoptic scopes, secretions,[35] fogging,[35] elevation of the epiglottis, and difficulty directing or advancing the ETT[35,37,47] through the vocal folds are the major obstacles to success.[47] Secretions can be dealt with using a Yankauer sucker or by attaching suction to the working channel. Fogging can be reduced by warming, or applying an antifogging agent to the optical bundle immediately prior to use. In addition, use of the working channel to insufflate oxygen (2.0–4.0 L·min^{-1}) may also reduce fogging and the effect of secretions on the view. Elevation of the epiglottis can

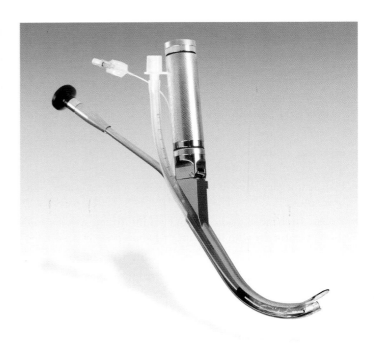

FIGURE 9-8. The Upsherscope Ultra™ is shown with a battery handle and an endotracheal tube residing in the tube slot. An external fiberoptic light source is advised when a video camera is attached to the eyepiece. Supplemental oxygen can be introduced through the endotracheal tube. (*Reproduced with permission from Mercury Medical.*)

frequently be further assisted by performing a mandibular thrust or pulling the tongue forward. If the operator chooses to use a video attachment, an external fiberoptic light source is also recommended, although this entire assembly becomes rather bulky.

Another disadvantage of the BL is the cost of the device. The BL Elite adult and pediatric models sell for $5500 and $5700, respectively. The multifunctional and dedicated stylets are $600 and $400. The cost of the fiberoptic adapter, necessary if the device is to be connected to an external light source, is $495.

9.3.2.1.8   How Should the BL Be Disinfected?[‡]

After removing the light source (bulb or fiberoptic adapter) and blade extender (if used), the device and the working channel should be washed, brushed, and flushed with soap and water. The Bullard Elite can be disinfected with ETO or immersed in a high-level disinfectant.

9.3.2.2   UpsherScope (UL)

9.3.2.2   Discuss the Characteristics of the UL

This rigid fiberoptic laryngoscope was developed by Michael Upsher and is manufactured by Mercury Medical (Clearwater, FL). It is available only in an adult size. It consists of a J-shaped blade with an incorporated C-shaped channel or "tube guide" through which an ETT, up to 8.5-mm ID in size, may be advanced (Figure 9-8). Light and image bundles run along the left side of the device. The light bundle may be connected either to a battery handle or an external halogen source. The image is conveyed to an eyepiece for direct viewing with a built-in focusing ring. Alternatively, the device can be fitted with a video camera system for display on a remote

---

[‡]Please consult with the manufacturer for detailed cleaning instructions.

monitor. An external light source is recommended if a video camera is used. Unlike the BL, there is neither a working channel nor a dedicated stylet.

An antisialagogue should be administered and the UL should be warmed or the image bundle should be sprayed with antifogging fluid. A lubricated ETT is introduced into the tube guide and advanced until the tip of the ETT can be seen through the eyepiece. Oxygen insufflation and suctioning may be achieved via the ETT.

Like the BL, the device is introduced in the midline and rotated around the tongue. In so doing, the handle of the device progresses from a horizontal to a vertical plane. A mandibular lift will help create space in the oropharynx and elevate the epiglottis. The blade of the UL should pass posterior to the epiglottis. Even when the larynx is well seen, it may be difficult to pick up the epiglottis or direct the ETT into the glottis. A coudé-tipped suction catheter, an Eschmann Introducer (gum-elastic bougie), or Frova Intubating Catheter (Cook Critical Care, Bloomington, IN) inserted through the ETT may be helpful.[48] This is advanced beyond the vocal folds and the ETT is railroaded over it. Following successful endotracheal intubation, the ETT is held securely and the device is rotated in the reverse direction, extracting the tube from the tube guide.

9.3.2.2.2 What Is the Clinical Experience of the UL?

Although simpler in design than the BL, published clinical experience using the UL has been disappointing. Pearce et al. used the UL successfully in 191 of 200 (95%) adults with an average intubation time of 38 seconds, though its use was considered straightforward in fewer than half the patients.[49] Fridrich et al. randomized 300 elective surgical adult patients requiring tracheal intubation using either the UL or DL. The UL was successful in 87% compared with DL (97%). UL success was achieved in 50 ± 41 seconds compared to 23 ± 13 seconds with DL. They identified no advantages of the UL over DL in routine or difficult airway management.[50] Others report a similar experience.[51–53] Using an in vitro model, Yeo and coworkers found that the tube guide directed the ETT downward and to the right of its intended target but use of an Eschmann Tracheal Introducer increased the success of tube placement in 53 of 56 patients.[53] Secretions, fogging, difficulty elevating the epiglottis, and misalignment of the tube guide were common problems.

Recently, the manufacturer has modified the original UL. This device, known as the UpsherScope Ultra™, has an increased fiberoptic bundle density (30,000 pixels) and an extended flange to the tube guide inferiorly. When this extension is aligned with the arytenoid cartilages, improved directional control of the ETT during advancement is allegedly achieved. Although users have reported its significantly improved performance, there are no published clinical reports (M.D. Carin Hagberg, personal communication, December 2004).

9.3.2.2.3 What Are the Advantages and Disadvantages of the UL?

It is simple in its design and operation. It is compact, and easily cleaned. The fiberoptic bundle provides a high-resolution image. It is reasonably priced and the Upsherscope Ultra™ with battery handle sells for $5275. An Upsherscope Ultra™ with a power handle, enabling connection to an external light source costs $5800. There is no need for specialized stylets.

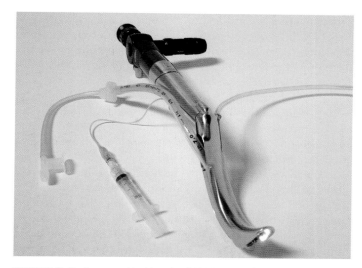

FIGURE 9-9. An assembled bivalved WuScope™ laryngoscope is shown with an attached battery-powered flexible fiberoptic bronchoscope, an endotracheal tube, and a suction catheter within the ETT. Intubation usually involves the passage of the suction catheter into the glottis and railroading of the ETT over the former. Oxygen is shown connected to a nipple on the right side of the device. (*Reproduced with permission from Achi Corporation.*)

The UL, like all fiberoptic laryngoscopes, is subject to the same challenges presented by secretions, fogging, and control of the epiglottis. The tube guide potentially provides for easier ETT advancement, compared with the BL, but it also increases its vertical profile. In addition, since the blade is narrower and more rounded than that of the BL, greater difficulty may occur in controlling the tongue, or elevating the mandible and epiglottis. Although simple in design, the original version did not perform well in tracheal intubation. The redesigned Upsherscope Ultra™ apparently corrects the misalignment of the ETT and the glottis. However, there are no peer-reviewed publications establishing improved performance.

9.3.2.2.4 How Should the UL be Disinfected?[§]

The manufacturer recommends that the Upsherscope Ultra™ be first cleaned with a mild soap solution and rinsed well with clean water. High-level disinfection or sterilization can then be performed with 2% glutaraldehyde, Steris®, or ETO (at <60°C, 25 PSI). The power handle is disinfected with 2% glutaraldehyde or wiped with 70% isopropyl alcohol or accelerated hydrogen peroxide.

9.3.2.3 WuScope (WS) System™

9.3.2.3.1 What Are the Characteristics of the WS and How Is It Used?

The WS, developed by Hsiu-chin Chou and Tzu-lang Wu (Achi Corporation, San Jose, CA) is available in two adult sizes.[54,55] It consists of two semicircular rigid blades that articulate, creating a tubular space to accommodate the ETT. A handle-to-blade angle of 110 degrees minimizes the need for head extension, tongue lifting, or physical alignment of the airway axes (Figure 9-9). A customized flexible fiberoptic scope is mounted atop the rigid blades and its

---

§ Please consult with the manufacturer for detailed cleaning instructions.

insertion cord is secured within a channel. (The dedicated Achi FA-10WUBS is a battery-operated nasopharyngoscope lacking an angulation controller. These modifications reduce the complexity and cost of the fiberoptic scope.) Like the BL and UL, a video camera can be attached to the eyepiece, allowing the image to be remotely displayed and/or recorded.

The patient may be awake or anesthetized and paralyzed as clinical circumstances dictate. The patient should be prepared with an antisialogogue and the fiberoptic scope should be warmed and/or pretreated with an antifog spray. The proper size WS blades are selected and the main blade is inserted into the handle. (If the smaller adult blades are used, a "blade extender" is required to ensure that the FFB does not protrude beyond the blades.) The fiberoptic scope is then secured within the main blade and the second blade is attached and locked into place. A lubricated ETT is introduced into the tubular space created by the two articulated blades and a suction catheter or other intubation guide (e.g., the Eschmann [Smith Medical] or Frova Intubating Introducer [Cook Critical Care]) is introduced into the ETT. It is prudent to confirm the integrity of the cuff after insertion into the tubular channel since it can become damaged during passage between the two blades. Oxygen can be administered via a nipple. This assembly and disassembly are somewhat complex and should be well rehearsed prior to clinical use.

If possible, the patient's head and neck are placed in a neutral position. The WS is introduced into the midline and rotated around the tongue. Elevation of the tongue with a tongue depressor or a jaw lift may prove helpful. As the WS is rotated, the uvula and the epiglottis come into view. Usually, the WS is advanced into the vallecula, although the epiglottis can be lifted if the view of the laryngeal inlet is obscured. The WS is aligned with the vocal folds, whereupon the suction catheter or intubation guide is advanced into the glottis. The ETT is then advanced over the guide under visual control. The bivalved blade is unlocked and removed. After securing the ETT, the main blade is disengaged from the ETT and is rotated out of the mouth.

The WS can also be used for nasotracheal intubations. In this case, the ETT is introduced through the nares into the oropharynx. Only the main blade and the dedicated fiberoptic scope are used. The assembly is introduced into the oropharynx and enables the practitioner to observe the advancement of the nasotracheal tube, as can be done with the BL.

9.3.2.3.2   Discuss the Clinical Experience of the WS

The developers described WS intubations in settings in which DL had proven unsuccessful. Anatomical features such as a receding jaw, limited temporomandibular joint mobility, a small atlanto-occipital gap, and a short mandibular ramus did not interfere with success.[54] Despite limited prior experience, Smith and coworkers enjoyed success in 45 patients with normal airways and 24 with factors predictive of difficulty had DL been used. Ideal intubating conditions (intubation difficulty score = 0) existed in 38/45 (84%) of patients without and 17/24 (71%) with predictors of difficulty.[56] The mean TTI was 50 and 31 seconds in patients with and without predictors of difficulty. A C/L Grade 1 view was obtained in 97% of the patients.

Smith and coworkers randomized 87 patients with normal airways to laryngoscopy with a Macintosh blade or WS while in-line cervical stabilization was applied.[57] There was no difference in successful tracheal intubation between the groups; however, optimal conditions were achieved in 18% of the DL versus 79% of the WS groups. More

patients had C/L Grade 3 and 4 views with DL compared with WS (39% vs. 2%); however, when only one attempt was required for DL, intubation was achieved more quickly. They concluded that the WS was associated with lower intubation difficulty scores compared with DL when cervical immobilization was applied.

Sprung et al. presented two very complex cases in which intubation could not be achieved by DL.[58] The first involved a morbidly obese patient who developed an expanding hematoma several days following a carotid endarterectomy. Failure to intubate or ventilate led to asystole shortly after a cricothyrotomy was performed. Following resuscitation, WS laryngoscopy and intubation were accomplished with minimal difficulty. Their second patient had laryngeal papillomatosis. Two previous attempts at intubation, the first by DL and the second with an FFB, were traumatic. While the FFB could be introduced into the trachea, passage of the ETT resulted in bleeding and necessitated an emergency surgical airway. On the third presentation, awake WS laryngoscopy and intubation were achieved atraumatically.

The WS has been used to perform visually guided exchange of ETTs, including nasal to oral conversion[59] and replacement of a damaged ETT in a patient with a difficult airway who was unable to tolerate interruption of ventilation.[60]

Smith and Kareti described the use of the WS in two patients in whom tracheal intubation using a conventional and Heine Corazzelli-London articulated laryngoscope (curved blade with a distal articulating tip) was unsuccessful or resulted in rupture of a cuff of a double-lumen tube. They were able to intubate the trachea of these patients using the larger size WS and a 35-F DLT.[61] This solution is not ideal since most patients who are able to accommodate the large WS blade will require a larger sized DLT.

Successful use of the WS was described in two patients with a difficult airway secondary to lingual tonsillar hypertrophy (LTH).[62] The first patient was morbidly obese and had a Mallampati III oropharyngeal view. Following the induction of anesthesia and muscle relaxation, mask ventilation was difficult but WS laryngoscopy with oxygen insufflation and tracheal intubation was easily achieved. The diagnosis of LTH was later confirmed. The second patient was known to have LTH, obstructive sleep apnea, and a Mallampati III airway. WS laryngoscopy and nasal intubation were easily achieved and a tonsillectomy was performed.

9.3.2.3.3   How Easy Is It to Learn WS Use?

No formal studies have evaluated the time investment or the number of procedures required to acquire proficiency with the WS. Although the device has been available for approximately a decade and despite its apparent advantages and utility in a wide variety of challenging settings, it does not appear to enjoy widespread use.[32,33]

9.3.2.3.4   What Are the Advantages and Disadvantages of the WS?

The WS is the only device that creates a tubular space through which the ETT is advanced. This requires a larger oropharyngeal volume for insertion; however, if the WS can be accommodated, ETT advancement is more easily achieved. The use of a diagnostic quality FFB provides excellent image quality.

The articulated bitubular construction is relatively complex to assemble and disassemble. The operation of the WS is generally more complex than the other rigid fiberoptic scopes. It can also result in entrapment of or damage to the ETT cuff. The profile of the WS requires a mouth opening of >20–25 mm and may limit its

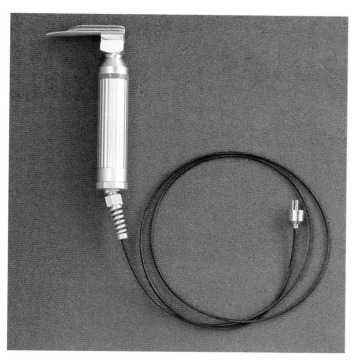

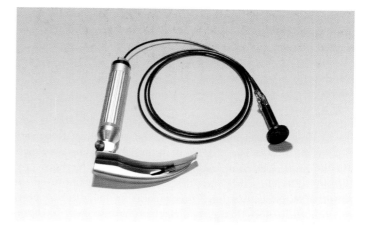

FIGURE 9-11. This shows an adult Acutronic Angulating Videointubating laryngoscope with a 25-degree anterior angulation of the distal tip. Note that the eyepiece can be viewed directly or connected to a video camera. (*Reproduced with permission from Dr. Markus Weiss.*)

FIGURE 9-10. A pediatric Acutronic Video Intubating laryngoscope is shown. Various blades are available. The image can be viewed on an external monitor. The video cable is attached to an external monitor. (*Reproduced with permission from Acutronic Medical Systems AG.*)

usefulness in patients with temporomandibular dysfunction. It incorporates a flexible fiberoptic scope that is protected by its placement within the WS; however, this increases the cost and the possibility of damage to the bundles during handling. Like the other scopes, it is subject to fogging and problems from oral secretions.

Another disadvantage of the WS is the substantial cost. The current price of the complete WS is $9700.** This includes the Wu-fiberscope with battery unit and both sizes of adult blades. A detachable light cable ($700) is desirable if the practitioner intends to connect the eyepiece to a video camera. This pricing represents a substantial reduction compared with earlier versions but this device remains one of the most costly.

9.3.2.4 What Is the Acutronic Fiberoptic Laryngoscope?

The Acutronic fiberoptic laryngoscope[6] (Acutronic Medical Systems, Switzerland), developed by Swiss pediatric anesthesiologist Marcus Weiss, consists of a modified Macintosh laryngoscope (sizes 2, 3, 4, and 5) with a fiberoptic bundle 3.9 mm in diameter and 200 cm in length (Figure 9-10). An eyepiece can be coupled to a video camera providing an image with 10,000 pixels. When approved for sale in North America, the estimated cost will be approximately $3400 for the laryngoscope and fiberoptic bundle.

9.3.2.5 What Is the Angulated Video-Intubation Laryngoscope (AVIL)?

The AVIL (Acutronic Medical Systems) is a modified plastic Macintosh laryngoscope (size #4), the distal 3.0 cm of which is

angulated upward about 25 degrees, resembling a McCoy (CLM; levering tip) blade (Figure 9-11). The vertical flange is also flattened, enabling it to be used in children. A thin fiberoptic bundle passes through the body of the laryngoscope, providing illumination and transmitting an image that can be viewed directly through an eyepiece or on a monitor via an attached video camera.

Use of the AVIL has been described in two children with Morquio's syndrome (hypoplasia of the odontoid process) in whom cervical extension posed a risk of spinal cord compression.[63] The device has been compared with the VOIS.[6,23,64] In this study, head extension of an intubation manikin was modified so that only a C/L Grade 3 view could be obtained by DL. Thirty endoscopists, previously unfamiliar with both devices, performed five intubations with each. Although the trachea was successfully intubated, in four early cases, AVIL intubation required multiple attempts and took longer than 60 seconds. Slightly less time was required for intubation using the VOIS (17.4 ± 6.8 seconds) compared with the AVIL (22.8 ± 13.4 seconds; $p = 0.027$), although greater improvement occurred with subsequent AVIL use compared to that with VOIS. Skill was easily achieved with both devices and they were highly rated by anesthesiologists and nurse anesthetists. The authors of this study concluded that both techniques were well suited to high-risk situations such as a rapid sequence induction with cervical immobilization or rescue of a failed conventional DL. Each device is estimated to cost €2000 (approximately US$2700) though this does not include the video camera, light source, or monitor.

9.3.2.6 What Is the Viewmax® or Truview®?

The Viewmax® or Truview® (Truphatek; North American Distributor: Rusch, Duluth, GA) is neither a rigid fiberoptic nor a video laryngoscope. It consists of an inexpensive proprietary lens inserted into the blade of a modified Macintosh laryngoscope. The lens refracts the viewing angle approximately 20 degrees anteriorly, allegedly improving the laryngeal view. The view is observed through a small eyepiece, though with a specialized adapter, it can be enlarged and displayed on a video monitor.

** All prices are in US dollars unless otherwise stated. All prices were accurate at the time of publication but may be subject to change.

The product is analogous to a modern Huffman prism. For a practitioner comfortable with DL, the Viewmax® requires no specialized training. It is available in two sizes, corresponding to Macintosh 2.5 for children and 3.5 for adults. The Viewmax® blade retails for approximately $150 and is compatible with any Green coded ISO laryngoscope handle.

If a video camera is to be used, a special adapter is required to fit its 22 mm eyepiece. When not used, the small eyepiece is similar to a camera's viewfinder, requiring the practitioner to be very close to the airway. The image is nonetheless small and only marginally improved compared with line-of-sight laryngoscopy, though the product brochures describe a consistent improvement of one C/L grade. We have been unable to identify any peer-reviewed evaluations though four abstracts have recently been presented. Compared with DL, these studies, using manikins and patients, generally describe a modestly improved laryngeal view despite a trend toward less force (not statistically significant), shorter time to obtain the optimal view, and slightly greater practitioner satisfaction.

The manufacturer does not expect this device to compete with more elaborate video laryngoscopy systems. Rather, it is conceived as an evolutionary product, attractively priced and similar enough to conventional laryngoscopy, which is accessible with virtually no additional training. It therefore competes with DL. A newer model, known as EVO II, has recently been released (Figure 9-12), at a higher price, designed to provide a view superior to the existing device. It incorporates an improved eyepiece and an optional

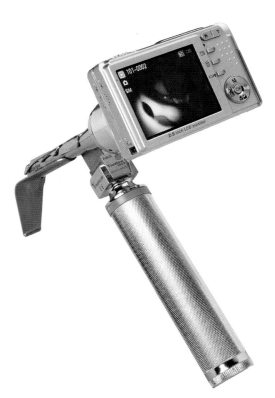

FIGURE 9-12. The new EVO video laryngoscope is shown connected to an optional, dedicated digital camera. The image is angulated upward approximately 45 degrees and enlarged on the camera's LCD. Alternatively, an existing operating room video camera can be attached to the eyepiece.

dedicated digital camera (David Grey, personal communication, June 2006).

After use, the view tube is rinsed in clean water and gently scrubbed in soapy water. The Viewmax® view tube and laryngoscope blade should be further disinfected by ETO, Steris®, or Sterrad® systems cold soaks.

9.4   RIGID VIDEO LARYNGOSCOPES

9.4.1   What are the characteristic features of rigid video laryngoscopes?

The rigid fiberoptic laryngoscopes convey their image along a bundle of glass fibers to an eyepiece. If the eyepiece is connected to a video camera, the benefits of video laryngoscopy are achieved, albeit with somewhat greater complexity. The fiberoptic stylets, BL, UL, WS, and Viewmax® can all be connected to a video camera in this way. As previously mentioned, video laryngoscopy can also be achieved using a conventional laryngoscope and an Airway Cam®. An integrated video laryngoscope incorporates a video camera into its design. This has been achieved in various ways. The Storz Video Macintosh is a hybrid, combining a distal fiberoptic bundle and a video camera within the handle. The GlideScope® dispenses with the fiberoptic bundle entirely, relying exclusively on video technology.

At the moment, there are two video laryngoscopes and both resemble curved blades of conventional laryngoscopes. It is expected that a practitioner with experience performing DL will find the operation of these devices easier than that of the rigid fiberoptic devices or FFBs, but comparative studies have not been conducted.

9.4.2   Video Macintosh (Storz)

9.4.2.1   Describe the Unique Features of the Video Macintosh

A standard Storz Macintosh laryngoscope was modified to accommodate a fiberoptic bundle that passes through a metal channel, terminating approximately 4.0 cm from the tip of the blade (Figure 9-13A). The bundle passes through the heel of the blade into the handle where the battery has been replaced with a concealed video camera. The video cable emerges from the proximal end of the handle, along with a power supply, and passes to a video cart housing a light source, video system, and video monitor (Figure 9-13B).[65] The Video Macintosh system (VMS) is used like a conventional laryngoscope. However, the ETT does not obscure the practitioner's view since its advancement is monitored on the video display. This enables the practitioner (and mentor) to have an identical view of the airway. Recently, the manufacturer has released three compatible blades, corresponding to a Macintosh #3, #4, and Dörges blades. A focusing wheel and programmable buttons have been added to the handle.

9.4.2.2   What Is the Clinical Utility of the VMS?

Kaplan and coworkers evaluated the VMS on 235 patients, 18 of whom had features suggesting a difficult conventional DL. In 22

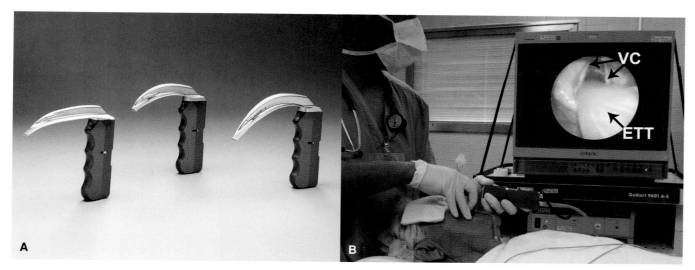

FIGURE 9-13. (A) This photograph shows three Storz blades attached to a Storz video laryngoscope handle. These blades, from left to right, are the Dorges Universal laryngoscope, a pediatric, and an adult Macintosh blade. The external light source and the video attachment are not shown. (*Reproduced with permission.*) (B) This photograph shows a Storz Video Macintosh laryngoscope connected to a proprietary video display. The vocal cords (VC) and the endotracheal tube (ETT) can be clearly visualized on the video monitor during tracheal intubation.

of the 217 (10%) patients in whom no difficulties were anticipated, external laryngeal manipulation (ELM) was required and the video system enabled the assistant to evaluate its effect making the appropriate adjustments. All but one of these intubations was successful. ELM was required in the patients predicted to be difficult and all these intubations were also successful.[65] They concluded that the VMS had a very short learning curve and provided a larger, brighter image that could be viewed by the practitioner and instructor. It was therefore a useful device for teaching. Unfortunately, they did not compare the laryngeal views with DL, making it difficult to determine whether this device provides a different view or simply a bigger, brighter one. While it is useful for an assistant to be able to make adjustments to the location, direction, and force of ELM, the need to apply it in 40/238 (17%) cases suggests that the VMS does not provide better glottic exposure in challenging airways. On the other hand, a recently reported abstract compared laryngeal views seen by direct viewing with those displayed on the VMS video monitor. In 308 anesthetized and paralyzed patients, the video display using VMS improved the laryngeal view by one or more grades in 72% of patients compared with direct viewing. The authors did state that ELM was required in 25% of their patients to improve the laryngeal view.[66] However, they did not indicate whether ELM was also applied when conventional DL yielded a suboptimal view.

This device appears to offer modest advantages in the management of the difficult airway though it may be the best system currently available for teaching laryngoscopy, since the technique is identical to DL and the laryngoscopist and mentor have very similar laryngeal views. Laryngoscopy can be recorded and replayed for feedback and the effects of either ELM or cricoid pressure can be assessed and modified as required.

9.4.2.3   What Are the Advantages and Disadvantages of the VMS?

The VMS results in a large, high resolution, and colored image. Since its operation is the same as DL and the laryngeal view is virtually identical to that seen by the laryngoscopist with the naked eye, it is very well suited to teaching DL. Laryngoscopy can be recorded as still or video images. These features are desirable for teaching, documenting, and research. As previously mentioned, it enables an assistant to make modifications to ELM to improve the laryngeal view.

The cost of the components is a significant deterrent for a device that may not improve laryngeal exposure. The VMS handle costs $8,000, while each blade costs $220.[††] A video system and cart are also required to power, illuminate, and display the image. The cost of this additional equipment, sold by Karl Storz, is $25,000, though it can also be used with the Storz flexible fiberoptic scope or Bonfils fiberoptic stylet. The VMS can be used with most xenon light sources; however, it requires a proprietary (Karl Storz) video camera to view the image.

9.4.2.4   How Is the VMS Disinfected?[‡‡]

The video laryngoscope can be disinfected with ETO, Steris® System1, Sterrad®, Cidex, and Cidex OPA. The camera head can be cleaned in all of the above with the exception of Cidex OPA.

9.4.3   Glidescope® video laryngoscope

9.4.3.1   What Are the Characteristics of the GlideScope® Video Laryngoscope?

The GlideScope® video laryngoscope (GVL) was developed by a Canadian surgeon, John A. Pacey (Saturn Biomedical Systems,[§§] Burnaby, British Columbia). It consists of a plastic modified Macintosh-type laryngoscope blade, the distal half of which is angled

---

[††] All prices are in US dollars unless otherwise stated. All prices were accurate at the time of publication but may be subject to change.

[‡‡] Please consult with the manufacturer for detailed cleaning instructions.

[§§] Richard Cooper is a consultant to and investor in Saturn Biomedical Systems, Burnaby, BC.

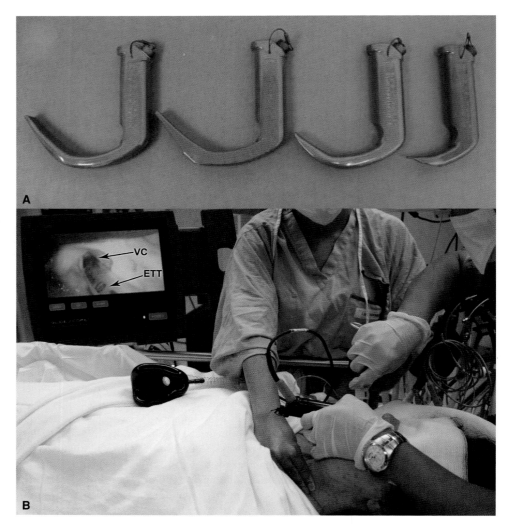

FIGURE 9-14. (A) This photograph shows four GlideScope® video laryngoscopes. From left to right, these are the new adult Lo-Pro (14.5 mm profile), the discontinued Classic (monochrome, 18 mm), the pediatric, and the neonatal models. The integrated power supply/video cable and proprietary LCD video display are not shown. (*Reproduced with permission from* Saturn Medical Systems) (B) This photograph shows a laryngoscopy being performed while the image is displayed on the dedicated GlideScope® 7′ LCD video monitor. During tracheal intubation, the vocal cords (VC) and the endotracheal tube (ETT) can be visualized on the video monitor.

this to 14.5 mm and provides a color image. Pediatric, neonatal, and battery-powered portable versions became available in 2005. The 18-mm black and white devices are no longer manufactured.

9.4.3.2 How Is the GVL Used?

The technique is similar to DL yet it differs in a few important respects. We recommend the following steps to facilitate tracheal intubation using the GVL:

- A malleable (or dedicated rigid) stylet is recommended since the larynx is not in the line-of-sight. Alternatively, a "dynamic stylet" such as the Parker Flex-it® (Parker Medical, Englewood, CO) can be used.

- Various stylet shapes have been described but Cooper et al. suggested that it resemble the distal aspect of the GlideScope® blade.[67,68]

- An antifogging solution is not required.

- Special positioning is not required.

- The laryngoscope should be introduced into the mouth in the midline and maintained in the midline as it is rotated around the tongue. Care should be taken to avoid injury to the lips and teeth during laryngoscope insertion. It is also necessary to insert the ETT with care to avoid patient injury or damage to the ETT cuff.

- The uvula, base of tongue, and epiglottis should be seen in succession to ensure proper midline orientation. The blade is preferentially introduced into the vallecula; however, if the epiglottis obscures the laryngeal view, the GVL can be used like a straight blade, picking up the epiglottis. It is important to introduce the laryngoscope blade under direct vision to ensure that the lips and teeth are not injured.

- If the ETT does not contact the teeth, the shape of the stylet should allow it to be directed anteriorly toward the larynx. Alternatively, the ETT can be introduced into the mouth prior to insertion of the GVL.

- Optimizing laryngeal exposure does not necessarily result in easier intubation. In fact, seeking optimal exposure can actually make intubation more difficult in two ways:

  ○ Rotation of the wrist producing a more vertical orientation of the handle tilts the laryngeal axis upward. This increases the angle of incidence created between the advancing ETT and the trachea, making intubation more difficult than it need be. The handle of the GVL should be oriented approximately 20 degrees from horizontal.

upward approximately 60 degrees (Figure 9-14A). The blade incorporates a charge coupled device (CCD, a miniature video chip) and light-emitting diodes that provide adjustable illumination and contrast. The video chip is covered by a heated glass window making it fog resistant. The video image is conveyed from the laryngoscope blade via a cable to a dedicated LCD video display. The image can be displayed or recorded on external devices (Figure 9-14B) using a standard video output cable (NTSC). The object seen on the monitor may be quite different from that in the line-of-sight. For example, with minimal lifting of the laryngoscope, the line-of-sight view may be limited to the uvula while complete laryngeal exposure is seen on the monitor. Cooper was involved in the development of this device and had extensive experience with it prior to its commercial release. The GVL has been commercially available since early 2002.

The original adult version required an inter-incisor gap of 18 mm. A new lower profile laryngoscope, released in 2005, reduces

○ When the GVL is too close to the larynx, there is less tolerance for lateral displacement of the ETT as it is advanced. It is not necessary to fully introduce the GVL; frequently it can be retracted providing a broader field of view and making ETT insertion easier.

• Occasionally, despite excellent laryngeal exposure the ETT cannot be directed through the glottis. After confirming that the angle of the GVL and depth of insertion (see above) are appropriate, external laryngeal pressure may "bring the glottis to the ETT" although this is rarely necessary. The shape of the stylet can also be altered. Alternatively, under visual control, a coudé-tipped Eschmann Tracheal Introducer can be introduced into the trachea following which the ETT is visually advanced over the bougie.

• Saturn Biomedical Systems makes a dedicated metal stylet that can be used to introduce the ETT. This has not undergone controlled clinical evaluation.

9.4.3.3   What Is the Clinical Utility of the GVL?

Sun and colleagues recently compared laryngeal exposure and TTI in 200 adult patients, randomized to GVL or DL using a #3 Macintosh blade.[69] All patients first underwent DL and the C/L view was scored. Subsequently, a second practitioner, unaware of the previous view, performed laryngoscopy and intubation. Among patients with a C/L Grade > 1, use of the GVL significantly improved the view in 68% of patients ($p < 0.001$). Of the 15 patients with C/L Grade 3, 8 and 6 were converted to Grade 1 and 2 views, respectively, when the GVL was used. TTI was longer in the GVL group (30 seconds for DL vs. 46 seconds for GVL); however, the time required increased as the laryngeal view deteriorated in the DL but not in the GVL group. There was no difference in the TTI between the two techniques in patients with C/L Grade 3. There was one failed intubation in the DL group (and the trachea of this patient was intubated after one attempt using the GVL). Multiple attempts were more frequently required in the DL group.

To date, the largest series reported the early experience of 133 users at five centers, involving 728 consecutive uses.[67] Use of the device was at the discretion of the anesthesiologist. Failure was defined as abandonment of the device in favor of an alternative. Since many of the practitioners had very limited or no prior experience and there was no formal training prior to its use, this abandonment may have occurred after a single attempt. The investigators found that C/L Grade 1 or 2 views were obtained in 92% and 7% of patients, respectively. A subset of these patients (133) underwent both DL and GVL. No laryngeal structures (C/L ≥ 3) could be seen by DL in 35 patients whereas GVL resulted in a C/L Grade 1 or 2 view in 77% of these patients. Intubation could not be achieved in 3.7% of the patients despite a C/L Grade 1 view in 14/26 of these patients. In contrast to DL, where intubation is frequently successful despite not seeing the larynx, the early experience with GVL showed that intubation occasionally failed *despite* good laryngeal exposure.[68] The authors believed that this reflected the additional skill of manipulating the ETT while viewing it on a monitor.[67]

The GVL has been used for both routine and complex airway management. As with the rigid fiberoptic scopes, it is speculated that not needing to deflect and compress the tongue, elevate the mandible, or apply force to the hyoepiglottic ligament might result in reduced hemodynamic stress associated with laryngoscopy using the GVL. This is currently under investigation.

9.4.3.4   How Effective Is the GVL for Tracheal Intubation in Patients with a Difficult Airway?

Agrò et al. simulated a difficult airway by applying a cervical collar to the necks of 15 surgical patients.[70] Each patient was subjected to both DL and GVL. The C/L view was improved by an average of one grade in 14 of 15 patients. One of 15 patients remained unchanged as a C/L Grade 3 but the trachea was intubated successfully using an Eschmann Tracheal Introducer under GVL visual control.

Turkstra et al. compared the GVL, Macintosh #3, and the Trachlight™ in 36 healthy adults with in-line cervical stabilization.[71] They evaluated tracheal intubation and assessed C-spine movement under fluoroscopy. Compared with DL, C-spine movement was reduced by 50% but only at the C2−5 segment. Elsewhere in the C-spine, there was no difference and GVL prolonged intubation time.

Cooper has described a patient at risk of regurgitation who could not be intubated by DL on repeated presentations. The patient had refused awake intubation using a flexible FOB. GVL was performed with a rapid sequence induction and successful intubation was achieved on the first attempt (within 15 seconds); the patient presented on two subsequent occasions with the same outcome.[72] The large series of consecutive uses, described above, included several patients in whom the GVL was used as a rescue device. At Cooper's institution, the GVL is frequently the first device selected to perform intubation when DL fails.[67]

Doyle described the use of the GVL in three morbidly obese patients and one with reduced mouth opening.[73] He elected to use the device in the first two patients because an FFB was unavailable. In the subsequent cases, the GVL became his device of choice. In all cases, laryngoscopy was performed on sedated patients, with topical airway anesthesia. He stated that this technique offered the following advantages: an excellent view unaffected by secretions or blood, provision for everyone to view the laryngoscopy and intubation, and events are readily recorded and the device is more robust and less susceptible to damage than the more delicate FFB. Finally, the passage of the ETT could be observed. The GVL has been described in a patient with ankylosing spondylitis.[74]

9.4.3.5   What Is the Learning Curve for the GVL?

Cooper and colleagues stated that novice laryngoscopists appeared just as capable of obtaining C/L 1 views as experienced practitioners[67] although they did not specifically study this. Unlike conventional DL, when video feedback can be provided, the learning experience is most likely to be of greater value. Thus, video laryngoscopes are likely to be associated with a faster, steeper learning curve when compared with DL. Using an intubation manikin, Chua and coworkers found that experienced laryngoscopists could complete intubation more quickly than inexperienced practitioners. Time to complete intubation improved between the first and second use of the GVL but subsequent improvements were not significant.[75] In demonstrating this device on a variety of manikins, Cooper has found that there are significant differences between intubation simulators, though these have not been systematically investigated. These differences not only pertain to the GVL but also to all the intubating devices discussed above. Though with any new airway device, manikin practice should precede clinical use, it is difficult to know how well this surrogate experience will translate into clinical practice. It also presents a problem in interpreting manikin-based studies.

9.4.3.6   What Is the Clinical Experience of the GVL?

The GVL has not been in widespread use long enough for its role to be properly defined. Enthusiastic early users advocate its purported advantages for routine and complex airway management. For routine airway management, like other video laryngoscope systems, it facilitates teaching and encourages the involvement of other personnel. This may enable them to anticipate problems and participate more effectively in their solution. If the GVL proves to require less force to achieve a laryngeal view, this in turn may reduce the stimulation and trauma associated with laryngoscopy.[76] If the GVL (or rigid fiberoptic and video laryngoscopes) results in a higher percentage of visualized intubations, this too will be advantageous. Like other video laryngoscopy systems, and in contrast to FFB, the introduction and advancement of the ETT through the glottis is performed under visual control. This may be less stressful and injurious to the patient, particularly if the procedure is performed without neuromuscular blockade. Studies have shown that FFB is associated with some difficulty advancing the ETT ranging from 0% to 90% and blind passage may occasionally be associated with significant complications.[77,78] Visualized tube insertion and advancement, particularly when muscle relaxants are avoided, offers at the very least a significant theoretical advantage.

Pediatric and neonatal devices are now available but experience is limited. In contrast to the original 18 mm GVL, the newer models have a 14.5 mm profile blade and this may extend the utility of this device, particularly when access to the oropharynx is reduced or tube size is increased (e.g., double-lumen tubes).

The use of a compact device with recording capabilities may be of value in the pre-hospital arena, emergency departments, and critical care units, particularly if skill can be easily acquired and maintained.[79] Ideally, video capture could be integrated with time annotation and possibly oximetry.

The role of the GVL in managing complex airway problems will likely be better defined in the coming years. It has been used to introduce double-lumen tubes in difficult airways, in patients with unstable or fused cervical spines, morbid obesity, limited mouth opening, failed DL, ETT exchanges, emergency obstetrical airways and patients in whom blood, secretions, fogging, or oxygen desaturation limit the practicality of more traditional methods. The GVL is enjoying limited use in emergency departments and intensive care units where significant airway challenges may be encountered and are often managed by "occasional endoscopists." Cooper has also found the GVL very useful in inserting difficult nasogastric tubes and transesophageal echocardiac probes.

9.4.3.7   What Are the Advantages and Disadvantages of the GVL?

The GVL is similar enough to DL that an experienced laryngoscopist can easily learn the technique. Even novice laryngoscopists have been able to obtain excellent glottic exposure. The device is relatively portable and requires virtually no setup time, making it useful in the unanticipated difficult airway. The portable version is even more suitable for use outside of the operating room. The GVL is very resistant to fogging. Secretions or blood in the oropharynx do not significantly interfere with visualization. The image is of very high resolution and contrast and brightness can be easily adjusted. The image can be exported to a larger (or smaller[80]) video display and/or recorded. It is constructed of an impact resistant medical grade plastic and there are no fragile fiberoptic bundles. It provides non line-of-sight laryngeal exposure even in circumstances where DL has proven unsuccessful. Like the other rigid fiberoptic and video laryngoscopes, it permits visualized control of ETT insertion and advancement.

Although laryngeal exposure was significantly improved compared with DL, more than half of the failed intubations occurred despite a C/L Grade 1 view.[67] Controlled ETT delivery and advancement requires a different set of skills that must be acquired. Krasser and colleagues have demonstrated prior training is associated with a better laryngeal view and more consistently successful endotracheal intubation compared with conventional DL.[81]

The GVL is more expensive than DL and many of the rigid fiberoptic devices; however, the cost includes the required proprietary LCD video display. The anterior angulation of the laryngoscope blade occasionally results in the handle impacting upon the patient's chest, particularly when cervical extension is reduced or the chest is prominent. The relatively high profile of the flange requires an inter-incisor distance of approximately 15 mm.

The GVL system includes a laryngoscope, monitor, connector and power cables, and a stand (or pole mount) and sells for $9,200.*** A battery-operated GVL and monitor packed in a rugged plastic Pelican™ case (mobile stand or pole mount) is also available. Additional GlideScope® video laryngoscopes in adult, pediatric, or neonatal configurations sell for $4,500.

9.4.3.8   How Is the GVL Disinfected?[†††]

Following tracheal intubation, the video/power cable should be detached from the laryngoscope, and the port be covered by a protective cap. The GVL should then be cleaned with a soapy solution to remove biological debris. The entire scope can then be disinfected by immersing in bleach, Cidex, Metricide, Steris®, or Sterrad® solutions.

9.5   SUMMARY

Traditionally, laryngoscopy has been dependent upon line-of-sight devices. Despite a variety of laryngoscope blades, it is not always possible to visualize the larynx despite our best efforts to anatomically align the axes of the mouth, pharynx, and larynx. Fiberoptic and video technology now make it feasible to look around those corners that are concealed from our line-of-sight. Traditional predictors of difficulty, developed for DL, may have limited relevance

---

*** All prices are in US dollars unless otherwise stated. All prices were accurate at the time of publication but may be subject to change.

[†††] Please consult with the manufacturer for detailed cleaning instructions.

to our success or failure with these alternative devices. This chapter has reviewed some of the specific devices now available.

Fiberoptic stylets (Bonfils Retromolar Intubation Fiberscope, Shikani Seeing Optical Stylet, Levitan FPS Scope, StyletScope, VOIS) require relatively limited space for insertion but provide a restricted visual field. Rigid fiberoptic laryngoscopes (Bullard Elite Laryngoscope, WS, Uspherscope Ultra™, Acutronic Fiberoptic Laryngoscope, Angulated Video-Intubation Laryngoscope, Truview®) and video laryngoscopes (VMS and GlideScope®) tend to provide a wider visual field and, space permitting, more readily identifiable anatomical identification. As the name suggests, the fiberoptic stylets are placed within the ETT and may be positioned at the laryngeal inlet or beyond, following which the ETT is advanced over the stylet. The fiberoptic and video laryngoscopes have a viewing channel adjacent to the ETT and remain outside the trachea. Advancement of the ETT toward and through the vocal folds is under visual control. The contrast between the latter technique and that of flexible fiberoptic- or video-bronchoscopic intubation is also worth emphasizing. The FFBs identify the larynx but ETT advancement is essentially a blind procedure.

This is a rapidly changing area with new products being added and older ones being modified. A user should not expect to reproduce the findings of experienced practitioners without an investment of some time and effort. Though this may be associated with early failures, we are of the belief that this investment will ultimately pay dividends. Familiarity with a technique should be obtained in patients with relatively normal airway features so that confidence is acquired and the benefits and limitations of specific devices are appreciated.

REFERENCES

1. Adnet F, Baillard C, Borron SW, et al.: Randomized study comparing the "sniffing position" with simple head extension for laryngoscopic view in elective surgery patients. *Anesthesiology.* 2001;95:836–841.
2. Adnet F, Borron SW, Dumas JL, et al.: Study of the "sniffing position" by magnetic resonance imaging. *Anesthesiology.* 2001;94:83–86.
3. Adnet F, Borron SW, Lapostolle F, Lapandry C: The three axis alignment theory and the "sniffing position": perpetuation of an anatomic myth? *Anesthesiology.* 1999;91:1964–1965.
4. Levitan RM, Mechem CC, Ochroch EA, Shofer FS, Hollander JE: Head-elevated laryngoscopy position: improving laryngeal exposure during laryngoscopy by increasing head elevation. *Ann Emerg Med.* 2003;41:322–330.
5. Rose DK, Cohen MM: The airway: problems and predictions in 18500 patients. *Can J Anaesth.* 1994;41:372–383.
6. Weiss M, Schwarz U, Dillier CM, Gerber AC: Teaching and supervising tracheal intubation in paediatric patients using videolaryngoscopy. *Paediatr Anaesth.* 2001;11:343–348.
7. Levitan RM: A new tool for teaching and supervising direct laryngoscopy. *Acad Emerg Med.* 1996;3:79–81.
8. Levitan RM: *The Airway Cam Guide to Intubation and Practical Emergency Airway Management.* Wayne, PA: Airway Cam Technologies, 2004.
9. Liem EB, Bjoraker DG, Gravenstein D: New options for airway management: intubating fiberoptic stylets†. *Br J Anaesth.* 2003;91:408–418.
10. Kitamura T, Yamada Y, Du HL, Hanaoka K: Efficiency of a new fiberoptic stylet scope in tracheal intubation. *Anesthesiology.* 1999;91:1628–1632.
11. Bein B, Yan M, Tonner PH, et al.: Tracheal intubation using the Bonfils intubation fibrescope after failed direct laryngoscopy. *Anaesthesia.* 2004;59:1207–1209.
12. Halligan M, Charters P: A clinical evaluation of the Bonfils intubation fibrescope. *Anaesthesia.* 2003;58:1087–1091.
13. Aoyama K, Takenaka I, Nagaoka E, Kadoya T: Jaw thrust maneuver for endotracheal intubation using a fiberoptic stylet. *Anesth Analg.* 2000;90:1457–1458.
14. Shikani AH: New "seeing" stylet-scope and method for the management of the difficult airway. *Otolaryngol Head Neck Surg.* 1999;120:113–116.
15. Rudolph C, Schlender M: Clinical experiences with fiber optic intubation with the Bonfils intubation fiberscope. *Anaesthesiol Reanim.* 996;21:127–130.
16. Halligan M, Charters P: Learning curve for the Bonfils intubation fibrescope. *Br J Anaesth.* 2003;90:826P.
17. Pfitzner L, Cooper MG, Ho D: The Shikani Seeing Stylet for difficult intubation in children: initial experience. *Anaesth Intensive Care* 2002;30:462–466.
18. Nagashima M, Saito T, Takahata O, Sengoku K, Iwasaki H: Orotracheal intubation using a StyletScope in a patient with restricted opening of the mouth. *Masui.* 2002;51:775–776.
19. Hamada T, Morokura N, Suzuki Y, et al.: Orotracheal intubation using a StyletScope in a patient to avoid neck recurvation. *Masui.* 2001;50:519–520.
20. Bein B, Worthmann F, Scholz J, et al.: A comparison of the intubating laryngeal mask airway and the Bonfils intubation fibrescope in patients with predicted difficult airways. *Anaesthesia.* 2004;59:668–674.
21. Humphries RL, Stone CK, Short JH, Weaver JD, Parks RA: Performance of the Shikani Seeing Stylet in a difficult airway model. *Ann Emerg Med.* 2002;40(II)(4):230.
22. Evans A, Morris S, Petterson J, Hall JE: A comparison of the Seeing Optical Stylet and the gum elastic bougie in simulated difficult tracheal intubation: a manikin study. *Anaesthesia.* 2006;61:478–481.
23. Biro P, Weiss M, Gerber A, Pasch T: Comparison of a new video-optical intubation stylet versus the conventional malleable stylet in simulated difficult tracheal intubation. *Anaesthesia.* 2000;55:886–889.
24. Weiss M, Schwarz U, Gerber AC: Difficult airway management: comparison of the Bullard laryngoscope with the video-optical intubation stylet. *Can J Anaesth.* 2000;47:280–284.
25. Weiss M, Hartmann K, Fischer J, Gerber AC: Video-intuboscopic assistance is a useful aid to tracheal intubation in pediatric patients. *Can J Anaesth.* 2001;48:691–696.
26. Kihara S, Yaguchi Y, Taguchi N, Brimacombe JR, Watanabe S: The StyletScope™ is a better intubation tool than a conventional stylet during simulated cervical spine immobilization. *Can J Anaesth.* 2005;52:105–110.
27. Wahlen BM, Gercek E: Three-dimensional cervical spine movement during intubation using the Macintosh and Bullard laryngoscopes, the bonfils fibrescope and the intubating laryngeal mask airway. *Eur J Anaesthesiol.* 2004;21:907–913.
28. Rudolph C, Schneider JP, Wallenborn J, Schaffranietz L: Movement of the upper cervical spine during laryngoscopy: a comparison of the Bonfils intubation fibrescope and the Macintosh laryngoscope. *Anaesthesia.* 2005;60:668–672.
29. Kimura A, Yamakage M, Chen X, Kamada Y, Namiki A: Use of the fibreoptic stylet scope (StyletScope) reduces the hemodynamic response to intubation in normotensive and hypertensive patients. *Can J Anaesth.* 2001;48:919–923.
30. Kitamura T, Yamada Y, Chinzei M, Du HL, Hanaoka K: Attenuation of haemodynamic responses to tracheal intubation by the StyletScope. *Br J Anaesth.* 2001;86:275–277.
31. Ezri T, Szmuk P, Warters RD, Katz J, Hagberg CA: Difficult airway management practice patterns among anesthesiologists practicing in the United States: have we made any progress? *J Clin Anesth.* 2003;15:418–422.
32. Jenkins K, Wong DT, Correa R: Management choices for the difficult airway by anesthesiologists in Canada. *Can J Anaesth.* 2002;49:850–856.
33. Rosenblatt WH, Wagner PJ, Ovassapian A, Kain ZN: Practice patterns in managing the difficult airway by anesthesiologists in the United States. *Anesth Analg.* 1998;87:153–157.
34. Hung OR, Tibbet JS, Cheng R, Law JA: Proper preparation of the Trachlight and endotracheal tube to facilitate intubation. *Can J Anaesth.* 2006;53:107–108.
35. MacQuarrie K, Hung OR, Law JA: Tracheal intubation using Bullard laryngoscope for patients with a simulated difficult airway. *Can J Anaesth.* 1999;46:760–765.
36. Cohn AI, Hart RT, McGraw SR, Blass NH: The Bullard laryngoscope for emergency airway management in a morbidly obese parturient. *Anesth Analg.* 1995;81:872–873.
37. Gorback MS: Management of the challenging airway with the Bullard laryngoscope. *J Clin Anesth.* 1991;3:473–477.
38. Midttun M, Laerkholm HC, Jensen K, Pedersen T: The Bullard laryngoscope. Reports of two cases of difficult intubation. *Acta Anaesthesiol Scand.* 1994;38:300–302.
39. Cohn AI, Zornow MH: Awake endotracheal intubation in patients with cervical spine disease: a comparison of the Bullard laryngoscope and the fiberoptic bronchoscope. *Anesth Analg.* 1995;81:1283–1286.
40. Hastings RH, Vigil AC, Hanna R, Yang BY, Sartoris DJ: Cervical spine movement during laryngoscopy with the Bullard, Macintosh, and Miller laryngoscopes. *Anesthesiology.* 1995;82:859–869.

41. Watts ADJ, Gelb AW, Bach D, Pelz DM: Comparison of the Bullard and Macintosh laryngoscopes for endotracheal intubation in patients with a potential cervical spine injury. *Anesthesiology.* 1997;87:1335–1342.

42. Shulman GB, Connelly NR: Double lumen tube placement with the Bullard laryngoscope. *Can J Anaesth.* 1999;46:232–234.

43. Ovassapian A, Glassenberg R, Randel GI, et al.: The unexpected difficult airway and lingual tonsil hyperplasia: a case series and a review of the literature. *Anesthesiology.* 2002;97:124–132.

44. Crosby E, Skene D: More on lingual tonsillar hypertrophy. *Can J Anaesth.* 2002;49:758.

45. Shulman GB, Nordin NG, Connelly NR: Teaching with a video system improves the training period but not subsequent success of tracheal intubation with the bullard laryngoscope. *Anesthesiology.* 2003;98:615–620.

46. Maktabi MA, Hoffman H, Funk G, From RP: Laryngeal trauma during awake fiberoptic intubation. *Anesth Analg.* 2002;95:1112–1114.

47. Katsnelson T, Farcon E, Schwalbe SS, Badola R: The Bullard laryngoscope and the right arytenoid. *Can J Anaesth.* 1994;41:552–553.

48. Zadrobilek E: Upsher laryngoscope (original version). In: *Airway Management Guide.* Zadrobilek E, ed. Vienna: Austrian Difficult Airway/Intubation Registry. Available at: http://www.adair.at/eng/manguide/intubation/upsheroriginal. htm.

49. Pearce AC, Shaw S, Macklin S: Evaluation of the Upsherscope. A new rigid fibrescope. *Anaesthesia.* 1996;51:561–564.

50. Fridrich P, Frass M, Krenn CG, et al.: The UpsherScope in routine and difficult airway management: a randomized, controlled clinical trial. *Anesth Analg.* 1997;85:1377–1381.

51. Andueza AA, Rivera GC, Trigo DC, et al.: Evaluation of the UpsherScope laryngoscope in routine intubation with no expected difficulties. *Rev Esp Anestesiol Reanim.* 2002;49:350–355.

52. Dounas M, Mercier FJ, Valmier M, Laboutique X, Benhamou D: Evaluation of training on intubation with a rigid fiber optic laryngoscope (UpsherScope). *Ann Fr Anesth Reanim.* 1998;17:669–673.

53. Yeo V, Chung DC, Hin LY: A bougie improves the utility of the UpsherScope. *J Clin Anesth.* 1999;11:471–476.

54. Wu TL, Chou HC: A new laryngoscope: the combination intubating device. *Anesthesiology.* 1994;81:1085–1087.

55. Wu TL, Chou HC: The WuScope System: a new combination intubating device Instruction Manual. Available at: http://www.achi.com/support/manual/wsmanual.pdf. 2003.

56. Smith CE, Sidhu TS, Lever J, Pinchak AB: The complexity of tracheal intubation using rigid fiberoptic laryngoscopy (WuScope). *Anesth Analg.* 1999;89:236–239.

57. Smith CE, Pinchak AB, Sidhu TS, et al.: Evaluation of tracheal intubation difficulty in patients with cervical spine immobilization: fiberoptic (WuScope) versus conventional laryngoscopy. *Anesthesiology.* 1999;91:1253–1259.

58. Sprung J, Weingarten T, Dilger J: The use of WuScope fiberoptic laryngoscopy for tracheal intubation in complex clinical situations. *Anesthesiology.* 2003;98:263–265.

59. Andrews SR, Norcross SD, Mabey MF, Siegel JB: The WuScope technique for endotracheal tube exchange. *Anesthesiology.* 1999;90:929–930.

60. Sprung J, Wright LC, Dilger J: Use of WuScope for exchange of endotracheal tube in a patient with difficult airway. *Laryngoscope.* 2003;113:1082–1084.

61. Smith CE, Kareti M: Fiberoptic laryngoscopy (WuScope) for double-lumen endobronchial tube placement in two difficult-intubation patients. *Anesthesiology.* 2000;93:906–907.

62. Andrews SR, Mabey MF: Tubular fiberoptic laryngoscope (WuScope) and lingual tonsil airway obstruction. *Anesthesiology.* 2000;93:904–905.

63. Dullenkopf A, Holzmann D, Feurer R, Gerber A, Weiss M: Tracheal intubation in children with Morquio syndrome using the angulated video-intubation laryngoscope. *Can J Anaesth.* 2002;49:198–202.

64. Biro P, Weiss M: Comparison of two video-assisted techniques for the difficult intubation. *Acta Anaesthesiol Scand.* 2001;45:761–765.

65. Kaplan MB, Ward DS, Berci G: A new video laryngoscope—an aid in intubation and teaching. *J Clin Anes.* 2002;14:620–626.

66. Hagberg CA, Kaplan M B, Lazada L, Ward D, Berci G: The experience of four American clinics with the Macintosh videolaryngoscope. *Eur J Anaesthesiol.* 2003;20(4):A-164.

67. Cooper RM, Pacey JA, Bishop MJ, McCluskey SA: Early clinical experience with a new videolaryngoscope (GlideScope). *Can J Anaesth.* 2005;52:191–198.

68. Cooper RM: The GlideScope® videolaryngoscope. *Anaesthesia.* 2005; 60:1042.

69. Sun DA, Warriner CB, Parsons DG, et al.: The GlideScope® video laryngoscope: randomized clinical trial in 200 patients. *Br J Anaesth.* 2005;94: 381–384.

70. Agro F, Barzoi G, Montecchia F: Tracheal intubation using a Macintosh laryngoscope or a GlideScope® in 15 patients with cervical spine immobilization. *Br J Anaesth.* 2003;90:705.

71. Turkstra TP, Craen RA, Pelz DM, Gelb AW: Cervical spine motion: a fluoroscopic comparison during intubation with lighted stylet, GlideScope, and Macintosh laryngoscope. *Anesth Analg.* 2005;101:910–915, table.

72. Cooper RM: Use of a new videolaryngoscope (GlideScope®) in the management of a difficult airway. *Can J Anaesth.* 2003;50:611–613.

73. Doyle DJ: Awake intubation using the GlideScope video laryngoscope: initial experience in four cases. *Can J Anaesth.* 2004;51:520–521.

74. Gooden CK: Successful first time use of the portable GlideScope® videolaryngoscope in a patient with severe ankylosing spondylitis. *Can J Anaesth.* 2005;52:777–778.

75. Chua NHL, Hwang N-C, Ng JM: The Glidescope®—A familiarisation study on an intubating mannequin [abstract]. *Anesthesiology.* 2004;101:A608.

76. Maktabi MA, Smith RB, Todd MM: Is routine endotracheal intubation as safe as we think or wish? *Anesthesiology.* 2003;99:247–248.

77. Asai T, Shingu K: Difficulty in advancing a tracheal tube over a fibreoptic bronchoscope: incidence, causes and solutions. *Br J Anaesth.* 2004;92: 870–881.

78. Johnson DM, From AM, Smith RB, From RP, Maktabi MA: Endoscopic study of mechanisms of failure of endotracheal tube advancement into the trachea during awake fiberoptic orotracheal intubation. *Anesthesiology.* 2005;102:910–914.

79. Dunford JV, Davis DP, Ochs M, Doney M, Hoyt DB: Incidence of transient hypoxia and pulse rate reactivity during paramedic rapid sequence intubation. *Ann Emerg Med.* 2003;42:721–728.

80. Doyle DJ: Miniaturizing the GlideScope® video laryngoscope system: a new design for enhanced portability. *Can J Anaesth.* 2004;51:642–643.

81. Krasser K, Missaghi-Berlini SM, MoserA, Zadrobilek E: Evaluation of the standard adult glidescope videolaryngoscope: orotracheal intubation performed by novice users after formal instruction. *Internet J Airway Manag.* 2006 3(1).

SELF-EVALUATION QUESTIONS

9.1. Which of the following statements about video laryngoscopes is **TRUE**?

A. The video laryngoscopes facilitate the recording of the laryngoscopy.

B. The technique for using the GlideScope® makes it well suited for teaching direct laryngoscopy.

C. The laryngeal view obtained using the Storz Video Macintosh makes it well suited for managing the difficult airway.

D. The laryngeal view is essentially the same as the line-of-sight view.

E. The images obtained using any of the video laryngoscopes is hampered by fogging.

9.2. Which of the following statements about optical/fiberoptic stylets (e.g., The Bonfils, Shikani Optical Stylet, or Levitan FPS Scope) is **TRUE**?

A. Fiberoptic stylets should generally be used as stand-alone tools.

B. Once the tube is loaded, fiberoptic stylets have the advantage of requiring no other preparation of patient or instrument.

C. Fiberoptic stylets have been proven to be effective in awake intubations.

D. Fiberoptic stylets can be used as an adjunct to direct laryngoscopy.

E. The learning curve of these devices is such that novices can be expected to have a good chance at a successful intubation using a fiberoptic stylet.

9.3. Which of the following regarding rigid fiberoptic laryngoscopes is **FALSE**?

A. The rigid fiberoptic laryngoscopes are delicate and are easily damaged.

B. The laryngeal view may be obscured by fogging or the presence of blood and secretions.

C. Advancement of the endotracheal tube can be observed.

D. All of these devices require wider mouth opening than is required for direct laryngoscopy.

E. These devices are well suited for managing difficult airways.

CHAPTER (10)

Blind Intubation Techniques

Chris C. Christodoulou and Orlando R. Hung

10.1 INTRODUCTION

10.1.1 Why do we need blind intubating techniques?

Over the years, laryngoscopic intubation has been shown to be an effective and safe technique that is relatively easy to perform. It has become the standard method of tracheal intubation in operating rooms, intensive care units, and emergency departments. Unfortunately, even in the hands of experienced laryngoscopists, the rapid and accurate placement of an endotracheal tube (ETT) remains a significant challenge in some patients. This is particularly true in "unprepared" patients, or patients requiring emergency intubation.

Because of these difficulties, alternative intubation techniques, such as fiberoptic intubation, have gained a measure of popularity over the past several decades. While effective and reliable, this technique requires expensive equipment and special skill and training. Additionally, fiberoptic intubation is difficult in emergency situations in which "unprepared" or uncooperative patients may have copious secretions or blood in the oropharynx. One large study involving more than 1,600 fiberoptic intubations recorded a success rate of approximately 94%.[1]

Because of the difficulties posed by laryngoscopic intubation under direct vision, particularly under emergency conditions, the search for other techniques has led to the development of blind techniques using a variety of devices. During the last few decades, intubating guides and light-guided intubation using the principle of transillumination have proven to be effective, safe, and simple.

10.1.2 Would it not be safer to place a tracheal tube using a technique that is under direct vision?

One would anticipate that the placement of an ETT into the trachea under direct vision using a laryngoscope ought to be safer and achieve higher success rates than non-direct-vision techniques. Such is not the case; success and complication rates are not substantially different with blind techniques performed by skilled practitioners elaborated below. Furthermore, the technique of direct vision can be very difficult or even impossible because of distorted anatomy or the patient's disease. Several factors influence the success rates for laryngoscopic intubation including the inability to visualize the passage of the ETT through the glottic opening in the presence of copious amounts of blood, secretions, and vomitus.

Many practitioners fail to understand that having placed the flexible fiberoptic bronchoscope into the trachea under vision (indirect vision), the actual passage of the ETT over the bronchoscope is done blindly employing the scope as a guide. In other words, during fiberoptic intubation, after advancing the tip of the bronchoscope to a position slightly above the carina, the function of the bronchoscope is to provide a conduit to facilitate and guide the ETT into the trachea similar to that of an Eschmann Introducer (EI). Following tracheal intubation, the fiberoptic bronchoscope can be used to confirm the appropriate position of the tracheal tube in the trachea.

Many other procedures performed in medicine are in fact *blind* techniques including the placement of pulmonary arterial catheters, arterial cannulas, epidural catheters, and femoral nerve sheath catheters as examples. All of these procedures demand placement blindly under the guidance of anatomical landmarks and physiological responses.

Blind intubating techniques have been shown to be effective and safe, and in the absence of abnormalities of the upper airway, these techniques are acceptable methods of airway management.

10.2   INTUBATING STYLETS OR GUIDES

10.2.1   What is the Eschmann tracheal tube introducer? How does it facilitate the placement of an endotracheal tube?

In 1949, Macintosh reported the use of an introducer (gum-elastic bougie) to facilitate orotracheal intubation under direct laryngoscopy.[2] Using the concept of the introducer, Venn designed the Eschmann Introducer (Eschmann Tracheal Tube Introducer, Portex Limited, Hythe, UK), a tubelike core woven from polyester threads covered with a resin layer.[3] The EI is 60 cm long, with a J (coudé) tip (a 35-degree angle bend) at the distal end to facilitate advancement anteriorly underneath the epiglottis into the trachea and to provide tactile tracheal confirmation (Figure 10-1). Centimeter markings designate the distance from the tip. The EI is often referred to as the "gum-elastic bougie" or "bougie." However, to avoid confusion, historically the "gum-elastic bougie" has been used to refer to a shorter urinary catheter made of different material and without a curved tip.[4]

The EI is particularly useful when the glottic opening cannot be clearly seen using a laryngoscope (e.g., Grade 3 laryngoscopic view as described by Cormack).[5] Under these circumstances, the EI can be "hooked" underneath the epiglottis and advanced into the trachea. If it is correctly placed in the trachea, a subtle tactile "clicking" sensation can be felt as the tip of the EI slides over the tracheal rings while advancing into the trachea. Furthermore, if the EI correctly enters the trachea, as it is gently advanced it will eventually be lodged (or "holdup") in a distal airway and cannot advance beyond the 30–35 cm mark. In contrast, if it is placed in the

esophagus, the entire EI can be advanced into without encountering resistance. With the EI in place and positioned to 20 cm at the teeth, the ETT can then be advanced over the EI into the trachea. To facilitate the advancement of the ETT over the EI, the tongue and epiglottis must be elevated by a gentle jaw lift, a jaw thrust, or preferably, by the laryngoscope already in place. If difficulty persists while advancing the ETT, rotating the ETT 90 degrees counterclockwise will turn the ETT bevel posteriorly and minimize the risk of catching on the structures of the glottic opening.[6] Following intubation, the position of the ETT is confirmed using conventional methods, such as end-tidal CO_2 and auscultation.

10.2.2   What are other commercially available intubating guides or introducers?

Since the introduction of the EI, many intubating guides of different sizes, shapes, lengths, and materials have been developed. All of the designs serve a function similar to the EI but many have some additional features.

(a) The Flex-Guide ETT introducer (Green Field Medical Sourcing, Inc., Northborough, MA) is a flexible plastic introducer with a distal tip that can be bent by means of a proximal handle.[7]

(b) The Sheridan Tube Exchanger (Sheridan Catheter Corp., Oregon, NY) is a hollow flexible straight tube designed as a tube exchanger for patients with difficult airways. It can be used to ventilate patients under difficult circumstances through the inner lumen, distal ports, and an adapter at the proximal end.

(c) The Cook Airway Exchange Catheter (Cook® Critical Care, Inc., Bloomington, IN) serves a similar function as the Sheridan Tube Exchanger (Figure 10-1).

(d) Frova Intubation Introducer (Cook® Critical Care Inc., Bloomington, IN) is an intubating catheter with a coudé tip at the distal end (Figures 10-1 and 10-2).[8] It has a hollow

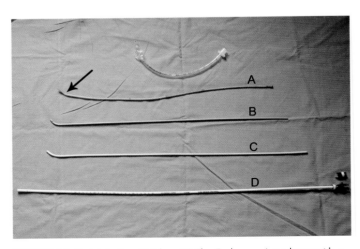

FIGURE 10-1. Intubating Guides: (A) The Eschmann Introducer with a coudé tip (arrow) at the distal end; (B) Frova Intubation Introducer is an intubating catheter with a hollow lumen and a coudé tip at the distal end; (C) The Endotracheal Tube Introducer is similar to the Eschmann Introducer in size and shape with a coudé tip, but it is 10 cm longer; and (D) The Cook Airway Exchange Catheter with an inner lumen, distal ports, and an adapter at the proximal end.

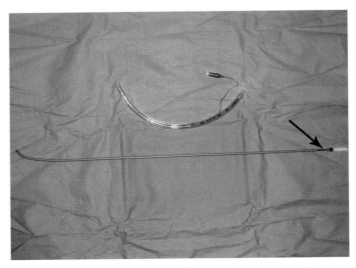

FIGURE 10-2. Frova Intubation Introducer is an intubating catheter with a hollow lumen and a coudé tip at the distal end. It also has a removable internal metal stylet (arrow) to increase stiffness to facilitate tracheal placement and ETT passage.

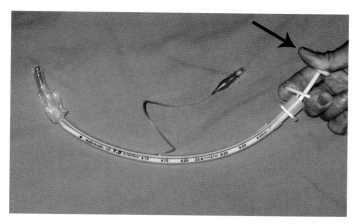

FIGURE 10-3. The Schroeder (Parker Flex-It™ Directional Stylet) Oral/Nasal Directional Stylet. Elevation of the tip of the ETT can be achieved by wrapping the index and middle fingers around the proximal tracheal tube and using the thumb to depress the proximal end of the stylet (arrow).

lumen with side ports distally; Rapi-Fit® adapters (luer lock and standard 15/22 mm) come with the device to permit oxygen insufflation in the event intubation cannot be achieved. It also has a removable internal metal stylet to prevent kinking and damage during shipping and to increase stiffness facilitating tracheal placement and ETT passage (Figure 10-2). The Frova introducer has two sizes: the adult version for ETT with greater than 5.5 mm inner diameter (ID) and the pediatric version for ETTs 3–5 mm ID.

(e) The Schroeder (Parker Flex-It™ Directional Stylet) Oral/Nasal Directional Stylet (Parker Medical, Englewood, CO) is a disposable articulating stylet that requires no bending prior to intubation (Figure 10-3). Inserting the stylet into an ETT allows the clinician to elevate the tip of the ETT by wrapping the index and middle fingers around the proximal tracheal tube and using the thumb to depress the proximal end of the stylet. Although the stylet is suitable for both oral and nasal intubation, it has been reported to be somewhat awkward to use and the curvature created is not at the tip, but rather over the distal half of the tube.[9] However, it has been reported to be effective for difficult as well as blind intubations.[10]

(f) Endotracheal Tube Introducer (Sun Med, Largo, FL) is similar to the EI in size and shape, but it is 10 cm longer. This confers some advantage in employing the device as more of the device protrudes from the mouth making it easier to thread a 30 cm ETT and capture the proximal end of the introducer. It is stiffer than the EI conferring an advantage in guiding the ETT, but at the same time, emphasizing the importance of gentle maneuvers to prevent airway injury. There are 10 cm markings on the device to indicate the depth of insertion. It is a single use disposable device, though resterilization is possible (Figure 10-1).

10.2.3   Is there any clinical evidence to support the widespread use of these intubating introducers?

Over the last several decades, numerous studies have reported the effectiveness and safety of the EI in facilitating tracheal intubation

in patients with difficult laryngoscopy.[11–14] The EI has been well accepted by most practitioners in the UK, and it continues to play an important role in the management of the difficult intubation. According to a recent survey in the UK, 100% of the respondents reported the use of the EI as their technique of choice when faced with an unanticipated difficult laryngoscopic intubation.[15] Though primarily a device used by the anesthesia practitioners in the past, over the past decade this relatively inexpensive and simple device has found its way to the hands of emergency practitioners and prehospital health care practitioners as an adjunct in airway management.[16–18] A telephone survey of emergency departments in England revealed that 99% of the respondents stocked the EI on their difficult airway carts.[19]

Following a recent review of the evidence related to the management of unanticipated difficult laryngoscopy, the Difficult Airway Society Guidelines for Management of the Unanticipated Difficult Intubation in the UK recommends the use of the EI as the initial device to facilitate a difficult laryngoscopy.[20] Many authorities recommend that this device be a standard piece of equipment for every laryngoscopic intubation.

While the EI has been accepted by the most as a useful adjunct for tracheal intubation, other types of introducers bearing similar features do not appear to share the same popularity. It is possible that there is a general lack of clinical evidence for their uses compared to the EI. In addition, most of these new intubating guides and stylets are disposable devices designed for a single use. Therefore, in some situations, particularly in the operating room setting, they may not be as cost-effective as the reusable EI.

10.2.4   What are the potential limitations of these intubating guides and introducers?

The popularity of the EI rests on its simplicity, ease of use, high success rates, and relatively few complications. However, it does have limitations. The much-anticipated "clicks" and the "holdup" as described by many may not be present. In 1988, Kidd et al. studied the reliability of these signs.[21] They found that the "holdup" was observed in 100% of tracheal placements of the EI, whereas the "clicks" were present only in 90%. Importantly, both were absent in all 22 esophageal placements. It is also possible, although rare, that "holdup" might occur with esophageal placement of the EI in cases of esophageal stenosis, pharyngeal pouch or diverticulum, or with cricoid pressure. Practitioners should be aware of these limitations, particularly where "holdup" can occur without the presence of "clicks." It is the opinion of the author (ORH) that the probability of feeling the "clicks" with EI placement into the trachea depends largely on the angle of insertion of the EI relative to the trachea. It is unlikely that the tip of the EI will "rub" against the tracheal rings if the EI is advancing into the trachea from a more vertical position. It is also related to the degree to which the EI contacts other soft tissues in the airway (e.g., tongue) insulating against the transmission of the subtle tactile sensation.

Although complications are rare with these devices, they tend to occur when these introducers are used improperly. Lacerations of the soft tissue, perforation of the esophagus, and injury to the bronchial tree have been reported with aggressive insertion of the

EI and forceful "railroading" of the ETT over the EI.[22,23] The incidence of these complications can be minimized by employing gentle advancement techniques and using the laryngoscope to move soft tissues out of the way to improve the angle of insertion of the ETT over the EI. Tip detachment has also been reported. Gardner et al. reported a detachment of the tip of the EI following its withdrawal.[24] The tip was initially identified just above the bifurcation of the trachea, though it was later documented to have moved into the right middle lobe bronchus. Manually checking the integrity of the tip of the EI prior to use is recommended.

10.2.5 Are there any clinical differences between the EI and other introducers with identical features?

Inspired by the simplicity and effectiveness of the EI, many newer introducers (the Frova Intubation Introducer, and the Endotracheal Tube Introducer) share similar characteristics such as the J (coudé) tip at the distal end. By and large, these newer devices are made of different materials and designed for single use. The Frova Intubation Introducer and the Cook Airway Exchange Catheter are hollow intubating introducers that permit urgent oxygenation and ventilation should the tracheal tube fail to advance into the trachea over the introducers. In addition to the "tracheal clicks" and "holdup" of the introducers during the insertion into the trachea, an aspiration test using a self-inflating bulb (SIB) can also be used with the hollow intubating introducers to further confirm tracheal placement. Tuzzo et al. recently reported that a prompt and complete reinflation of the SIB did not occur when the hollow intubating introducer was placed accidentally into the esophagus with 100% sensitivity and at a 3.5% false positive rate.[25]

While these newer devices appear to function similarly in facilitating tracheal intubation, they may not have comparable success rates. Using a simulated Grade 3 laryngoscopic view in a manikin, a recent comparative study showed that successful placement of the Frova Introducer (65%) and the EI (60%) was significantly higher than with the Portex Introducer (8%).[8] A separate experiment also revealed that the peak force exerted by the Frova and Portex introducers was two to three times greater than that which could be exerted by the EI, suggesting that placement of the single-use introducers may be more traumatic.

10.3 LIGHTWANDS

10.3.1 What is a lightwand? How does it help with the placement of an endotracheal tube?

The technique of transillumination using a lightwand (lighted-stylet) was first described by Yamamura et al. in 1959 with naso-tracheal intubation.[26] The lightwand employs the principle of

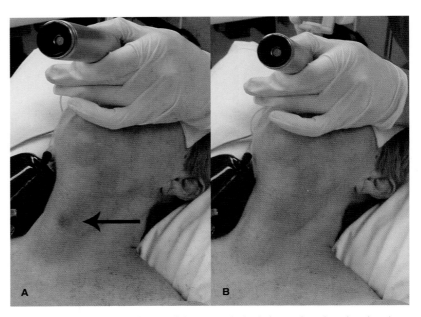

FIGURE 10-4. (A) When the tip of the ETT with the lightwand is placed at the glottic opening under direct laryngoscopy, a well-defined circumscribed glow (arrow) in the anterior neck just below the thyroid prominence can be readily seen. (B) When the tip of the endotracheal tube is placed in the esophagus under direct laryngoscopy, transillumination is poor and the transmitted glow is diffuse in the anterior neck and cannot be seen easily under ambient lighting condition.

transillumination of the soft tissues of the anterior neck to guide the tip of the lightwand, and the mounted ETT, into the trachea. It also takes advantage of the anterior (superficial) location of the trachea relative to the esophagus.

When the tip of the ETT/lightwand (ETT/LW) combination enters the glottic opening, a well-defined circumscribed glow can be readily seen slightly below the thyroid prominence (Figure 10-4A). However, if the tip of the ETT/LW is in the esophagus, the transmitted glow is diffuse and cannot be readily detected under ambient lighting conditions (Figure 10-4B). If the tip of the ETT/LW is placed in the vallecula, the light glow is diffuse and appears slightly above the thyroid prominence. Using these landmarks and principles, the practitioner can guide the tip of the ETT easily and safely into the trachea without the use of a laryngoscope.

10.3.2 Are all lightwands the same?

Through the 1970s and 1980s, many versions of a lighted stylet had been introduced, including the Fiberoptic Malleable Lighted Stylette (Metropolitan Medical Inc., Winchester, VA), Fiberoptic Lighted-Intubation Stylette (Anesthesia Medical Specialties, Santa Fe, CA), Lighted Intubation Stylet (Aaron Medical, St. Peterborough, FL), Flexilum™ (Concept Corporation, Clearwater, FL), Tubestat™ (Xomed, Jacksonville, FL) (Figure 10-5), and Imagica Fiberoptic Lighted Stylet (Fiberoptic Medical Products, Inc., Allentown, PA). Some of these devices have proven to be effective and safe in placing the ETT both orally and nasally.[27–29] Even though favorable results had been reported with these devices, they had substantial limitations: (1) poor light intensity; (2) short length, limiting the use of the lightwand device to short or cut ETT; (3) absence of a connector to secure the ETT to the lightwand device; (4) rigidity of the lightwand, hampering use of the devices with other techniques, such as

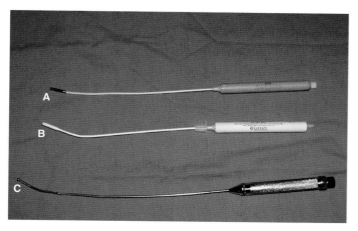

FIGURE 10-5. Commercially available lighted-stylets: (A) Flexilum™, (B) Tubestat™, and (C) Fiberoptic Malleable Lighted Stylette.

light-guided nasal intubation; and (5) most lightwands were designed for single use, increasing the cost per intubation. For these reasons and others, intubation using a lightwand did not receive widespread popularity until a novel commercial lightwand (Trachlight™, Laerdal Medical, Wappingers Falls, NY) device became available.

10.3.3   What are some of the unique characteristics of the Trachlight™ compared to other lightwand devices?

The Trachlight™ (TL) consists of three parts: a reusable handle, a flexible wand, and a stiff retractable wire stylet (Figure 10-6). The power control circuitry and three triple "A" alkaline batteries are encased in the handle. A locking clamp located on the handle accepts and secures a standard 15-mm ETT connector. The stylet or "wand" consists of a durable, flexible plastic shaft with a bright light bulb affixed at the distal end, permitting intubation under ambient lighting conditions. After 30 seconds of illumination, the

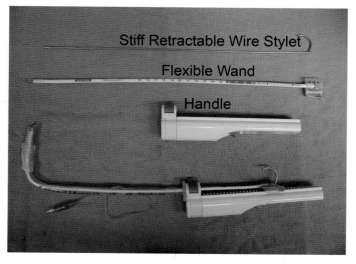

FIGURE 10-6. The Trachlight™ consists of three parts: a handle, a flexible wand, and a stiff retractable stylet wire. With the TL in place, the ETT-TL unit is bent at a 90-degree angle just proximal to the cuff of the tube in the shape of a "field-hockey stick."

light bulb blinks to minimize heat production and provide a convenient reminder of elapsed time. Ensuring that the tip of the stylet is inside the distal tip of ETT enhances its heat safety profile. A recent animal study confirmed an absence of histopathological changes suggesting that it is unlikely to have thermal injury following the use of the TL.[30]

A rigid plastic connector with a release arm at the proximal end of the TL handle allows adjustment of the wand along the handle and into the ETT when the release arm is depressed. Enclosed within the wand is a stiff but malleable, retractable wire stylet. When the wire stylet is retracted, the wand becomes pliable, permitting the ETT to advance easily into the trachea. This may well be the most important feature of this lightwand device, since it significantly improves its ease of use.

The retractable wire stylet stiffens the wand sufficiently so that it can be shaped in the form of a "field-hockey stick" (Figure 10-6). This configuration directs the bright light of the bulb against the anterior wall of the larynx and trachea. In addition, the "hockey stick" configuration enhances maneuverability during intubation and facilitates the placement of the ETT through the glottic opening. However, once through the glottis, the "field hockey stick" configuration can impede further advancement of the tube into the trachea. Retraction of the wire stylet produces a pliable ETT-TL unit, permitting its advancement into the trachea until the transilluminated glow reaches the sternal notch, a point known to be midtrachea.

10.3.4   How do you prepare the Trachlight™ device?

One of the authors (ORH) had significant involvement in the development of the TL, as reflected in the following narrative describing intubation technique using the TL. The technique described can be applied to any device that employs the concept of intubation using transillumination. As with any intubation technique, regular use of a TL will improve the clinician's performance and intubation success rates, and it reduces the possibility of complications.

Lubrication of the internal wire stylet of the wand using silicone fluid (Endoscopic Instrument Fluid, ACMI, Southborough, MA) ensures its easy retraction during intubation. The wand should also be lubricated with the same silicone fluid to facilitate retraction of the wand following the ETT placement. Cutting the ETT to 26 cm in length for easy maneuvering during oral tracheal intubation is recommended. The wand is then inserted into the ETT and the tube attached to the handle. The length of the wand is adjusted by sliding the wand along the handle to position the light bulb close to, but not protruding beyond, the tip of the ETT. With the TL in place, the ETT-TL unit is bent to a 90 degree angle just proximal to the cuff of the tube in the shape of a "field hockey stick" (Figure 10-6). Even though the degree of bend should be individualized to the patient, the 90 degree angle bend generally makes the intubation considerably easier. When the tip of the ETT is in the glottic opening, the 90 degree angle bend projects the maximum light intensity toward the surface of the skin, producing a well-defined exterior circumscribed glow. If the TL is bent to 45 degrees, the maximum light intensity will be directed down the trachea. For obese patients or patients with short necks, a more acute bend (greater than 90 degrees) provides better transillumination. Although it is the author's experience that the recommended length of the TL from bend to tip of 6.5–8.5 cm is suitable for most patients, some investigators have suggested that the length from bend to tip is best established by matching it to the patient's thyroid prominence-to-mandibular angle distance.[31]

10.3.5 How do you use the Trachlight™ to perform tracheal intubation?

Although the practitioner usually stands at the head of the table or bed during lightwand intubation, it is also possible to employ this technique from the front or side of the patient, in the prehospital environment for instance. When the head is in the sniffing position, the epiglottis is in close contact with the posterior pharyngeal wall making it more difficult for the TL to advance behind the epiglottis. It is preferable that the patient's head and neck be positioned in a neutral or slightly extended position.

In most cases, patients can be intubated easily under ambient lighting conditions.[32] In very thin patients, the light intensity is so bright that it is possible to mistakenly interpret an esophageal intubation as an intratracheal placement. It is therefore recommended that intubations using the TL in otherwise normal individuals be carried out under ambient light. Dimming room lights may be advantageous in obese patients, patients with thick necks or dark skin, or when the technique is being learned. In settings where controlling the ambient lighting is not possible (e.g., prehospital), it may be helpful to shade the neck with a towel or a hand.

Denitrogenation of the patient should precede all light-guided intubations. In an unconscious patient lying supine, the tongue falls posteriorly, pushing the epiglottis against the posterior pharyngeal wall (Figure 10-7). In order to have clear access to the glottic opening during intubation, it is necessary for the practitioner to grasp the jaw and lift it upward using the thumb and index finger of the nondominant hand. This lifts the tongue and epiglottis

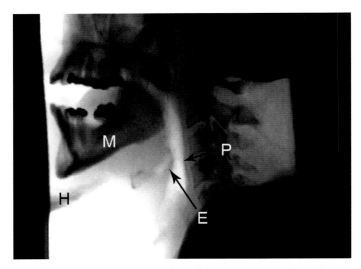

FIGURE 10-8. This radiological film of the upper airway shows that the jaw or mandibular (M) lift by the nondominant hand (H) can elevate the tongue and epiglottis (E) off the posterior pharyngeal wall (P), thus providing a clear passage for the endotracheal tube to enter the glottic opening.

away from the posterior pharyngeal wall to facilitate placement of the tip of the ETT posterior to the epiglottis and into the glottic opening (Figure 10-8). The ETT-TL unit is then inserted into the midline of the oropharynx. The midline position of the ETT-TL is maintained while the device is advanced gently in a rocking motion along an imaginary anterior–posterior arc. When resistance to cephalad rocking of the handle is felt, the ETT-TL handle should be "rocked" forward (toward the feet) and the tip redirected toward the laryngeal prominence using the glow of the light as a guide. A faint glow seen above the laryngeal prominence indicates that the tip of the ETT-TL is located in the vallecula. When the tip of ETT-TL enters the glottic opening, a well-defined circumscribed glow can be seen in the anterior neck slightly below the laryngeal prominence (Figure 10-9). Retracting the wire inner

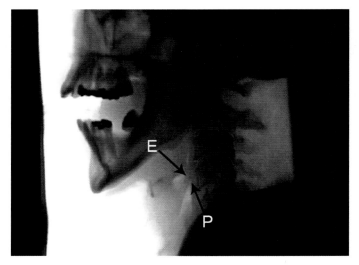

FIGURE 10-7. This radiological film of the upper airway shows that under anesthesia and with the patient lying supine, the tongue falls posteriorly, pushing the epiglottis (E) against the posterior pharyngeal wall (P).

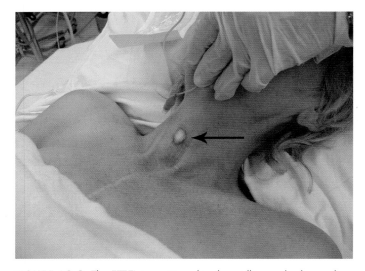

FIGURE 10-9. The ETT-TL is positioned in the midline and advanced gently in a rocking motion along an imaginary anterior–posterior arc. A bright, well-defined, circumscribed glow (arrow) is seen below the thyroid prominence when the ETT-TL enters the glottic opening.

stylet approximately 10 cm makes the ETT-TL more pliable, allowing advancement into the trachea with reduced risk of trauma. The ETT-TL is then advanced until the glow begins to disappear at the sternal notch indicating that the tip of the ETT is approximately 5 cm above the carina in the average adult.[33] Following release of the locking clamp, the TL wand can be removed from the ETT.

Occasionally, the circumscribed glow cannot be readily seen in the anterior neck due to anatomical features such as morbid obesity or a short neck. Neck extension as described above may be helpful. Retraction of the breast or chest wall tissues together with "spreading" of the tissues around the trachea by an assistant enhances transillumination of the soft tissues in the anterior neck. Dimming the ambient light is uncommonly required.

Occasionally, following retraction of the wire stylet, the tip of the tube and lightwand can "hang up" on laryngeal structures or the cricoid ring and cannot be advanced into the trachea readily. While maintaining the tube tip in contact with the anterior airway, the clinician should rotate the ETT-TL 90 degrees or more to the right or the left side permitting the tip of the ETT to point sideways or downward enhancing the chance that the ETT will enter the trachea. Alternatively, one may grasp the anterior larynx with the nondominant hand and lift it upward.

10.3.6 Can the Trachlight™ be used for nasotracheal intubation? How do you use the TL to perform a nasotracheal intubation?

In contrast to other commercially available lighted stylets, once the internal wire stylet is removed, the wand of the TL becomes pliable and able to facilitate a light-guided nasotracheal intubation. When used with a nasal RAE (Ring, Aldair, & Elwyn) ETT, the wire stylet should be retracted halfway (about 15 cm) to allow unbending of the proximal curvature of the nasal RAE tube (Figure 10-10). Application of a vasoconstrictor nasal spray to the nasal mucosa prior to intubation minimizes bleeding. The ETT-TL should be immersed in a bottle of warm sterile water or saline to soften the ETT to reduce the risk of mucosal damage during nasal intubation. Water-soluble lubricant is applied to the nostril to facilitate entry of the ETT-TL through the nose. As with oral intubation, a jaw lift during intubation will elevate the tongue and epiglottis away from the posterior wall of the pharynx, facilitating the placement of the tip of the ETT behind the epiglottis and into the glottic opening. The TL is switched on once the tip of the ETT-TL has advanced into the oropharynx, positioned in the midline and advanced gently using the light glow as a guide. A faint glow seen above the laryngeal prominence indicates that the tip of the ETT-TL is located in the vallecula. A jaw lift and slight withdrawal of the ETT-TL will help to elevate the epiglottis and enhance the passage of the ETT-TL under it. When the ETT-TL enters the glottic opening, a well-defined circumscribed glow is seen in the anterior neck just below the thyroid prominence (Figure 10-11). Following the release of the locking clamp, the TL is withdrawn from the ETT. Correct tube placement should be confirmed using end-tidal CO_2 and auscultation.

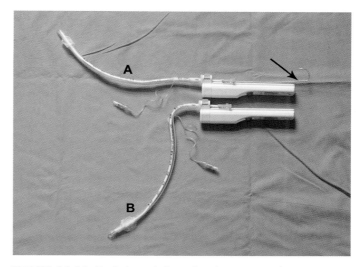

FIGURE 10-10. For light-guided nasal intubation using the Trachlight™, the internal wire stylet is generally removed so that the wand of the TL becomes pliable to facilitate nasotracheal intubation. However, if a nasal RAE tube is used, the proximal curvature of the nasal RAE Tracheal Tube will bend the pliable wand of the TL (B), making it difficult to control the tip of the tracheal tube during intubation. When the TL is used with a nasal RAE ETT, the wire stylet (arrow) should be retracted only halfway (about 15 cm) to allow unbending of the proximal curvature of the nasal RAE tube (A) to facilitate light-guided nasal intubation.

10.3.7 What are the common problems with a blind or light-guided nasotracheal intubation? How do you overcome these problems?

Due to the natural curvature of the ETT, the tip of the tube often goes posteriorly into the esophagus during a "blind" or light-guided nasal intubation. To elevate the tip of the ETT anteriorly during intubation, it is sometimes necessary to flex the neck of the patient while advancing the ETT-TL slowly. In the event that flexing the neck of the patient is contraindicated, inflating the

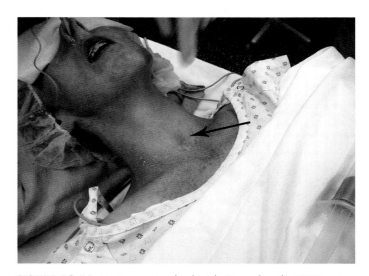

FIGURE 10-11. During nasotracheal intubation, when the ETT-TL enters the glottic opening, a well-defined circumscribed glow (arrow) is seen in the anterior neck just below the thyroid prominence.

ETT cuff completely with 20 mL of air will help to elevate the ETT tip and align it with the glottis during intubation.[34–36] Alternatively, the use of a directional-tip tube, Endotrol™ tube (Mallinckrodt Critical Care, Inc., St. Louis, MO), will facilitate directing the tip of the ETT anteriorly during nasal intubation.[37] In some difficult circumstances, nasotracheal intubation using the TL can be performed safely with the internal stiff stylet in place.[38] Although there may be an increased risk of nasal trauma with the stylet in place, this technique may be associated with fewer head–neck manipulations and perhaps deliver better control of the tip of the ETT.

10.3.8   What are the limitations of the Trachlight™ intubating technique?

The TL intubating technique requires transillumination of the soft tissues of the anterior neck without visualization of the laryngeal structure. Therefore, TL should not be used in patients with known abnormalities of the upper airway, such as tumors, polyps, infection (e.g., epiglottitis, retropharyngeal abscess), and trauma of the upper airway, or if there is a foreign body in the upper airway. In these cases, alternative intubating techniques using direct or indirect vision, such as fiberoptic intubation, should be considered. TL should also be used with caution in patients in whom transillumination of the anterior neck may not be adequate, such as patients who are grossly obese or with a limited neck extension. However, these contraindications and precautions must be weighed in the light of the urgency of achieving a patent airway in any patient whose ventilation may be compromised and urgent intubation is required. Clearly, this light-guided technique should not be attempted with an awake uncooperative patient unless a bite block is used to prevent damage to the device or injury to the clinician.

Since its introduction in 1995, the TL has been used extensively in many countries. While the potential risks of damage to the glottic opening during tracheal intubation using a "nonvisual" intubating technique is real, there have been no serious complications reported. Aoyama et al. used a nasally placed fiberoptic bronchoscope to visualize the airway during TL intubation. They reported that the epiglottis may be pushed into the laryngeal inlet by the ETT-TL during a TL intubation.[39] Fortunately, the epiglottis usually spontaneously returned to the correct position. They also reported that structures around the glottic opening, including the epiglottis and the arytenoids, can be transiently displaced during the placement of the ETT using the TL. The investigators concluded that there are potential risks of laryngeal damage in addition to the down folding of the epiglottis during the ETT placement using the TL, but such occurrences do not appear to cause permanent damage. Other investigators have identified a reduced incidence of sore throat in patients intubated using the TL compared to laryngoscopic intubation.[32]

Intubation using the TL has other potential risks. Stone and other investigators reported disconnection of the light bulb from a lightwand requiring retrieval from a major bronchus.[40] However, the lightwand device (Flexilum™) was not designed nor recommended for tracheal intubation. A later version of the same design solved the problem of bulb loss into the trachea by encasing stylet and bulb in a tough plastic sheath (Tubestat™). In contrast to the older lightwand devices, it is extremely unlikely that the light bulb will be detached from the TL, since the light bulb is firmly attached to the durable plastic sheath of TL. In fact, since its introduction in 1995, there have been no reported cases of detached light bulb from the TL. Although rare, subluxation of the cricoarytenoid cartilage has been reported in a study using an older version of a lightwand (Tubestat™).[41] However, with the retractable wire stylet, the risk of damaging the arytenoid cartilage during TL intubation would be low.

10.3.9   Is there any clinical evidence to suggest that the Trachlight™ is an effective and safe intubating device?

A large clinical study involving 950 elective surgical patients was conducted to determine the effectiveness and safety of orotracheal intubation using either the TL or direct-vision intubation using a laryngoscope.[32] There was a statistically significant difference in the total intubation time between the groups (15.7 ± 10.8 vs. 19.6 ± 23.7 seconds for TL and laryngoscopy, respectively). However, such a small difference is probably of little clinical importance. There was a 1% failure rate with the TL and 92% success rate on the first attempt, compared with a 3% failure rate and an 89% success rate on the first attempt using the laryngoscope. There were significantly fewer traumatic events and sore throats in the TL group compared to laryngoscopy patients. Tsutsui et al. reported similar findings in a study with 511 patients.[42] TL intubation appears to be highly successful (99%) with the majority of the successful intubations (93%) being accomplished after one attempt. Unsuccessful intubation even at the third attempt occurred in three patients (1%).

In 1995, Hung et al. reported the effectiveness of the TL intubation in 265 patients with a "difficult" airway (206 patients with a documented history of difficult intubation or anticipated difficult airways and 59 anesthetized patients with an unanticipated failed laryngoscopic intubation).[43] Tracheal intubation was successful in all patients except two in the anticipated difficult laryngoscopic intubation group. Apart from minor mucosal bleeding (mostly from nasal intubation), no serious complications were observed in any of the study patients. The results of this study indicate that TL is a useful and effective technique for placement of ETT both nasally and orally for patients with an anticipated as well as unanticipated difficult airway. Other investigators have also reported successful use of the TL in patients with a difficult airway. These include patients with a history of limited mouth opening,[44] cervical spine abnormality,[45] Pierre-Robin Syndrome,[46] and cardiac patients with a difficult airway.[47]

10.3.10   What are some of the potential uses of the Trachlight™?

Tracheal intubation can fail with TL as well as with the laryngoscope. However, in one study with 950 patients showed that all TL failures were resolved with direct laryngoscopy.[32] Similarly, all failures of direct laryngoscopy were resolved with TL. These results suggest that a success rate approaching 100% can be achieved in tracheal intubation with the use of a technique combining the two methods. This combined approach may be particularly useful for the unanticipated difficult laryngoscopic intubation, such as patients with Cormack/Lehane (C/L) Grade 3 laryngoscopic views.[5] Instead of using a styletted ETT with a 90-degree bend, one might employ an ETT-TL with the same bend. Under direct laryngoscopy, the tip of the ETT-TL can be "hooked" under the epiglottis. A well-defined circumscribed glow seen in the anterior neck slightly below the laryngeal prominence indicates that the tip of the ETT is placed at the glottic opening. In the event that such a glow is not seen, the ETT-TL can be repositioned until it can be seen. The effectiveness of this combined technique has been reported by Agro et al.[48] In this study, the investigators successfully performed tracheal intubation in all 350 surgical patients studied with a simulated difficult airway using a combined laryngoscope/TL approach.

The TL has been combined successfully with other intubating techniques including intubation through the LMA Classic™,[49,50] use in conjunction with the intubating LMA (Fastrach™),[51] with the Bullard laryngoscope,[52,53] and with a retrograde intubating[54] technique.

Recently, the TL has been shown to be useful in identifying the intratracheal position of the ETT tip during percutaneous tracheotomy.[55] The TL wand without the stiffening wire is passed through the in situ ETT matching the length numbers on the ETT to position the TL tip at the ETT tip. This simple technique may help to prevent inadvertent punctures of the ETT and/or its cuff, thus ensuring that adequate ventilation and oxygenation can be reinstituted during the percutaneous tracheotomy if required. This technique is also inexpensive and minimizes the risk of damaging expensive equipment ordinarily used during such procedures such as the fiberoptic bronchoscope. Used properly, it is possible that this simple light-guided technique can also be used to accurately determine when the tip of the ETT is above the surgical tracheotomy site as the tube is pulled back during surgical tracheotomy.

10.4   DIGITAL INTUBATION

10.4.1   What is digital intubation? When was it introduced?

Airway management has been revolutionized by the abundance of extraglottic devices that not only facilitate effective ventilation but also aid tracheal intubation. Despite these advances, certain situations may prevail that make blind insertion of an ETT into the trachea using the digits of the hand (digital intubation or tactile orotracheal intubation) a suitable alternative method of establishing a secure airway.

It is believed that this technique was first described by Herholt and Rafn in 1796 for the management of drowning victims. It surfaced as a viable method of intubation in the emergency medicine literature in the mid 1980s.[56,57] Blind digital intubation has also been used to establish an airway during neonatal resuscitation[58] and as an adjunct in blind nasotracheal intubation.[59]

10.4.2   What are the indications for digital intubation?

The skill levels of the operator, coupled with previous experience in using the technique of blind digital intubation are important prerequisites for success. The importance of practicing this technique in nonemergency situations cannot be overemphasized. The risk of infectious disease transmission must always be borne in mind. Awake patients with an active gag reflex are not suitable for this technique. Muscle paralysis may be helpful in certain situations. The following list briefly describes the clinical situations where blind digital intubation may be used to establish a patent airway:

(a) Inadequate access to a patient that prevents standard laryngoscopic techniques from being used.

(b) Lack or failure of other airway management devices.

(c) Inability to secure an airway with laryngoscopic techniques or extraglottic devices.

(d) In the setting of cervical spine instability in an unconscious patient.

(e) When blood, secretions, vomitus, or pus make adequate visualization of the glottis impossible.

10.4.3   How do you perform digital intubation?

A skilled operator will always ensure that an oxygen source, rescue airway devices, suction, and emergency drugs are always at hand. Appropriate in-line stabilization maneuvers should always be performed in the setting of cervical spine instability. Cricoid pressure should be applied where clinically indicated. Although digital intubation can usually be performed without other adjuncts (Figure 10-12), the classic description of blind digital intubation required a malleable stylet to be inserted into the ETT.[60] The ETT is bent into a curve conducive to accessing the trachea by elevating the epiglottis. However, the authors believe that using an intubating guide (e.g., the EI) together with an appropriately sized ETT is a simpler technique. The advantage of this technique is that it is far easier to guide the intubating guide through the glottic opening,

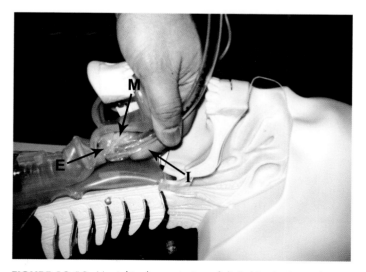

FIGURE 10-12. Maninkin demonstration of digital intubation without using a stylet or intubating guide: the index and middle fingers of the nondominant hand are inserted into the mouth. Once the epiglottis (E) is palpated by the middle finger (M), it is lifted in an anterior direction. The index finger (I) of the nondominant hand is then flexed to guide the tracheal tube under the epiglottis and into the trachea.

and then railroad the ETT over the intubating guide into the trachea. The intubating guide is of a small external diameter and is easily manipulated with the fingers to enable passage through the vocal cords. In addition, the clicks felt as the intubating guide (e.g., EI) advances over the tracheal rings combined with "holdup" can confirm the entrance into the trachea. The ETT with the malleable stylet is rigid and perhaps more likely to cause blunt trauma to the airway structures, especially if repeated manipulation is necessary for successful entry into the trachea. To perform the procedure:

(a) The patient's head should be placed in the sniffing position as for standard laryngoscopic intubation except in situations where cervical instability exists.

(b) The practitioner stands or kneels adjacent to the patient (facing the patient) so that the nondominant side of the intubator is closest to the patient (Figure 10-13).

(c) If an assistant is available, they can then grasp and pull the tongue forward using gauze. This maneuver helps to lift the epiglottis anteriorly and makes palpation of the structures of the upper airway easier.

(d) The practitioner then places the index and middle fingers of his nondominant hand into the patient's mouth. Once the epiglottis is palpated by the middle finger, it is lifted in an anterior direction.

(e) The intubating guide is then guided into the mouth along the palmar surface of the index finger of the nondominant hand.

(f) The index finger of the nondominant hand is then flexed to guide intubating guide under the epiglottis and into the trachea (Figure 10-13). Occasionally the middle finger of the nondominant hand lifting the epiglottis has to be moved slightly laterally to allow successful passage of the intubating guide.

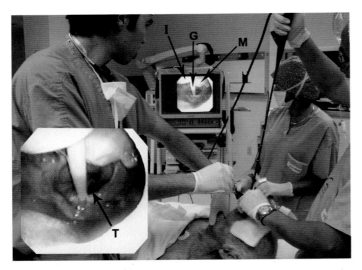

FIGURE 10-13. Digital intubation using an intubating guide: to visualize the technique of digital intubation, a flexible fiberoptic bronchoscope was placed through the right nostril into the nasopharynx of the patient. During the digital intubation, the index and middle fingers of the nondominant hand are inserted into the mouth. As shown in the monitor (and the enlarged insert), once the epiglottis is palpated by the middle finger (M), it is lifted in an anterior direction. The index finger (I) is then flexed to guide the Intubating Guide (G) under the epiglottis and into the trachea (T).

(g) The clicks on the tracheal rings and holdup of the intubating guide on the lower bronchial tree serve as indicators of correct tracheal placement.

(h) The ETT is then railroaded over the intubating guide into the trachea. Maintaining anterior traction on the epiglottis facilitates ETT passage through the vocal cords.

(i) Confirmation of successful tracheal intubation should be determined clinically with devices able to measure end-tidal CO_2.

10.4.4 Can digital intubation be performed on a child?

Although the principles and techniques of digital intubation are similar, digital intubation can readily be performed without the use of a stylet or the EI in children. Hancock et al. have employed this technique during neonatal resuscitation and accidental extubation scenarios.[58] Blind digital intubation of neonates and infants can be considered in situations where direct laryngoscopic techniques have failed, airway equipment failure has occurred, or during transport when inadequate access may preclude conventional techniques.

10.4.5 What are the limitations of digital intubation?

Although digital intubation is a simple and easy to learn technique, it is difficult to perform when the epiglottis cannot be identified or felt during intubation. This is particularly true for the patients who are excessively tall or with a full set of teeth and a small mouth opening. The procedure can also be difficult to perform if the practitioner has short or large fingers in relation to the patient's anatomy.

To minimize the risk of injury to the practitioner's fingers, digital intubation is generally contraindicated for patients who are awake and uncooperative. However, in emergency situations when limited equipment is available, a digital intubation can be safely performed with a bite block in place.

10.5 BLIND NASAL INTUBATION

10.5.1 What are the indications for blind nasal intubation?

The technique of blind nasal intubation was first popularized by Sir Ivan Magill and Stanley Rowbotham in the 1920s. This method of tracheal intubation has proved life-saving in many difficult airway situations. Maintenance of spontaneous ventilation facilitates blind nasal intubation. The experience and skill of the operator are key determinants for success with this technique. The following is a list of indications for blind nasal intubation:

(a) elective oral, pharyngeal, and dental surgery

(b) any indication for tracheal intubation where the oral route is difficult or impossible (e.g., limited mouth opening or severe masseter spasm)

(c) difficult airway—elective or unanticipated

10.5.2   What are the contraindications of blind nasal intubation?

The following is a list of contraindications for blind nasal intubation:

  (a) inadequate experience or skill of the operator

  (b) base of the skull cranial fractures

  (c) severe maxillofacial fractures with distorted nasal or midface anatomy

  (d) known or suspected nasal obstruction secondary to pathology (e.g., massive nasal polyps or tumors)

  (e) bleeding diathesis secondary to hematological disease or anticoagulant medication

10.5.3   Which nostril should be used for blind nasal intubation?

As most practitioners are right handed, naturally, most would favor the use of the right hand to advance the ETT through the right nostril while using the left hand to feel the anterior neck to assess the position of the tip of the ETT during blind nasal intubation. In the absence of a septal abnormality (e.g., a septal deviation), traditional teaching also suggests that the right nostril is better than the left for nasal intubation.[61] It is generally felt that the left-facing bevel of the tracheal tube is the main cause of nasal trauma. The mucosa over the turbinates is highly vascular and can be easily traumatized. It is likely that the mucosa over the left turbinate is particularly at risk during left-sided intubation since the bevel tends to impact directly against it. So, to minimize trauma, most practitioners would insert the ETT with the bevel facing the flat nasal septum rather than facing the irregularly shaped turbinates along the lateral wall of the nasal cavity. However, others consider that the tip of the tracheal tube is more likely to cause nasal trauma than the bevel and therefore it is more reasonable to have the tip of the ETT to advance alongside the septal mucosa during intubation. Hence, some practitioners choose to advance the ETT through the left nostril during nasal intubation. Unfortunately, there is currently no scientific evidence to suggest that one nostril is safer than the other for nasal intubation in patients with a normal nasal anatomy.[62] Instead of debating which is the preferred nostril to minimize the risk of injury, it is perhaps more important to properly prepare the ETT (e.g., selecting an appropriate size ETT and softening the ETT in warm saline or water) and the patient (e.g., apply vasoconstrictor to the nostrils prior to performing the nasal intubation), resist excessive force during intubation, and change to a different nostril or use a smaller ETT when it becomes necessary.

10.5.4   How do you perform a blind nasal tracheal intubation?

The answer to this question is largely determined by the indication for tracheal intubation. In elective situations, the nares are best prepared with a vasoconstrictor and a local anesthetic of choice. In emergency situations with life-threatening hypoxemia, this may not be possible. The potential for severe epistaxis with airway hemorrhage must always be borne in mind. Rescue airway equipment

including extraglottic ventilation devices and surgical airway access kits should be available. Vital sign monitors are attached and the patient is fully denitrogenated if practical prior to the procedure being undertaken. Cervical spine precautions and cricoid pressure should be instituted as indicated. Maintenance of spontaneous ventilation is crucial to identifying successful tracheal intubation. Confirmation of tracheal tube placement is obtained by the usual clinical criteria as well as CO_2 detection methods. To perform the procedure:

  (a) Insert the appropriate size ETT into the naris.

  (b) Gently advance the ETT. If resistance is met do not use excessive force. Consider switching to the alternative nostril.

  (c) Listen for breath sounds as you advance the ETT. The author has successfully used a stethoscope attached to the ETT adaptor to auscultate for breath sounds during the procedure. Careful inspection of the neck can provide useful clues to the location of the tip of the ETT.

  (d) In the event that esophageal entry occurs repeatedly, the ETT can be withdrawn to the hypopharynx and the cuff of the ETT inflated to produce anterior displacement of the ETT toward the glottic opening. Neck flexion is a commonly used maneuver to aid in passage of the ETT into the trachea. Clearly, this maneuver should not be performed in patients with known or suspected cervical pathology.

  (e) Confirm ETT placement once tracheal entry is suspected.

The BAAM Whistle (*B*eck *A*irway *A*irflow *M*onitor, Great Plains Ballistics, Inc., Lubbock, TX) and Endotrol (Mallinckrodt Medical Inc. Argyle, NY) tube can be used to provide an auditory cue in the form of a to and fro whistle to facilitate nasotracheal intubation.[63]

10.6   SUMMARY

While tracheal intubation under direct vision using a laryngoscope has been considered to be the conventional method of intubation, a small percentage of the population remains a challenge to all practitioners. Many alternative techniques of tracheal intubations have been developed over the last several decades to overcome these difficulties. However, these techniques often require expensive equipment, specialized skills, and are sometimes not particularly useful for patients in an emergency situation with limited resources.

Blind intubating techniques occupy an important role in airway management. Over the last several decades, these blind techniques have been shown to be effective and safe in securing an airway. However, as with all technical skills, one has to recognize that there is a learning curve and a skills maintenance requirement for all of these techniques to be of clinical utility.

REFERENCES

1. Heidegger T, Gerig HJ, Ulrich B, Schnider TW: Structure and process quality illustrated by fibreoptic intubation: analysis of 1,612 cases. *Anaesthesia.* 2003;58:734–739.
2. Macintosh RR: An aid to oral intubation (Letter). *BMJ.* 1949;1:28.
3. Venn PH: The gum elastic bougie. *Anaesthesia.* 1993;48:274–275.

4. El-Orbany MI, Salem MR, Joseph NJ: The Eschmann tracheal tube introducer is not gum, elastic, or a bougie. *Anesthesiology*. 2004;101:1240.

5. Cormack RS, Lehane J: Difficult tracheal intubation in obstetrics. *Anaesthesia*. 1984;39:1105–1111.

6. Hagberg CA: Special devices and techniques. *Anesthesiol Clin North America*. 2002;20:907–932.

7. Moscati R, Jehle D, Christiansen G, et al.: Endotracheal tube introducer for failed intubations: a variant of the gum elastic bougie. *Ann Emerg Med*. 2000;36:52–56.

8. Hodzovic I, Latto IP, Wilkes AR, Hall JE, Mapleson WW: Evaluation of Frova, single-use intubation introducer, in a manikin. Comparison with Eschmann multiple-use introducer and Portex single-use introducer. *Anaesthesia*. 2004;59:811–816.

9. Levitan R, Ochroch EA: Airway management and direct laryngoscopy a review and update. *Crit Care Clin*. 2000;16:373–388.

10. Weiss M: Management of difficult tracheal intubation with a video-optically modified Schroeder intubation stylet. *Anesth Analg*. 1997;85:1181–1182.

11. Combes X, Le Roux B, Suen P, et al.: Unanticipated difficult airway in anesthetized patients: prospective validation of a management algorithm. *Anesthesiology*. 2004;100:1146–1150.

12. Bokhari A, Benham SW, Popat MT: Management of unanticipated difficult intubation: a survey of current practice in the Oxford region. *Eur J Anaesthesiol*. 2004;21:123–127.

13. Nolan JP, Wilson ME: Evaluation of the gum elastic bougie. *Anaesthesia*. 1992;47:878–881.

14. Nolan JP, Wilson ME: Orotracheal intubation in patients with potential cervical spine injury. *Anaesthesia*. 1993;48:630–633.

15. Annamaneni R, Hodzovic I, Wilkes AR, Latto IP: A comparison of simulated difficult intubation with multiple-use and single-use bougies in a manikin. *Anaesthesia*. 2003;58:45–49.

16. Phelan MP: Use of the endotracheal bougie introducer for difficult intubations. *Am J Emerg Med*. 2004;22:479–482.

17. Jones I, Roberts K: Towards evidence based emergency medicine: best BETs from the Manchester Royal Infirmary. Difficult intubation, the bougie and the stylet. *Emerg Med J*. 2002;19:433–434.

18. Nocera A: A flexible solution for emergency intubation difficulties. *Ann Emerg Med*. 1996;27:665–667.

19. Morton T, Brady S, Clancy M: Difficult airway management in english emergency departments. *Anaesthesia*. 2000;55:485–488.

20. Henderson JJ, Popat MT, Latto IP, Pearce AC: Difficult airway society guidelines for management of the unanticipated difficult intubation. *Anaesthesia*. 2004;59:675–694.

21. Kidd JF, Dyson A, Latto IP: Successful difficult intubation. Use of the gum elastic bougie. *Anaesthesia*. 1988;43:437–438.

22. Smith BL: Haemopneumothorax following bougie-assisted tracheal intubation. *Anaesthesia*. 1994;48:91.

23. Kadry M, Popat M: Pharyngeal wall perforation—an unusual complication of blind intubation with a gum elastic bougie. *Anaesthesia*. 1999;54:393–408.

24. Gardner M, Janokwski S: Detachment of the tip of a gum-elastic bougie. *Anaesthesia*. 2002;57:88–89.

25. Tuzzo DM, Frova G: Application of the self-inflating bulb to a hollow intubating introducer. *Minerva Anestesiol*. 2001;67:127–132.

26. Yamamura H, Yamamoto T: Device for blind nasal intubation. *Anesthesiology*. 1959;20:221.

27. Ellis DG, Stewart RD, Kaplan RM, et al.: Success rates of blind orotracheal intubation using a transillumination technique with a lighted stylet. *Ann Emerg Med*. 1986;15:138–142.

28. Ainsworth QP, Howells TH: Transilluminated tracheal intubation. *Br J Anaesth*. 1989;62:494–497.

29. Vollmer TP, Stewart RD, Paris PM, Ellis D, Berkebile PE: Use of a lighted stylet for guided orotracheal intubation in the prehospital setting. *Ann Emerg Med*. 1985;14:324–328.

30. Nishiyama T, Matsukawa T, Hanaoka K: Safety of a new lightwand device (Trachlight): temperature and histopathological study. *Anesth Analg*. 1998;87:717–718.

31. Chen TH, Tsai SK, Lin CJ, et al.: Does the suggested lightwand bent length fit every patient? The relation between bent length and patient's thyroid prominence–to–mandibular angle distance. *Anesthesiology*. 2003;98:1070–1076.

32. Hung OR, Pytka S, Morris I, et al.: Clinical trial of a new lightwand (TL) to intubate the trachea. *Anesthesiology*. 1995;83:509–514.

33. Stewart RD, LaRosee A, Kaplan RM, Ilkhanipour K: Correct positioning of an endotracheal tube using a flexible lighted stylet. *Crit Care Med*. 1990;18:97–99.

34. Gorback MS: Inflation of the endotracheal tube cuff as an aid to blind nasal endotracheal intubation (Letter). *Anesth Analg*. 1987;66:913.

35. Hung OR: Nasal intubation with the Trachlight. *Can J Anaesth*. 1999;46:907–908.

36. Chung YT, Sun MS, Wu HS: Blind nasotracheal intubation is facilitated by neutral head position and endotracheal tube cuff inflation in spontaneously breathing patients. *Can J Anaesth*. 2003;50:511–513.

37. Asai T: Endotrol tube for blind nasotracheal intubation (Letter). *Anaesthesia*. 1996;50:507.

38. Agro F, Brimacombe J, Marchionni L, Carassiti M, Cataldo R: Nasal intubation with the Trachlight. *Can J Anaesth*. 1999;46:907–908.

39. Aoyama K, Takenaka I, Nagaoka E, et al.: Potential damage to the larynx associated with light-guided intubation: a case and series of fiberoptic examinations. *Anesthesiology*. 2001;94:165–167.

40. Stone DJ, Stirt JA, Kaplan MJ, McLean WC: A complication of lightwand-guided nasotracheal intubation. *Anesthesiology*. 1984;61:780–781.

41. Debo RF, Colonna D, Dewerd G, Gonzalez C: Cricoarytenoid subluxation: complication of blind intubation with a lighted stylet. *Ear Nose Throat J*. 1989;68:517–520.

42. Tsutsui T, Setoyama K: A clinical evaluation of blind orotracheal intubation using Trachlight in 511 patients. *Masui*. 2001;50:854–858.

43. Hung OR, Pytka S, Morris I, Murphy M, Stewart RD: Lightwand intubation: II. Clinical trail of a new lightwand to intubate patients with difficult airways. *Can J Anaesth*. 1995;42:826–830.

44. Favaro R, Tordiglione P, Di Lascio F, et al.: Effective nasotracheal intubation using a modified transillumination technique. *Can J Anaesth*. 2002;49:91–95.

45. Inoue Y, Koga K, Shigematsu S: A comparison of two tracheal intubation techniques with Trachlight and Fastrach in patients with cervical spine disorders. *Anesth Analg*. 2002;94:667–671.

46. Iseki K, Watanabe K, Iwama H: Use of the Trachlight for intubation in the Pierre-Robin syndrome. *Anaesthesia*. 1997;52:801–802.

47. Gille A, Komar K, Schmidt E, Alexander T: Transillumination technique in difficult intubations in heart surgery. *Anasthesiol Intensivmed Notfallmed Schmerzther*. 2002;37:604–608.

48. Agro F, Benumof JL, Carassiti M, et al.: Efficacy of a combined technique using the Trachlight together with direct laryngoscopy under simulated difficult airway conditions in 350 anesthetized patients. *Can J Anaesth*. 2002;49:525–526.

49. Asai T, Latto IP: Use of the lighted stylet for tracheal intubation via the laryngeal mask airway. *Br J Anaesth*. 1995;75:503–504.

50. Asai T, Latto IP: Unexpected difficulty in the lighted stylet-aided tracheal intubation via the laryngeal mask. *Br J Anaesth*. 1996;76:111–112.

51. Fan KH, Hung OR, Agro F: A comparative study of tracheal intubation using an intubating laryngeal mask (Fastrach) alone, or together with a lightwand (Trachlight). *J Clin Anesth*. 2000;12:581–585.

52. Gutstein HB: Use of the bullard laryngoscope and lightwand in pediatric patients. *Anesthesiol Clin North America*. 1998;16:795–812.

53. McGuire G, Krestow M: Bullard assisted trachlight technique. *Can J Anaesth*. 1999;46:907.

54. Hung OR, Al-Qatari M: Light-guided retrograde intubation. *Can J Anaesth*. 1997;44:877–882.

55. Addas BM, Howes WJ, Hung OR: Light-guided tracheal puncture for percutaneous tracheostomy. *Can J Anaesth*. 2000;47:919–922.

56. Stewart RD: Digital intubation. In: *The Airway: Emergency Management*. Dailey RH, Simon B, Young GP, Stewart RD, eds. St. Louis: Mosby, 1992.

57. Stewart RD: Tactile orotracheal intubation. *Ann Emerg Med*. 1984;13:175.

58. Hancock PJ, Peterson G: Finger intubation of the trachea in newborns. *Pediatrics*. 1992;89:325–327.

59. Korber TE, Henneman PL: Digital nasotracheal intubation. *J Emerg Med*. 1989;7.

60. Murphy MF, Hung OR: Blind digital intubation. In: *Airway Management: Principles and Practice*, 1st edn. Benumof JL, ed. Philadelphia: Mosby-Year Book Inc., 1996:277–281.

61. Aitkenhead AR, Smith G: *Textbook of Anaesthesia*. Edinburg: Churchhill Livingstone, 1998.

62. Smith JE, Reid AP: Identifying the more patent nostril before nasotracheal intubation. *Anaesthesia*. 2001;56:258–262.

63. Cook RT, Jr, Stene JK, Marcolina B, Jr: Use of a beck airway airflow monitor and controllable-tip endotracheal tube in two cases of nonlaryngoscopic oral intubation. *Am J Emerg Med*. 1995;13(2):180–183.

SELF-EVALUATION QUESTIONS

10.1. Light-guided intubation using a lightwand should be used with great caution in all of the following conditions **EXCEPT**

A. morbid obesity

B. foreign body in the upper airway

C. retropharyngeal abscess

D. blood and secretion in the oropharynx

E. trauma to the anterior neck

10.2. Which of the following statements regarding the light-guided intubation using the Trachlight™ is **NOT** correct?

A. Trachlight™ can be used for both oral and nasal intubation.

B. Trachlight™ can be used for pediatric and adult patients.

C. Trachlight™ can be used effectively with cricoid pressure.

D. Trachlight™ is designed for a single use.

E. Light-guided intubation using a Trachlight™ can be used in a patient with dark skin.

10.3. Which of the following is **NOT** a characteristic feature of the Eschmann Tracheal Tube Introducer ("gum-elastic bougie")?

A. The Eschmann Introducer is 60 cm long.

B. The Eschmann Introducer has a J (coudé) tip (a 35-degree angle bend) at the distal end.

C. The Eschmann Introducer has two side ports and a hollow lumen.

D. The Eschmann Introducer is a reusable device.

E. The Eschmann Introducer consists of a core of tube woven from polyester threads covered with a resin layer.

CHAPTER (11)

Extraglottic Devices for Ventilation and Oxygenation

Felice E. Agrò, D. John Doyle, Orlando R. Hung, Thomas J. Coonan, Rita Cataldo, and Benedetta Gallì

11.1 INTRODUCTION

11.1.1 What are extraglottic devices? Why do we need these devices?

As opposed to a mask placed on the face to effect bag-mask-ventilation (BMV), an extraglottic device (EGD) establishes a direct conduit for air to flow when placed in the periglottic area. The terminology has been confusing. For instance, some have referred to these devices as "supraglottic airway devices," though many devices have components that are infraglottic.[1]

Difficulties in airway management are associated with significant morbidity and mortality.[2] Therefore, it is crucial that practitioners responsible for airway management continue to refine existing skills and acquire new knowledge and skills as they become available. Two decades ago, ventilation and oxygenation were achieved primarily via a facemask or an endotracheal tube (ETT).

While BMV is relatively simple, it has limitations.[3] Tracheal intubation has been considered to be the "gold standard" for providing effective ventilation, while at the same time providing protection from the aspiration of gastric content. However, tracheal intubation is a skill that is not easily mastered[4] and regular practice is necessary to maintain the skill. Employing an EGD to successfully facilitate gas exchange may well be a more easily acquired skill for the nonexpert airway practitioner.

EGDs vary in size and shape. Most have balloons or cuffs that upon inflation can provide a reasonably tight seal in the upper airway.

There is clear evidence of their effectiveness and safety in providing ventilation and oxygenation. These devices have changed the landscape of contemporary airway management securing a place in the most recent iteration of the American Society of Anesthesiologists (ASA) Difficult Airway Management Algorithm.[5]

11.1.2 Do manufacturing standards exist for EGDs to ensure patient safety?

The American Society for Testing and Materials Standards (ASTM) Committee F29 on Anesthetic and Respiratory Equipment has proposed the establishment of standards related to EGDs used in human subjects. A task group has proposed the standardization of terminology, design, production, manufacturing, testing, labeling, and promotion. Devices produced according to the proposed ASTM standard will:

- facilitate unobstructed access of respiratory gases to the glottic inlet by displacing tissue;
- not require a (external) facial seal to maintain airway patency;
- terminate in a 15/22-mm connector to facilitate positive-pressure ventilation (PPV) via an anesthetic breathing system;
- be capable of maintaining airway patency when the (15/22 mm) airway connector is open to ambient atmosphere; and
- minimize the escape of airway gases to the atmosphere.

11.1.3 What EGDs are commercially available?

Many EGDs have been introduced.[1] The best known are the Laryngeal Mask Airway (LMA) Classic™, LMA ProSeal™ (PLMA), LMA Fastrach™ (LMA-FT), and Combitube™ (CBT). A number of more recently developed EGDs such as the Laryngeal Tube (LT), CobraPLA™ (CPLA), Airway Management Device

(AMD), LaryVent™ (LV), Cuffed Oropharyngeal Airway (COPA), and PAxpress™ (PAX) are also gaining acceptance. This is an evolving field with many new reusable and disposable EGDs introduced every year. This chapter will review the commonly used EGDs but should not be considered as an exhaustive review of all available devices. It should be emphasized that some devices (e.g., the COPA and PAxpress™) are no longer being manufactured. However, the authors have elected to include them, as these devices have participated materially in the evolution of EGDs as we know them today.

11.2   LARYNGEAL MASK AIRWAY (LMA) CLASSIC™

11.2.1   What is the LMA? When was it introduced?

The LMA (LMA North America Inc., San Diego, CA) (Figure 11-1) was designed in 1981 by Dr. Archie Brain as he searched for a device that was easier to use and more effective than the face mask and less invasive than an ETT. The LMA is designed to surround and cover the periglottic area to provide continuity of airflow between the environment and the lungs. The device has a wide-bore tube connecting to an oval inflatable cuff that seals around the larynx. It is currently available in eight different sizes for use in patients ranging in size from neonates to large adults. Typically, a #3 LMA is used in teenagers and small adult females, while #4, #5, and #6 in average and large size adults.

Published data from large studies and reports (>1,000 publications) have confirmed the safety and efficacy of the device for difficult airway management, both as a substitute airway and as an intubation aid.[6] The LMA is specified in the ASA's Difficult Airway Management Algorithm.[5] Moreover, the LMA has a role in emergency airway management during cardiopulmonary resuscitation (CPR), the transport of the critically ill patient, and in the ICU.[7–9] Although the LMA is a potentially useful device in situations in which mask ventilation or tracheal intubation are not possible ("can't intubate, can't ventilate," or CICV),[5] it should never be used as a substitute for a surgical airway. While this device can provide adequate ventilation and oxygenation, it does not protect the airway from aspiration and does not easily allow for the removal of pulmonary secretions. Therefore, when

employed as a rescue device, the LMA can only be considered a temporizing measure, until a more definitive and protective airway is secured.

11.2.2   What is the proper way to insert the LMA?

While many techniques have been suggested for the insertion of the device, including the midline approach, the lateral approach, and the thumb technique,[10] the authors recommend the following steps:

1. Following complete deflation of the cuff, the LMA (posterior side) is lubricated with a water-soluble lubricant.

2. Provided that there is no contraindication to moving the cervical spine, the patient's head and neck should be placed in a sniffing position. A head tilt will help to open the mouth.

3. In order to have clear access to the glottic opening and minimize down folding of the epiglottis, it is recommended that the practitioner perform a jaw lift using the thumb and index finger of the nondominant hand. This lifts the tongue and epiglottis away from the posterior pharyngeal wall to facilitate placement of the LMA. The LMA should be inserted into the mouth with the index finger placed between the mask–tube junction, pressing the cuff against the hard palate and advancing the LMA into the oropharynx following the natural curve of the posterior pharyngeal wall. The dimensions and design of the device allow the tip of the LMA to wedge into the hypopharynx. A definite resistance should be felt when the tip of the LMA enters the hypopharynx. Occasionally, resistance is encountered during insertion because of backward folding of the cuff. Sweeping a finger behind the cuff to redirect it inferiorly into the laryngopharynx can easily overcome this problem.[11]

4. Following placement, the cuff should be inflated with the minimal volume of air necessary to achieve an adequate seal. However, this "just-seal" volume may not be adequate to seal the hypopharynx from the esophagus.[10] Therefore, most practitioners commonly inflate the cuff with more volume. In general, approximately 20 mL is required for #3, 30 mL for #4, and 40 mL #5 LMA. Seal characteristics may be improved by ensuring that the LMA is secured in the midline of the mouth.

5. The LMA should be fixed in position by taping it to the face or by bonding it to the anesthesia breathing circuit.[12]

11.2.3   What is the proper way to remove the LMA?

In its normal position, the LMA is less stimulating than an ETT and is generally well tolerated by most patients on emergence. Many studies have compared removal under deep anesthesia versus while awake. Though airway obstruction appears to be less frequent if the device is removed with the patient awake, this technique is associated with more coughing, laryngospasm, biting, and hypersalivation.[13] While much controversy remains, it is the opinion of the authors that in adults, the LMA should be removed awake. This is particularly true if mask ventilation is expected to be difficult. Many pediatric airway practitioners prefer removal under deep anesthesia, as children are more prone to laryngospasm.

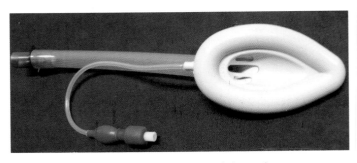

FIGURE 11-1. The LMA Classic™ has a wide-bore tube connecting to an oval inflatable cuff which seals around the larynx.

It is unclear whether the LMA should be removed with the cuff deflated or inflated. Some recommend an inflated cuff because of its capacity to remove secretions that accumulate above the device from the oral cavity.[14] Others argue that the cuff should be deflated to minimize trauma and damage to the cuff. Brimacombe recommends the removal of the LMA with the cuff partially deflated.[13]

11.2.4 What are the advantages and disadvantages of using the LMA as opposed to an ETT?

Brimacombe conducted a meta-analysis on randomized prospective trials involving 2,440 patients comparing the LMA with other forms of airway management, including tracheal intubation.[15] He reported many advantages of the LMA including rapidity and ease of placement, particularly for inexperienced operators; improved hemodynamic stability on induction and during emergence; minimal rise in intraocular pressure following insertion; reduced anesthetic requirements for airway tolerance; lower frequency of coughing during emergence; improved oxygen saturation during emergence; and lower incidence of sore throat in adults.

An additional advantage of the device is its utility as a rescue device and during resuscitation.[16] Further studies have shown that the LMA has less impact on mucociliary clearance than an ETT and may reduce the risk of retention of secretions, atelectasis, and pulmonary infection.[17]

The major disadvantage of the LMA is its inability to seal the larynx and protect against aspiration. The mask is designed in such a way that the distal end of the device is intended to become wedged into the upper esophageal sphincter. However, in reality the distal end may lie anywhere from the nasopharynx to the hypopharynx. In a meta-analysis, Brimacombe found that an additional disadvantage of the LMA was related to poor seal leading to air leak on PPV and gastric insufflation.[15]

The magnitude of the insufflation probably depends on the airway pressure generated and the position of the LMA. While it is possible that this gastric insufflation could increase the risk of gastric aspiration, very large series have shown that PPV with the LMA is both safe and effective with no episodes of gastric dilatation in 11,910 LMA anesthetics under both spontaneous and PPV.[18]

According to a meta-analysis involving 547 LMA publications, the incidence of gastric aspiration associated with the use of LMA is rare (0.02%),[19] and most of these cases had predisposing risk factors for pulmonary aspiration. However, fatal aspiration of gastric content has recently been reported.[20] Therefore, a proper assessment of aspiration risk prior to the use of the LMA is imperative. Most airway practitioners would probably avoid the use of the LMA in patients with a history of hiatal hernia, gastroesophageal reflux, in obstetrical patients, or in patients with a bowel obstruction. Careful placement of the device and maintenance and emergence of anesthesia may attenuate the risk of gastric aspiration.

11.2.5 Is it safe to use the LMA for positive-pressure ventilation?

Over the last two decades, the use of a face mask to facilitate the administration of anesthesia has largely been replaced by the LMA, particularly in the United Kingdom. Originally felt to be most appropriate for nonparalyzed patients with spontaneous ventilation, a survey in the United Kingdom in the mid 1990s showed that 5,236 of 11,910 patients (44%) underwent PPV through the LMA.[18] While a few studies reported the successful use of the LMA for PPV for a variety of patient populations and procedures,[21–23] they involved mostly small numbers of patients, with few large prospective randomized trials.[24] Based on the current evidence, the LMA appears to be effective and probably safe for PPV in patients with normal airway resistance and compliance, and normal tidal volumes. However, gastroesophageal insufflation may occur when the LMA is used in conjunction with, and in the presence of, decreased pulmonary or chest wall compliance.[25,26]

Pressure-controlled ventilation (PCV) rather than volume-controlled ventilation (VCV) may improve the effectiveness of mechanical ventilation in patients with high airway pressure, or reduced lung compliance, thus minimizing the risk of gastric insufflation with the LMA.[27] It should be emphasized that while rare, cases of serious and even fatal gastric aspiration associated with the use of LMA have been reported.[20,28–30] Because of the potential for serious complications, an editorial published in the *British Journal of Anesthesia* in 2001 cautioned anesthesia practitioners on the use of the LMA for PPV and suggested that more evidence was needed before valid conclusions on the safety of the practice could be made.[24]

11.2.6 How are LMAs used appropriately in clinical practice?

Since its introduction in 1988, the LMA has been used in more than 150 million patients worldwide[20] and it has largely replaced the ETT and face mask for patients undergoing simple and uncomplicated surgical procedures. The extensive use of the LMA is a reflection of its overwhelming effectiveness and safety in a variety of age groups and surgical procedures. The LMA has also been shown to be effective and safe for elective caesarean section in nonobese parturients, though its use for this indication is controversial.[31]

A meta-analysis of currently available data shows that the LMA is safe and effective for pediatric airway management.[32] Furthermore, the LMA has been used successfully in the management of large numbers of difficult pediatric airways associated with a variety of congenital anomalies.

The LMA was approved for resuscitation by the European Resuscitation Council in 1996[33] and the American Heart Association (AHA) in 2000.[34] However, the possibility of gastric insufflation, related to high peak airway pressure, continues to be a concern in these patient populations.

In a prospective study, inspiratory pressures, air leak, and signs of gastric insufflation using an LMA were compared using VCV and PCV in children. The results show that during general anesthesia, PCV offers lower peak inspiratory airway pressures while maintaining equal ventilation. Although no signs of gastric insufflation were detected in either group, the lower pressures might be significant in patients with reduced chest wall or lung compliance.[35]

Brimacombe summarized the current evidence with respect to the use of the LMA in the management of the difficult and failed airway.[36] With the exception of airway pathology that may interfere with the LMA placement, there is a considerable body of evidence to support the use of the LMA in both predicted and unpredicted difficult airway.[5]

The LMA also provides a conduit for tracheal intubation using either a blind technique, a transillumination technique (using the Trachlight™ without the stylet),[37,38] or a flexible fiberoptic bronchoscope (FFB). Intubation success rates through the LMA have been found to be similar for patients with normal and abnormal airways, respectively.[39]

The flexible laryngeal mask airway (FLMA) was specifically designed for use in ear, nose and throat, head and neck, and dental surgery. It has been used for adenotonsillectomy,[40] laser pharyngoplasty,[41] and dental extraction.[42] The device consists of a normal LMA bowl connected to a floppy, wire-reinforced tube that has a narrower bore than the LMA. The long flexible, narrow bore tube provides better surgical access to the oropharyngeal cavity than the standard LMA. The technique for placement of the FLMA is similar to that for the LMA.

The reusable LMA Classic™ is the original LMA. Variations on the original include:

- LMA Fastrach™, also known as the Intubating LMA (ILMA), also available in a disposable form (Figure 11-2).

- LMA Flexible™, similar in design to the Classic but incorporating a non-kinkable, wire-reinforced tube.

- LMA ProSeal™, a device that has improved seal characteristics and incorporates a gastric drainage capability (Figures 11-3 and 11-4).

- LMA Unique™, a single use device virtually identical to the Classic (Figure 11-5).

- LMA Supreme™, a new disposable device that incorporates the insertion advantages of the Fastrach™ and the seal characteristics of the LMA ProSeal™ (Figure 11-6).

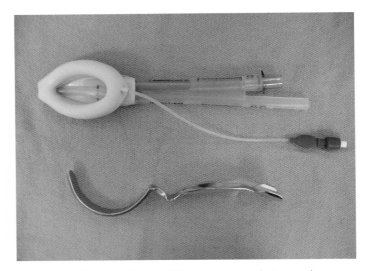

FIGURE 11-3. The LMA ProSeal™ incorporates a drainage tube placed lateral to the airway tube and a second dorsal cuff. The drainage tube travels from the proximal end of the device through the bowl opening into the upper esophagus. It permits the insertion of standard nasogastric tubes to facilitate the drainage of gastric contents. Also shown is the metal introducer employed to facilitate placement of the PLMA.

11.3 FASTRACH™ INTUBATING LARYNGEAL MASK AIRWAY (ILMA)

11.3.1 What is the LMA Fastrach™, or ILMA, and why was it developed?

While it is possible to intubate the trachea through an LMA, success rates are variable and generally unreliable. Accordingly, an intubating LMA (LMA Fastrach™ or ILMA, LMA North America Inc., San Diego, CA) (Figure 11-2) was designed by Dr. Brain.

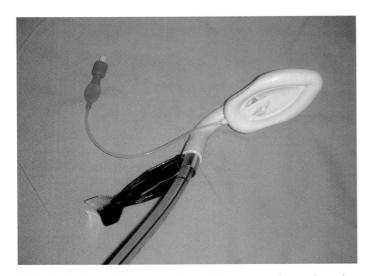

FIGURE 11-2. The LMA Fastrach™ or ILMA has a rigid curved metal airway tube with a manipulating handle, an epiglottic elevating bar, a deeper bowl, and a ramp that directs an ETT up and into the larynx, enhancing the success rate of blind intubation. In this figure, a dedicated wire-reinforced silicone tipped tracheal tube (TT) is inserted into the metal lumen of the ILMA. When the horizontal black line on the TT meets the proximal end of the ILMA, the tip of the TT will emerge from beneath the epiglottic elevating bar.

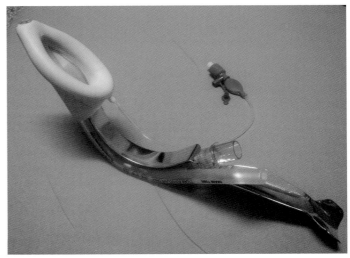

FIGURE 11-4. This figure shows the LMA ProSeal™ loaded onto the introducer. The distal end of the metal introducer is placed in an "insertion strap" on the PLMA and the airway tube is folded around the introducer and "clipped" into a proximal matching slot.

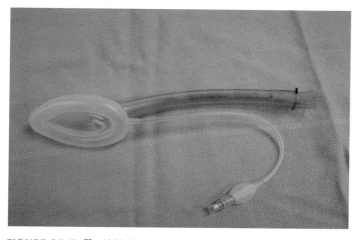

FIGURE 11-5. The LMA Unique™ is a single use device virtually identical to the Classic with aperture bars.

The device has a rigid metal curved airway tube with a guiding handle, an epiglottic elevating bar, a deeper bowl, and ramp that directs an ETT up and into the larynx. The device is easy to use, is associated with high success rates of intubation, and has received widespread acceptance. The ILMA is a reusable device, which can be cleaned and sterilized using an autoclave. A disposable device has also recently been introduced.

11.3.2 How is tracheal intubation performed using the ILMA?

Tracheal intubation through the ILMA can be achieved with a blind, light-guided (with a lightwand, Trachlight™), or fiberoptic-guided technique. To facilitate the insertion of an ETT through the ILMA, the following steps are recommended:

1. Lubricate the posterior side of the ILMA and the ETT (including the connector of the ETT) with a water-soluble lubricant. Ensure that the ETT slides easily through the ILMA.

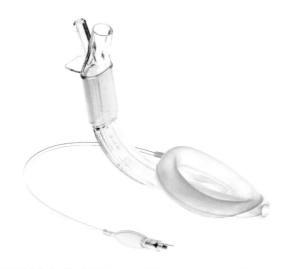

FIGURE 11-6. The LMA Supreme™ is a new disposable device that incorporates the insertion advantages of the Fastrach™ and the seal characteristics of the LMA ProSeal™.

2. Open the airway by using a head tilt, with a sniffing position, if possible.

3. Grasp the metal handle of the ILMA and insert the device straight back over the tongue to the back of the oropharynx. Then advance the cuff into the hypopharynx by rotating the device using the metal handle while maintaining pressure against the palate and following the palatopharyngeal curve. Once in place, inflate the cuff to achieve a seal for manual ventilation. The metal handle may be used to manipulate the device to achieve a seal to ensure adequate ventilation and oxygen saturation. The Chandi maneuver described as optimizing the seal by lifting the handle may be necessary.[43]

While a number of ETTs, including the Mallinckrodt Hi-Lo PVC tube,[44] can be used for tracheal intubation, the dedicated wire-reinforced silicone tipped ETT supplied with the ILMA has been shown to give the highest success rates. With the black vertical line on the tube facing the operator, insert the tube into the metal lumen of the ILMA, until the horizontal black line on the ETT meets the proximal end of the ILMA (see Figure 11-2). At this point, the tip of the ETT is just emerging from beneath the epiglottic elevating bar. Resistance will be felt as the ETT elevates this bar and exits the distal end of the ILMA and enters the patient's glottis. Tracheal placement is confirmed by end-tidal CO_2 detection and other clinical means as indicated. Manipulation of the ILMA by the metal handle may enhance successful passage in the event of failure.

Recent evidence suggests that the ILMA in situ produces sufficient pressure on the posterior hypopharyngeal wall to potentially compromise mucosal blood flow.[45] For this reason, except perhaps in an airway rescue or resuscitation situation, it is recommended that the device be withdrawn over the ETT. A stabilizing rod is provided with the ILMA to hold the ETT in position while the ILMA is withdrawn.

It should be emphasized that the insertion of an ILMA may be difficult if the interdental gap is less than 20 mm. Furthermore, the rigidity of the airway limits any adjustment to neck position. Many investigators have studied the effectiveness of the blind intubating technique through the ILMA. The reported mean (range) first-time and overall success rate is 73% (53–100) and 90% (44–100), respectively.[36] Several factors that decrease success rates of the blind intubation through the ILMA technique have been identified: the use of a #3 ILMA instead of a #4 or #5 ILMA for adult male patients, the application of cricoid pressure, lifting the ILMA handle, the use of a collar, and an inexperienced user.[36]

11.3.3 What other techniques have been described to enhance success rates for tracheal intubation through the ILMA?

Several studies have been published evaluating the effectiveness of a laryngoscope to assist ILMA intubation. The overall success rate appears to be no better than the blind technique. Light-guided techniques employing a flexible lightwand (Trachlight™) have also been investigated and have demonstrated improved success rates.[46,47] Lightwand-guided intubation through the ILMA has a first-time and overall success rate of 84% and 99%, respectively.[36]

Fiberoptic-guided intubation through the ILMA has a first time and overall success rate of 87% and 96%, respectively. However, following a failed blind technique, fiberoptic-guided intubation through the ILMA has a success rate of only 86%.[36]

11.3.4 What are the indications for the ILMA?

The ILMA alone does not prevent the aspiration of gastric contents and may produce hypopharyngeal mucosal ischemia if it is left in place for a prolonged duration. Therefore, its role in routine airway management may be limited. However, when used as a temporizing maneuver, it is a highly effective device in the emergency environment as an adjunct to failed or difficult BMV, and as a rescue device in the failed airway. Brain has suggested that the ILMA may not be indicated when the patient is anticipated to be an easy intubation (easy direct laryngoscopy), but may be of considerable benefit when the glottis is high and anterior (difficult direct laryngoscopy).

With respect to Emergency Medical Services (EMS) and prehospital care, the importance of early and effective airway control in trauma is universally acknowledged. Tracheal intubation under direct laryngoscopy is associated with a number of practical problems in prehospital trauma care and, there is evidence to suggest that the ILMA can play an important role in the prehospital setting in securing the airway of trauma patients with a head injury.[48,49]

The prime role of the ILMA lies in managing the airway for patients with a difficult or a failed airway. A retrospective study involving 254 patients with a difficult airway included patients with

- Cormack/Lehane (C/L) Grade 4 views,
- patients with immobilized cervical spines,
- patients with airways distorted by surgery or radiation therapy, and
- patients wearing stereotactic frames.

In these patients, the clinical experience with the ILMA (both elective and emergency use) was largely positive.[50,51] The Difficult Airway Society guidelines for management of the unanticipated difficult tracheal intubation in the nonobstetric adult patient without upper airway obstruction now include the ILMA.[52]

Further, recent studies have confirmed earlier findings that ventilation and intubation through the LMA Fastrach™ can be successfully achieved in obese patients with BMI >30.[53,54]

11.4 PROSEAL™ LARYNGEAL MASK AIRWAY (PLMA)

11.4.1 What is the PLMA? How does it differ from the LMA?

The PLMA (Intavent Orthofix, Maidenhead, UK, Figure 11-3) is a laryngeal mask variant that incorporates several modifications to the LMA:

- An esophageal conduit is incorporated to provide access to the esophagus and the gastrointestinal tract to minimize the risk of aspiration. This incorporated conduit renders a "dual tube" look to the device.

- A second cuff on the "dorsal" aspect of the PLMA is intended to enhance the seal characteristics of the device.
- The PLMA lacks mask aperture bars and (like the ILMA) has a deeper bowl, which makes the migration of the epiglottis into the distal lumen of the device less likely.
- The PLMA also has a flexible wire-reinforced airway tube to improve flexibility and minimize kinking, and a bite-block to reduce the danger of airway obstruction, or tube damage due to biting.

The drainage conduit traverses the bowl of the cuff on its way to the upper esophagus in an effort to reduce the risk of gastric insufflation when positive pressure is applied to the airway. Standard gastric tubes (≤18 French [Fr] gauge) can be accommodated by the conduit to facilitate the gastric decompression and aspiration. An accessory vent under the drain tube is intended to prevent the pooling of secretions and can act as an accessory ventilation port.[55]

Employing moderate force to advance the laryngeal cuff forward into the periglottic tissues may improve the airway seal. The dual tube arrangement seems to reduce the incidence of accidental device rotation occurring during anesthesia. This feature enhances the ability to secure the device in position giving greater confidence for use in longer procedures.

11.4.2 How is the PLMA placed?

The PLMA is inserted similarly to the LMA. While there is no randomized controlled study comparing the placement technique of the PLMA with or without a muscle relaxants, it has recently been shown that successful placement of the PLMA requires deeper anesthesia when compared with the LMA.[56]

Three insertion techniques for the PLMA have been advocated:

1. The Introducer Assisted Insertion Technique: Prior to its placement, the PLMA is loaded onto an introducer by placing the distal end of a metal introducer in an 'insertion strap' on the PLMA (Figure 11-4). The airway tube is folded around the introducer and 'clipped' into a proximal matching slot. The head and neck of the patient should be placed in a sniffing position. Following the placement of the PLMA, the introducer is removed as the PLMA is held in position.

2. The Digital Technique: Similar to the LMA, the digital technique involves the placement of the index finger under the insertion strap during the insertion of the PLMA.

3. The Tracheal Introducer Guided Insertion Technique: This is probably the most reliable technique to optimally place the tip of the PLMA cuff in the hypopharynx.[57] Following the placement of the tracheal introducer (e.g., the Eschmann Tracheal Introducer) into the esophagus under direct vision with a laryngoscope, the PLMA is guided into position by placing the tracheal introducer through the esophageal conduit (Figure 11-7). While this is technique enjoys a high success rate, it is probably more stimulating and traumatic.

Proper placement of the PLMA can be confirmed by a number of techniques. Air leaks through the drainage tube at low airway pressures suggest malposition of the PLMA. Though air leaks are

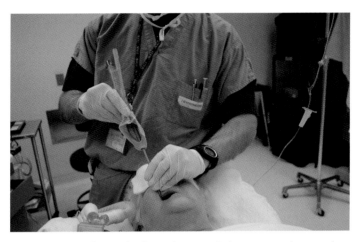

FIGURE 11-7. The Tracheal Introducer guided insertion technique of the LMA ProSeal™. Following the placement of the tracheal introducer into the esophagus under direct vision with a laryngoscope the PLMA is guided into position by placing the tracheal introducer through the esophageal conduit.

ordinarily easily detected by auscultating or by feeling air exiting the drainage tube, a small volume leak is probably best detected by the soap bubble test.[58] Three other tests have been suggested to check the patency of the drainage tube including passing a gastric tube though the drainage tube; passing a FFB through the drainage tube; and performing a suprasternal notch tap while observing the soap bubble or lubricant at the proximal end of the drainage tube for movement.[59]

11.4.3 What are the advantages of the PLMA compared to the LMA?

In principle, the PLMA would be expected to reduce the aspiration risk compared to the LMA. Laboratory (and cadaver) evidence are supportive of the theoretical efficacy of the PLMA.[60] However, clinical evidence is lacking, largely because the incidence of aspiration of gastric contents with the LMA is so low that it is difficult to demonstrate an improvement (0.02%). Aspiration of gastric contents has been reported with the PLMA.[61] Malposition of the PLMA has been identified as a cause of the aspiration.[62]

The design of the PLMA cuff significantly improves airway seal when compared to the LMA. The larger, softer, wedge-shaped PLMA cuff enables the anterior cuff to better adapt to the shape of the pharynx.[60] Most believe that pressure exerted on the pharyngeal mucosa by the cuffs of LMAs is the cause of sore throat seen with the device. Compared to the LMA, PLMA intracuff pressures are lower and airway seal pressure higher for any given intracuff volume.[63] Moreover, pressure exerted on the hypopharyngeal mucosa has been found to be below that considered critical for mucosal perfusion.

Perhaps the greatest limitation of the use of the LMA in small children is that the seal is often inadequate for PPV, even at high intracuff pressures. This does not appear to be as significant a limitation when the PLMA is used in these patients. Goldmann and Jakob showed that the first-time insertion of the PLMA in 30 children weighing 10–21 kg was always successful, associated with a seal sufficient to permit maximal tidal volume with PPV, produced

less gastric insufflation, and provided an improved bronchoscopic laryngeal view compared to the LMA.[64]

11.4.4 What are the disadvantages of the PLMA?

It is generally felt that the PLMA is more difficult to place than the LMA. The success rate for first-time PLMA insertion is lower than the first time insertion success rate for the LMA (average success rate of 85% with a range from 81 to 100% for the PLMA vs. average success rate of 93% with a range of 89–100% for LMA).[60] It is possible that the insertion difficulty may in part be related to the larger, deeper, and softer cuff of the PLMA. Although the learning curve for the insertion of the PLMA has not been studied, it has been suggested that 20–30 insertions of the PLMA are required before competency is achieved.[60]

11.4.5 What are the potential clinical uses of the PLMA?

The improved airway seal characteristics and touted lower risk of gastric aspiration of the PLMA compared to the LMA has expanded its applicability to surgical procedures that would not have been considered safe had an LMA been employed. These procedures include laparoscopy,[65] open abdominal surgery, surgery in patients with obesity, and in patients with gastroesophageal reflux.[60]

The PLMA has been used to provide ventilation and oxygenation in patients with a history of difficult laryngoscopic intubation.[66,67] Recently, a number of investigators reported the successful use of the PLMA to rescue a failed airway in obstetrical patients after a failed intubation.[61,68–72]

A number of studies involving volunteers under general anesthesia[73] and manikins have shown that the PLMA may play an important role in airway management in the trauma setting. Although supported by laboratory evidence,[74] there are no clinical case reports of the use of the PLMA in the trauma setting.

11.5 THE COMBITUBE™ (CBT)

11.5.1 What is CBT and how does it differ from the LMA?

The CBT (Tyco-Healthcare-Kendall-Sheridan, Mansfield, MA) (Figure 11-8) is an easily inserted and highly efficacious EGD. It is specified in the ASA Difficult Airway Algorithm as a primary rescue device in CICV situations. It also has been used successfully during CPR and in trauma patients.[5]

The CBT is a double-lumen airway which at the distal end has a proximal open-ended (tracheoesophageal) lumen and a distal-blocked lumen resembling an esophageal obturator airway.[75–79] The device has two balloons designed to trap the glottis between them. An oropharyngeal balloon is designed to be positioned just behind the posterior part of the hard palate. Once inflated, this balloon presses the base of the tongue in a ventrocaudal direction and the soft palate in a dorsocranial direction sealing the oral and

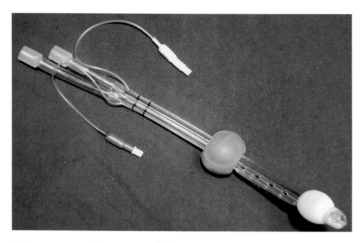

FIGURE 11-8. The combitube™ is a double-lumen airway, one open distally and the other closed distally (the former being more distal on the distal end of the device). The oropharyngeal balloon is designed to be positioned just behind the posterior part of the hard palate sealing both the mouth and nose. A smaller cuff seals the esophagus. Two printed ring marks at the proximal end of the tube indicate appropriate depth of insertion when the upper teeth or alveolar ridges are situated between these two marks.

nasal airways from behind. Another smaller cuff seals the esophagus once inflated. Perforations between the two balloons permit the egress of air or oxygen when PPV is applied to a proximal port. Two circumferential rings printed on the proximal end of the tube indicate proper depth of insertion when the upper teeth or alveolar ridges are situated between these two marks. The CBT is available in two sizes: the CBT 37F SA (Small Adult), to be used in patients 4–6 ft in height (approximately 120–180 cm), and the CBT 41 F, for patients taller than 6 ft (approximately >180 cm).

11.5.2   How is the CBT inserted?

Insertion is facilitated by bending the CBT between the balloons for a few seconds before insertion. It is made more pliable if heated to body temperature, attenuating its blunt trauma potential. Placement of the CBT is most readily performed with the patient's head placed in a neutral position,[78] although some clinicians prefer slight extension or flexion. The classical sniffing position is usually not helpful. In the fully awake patient, sedation and topical anesthesia may be necessary to ensure that the patient does not react to the insertion. To elevate the tongue and epiglottis, a jaw lift is performed by grasping the lower jaw with the thumb and forefinger. The CBT is inserted blindly along the surface of the tongue with initial gentle downward, curved, dorsocaudal movement and then directed parallel to the patient's horizontal plane until the printed ring marks lie between the upper and lower teeth, or alveolar ridges in edentulous patients. After insertion, the oropharyngeal balloon of the CBT 37 F is inflated with 85 mL of air through a blue pilot balloon. The corresponding filling volume for the CBT 41 F is 100 mL. Then, the distal balloon is inflated with approximately 10 mL of air.

With blind insertion, the CBT is successfully placed in the esophagus in more than 95% of cases. Ventilation is achieved via a longer blue connector (No. 1), leading to the proximal lumen, which is contiguous with pharyngeal perforations between the two

balloons. The trachea is effectively ventilated because the nose, mouth, and esophagus are sealed by the two balloons. The second "tracheoesophageal" lumen of the CBT can be used for decompression of the esophagus and stomach, thereby minimizing the risk of aspiration.

Auscultation of breath sounds over the chest, the absence of gastric insufflation, end-tidal CO_2 detection, and esophageal detection devices can all assist to confirm correct positioning.[80,81]

Should the CBT enter the trachea on blind insertion, it can function like a standard ETT and there will be no need for inflation of the pharyngeal cuff. Ventilation can be achieved through the shorter clear tube (No. 2) leading to the tracheal lumen.

Although it is rare, ventilation may be impossible through either the proximal or distal lumen. This usually signifies that the CBT has been placed too deeply, with the proximal lumen positioned in the esophagus and the oropharyngeal balloon obstructing the entrance to the larynx. After deflation of the balloons, the CBT should be withdrawn approximately 2–3 cm. While the CBT may be inserted blindly, the use of a laryngoscope is recommended, whenever possible.

11.5.3   What are the advantages of the CBT, compared to the LMA?

The CBT was designed primarily for the use in CPR,[76,82] even by nonmedical personnel. It has been demonstrated to permit effective ventilation during routine surgery, as well as in the ICU.[83] Most believe that the principal role of the CBT is in emergency airway control when endotracheal intubation is not immediately possible.[84–87] The CBT may be kept in situ for up to 8 hours, and it allows controlled mechanical ventilation at inflating pressures as high as 50 cm H_2O (see aspiration potential below). The CBT can be replaced by deflation of the oropharyngeal balloon and insertion of an ETT either under direct laryngoscopy or indirect view using a FFB, placed anteriorly or laterally to the CBT.

Several case reports describe the successful use of the CBT in cases of unanticipated difficult airways.[88–90] Thus, it is not surprising that the ASA task force on difficult airway management lists the CBT, along with the LMA and transtracheal jet ventilation, as CICV rescue methods.[5,91] Consequently, the CBT should be part of a portable kit for the management of difficult airways.

A major advantage of the CBT over conventional endotracheal intubation is that the device can be inserted with the head and neck in a neutral position. Additionally, it requires only modest mouth opening for insertion, and its tubular profile permits insertion in situations that cannot be negotiated by more bulky devices. The CBT can be inserted from a variety of angles making it useful in awkward environments (e.g., a patient who is trapped in a vehicle, see Chapter 30). The CBT may be of special benefit in patients with massive bleeding or regurgitation, when visualization of the vocal cords is impossible. While protection from aspiration is not absolute, the CBT seems to be relatively effective in this regard.

11.5.4   What are the disadvantages of the CBT?

While the esophageal cuff offers some protection against the reflux of gastric contents into the periglottic area, the level of protection against aspiration does not approach that of a cuffed ETT.

The suctioning of tracheal secretions is impossible when the CBT is in the esophageal position. To address the issue of secretions and suctioning, Krafft et al. proposed a modification in the CBT in which the two anterior, proximal perforations of the CBT are replaced by a single, larger, ellipsoid-shaped hole that allows for fiberoptic access of the trachea, tracheal suctioning, and tube exchange over a guide wire.[92] It should be noted that recently developed FFBs (e.g., Storz, Tuttlingen, Germany) with a small outer diameter (3 mm OD) allow passage through the unmodified pharyngeal perforations.

Contraindications to the use of the CBT include an intact gag reflex, airway obstruction by foreign bodies, tumors or swelling, the presence of known esophageal disease, and the prior ingestion of caustic substances.

Complications associated with the use of the CBT have been reported.[93,94] In a 1998 study of cardiac arrest patients, four cases of subcutaneous emphysema, pneumomediastinum, and pneumoperitoneum associated with the CBT during prehospital management were reported.[94] The reason for these complications appeared to be hyperinflation of the distal balloon (20–40 mL), although external chest compression and continuous PPV may also have been factors.

11.5.5 What are the potential clinical uses of the CBT?

The CBT is an easy-to-use, rapidly inserted emergency airway device that has performed satisfactorily in many circumstances. It is accepted as a primary rescue device in CICV situations, as well as for CPR, and in trauma patients. The CBT has been recommended in "Practice Guidelines for Management of the Difficult Airway" of the ASA.[5] It has also been recommended in the "Guidelines for Cardiopulmonary Resuscitation and Emergency Cardiac Care" of the AHA. In 2000, the CBT was upgraded by the AHA as a class II device. Furthermore, the CBT may provide an element of protection in patients at risk for aspiration, and it may be of benefit for patients in whom manipulation of the cervical spine is hazardous or impossible. Successfully placed, the device is capable of facilitating adequate sufficient ventilation and oxygenation and in most instances is as effective as endotracheal intubation.[95]

11.6 LARYNGEAL TUBE (LT)

11.6.1 What is the LT and how does it differ from the LMA?

The laryngeal tube airway (VBM Medizintechnik, Sulz am Neckar, Germany) (Figure 11-9), also known as the King LT™ in North America, is an EGD, which was introduced to the European market in 1999.[96] It is similar in appearance and function to the CBT and is available in three configurations (see below). The fundamental configuration of the LT is a silicone airway tube with ventilation outlet perforations lying between two cuffs, pharyngeal and esophageal. As opposed to the CBT, the LT has a single pilot balloon connected to both cuffs and a single 15-mm standard male adapter. The airway tube is short and "J" shaped with an average diameter of 1.5 cm leading to a blind tip.

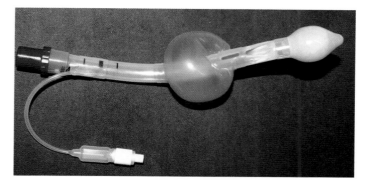

FIGURE 11-9. The King LT™ Airway consists of a silicone airway tube with two ventilation outlet perforations lying between two cuffs, a single pilot balloon, and a 15 mm male adapter.

The device requires a mouth opening of at least 23 mm for its insertion. After device placement, the proximal cuff should lie in the hypopharynx and the distal cuff in the upper esophagus. Both cuffs are high volume–low pressure in design to establish an adequate seal while minimizing the risk for ischemic mucosal damage. Two ventilation outlets are located between the two cuffs, in the anterior aspect of the tube. The proximal outlet is "protected" by a "V" shaped deflection in the pharyngeal cuff such that when the cuff is inflated soft tissue is deflected from this opening, helping to maintain a patency. There are two side holes near the distal outlet.

The design of the inflation system allows the pharyngeal cuff to be filled first stabilizing the position of the tube.[96] Once it has molded to the anatomy of the patient, the esophageal cuff inflates. Six sizes, suitable for neonates up to large adults, are available. Safe inflation of the dual cuffs may be enhanced with the aid of a cuff pressure gauge and limited to 60 cm H_2O.

There are three versions of the laryngeal tube: single-use laryngeal tube, laryngeal tube-Suction II, and single-use laryngeal tube-Suction II.[97] Similar to the PLMA, the laryngeal tube-Suction has two lumens: one for ventilation and the other serves as a conduit to the esophagus and stomach.

11.6.2 How is an LT inserted?

An appropriately sized LT should be selected based on the patient's weight and height. Prior to insertion, the cuffs should be completely deflated and well lubricated. The device should be inserted with the patient's head and neck in a "sniffing" or neutral position.[97] The head is extended on the neck with the nondominant hand to open the mouth. The LT is then inserted blindly in the midline, with the tip pressed against the hard palate. The LT is then advanced along the palate into the hypopharynx until resistance is felt at a point where a middle, proximal horizontal black line is aligned with the front teeth. The device is usually easily inserted with insertion times being comparable to those reported for the LMA.[98]

The device provides a patent airway in the majority of patients following the first insertion attempt. Success does not require extensive training.[99] Indicators of correct placement include end-tidal CO_2 detection, auscultation of the bilateral breath sounds, absence of gastric insufflation, and adequate chest movement. Capnographic waveform analysis may also be of use in confirming proper positioning of the LT. A brief period of PPV may also confirm proper alignment of the LT and the absence of obstruction. As with the other EGDs, it is important to become familiar with employing the LT in spontaneously ventilating patients prior to using it with prolonged PPV.

The LT should be removed with the patient either deeply anesthetized or totally awake. In an awake patient, the LT should be removed only when airway protective reflexes have completely returned.

Correct placement of the LT may also be verified using a lightwand (Trachlight™). The Trachlight™ (without the internal stiff wire stylet) is inserted into the LT and advanced until a faint glow can be seen above the thyroid prominence. This indicates that the tip of the lightwand is just above the laryngeal inlet. The lightwand is then advanced further until a well-defined circumscribed glow is seen in the anterior neck slightly below the thyroid prominence, indicating entrance into the glottis and correct positioning of the LT. Incorrect positioning would involve a lateral glow, or a glow with a halo, indicating malpositioning of the ventilation orifice.

11.6.3   What are the advantages of the LT compared to the LMA?

Insertion of this device is relatively easy and successful in most patients on the first attempt. It is simple to use and insertion is rapidly learned. The soft tip minimizes mechanical trauma on insertion and high-volume/low-pressure cuffs provide a good seal and protection against mucosal ischemic damage. A single pilot balloon confers an element of simplicity and speed in emergency situations. Other advantages of LT include:

1. The adequacy of ventilation with the LT is comparable to that obtained with other EGDs. The ease of insertion and high quality of the seal achieved may confer a preferred role for the LT in airway management during CPR.[99]

2. The esophageal cuff of the laryngeal tube may provide an element of protection against the reflux of gastric contents into the periglottic area, and the LT suction devices permit gastric decompression. Both of these features may reduce the risk of aspiration, relative to the LMA.[100,101]

3. Compared to the LMA, placement of an ETT through an LT with a FFB is substantially easier.[102]

4. Due to the form and length of the tube, an unintended tracheal intubation should not occur.

5. As compared to the face mask, like most EGDs the LT allows a better airway patency, reduced dead space, a "free hand" and reduced environmental pollution from waste anesthetic gases and vapors.

11.6.4   What are the disadvantages of the LT?

1. Protection from aspiration is less than that offered by a cuffed ETT and in high aspiration-risk situations tracheal intubation remains necessary.

2. The intracuff pressure may increase by as much as 15 cm H_2O within 30 minutes after its insertion if nitrous oxide is employed in the anesthetic technique related to the diffusion of this gas into the cuff. Manometric monitoring of the cuff pressure has been suggested.[103]

3. Position adjustments to ensure airflow continuity may be required more frequently in obese patients.[104]

4. PPV through the LT may provide inadequate ventilation in patients who require high pulmonary inflation pressures.

5. The mouth opening required for LT insertion is at least 23 mm.

6. As with any EGD, the LT cannot be used in the presence of anatomic distortion of the upper airway, such as lesions of the epiglottis or laryngopharynx.

11.6.5   What are the potential clinical uses of the LT?

In anesthetic practice, the LT can be used in patients who are candidates for face-mask- or LMA-delivered anesthesia. It may also find a role in the failed airway, similar to that of the LMA and the CBT.

The dimension and position of the ventilation holes and the protection offered by the overhanging cuff block permit the insertion of a suction catheter, ETT exchange device, an FFB, or an Eschmann Introducer over which an ETT may be passed.[102]

11.6.6   How should the LT be disinfected?

A reusable LT should be cleaned and sterilized before use. It can be washed with soap and warm water, or with an 8–10% sodium bicarbonate solution. Exposure chemicals, disinfectants, or cleaning agents are not recommended for silicone devices. Prior to sterilizing the LT, all air must be removed from the cuffs. With the cuffs deflated, the device may be steam autoclaved. The maximum autoclave temperature should not exceed 134°C at 35 psi for 10 minutes. After autoclaving, and before each use, the LT must be tested.

11.7   LARYVENT™ (LV)

11.7.1   What is the LV and how does it differ from the LMA?

The LV (B+P Beatmungs-Produkte GmbH, Seelscheid, Germany) consists of a single tube with a standard male connector, two cuffs with a single pilot balloon, and a ventilation outlet. The superior cuff lies in the hypopharynx and in the ventral part, and the cuff contains the orifice for ventilation. The inferior cuff is smaller and should lie at the level of the upper esophageal sphincter. As with other EGDs, the insertion of the LV is a blind technique and appears to have a rapid learning curve, similar to that of the LT.

11.7.2   How do you insert the LV?

Prior to the use of the LV, the cuffs should be tested by inflating 50 mL of air. During insertion, the tip of the LV should be introduced along the posterior wall of pharynx and advanced until resistance is felt. The cuffs should then be inflated with 50 mL of air. There should be little resistance to filling. If there is resistance, the LV has been introduced too deeply and should be retracted 2–3 cm before reattempting cuff inflation.

11.7.3   What are the advantages of the LV compared to the LMA?

The advantages of the LV are similar to those of the LT. In their early clinical experience, Dörges et al. reported that the device provided ventilation and oxygenation comparable to the LT.[105]

11.7.4   What are the disadvantages of the LV?

The more complex handling, resulting in a significantly higher failure rate, and postoperative patient discomfort suggest that the LV may not be the first choice in routine anesthesia practice.[105]

11.7.5   What are the potential clinical uses of the LV?

The role and advantage of the LV are similar to those of the LT. The precise advantages have not yet been defined by clinical trials.

11.8   AIRWAY MANAGEMENT DEVICE™ (AMD)

11.8.1   What is the AMD and how does it differ from the LMA?

The AMD (Nagor Limited, Isle of Man; manufactured by Biosil Ltd, Cumbernauld, UK, Figure 11-10) is a newly introduced EGD.[106] The AMD consists of a clear silicone dual lumen tube that is concave ventrally with inflatable oropharyngeal and hypopharyngeal cuffs. An oval ventilation port is located in the ventral part of the device opposite the laryngeal inlet. The connector at the proximal end of the tube is Y shaped incorporating ports for anesthetic gas delivery and providing access for suction catheters, an FFB, or an Eschmann Introducer. One lumen provides a channel into the esophagus for suction. When fully inflated, the upper cuff fills elevating the tongue and epiglottis in a manner similar to the CBT. The cuffs have independent, color-coded inflation controls. The shape of the cuffs ensures correct orientation in the airway and prevents both lateral movement and rotation of the tube. The AMD is available in several sizes: 3–3.5 for patients weighing 30–60 kg and size 4–5 for patients more than 60 kg.

11.8.2   How is the AMD inserted?

The insertion technique is similar to other EGDs. Both cuffs of the AMD should be well lubricated, the pharyngeal cuff should be fully deflated, and the esophageal cuff should have 5–9 mL of air.

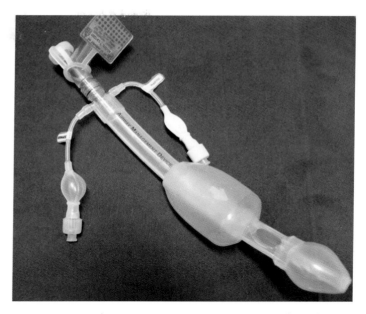

FIGURE 11-10. The Airway Management Device™ is a clear silicone tube with hypopharyngeal and oropharyngeal cuffs. An oval hole located between the two cuffs in the ventral part of the device allows ventilation.

This closes the esophageal cuff channel and permits atraumatic insertion. The AMD, held in the dominant hand, is inserted in the midline of the mouth in a caudal direction until it seats properly in the hypopharynx. The pharyngeal cuff is then inflated with 50–80 mL of air. Like other EGDs, proper placement should be confirmed by end-tidal CO_2, auscultation, and other clinical signs.

11.8.3   What are the advantages of the AMD compared to the LMA?

A key feature of this device lies in the access it provides to the esophagus when the esophageal cuff is partially deflated. A suction catheter can be introduced through the device without interrupting ventilation after deflating the lower cuff to aspirate the esophagus. As with the LT, the device is relatively easy to use and it provides an element of protection against aspiration.

11.8.4   What are the disadvantages of the AMD?

The device is somewhat difficult to insert and airway trauma is possible.[106–108] Cook et al. reported a first-time success rate of 66% in establishing the airway with an average of 0.56 manipulations per patient and a primary failure rate of 11%.[107] While the AMD may provide protection against aspiration, presently there are no data to support the claim.

11.8.5   What are the potential clinical uses of the AMD?

While the dynamic relationship between the hypopharyngeal cuff and the esophageal suction port is interesting, the precise advantage of the AMD is difficult to define at this time.

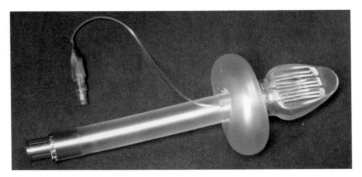

FIGURE 11-11. The CobraPLA™ consists of a breathing tube with a circumferential inflatable cuff proximal to the ventilation outlet portion, a 15-mm standard adapter, and a distal widened "Cobra head" designed to separate the soft tissues of the hypopharynx and permit ventilation.

11.9   CobraPLA™ PERILARYNGEAL AIRWAY (CPLA)

11.9.1   What is the CPLA and how does it differ from the LMA?

The CPLA (Engineered Medical Systems, Inc., Indianapolis, IN, Figure 11-11) consists of a breathing tube with a circumferential inflatable cuff proximal to a ventilation outlet, a 15 mm standard adapter, and a distal widened cobra-shaped head designed to separate soft tissues and to allow ventilation of the trachea. Once in place, the cobra head lies in front of the laryngeal inlet. Internal to the cobra head, a ramp directs ventilation into the trachea. A soft grille shields the inferior aperture of the device in an attempt to deflect the epiglottis anteriorly off the cobra head. The bars of the grill are sufficiently flexible to permit an ETT to pass easily. The cuff is shaped such that it resides in the hypopharynx at the base of the tongue and when inflated, raises the base of the tongue exposing the laryngeal inlet and effects an airway seal. The unique shape of the distal part of the device allows it to slide easily along the hard palate during insertion, and moves soft tissues away from the laryngeal inlet once in place.

The CPLA is available in eight sizes. Size selection is governed by the weight of the patient. Generally, a #3 is used in most female

TABLE 11-1

Size Selection of CobraPLA™ as Suggested by the Manufacturer

SIZE	WEIGHT (kg)
½	2.5–7.5
1	5–15
1½	10–35
2	20–60
3	40–100
4	70–130
5	100–160
6	Over 130

TABLE 11-2

Cuff Inflation Volumes for the CobraPLA™ as Suggested by the Manufacturer

SIZE	MILLILITERS
3	<65
4	<70
5	<85

patients, a #4 for most men, and a #5 for larger men. When one is unsure which size is best, or when learning placement technique, selecting the lower size is recommended. The manufacturer's size selection and cuff inflation volume guidelines are shown in Tables 11-1 and 11-2. Agrò et al.[109] suggested alternative size selection using weight intervals (Table 11-3) and alternative cuff inflation volumes (Table 11-4). They found that in general, larger sizes required considerably higher cuff pressures to produce an acceptable seal compared to the smaller sizes.

11.9.2   How do you insert the CPLA?

The CPLA is simple to insert, though somewhat more difficulty is encountered in the obese.[110,111] Prior to insertion, the pharyngeal cuff is fully deflated and folded back against the breathing tube. The back of the cobra head and cuff are lubricated, taking care that the lubricant does not obstruct the grille. The patient's head is placed in the sniffing position. A jaw lift is performed and the distal end of the CPLA is directed straight back through the mouth between the tongue and hard palate. Modest neck extension (without a jaw lift maneuver) may aid the passage of the device as it turns toward the glottis at the back of the mouth. Once the CPLA traverses the back of the mouth, it usually turns caudally toward the larynx with minimal resistance as the flexible distal tip guides the device downward. The CPLA is properly seated above the glottis when modest resistance to further distal passage is encountered. Once inserted, the flexible tip lies behind the arytenoids, the cuff lies in the hypopharyx at the base of the tongue, and the ramp lifts the epiglottis. Then the cuff is inflated until the leak with PPV disappears. Indicators of correct placement are absence of leak on auscultation of the neck, bilateral breath sounds, absence of gastric insufflation, easily accomplished chest movement, and positive CO_2 detection. Exceeding a peak airway pressure of 25 cm H_2O of airway pressure with PPV is not recommended, even when

TABLE 11-3

Size Selection of CobraPLA™ for Adults as Suggested by Agrò et al.[110]

SIZE	WEIGHT (kg)
3	<60
4	60–80
5	>80

TABLE 11-4

Cuff Inflation Volumes for the CobraPLA™ as Suggested by Agrò et al.[110]

SIZE	MILLILITERS
3	26.5 ± 2.1
4	31.9 ± 4.0
5	40.0 ± 4.1

testing for ventilation and cuff seal, because of the risk of gastric insufflation.

If the CPLA is not inserted far enough, inflation of the cuff may cause the tongue to protrude from the mouth of the patient. In this situation, the cuff should be deflated and the device advanced further or a smaller sized CPLA selected. It is possible to advance the cobra head beyond the laryngeal inlet, in which case ventilation will not be possible. The CPLA should be removed awake with the airway protective reflexes intact.

11.9.3   What are the advantages of the CPLA compared to the LMA?

The tube of the CPLA has a larger lumen than most EGDs and may be particularly useful in directing fiberoptic-assisted tracheal intubation,[112] especially when larger ETTs are indicated (Table 11-5). In addition, it has been made short enough that its removal after insertion of an ETT is greatly facilitated.

The CPLA can be used as a "rescue airway" in CICV or "can't intubate/difficult to ventilate" scenarios. As with similar EGDs, a Trachlight™ with the rigid internal stylet removed can be used in lieu of an FFB to facilitate tracheal intubation. Although less reliable, blind tracheal intubation through the CPLA using a generic tracheal tube introducer (e.g., the Eschmann Introducer) may be possible.

Like many other EGDs, the insertion technique is simple and has been accomplished by personnel with little or no experience. The airway sealing characteristics seem to be superior to the LMA.[111]

TABLE 11-5

Endotracheal Tube Size Selection for Different Sizes of CobraPLA™

SIZE	ETT
½	3.0
1	4.5
1½	4.5
2	6.5
3	6.5
4	8.0
5	8.0
6	8.0

A number of reports have supported the use of the CPLA in the CICV situation, a factor related to the unique design of the device.[110,113]

11.9.4   What are the disadvantages of the CPLA?

The CPLA is not appropriate for patients with low lung compliance or increased airway resistance. The major disadvantage of the device is that it does not protect against aspiration and does not secure the airway as effectively as an ETT.[114] Until more clinical studies become available, it is difficult to determine the role of the CPLA in airway management.

11.10   THE STREAMLINED PHARYNX AIRWAY LINER (SLIPA™)

11.10.1   What is the SLIPA and how does it differ from the LMA?

The SLIPA (SLIPA Med, Cape Town, South Africa), (Figure 11-12) is a relatively new disposable EGD. It is designed for airway management during controlled ventilation.[115,116] The peculiar shape of the device provides a seal without the use of a inflatable cuff.

The body of the SLIPA is shaped like a hollow boot with "toe," "bridge," and "heel" prominences, designed to engage the mucosal lining of the patient's pharynx. Its hollow configuration and shape permits the entrapment of secretions, blood, or gastric contents in the device should they find themselves to the hypopharynx, reducing the risk of aspiration. The device is formed from soft plastic material, flexible enough to allow easy insertion. The hollow chamber flattens to facilitate insertion. After the placement, the "toe" should sit in hypopharynx, the "bridge" in the pyriform fossae, and the "heel" should slide into the nasopharyngeal opening and soft palate. The bridge, with its two lateral bulges, fits into the pyriform fossae, displacing tissue away from the posterior pharyngeal wall. The heel of the chamber anchors the SLIPA in position by sliding over the soft palate and nasopharyngeal opening. Toward the toe side of the bridge, are smaller lateral bulges that coincide with the inferior cornus of the hyoid bone designed to relieve pressure on relevant nervous tissues such as the superior laryngeal branch of the vagus.

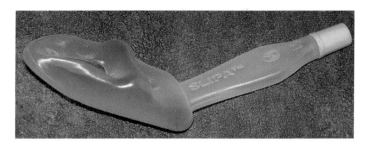

FIGURE 11-12. The SLIPA™ is shaped like a hollow boot with "toe," "bridge" and "heel" prominences, designed to engage the patient's pharynx. The hollow design feature permits the entrapment of liquids such as secretions, blood, and gastric fluids preventing aspiration.

11.10.2   How is the SLIPA inserted?

The SLIPA is inserted similarly to the LMA. Held in the dominant hand, it is inserted in the midline of the mouth, pressed against hard palate, and advanced until resistance is felt. A jaw lift may facilitate placement. The crescent shape of the toe minimizes the risk of downward folding of the epiglottis which may lead to airway obstruction. The toe of the device slips easily into the esophagus, where it creates a seal. After placement, the SLIPA returns to its preinsertion shape.

11.10.3   What are the advantages and disadvantages of the SLIPA compared to the LMA?

There may be a lower risk of gastric insufflation relative to the LMA, reducing the risk of regurgitation and aspiration, should reflux occur. However, currently there are no data to support this assertion.

Problems with the device have yet to be reported.

11.10.4   What are the potential clinical uses of the SLIPA device?

While the SLIPA may have a lower risk of aspiration in the presence of PPV, there are few clinical trials in this regard.

11.11   CUFFED OROPHARYNGEAL AIRWAY (COPA)

11.11.1   What is the COPA and how does it differ from the LMA?

The COPA (Mallinckrodt Medical, Athlone, Ireland), Figure 11-13) was first described in 1992 by Greenberg.[117] It was intended for use during anesthesia in spontaneously breathing patients. The device is a modified Guedel airway, with an inflatable distal cuff and a proximal 15 mm connector. The flange at the proximal end is fitted with two posts for securing a strap, which is used to stabilize the device in the mouth against the upper teeth or gums.

The COPA is available in four sizes: 8, 9, 10, and 11 (the numbers refer to the length of the shaft of the device, i.e., the distance in centimeters between the flange and the distal tip).

11.11.2   How is the COPA inserted?

The COPA is inserted in the same fashion as a Guedel airway, with a rotating movement.

11.11.3   What are the advantages of the COPA compared to the LMA?

Agrò et al.[118] demonstrated the ability of the COPA to guide an ETT into the trachea employing a light-guided technique with a lightwand. In that study, a lightwand (Trachlight™) was inserted into the COPA to confirm proper placement. The lightwand was then removed and a tube exchange catheter (TE) was inserted

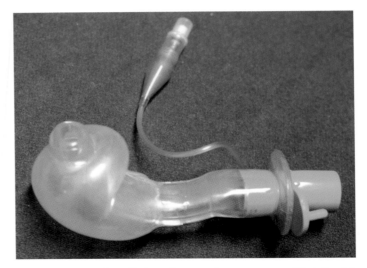

FIGURE 11-13. The cuffed oropharyngeal airway is a modified Guedel airway with an inflatable distal cuff and a proximal 15 mm connector. The flange at the proximal end is fitted with two posts for a securing strap to stabilize the device in the mouth against the upper teeth or gums.

through the COPA into the trachea. The proximal end of the TE was connected to a 15 mm connector. The TE's position in the trachea is confirmed by the presence of end-tidal CO_2 during ventilation. The patients were then paralyzed and ventilation through the TE reconfirmed. The COPA was removed leaving the TE in situ for the ETT to be guided into place. This combined technique was successful in 6 out of 10 patients.

11.11.4   What are the disadvantages of the COPA?

The COPA is contraindicated in patients at risk for aspiration. Compared to LMA, the COPA appears to have a higher incidence of postoperative sore throat and jaw and neck pain.[119]

11.11.5   What are the potential clinical uses of the COPA?

The simplicity of the COPA is its most compelling feature, enhancing its utility in many environments. It is smaller than most other devices and therefore may be particularly useful in patients with a restricted mouth opening. The COPA can be used to assist with the placement of an ETT, though the success rate is low.

11.12   PHARYNGEAL AIRWAY EXPRESS (PAXPRESS™—PAX)

11.12.1   What is the PAX and how does it differ from the LMA?

The PAX (Vital Signs, Totowa, NJ) is an EGD invented by Douglas Mongeon of Orange Park Acres, California. The PAX is made from polyvinyl chloride and intended for single use. It consists of a single curved tube with an inflatable cuff to be positioned in the proximal pharynx and a noninflatable, gilled, conical tip at the distal end. The tip forms a no-pressure seal in the hypopharynx that may minimize gastric insufflation and regurgitation. Between the cuff and tip on the inner curve is a rectangular vent that faces anteriorly toward the glottic inlet. The distal half of the vent has three vertical gills to prevent epiglottic intrusion and device obstruction. The internal diameter of the airway tube is about 12 mm. The maximum recommended cuff inflation volume is 60 mL. There is only one size for adults weighing >41 kg.

11.12.2 How is the PAX inserted?

Prior to insertion, the cuff is deflated and lubricated. During insertion, the PAX is held in the dominant hand like a pen. The mouth is opened with the nondominant hand and the PAX is advanced into the pharynx until resistance is felt. The cuff is then inflated with the pilot balloon until a seal sufficient to permit ventilation is achieved, or the maximum cuff inflation volume is reached.

11.12.3 What are the advantages of the PAX compared to the LMA?

The insertion success rate for the PAX is high and it is an effective ventilatory device with a low risk of gastric insufflation.[120] Mondello and Casati[121] evaluated the PAX in 91 patients undergoing surgery and demonstrated that the device provided safe and effective airway control during mechanical ventilation in all but one case (98% success).

11.12.4 What are the disadvantages of the PAX?

This device has been associated with a relatively high incidence of mucosal trauma. Further, mucosal pressures with the device in place may exceed pharyngeal perfusion pressure.

The PAX has a moderately high failure rate and produces more marked changes in hemodynamic variables when compared with those produced by the LMA.[122] However, further studies are required to evaluate safety and the incidence of airway trauma with this new extraglottic airway.

11.12.5 What are the potential clinical uses of the PAX?

Information about this device currently available would suggest that the PAX has limited applicability. However, its novel design characteristics may be of use in yet to be determined ways.

11.13 SUMMARY

During the last two decades, EGDs, such as the LMA™ and the CBT, have been shown to be effective and safe devices for delivering effective oxygenation and ventilation. In addition, many studies have shown that these devices can be used successfully to "rescue" patients with a failed airway. These devices are now recommended by authorities such as the ASA (Difficult Airway Management Algorithm) and the Difficult Airway Society (UK).

As a result of the widespread acceptance and popularity of EGDs, many newly designed reusable and disposable devices have been introduced. Preliminary clinical studies have demonstrated that these devices compare favorably with reusable counterparts. However, more studies are needed to confirm the safety and efficacy of these newer devices.

REFERENCES

1. Brimacombe J: A proposed classification system for extraglottic airway devices. *Anesthesiology.* 2004;101:559.
2. Caplan RA, Posner KL, Ward RJ, et al.: Adverse respiratory events in anesthesia: a closed claims analysis. *Anesthesiology.* 1990;72:828–833.
3. Langeron O, Masso E, Huraux C, et al.: Prediction of difficult mask ventilation. *Anesthesiology.* 2000;92:1229–1236.
4. Mulcaster JT, Mills J, Hung OR, et al.: Laryngoscopic intubation: learning and performance. *Anesthesiology.* 2003;98:23–27.
5. American Society of Anesthesiologists Task Force on Management of the Difficult Airway: Practice guidelines for management of the difficult airway: an updated report by the American Society of Anesthesiologists Task Force on Management of the Difficult Airway. *Anesthesiology.* 2003;98:1269–1277.
6. Bogetz MS: Using the laryngeal mask airway to manage the difficult airway. *Anesthesiol Clin North America.* 2002;20:863–870.
7. Brimacombe J, De Maio B: Emergency use of laryngeal mask airway during helicopter transfer of a neonate. *J Clin. Anaesthesia.* 1993;7:689–690.
8. Kokkinis K: The use of laryngeal mask airway in CPR. *Resuscitation.* 1994;27:9–12.
9. The use of laryngeal mask airway by nurses during cardiopulmonary resuscitation-results of multicenter trial. *Anaesthesia.* 1994;49:3–7.
10. Brimacombe JR: *Placement Phase, Laryngeal Mask Anesthesia*, 2nd edn. Brimacombe JR, ed. Philadelphia: Saunders, Elsevier Ltd., 2005: 191–240.
11. Garcia-Pedrajas F, Monedero P, Carrascosa F: Modification of Brain's technique for insertion of laryngeal mask airway. *Anesth Analg.* 1994;79:1024–1025.
12. Bignell S, Brimacombe J: LMA stabilization and fixation. *Anaesth Intens Care.* 1994;22:745.
13. Brimacombe JR: *Emergence Phase, Laryngeal Mask Anesthesia*, 2nd edn. Brimacombe JR, ed. Philadelphia: Saunders, Elsevier Ltd., 2005: 265–280.
14. Deakin CD, Diprose P, Majumdar R, Pulletz M: An investigation into the quantity of secretions removed by inflated and deflated laryngeal mask airway. *Anaesthesia.* 2000;55:478–480.
15. Brimacombe J: The advantages of the LMA over the tracheal tube or facemask: a meta-analysis—Clinical Report. *Can J Anesth.* 1995;42:1017–1023.
16. Benumof JL: Laryngeal mask airway and the ASA difficult airway algorithm. *Anesthesiology.* 1996;84:686–699.
17. Keller C, Brimacombe J: Bronchial mucus transport velocity in paralyzed anesthetized patient a comparison of the laryngeal mask airway and cuffed tracheal tube. *Anesth Analg.* 1998;86:1280–1282.
18. Verghese C, Brimacombe J: Survey of laryngeal mask airway usage in 11,910 patients: safety and efficacy for conventional and nonconventional usage. *Anesth Analg.* 1996;82:129–133.
19. Brimacombe J, Berry A: The incidence of aspiration associated with the laryngeal mask airway—a meta-analysis of published literature. *J Clin Anesth.* 1995;7:297–305.
20. Keller C, Brimacombe J, Bittersohl J, Lirk P, von Goedecke A: Aspiration and the laryngeal mask airway: three cases and a review of the literature. *Br J Anaesth.* 2004;93:579–582.
21. Keller C, Sparr HJ, Brimacombe JR: Positive pressure ventilation with the laryngeal mask airway in non-paralysed patients: comparison of sevoflurane and propofol maintenance techniques. *Br J Anaesth.* 1998;80:332–336.
22. Keller C, Sparr HJ, Luger TJ, Brimacombe J: Patient outcomes with positive pressure versus spontaneous ventilation in non-paralysed adults with the laryngeal mask. *Can J Anesth.* 1998;45:564–567.
23. Maltby JR, Beriault MT, Watson NC, Fick GH: Gastric distension and ventilation during laparoscopic cholecystectomy: LMA-Classic vs. tracheal intubation. *Can J Anesth.* 2000;47:622–626.
24. Sidaras G, Hunter JM: Is it safe to artificially ventilate a paralysed patient through the laryngeal mask? The jury is still out. *Br J Anaesth.* 2001;86:749–753.

25. Devitt JH, Wenstone R, Noel AG, O'Donnell MP: The Laryngeal Mask Airway and Positive-pressure Ventilation. *Anesthesiology*. 1994;80:550–555.

26. Johannigman JA, Branson RD, Davis K, Hurst JM: Techniques of emergency ventilation: A method to evaluate tidal volume, airway pressure and gastric insufflation. *J Trauma*. 1991;31:93–98.

27. Natalini G, Facchetti P, Dicembrini MA, et al.: Pressure controlled versus volume controlled ventilation with laryngeal mask airway. *J Clin Anesth*. 2001;13:436–439.

28. Griffin RM, Hatcher IS: Aspiration pneumonia and the laryngeal mask airway. *Anaesthesia*. 1990;45:1039–1040.

29. Ismail-Zade IA, Vanner RG: Regurgitation and aspiration of gastric contents in a child during general anaesthesia using the laryngeal mask airway. *Paediatr Anaesth*. 1996;6:325–328.

30. Nanji GM, Maltby JR: Vomiting and aspiration pneumonitis with the laryngeal mask airway. *Can J Anesth*. 1992;39:69–70.

31. Han TH, Brimacombe J, Lee EJ, Yang HS: The laryngeal mask airway is effective (and probably safe) in selected healthy parturients for elective Cesarean section: a prospective study of 1,067 cases. *Can J Anesth*. 2001;48:1117–1121.

32. Brimacombe JR: *Pediatrics, Laryngeal Mask Anesthesia*, 2nd edn. Brimacombe JR, ed. Philadelphia: Saunders, Elsevier Ltd., 2005: 357–389.

33. Basket P, Bossaert L, Carli P, et al.: Guidelines for the advanced airway management of the airway and ventilation during resuscitation. A statement by the Airway and Ventilation Management of the Working Group of the European Resuscitation Council. *Resuscitation*. 1996;31:187–200.

34. The American Heart Association: Guidelines 2000 for cardiopulmonary resuscitation and emergency cardiovascular care. Part 11: Neonatal resuscitation. *Circulation*. 2000;102:1343–1357.

35. Keidan I, Berkenstadt H, Segal E, Perel A: Pressure versus volume-controlled ventilation with a laryngeal mask airway in paediatric patients. *Paediatr Anaesth*. 2001;11:691–694.

36. Brimacombe JR: Intubating LMA for airway intubation. In: *Laryngeal Mask Anesthesia*, 2nd edn. Brimacombe JR, ed. Philadelphia: Saunders, Elsevier Ltd., 2005: 469–504.

37. Hung OR: Light-guided tracheal intubation through the laryngeal mask airway. *Anesth Analg*. 1997;85:1415.

38. Agro F, Brimacombe J, Berry A, et al.: Use of a lighted stylet for intubation via the laryngeal mask airway. *Can J Anaesth*. 1998;45:556–560.

39. Langenstein H: The laryngeal mask for difficult intubation. The results of a prospective study. *Anesthetists*. 1995;44:712–718.

40. Williams PJ, Bailey PM: Comparison of the reinforced laryngeal mask airway and tracheal intubation for adenotonsillectomy. *Br J Anaesth*. 1993;70:30–33.

41. Sher M, Brimacombe J, Laing D: Anaesthesia for laser pharyngoplasty: a comparison of the tracheal tube verses reinforced laryngeal mask airway. *Anaesth Intens Care*. 1995;23:149–154.

42. Quinn AC, Samaan A, McAteer EM, et al.: The reinforced laryngeal mask airway for dento-alveolar surgery. *Br J Anaesth*. 1996;77:185–188.

43. Brain AIJ, Verghese C, Addy EV, Kapila A, Brimacombe J: The intubating laryngeal mask. II: A preliminary clinical report of a new means of intubating the trachea. *Br J Anaesth*. 1997;79:704–709.

44. Wong JK, Tongier WK, Armbruster SC, White PF: Use of the intubating laryngeal mask airway to facilitate awake orotracheal intubation in patients with cervical spine disorders. *J Clin Anesth*. 1999;11:346–348.

45. Ulrich-Pur H, Hrska F, Krafft P, et al.: Comparison of mucosal pressures induced by cuffs of different airway devices. *Anesthesiology*. 2006;104:933–938.

46. Chan PL, Lee TW, Lam KK, Chan WS: Intubation through intubating laryngeal mask with and without a lightwand: a randomized comparison. *Anaesth Intens Care*. 2001;29:255–259.

47. Fan KH, Hung OR, Agro F: A comparative study of tracheal intubation using a fastrach alone or together with a lightwand. *J Clin Anesth*. 2000;12:581–585.

48. Asai T, Matsumoto H, Shingu K: Awake tracheal intubation through the intubating laryngeal mask. *Can J Anaesth*. 1999;46:182–184.

49. Mason AM: Use of the intubating laryngeal mask airway in pre-hospital care: a case report. *Resuscitation*. 2001;51:91–95.

50. Ferson DZ, Rosenblatt WH, Johansen MJ, Osborn I, Ovassapian A: Use of the intubating LMA-Fastrach in 254 patients with difficult-to-manage airways. *Anesthesiology*. 2001;95:1175–1181.

51. Langeron O, Semjen F, Bourgain JL, Marsac A, Cros AM: Comparison of the intubating laryngeal mask airway with the fiberoptic intubation in anticipated difficult airway management. *Anesthesiology*. 2001;94:968–972.

52. Henderson JJ, Popat MT, Latto IP, Pearce AC: Difficult Airway Society guidelines for management of the unanticipated difficult intubation. *Anaesthesia*. 2004;59:675–694.

53. Frappier J, Guenoun T, Journois D, et al.: Airway management using the intubating laryngeal mask airway for the morbidly obese patient. *Anesth Analg*. 2003;96:1510–1515.

54. Roblot C, Ferrandiere M, Bierlaire D, et al.: Impact of Cormack and Lehane's grade on Intubating Laryngeal Mask Airway Fastrach using: a study in gynaecological surgery. *Ann Fr Anesth Reanim*. 2005;24:487–491.

55. Keller C, Brimacombe J, Kleinsasser A, Loeckinger A: Does the ProSeal laryngeal mask airway prevent aspiration of regurgitated fluid? *Anesth Analg*. 2000;91:1017–1020.

56. Kodaka M, Okamoto Y, Koyama K, Miyao H: Predicted values of propofol EC50 and sevoflurane concentration for insertion of laryngeal mask Classic™ and ProSeal™. *Br J Anaesth*. 2004;92:242–245.

57. Howarth A, Brimacombe J, Keller C: Gum elastic bougie-guided placement of the ProSeal LMA. *Can J Anaesth*. 2002;49:528–529.

58. O'Connor CJ, Stix MS: Place the bubble solution with your fingertip. *Anesth Analg*. 2002;94:763–764.

59. O'Connor CJ, Borromeo CJ, Stix MS: Assessing ProSeal laryngeal positioning: the suprasternal notch test. *Anesth Analg*. 2002;94:1374–1375.

60. Cook TM, Gene L, Nolan JP: The ProSeal™ laryngeal mask airway: a review of the literature. *Can J Anaesth*. 2005;52:739–760.

61. Cook TM, Brooks TS, Van der Westhuizen J, Clarke M: The Proseal LMA is a useful rescue device during failed rapid sequence intubation: two additional cases. *Can J Anaesth*. 2005;52:630–633.

62. Brimacombe J, Keller C: Aspiration of gastric contents during use of a ProSeal™ laryngeal mask airway secondary to unidentified foldover malposition. *Anesth Analg*. 2003;97:1192–1194.

63. Keller C, Brimacombe J: Mucosal pressure and oropharyngeal leak pressure with the ProSeal versus laryngeal mask airway in anaesthetized paralysed patients. *Br J Anaesth*. 2000;85:262–266.

64. Goldmann K, Jakob C: Size 2 ProSeal™ laryngeal mask airway: a randomized, crossover investigation with the standard laryngeal mask airway in paediatric patients. *Br J Anaesth*. 2005;94:385–389.

65. Maltby JR, Beriault MT, Watson NC, Fick LD, Fick GH: The LMA-ProSeal™ is an effective alternative to tracheal intubation for laparoscopic cholecystectomy. *Can J Anaesth*. 2002;49:857–862.

66. Brimacombe J, Keller C: Awake fibreoptic-guided insertion of the ProSeal Laryngeal Mask Airway™. *Anesthesia*. 2002;57:719.

67. Ivascu BN, Fogarty MP, Mitera DM, Dhar P: Use of the ProSeal™ laryngeal mask airway in a pregnant patient with a difficult airway during electroconvulsive therapy. *Br J Anaesth*. 2003;91:752–754.

68. Awan R, Nolan JP, Cook TM: Use of a ProSeal laryngeal mask airway for airway maintenance during emergency Caesarean section after failed tracheal intubation. *Br J Anaesth*. 2004;92:144–146.

69. Bullingham A: Use of the ProSeal laryngeal mask airway for airway maintenance during emergency Caesarean section after failed intubation. *Br J Anaesth*. 2004;92:903.

70. Cook TM, Nolan JP: Failed obstetric tracheal intubation and postoperative respiratory support with the proseal laryngeal mask airway. *Anesth Analg*. 2005;100:290–291.

71. Keller C, Brimacombe J, Lirk P, Puhringer F: Failed obstetric tracheal intubation and postoperative respiratory support with the ProSeal laryngeal mask airway. *Anesth Analg*. 2004;98:1467–1470.

72. Vaida SJ, Gaitini LA: Another case of use of the ProSeal laryngeal mask airway in a difficult obstetric airway. *Br J Anaesth*. 2004;92:905.

73. Asai T, Murao K, Shingu K: Efficacy of the ProSeal™ laryngeal mask airway during manual in-line stabilisation of the neck. *Anaesthesia*. 2002;57: 918–920.

74. Genzwuerker H, Hundt A, Finteis T, Ellinger K: Comparison of different laryngeal mask airways in a resuscitation model. *Anasthesiol Intensivmed Notfallmed Schmerzther*. 2003;38:94–101.

75. Agro F, Frass M, Benumof JL, Krafft P: Current status of the Combitube: a review of the literature. *J Clin Anesth*. 2002;14:307–314.

76. Frass M, Frenzer R, Zdrahal F, et al.: The esophageal tracheal combitube: preliminary results with a new airway for CPR. *Ann Emerg Med*. 1987;16:768–772.

77. Urtubia R, Aguila C: Combitube: a new proposal for a confusing nomenclature. *Anesth Analg*. 1999;89:803.

78. Urtubia R, Aguila C: Combitube: a study for proper use. *Anesth Analg*. 2000;90:958–962.

79. Walz R, Davis S, Panning B: Is the Combitube a useful emergency airway device for anesthesiologists? (Letter). *Anesth Analg*. 1998;88:233.

80. Butler BD, Little T, Drtil S: Combined use of the esophageal-tracheal Combitube with a colorimetric carbon dioxide detector for emergency intubation/ventilation. *J Clin Monit*. 1995;11:311–316.

81. Wafai Y, Salem MR, Baraka A, et al.: Effectiveness of the self-inflating bulb for verification of proper placement of the Esophageal Tracheal Combitube. *Anesth Analg*. 1995;80:122–126.

82. Frass M, Frenzer R, Rauscha F, Schuster E, Glogar D: Ventilation with the esophageal tracheal combitube in cardiopulmonary resuscitation. Promptness and effectiveness. *Chest*. 1988;93:781–784.

83. Frass M, Frenzer R, Mayer G, Popovic R, Leithner C: Mechanical ventilation with the esophageal tracheal Combitube (ETC) in the ICU. *Arch Emerg Med*. 1987;4:219–225.

84. Bishop MJ, Karasch ED: Is the Combitube a useful emergency airway device for anesthesiologist? *Anesth Analg*. 1998;86:1141–1142.

85. Brimacombe J: The oesophageal tracheal Combitube for difficult intubation. *Can J Anaesth*. 1994;41:656.

86. Mercer M: The role of the Combitube in airway management. *Anaesthesia*. 2000;55:394–395.

87. Staudinger T, Tesinsky P, Klappacher G: Emergency intubation with the Combitube in two cases of difficult airway management. *Eur J Anaesthesiol*. 1995;12:189–193.

88. Banyai M, Falger S, Roggla M: Emergency intubation with the Combitube in a grossly obese patient with bull neck. *Resuscitation*. 1993;26:271–276.

89. Deroy R, Ghoris M: The Combitube elective anesthetic airway management in a patient with cervical spine fracture. *Anesth Analg*. 1998;87:1441–1442.

90. Klauser R, Roggla G, Pidlich J, Leithner C, Frass M: Massive upper airway bleeding after thrombolytic therapy: successful airway management with the Combitube. *Ann Emerg Med*. 1992;21:431–433.

91. American Society of Anesthesiologists Task Force on Management of the Difficult Airway: Practice guidelines for the difficult airway. *Anesthesiology*. 1993;78:597–602.

92. Krafft P, Roggla M, Fridrich P, et al.: Bronchoscopy via a redesigned Combitube in the esophageal position. A clinical evaluation. *Anesthesiology*. 1997;86:1041–1045.

93. Calkins TR, Miller K, Langdorf MI: Success and complication rates with prehospital placement of an esophageal-tracheal combitube as a rescue airway. *Prehospital Disaster Med*. 2006;21:97–100.

94. Vezina D, Lessard MR, Bussieres J, Topping C, Trepanier CA: Complications associated with the use of the Esophageal-Tracheal Combitube. *Can J Anaesth*. 1998;45:76–80.

95. Frass M, Rodler S, Frenzer R, et al.: Esophageal tracheal combitube, endotracheal airway, and mask: comparison of ventilatory pressure curves. *J Trauma*. 1989;29:1476–1479.

96. Agrò F, Cataldo R, Alfano A, Gallì B: A new prototype for airway management in an emergency: the Laryngeal Tube. *Resuscitation*. 1999;41:284–286.

97. Asai T, Shingu K: The laryngeal tube. *Br J Anaesth*. 2005;95:729–736.

98. Doerges V, Ocker H, Wenzel V, Schmucker P: The laryngeal tube: a new simple airway device. *Anesth Analg*. 2000;90:1220–1222.

99. Finteis T, Genzwuerker H, Blankenburg A, Ellinger K, Kuhnert-Frey B: Airway management by nonmedical personnel: a prospective, randomized comparison of laryngeal masks, combitubes, and laryngeal tubes (German). *Notfall Rettungsmed*. 2001;4:327–334.

100. Asai T, Murao K, Shingu K: Efficacy of the laryngeal tube during intermittent positive-pressure ventilation. *Anaesthesia*. 2000;55:1099–1102.

101. Marquez X, Marquez A: A new laryngeal tube. *Anesth Analg*. 2003;96:1842.

102. Genzwuerker HV, Vollmer T, Ellinger K: Fibreoptic tracheal intubation after placement of the laryngeal tube. *Br J Anaesth*. 2002;89:733–738.

103. Asai T, Kawachi S: Pressure exerted by cuff of laryngeal tube on the oropharynx. *Anaesthesia*. 2001;56:912.

104. Agro FE, Galli B, Cataldo R, et al: Relationship between body mass index and ventilation with the Laryngeal Tube® in 228 anesthetized paralyzed patients: a pilot study. *Can J Anaesth*. 2002;49:641–642.

105. Dörges V, Francksen H, Bein B, Moikow L, Steinfath M: Disposable Laryngeal Tube vs. Laryvent. *Anesthesiology*. 2004;101:A568.

106. Johnson R, Bailie R: Airway Management Device AMD™ for airway control in percutaneous dilatational tracheostomy. *Anaesthesia*. 2000;55:596–597.

107. Cook T, Nolan JP, Gupta KJ, Gabbott DA: The Airway Management Device (AMD) is not 'reliable and safe'. *Anaesthesia*. 2002;3:291.

108. Mandal NG: A new device has to be safe and reliable too. *Anaesthesia*. 2001;56:382.

109. Agrò F, Barzoi G, Carassiti M, Gallì B: Getting the tube in the oesophagus and oxygen in the trachea: preliminary results with the new extraglottic device (Cobra) in 28 anaesthetised patients. *Anaesthesia*. 2003;58:920–921.

110. Agrò F, Barzoi G, Carassiti M, Gallì B: The Cobra PLA™ in 110 anaesthetized and paralysed patients: what size to choose? *Br J Anaesth*. 2004;92:777–778.

111. Akca O, Wadhwa A, Sengupta P, et al.: The Perilaryngeal Airway (Cobra-PLA™) provides better airway sealing pressures than the laryngeal mask airway (LMA®). *Anesthesiology*. 2003;99:A566.

112. Gaitini LA, Somri MJ, Kersh K, Yanovski B, Vaida S: A comparison of the Laryngeal Mask Airway Unique™, Pharyngeal Airway Xpress™ and Perilaryngeal Airway Cobra™ in paralysed anesthetized adult patients. *Anesthesiology*. 2003;98:1495.

113. Agrò F, Carassiti M, Barzoi G, Millozzi F, Gallì B: Diagnosis and treatment of acute post-operative airway obstrucion with CobraPLA: a first case report. *Can J Anaesth*. 2004;51:640–641.

114. Cook TM, Lowe JM: An evaluation of the Cobra Perilaryngeal Airway™: study halted after two cases of pulmonary aspiration. *Anaesthesia*. 2005;60:791–796.

115. Miller DM, Lavelle M: A streamlined Pharynx Airway Liner: a pilot study in 22 patients in controlled and spontaneous ventilation. *Anesth Analg*. 2002;94:759–761.

116. Miller DM, Light D: Laboratory and clinical comparisons of the Streamlined Liner of the Pharynx Airway with the laryngeal mask airway. *Anaesthesia*. 2003;58:136–142.

117. Greenberg RS, Toung T: The cuffed oropharyngeal airway—a pilot study. *Anesthesiology*. 1992;77:A558.

118. Agrò F, Cataldo R, Carassiti M, Giuliano I, Sarubbi D: COPA as an aid for tracheal intubation. *Resuscitation*. 2000;44:181–185.

119. Brimacombe JR, Brimacombe JC, Berry AM, et al.: A comparison of the laryngeal mask airway and cuffed oropharyngeal airway in anesthetized adult patients. *Anesth Analg*. 1998;87:147–152.

120. Dimitriou V, Voyagis GS, Iatrou C, Brimacombe J: The PAxpress is an effective ventilatory device but has an 18% failure rate for flexible lightwand-guided tracheal intubation in anesthetized paralyzed patients. *Can J Anaesth*. 2003;50:495–500.

121. Mondello E, Casati A: A prospective, observational evaluation of a new supraglottic airway: the PAXpress. *Minerva Anestesiol*. 2003;69:517–525.

122. Casati A, Vinciguerra F, Spreafico E, et al.: The new PA(Xpress) airway device during mechanical ventilation in anaesthetized patients: a prospective, randomized comparison with the laryngeal mask airway. *Eur J Anaesthesiol*. 2004;21:667–669.

SELF-EVALUATION QUESTIONS

11.1. Which of the following is **NOT** true about the Laryngeal Tube?

A. It cannot be used in patients with a history of latex allergy.

B. The LT has two cuffs (pharyngeal and esophageal) but a single balloon for pressure control.

C. The LT requires a mouth opening of at least 23 mm for its insertion.

D. The LT cuffs should be inflated to a pressure up to 60 cm H_2O using a manometer if possible.

E. A well-lubricated ETT can be passed blindly through the airway lumen of the LT.

11.2. Which of the following is **NOT** true with the use of the Laryngeal Mask Airway?

A. In general, approximately 20 mL is required to inflate the cuff for a #3, 30 mL for a #4, and 40 mL for a #5 LMA.

B. The LMA should be inserted into the mouth with the index finger placed between the mask–tube junction.

C. The LMA cuff should be pressed against the hard palate during the insertion into the oropharynx.

D. Prior to insertion, the cuff should be completely deflated.

E. To facilitate placement, the LMA should be lubricated using lidocaine gel.

11.3. Which of the following factors would suggest difficulties in using the Laryngeal Mask Airway?

A. Obese patient

B. Patients with Mallampati III or IV pharyngeal view

C. Cricoid pressure

D. Edentulous patient

E. Pediatric patient

CHAPTER (12)

Surgical Airway

Gordon O. Launcelott and Liane B. Johnson

12.1 INTRODUCTION

In 1799, as George Washington lay dying of life-threatening upper-airway obstruction, one of his physicians, Elisha Cullen Dick, argued against further blood letting and for tracheotomy. In retrospect, this was the only life-saving option available. It was not attempted and the President succumbed.[1]

Indications for surgical airway access vary from the elective through to impending airway compromise, and finally to the true emergency "can't intubate, can't ventilate" scenario. This chapter will deal primarily with techniques of surgical airway access that the practitioner can use to deal with the difficult airway that presents either in the form of impending airway compromise or, the life-threatening emergency.

12.1.1 Why cricothyrotomy and not tracheotomy?

The higher complication rate of emergency tracheotomy, compared to cricothyrotomy,[2] results from the fact that the trachea is situated deeper in the neck, the posterior tracheal wall lacks the protection of a circumferential cricoid cartilage (increasing the risk of esophageal perforation), there is a greater abundance of adjacent vascular structures, and there is a proximity of the thyroid gland and lung. The palpable, often visible, surface landmarks of the thyroid and cricoid cartilages and the ability to accomplish the task faster, and with a minimum of equipment, make emergency cricothyrotomy more attractive than tracheotomy, for the surgeon and nonsurgeon alike.[3]

As a consequence, all of the techniques to be discussed with the exception of percutaneous dilational tracheotomy (PDT) and possibly needle insufflation in children will involve access to the airway through the cricothyroid membrane (CTM).

12.1.2 What is the history of cricothyrotomy?

Surgical access to the airway has its origins in ancient times, but it was the pandemic of "morbus strangulatorius" in Europe at the beginning of the nineteenth century that began its modern evolution. The French surgeon Pierre Bretonneau first attempted to relieve the laryngeal obstruction of this infectious laryngotracheal bronchitis by tracheotomy in 1818, and he was finally successful in 1825.[4] His paper, published in 1826, gave the disease entity the name diphtheria,[5] from the Greek "*diphthera*" meaning leather. This was in recognition of the thick, leathery, blue white upper respiratory tract membranes characteristic of the disease (see Merriam-Webster Online Dictionary available at www.m-w.com/ cgi-bin/dictionary?book=Dictionary&va=diphtheria&x=14&y=16). In the 20 years that followed, Armand Trousseau, Joseph Récamier, and M. P. Guersant honed the technical aspects of "bronchotomy"[6]—laryngotomy and tracheotomy—and by 1851 Trousseau published his experience in 222 cases, 127 of whom survived.[7]

In the United States, Chevalier Jackson published further refinements to the technique in 1909.[8] After 10 years (1921), he published a paper attributing the devastating complication of subglottic stenosis to "high" tracheotomy. Jackson concluded that the only acceptable point of access to the airway was below the first tracheal ring and "high" tracheotomy should be abandoned.[9] Jackson was a figure of immense authority,[10] and it is not surprising that "high" tracheotomy, or cricothyrotomy, was relegated to almost total obscurity for close to five decades.

Brantigan and Grow[11] renewed interest in the approach following publication of their 1976 paper. The impetus for the study came from the anecdotal experience, during the early days of cardiac surgery. Grow, a student of Chevalier Jackson, looked to cricothyrotomy as a way to avoid contamination of median sternotomy wounds by pathogens tracking down the shared mediastinal tissue planes from open tracheotomy sites. He began performing cricothyrotomy, initially in emergency situations, and later electively when it was evident to him that subglottic stenosis did not appear to be a problem.

Grow and Brantigan reported their experience in 655 cricothyrotomies performed over an 8-year period. Duration of intubation ranged from 1 to less than 40 days, with an average of 7 days. Their results showed minimal complications and no cases of subglottic stenosis. Subsequently, several authors,[12–14] including a recent prospective study,[15] reported similar findings in patients not previously subjected to prolonged endotracheal intubation, or suffering from any acute laryngeal pathology.

The discrepancy between the observations of Jackson in the 1920s and the modern authors results from several factors that reflect the two eras, separated by over half a century. Most of the surgical indication in Jackson's era was inflammatory in nature, and it is now recognized that this predisposes to subglottic stenosis. In addition, "high" tracheotomy was a much more complex procedure than the modern cricothyrotomy, involving division of the cricoid or thyroid cartilages. The lack of antibiotics, and the primitive design of the tracheotomy tubes available in the 1920s, undoubtedly compounded the situation.[16]

As rapid airway control and its subsequent management is rarely associated with subglottic stenosis, and there are major advantages in simplicity, speed, and safety,[17] access through the CTM has become the technique of choice in emergency surgical airway management.

In spite of literature to the contrary, the devastating complication of subglottic stenosis associated with cricothyrotomy still compels most clinicians to convert to tracheotomy as soon as possible.

12.1.3   What anatomy do I have to know to perform these procedures?

Access to the airway through the CTM requires a practical knowledge of the anatomy of the larynx, particularly the surface landmarks, as well as the important adjacent structures in the neck.

In most adult males, the thyroid notch ("Adam's apple") is a prominent feature, which identifies the superior aspect of the thyroid cartilage. With the neck extended, palpation inferiorly from this point will often allow the operator to identify the inferior margin of the thyroid cartilage and the ring-shaped cricoid cartilage below (Figure 12-1). Between the inferior margin of the thyroid and cricoid cartilages is the CTM. The size of the membrane in adults is 22–33 mm wide and 9–10 mm high.[18] The vocal cords are attached to the internal, anterior surface of the thyroid cartilage approximately 1 cm above the upper border of the CTM.[19] Care should be exercised in placing instruments superior to the cricothyroid incision for this reason. The only important vascular structure in the vicinity of the CTM is the superior thyroid artery, which, in 54% of people, courses on its lateral border.[20] The left and right cricothyroid arteries, branches of their respective superior thyroid arteries, course medially and traverse the upper half of the CTM,[21] anastomosing in the midline. Injury to this vessel can be avoided by entering the CTM in its inferior half. Caution also dictates that the incision should not extend laterally greater than 1 cm.[16]

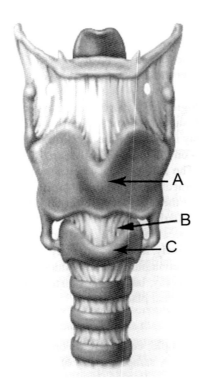

FIGURE 12-1. Anatomy of the larynx and trachea: (A) the larynx, (B) the CTM, and (C) the cricoid cartilage.

Other important anatomical structures include the hyoid bone and the thyroid gland and isthmus. The airway itself is suspended by the hyoid bone lying superior to the thyroid cartilage. Identifying the hyoid bone is important to avoid mistaking the thyrohyoid space for the CTM. In patients with poorly palpable surface anatomy, the location of the hyoid bone can be estimated by extending a line from the mentum posteriorly, half the distance between the mentum and the angle of the mandible.[22]

The thyroid gland has a pyramidal lobe, in 40% of patients[23] who may extend as high as the hyoid bone and could be at risk of injury during cricothyrotomy.

12.1.4   How can I predict whether access through the CTM will be difficult?

Although there is no formal evidence, it is intuitive that anything interfering with either physical access to the larynx, or the ability to appreciate the landmarks of the larynx, will make CTM puncture difficult. This includes factors such as previous surgery, fixed cervical spine flexion deformity, hematoma, obesity, radiation to the neck, laryngotracheal malignancy, or tumor. SHORT (Surgery/Spine, Hematoma, Obesity, Radiation, and Tumor) is a useful mnemonic to remind practitioners of the factors that may be associated with a difficult surgical airway (see Section 1.6.4).

12.1.5   So, what do I need to do to get ready?

The following are common to all techniques of surgical access by way of the CTM:

1. Antisepsis and local anesthetic infiltration. If time permits, every effort should be made to use aseptic technique and infiltrate the proposed surgical site with local anesthetic.

2. Positioning the patient. The patient is ideally placed in the supine sniffing position, with the head extended to best expose the surface landmarks of the larynx. In an emergency situation, particularly in the setting of severe upper-airway obstruction, it may be necessary to position the patient semirecumbent, or fully erect.

3. Immobilization of the larynx and identification of the CTM. Immobilization of the larynx and identification of the CTM is most effectively accomplished by the right-handed operator standing on the right side of the patient. The left (nondominant) hand is used to stabilize the larynx by grasping the body of the thyroid cartilage between the thumb and middle finger leaving the index finger free to palpate the cartilaginous structures (Figure 12-2). If the laryngeal notch is palpable, the index finger is moved caudad along the thyroid cartilage, in the midline, until the fingertip dips off its inferior aspect. Should surface landmarks be difficult to appreciate, the level of the CTM can be estimated as follows: with the head in neutral position, the fifth finger is placed in the suprasternal notch; with all fingers in juxtaposition, the location of the index finger will approximate the level of the CTM.[24]

For transtracheal catheter and Seldinger techniques, some right-handed operators will choose to stand over the right shoulder or at the head of the patient, immobilizing the larynx and identifying the CTM, as described above. Others will choose to stand on the left side of the patient for these techniques, immobilizing the larynx and identifying the CTM with the left hand from below. This permits the operator to use the right hand to pass implements through the CTM in a caudad direction and in a more dextrous fashion. Primary immobilization of the larynx by the left hand, from below, also minimizes trauma to the thyroid cartilage by promoting retraction of the cricoid ring inferiorly, rather than superior retraction on the thyroid cartilage.

12.2   TECHNIQUES

Five methods of surgical access to the airway will be outlined:

1. open cricothyrotomy
2. Seldinger cricothyrotomy
3. retrograde intubation (RI)
4. transtracheal catheter ventilation
5. PDT

12.2.1   Can you walk me through each method . . . step by step?

12.2.1.1   Open Cricothyrotomy

Equipment. The instruments required are a scalpel with a #11 blade; a tracheal hook; Armand Trousseau dilator; and a 5 mm ID cuffed endotracheal tube (ETT), or a small, cuffed tracheotomy tube (Figure 12-3).

Technique. It should be clearly appreciated by the operator, that the technique of emergency cricothyrotomy is primarily a tactile and *not* a visual technique. With the patient positioned and landmarks identified, the following are steps to a successful standard surgical cricothyrotomy technique:

1. A 4 cm vertical, midline skin incision (Figure 12-4);
2. A transverse incision of the CTM at the superior border of the cricoid cartilage;
3. Retraction with a tracheal hook (Figure 12-5). Either superiorly, with potential trauma to the vocal cords or thyroid cartilage, or inferiorly, with less risk and perhaps better exposure;

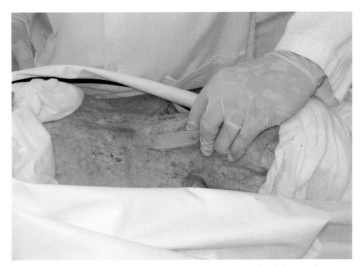

FIGURE 12-2. Open cricothyrotomy in a cadaver: the left (nondominant) hand is used to stabilize the larynx by grasping the body of the thyroid cartilage between the thumb and middle finger leaving the index finger free to palpate the cartilaginous structures.

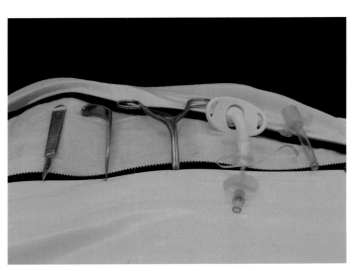

FIGURE 12-3. Equipment required for an open cricothyrotomy: a scalpel with a #11 blade; a tracheal hook; Armand Trousseau dilator; and a small, cuffed tracheotomy tube.

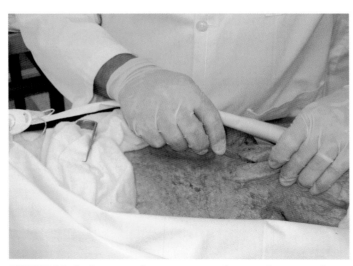

FIGURE 12-4. Open cricothyrotomy in a cadaver: a 4 cm vertical, midline skin incision is made followed by a transverse incision of the CTM at the superior border of the cricoid cartilage.

4. Insertion of the Trousseau dilator (Figure 12-6);
5. Caudal placement of a 5 mm ID cuffed ETT, or a small, cuffed tracheotomy tube (Figure 12-7);
6. Inflation of the cuff, ensuring the proper position and removal of the hook and dilator.

Prior to securing the tube, it is important to confirm proper placement by ETCO$_2$ and by auscultation. An X-ray should be obtained, as soon as conveniently possible, to determine adequate tube position and to rule out any parenchymal lung injury, or pneumothorax. Current recommendations view a cricothyrotomy as a temporizing, life-saving measure. The patient should undergo conversion to a traditional tracheotomy once stabilized.

12.2.1.2 Seldinger Cricothyrotomy Technique

The majority of practitioners are familiar with the Seldinger technique and most will be more comfortable with this approach.

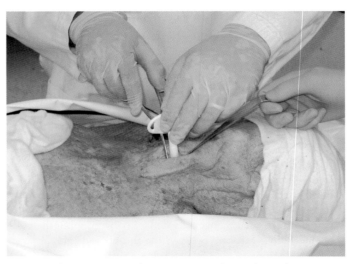

FIGURE 12-6. Open cricothyrotomy in a cadaver: the tracheotomy tube is inserted into the trachea through the Trousseau dilator.

Equipment: There are several cricothyrotomy kits designed with this technique in mind and all with similar contents. They contain a scalpel blade, a syringe, an 18-gauge catheter over needle and/or a thin walled introducer needle, a guidewire, a dilator and a cuffed airway catheter (Figure 12-8).

Technique: As access to the airway is achieved through the CTM, the anatomic considerations and patient positioning are the same as for open cricothyrotomy. The technique is summarized as follows:

1. Vertical midline stab incision through the skin overlying the CTM;
2. Caudal insertion of an 18-gauge needle attached to a syringe (Figure 12-9);
3. Confirmation of needle placement by aspirating air, followed by removal of the needle and syringe;
4. Insertion of the guidewire and removal of the catheter (Figure 12-10), leaving the guidewire in the trachea;

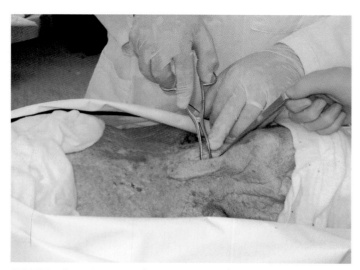

FIGURE 12-5. Open cricothyrotomy in a cadaver: retraction with a tracheal hook and the insertion of the Trousseau dilator.

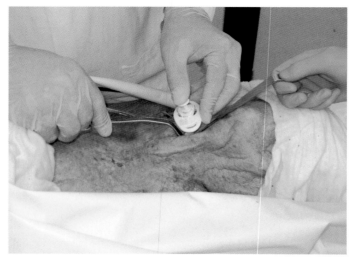

FIGURE 12-7. Open cricothyrotomy in a cadaver: caudal placement of the cuffed tracheotomy tube.

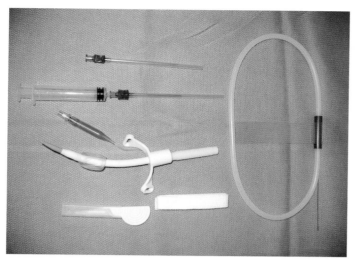

FIGURE 12-8. Equipment for Seldinger cricothyrotomy: a scalpel blade, a syringe, an 18-gauge catheter over needle and/or a thin-walled introducer needle, a guidewire, a dilator, and a cuffed airway catheter.

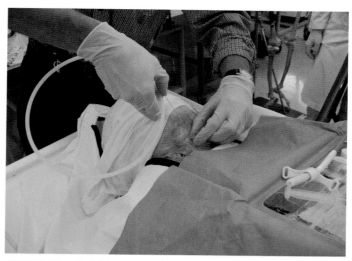

FIGURE 12-10. Seldinger cricothyrotomy in a cadaver: after confirming accurate needle placement by aspirating air, the needle and syringe are removed. A guidewire is inserted into the trachea through the catheter.

5. After making a small cut of the CTM along the guidewire (Figure 12-11), the cuffed airway catheter loaded onto the dilator is advanced as a single unit, over the wire and into the airway (Figures 12-12 and 12-13);

6. Removal of the dilator and securement of the tube;

7. Confirmation of proper tube placement by $ETCO_2$ and/or by auscultation.

It should be noted that the Cook® Critical Care "Melker" Cricothyrotomy kit contains devices to perform both open and Seldinger techniques. Once again, current teaching recommends securing a formal tracheotomy, once the patient is stabilized.

12.2.1.3   Retrograde Intubation

The term "retrograde intubation," coined by Butler and Cirillo[25] in 1960, is a misnomer for what, in fact, is a translaryngeal-guided

intubation. Waters first reported the basic technique that is presently referred to as RI in 1963.[26] In patients with limited mouth opening, he used a Tuohy needle to direct an epidural catheter cephalad through the CTM into the nasopharynx. The catheter was then retrieved through a naris and was used to guide a nasotracheal tube into the airway.

RI is most useful in elective, or semiurgent intubation, in patients with unstable cervical spine injuries, or in those with maxillofacial trauma. In a series of patients with maxillofacial trauma, Barriot reported times of less than 5 minutes for securing an emergency airway with RI.[27] Although the authors claim RI as a rapid, efficacious method of establishing an airway, it is more complex, time consuming, and has more potential complications than other surgical airway access techniques. Bleeding (puncture site and peritracheal hematoma), subcutaneous emphysema, pneumothorax, pneumomediastinum, and trigeminal nerve trauma have all been reported with RI.

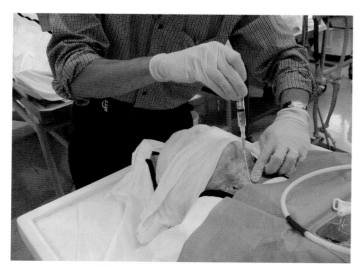

FIGURE 12-9. Seldinger cricothyrotomy in a cadaver: following a vertical midline stab incision through the skin overlying the CTM, an 18-gauge needle attached to a syringe is inserted through the CTM.

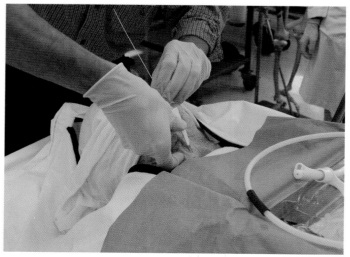

FIGURE 12-11. Seldinger cricothyrotomy in a cadaver: A small cut of the CTM is made along the guidewire.

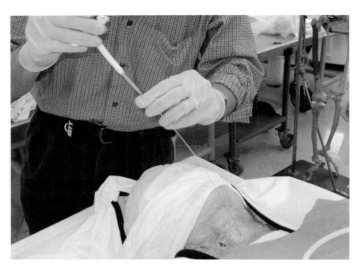

FIGURE 12-12. The airway catheter loaded onto the dilator is advanced as a single unit through the guidewire.

Guidewire and antegrade guide catheter technique. The Cook Critical Care retrograde guidewire kit contains a syringe, a #18 catheter over the needle introducer, a thin-walled #18-gauge introducer needle, a J wire guidewire with positioning marks, and a tapered guide catheter. The procedure is as follows:

1. Unlike cricothyrotomy and Seldinger techniques, no incision is needed for RI. A CTM puncture is performed using the #18 introducer needle in the midline at a 90 degree angle.

2. The guidewire is advanced cephalad through the introducer until it can be retrieved from the oropharynx with a Magill forceps.

3. The wire is pulled antegrade through the mouth until the neck-positioning mark appears flush with the site of insertion. It is then secured with a hemostat.

4. The tapered catheter is inserted over the guidewire until it abuts the CTM.

5. An ETT is fed over the catheter and advanced into the airway, as the wire and catheter are removed.

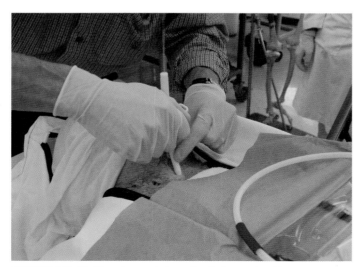

FIGURE 12-13. The airway catheter loaded onto the dilator is advanced through the guidewire into the trachea.

When the distal end of the catheter abuts the CTM, it is only 1 cm below the vocal cords and may cause the ETT to snag on the supraglottic or glottic structures during insertion. This may be minimized by choosing an ETT with a diameter only slightly larger than that of the guide catheter.

Modifications of the retrograde intubating technique have been developed over the past several decades to improve its effectiveness. King et al.[28] recommend removing the J guidewire and advancing the guide catheter distally into the airway, prior to passing the ETT antegrade.

Bourke suggested that the guidewire should be inserted through the "Murphy's" eye of the ETT.[29] Others have suggested the use of subcricoid puncture,[30] in conjunction with a pulling rather than guided technique,[31] and a multilumen catheter guide[32] to improve the success rate of the RI.

Fiberoptic-assisted RI. Much of the advantage of using the flexible fiberoptic bronchoscope (FFB) in conjunction with RI is that it adds a visual dimension to an otherwise blind technique.

The bronchoscope, armed with an ETT of appropriate internal diameter, is passed antegrade over a J wire that has been passed through the suction port of the bronchoscope, and the bronchoscope is advanced until it reaches the CTM. Should there be difficulty in negotiating the glottis, the scope can be maneuvered under direct vision. Upon reaching the CTM, the J guidewire is removed distally and the bronchoscope is advanced toward the carina, under indirect vision.

Some practitioners recommend pulling the J wire through into the airway, under indirect vision, then advancing the J wire toward the carina in order to guide the bronchoscope distally. Others recommend that, once the progress of the FFB is halted at the CTM, the J wire should be allowed to relax and the FFB and J guidewire should be advanced together, distally into the airway, prior to removing the J wire.[33]

Light-guided RI. As transillumination of the soft tissues of the anterior neck can help to identify the location of the tip of the ETT during intubation, the use of a lightwand has been reported to facilitate the retrograde intubating technique.[34] Instead of using a guidewire, Hung and Al-Qatari used a #21 gauge epidural catheter. The epidural catheter is relatively inexpensive and readily available in most operating rooms. In addition, the flexible epidural catheter can bend easily to facilitate ETT advancement into the trachea, past the puncture site at the CTM. Furthermore, the flexible epidural catheter easily fits between the connector of the ETT and the anesthetic circuit.

Following CTM puncture using a #18-gauge intravenous catheter over needle (Jelco™, Critikon, Tampa, FL), a #21-gauge epidural catheter (Concord Portex, Keene, New Hampshire) is inserted through the intravenous catheter and advanced cephalad into the oropharynx. The epidural catheter can be readily retrieved from the mouth.

After removal of the intravenous catheter, the epidural catheter is then inserted into the ETT. A flexible lightwand, such as the Trachlight™ without the internal stiff stylet, is then inserted into the ETT alongside the epidural catheter, until the light bulb is positioned close to the tip of the ETT. While pulling the epidural catheter taut from both ends, the ETT and Trachlight™ assembly is inserted into the oropharynx. When the tip of the ETT enters the glottic opening and reaches the CTM, a bright circumscribed glow is readily seen in the anterior neck at the puncture site. While relaxing the tension of the epidural catheter at the distal end, the ETT is advanced gently into the trachea. Following confirmation of intratracheal placement of the ETT using end-tidal CO_2, the epidural catheter can then be removed through the mouth.

Hung and Al-Qatari have shown that this light-guided RI was effective and safe in 27 patients with cervical spine instability.[34]

12.2.1.4 Transtracheal Catheter Ventilation

The passage of a 12–14-gauge catheter through the CTM for the purposes of establishing an emergency airway is a temporizing method at best. It provides short-term oxygenation until a definitive airway can be established. Many variations on this technique have been used in general relation to availability of equipment. One such technique is summarized as follows:

1. Caudal insertion of 14-gauge intravenous catheter, with syringe attached, through the CTM;

2. Confirmation of position by aspiration air, and advancement of the catheter to its hub, while removing the needle and syringe;

3. Oxygenation using one of several options;

4. Insurance that there is sufficient time for egress of gas, in order to prevent hypercapnea/hypoxia and air trapping.

Options that are available for delivery of O_2 include jet ventilation, the O_2 flush valve on the anesthetic machine, and the anesthesia circuit itself. As mentioned, it is essential that there is sufficient time and an available route for egress of gas. An assistant should be instructed to manage the upper airway with all necessary maneuvers, including LMA, or other airway, and appropriate airway maneuvers.

Gaufberg and Workman recommend that ventilation with this technique should not exceed 20 minutes in adults and 40 minutes in children.[35] It is also the only recommended emergency surgical airway, other than tracheotomy, in children under the age of 12 years.

Trans tracheal jet ventilation. For the purposes of simplicity, only classic transtracheal jet ventilation (TTJV) and TTJV with the ENK oxygen flow modulator will be considered here.

Many operating rooms have access to a commercially available jet ventilator, consisting of a high-pressure connector, high-pressure hosing, an in-line regulator, a jet ventilation toggle switch, and a Luer-Lock connector. This device is powered by central wall oxygen at 50 psi (15 $L \cdot min^{-1}$) and subject to an in-line regulator. Activation of the toggle switch, in a controlled fashion, allows oxygen to be safely jetted through the transtracheal catheter into the airway.

An O_2 tank regulator powers another form of TTJV system, with similar high-pressure hosing, jet injector and Luer Lock connector. A low flow tank regulator, as on the E cylinder O_2 transport tanks, can achieve a maximum pressure of 120 psi with the flow meter set at 15 $L \cdot min^{-1}$. When the jet is activated briefly, very high flows are generated and can result in satisfactory tidal volumes through 14 gauge catheters over 0.5 seconds.[36]

For all systems, chest rise and fall, and the pulse oximeter response, are noted as a measure of ventilatory adequacy.

ENK Oxygen Flow Modulator. The ENK Flow Modulator permits transtracheal ventilation by tubing connected to the O_2 flush valve on an anesthesia machine, or on a wall-mounted flow meter. The device is equipped with a series of five holes that can be occluded in a measured fashion to direct flow through the device to the patient. As with TTJV, chest rise and fall is noted as a measure of ventilatory adequacy.

12.2.1.5 Percutaneous Dilational Tracheotomy

There is an increase in popularity of using PDT following Ciaglia's[37] 1985 publication. Limited to elective, bedside procedures, the current widespread use of this technique has revealed it to be safe, rapid, with minimal overall procedural morbidity.[38] In fact; the overall complication rate is low and comparable to traditional surgical tracheotomy.[39]

The procedure was initially performed as a blind technique relying on knowledge of surface landmarks. Adjuncts, such as the lightwand[40] (Trachlight™, Laerdal Medical Inc., Wappingers Falls, NY) and the FFB, can enhance the ease of the procedure while minimizing complications, such as paratracheal placement of the tracheotomy tube, pneumothorax, and loss of airway control upon withdrawal of the ETT.[41]

A summary of yet another Seldinger-based procedure with the Ciaglia Blue Rhino (Cook Inc., Bloomington, IN) is as follows:

1. skin incision and palpation of cricoid and proximal trachea

2. FFB visualization to retract the ETT and monitor insertion of a catheter over needle device between the second and third, or third and fourth, tracheal rings

3. application of the Seldinger technique with J guidewire and a single tapered dilator

4. insertion of a size-appropriate tracheotomy tube

5. confirmation of the intratracheal placement with the FFB

PDT should be performed by a team of experienced operators familiar with the use of the FFB and with the traditional surgical approach. Avoidance of the obese patient with poorly defined neck anatomy, acute laryngeal pathology, complete airway obstruction, previous neck surgery, or C-spine flexion deformity will increase the overall success rate of the procedure. For a complete review, and application of the technique, please refer to Chapter 32.

12.3 OTHER CONSIDERATIONS

12.3.1 Are there any contraindications in performing a surgical airway?

In the emergency situation when gas exchange cannot be established, a surgical airway is mandatory to prevent catastrophe. As such, there are no contraindications to a surgical airway. There are, however, certain issues that deserve consideration.

In acute or chronic inflammatory laryngeal pathology, and neoplastic disease, cricothyrotomy will likely be more difficult to perform and be subject to a greater incidence of subglottic stenosis. Obesity, injuries, and deformities of the neck may either distort the anatomy and/or render surface landmarks difficult to palpate, and uncontrolled hemorrhage may complicate the situation in the anticoagulated patient. Cricotracheal separation is an absolute contraindication to any procedures that use the CTM.

12.3.2   What are the concerns in establishing a surgical airway in patients with a deep neck infection?

Deep space neck infections are most common in the extremes of age. Underlying medical problems often accompany the afflicted elderly patient. Deep space infections can either variably occlude, or shift the airway, rendering what should be an easily managed airway into an emergency. Caution dictates that airway management should be performed in a controlled environment, preferably the operating room. A CT scan, if feasible, would greatly facilitate understanding of the altered anatomy but this may not be feasible in the severely compromised airway.

In the moderately affected airway, topical anesthesia and "awake" FFB-assisted intubation is the method of choice. If the airway is severely compromised, with total airway obstruction a possibility, an "awake" surgical airway is the procedure of choice to ensure a secure airway until the infection and its source can be treated.

12.3.3   Do you have any concerns in establishing a surgical airway in children?

In children, as the laryngeal prominence does not develop until adolescence, surface landmarks are more difficult to palpate. The vertical dimension of the CTM is considerably smaller in children than adults, with the result that an ETT may permanently damage the cartilaginous structures. There is an increased risk that the cricoid cartilage, the only completely circumferential supporting laryngeal structure and the narrowest part of the airway in the child, may be damaged. In addition, the airway of the child is more malleable, making posterior perforation a greater risk and the laryngeal mucosa more vulnerable to injury and subglottic stenosis.[42] For all of these reasons, in an emergency situation, if transglottic tracheal tube placement cannot be accomplished, needle cricothyrotomy, or tracheotomy, is the method of choice in children 12 years of age or younger.[43]

12.3.4   What are the pros and cons of using noncuffed and cuffed tracheal tube for surgical airway?

The greatest risk of prolonged cricothyrotomy intubation is the development of subglottic stenosis. Underlying medical illness and/or an element of gastroesophageal reflux, in conjunction with the mechanical disruption of intubation, may contribute to the development of subglottic stenosis. Modern tracheotomy tubes are less likely to produce an inflammatory response in the mucosal airway, while low-pressure cuffs reduce mechanical trauma and its sequelae.

Cuffed tubes provide a seal in the airway to allow delivery of larger tidal volumes with lower airway pressures. However, cuffed tubes may be more difficult to insert in an emergency situation,

due to their bulk and the risk of snagging the cuff on the edge of the surgical incision. This may tear the cuff and prevent an effective seal. It is critical that the simplest, safest, speediest, and most effective technique be used to reestablish a lost airway. Thus a small, noncuffed tube would be adequate for the primary goal of salvage and provision of oxygenation.

As patients requiring a surgical airway may have decreased lung compliance, positive pressure ventilation through a noncuffed ETT can result in gas escaping from the proximal airway, resulting in inadequate ventilation. For this reason, either the Cook cuffed airway catheter or #5-cuffed ETT are the tracheal tubes of choice when establishing an emergency surgical airway.

12.4   COMPLICATIONS

12.4.1   What immediate and delayed complications should I be aware of?

In most studies, complication rates are higher for emergency than elective cricothyrotomy. In a series of 38 emergency cricothyrotomies, McGill et al.[44] reported an overall complication rate of 40%. The most frequent complication identified by this group was misplacement of the ETT through the thyrohyoid membrane (i.e., above the larynx), instead of through the CTM. Other complications included execution time greater than 3 minutes, unsuccessful tube placement, and significant hemorrhage. One patient suffered a longitudinal fracture of the thyroid cartilage due to attempted placement of an 8-mm ID tube, resulting in significant long-term morbidity. In a similar series in 1989, Erlandson et al.[45] reported a complication rate of 23%, related primarily to incorrect tube placement (10%) and hemorrhage (8%). Miklus et al.[46] reported on 20 patients requiring emergency cricothyrotomy in the field. In this study, there were no complications of tube misplacement, significant hemorrhage, or long-term morbidity in survivors. Gillespie and Eisele reviewed 35 patients requiring emergency surgical airway over a 6-year period and noted no differences in the overall complication rate between emergency tracheotomy and cricothyrotomy. Note that there were no long-term complications in the patients who received cricothyrotomy and were not subsequently converted to tracheotomy.[47]

Although rare, fatal hemorrhages have been reported as a result of laceration of the cricothyroid artery.[48] As this artery courses closer to the thyroid cartilage, there is a greater risk of hemorrhage if the incision is made in the upper half of the CTM.

Other complications include subglottic stenosis, dysphonia due to laryngeal damage, tracheal cartilage fracture, endobronchial intubation, pulmonary aspiration, recurrent laryngeal nerve injury, esophageal perforation, and tracheoesophageal fistula.[49]

Tissue emphysema (including subcutaneous and mediastinal emphysema) and barotrauma (including tension pneumothorax) have been reported as complications of jet ventilation and establishment of a surgical airway.[50,51] Weymuller et al.[52] caution that only clinicians experienced with TTJV should attempt it in emergency airway management. They describe kinked or displaced transtracheal catheters, incoordination of respiratory effort, outlet obstruction, and distal airway secretions as the major problems encountered.

12.5 SUMMARY

When confronted with the difficult airway, it should be recognized that there are a multitude of techniques available to the practitioner. The wise practitioner is intimately familiar with the noninvasive techniques of difficult airway management and avoids the temptation to unnecessarily substitute surgical methods for the less invasive approaches.

Even within the parameters of the techniques of surgical airway access, it is evident that the practitioner needs to decide which is most appropriate for the clinical situation at hand. Dilational percutaneous tracheotomy is an elective technique, whereas cricothyrotomy is a technique designed to address the true airway emergency. Some catheter insufflation techniques have the advantage of simplicity but all are temporizing at best. This remains the procedure of choice in children under 12 years, where cricothyrotomy is considered a relative contraindication. RI is a technique that can be used in adults and children. It is more applicable to the impending airway obstruction, or the difficult direct laryngoscopy/easy BMV scenarios, where less-invasive techniques are often appropriate.

What is of vital importance for the practitioner is to recognize that "can't intubate, can't ventilate" scenario can occur in a variety of clinical settings. As such, the practitioner needs to have in place the necessary knowledge, the necessary equipment, and the clinical confidence to act.

As it is unlikely that sophisticated gadgetry will be available in all circumstances, it is vital for the practitioner to be familiar with the technique that will most likely be successful with the minimum of equipment; this technique is undoubtedly cricothyrotomy. Commercial kits are now available that can be used for either open or Seldinger techniques, packaged as one. These kits, or a suitable facsimile, should be available in all areas where the expert airway practitioner may be called upon to provide airway management, whether in the operating room, the emergency department, the Intensive Care Unit, or the hospital ward.

REFERENCES

1. Morens DM: Death of a president. *N Engl J Med*. 1999;341:1845–1849.
2. Ger R, Evans JT: Tracheostomy: an anatomico-clinical review. *Clin Anat*. 1993;6:337–341.
3. Brantigan CO, Grow JB, Sr: Cricothyroidotomy: elective use in respiratory problems requiring tracheotomy. *J Thorac Cardiovasc Surg*. 1976;71:72–81.
4. Salmon LF: Tracheostomy. *Proc R Soc Med*. 1975;68:347–356.
5. Brettoneau P: Des inflammations speciales du tissu muquex. Paris 1826.
6. Alberti PW: Tracheotomy versus intubation. A 19th century controversy. *Ann Otol Rhinol Laryngol*. 1984;93:333–337.
7. Trousseau A: Recherches sur la tracheotomie. Paris 1851.
8. Jackson C: Tracheotomy. *Laryngoscope*. 1909;19:285–290.
9. Jackson C: High tracheotomy and other errors: The chief cause of chronic laryngeal stenosis. *Surg Gynaecol Obstet*. 1921;32:392.
10. Clerf LH: Chevalier Jackson. *Arch Otolaryngol*. 1966;83:292–296.
11. Brantigan CO, Grow JB Sr: Cricothyroidotomy: elective use in respiratory problems requiring tracheotomy. *J Thorac Cardiovasc Surg*. 1976;71:72–81.
12. Boyd AD, Romita MC, Conlan AA, Fink SD, Spencer FC: A clinical evaluation of cricothyroidotomy. *Surg Gynecol Obstet*. 1979;149:365–368.
13. Greisz H, Qvarnström O, Willen R: Elective cricothyroidotomy: a clinical and histopathological study. *Crit Care Med*. 1982;10:387–389.
14. Holst M, Hedenstierna G, Kumlien JA, et al.: Elective cricothyroidotomy: a prospective study. *Acta Otolaryngol*. 1983;96:329–335.
15. Francois B, Clavel M, Desachy A, et al.: Complications of tracheostomy performed in the ICU: subthyroid tracheostomy vs surgical cricothyroidotomy. *Chest*. 2003;123(1):151–158.
16. Boon JM, Abrahams PH, Meiring JH, Welch T: Cricothyroidotomy: A clinical anatomy review. *Clin Anat*. 2004;17:478–486.
17. Mace SE: Cricothyrotomy. *J Emerg Med*. 1988;6:309–319.
18. Kress TD, Balasubramaniam S: Cricothyroidotomy. *Ann Emerg Med*. 1982;11:197–201.
19. Bennett JD, Guha SC, Sankar AB: Cricothyrotomy: the anatomical basis. *J R Coll Surg Edinb*. 1996;41:57–60.
20. Dover K, Howdieshell TR, Colborn GL: The dimensions and vascular anatomy of the cricothyroid membrane: relevance to emergent surgical airway access. *Clin Anat*. 1996;9:291–295.
21. Dover K, Howdieshell TR, Colborn GL: The dimensions and vascular anatomy of the cricothyroid membrane: relevance to emergent surgical airway access. *Clin Anat*. 1996;9:291–295.
22. McGill J, Clinton JE, Ruiz E: Cricothyrotomy in the emergency department. *Ann Emerg Med*. 1982;11:361–364.
23. Blumberg NA: Observations on the pyramidal lobe of the thyroid gland. *S Afr Med J*. 1981;59:949–950.
24. Walls RM: Cricothyroidotomy. *Emerg Med Clin North Am*. 1988;6:725–736.
25. Butler FS, Cirillo AA: Retrograde tracheal intubation. *Anesth Analg*. 1960;39:333–338.
26. Waters DJ: Guided blind endotracheal intubation. For patients with deformities of the upper airway. *Anaesthesia*. 1963;18:158–162.
27. Barriot P, Riou B: Retrograde technique for tracheal intubation in trauma patients. *Crit Care Med*. 1988;16:712–713.
28. King HK, Wang LF, Khan AK, Wooten DJ: Translaryngeal guided intubation for difficult intubation. *Crit Care Med*. 1987;15:869–871.
29. Bourke D: Modification of retrograde guide for endotracheal intubation. *Anesth Analg*. 1974;53:1013–1014.
30. Shantha TR: Retrograde intubation using the subcricoid region. *Br J Anaesth*. 1992;68:109–112.
31. Abou-Madi MN, Trop D: Pulling versus guiding: a modification of retrograde guided intubation. *Can J Anaesth*. 1989;36:336–339.
32. Dhara SS: Retrograde intubation-A facilitated approach. *Br J Anaesth*. 1992;69:631–633.
33. Antonio Sanchez: Retrograde Intubation Techniques. In: *Airway Management Principles and Practice*. Benumof JL, ed. St. Louis: Mosby-Year Book Inc., 1996.
34. Hung OR, Al-Qatari M: Light-guided retrograde intubation. *Can J Anaesth*. 1997;44:877–882.
35. Gaufberg SV, Workman TP: New needle cricothyroidotomy setup. *Am J Emerg Med*. 2004;22:37–39.
36. Gaughan SD, Ozaki GT, Benumof JL: A comparison in a lung model of low- and high-flow regulators for transtracheal jet ventilation. *Anesthesiology*. 1992;77:189–199.
37. Ciaglia P, Firsching R, Syniec C: Elective percutaneous dilatational tracheostomy. A new simple bedside procedure; preliminary report. *Chest*. 1985;87:715–719.
38. Francois B, Clavel M, Desachy A, et al.: Complications of tracheostomy performed in the ICU: Subthyroid tracheostomy vs. surgical cricothyroidotomy. *Chest*. 2003;123:151–158.
39. Feller-Kopman D: Acute complications of artificial airways. *Clin Chest Med*. 2003;24:445–455.
40. Addas BA, Howes WJ, Hung OR: Light-guided tracheal puncture for percutaneous tracheostomy. *Can J Anesth*. 2000;47:919–922.
41. Freeman BD, Isabella K, Lin N, et al.: A meta-analysis of prospective trials comparing percutaneous and surgical tracheostomy in critically ill patients. *Chest*. 2000;118:1412–1418.
42. Boon JM, Abrahams PH, Meiring JH, Welch T: Cricothyroidotomy: a clinical anatomy review. *Clin Anat*. 2004;17:478–486.
43. Elliott WG: Airway management in the injured child. *Int Anesthesiol Clin*. 1994; 32:27.
44. McGill J, Clinton JE, Ruiz E: Cricothyrotomy in the emergency department. *Ann Emerg Med*. 1982;11:361–364.
45. Erlandson MJ, Clinton JE, Ruiz E, Cohen J: Cricothyrotomy in the emergency department revisited. *J Emerg Med*. 1989;7:115–118.
46. Miklus RM, Elliott C, Snow N: Surgical cricothyrotomy in the field: experience of a helicopter transport team. *J Trauma*. 1989;29:506–508.
47. Gillespie MB, Eisele DW: Outcomes of emergency surgical airway procedures in a hospital-wide setting. *Laryngoscope*. 1999;109:1766–1769.
48. Schillaci CR, Iacovoni VF, Conte RS: Transtracheal aspiration complicated by fatal endotracheal hemorrhage. *N Engl J Med*. 1976;295:488–490.

49. Boon JM, Abrahams PH, Meiring JH, Welch T: Cricothyroidotomy: a clinical anatomy review. *Clin Anat.* 2004;17:478–486.
50. Smith RB, Schaer WB, Pfaeffle H: Percutaneous transtracheal ventilation for anaesthesia and resuscitation: a review and report of complications. *J Can Anaesth Soc.* 1975;22:607–612.
51. Sanchez TF: Retrograde intubation. *Anesthesiol Clin North America.* 1995;13:439–476.
52. Weymuller EA, Jr, Pavlin EG, Paugh D, Cummings CW: Management of difficult airway problems with percutaneous transtracheal ventilation. *Ann Otol Rhinol Laryngol.* 1987;96:34–37.

SELF-EVALUATION QUESTIONS

12.1. All of the following are reported complications of a surgical airway **EXCEPT**

  A. hemorrhage

  B. fracture of the thyroid cartilage

  C. subglottic stenosis

  D. vocal cord damage

  E. mediastinal emphysema

12.2. Which of the following is **NOT** a useful predictor of a difficult cricothyrotomy?

  A. fixed cervical spine flexion deformity

  B. previous surgery of the neck

  C. previous radiation to the neck

  D. neck hematoma

  E. female gender

12.3. Which of the following is **NOT** true about establishing a surgical airway in children?

  A. A greater risk of posterior perforation while performing a surgical airway in children.

  B. A greater incidence of subglottic stenosis.

  C. The laryngeal prominence does not develop until adolescence.

  D. The height of the cricothyroid membrane is considerably larger in children than adults.

  E. Increase risk of cricoid cartilage damage.

SECTION 3

Case Studies in Difficult and Failed Airway Management

CHAPTER (13)

What Is Unique About Airway Management in the Prehospital Setting?

David Petrie, John M. Tallon, and Michael F. Murphy

13.1 CASE PRESENTATION

On a dark and stormy night in the countryside, a 72-year-old male driver falls asleep at the wheel and strays into on-coming traffic. A transport truck trying to turn to avoid him strikes his small car. The car is crushed with the patient trapped inside. Emergency medical service (EMS) is activated. Firefighters and basic life support (BLS) medics arrive on scene within 10 minutes. The patient is conscious, Glasgow Coma Score 13, BP 80/40 mm Hg, HR 100 bpm, RR 26 breaths per minute, and O_2 saturations of 82% prior to oxygen therapy.

13.2 UNIQUE PREHOSPITAL ISSUES

13.2.1 What level of airway management can we expect from prehospital care providers?

"A" is the flagship of the ABCs that form the foundation for BLS training for all prehospital care providers. The type of training and categorization of skill sets varies significantly from country to country and the provider mix varies from one jurisdiction to the next in any country. For the purposes of simplicity, we will define four discrete levels of care with regard to airway management provided in an EMS system. Each subsequent level assumes proficiency in the skills of the previous:

- First aid providers or first responders—able to apply supplemental O_2 by face mask and perform artificial respiration, typically bag-mask-ventilation (BMV), though in some juris-

dictions extraglottic devices (EGDs) are employed at this level as first-line devices over BMV.

- BLS providers—a moderate degree of proficiency with BMV though again, in some systems, these providers use EGDs, particularly Combitube™ and Laryngeal Mask Airways (LMA).

- Advanced life support (ALS) providers—typically perform laryngoscopy and endotracheal intubation with or without the use of facilitating drugs such as sedative hypnotics and neuromuscular blocking agents.

- Critical care providers (e.g., Air Medical Transport team members)—are ordinarily permitted to perform rapid sequence intubation (RSI) using a laryngoscope and, usually, other advanced airway techniques such as cricothyrotomy.

13.2.2 How are airway management protocols and equipment determined in prehospital care systems?

In most North American systems, prehospital care providers perform delegated medical acts based on preestablished, standardized medical protocols. In many European systems, physicians may be the primary prehospital care providers and, therefore, are less protocol driven. While protocols ought to reflect best clinical evidence, from a practical perspective they are limited by cost, training, competency maintenance, and space constraints.

Equipment availability is driven by the protocols approved by the medical director of the system. The type and range of equipment available for managing the difficult airway in the prehospital setting is limited compared to emergency department (ED) and operating room settings. Even basic equipment such as the

Eschmann Tracheal Introducer (commonly known as the "gum-elastic bougie"),[1] laryngoscope blades, and endotracheal tubes (ETT) in an array of types and sizes may be limited in availability. Alternate intubating devices such as the Intubating Laryngeal Mask Airway (ILMA or LMA Fastrach™) or lightwands (e.g., Trachlight™) often are not available due to cost and skills maintenance issues. Rescue devices such as the esophageal–tracheal Combitube™, Laryngeal Mask Airway (LMA), and the LMA Unique™ (the disposable LMA) are becoming more popular because they are relatively inexpensive and easy to use.[2,3] However, as nontracheal ventilation devices they may not be appropriate in some clinical situations, particularly if adequate ventilation calls for an increase in peak airway pressure beyond the seal capabilities of the device, if the patient is sufficiently responsive to reject the device or if protection against aspiration is mandatory.[4] Surgical airway management devices[5] must be available in any system considering RSI.

13.2.3 What unique environmental considerations do prehospital care providers face when managing the airway?

The prehospital environment presents an array of unique circumstances to the airway practitioner:

- chaotic scene;
- dangerous scene (e.g., flood, fire, radiation, electrical wires down, toxic environment, assailant on the loose, etc.);
- access to the patient and the airway may be challenging due to a variety of factors:
  - extrication is under way;
  - position of the patient (e.g., seated, upside down, etc). In non-trauma airway management, positioning may also be problematic (e.g., intubation performed lying prone and leaning on the elbows). Even with the patient on a stretcher in an ambulance or helicopter, it is difficult to achieve an ideal position for managing the airway of the patient.
- other uncontrollable environmental conditions:
  - darkness inhibits full preintubation airway assessment and obscures subtle nonverbal communication cues between providers and assistants;
  - bright sunlight may do the same or make tools such as the lighted stylet difficult to use;
  - extremes of weather may impede performance.
- lack of other essential equipment for airway management, e.g., suction;
- uncontrolled human behavior in the prehospital setting may further distract airway management decisions and procedures:
  - distraught relatives challenge the focus of prehospital care providers;
  - knowledgeable and skilled assistants are rarely available;
  - even well-meaning first aiders or bystander physicians may hamper efforts with inappropriately timed comments or over vigorously applied "cricoid pressure."

Finally, prehospital airway management may have to take place in a recently secured crime scene or in front of a crowd of morbidly curious supermarket shoppers.

ALS responders arrive on the scene 15 minutes later. The patient's level of consciousness is falling and he remains hypotensive. BLS providers have skillfully assisted ventilations with the BMV while the firefighters try to extricate the patient from the wreckage. The GCS is now 9, BP 80/40, HR 120, and O_2 saturation 88%.

13.3 AIRWAY CONSIDERATIONS

13.3.1 What are the patient factors that influence airway management decisions of a prehospital care provider?

There are three interrelated considerations governing airway management in the prehospital environment: time factors, anatomic factors, and clinical factors.

13.3.1.1 Time Factors: When Is It Better to Wait?

All emergency airway management situations share this feature. Consider, for example, the following two cases:

- A 40-year-old male with sudden collapse, GCS 6, with no cough or swallowing reflex, O_2 saturations of 99%, and normal airway anatomy.
- The same 40-year-old man in a house fire who has stridor, O_2 saturations of 70, and evidence of upper airway burns.

Both patients have clear indications for securing the airway, though the approach in the prehospital setting should be quite different.

- For the first case, the decision to intubate immediately will depend upon the anatomical assessment and time considerations. For example, if the transport time to a hospital is very short it might be prudent to wait (i.e., maximize O_2 with BMV, protect with suction) until arrival at the ED where a more formal and controlled neuroprotective RSI can be done. Training must emphasize that airway management means gas exchange and it does not always require intubation. We must avoid the trap of the technical imperative—*just because it can be done, it should be done*. In fact, there is growing evidence that in certain situations prehospital intubation may not necessarily improve outcomes[6,7];
- On the other hand, in the second case, despite predicted difficulty with laryngoscopy, time is of the essence. A quick decision must be made and the provider must proceed with confidence down the Emergency Difficult Airway Algorithm (Figure 2-5, Chapter 2).

13.3.1.2 Anatomic Factors: Predicting the Difficult Airway

The airway assessment is essentially an attempt to predict difficult laryngoscopy and intubation, difficult bag-mask-ventilation, difficult EGD, and difficult cricothyrotomy based on an examination of external anatomic features (see Sections 1.6.1, 1.6.2, 1.6.3, and 1.6.4). This evaluation is as crucial a component of prehospital airway management as it is in hospital, in that it permits one to make appropriate airway management plans (Plans A, B, and C) that are most likely to be successful.

The patient with acceptable oxygen saturations and a short transport time displaying predictors of difficult laryngoscopy and intubation might be better served by a timely transport to the nearest ED equipped with more resources. Should clinical or time considerations work against this plan, the Emergency Difficult Airway Algorithm directs one to weigh carefully the RSI versus sedation and "awake" intubation decision. If this is unsuccessful, one should move promptly to the Failed Airway Algorithm (Chapter 2, Figure 2-6). In situations where difficulty is predicted and airway management is urgently indicated, an early call for scene backup (if available) ought to be made through dispatch.

Most ALS and critical care prehospital providers are familiar with the necessity for an airway evaluation prior to each intubation, particularly if medications are to be administered to facilitate the procedure. However, this may be limited to predictors of difficult laryngoscopy and intubation rather than difficulty in other airway techniques (see Chapter 1), such as difficult mask-ventilation and difficult surgical airway.

13.3.1.3 Clinical Factors: How Does the Clinical Condition and Presumed Diagnosis Affect Airway Management Decisions?

There are two clinical factors: the indication for intubation and the underlying pathology.

Indications The indications for endotracheal intubation in the prehospital environment are no different than those in any other emergency.[8]

• Failure to maintain adequate oxygenation;
• failure to maintain adequate ventilation (CO_2 removal);
• failure to protect the airway;
• the need for neuromuscular blockade;
• the anticipated clinical course.

In practice, many patients may have more than one indication for intubation.

Underlying Pathology The pathologic conditions producing the indication for intubation differ among EMS systems. The most common precipitating event (up to two-thirds of all intubations) in a typical ground EMS system is cardiac arrest.[9] The remainder tend to be split evenly among respiratory failure (asthma, chronic obstructive lung disease, congestive heart failure, pulmonary embolism, pneumonia, anaphylaxis), non-trauma CNS conditions (coma, intracranial bleed/stroke, seizure, overdose), trauma (head injury, chest injury, neck injury, blood loss causing shock), and shock states (sepsis, cardiogenic, hypovolemic).

Helicopter EMS (HEMS) (also called rotorcraft Air Medical Transport (AMT)) operations rarely respond to primary cardiac arrest victims and, therefore, are likely to see the other causes more frequently.

In certain circumstances, a patient may have an indication for intubation but circumstances (e.g., predicted difficult airway and a short transport time to the ED) may sanction BMV and suction until more optimal conditions for intubation are met. This balancing of risks and benefits is illustrated in the example above (40-year-old man with a collapse and a short transport time versus burn with long prehospital time). Even in the face of an accepted indication for intubation, the potential benefits of prehospital intubation must be weighed against the risks in the context of time, anatomic, and clinical factors.

13.3.2 What alternatives do prehospital providers have in managing a difficult airway?

Consummate BMV technique (including two-handed mask hold requiring two providers if available or necessary) is essential to the prehospital care provider, particularly where the airway is predicted to be difficult and the transport time is relatively brief.

Despite considerable controversy in the literature, the gold standard for definitive airway control remains the correct tracheal placement of a cuffed ETT. According to the "Recommended Guidelines for Uniform Reporting of Data from Out-Of-Hospital Airway Management"[10] there are four methods by which this can be achieved: direct oral laryngoscopy and intubation, nasotracheal intubation, oral rescue techniques (BMV, Combitube™), and surgical rescue techniques (transtracheal jet ventilation and cricothyrotomy). These four methods may each be modified by five variables:

1. oral approach—no facilitating sedative drugs or paralytics;
2. nasal approach—no facilitating sedative drugs or paralytics;
3. sedation-facilitated intubation;
4. RSI, i.e., the use of paralytics ± induction agents;
5. other intubation techniques (e.g., digital, lighted stylet, etc.).

The *actual* number of alternatives available to a specific EMS system is limited by protocols, training, and equipment.

There is ample evidence that endotracheal intubation is not a benign intervention in the hands of inexperienced personnel who apply the technique infrequently.[11–13] New, simple-to-use devices such as the LMA and the Combitube™ have been introduced and validated into this prehospital care setting.[4,14–20] These devices may be employed in two ways: as an alternative to endotracheal intubation in the cardiac arrest (or deeply comatose) patient by BLS providers[4,14,17,21] or as a rescue device in the setting of failed intubation by ALS or critical care providers.[16,18]

An emerging alternative to endotracheal intubation in the respiratory failure patient is prehospital noninvasive ventilation. Several case series have shown continuous positive airway pressure (CPAP) or bi-level ventilation to be feasible and potentially beneficial in the prehospital setting.[22–24] Further study is necessary to validate its effectiveness and safety.

13.3.3 Should tracheal intubation be performed in the field at all?

Inadequate ventilation and oxygenation have been identified as primary contributors to preventable mortality, both in and out of the hospital. It would seem intuitive that successful endotracheal intubation ought to mitigate these deaths, and because of this thinking, endotracheal intubation became the gold standard in prehospital airway management. However, there has been considerable controversy as to whether patients requiring endotracheal intubation should have tracheal intubation in the field or have tracheal intubation deferred until hospital arrival. There are several dimensions to this controversy:

- *Trauma victims.* There continues to be skepticism as to whether the intubation of trauma victims in the field improves survival or not. During the 1980s it was generally felt that invasive airway management was ineffective in improving survival in urban environments but might be effective in longer transport environments.[25] Many studies with conflicting results populated the literature during the 1990s.[26–31] It might, at the very least, be anticipated that endotracheal intubation would be advantageous in patients with acute, severe head injury. Early studies provided no clear direction[7,32–37] and a recent large trauma registry study found that prehospital intubation was associated with adverse outcomes after severe head trauma.[7] However, covariate adjustment in the same study suggests that involvement of the air medical team may improve outcomes. Unfortunately, as Zink and Maio pointed out in an accompanying editorial, this is a retrospective association rather than a causation study.[38]

- *Cardiac Arrest.* In cardiac arrest patients, the issue of efficacy remains unresolved.[39–43] To fuel the controversy further, a recent study involving out-of-hospital cardiac arrest victims showed that patients who received only CPR with chest compressions had comparable survival outcome compared to those who received chest compression and mouth-to-mouth ventilation.[44] A large prospective before/after study to determine the incremented benefit to introducing ALS (including intubation) to a previously optimized system did not show a mortality benefit[45] in cardiac arrest patients.

- *Children.* Early studies showed that tracheal intubation in children by paramedics was associated with higher failure and complication rates than that in adults.[46] Subsequent studies have challenged these early findings without success.[6,29,47–50] The only prospective, pseudorandomized trial to investigate the effectiveness of ground paramedic in performing tracheal intubation in children showed that there was no demonstrable advantage in survival outcome following endotracheal intubation (ETI) as compared to that in the group treated with BMV.[6] This same study revealed concerns about ETI displacement and lack of recognition thereof.[6] Many authorities maintain that the results of these latter studies reflect a deficiency in tracheal intubation training in the pediatric population. Furthermore, the literature does not resolve whether the prehospital intubation of head injured children improves their outcome.[51,52] In the final analysis, the emergency intubation of children is an uncommon and anxiety-provoking event for most paramedics. Both of these factors are likely to increase performance stress and failure rates, compared to the intubation in adults.

Recent studies have presented data and conclusions that challenge the basic, time-honored dogma of EMS airway management and question the best approach to the compromised airway in the prehospital environment. Furthermore, the development of other airway adjuncts (e.g., Combitube™, LMA™, and CPAP) coupled with a reemphasis on standard BMV has attenuated the imperative for prehospital endotracheal intubation and is a clear sign of EMS system maturity and success.

It is becoming clear that airway management training and maintenance of competency programs are vital, as they will affect both the psychomotor skill development and the cognitive decision making. Other issues such as equipment availability, the air versus ground environment, and the logistics associated with rural versus urban critical care transport/EMS suggest that a single, rigid approach to EMS airway management is inappropriate and cannot be supported.

ALS medics are unsuccessful in obtaining a definitive airway. Two IVs have been started and a normal saline (NS) bolus administered. The patient has just been extricated (30 minutes later), boarded, and collared. The HEMS critical care crew has just landed at the scene. The patient now has a GCS of 7, a clenched jaw, BP 90/60, HR 120, and an O_2 saturation of 90% with assisted BMV.

13.4 MANAGEMENT OF THE AIRWAY IN THIS CASE

13.4.1 Prehospital RSI—what does the evidence show?

The HEMS crew on the scene has the training and capability to perform an RSI on appropriate patients as part of their clinical mandate. This includes the use of an induction agent, followed in rapid sequence by a neuromuscular blocking agent in order to optimize intubating conditions to promote successful insertion of an ETT.[53]

The evidence in the EMS literature supporting the use of RSI is, until most recently, nonsupportive except in very specific circumstances. For ground EMS systems, several recent, well-designed studies have consistently shown suboptimal outcomes, or no difference in outcome, in patients suffering acute severe head injury where RSI is used to facilitate endotracheal intubation.[6,7,12,32,54] Head injury was deliberately chosen in these studies because prior studies have suggested that optimal oxygenation and ventilation of these patients improve outcomes. Therefore, it was assumed that successful endotracheal intubation would demonstrate benefit.[55] A case-control study of prehospital RSI of the severely head injured patients in 2003 identified increased mortality and morbidity in the RSI group versus those patients transported without this intervention, and subsequently had tracheal intubation in the ED.[54]

There have been attempts to determine the reasons for the poor outcomes associated with RSI in ground EMS services. These explanations have included:

- increased on-scene time (average 15 minutes in one study[56]);
- lack of adequate training of the paramedics[6,36,54];
- inappropriate hyperventilation and nonrecognition of hypoxia during induction;
- paralysis and attempts at intubation.[57]

Despite recent studies showing the lack of efficacy of RSI in the ground EMS systems, a distinct pattern of improved outcomes has emerged in the subpopulation of those patients where air medical transport (HEMS) had been utilized.[7,58–61] It would appear that the key to improved outcomes lies in the initial training and maintenance of competence programs (cognitive and psychomotor skills) for the prehospital providers.

13.4.2 How should a critical care transport team proceed with the management of the airway in this patient?

The HEMS crew elects to perform RSI using succinylcholine (1.5 mg·kg^{-1}) as the muscle relaxant and etomidate (0.2 mg·kg^{-1}) as the induction agent. A Grade 3 view of the laryngeal structures is obtained with no improvement with the use of laryngeal manipulation. An Eschmann Introducer is placed into the trachea and a 7.5-mm ID ETT is passed over it. A colorimetric end-tidal CO_2 (ETCO$_2$) detector confirms tracheal tube placement. Oxygen saturation is continuously monitored (without desaturation) during the procedure, post intubation systolic blood pressure is 90. Other options for the pharmacologic approach to RSI in this patient could include rocuronium as the paralytic (1.0 mg·kg^{-1}); ketamine (relatively contraindicated in head injury) and propofol (relatively contraindicated in hypovolemic compromise) as the induction agents; or a 50–50 mixture of these two induction agents.

Because of its slow onset of drug effect and associated hypotensive side effects, midazolam is not recommended as an induction agent in EMS. Although the concept of "nonparalytic RSI" has been enshrined in some EMS systems, tracheal intubation after the administration of an induction agent alone (without paralytic agent) is not supported by the literature and is not generally recommended.[62] In fact, success rates in intubation are generally lower and complications are higher with deep sedation versus those employing true RSI.[63–65]

It should be emphasized that full C-spine immobilization ought to be maintained during the intubation procedure. Plan B for most EMS providers in this setting would be an EGD (e.g., LMA, Combitube™) in the event oral intubation failed. Cricothyrotomy (or an alternative percutaneous technique in young children) is a technique in the armamentarium of most advanced EMS providers, though rarely employed. Continuous monitoring of oxygen saturation and ETCO$_2$ should be maintained during transport in order to prevent hypoxemia, inadvertent hyperventilation, or inadvertent extubation.

13.4.3 How do prehospital providers confirm and maintain intratracheal placement of the ETT?

The consequences of an unrecognized, misplaced ETT may be devastating. Given the chaotic environment, the difficulty in employing the usual clinical verification signs, and the increased movement and transfer of the patient, failing to recognize an esophageal intubation is more likely to occur in the prehospital setting than in some others. The exact number of unrecognized esophageal intubations is uncertain since many EMS systems do not systematically gather these data. Inadvertent esophageal intubation rates in EMS have ranged from 1%[66] up to 25%[67] based on tube position verification by emergency physicians on arrival at the hospital. Very low rates are found in systems with specific tube verification protocols, ETCO$_2$ monitoring, and ongoing performance improvement to ensure compliance. Unacceptably high rates are found when no such protocols or tube placement verification devices are available.

Prehospital care providers can confirm correct placement of the ETT in three ways: clinically, with mechanical esophageal detector devices (EDD), or with an ETCO$_2$ detector. Clinical signs include visualization of the tube going through the vocal cords, auscultation of lungs and stomach, mist condensation on the ETT, etc. Esophageal detection devices (EDDs) may take the

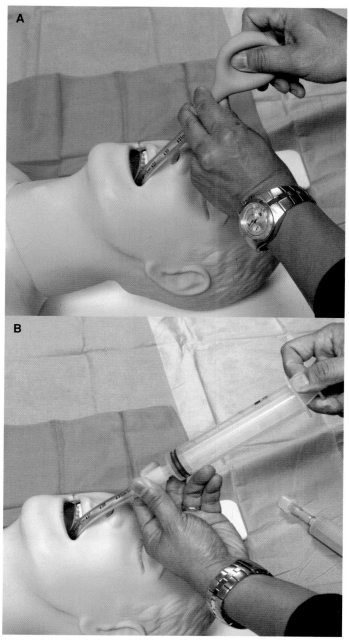

FIGURE 13-1. Esophageal detection devices (EDD): (A) The bulb type of EDD and (B) the syringe type of EDD.

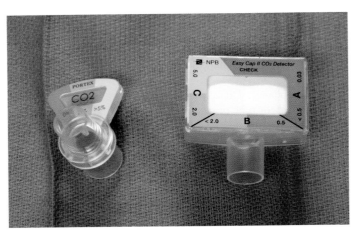

FIGURE 13-2. This figure depicts typical qualitative end-tidal carbon dioxide detection devices.

form of a bulb or syringe aspiration device (Figure 13-1A and B). CO_2 detectors may be from colorimetric (Figure 13-2) or digital capnometers, or continuous graphic display capnographs. End-tidal CO_2 verification of correct ETT placement is the standard of care in EMS.[68]

The limitations of each of these techniques must be recognized. Carbon dioxide detection techniques tend to be less accurate in identifying correct placement of the ETT in patients with circulatory arrest, with reported false negative rates (carbon dioxide not detected, tube in the trachea) as high as 30–35%.[69] In nonarrested patients, carbon dioxide detection is highly reliable indicating correct placement 99–100% of the time.[69–73]

Unlike carbon dioxide detection techniques, the EDD is not dependent on the presence of pulmonary blood flow. While some prehospital care systems use this device instead of carbon dioxide detection, the failure to detect esophageal intubation can be as high as 20%, suggesting that it should not be the only verification method used.[74] Physical examination techniques to verify placement of an ETT in the trachea while neither sensitive nor specific, remain important adjuncts to carbon dioxide detection and EDD, particularly in the arrested patient.

Finally, the migration of an ETT from the trachea to the esophagus during transport is an ever-present hazard. It has been demonstrated that the continuous monitoring of exhaled carbon dioxide during the prehospital phase of care minimizes the risk of unrecognized displacement.[75] In summary, while carbon dioxide detection remains the most reliable method of verifying tracheal placement of the ETT in prehospital care, the incorporation of multiple methods of confirmation are superior to any single method.

13.5   SUMMARY

Airway management in the prehospital arena is difficult and fraught with realities that are unique to the environment. Individuals that provide prehospital airway management vary widely in their training and experience. Although BMV is difficult to perform and may be supplanted by EGD techniques that are easier to perform and equally as effective, BMV will continue to play a crucial role in prehospital airway management for the foreseeable future.

Induction and neuromuscular blocking agents are widely used in prehospital care. It would appear that individuals (and systems) that have extensive training in airway management, intubate frequently, and participate in intensive skills maintenance and quality programs have improved intubation success rates and patient outcomes compared to those who do not embrace these factors. As with any airway practitioner employing these techniques, it is crucial that the medications are used correctly in appropriate patients (i.e., not in patients predicted to have a difficult airway) and the airway practitioner is capable of rescuing the airway (Plan B and Plan C) should Plan A fail (the Failed Airway).

Finally, initial and continuous confirmation of ETT placement by capnometry, the use of EDDs, and clinical methods is the standard of care in the prehospital arena.

REFERENCES

1. Phelan MP, Moscati R, D'Aprix T, Miller G: Paramedic use of the endotracheal tube introducer in a difficult airway model. *Prehosp Emerg Care.* 2003;7(2): 244–246.
2. Davis DP, Valentine C, Ochs M, Vilke GM, Hoyt DB: The Combitube as a salvage airway device for paramedic rapid sequence intubation. *Ann Emerg Med.* 2003;42(5):697–704.
3. Swanson ER, Fosnocht DE, Matthews K, Barton ED: Comparison of the intubating laryngeal mask airway versus laryngoscopy in the Bell 206-L3 EMS helicopter. *Air Med J.* 2004;23(1):36–39.
4. Rumball CJ, MacDonald D: The PTL, Combitube, laryngeal mask, and oral airway: a randomized prehospital comparative study of ventilatory device effectiveness and cost-effectiveness in 470 cases of cardiorespiratory arrest. *Prehosp Emerg Care.* 1997;1(1):1–10.
5. Marcolini EG, Burton JH, Bradshaw JR, Baumann MR: A standing-order protocol for cricothyrotomy in prehospital emergency patients. *Prehosp Emerg Care.* 2004;8(1):23–28.
6. Gausche M, Lewis RJ, Stratton SJ, et al.: Effect of out-of-hospital pediatric endotracheal intubation on survival and neurological outcome: a controlled clinical trial. *JAMA.* 2000;283(6):783–790.
7. Wang HE, Peitzman AB, Cassidy LD, Adelson PD, Yealy DM: Out-of-hospital endotracheal intubation and outcome after traumatic brain injury. *Ann Emerg Med.* 2004;44(5):439–450.
8. Walls RM: The decision to intubate. In: *Manual of Emergency Airway Management*, 2nd edn. Walls RM, Murphy MF, Luten RC, Schneider R, eds. Philadelphia, PA: Lippincott Williams and Wilkins, 2004:1–7.
9. Wang HE, Kupas DF, Paris PM, Bates RR, Yealy DM: Preliminary experience with a prospective, multi-centered evaluation of out-of-hospital endotracheal intubation. *Resuscitation.* 2003;58(1):49–58.
10. Wang HE, Domeier RM, Kupas DF, Greenwood MJ, O'Connor RE: Recommended guidelines for uniform reporting of data from out-of-hospital airway management: position statement of the national association of EMS physicians. *Prehosp Emerg Care.* 2004;8(1):58–72.
11. Deakin CD: Prehospital management of the traumatized airway. *Eur J Emerg Med.* 1996;3(4):233–243.
12. Dunford J, Davis D, Ochs M, Doney M, Hoyt D: Incidence of transient hypoxia and pulse rate reactivity during paramedic rapid sequence intubation. *Ann Emerg Med.* 2003;42(6):721–728.
13. Nolan JD: Prehospital and resuscitative airway care: should the gold standard be reassessed? *Curr Opin Crit Care.* 2001;7(6):413–421.
14. Genzwuerker HV, Dhonau S, Ellinger K: Use of the laryngeal tube for out-of-hospital resuscitation. *Resuscitation.* 2002;52(2):221–224.
15. Doerges V, Sauer C, Ocker H, Wenzel V, Schmucker P: Airway management during cardiopulmonary resuscitation—a comparative study of bag-valve-mask, laryngeal mask airway and combitube in a bench model. *Resuscitation.* 1999;41(1):63–69.
16. Della Puppa A, Pittoni G, Frass M: Tracheal esophageal combitube: a useful airway for morbidly obese patients who cannot intubate or ventilate. *Acta Anaesthesiol Scand.* 2002;46(7):911–913.
17. Calkins MD, Robinson TD: Combat trauma airway management: endotracheal intubation versus laryngeal mask airway versus combitube use by Navy SEAL and Reconnaissance combat corpsmen. *J Trauma.* 1999;48(2): 362–363.

18. Blostein PA, Koestner AJ, Hoak S: Failed rapid sequence intubation in trauma patients: esophageal tracheal combitube is a useful adjunct. *J Trauma.* 1998;44(3):534–537.

19. Tanigawa K, Shigenmatsu A: Choice of airway devices for 12,020 cases of non-traumatic cardiac arrest in Japan. *Prehosp Emerg Care.* 1998;2:96–100.

20. Dorges V, Ocker H, Wenzel V, Sauer C, Schmucker P: Emergency airway management by non-anaesthesia house officers—a comparison of three strategies. *Emerg Med J.* 2001;18(2):90–94.

21. Tanigawa K, Takeda T, Goto E, Tanaka K: Accuracy and reliability of the self-inflating bulb to verify tracheal intubation in out-of-hospital cardiac arrest patients. *Anesthesiology.* 2000;93(6):1432–1436.

22. Mosesso V, Dunford J, Blackwell T, Griswell JK: Prehospital therapy for acute congestive heart failure: state of the art. *Prehosp Emerg Care.* 2003;7(1):13–23.

23. Kallio T, Kuisma M, Alaspaa A, Rosenberg PH: The use of prehospital continuous positive airway pressure treatment in presumed acute severe pulmonary edema. *Prehosp Emerg Care.* 2003;7(2):209–213.

24. Craven RA, Singletary N, Bosken L, et al.: Use of bilevel positive airway pressure in out-of-hospital patients. *Acad Emerg Med.* 2000;7(9):1065–1068.

25. Pepe PE, Stewart RD, Compass MK: Prehospital management of trauma: a tale of three cities. *Ann Emerg Med.* 1986;15:1484–1490.

26. Ruchholtz S, Waydhas C, Ose C, Lewan U, Nast-Kolb D, Working Group on Multiple Trauma of the German Trauma Society: Prehospital intubation in severe thoracic trauma without respiratory insufficiency: a matched-pair analysis based on the Trauma Registry of the German Trauma Society. *J Trauma.* 2002;52(5):879–886.

27. Karch SB, Lewis T, Young S, Hales D, Ho CH: Field intubation of trauma patients: complications, indications, and outcomes. *Am J Emerg Med.* 1996;14(7):617–619.

28. Frankel H, Rozycki G, Champion H, Harviel JD, Bass R: The use of TRISS methodology to validate prehospital intubation by urban EMS providers. *Am J Emerg Med.* 1997;15(7):630–632.

29. Eckstein M, Chan L, Schneir A, Palmer R: Effect of prehospital advanced life support on outcomes of major trauma patients. *J Trauma.* 1996;48(4):643–648.

30. Adnet F, Lapostolle F, Ricard-Hibon A, Carli P, Goldstein P: Intubating trauma patients before reaching hospital—revisited. *Crit Care.* 2001;5(6):290–291.

31. Liberman M, Mulder D, Sampalis J: Advanced or basic life support for trauma: meta-analysis and critical review of the literature. *J Trauma.* 2000;49(4):584–599.

32. Bochicchio GV, Ilahi O, Joshi M, Bochicchio K, Scalea TM: Endotracheal intubation in the field does not improve outcome in trauma patients who present without an acutely lethal traumatic brain injury. *J Trauma.* 2003;55(6):1184.

33. Garner A, Rashford S, Lee A, Bartolacci R: Addition of physicians to paramedic helicopter services decreases blunt trauma mortality. *Aust N Z J Surg.* 1999;69(1069):697–701.

34. Garner A, Crooks J, Lee A, Bishop R: Efficacy of prehospital critical care teams for severe blunt head injury in the Australian setting. *Injury.* 2001;32(6):455–460.

35. Murray JA, Demetriades D, Berne TV, et al.: Prehospital intubation in patients with severe head injury. *J Trauma.* 2000;49(6):1065–1070.

36. Ochs M, Davis DP, Hoyt DB: Lessons learned during the San Diego paramedic RSI trial. *J Emerg Med.* 2003;24(3):343–344.

37. Winchell RJ, Hoyt DB: Endotracheal intubation in the field improves survival in patients with severe head injury. Trauma Research and Education Foundation of San Diego. *Arch Surg.* 1997;132(6):592–597.

38. Zink BJ, Maio RF: Out-of-hospital endotracheal intubation in traumatic brain injury: outcomes research provides us with an unexpected outcome. *Ann Emerg Med.* 2004;44(5):451–453.

39. Rainer TH, Marshall R, Cusack S: Paramedics, technicians, and survival from out of hospital cardiac arrest. *J Accid Emerg Med.* 1997;14(5):278–282.

40. Mitchell RG, Guly UM, Rainer TH, Robertson CE: Can the full range of paramedic skills improve survival from out of hospital cardiac arrests? *J Accid Emerg Med.* 1997;14(5):274–277.

41. Eisen JS, Dubinsky I: Advanced life support vs basic life support field care: an outcome study. *Acad Emerg Med.* 1998;5(6):592–598.

42. Bissell RA, Eslinger DG, Zimmerman L: The efficacy of advanced life support: a review of the literature. *Prehosp Disaster Med.* 1998;13(1):77–87.

43. Adnet F, Jouriles N, Le Toumelin P, et al.: Survey of out-of-hospital emergency intubations in the French prehospital medical system: a multicenter study. *Ann Emerg Med.* 1998;32(4):454–460.

44. Hallstrom A, Cobb L, Johnson E, Copass M: Cardiopulmonary resuscitation by chest compression alone or with mouth-to-mouth ventilation. *N Engl J Med.* 2000;342(21):1546–1553.

45. Stiell IG, Wells GA, Field B, et al.: Advanced cardiac life support in out-of-hospital cardiac arrest. *N Engl J Med.* 2004;351(7):647–656.

46. Aijian P, Tsai A, Knopp R, Kallsen GW: Endotracheal intubation of pediatric patients by paramedics. *Ann Emerg Med.* 1989;18(5):489–494.

47. Vilke GM, Steen PJ, Smith AM, Chan TC: Out-of-hospital pediatric intubation by paramedics: the San Diego experience. *J Emerg Med.* 2002;22(1):71–74.

48. Brownstein D, Shugerman R, Cummings P, Rivara F, Copass M: Prehospital endotracheal intubation of children by paramedics. *Ann Emerg Med.* 1996;28(1):34–39.

49. Su E, Mann NC, McCall M, Hedges JR: Use of resuscitation skills by paramedics caring for critically injured children in Oregon. *Prehosp Emerg Care.* 1997;1(3):123–127.

50. Boswell WC, McElveen N, Sharp M, Boyd CR, Frantz EI: Analysis of prehospital pediatric and adult intubation. *Air Med J.* 1995;14(3):125–128.

51. Suominen P, Baillie C, Kivioja A, Ohman J, Olkkola KT: Intubation and survival in severe paediatric blunt head injury. *Eur J Emerg Med.* 2000;7(1):3–7.

52. Cooper A, DiScala C, Foltin G, et al.: Prehospital endotracheal intubation for severe head injury in children: a reappraisal. *Semin Pediatr Surg.* 2001;10(1):3–6.

53. Walls RM: Rapid sequence intubation. In: *Manual of Emergency Airway Management,* 2nd edn. Walls RM, Murphy MF, Luten RC, Schneider R, eds. Philadelphia, PA: Lippincott Williams and Wilkins, 2004:22–32.

54. Davis DP, Hoyt DB, Ochs M, et al.: The effect of paramedic rapid sequence intubation on outcome in patients with severe traumatic brain injury. *J Trauma.* 2003;54(3):444–453.

55. Chesnut RM, Marshall LF, Klauber MR, et al.: The role of secondary brain injury in determining outcome from severe head injury. *J Trauma.* 1993;34(2):216–222.

56. Ochs M, Davis D, Hoyt D, et al.: Paramedic-performed rapid sequence intubation of patients with severe head injuries. *Ann Emerg Med.* 2002;40(2):159–167.

57. Dunford JV, Davis DP, Ochs M, Doney M, Hoyt DB: Incidence of transient hypoxia and pulse rate reactivity during paramedic rapid sequence intubation. *Ann Emerg Med.* 2003;42(6):721–728.

58. Ma OJ, Atchley RB, Hatley T, et al.: Intubation success rates improve for an air medical program after implementing the use of neuromuscular blocking agents. *Am J Emerg Med.* 1998;16(2):125–127.

59. Murphy-Macabobby M, Marshall WJ, Schneider C, Dries D: Neuromuscular blockade in aeromedical airway management. *Ann Emerg Med.* 1992;21(6):664–668.

60. Sing RF, Rotondo MF, Zonies DH, et al.: Rapid sequence induction for intubation by an aeromedical transport team: A critical analysis. *Am J Emerg Med.* 1998;16(6):598–602.

61. Slater EA, Weiss SJ, Ernst AA, Haynes M: Preflight versus en route success and complications of rapid sequence intubation in an air medical service. *J Trauma.* 1998;45(3):588–592.

62. Werman HA, Schwegman D, Gerard JP: The effect of etomidate on airway management practices of an air medical transport service. *Prehosp Emerg Care.* 2004;8(2):185–190.

63. Lieutaud T, Billard V, Khalaf H, Debaene B: Muscle relaxation and increasing doses of propofol improve intubating conditions. *Can J Anesth.* 2003;50(2):121–126.

64. McKeating K, Bali IM, Dundee JW: The effects of thiopentone and propofol on upper airway integrity. *Anaesthesia.* 1988;43(8):638–640.

65. McNeil IA, Culbert B, Russell I: Comparison of intubating conditions following propofol and succinylcholine with propofol and remifentanil 2 $\mu g \cdot kg^{-1}$ or 4 $\mu g \cdot kg^{-1}$. *Br J Anaesth.* 2000;85(4):623–625.

66. Bozeman W, Hexter D, Liang H, Kelen G: Esophageal detector device versus detection of end-tidal carbon dioxide level in emergency intubation. *Ann Emerg Med.* 1996;27(5):595–599.

67. Katz S, Falk J: Misplaced endotracheal tubes by paramedics in an urban emergency medical services system. *Ann Emerg Med.* 2001;37(1):32–37.

68. O'Connor RE, Swor RA: Verification of endotracheal tube placement following intubation. National Association of EMS Physicians Standards and Clinical Practice Committee. *Prehosp Emerg Care.* 1999;3(3):248–250.

69. MacLeod BA, Heller MB, Gerard J, Yealy DM, Menegazzi JJ: Verification of endotracheal tube placement with colorimetric end-tidal CO_2 detection. *Ann Emerg Med.* 1991;20(3):267–270.

70. Takeda T, Tanigawa K, Tanaka H, Hayashi Y, Goto E, Tanaka K: The assessment of three methods to verify tracheal tube placement in the emergency setting. *Resuscitation.* 2003;56(2):153–157.

71. Ornato JP, Shipley JB, Racht EM, et al.: Multicenter study of a portable, hand-size, colorimetric end-tidal carbon dioxide detection device. *Ann Emerg Med.* 1992;21(5):518–523.

72. Li J: Capnography alone is imperfect for endotracheal tube placement confirmation during emergency intubation. *J Emerg Med.* 2001;20(3):223–229.

73. Grmec S: Comparison of three different methods to confirm tracheal tube placement in emergency intubation. *Intensive Care Med.* 2002;28(6):701–704.

74. Hendey GW, Shubert GS, Shalit M, Hogue B: The esophageal detector bulb in the aeromedical setting. *J Emerg Med.* 2002;23(1):51–55.

75. Silvestri S, Ralls G, Carter E, Senn A, et al.: Improvement in misplaced endotracheal tube recognition within a regional emergency medical services system. *Acad Emerg Med.* 2003;10(5):445.

SELF-EVALUATION QUESTIONS

13.1. Rapid sequence intubation by nonphysician prehospital care providers

   A. is regulated by federal statute

   B. is safe in adults but not children

   C. is well established for paramedics

   D. is supported by the available evidence for critical care prehospital providers

   E. will replace EGDs in the foreseeable future

13.2. All of the following statements about "nonparalytic RSI" are correct **EXCEPT**

   A. some jurisdictions permit paramedics to employ this technique

   B. it has been proven to be safer than "paralytic RSI"

   C. it employs an induction agent at full dose but no neuromuscular blocking agent

   D. it provides an inferior view of the glottis

   E. it is felt to be more humane than intubating patients awake

13.3. All of the following statements regarding qualitative, colorimetric end-tidal carbon dioxide determination in EMS are correct **EXCEPT**

   A. continuous monitoring is indicated to identify inadvertent extubation during transport.

   B. these devices enable one to adhere to the standard of care for confirmation of endotracheal intubation.

   C. these devices are almost totally unreliable in patients having suffered a cardiac arrest.

   D. they are more effective than esophageal detector devices in confirming endotracheal placement.

   E. they are neither better nor worse than capnograpy in confirming correct endotracheal tube placement.

CHAPTER (14)

Airway Management of a Patient with Traumatic Brain Injury

J. Adam Law, Edward T. Crosby, and Andy Jagoda

14.1   CASE PRESENTATION

An advanced life-support emergency services unit brought a 35-year-old male in to the emergency department (ED) "backboarded and collared". The patient was an unrestrained driver who was ejected from his car when it ran off the road and hit a tree. When the paramedic team arrived 10 minutes after the crash, the patient had a Glasgow Coma Scale (GCS) score of 7 (opened eyes to pain − 2, moaned − 2, abnormal flexion − 3). He had a blood pressure (BP) of 90/50 mm Hg, pulse rate (PR) 100 bpm, respiratory rate (RR) 20 breaths per minute, and oxygen saturation (SpO_2) 96% on room air. Pupils were equal and reactive, and his mouth was clenched closed. The patient was given oxygen via a non-rebreathing face mask. Although the patient exhibited periods of extreme agitation with combative behavior during transport, an IV with lactated Ringers was successfully started.

14.2   PREHOSPITAL CARE

After ensuring safety of the field environment, the immediate management of the patient with traumatic brain injury (TBI) in a field setting should focus on stabilizing and maintaining oxygenation and BP. All head-injured patients have potential cervical injury and should be immobilized. A fundamental premise in prehospital care is to anticipate and prepare for eventualities such as vomiting, seizures, and aberrations of BP or oxygenation.

14.2.1   Should tracheal intubation be performed in the field for a patient with TBI?

In a patient with TBI, ensuring oxygenation via a patent airway is of paramount importance. Indications for a field intubation include inadequate ventilation or oxygenation despite supplemental oxygen administration or the inability of the patient to protect the airway. A relative indication for intubation is the risk of losing the airway during transport. Transport time and type of transport, i.e., ground versus aeromedical, must be taken into consideration. Studies of the outcome of prehospital intubations have yielded conflicting results[1–3] and, as discussed in Chapter 13, prehospital airway management protocols are currently being further investigated. In the case presented, the patient was maintaining oxygenation and ventilation. His clinical course could not be certain, and it was reasonable for the field team to consider tracheal intubation. However, the patient had clenched teeth and was predicted to pose a difficult laryngoscopic intubation based on his short neck and cervical-spine (C-spine) immobilization. A decision to intubate would involve the use of a rapid sequence intubation (RSI) protocol: considering the short transport time, RSI was not indicated.

14.2.2   What additional considerations are imposed by field conditions?

Several other priorities in clinical care must be addressed by the field team after initial scene securing and patient stabilization.

14.2.2.1 Circulation

As with the detrimental effects of hypoxemia, hypotension is a critical factor associated with an increased morbidity and mortality in head-injured patients.[4] BP in the field should be monitored closely with the goal of avoiding hypotension (systolic BP < 90 mm Hg in adults): if present, it should be corrected immediately. This patient presented with a field BP of 90/60 mm Hg. As hypotension is strongly associated with poor outcomes in TBI patients, fluid resuscitation becomes a priority. However, the field team must weigh the benefit of delaying transport from the field to secure an IV with the risk of delayed transport to a trauma center. Ideally, IV access should be attempted as the patient is expeditiously transported to the trauma center. Note that isolated brain injury rarely accounts for hypotension in trauma patients with multisystem injury[5]: rather, if present, hemorrhage must always be suspected.

14.2.2.2 Neurologic Disability: Intracranial Pressure (ICP) and C-Spine

ICP: The GCS of 7, 10 minutes after the injury, is not predictive of the patient's clinical course or prognosis (other than the increased likelihood of C-spine injury (CSI)). The patient did not have unequivocal evidence of increased intracranial pressure (ICP) since the pupils were equal and reactive and the motor response was decorticate, not decerebrate. As such there was no indication for paramedics to provide any intervention for managing elevated ICP with modalities such as intubation/hyperventilation, mannitol, or hypertonic saline.[6]

A potential pitfall in the management of the head-injury patient is to assume that trauma is entirely responsible for altered mental status. Consideration must be given to the reversible causes of altered mental status, e.g., hypoglycemia and drug toxicity, in addition to hypoxemia and hypotension.

C-spine immobilization: All patients with blunt trauma to the torso or neurological dysfunction should be suspected of having spinal cord injury until proven otherwise. Although neurologic impairment is fully manifest at the time of injury in most patients with vertebral injury,[7] the implications of an unidentified spine injury are such that routine use of immobilization devices is indicated. Secondary neurological injuries are reported to occur in 10–30% of patients with delayed diagnosis who are not immobilized at time of entry into care[8,9] and in 2–10% of those who are immobilized.[10] Two recent studies suggest that the probability of associated CSI is at least tripled with GCS scores of 8 or less.[11,12] Studies of techniques for optimal cervical immobilization have supported the use of a rigid cervical collar that incorporates the upper thorax, stabilization blocks on either side of the head, and a long spine board for transport.[13,14] Spinal immobilization is not without consequence in that patients are at risk of aspirating if they seize, vomit, or lose protective airway mechanisms. In addition, collars have been consistently demonstrated to increase ICP and may worsen ICP dynamics in patients with head injury.[15,16] With the history of TBI and GCS of 7, the presented patient was at significant risk of C-spine trauma and required full C-spine immobilization.

14.2.2.3 Analgesia/Sedation

Patients with severe head injuries can experience episodes of agitation and combativeness, both of which tend to increase ICP and can pose safety risks to both the patient and the field paramedic

crew. Although sedatives such as benzodiazepines and opioid analgesics are typically employed, if given, the GCS score should first be determined, and the status of oxygenation and ventilation closely monitored after administration.

14.2.2.4 Transport Decisions

A priority in the early management of patients with moderate or severe brain injuries is transportation to the closest facility providing immediate access to neuroimaging and neurosurgical services. Severe TBI patients transported to trauma centers without the availability of prompt neurosurgical care or ICP monitoring are at risk of a poor outcome. Acute subdural hematomas in patients with severe TBI are associated with a 90% mortality if evacuated more than 4 hours after injury, but only 30% mortality if evacuated earlier.[17,18] Consequently, it is recommended that field emergency medical services (EMS) systems operate under strict ground and aeromedical trauma transport protocols. Commonly accepted criteria for transport of head-injured patients to a trauma center include severity of injury, an RR < 10 breaths per minute, systolic BP < 90 mm Hg, and a GCS score < 12.

14.3 EMERGENCY DEPARTMENT MANAGEMENT

The ambulance arrived in the ED after a 15 minute transport. While the patient was being transferred onto the gurney in the trauma bay, it was noted that he was obese, 5' 8'' (172 cm), 275 lbs (125 kg); he had blood coming out of his right ear, and his cervical collar was riding high up over his short neck. His BP was now 130/80 mm Hg, PR 110 bpm, RR 24 breaths per minute, SpO$_2$ 90% on a non-rebreathing face mask, and he had snoring respirations. His blood sugar was 110 mg/dL (6.1 mmol·L^{-1}). His GCS score had decreased to 6 (opened eyes to pain only −2, moaned −2, intermittent decerebrate posturing −2). At this point, it was noted that his right pupil was 8 mm and unreactive and his left pupil was 4 mm and reacted sluggishly. He moved all four extremities with no asymmetry. A quick airway evaluation revealed that his teeth were still clenched; he had a 6 cm thyromental span and 4 cm hyothyroid distance. There was no evidence of blunt trauma to the neck and the cricothyroid membrane was identifiable and palpable in the midline. Two large-bore IVs were secured, blood was drawn and sent for chemistries and type and cross match. Spun hematocrit was 45%. Portable chest and pelvis radiographs in the trauma bay were normal. Cross-table lateral x-rays of the C-spine showed good alignment and no prevertebral soft tissue swelling. An abdominal ultrasound (FAST examination) was performed, which showed no free fluid in the abdomen. A stat neurosurgery consult was ordered. Radiology called, saying that they were ready to image the patient once he was stabilized. While deciding the best approach to securing the airway and managing the suspected increased ICP, the patient had a 30 second tonic-clonic seizure and desaturated to a SpO$_2$ of 80%.

14.3.1 What elements of airway management must be considered in this patient?

The immediate priority in this patient is re-oxygenation, as available evidence suggests that even a single episode of hypoxemia can worsen the prognosis in the patient with TBI.[4] The patient should receive assisted bag-mask-ventilation (BMV) with 100% O_2. Once the SpO_2 is again well above 90%, attention can be turned to formulating a plan for intubation. Concomitant application of cricoid pressure should be considered as he is clearly too obtunded to protect his airway, and a suction apparatus should be immediately available.

Trauma patients secured on a backboard with cervical immobilization can look very intimidating from an airway management perspective. However, formal airway assessment may in fact point to little anticipated difficulty (see Sections 1.6.1–1.6.4). In this patient's case, his obesity predicts an increased likelihood of difficult BMV. A history of obstructive sleep apnea would also suggest higher risk.[19,20] Any trismus may be managed with muscle relaxant administration. Direct laryngoscopy may be difficult due to the patient's short neck and the C-spine immobilization: manual in-line immobilization (MILI) by itself increases the likelihood of obtaining an obscured (e.g., Grade 3) view at laryngoscopy.[21] Finally, while obesity can make transtracheal access difficult, in this patient, the cricothyroid membrane was easily palpable, suggesting easy access.

14.3.2 How are you going to proceed with the intubation?

With a reasonable expectation of successful laryngoscopic intubation and the availability of a backup plan "B" (e.g., BMV, extraglottic device use, or cricothyrotomy) should intubation fail, RSI should be used in this patient. This route confers the advantages of optimal intubating conditions with skeletal muscle relaxation while helping to offset, through the use of pretreatment and induction agents, any laryngoscopic and intubation-induced increases in ICP.

14.3.3 What are your goals during intubation of the TBI patient with C-spine precautions?

Quite simply, our goals are: (1) to achieve intubation expeditiously while avoiding secondary neurologic injury; (2) to maintain oxygenation; (3) to avoid decreases in cerebral perfusion pressure (CPP); (4) to minimize movement of the head and neck; and (5) to avoid aspiration of gastric contents.

14.3.4 How are CPP, ICP, cerebral blood flow, and autoregulation related? What changes occur in TBI and how can we modify these changes?

Elevated ICP is associated with worse outcomes in TBI. While its early recognition and management have not been conclusively linked to improved outcome, it at least seems logical to avoid any further increases in ICP in the brain-injured patient.

ICP reflects the state of the contents of the fixed housing of the intracranial vault. The three normal contents of the vault are brain tissue, cerebrospinal fluid (CSF), and blood. Intracranial blood volume is directly related to cerebral blood flow (CBF). This flow is normally kept reasonably constant over a wide range of BPs by cerebral autoregulation, whereby as BP varies, cerebral vasoconstriction or vasodilatation occurs to maintain constant blood flow,

and in turn volume. However, the brain's ability to autoregulate blood flow over a range of BPs is often lost in TBI.

A second mediator of cerebral blood flow is blood carbon dioxide tension. As blood carbon dioxide tension rises, so will cerebral blood flow, leading to increased intracranial blood volume and thereby pressure. While aggressive hyperventilation in the patient with TBI is no longer recommended in the absence of signs of brain herniation,[6] attention should be paid throughout the airway management process to maintaining the lower limits of normocarbia.

Cerebral perfusion pressure (CPP) is the driving force for blood flow to the brain, and is measured by the difference between the mean arterial blood pressure (MAP) and the ICP, so that CPP = MAP − ICP. In the patient with disrupted autoregulation, decreases in MAP will decrease CPP while increases in MAP, if not accompanied by equivalent increases in ICP, may be beneficial because of the increase in the driving pressure for oxygenation of brain tissue. It is generally recommended that the ICP be maintained below 20 mm Hg, the MAP between 100 and 110 mm Hg, and the CPP at or above 70 mm Hg. Hypotension leading to a decrease in CPP, even for a very brief period, is especially harmful, and along with hypoxia, has been shown to be an independent predictor of an increased rate of mortality and morbidity in patients with a TBI.[4]

14.3.5 How does airway management affect ICP dynamics?

Laryngoscopy and intubation may cause an increase in ICP indirectly through an increase in BP (with disrupted autoregulation) or through a direct effect on ICP. Both laryngoscopy and placement of an endotracheal tube (ETT) result in afferent discharges that increase sympathetic activity and release of catecholamines, i.e., the reflex sympathetic response to laryngoscopy (RSRL). With multiple attempts at laryngoscopy especially, a catecholamine surge may occur, potentially leading to increased heart rate and BP. In the patient with TBI, who has impaired autoregulation, such a BP surge may contribute to an increase in ICP. This fact underscores the importance of using drugs to mitigate this RSRL.

14.3.6 What effects can be expected on ICP from medications commonly used during airway management in the ED?

Pharmacologic agents used to aid in airway management must be selected with consideration of their effects on CPP. Prior to intubation, a modest fluid bolus will help maintain BP, while vasopressors such as ephedrine or phenylephrine should also be immediately available to treat postintubation hypotension. Pretreatment, induction, and paralytic agents used to attenuate a rise in ICP and/or facilitate intubation in the patient with TBI have been discussed in detail in Chapter 4.

14.4 CERVICAL-SPINE CONSIDERATIONS

Victims of major trauma often require several interventions including definitive airway control before a full assessment of the

C-spine is possible. Without radiologic evidence of an intact C-spine, an unstable injury should be assumed and airway management undertaken accordingly.

14.4.1   What effects do direct laryngoscopy and intubation have on the normal C-spine?

Sawin et al. determined the nature, extent, and distribution of segmental cervical motion produced by direct laryngoscopy and orotracheal intubation in subjects without cervical abnormality.[22] Extension was noted at each motion segment; the most significant motion was measured at the atlanto-occipital and atlanto-axial joints. Intubation created slight additional superior rotation at the occiput and C1, but little other movement. Horton et al. conducted a similar experiment in volunteers under topical anesthesia only and also concluded that extension in the atlanto-axial-occipital complex was near maximal but that there was much less extension in the subaxial spine.[23] Similar findings have been reported in a cadaver model subjected to direct laryngoscopy.[24]

14.4.2   What are the effects of basic airway maneuvers and direct laryngoscopy in models of an injured C-spine?

Donaldson et al. studied the motion that occurred during various airway maneuvers in a cadaver series with an unstable C1–2 segment.[25] Chin lift (1 mm) and jaw thrust (2.5 mm) caused the most narrowing of the space available for the spinal cord (SAC). Direct laryngoscopic oral and blind nasal intubation caused similar reductions in the SAC (1.6 mm). In the unstable cadaver, chin lift, jaw thrust, and crash intubation resulted in similar distraction at the injured level (1–2 mm). Donaldson concluded that (1) preintubation maneuvers produced more narrowing of the SAC than did the actual intubation techniques; (2) nasal techniques resulted in SAC narrowing similar to that caused by oral intubation techniques, and (3) application of cricoid pressure produced no significant movement at a C1–2 site of injury.

Aprahamian et al. concluded from his study of a posteriorly destabilized C5–6 segment in a cadaver model that preintubation maneuvers (chin lift, jaw thrust) caused as much or more movement (>5 mm) at the site of injury as did oral or nasal intubation.[26] Hauswald et al. also reported that BMV caused more spinal movement than did either nasal or oral intubation and that intubation caused movements of similar magnitude irrespective of the technique used.[27] Brimacombe et al. determined C-spine motion for six airway management techniques in 10 human cadavers with a posteriorly destabilized third cervical (C3) vertebra. Displacement of the injured segment occurred during airway management with the face mask, laryngoscope-guided oral intubation, insertion of the Combitube™ as well as the standard and intubating laryngeal mask airways, but not with fiberscope-guided nasal intubation.[28] Together these studies provide reassuring evidence that laryngoscopic intubation causes no more movement than do preintubation airway maneuvers, yet also underscores the importance of in-line stabilization starting well before intubation and continuing during all aspects of airway management.

14.4.3   How effective is manual in-line stabilization (MILI) in preventing movement in models of an injured C-spine?

MILI appears to restrain spinal movements occurring during airway interventions to within physiological levels and has less impact on airway interventions than do other forms of immobilization. Lennarson et al. reported that MILI did not completely eliminate movement during intubation in a cadaver model with either posterior injury or complete ligamentous disruption; however, the movements recorded during interventions were within physiological limits.[24,29] Lennarson et al. conducted a similar experiment assessing the efficacy of immobilization maneuvers in the setting of complete segmental instability at the C4–5 level.[29] Despite allowing some subluxation, MILI permitted oral tracheal intubation while restraining cervical movements to levels that were well within physiological limits and thus unlikely to cause harm. Gerling evaluated the effect of MILI as well as cervical collar immobilization on spinal movement during direct laryngoscopy in a cadaver model with a C5–6 transection injury. Although there was less displacement (2 mm) measured with application of MILI compared with collars, the magnitude of movement was small overall and within physiological ranges.[28,30] Majernick et al. demonstrated that MILI reduced total spinal movement during the process of intubation; movement was not reduced to the same extent by either soft or hard collars.[31]

14.4.4   Why is traction no longer used during MILI?

Older publications make reference to using in-line traction during C-spine precautions. However, avoiding traction forces during the application of MILI may be particularly important when there is a serious ligamentous injury, whether recognized initially or not. Lennarson et al. noted excess distraction at the site of a complete ligamentous injury when traction forces were applied for the purposes of spinal stabilization during direct laryngoscopy.[29] Similarly, Kaufmann et al. demonstrated that in-line traction applied for the purposes of radiographic evaluation resulted in spinal column lengthening and distraction at the site of injury in four patients with ligamentous disruptions.[32] Bivins et al. studied the effect of in-line traction during orotracheal intubation in four victims of blunt traumatic arrest with unstable spinal injuries.[33] Traction applied to reduce subluxation at the site of injury resulted in both distraction and posterior subluxation at the fracture site. Current recommendations promote the use of in-line immobilization and not traction during airway interventions requiring C-spine precautions.

14.4.5   How does applied MILI affect ease of direct laryngoscopy?

Many trauma patients presenting to the ED arrive on a backboard immobilized with rigid cervical collar, sandbags, and tape. Unfortunately, any immobilization technique that restricts mouth opening will make laryngoscopy more difficult.

A common pattern of practice is to remove the front of a rigid collar during laryngoscopy after the application of MILI. Heath examined the effect on laryngoscopy of two different C-spine immobilization techniques in 50 patients.[21] There was a poor view at laryngoscopy (Grade 3–4) in 64% of patients when immobilized with a collar, tape, and sandbags, compared to 22% of patients undergoing MILI. In 56% of patients the view of the larynx improved by one grade and in 10% the view improved by two grades when MILI was substituted for the collar, tape, and sandbags. Reduced mouth opening in the patients wearing cervical collars was the main factor contributing to the increased difficulty of laryngoscopy. Other studies in both elective surgical and cadaver series confirm that, during attempted direct laryngoscopy with an applied rigid collar, a Cormack Grade 3 or worse view can be anticipated in over 50% of cases.[30,34] When application of MILI is substituted for a rigid collar, the incidence of Grade 3 or 4 views will decrease to 20–25%. However, although MILI has the least impact of all immobilization techniques on airway management, it will still make direct laryngoscopy more difficult than if no immobilizing forces are being used.[35]

14.4.6 Does the choice of laryngoscope blade impact the degree of C-spine movement during laryngoscopy?

A number of studies have reported the influence of the type of laryngoscope blade on C-spine movements generated during direct laryngoscopy. Most studies measuring movement in normal C-spines found no significant differences in the amount of spinal movement recorded when Miller and Macintosh blades were compared.[27,31,36] In Gerling's study using a cadaver model with a surgically created C5–6 transection, the Miller blade resulted in less axial distraction at the level of the lesion than did the Macintosh.[30] However, Aprahamian's study of a single cadaver with a CSI reported no difference between Macintosh and Miller blades.[26] Studies with the levering tip McCoy/CLM-type blades have generated conflicting results: some have found significantly less movement with use of the activated blade when compared to a Macintosh[37,38] while others have not.[30,39] Laryngoscopy and intubation with the Bullard laryngoscope has been shown to result in significantly less C-spine movement than the Macintosh[36,40] or Miller blades.[36]

14.4.7 Is any blade particularly useful for attaining a view of the glottis during laryngoscopy with applied MILI?

To date, there is no convincing evidence that either curved or straight blades are superior to the other in exposing the laryngeal inlet during direct laryngoscopy with applied MILI. However, a number of studies suggest that laryngoscopy using the McCoy/CLM blade with the tip activated may be helpful when a poor view is obtained in the setting of cervical immobilization. Three studies report improvement of a Grade 3 view to 2 or better in 83% (with applied MILI),[41] 86% (MILI with cricoid pressure),[42] and 92% (rigid cervical collar) of cases, respectively.[43] Other studies have documented the significantly

improved view obtained by the Bullard laryngoscope compared to that obtained by the Macintosh[36,40] or Miller blades[36] during MILI.

14.4.8 Is cricoid pressure contraindicated in patients with potential CSI?

Helliwell reported a small cadaver series (with intact spines) in which lateral radiographs were taken before and during application of 40 N of single-handed cricoid pressure. Vertical displacement at C5 was minimal and unlikely to be clinically significant.[44] Separately, Donaldson et al. reported that application of cricoid pressure does not result in movement in an injured upper C-spine (with an unstable C1–2 segment).[25] In contrast, the same group had previously shown significant movement with application of cricoid pressure in a cadaver model with surgically created instability at C5–6.[45] However, we do not consider cricoid pressure to be contraindicated in a C-spine precaution situation.

14.4.9 Does administration of an induction agent and/or a muscle relaxant by itself have any effect on the C-spine?

Historically, concern has been raised that administration of an induction agent or muscle relaxant to the patient with a CSI could release any "splinting" of an unstable segment by adjacent muscle spasm. However, we could find no objective evidence for a clinically significant degree of cervical spinal movement due solely to induction agent or muscle relaxant administration.

14.4.10 Do flexible or rigid fiberoptic scopes have any advantage in tracheal intubation of a patient with C-spine precautions?

Reviewed in more detail in Chapters 8 and 9, respectively, tracheal intubation using a flexible fiberoptic bronchoscope or a rigid fiberoptic laryngoscope has generally been shown to cause less movement of the head and neck when compared to direct laryngoscopy. These data must be tempered with the appreciation that these devices are more expensive and can be more difficult to use, particularly in the presence of blood and secretions. Flexible fiberoptics are generally used if an awake intubation is elected, an option which retains the advantage of permitting postintubation neurologic reassessment.

14.4.11 Do nonlaryngoscopic techniques have any proven advantage over direct laryngoscopy for intubation in C-spine precaution situations?

L-shaped intubation devices such as the Trachlight™ version of the lightwand or the intubating laryngeal mask (LMA Fastrach™, ILMA) are reasonable alternatives[46,47] to direct laryngoscopy for patients with CSI for those familiar with their use. Theoretically, intubation using these devices should result in less cervical motion since their routine use is with the head and neck in the neutral position. In one study, the Trachlight™ was indeed found to cause less C-spine movement during intubation than did direct laryngoscopy.[48] Compared with the ILMA in a prospective study of elective surgical patients with applied MILI, intubation with the Trachlight™ was quicker and resulted in a significantly higher success rate.[49]

The effect of ILMA use on C-spine movement has been well studied, with most studies agreeing that ILMA intubation results in less upper C-spine extension than direct laryngoscopy.[46] Indeed, one study actually showed a small degree of flexion occurring during ILMA insertion and intubation.[50] A number of series evaluating ILMA use in patients with applied rigid collars have reported intubation success rates comparable to those obtained in elective surgical patients[51–53]; the one study reporting a poor success rate under these conditions had included cricoid pressure in the study protocol.[54] ILMA insertion, cuff inflation, and intubation exert significantly more pressure against C3 than other techniques, and may result in some posterior displacement of the upper C-spine.[55] This latter finding has been further confirmed in a cadaver study with a destabilized C2–3 segment, where ILMA intubation caused a significant posterior displacement of the destabilized segment (as was the case with face-mask-ventilation, direct laryngoscopic intubation, Combitube™ insertion, and LMA Classic™ insertion, but not flexible fiberoptic intubation).[28] The clinical significance of these studies remains to be determined.

14.4.12   What is the role of extraglottic ("rescue") ventilation devices or cricothyrotomy in the patient with C-spine precautions?

Available data suggest that the Combitube™ is difficult to insert with the neck held in-line[56] and is likely to cause spinal movement.[28] During insertion, the LMA Classic™ transiently exerts as much pressure on the upper cervical vertebrae as the ILMA.[55] In a cadaver model of a destabilized C3 segment, both the ILMA and LMA caused significant posterior displacement of the unstable segment, yet significantly less than that caused by Combitube™ insertion.[28] In a comparison with the ILMA, the Laryngeal Tube was found to have a lower first-time insertion success rate in a series of patients with in-line stabilization and required more time to successfully establish ventilation.[57] However, it must be recognized that extraglottic devices are vital rescue oxygenation tools in difficult situations, and the benefits of their use in re-oxygenating a hypoxemic patient will often outweigh the risk of C-spine movement, particularly if care is taken to minimize such movements with MILI.

Surgical cricothyrotomy was originally advocated as a preferred airway intervention in patients at risk for CSI, rather than orotracheal intubation, and is now deemed to be an appropriate alternative if oral or nasal routes cannot be used or are unsuccessful. Although long considered safe in the presence of a CSI, surgical cricothyrotomy has not been well studied. Gerling et al. used a cadaver model to quantify cervical movement during cricothyrotomy.[58] Peak axial distraction was measured at 4.5% of the C5 width, amounting to 1–2 mm of axial compression; peak AP displacement was measured at 6.3% of the C5 width, equivalent to 1–2 mm of displacement. Although these values were statistically significant, they would likely be clinically irrelevant, residing well within the physiological levels established by White and Panjabi.[59]

14.4.13   How safe is it to intubate the trachea of the patient with a potential CSI?

There is no evidence that endotracheal intubation using direct laryngoscopy with in-line stabilization increases the risk of neurologic injury in patients with unstable C-spine fractures.[60–62] Traditionally, oral intubation using direct laryngoscopy was deemed dangerous because it was thought to cause excessive spinal movement with the potential for secondary injury.[63] It was thought that such secondary injury could be avoided by the careful performance of nasotracheal intubation or cricothyrotomy. Although there were no data at that time to support this thesis and data collected since would seem to largely refute it, this hypothesis had achieved a sufficiently widespread acceptance as to be labeled a "therapeutic legend of emergency medicine" by Rosen and Wolfe.[64] McLeod and Calder reviewed the use of the direct laryngoscope in patients with spinal injury or pathology.[65] With the possible exception of one case,[66] they concluded after review and analysis of the case reports that it was unlikely that the use of the direct laryngoscope was the cause of the myelopathies reported. The potential for aggressive direct laryngoscopy with unrestricted spinal movement to cause neurological injury in spine-injured patients has been shown in two further case reports.[66-67] The message these reports deliver is the need for spine immobilization in at-risk patients until injury is ruled out or definitive therapy for diagnosed CSI is implemented.

14.4.14   Is direct laryngoscopy acceptable for intubation of the patient with a CSI?

There is clearly a difference of opinion in the literature regarding the optimal means of securing the airway in patients with CSI. Many authors have reported on the use of the direct laryngoscope in the management of patients with CSI for both elective and emergency intubations.[60–62,68–73] Most of these studies are limited both by their small sample size and their retrospective nature. However, they do reveal that neurological deterioration in spine-injured patients is uncommon after airway management when appropriate care is provided, even in high-risk patients undergoing urgent tracheal intubation. These studies are not sufficient to rule out the possibility that airway management provided in isolation or as part of a more complex clinical intervention, even provided with the utmost care, may rarely result in neurological injury.

The use of a direct laryngoscope following induction of anesthesia in the patient with a head injury is deemed an appropriate practice option by the American College of Surgeons as outlined in the manual of Advanced Trauma Life Support Program® (ATLS®, 1997) for doctors and by experts in trauma, anesthesia, and neurosurgery,[61,62,65,74–83] and by the Eastern Association for the Surgery of Trauma.[82] Advantages of the direct laryngoscope in this setting include its effectiveness, the ability to visualize and remove upper airway foreign bodies during use, and clinician familiarity: many anesthesia practitioners are not similarly skilled with other practice options.[84] Enthusiasm has been expressed by neuroanesthesia experts for the exclusive use of the flexible fiberoptic bronchoscope to facilitate tracheal intubation in spine-injured patients, citing this as the optimal practice option.[85] However, it is worth noting that over 40% of American anesthesiologists admit that they are not comfortable using a flexible fiberoptic bronchoscope for airway management.[84] Further, it should be recognized that significant difficulties may be experienced during the use of the bronchoscope, even by persons skilled in its use, during management of the airway in spine-injured patients.[86] Carefully performed direct laryngoscopy with appropriate MILI in the trauma patient at risk for a CSI can be considered a pattern of practice well within the standard of care.

14.4.15 Is there anything else that might make airway management more difficult in the patient with a CSI?

A small number of case reports and case series document the association of prevertebral retropharyngeal hematomas with some injuries of the upper C-spine, particularly with a hyperextension injury, as anterior elements of the spinal column such as the anterior longitudinal ligament are disrupted.[87–90] Such patients may present with symptoms of dysphagia and dyspnea, with the potential for difficult laryngoscopy due to anterior displacement of the laryngeal inlet.

14.5 POSTINTUBATION CONSIDERATIONS

14.5.1 What are the postintubation considerations in the head-injured patient?

Objective confirmation (e.g., with an end-tidal CO_2 monitor) of tracheal placement of the ETT is essential. Recognizing the importance of maintaining CPP, BP should be reassessed after airway interventions and any unacceptable drop corrected with fluid and/or vasopressors. Pupils should be reassessed. After checking for optimal position of the tip of the ETT, the tube should be firmly fixed to the patient, as a number of transfers, e.g., to the diagnostic imaging department and thereafter to the ICU or operating room, will occur. However, tight ties encircling the neck should be avoided. If the patient's BP permits, a slight head-up position can be achieved by placing the stretcher in the reverse Trendelenberg position. This will promote venous drainage and may reduce elevated ICP. Mechanical ventilation in the patient with elevated ICP is based on optimizing oxygenation and avoiding ventilation mechanics (e.g., positive end-expiratory pressure, PEEP; high peak inspiratory pressure, PIP) that would increase ICP.

Controlled hyperventilation to a $PaCO_2$ of approximately 30 mm Hg was formerly recommended for the early management of elevated ICP. It was believed that reduction in $PaCO_2$ tensions in the brain led to vasoconstriction, decreased cerebral blood flow, and therefore decreased ICP. However, a growing body of research provides evidence that routine hyperventilation results in worse outcomes in TBI patients, possibly due to alterations in regional cerebral blood flow resulting in accumulations of neurotoxic agents, e.g., lactate and glutamate.[91] The Brain Trauma Foundation Guidelines for the Management of Severe Traumatic Brain Injury now recommend that prophylactic hyperventilation be avoided, and that patients with severe TBI be ventilated in such a way as to target the lower limits of normocapnia ($PaCO_2$ of 35–40 mm Hg).[6] A similar approach seems prudent in patients with nontraumatic elevations of ICP (e.g., cerebral hemorrhage). Hyperventilation to a $PaCO_2$ of 30 mm Hg should be used only when osmotic agents and CSF drainage are not effective in managing an acute rise in ICP accompanied by patient deterioration, and utilized only until signs of herniation (e.g., decerebrate posturing or a fixed dilated pupil) resolve.

Unless early and frequent neurological examinations are required (e.g., by a neurosurgeon to decide whether there is sufficient persisting neurological functioning to warrant an attempt at surgical evacuation of a massive subdural hematoma), long-term sedation and paralysis will permit effective controlled mechanical ventilation and other necessary interventions. Sedation and paralysis can also help mitigate the stimulating effects of the tube in the trachea, eliminating any possibility of the patient coughing or "bucking." A full paralyzing dose of a competitive neuromuscular blocking agent, such as rocuronium 1 mg·kg^{-1}, may be given, along with an initial dose of a sedative agent such as a benzodiazepine. Subsequent doses of approximately one-third of the initial dose of both agents should be given if the patient shows evidence of increased sympathetic activity or initiating motor movement.

14.5.2 What happened to this patient?

As outlined in Section 14.3 above, the patient's airway was fully assessed. The decision was taken to perform RSI. Preparations included ensuring qualified help and requisite airway equipment were at hand, together with a briefing of the team about the "Plan B" approach should difficulty be encountered. An assistant was delegated to provide in-line immobilization of the C-spine, following which the front of the patient's rigid collar was removed. Denitrogenation was provided with a tightly fitting face mask, and the induction medication was administered, followed immediately by application of cricoid pressure and administration of the skeletal muscle relaxant. For intubation, direct laryngoscopy was performed with a Macintosh #4 blade, with the practitioner attempting to expose only the posterior-most aspect of the laryngeal inlet. A tracheal tube introducer was then placed above the exposed arytenoid cartilages,[92] followed by ETT passage over the introducer with the laryngoscope blade still in situ. Tracheal placement of the ETT was confirmed with a disposable end-tidal CO_2 detector, whereupon cricoid pressure was released. The anterior aspect of the rigid cervical collar was reapplied, and MILI was released. Vital signs were reassessed with particular reference to the BP. Decisions were then made about ongoing sedation and skeletal muscle relaxation, and arrangements were made for patient transfer to the diagnostic imaging department.

14.6 SUMMARY

Airway management of the patient with a head injury must be undertaken with an appreciation of the importance of avoiding secondary injury to both brain and C-spine. Hypoxia and hypotension must be avoided and formal C-spine precautions must be observed. However, apart from these directives, the practitioner should take comfort in the knowledge that as long as reasonable precautions are undertaken, familiar airway interventions are within the standard of care for the patient with potential CSI, including RSI, BMV, and intubation using careful direct laryngoscopy. To the practitioner experienced in their use, alternative intubation techniques (e.g., lightwand, rigid, and flexible fiberoptic scopes) may well permit intubation with less C-spine movement, although evidence is lacking of improved clinical outcome compared to the use of direct laryngoscopy with MILI. Awake intubation of the patient with a known CSI confers the opportunity to reevaluate the patient's neurologic status postintubation. Irrespective of technique chosen, airway management in this setting should not proceed before a formal airway evaluation has been performed, needed personnel have been assembled and briefed, and airway equipment for the chosen and "Plan B and C" approaches has been readied.

REFERENCES

1. Winchell RJ, Hoyt DB: Endotracheal intubation in the field improves survival in patients with severe head injury. Trauma Research and Education Foundation of San Diego. *Arch Surg.* 1997;132:592–597.
2. Davis DP, Hoyt DB, Ochs M, et al.: The effect of paramedic rapid sequence intubation on outcome in patients with severe traumatic brain injury. *J Trauma.* 2003;54:444–453.
3. Davis DP, Peay J, Serrano JA, et al.: The impact of aeromedical response to patients with moderate to severe traumatic brain injury. *Ann Emerg Med.* 2005;46:115–122.
4. Chesnut RM, Marshall LF, Klauber MR, et al.: The role of secondary brain injury in determining outcome from severe head injury. *J Trauma.* 1993;34:216–222.
5. Mahoney EJ, Biffl WL, Harrington DT, Cioffi WG: Isolated brain injury as a cause of hypotension in the blunt trauma patient. *J Trauma.* 2003;55:1065–1069.
6. *Guidelines for prehospital management of traumatic brain injury.* New York: Brain Trauma Foundation Press, 1998.
7. Colterjohn NR, Bednar DA: Identifiable risk factors for secondary neurologic deterioration in the cervical spine-injured patient. *Spine.* 1995;20:2293–2297.
8. Reid DC, Henderson R, Saboe L, Miller JD: Etiology and clinical course of missed spine fractures. *J Trauma.* 1987;27:980–986.
9. Davis JW, Phreaner DL, Hoyt DB, Mackersie RC: The etiology of missed cervical spine injuries. *J Trauma.* 1993;34:342–346.
10. Harrop JS, Sharan AD, Vaccaro AR, Przybylski GJ: The cause of neurologic deterioration after acute cervical spinal cord injury. *Spine.* 2001;26:340–346.
11. Holly LT, Kelly DF, Counelis GJ, et al.: Cervical spine trauma associated with moderate and severe head injury: incidence, risk factors, and injury characteristics. *J Neurosurg.* 2002;96:285–291.
12. Demetriades D, Charalambides K, Chahwan S, et al.: Nonskeletal cervical spine injuries: epidemiology and diagnostic pitfalls. *J Trauma.* 2000;48:724–727.
13. Rosen PB, McSwain NE, Jr., Arata M, Stahl S, Mercer D: Comparison of two new immobilization collars. *Ann Emerg Med.* 1992;21:1189–1195.
14. Graziano AF, Scheidel EA, Cline JR, Baer LJ: A radiographic comparison of prehospital cervical immobilization methods. *Ann Emerg Med.* 1987;16:1127–1131.
15. Davies G, Deakin C, Wilson A: The effect of a rigid collar on intracranial pressure. *Injury.* 1996;27:647–649.
16. Kolb JC, Summers RL, Galli RL: Cervical collar-induced changes in intracranial pressure. *Am J Emerg Med.* 1999;17:135–137.
17. Seelig JM, Becker DP, Miller JD, et al.: Traumatic acute subdural hematoma: major mortality reduction in comatose patients treated within four hours. *N Engl J Med.* 1981;304:1511–1518.
18. Haselsberger K, Pucher R, Auer LM: Prognosis after acute subdural or epidural haemorrhage. *Acta Neurochir (Wien).* 1988;90:111–116.
19. Langeron O, Masso E, Huraux C, et al.: Prediction of difficult mask ventilation. *Anesthesiology.* 2000;92:1229–1236.
20. Yildiz TS, Solak M, Toker K: The incidence and risk factors of difficult mask ventilation. *J Anesth.* 2005;19:7–11.
21. Heath KJ: The effect of laryngoscopy of different cervical spine immobilisation techniques. *Anaesthesia.* 1994;49:843–845.
22. Sawin PD, Todd MM, Traynelis VC, et al.: Cervical spine motion with direct laryngoscopy and orotracheal intubation. An in vivo cinefluoroscopic study of subjects without cervical abnormality. *Anesthesiology.* 1996;85:26–36.
23. Horton WA, Fahy L, Charters P: Disposition of cervical vertebrae, atlantoaxial joint, hyoid and mandible during x-ray laryngoscopy. *Br J Anaesth.* 1989;63:435–438.
24. Lennarson PJ, Smith D, Todd MM, et al.: Segmental cervical spine motion during orotracheal intubation of the intact and injured spine with and without external stabilization. *J Neurosurg.* 2000;92:201–206.
25. Donaldson WF, 3rd, Heil BV, Donaldson VP, Silvaggio VJ: The effect of airway maneuvers on the unstable C1–C2 segment. A cadaver study. *Spine.* 1997;22:1215–1218.
26. Aprahamian C, Thompson BM, Finger WA, Darin JC: Experimental cervical spine injury model: evaluation of airway management and splinting techniques. *Ann Emerg Med.* 1984;13:584–587.
27. Hauswald M, Sklar DP, Tandberg D, Garcia JF: Cervical spine movement during airway management: cinefluoroscopic appraisal in human cadavers. *Am J Emerg Med.* 1991;9:535–538.
28. Brimacombe J, Keller C, Kunzel KH, et al.: Cervical spine motion during airway management: a cinefluoroscopic study of the posteriorly destabilized third cervical vertebrae in human cadavers. *Anesth Analg.* 2000;91:1274–1278.
29. Lennarson PJ, Smith DW, Sawin PD, et al.: Cervical spinal motion during intubation: efficacy of stabilization maneuvers in the setting of complete segmental instability. *J Neurosurg.* 2001;94:265–270.
30. Gerling MC, Davis DP, Hamilton RS, et al.: Effects of cervical spine immobilization technique and laryngoscope blade selection on an unstable cervical spine in a cadaver model of intubation. *Ann Emerg Med.* 2000;36:293–300.
31. Majernick TG, Bieniek R, Houston JB, Hughes HG: Cervical spine movement during orotracheal intubation. *Ann Emerg Med.* 1986;15:417–420.
32. Kaufman HH, Harris JH, Jr, Spencer JA, Kopanisky DR: Danger of traction during radiography for cervical trauma. *JAMA.* 1982;247:2369.
33. Bivins HG, Ford S, Bezmalinovic Z, Price HM, Williams JL: The effect of axial traction during orotracheal intubation of the trauma victim with an unstable cervical spine. *Ann Emerg Med.* 1988;17:25–29.
34. MacQuarrie K, Hung OR, Law JA: Tracheal intubation using Bullard laryngoscope for patients with a simulated difficult airway. *Can J Anaesth.* 1999;46:760–765.
35. Wood PR: Direct laryngoscopy and cervical spine stabilisation. *Anaesthesia.* 1994;49:77–78.
36. Hastings RH, Vigil AC, Hanna R, Yang BY, Sartoris DJ: Cervical spine movement during laryngoscopy with the Bullard, Macintosh, and Miller laryngoscopes. *Anesthesiology.* 1995;82:859–869.
37. Sugiyama K, Yokoyama K: Head extension angle required for direct laryngoscopy with the McCoy laryngoscope blade. *Anesthesiology.* 2001;94:939.
38. Konishi A, Sakai T, Nishiyama T, Higashizawa T, Bito H: Cervical spine movement during orotracheal intubation using the McCoy laryngoscope compared with the Macintosh and the Miller laryngoscopes. *Masui.* 1997;46:124–127.
39. MacIntyre PA, McLeod AD, Hurley R, Peacock C: Cervical spine movements during laryngoscopy. Comparison of the Macintosh and McCoy laryngoscope blades. *Anaesthesia.* 1999;54:413–418.
40. Watts AD, Gelb AW, Bach DB, Pelz DM: Comparison of the Bullard and Macintosh laryngoscopes for endotracheal intubation of patients with a potential cervical spine injury. *Anesthesiology.* 1997;87:1335–1342.
41. Uchida T, Hikawa Y, Saito Y, Yasuda K: The McCoy levering laryngoscope in patients with limited neck extension. *Can J Anaesth.* 1997;44:674–676.
42. Laurent SC, de Melo AE, Alexander-Williams JM: The use of the McCoy laryngoscope in patients with simulated cervical spine injuries. *Anaesthesia.* 1996;51:74–75.
43. Gabbott DA: Laryngoscopy using the McCoy laryngoscope after application of a cervical collar. *Anaesthesia.* 1996;51:812–814.
44. Helliwell V, Gabbott DA: The effect of single-handed cricoid pressure on cervical spine movement after applying manual in-line stabilisation—a cadaver study. *Resuscitation.* 2001;49:53–57.
45. Donaldson WF, 3rd, Towers JD, Doctor A, Brand A, Donaldson VP: A methodology to evaluate motion of the unstable spine during intubation techniques. *Spine.* 1993;18:2020–2023.
46. Waltl B, Melischek M, Schuschnig C, et al.: Tracheal intubation and cervical spine excursion: direct laryngoscopy vs. intubating laryngeal mask. *Anaesthesia.* 2001;56:221–226.

47. Wong JK, Tongier WK, Armbruster SC, White PF: Use of the intubating laryngeal mask airway to facilitate awake orotracheal intubation in patients with cervical spine disorders. *J Clin Anesth.* 1999;11:346–348.

48. Konishi A, Kikuchi K, Sasui M: Cervival spine movement during light-guided orotracheal intubation with lightwand stylet (Trachlight). *Masui.* 1998;47:94–97.

49. Inoue Y, Koga K, Shigematsu A: A comparison of two tracheal intubation techniques with Trachlight and Fastrach in patients with cervical spine disorders. *Anesth Analg.* 2002;94:667–71.; table of contents.

50. Kihara S, Watanabe S, Brimacombe J, et al.: Segmental cervical spine movement with the intubating laryngeal mask during manual in-line stabilization in patients with cervical pathology undergoing cervical spine surgery. *Anesth Analg.* 2000;91:195–200.

51. Komatsu R, Nagata O, Kamata K, et al.: Intubating laryngeal mask airway allows tracheal intubation when the cervical spine is immobilized by a rigid collar. *Br J Anaesth.* 2004;93:655–659.

52. Moller F, Andres AH, Langenstein H: Intubating laryngeal mask airway (ILMA) seems to be an ideal device for blind intubation in case of immobile spine. *Br J Anaesth.* 2000;85:493–495.

53. Ferson DZ, Rosenblatt WH, Johansen MJ, Osborn I, Ovassapian A: Use of the intubating LMA-Fastrach in 254 patients with difficult-to-manage airways. *Anesthesiology.* 2001;95:1175–1181.

54. Wakeling HG, Nightingale J: The intubating laryngeal mask airway does not facilitate tracheal intubation in the presence of a neck collar in simulated trauma. *Br J Anaesth.* 2000;84:254–256.

55. Keller C, Brimacombe J, Keller K: Pressures exerted against the cervical vertebrae by the standard and intubating laryngeal mask airways: a randomized, controlled, cross-over study in fresh cadavers. *Anesth Analg.* 1999;89:1296–1300.

56. Mercer MH, Gabbott DA: Insertion of the Combitube airway with the cervical spine immobilised in a rigid cervical collar. *Anaesthesia.* 1998;53:971–974.

57. Komatsu R, Nagata O, Kamata K, et al.: Comparison of the intubating laryngeal mask airway and laryngeal tube placement during manual in-line stabilisation of the neck. *Anaesthesia.* 2005;60:113–117.

58. Gerling MC, Davis DP, Hamilton RS, et al.: Effect of surgical cricothyrotomy on the unstable cervical spine in a cadaver model of intubation. *J Emerg Med.* 2001;20:1–5.

59. White AI, Panjabi M: *Clinical Biomechanics of the Spine,* 2nd edn. Philadelphia, PA: JB Lippincott, 1990.

60. Talucci RC, Shaikh KA, Schwab CW: Rapid sequence induction with oral endotracheal intubation in the multiply injured patient. *Am Surg.* 1988;54:185–187.

61. Shatney CH, Brunner RD, Nguyen TQ: The safety of orotracheal intubation in patients with unstable cervical spine fracture or high spinal cord injury. *Am J Surg.* 1995;170:676–679; discussion 679–680.

62. Suderman VS, Crosby ET, Lui A: Elective oral tracheal intubation in cervical spine-injured adults. *Can J Anaesth.* 1991;38:785–789.

63. Walls RM: Orotracheal intubation and potential cervical spine injury. *Ann Emerg Med.* 1987;16:373–374.

64. Rosen P, Wolfe RE: Therapeutic legends of emergency medicine. *J Emerg Med.* 1989;7:387–389.

65. McLeod AD, Calder I: Spinal cord injury and direct laryngoscopy—the legend lives on. *Br J Anaesth.* 2000;84:705–709.

66. Hastings RH, Kelley SD: Neurologic deterioration associated with airway management in a cervical spine-injured patient. *Anesthesiology.* 1993;78:580–583.

67. Liang BA, Cheng MA, Tempelhoff R: Efforts at intubation: cervical injury in an emergency circumstance? *J Clin Anesth.* 1999;11:349–352.

68. Meschino A, Devitt JH, Koch JP, Szalai JP, Schwartz ML: The safety of awake tracheal intubation in cervical spine injury. *Can J Anaesth.* 1992;39:114–117.

69. Holley J, Jorden R: Airway management in patients with unstable cervical spine fractures. *Ann Emerg Med.* 1989;18:1237–1239.

70. Rhee KJ, Green W, Holcroft JW, Mangili JA: Oral intubation in the multiply injured patient: the risk of exacerbating spinal cord damage. *Ann Emerg Med.* 1990;19:511–514.

71. Scannell G, Waxman K, Tominaga G, Barker S, Annas C: Orotracheal intubation in trauma patients with cervical fractures. *Arch Surg.* 1993;128:903–905; discussion 905–906.

72. Wright SW, Robinson GG, 2nd, Wright MB: Cervical spine injuries in blunt trauma patients requiring emergent endotracheal intubation. *Am J Emerg Med.* 1992;10:104–109.

73. Norwood S, Myers MB, Butler TJ: The safety of emergency neuromuscular blockade and orotracheal intubation in the acutely injured trauma patient. *J Am Coll Surg.* 1994;179:646–652.

74. Richards CF, Mayberry JC: Initial management of the trauma patient. *Crit Care Clin.* 2004;20:1–11.

75. Ball PA: Critical care of spinal cord injury. *Spine.* 2001;26:S27–S30.

76. Urdaneta F, Layon AJ: Respiratory complications in patients with traumatic cervical spine injuries: case report and review of the literature. *J Clin Anesth.* 2003;15:398–405.

77. Ivy ME, Cohn SM: Addressing the myths of cervical spine injury management. *Am J Emerg Med.* 1997;15:591–595.

78. Gajraj NM, Chason DP, Shearer VE: Cervical spine movement during orotracheal intubation: comparison of the Belscope and Macintosh blades. *Anaesthesia.* 1994;49:772–774.

79. Crosby ET: Tracheal intubation in the cervical spine-injured patient. *Can J Anaesth.* 1992;39:105–109.

80. Abrams K, Grande C: Airway management of the trauma patient with cervical spine injury. *Curr Opin Anaesthesiol.* 1994;7:184–190.

81. Hastings RH, Marks JD: Airway management for trauma patients with potential cervical spine injuries. *Anesth Analg.* 1991;73:471–482.

82. Dunham CM, Barraco RD, Clark DE, et al.: Guidelines for emergency tracheal intubation immediately after traumatic injury. *J Trauma.* 2003;55: 162–179.

83. Gajraj N, Pennant J, Giesecke A: Cervical spine trauma and airway management. *Curr Opin Anaesthesiol.* 1993;6:369–374.

84. Ezri T, Szmuk P, Warters RD, Katz J, Hagberg CA: Difficult airway management practice patterns among anesthesiologists practicing in the United States: have we made any progress? *J Clin Anesth.* 2003;15:418–422.

85. Chesnut RM: Management of brain and spine injuries. *Crit Care Clin.* 2004;20:25–55.

86. McGuire G, el-Beheiry H: Complete upper airway obstruction during awake fibreoptic intubation in patients with unstable cervical spine fractures. *Can J Anaesth.* 1999;46:176–178.

87. Penning L: Prevertebral hematoma in cervical spine injury: incidence and etiologic significance. *AJR Am J Roentgenol.* 1981;136:553–561.

88. Biby L, Santora AH: Prevertebral hematoma secondary to whiplash injury necessitating emergency intubation. *Anesth Analg.* 1990;70:112–114.

89. Shiratori T, Hara K, Ando N: Acute airway obstruction secondary to retropharyngeal hematoma. *J Anesth.* 2003;17:46–48.

90. Myssiorek D, Shalmi C: Traumatic retropharyngeal hematoma. *Arch Otolaryngol Head Neck Surg.* 1989;115:1130–1132.

91. Marion DW, Puccio A, Wisniewski SR, et al.: Effect of hyperventilation on extracellular concentrations of glutamate, lactate, pyruvate, and local cerebral blood flow in patients with severe traumatic brain injury. *Crit Care Med.* 2002;30:2619–2625.

92. Nolan JP, Wilson ME: Orotracheal intubation in patients with potential cervical spine injuries. An indication for the gum elastic bougie. *Anaesthesia.* 1993;48:630–633.

SELF-EVALUATION QUESTIONS

14.1. Which of the following is contraindicated during intubation of the trauma patient undergoing C-spine precautions with manual in-line stabilization?

A. removal of the front of the cervical collar

B. oral intubation using direct laryngoscopy

C. cricoid pressure

D. external laryngeal manipulation

E. none of the above

14.2. Which of the following airway interventions results in the least movement of the cervical spine?

A. bag-mask-ventilation

B. laryngeal mask insertion

C. direct laryngoscopy

D. intubation by the nasal route

E. bullard laryngoscope intubation

14.3. Which of the following statements concerning the head-injured patient is **TRUE**?

A. Improved neurological outcome is associated with the avoidance of direct laryngoscopy for intubation in this population.

B. The unconscious head-injured patient (GCS < 8) has a threefold chance of cervical spine injury.

C. Avoidance of cervical spine movement during airway management is more important than avoiding transient hypoxia and hypotension.

D. The safest way of proceeding with intubation is proven to be the flexible fiberoptic bronchoscope.

E. The use of muscle relaxants for intubation of these patients is contraindicated because they will interfere with subsequent neurological evaluation.

CHAPTER (15)

Airway Management of an Unconscious Patient Who Remains Trapped Inside the Vehicle Following a Motor Vehicle Accident

Tom C. Phu, Orlando R. Hung, and Ronald D. Stewart

15.1 CASE PRESENTATION

A 23-year-old driver is involved in a motor vehicle accident (MVA). Her car had collided with an oncoming vehicle. On arrival at the scene, paramedics are unable to extricate her from the vehicle. The paramedics are concerned because the patient is unconscious and appears to have an obstructed airway. Assistance to extricate her from the vehicle is requested by the paramedic team. Upon arriving at the scene, you note that she appears to be unconscious inside the vehicle and is not making effective respiratory efforts. She is slumped back against her seat. You recognize that this patient requires her airway secured urgently and that there is not sufficient time to await the arrival of backup to remove her from the vehicle.

15.2 PATIENT CONSIDERATIONS

15.2.1 According to the advanced trauma life support (ATLS) guidelines, what are the immediate issues that need to be addressed?

ATLS suggests that, prior to the initiation of resuscitation protocols, scene safety first be assessed. Assessment and management of the airway, breathing, and then circulation (ABCs) follows.[1] The greatest priority, and challenge, in this patient will be airway

management. The patient is trapped in the vehicle, which will limit the trained responder's ability to access the patient and manage her airway appropriately. Thus, unless she can be removed from the vehicle fairly quickly, consideration to definitive airway management should be made immediately. Further management of the patient will require her extrication from the vehicle.

15.2.2 How does this setting affect your management of this patient?

Most trained responders will be familiar with airway management and resuscitation in a patient who is readily accessible. In the trapped, unconscious patient, access will be limited. This will necessitate airway management techniques other than direct laryngoscopy (DL). The responder should immediately relieve the airway obstruction by gently performing a jaw thrust (with minimal cervical movement), or by placing an oral or nasal airway. This should be followed by the application of a face mask with oxygen supplementation, if spontaneous ventilation is considered to be adequate. However, in the absence of adequate respiratory effort, ventilation and oxygenation must be provided to the patient immediately by bag-mask-ventilation (BMV), if possible, while planning for a more definitive airway.

Assessment of the patient will be made more difficult by limitations to patient access. It will be difficult to assess the patient for associated injuries, including injuries to the thorax, airway, and basal skull. All these factors will influence airway and postintubation management. Resources in the prehospital environment will not be as readily available as in the hospital environment, where access to more advanced airway tools, and trained personnel, would provide more options for airway control. Responders should focus on using those techniques that they are trained to perform.

15.2.3   What potential injuries could this patient have?

Although the trauma experienced by this patient may cause injuries to all organ systems, the systems that are of immediate interest to the health-care providers would be those which affect the airway. These include basal skull fractures (which can be present in the absence of traditional signs of basal fracture). The potential for basal skull injury implies a relative contraindication for nasotracheal intubation because of the risk of the endotracheal tube (ETT) penetrating the cranial vault. Injuries to the cervical spine (C-spine) are a constant risk in any trauma patient, and C-spine precautions should be taken, if possible, with manual in-line stabilization.

15.2.4   Are there any special considerations in this case?

There are several important considerations that should guide the prehospital practitioner in managing this patient's airway. These include scene safety, limited patient access, and an immediate need for securing the airway, potential for injuries to the head, cervical spine, basal skull, as well as risks to the responder. The fact that the patient is trapped and the confines of the vehicle restrictive will not allow for "controlled" intubation conditions. DL will be challenging because of the sitting position of the patient. Alternative intubating techniques should be considered. Securing an airway must be undertaken in an expeditious, yet strategic manner.

The fact that the patient is unconscious, obstructed, and perhaps hypoxic makes for a difficult clinical situation. One should avoid multiple attempts at managing the airway, which may potentially cause trauma. Therefore, if at all possible, the most experienced practitioner should manage the airway using the technique most familiar to them. Failure to rapidly secure the airway is an indication to proceed to surgical cricothyrotomy (SC).

Following an MVA, particularly when there is evidence of facial injury, there may be airway trauma with blood, secretions, and foreign bodies. There may be frank airway disruption. Each of these can make oxygenation, ventilation, and visualization of the laryngeal inlet difficult.

15.2.5   What are your immediate concerns regarding this patient's airway?

Management of this patient's airway will have to be expedited; there has already been a delay in relation to time elapsed between the injury and the arrival of the response team. Although not without controversy, there is evidence that an aggressive (in the field) approach to intubation of the trachea is associated with improved survival.[2] If tracheal intubation is not performed at the scene of trauma, expert management is required for the maintenance of airway patency and lung ventilation.

Unconsciousness in a patient raises concern regarding the severity of the trauma and the presence of associated injuries, including traumatic brain injury (TBI), C-spine injuries, and visceral/internal injuries. While immediate airway management is critical in every trauma patient, the presence or suspicion of a TBI would place an even greater imperative for expert airway management to avoid secondary brain injury related to hypoxia and intracranial pressure.

15.2.6   How would you alleviate the airway obstruction?

Several simple maneuvers can be used to alleviate an airway obstruction. These include a chin lift, jaw lift, jaw thrust, head tilt, and tongue protrusion. While all these maneuvers are effective, some of these simple steps may involve significant movement of the C-spine.

Although a jaw thrust, or pulling the tongue forward, is traditionally felt to be associated with the least cervical movement, cadaver studies have shown it is still associated with some C-spine movement and should be performed with circumspection.[3] An oral or nasal airway will often alleviate airway obstruction, and the risk of violation of the cranial vault is likely less with a nasal airway than with the longer, and larger, nasotracheal tube. The insertion of a nasal airway under these circumstances is a clinical decision based on situational risk/benefit and the experience of the practitioner.

15.2.7   How would you assess the patient's airway? Are traditional means of airway assessment valid in the unconscious patient?

A number of airway measurements exist as tools to predict a difficult laryngoscopy (see Chapter 1). Unfortunately, these assessment tools are less useful in an unconscious trauma patient.

The focus of airway assessment in this patient should be the recognition of external anatomical characteristics, as well as signs of trauma to the head and neck. Signs of basal skull fracture are unlikely to be immediately evident and a high index of suspicion should exist, based on the mechanism of injury, for the presence of basal skull and neck fractures.

15.3   AIRWAY MANAGEMENT

15.3.1   Is this patient likely to be difficult to oxygenate? Why?

This patient has the potential to be a case of difficult BMV because of potential trauma to the head and neck causing facial deformities. It is also possible that there are foreign bodies, such as fractured teeth and blood clots, in the upper airway. In the context of an upright position and limited facial access, these are likely to make oxygenation a challenging task. While the acronym "MOANS" (see Section 1.6.1) may be useful to predict difficulties with BMV in conscious cooperative patients, it is not useful for this patient. The effect of trauma to the head and neck on BMV can be unpredictable but does not preclude an initial attempt at BMV to oxygenate the patient. It is also reasonable to use an extraglottic device (EGD) such as the laryngeal mask airway (LMA) if the BMV fails. Unfortunately, the effectiveness of ventilating a patient using the LMA may be equally unpredictable following a facial trauma.

15.3.2 Would DL be successful in this patient? Why or why not?

DL is unlikely to be effective in this patient because of limitations resulting from patient access and patient positioning.[4] The "toma-hawk" frontal approach is used in some parts of the world and by some practitioners in cases such as these with some success. However, unless skilled in the technique, the focus for this patient should be alternate management strategies including digital intubation, lightwand-guided intubation, EGDs, and cricothyrotomy.

15.3.3 When assessing this patient, what are your considerations for a surgical airway?

A surgical airway is indicated when tracheal intubation is not possible, deemed to be possible and other methods of providing adequate gas exchange are not immediately possible or successful. Delay in proceeding to a surgical airway is an important cause of morbidity and mortality. Surgical airways, such as SC, should only be performed by those familiar with the techniques. Studies in prehospital airway management have reported success rates of 82–100% when performed by trained paramedics, nurses, or physicians. Complication rates vary from 0% to 27%.[4] It should be emphasized that to ensure adequate ventilation and oxygenation, a cricothyrotomy kit with a cuffed tube (e.g., Cook Critical Care, Bloomington, IN) should be used when an SC is performed.

15.3.4 What are your options for endotracheal intubation in this patient?

Laryngoscopic intubation will be virtually impossible unless the patient is extricated from the vehicle. In the clinical situation where the patient cannot be removed from the vehicle, the options for endotracheal intubation include lightwand-guided intubation, digital intubation, and intubation using the LMA.

15.3.4.1 Lightwand (Trachlight™) Intubation

Intubation using the lightwand (Trachlight™) is described in Chapter 10.[5,6] The lightwand is a light-guided intubating technique that depends on transillumination of the trachea to produce a well circumscribed light glow in the anterior neck to facilitate endotracheal intubation. As long as the anterior neck can be accessed and visualized, this light-guided technique should be easy to perform. Lightwand intubation can be performed from the head or the side of the patient (facing the patient),[7] making it a suitable technique for patients who are in a sitting position.

The lightwand has been shown to facilitate endotracheal intubation in the trauma setting.[8] It may be particularly advantageous in this patient because of her seated position, potential for limited mouth opening and C-spine injury.[8–10] If she is clenching her jaw, the lightwand can be used for intubation by inserting the light-wand behind the molars and directing it toward the trachea in a paramedian fashion,[11] or nasally (see Section 15.3.5 below). Other advantages of the lightwand include its effectiveness despite the presence of blood and secretions in the airway as these substances transilluminate as do tissues. Lightwand intubation using cricoid pressure (although the intubation time is longer with the application of cricoid pressure)[12,13] and combining it with other airway adjuncts, including lightwand-guided digital intubation, and intubation through an LMA (see Chapter 10) are also options.

One of the difficulties of the lightwand intubating technique is the effect of ambient lighting on visualization of the lighted stylet on the anterior neck. Using the Trachlight™, Hung et al. reported an 88% success rate without dimming the operating room lights, suggesting that the effect of ambient light is relatively minor.[10] However, if necessary, the anterior neck can be shaded to facilitate intubation with the lightwand.

15.3.4.2 Digital Intubation

Digital intubation (or tactile orotracheal intubation) describes the insertion of an ETT into the trachea using the fingers. Digital-guided intubation has been described previously (see Chapter 10). It is a safe and effective technique for airway management in the prehospital setting, requiring minimal equipment and patient access.[14,15]

While facing the patient, the clinician pulls the patient's tongue forward using the dominant hand. The nondominant hand is then inserted into the airway where the epiglottis can be palpated and lifted superiorly using the long finger. An Eschmann Introducer (if available) can then be inserted into the airway with the dominant hand. The Eschmann Introducer is then guided anteriorly into the trachea with the index finger of the nondominant hand. Confirmation of tracheal placement of the Eschmann Introducer can be done in the usual manner (e.g., tracheal clicks and the "hold up"). The ETT can then be loaded onto the Eschmann Introducer and advanced into the trachea employing the nondominant hand to guide the ETT over the tongue into the trachea. The Eschmann Introducer is then removed and positioning of the ETT in the trachea is confirmed. If an Eschmann Introducer is not available, a styletted ETT can be advanced into the airway and guided into the trachea as described in Chapter 10. Digital intubation can also be performed using the lightwand in lieu of the Eschmann Introducer. This allows the clinician to confirm placement using tactile and visual cues.

There are relatively few studies examining the role of digital intubation in the management of a patient's airway. Stewart reported that digital intubation is a simple and useful airway technique in the prehospital environment because it can be performed with minimal head and neck movement and with a cervical collar in place.[14] The presence of blood or secretions in the airway does not seem to influence its success. Similarly, Hardwick and Bluhm, in their series, report successful intubation in 58 out of 66 patients in the prehospital setting.[15]

15.3.5 Would nasotracheal intubation be suitable for this patient?

Blind nasal tracheal intubation would not be the first choice for endotracheal intubation in this patient because of potential basal skull fracture and lack of respiratory efforts. However, this alternative should be kept in mind if orotracheal intubation is difficult or unsuccessful. In the event that the patient's condition is deteriorating rapidly, and multiple attempts at the airway have been made, it may be more practical to proceed to an SC rather than persist in the struggle to secure a nasotracheal intubation. This, of course, requires a practitioner with the appropriate skills and equipment to perform an SC. In the absence of this, nasotracheal intubation could be considered.

If there are no spontaneous breathing efforts, and blind nasotracheal intubation is planned, it should be performed with a lightwand (Trachlight™).[7] The ETT is loaded onto the Trachlight™ (with the stylet removed) and inserted through the largest nostril. The ETT is guided into the trachea while watching the anterior neck for transillumination of the trachea. Once this is visualized, the ETT can be advanced into the trachea.

15.3.6 What are the alternative methods of airway management for this patient?

15.3.6.1 Extraglottic Devices

This is a rapidly expanding group of devices that can be used in this patient, as a rescue airway, in the event intubation and/or oxygenation are unsuccessful. EGDs include the LMA™ and its variations (such as the LMA Fastrach™ and the LMA ProSeal™), Combitube®, laryngeal tube (King LT™), and others.

Insertion and use of the LMA is described in Chapter 11. The LMA, and its variations, can be inserted by the practitioner while facing the patient; thus, providing an effective rescue airway to oxygenate the patient. While there are a host of other EGDs that can be used in this setting, the clinical experience has been primarily with the LMA and its variations. The LMA is also useful because it can act to subsequently facilitate endotracheal intubation (LMA Classic™ and LMA Fastrach™).

Although intubation using the LMA to guide the ETT into the trachea can be performed using either the LMA Classic™ or the LMA Fastrach™ (intubating LMA), it is substantially easier to advance the ETT through the LMA Fastrach™. See Table 15-1 for appropriate ETT sizes.

The LMA Fastrach™ is designed with a rigid handle to facilitate its insertion. Once positioned, the LMA Fastrach™ opening is designed to direct the ETT into the trachea. Reported intubation success rates using the LMA Fastrach™ range from 82% to 99.3%.[16] The LMA Fastrach™ comes with a specifically designed

silicone-wire-reinforced tracheal tube. However, a recent report comparing the specially designed silicone ETT for the LMA Fastrach™ with a traditional polyvinyl chloride ETT that has been warmed showed no difference in success rates,[17] although the practicality of warming an ETT in the prehospital environment makes this a less attractive option. When used together with the LMA Fastrach™, the Trachlight™ in the ETT has been shown to facilitate confirmation of tracheal placement of the ETT.[18]

The Combitube® is another EGD which can be easily inserted as a rescue device in this patient. Several reports suggested that it can play a significant role in the airway management of trauma patient.[19–21] Its use is described in detail in Chapter 11.

15.3.6.2 Surgical Cricothyrotomy

If the airway cannot be secured (either by endotracheal intubation or otherwise), and ventilation is unsuccessful or inadequate, securing the airway using a surgical technique is indicated. Details of performing SC are described in Chapter 12. The practitioner should be aware that obese patients, or those with abnormal anatomy (e.g., hematoma, trauma to the neck, previous surgery and radiation), might make identifying the cricothyroid membrane difficult. SC can be performed using either the open or Seldinger technique. There are a number of cricothyrotomy kits available (e.g., Cook Critical Care, Bloomington, IN) to facilitate SC. It should be emphasized that a cuffed cricothyrotomy tube should be used to ensure effective ventilation following its placement.

While SC may not be performed often in the prehospital environment, there is evidence that it can be performed, with reasonable success, should prehospital responders be appropriately trained.[4,22,23] In their retrospective review of SC performed by paramedics, Fortune et al. found that paramedics who were trained in SC were able to perform the technique with 64% of patients arriving in the emergency department with acceptable SC airways.[23] A further 16% required minor manipulation in the emergency department. Transtracheal jet ventilation has been touted by some as a reasonable alternative,[24] though success rates are low and the availability of such equipment in the field is unlikely.

15.4 OTHER CONSIDERATIONS

15.4.1 Discussion on the role of EGDs in the trauma patient

Increasingly, EGDs are gaining popularity in managing the airway of the trauma victim when the trachea cannot be intubated.[25–28] In their study, examining the use of the LMA in the prehospital environment, Martin et al. reported a success rate of 94% in trauma patients.[26] All successful insertions were performed in 10 seconds or less. The authors investigated the effectiveness of the LMA in providing adequate oxygenation and ventilation in these patients and found that, during transport, patient oxygen saturations ranged from 97% to 100% while the end-tidal CO_2 ranged from 24 to 35 mm Hg.[26] These data support a role for the LMA, and other EGDs (although most studies have examined the role of LMAs only), as tools for oxygenation and ventilation in trauma patients when tracheal intubation in the field was unsuccessful.

TABLE 15-1

Appropriate ETT Sizes for Intubation via LMA

LMA SIZE (in mm)	ENDOTRACHEAL TUBE SIZE (in mm ID)
4	6.0
5	7.0
LMA Fastrach™ (3, 4, and 5)	up to 8.0

To address the issue of aspiration with EGDs, multiple devices have been developed with alternate channels that should allow for drainage of regurgitated gastric contents.[29] The LMA ProSeal™ (see Chapter 11 for details) contains a drainage tube that extends into the upper esophagus at the distal end of the device.[29] Multiple case reports suggest that the LMA ProSeal™ is effective at minimizing aspiration risk,[30,31] although it does not eliminate it.[32,33]

The Combitube® also has the potential to protect the airway from aspiration of gastric contents. Using dye within the oropharynx, Mercer recently showed that the Combitube® could protect the airway in the majority of anesthetized patients. Unfortunately, tracheal soiling was seen in 7% (2/27) of the studied patients.[34] Similarly, using a pH probe in the trachea, Hagberg et al. reported evidence of low pH in the trachea in 1 of 25 anesthetized patients (4%) using a Combitube®, suggesting possible microaspiration of acidic gastric contents.[35]

In summary, while these EGDs are effective rescue devices to provide oxygenation and ventilation in trauma patients, they do not absolutely protect against the risk of aspiration of gastric contents.

15.4.2 What are your concerns with transporting this patient with an EGD as an airway?

EGDs are effective airway devices. Practitioners employing such devices as a rescue device must weigh the risks of removing a functioning EGD prior to transport, to attempt tracheal intubation rather than leave the EGD in situ and transport the patient immediately to a trauma center. Indeed, if the EGD is functioning well, it may be safer to leave it in place. There are a few considerations to keep in mind during transport.

First, these devices are not designed to protect the airway against the risks of aspiration, although multiple studies have not reported a significant incidence of aspiration.[25,26,36] At this time, the lack of well-designed studies of EGDs in the trauma setting suggests that they should be used as rescue devices in the event that the primary management plan (i.e., endotracheal intubation) fails.

A second concern regarding the use of EGDs in the transport of the trauma patient relates to the risk of malpositioning during patient transport. Any change in the positioning of the EGD may impair its ability to provide effective oxygenation and ventilation. The practitioner must continuously monitor the positioning and effectiveness of the EGD during transport. The application of cervical collars to maintain in-line cervical stabilization may also cause the EGDs to shift or cause airway obstruction during transport.[25]

15.5 SUGGESTED AIRWAY MANAGEMENT IN THE TRAPPED, UNCONSCIOUS PATIENT

The following is a suggested approach in managing the airway of an unconscious, nonbreathing patient trapped in a vehicle:

- 100% O_2.
- Attempts at BMV, with appropriate maneuvers to relieve airway obstruction (jaw thrust, oral/nasal airways). No pharmacological adjuncts should be necessary in this patient.

- Appropriate considerations to minimize C-spine movement should be taken, if possible.
- Depending on the skill of the practitioner, digital guided intubation will likely be the best option in this patient because it is rapid, requires minimal equipment, and can be used in conjunction with other adjuncts such as the lightwand to facilitate intubation.
- Light-guided intubation is an equally reasonable *alternative* to digital intubation because of its ease of use, portability, effectiveness with limited mouth opening, minimal C-spine movement, and compatibility with other techniques (digital intubation, nasotracheal intubation, LMA). The lightwand can also be used in the presence of a soiled airway (blood/secretions).
- The EGDs and SC are effective rescue devices/options should BMV and tracheal intubation fail.
- Confirm placement (auscultation, end-tidal CO_2 detectors).

15.6 SUMMARY

Prehospital airway management of an unconscious, nonbreathing patient trapped in a vehicle is one of the most challenging situations for airway practitioners. Options in airway management are generally limited. The selection of an airway technique must depend on the patient's condition, available resources, and the skills of the practitioner. Alternative intubating techniques such as light-guided intubation, digital intubation, and intubation through an LMA Fastrach™ are likely to be more successful than laryngoscopic intubation. The use of an EGD or SC are effective rescue options should BMV and tracheal intubation fail.

REFERENCES

1. Advanced Trauma Life Support® (ATLS®), American College of Surgeons.
2. Arbabi S, Jurkovich GJ, Wahl WL, et al.: A comparison of prehospital and hospital data in trauma patients. *J Trauma.* 2004;56:1029–1032.
3. Donaldson WF, 3rd, Heil BV, Donaldson VP, Silvaggio VJ: The effect of airway maneuvers on the unstable C1-C2 segment. A cadaver study. *Spine.* 1997;22:1215–1218.
4. Gerich TG, Schmidt U, Hubrich V, Lobenhoffer HP, Tscherne H: Prehospital airway management in the acutely injured patient: the role of surgical cricothyrotomy revisited. *J Trauma.* 1998;45:312–314.
5. Davis L, Cook-Sather SD, Schreiner MS: Lighted stylet tracheal intubation: a review. *Anesth Analg.* 2000;90:745–756.
6. Agro F, Hung OR, Cataldo R, Carassiti M, Gherardi S: Lightwand intubation using the Trachlight: a brief review of current knowledge. *Can J Anaesth.* 2001;48:592–599.
7. Hung OR, Stewart RD: Lightwand intubation: I – a new lightwand device. *Can J Anaesth.* 1995;42:820–825.
8. Vollmer TP, Stewart RD, Paris PM, Ellis D, Berkebile PE: Use of a lighted stylet for guided orotracheal intubation in the prehospital setting. *Ann Emerg Med.* 1985;14:324–328.
9. Hung OR, Pytka S, Morris I, Murphy M, Stewart RD: Lightwand intubation. II:Clinical trial of a new lightwand for tracheal intubation in patients with difficult airways. *Can J Anaesth.* 1995;42:826–830.
10. Hung OR, Pytka S, Morris I, et al.: Clinical trial of a new lightwand device (Trachlight™) to intubate the trachea. *Anesthesiology.* 1995;83:509–514.
11. Hartman RA, Castro T, Jr, Matson M, Fox DJ: Rapid orotracheal intubation in the clenched-jaw patient: a modification of the lightwand technique. *J Clin Anesth.* 1992;4:245–246.
12. Hodgson RE, Gopalan PD, Burrows RC, Zuma K: Effect of cricoid pressure on the success of endotracheal intubation with a lightwand. *Anesthesiology.* 2001;94:259–262.

13. Weis FR, Jr: Light-wand intubation for cervical spine injuries. *Anesth Analg.* 1992;74:622.
14. Stewart RD: Tactile orotracheal intubation. *Ann Emerg Med.* 1984;13:175–178.
15. Hardwick WC, Bluhm D: Digital intubation. *J Emerg Med.* 1984;1:317–320.
16. Nakazawa K, Tanaka N, Ishikawa S, et al.: Using the intubating laryngeal mask airway (LMA-Fastrach™) for blind endotracheal intubation in patients undergoing cervical spine operation. *Anesth Analg.* 1999;89:1319–1321.
17. Kundra P, Sujata N, Ravishankar M: Conventional tracheal tubes for intubation through the intubating laryngeal mask airway. *Anesth Analg.* 2005;100:284–288.
18. Fan KH, Hung OR, Agro F: A comparative study of tracheal intubation using an intubating laryngeal mask (Fastrach™) alone or together with a lightwand (Trachlight™). *J Clin Anesth.* 2000;12:581–585.
19. Blostein PA, Koestner AJ, Hoak S: Failed rapid sequence intubation in trauma patients: esophageal tracheal combitube is a useful adjunct. *J Trauma.* 1998;44:534–537.
20. Mercer MH, Gabbott DA: Insertion of the Combitube airway with the cervical spine immobilised in a rigid cervical collar. *Anaesthesia.* 1998;53:971–974.
21. Mercer MH, Gabbott DA: The influence of neck position on ventilation using the Combitube airway. *Anaesthesia.* 1998;53:146–150.
22. Bair AE, Panacek EA, Wisner DH, Bales R, Sakles JC: Cricothyrotomy: a 5-year experience at one institution. *J Emerg Med.* 2003;24:151–156.
23. Fortune JB, Judkins DG, Scanzaroli D, McLeod KB, Johnson SB: Efficacy of prehospital surgical cricothyrotomy in trauma patients. *J Trauma.* 1997;42:832–836; discussion 837–838.
24. Divatia JV, Bhadra N, Kulkarni AP, Upadhye SM: Failed intubation managed with subcricoid transtracheal jet ventilation followed by percutaneous tracheostomy. *Anesthesiology.* 2002;96:1519–1520.
25. Matioc AA, Wells JA: The LMA-unique in a prehospital trauma patient: interaction with a semirigid cervical collar: a case report. *J Trauma.* 2002;52:162–164.
26. Martin SE, Ochsner MG, Jarman RH, Agudelo WE, Davis FE: Use of the laryngeal mask airway in air transport when intubation fails. *J Trauma.* 1999;47:352–357.
27. Martin SE, Ochsner MG, Jarman RH, Agudelo WE: Laryngeal mask airway in air transport when intubation fails: case report. *J Trauma.* 1997;42:333–336.
28. Greene MK, Roden R, Hinchley G: The laryngeal mask airway. Two cases of prehospital trauma care. *Anaesthesia.* 1992;47:688–689.
29. Brain AI, Verghese C, Strube PJ: The LMA 'ProSeal'—a laryngeal mask with an oesophageal vent. *Br J Anaesth.* 2000;84:650–654.
30. Evans NR, Llewellyn RL, Gardner SV, James MF: Aspiration prevented by the ProSeal laryngeal mask airway: a case report. *Can J Anaesth.* 2002;49:413–416.
31. Mark DA: Protection from aspiration with the LMA-ProSeal™ after vomiting: a case report. *Can J Anaesth.* 2003;50:78–80.
32. Brimacombe J, Keller C: Aspiration of gastric contents during use of a ProSeal™ laryngeal mask airway secondary to unidentified fold over malposition. *Anesth Analg.* 2003;97:1192–1194.
33. Koay CK: A case of aspiration using the proseal LMA. *Anaesth Intensive Care.* 2003;31:123.
34. Mercer MH: An assessment of protection of the airway from aspiration of oropharyngeal contents using the Combitube airway. *Resuscitation.* 2001;51:135–138.
35. Hagberg CA, Vartazarian TN, Chelly JE, Ovassapian A: The incidence of gastroesophageal reflux and tracheal aspiration detected with pH electrodes is similar with the Laryngeal Mask Airway and Esophageal Tracheal Combitube—a pilot study. *Can J Anaesth.* 2004;51:243–249.
36. Rosenblatt WH: Airway management. In: *Clinical Anesthesia,* 4th edn. Barash PG, Cullen BF, Stoelting RK, eds. Philadelphia, PA: Lippincott Williams & Wilkins, 2001:601, 606–608.

SELF-EVALUATION QUESTIONS

15.1. How would you immediately manage this patient who is unconscious and not making effective respiratory efforts?

   A. him/her from the vehicle for definitive management.

   B. Insert a nasal/oral airway and attempt positive pressure ventilation.

   C. Obtain a definitive airway by intubating the patient.

   D. Scene survey, followed by maneuvers to relieve airway obstruction and attempts at BMV.

   E. This patient is impossible to intubate and surgical cricothyroidotomy is indicated.

15.2. Which of the following statements of the use of EGDs in managing the trauma airway is **INCORRECT?**

   A. Aspiration is a small risk and therefore EGDs are an effective first-line airway in trauma.

   B. EGDs are an effective rescue device should intubation be delayed or unsuccessful.

   C. EGDs can act as an adjunct to intubation.

   D. EGDs are effective airways in the trauma patient during transport.

   E. All EGDs (e.g., LMAs, Fastrach™, ProSeal™, Combitube®, Laryngeal Tubes) have been well studied in the trauma population and are proven to be effective.

15.3. The Lightwand/Trachlight™ can be used as an airway adjunct on its own or it can be combined with which one of the following techniques to facilitate intubation?

   A. direct laryngoscopy

   B. digital intubation

   C. intubation via an LMA

   D. nasotracheal intubation

   E. all of the above

CHAPTER (16)

Airway Management of a Motorcyclist with a Full Face Helmet Following an Accident

Mark P. Vu and Orlando R. Hung

16.1 CASE PRESENTATION

A 29-year-old male motorcyclist presents to the emergency department (ED) after being involved in a high-speed motor vehicle accident (MVA). The motorcyclist was traveling at approximately 65 km·h^{-1} (40 miles·h^{-1}) when he drove through an intersection and collided with a car. Although damage to the car was minimal, the motorcycle was severely damaged and the patient was found approximately 50 m (160 ft) from the point of impact. The patient's vital signs at the scene were heart rate 110 bpm, blood pressure 120/70 mm Hg, respiratory rate 24 breaths per min, SpO$_2$ 93% on room air. Paramedics placed the patient on a spine board and transferred him to the ED. In the ED, he complains of pain in his chest, difficulty breathing, and pain in his legs. He is wearing a nonmodular full-face helmet. His vital signs are found to be heart rate 120 bpm, blood pressure 110/50 mm Hg, respiratory rate 32 breaths per min, SpO$_2$ 89%, and he is becoming confused. There is clinical evidence of a compound fracture of his right femur.

16.2 PATIENT CONSIDERATIONS

16.2.1 What are the initial steps in the management of this patient?

The general principles of trauma care and resuscitation apply to this patient. An initial, rapid survey of the patient's vital functions including his airway, breathing, and circulation (the ABCs) should be undertaken.[1] Large bore intravenous access, oxygen, and basic monitoring (pulse oximetry, ECG, and serial blood pressure readings) should be instituted quickly. If the helmet cannot be easily or safely removed for the primary survey, supplemental oxygen may be provided by placing an inverted simple face-mask through the opening in the helmet. His airway assessment shows that he was wearing a full-face, nonmodular type motorcycle helmet, obscuring his mouth from view. His nose and nares are visible above the line of the face shield portion of the helmet, and his anterior neck is visible and displays normal anatomy. Rapid examination of his chest demonstrates equal air entry bilaterally, and his pulses are equal. Although this patient is protecting his airway, is breathing, and has an adequate blood pressure, he may require intervention to control his airway and breathing emergently after completion of the primary survey.

16.2.2 Are there recommendations in the advanced trauma life support (ATLS®) guidelines for the removal of helmets prior to transport?

There is currently no consensus regarding whether prehospital personnel should routinely remove a patient's helmet prior to transport to hospital. Individual patient factors and coexisting injuries should guide the decision to remove the patient's helmet. If possible, the helmet should remain in place unless emergent airway or respiratory support is needed in which case the helmet should be carefully removed in a manner that minimizes cervical spine motion. Most helmet removal techniques endorse a two-person approach: one person stabilizes the patient's head from below while another person carefully removes the helmet from above.[2] Prehospital personnel should be encouraged to consult with a hospital-based receiving physician if questions regarding patient care exist.

16.2.3   Are there recommendations in the ATLS® guidelines for the removal of helmets once the patient has arrived in hospital?

There is also no consensus on when or how a patient's helmet should be removed once the patient arrives in hospital. If the patient's condition permits, the helmet can remain in place during the trauma assessment to minimize the potential for cervical spine movement. After a careful neurological assessment, removal of the helmet under the fluoroscopy should be considered. If the patient's condition necessitates emergency airway or breathing support, the risks of providing airway management with the helmet in place should be carefully weighed against the risks of urgently removing the helmet. These issues will be discussed later in this chapter.

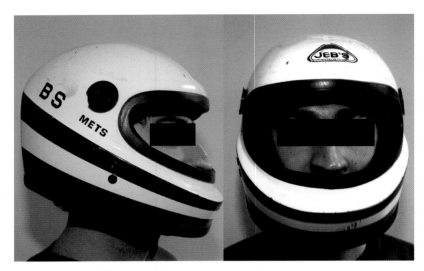

FIGURE 16-1. Full-face type helmets present a challenge to airway practitioners. The patient's mouth is completely obscured by the face-shield portion of the helmet. In general, the nose and neck are readily accessible (Right). However, in some types of full-face helmets, access to the nose may be limited.

16.2.4   Following a high-speed motorcycle crash, what other injuries might you anticipate for this patient?

Anticipating and identifying coexisting medical conditions in patients is important for practitioners. Alcohol is often a factor in motorcycle crashes and should be suspected in all cases.[3] A recent prospective study of 150 patients admitted to the emergency surgical service following an MVA showed that 37% were intoxicated with blood alcohol concentration greater than or equal to 100 mg·dL^{-1} (Ref. 4) (the blood alcohol concentration legal limit is between 0.08–0.1% depending on the province or state). Other causes for the crash should also be considered, including cerebrovascular accident, cardiac event, seizure, or intoxication from substances other than alcohol. A focused survey of the patient as suggested by the ATLS® guidelines will help to identify injuries that will significantly affect airway management. Airway practitioners should presume that this group of patients will have a full stomach and are at high risk for a cervical spine injury. Also, patients with open-face type helmets are at higher risk of sustaining facial injuries, but these injuries are still possible in patients wearing full-face helmets. A rigorous assessment of the oropharynx, nasal passages, and ears is often difficult in patients wearing helmets, and the benefits of a nasotracheal approach to endotracheal intubation should be weighed against the risks of this procedure in this population of patients.

16.3   AIRWAY CONSIDERATIONS

16.3.1   What types of helmets worn by motorcyclists are potentially problematic for airway management?

Motorcycle helmets can be grouped into two categories in the context of airway management: open-face and full-face. Open face helmets cover the cranium, sometimes the ears, but do not cover

the neck, chin, mouth, or nose. These features make them less protective to the patient in the event of a crash. There is an increase in the likelihood of serious anterior neck and facial injuries affecting airway anatomy, but concurrently renders airway assessment and intervention more straightforward. Full-face helmets are more protective to patients in the event of a crash, but are a major hindrance to airway assessment and intervention since access to the mouth is practically impossible (Figure 16-1). Moreover, removal of full-face helmets can be difficult, resulting in potentially significant cervical spine motion.[5,6] A recent study was conducted to evaluate the cervical spinal movement during the removal of a full-face helmet in 10 fresh cadavers with an experimental unstable fractured odontoid. Under fluoroscopy, there was significant movement of C1–2 during helmet removal and dislocation of C1–2 in two cases.[7] Although the clinical significance of these findings in live patients is unknown, this study suggests that there is a potential risk of spinal cord injury in a patient during the removal of a full-face helmet.

An important variation on the full-face helmet is the "modular" full-face helmet (Figure 16-2). The design of this helmet allows the movement of the face shield portion of the helmet away from the face. This helmet design allows the effective conversion of a full-face helmet into an open-face configuration, making airway management with the helmet in place more feasible.

16.3.2   Should helmets always be removed in order to provide airway management?

Removal of helmets for airway management is case dependent. There is currently no consensus on whether helmets should be routinely removed prior to airway management in trauma patients. There are concerns that cervical spine movement during helmet removal may be significant. Although the evidence of cervical spine movement during helmet removal has been supported by radiographic studies in cadavers, its clinical importance remains unknown. In prehospital care, removal of helmets by paramedics is

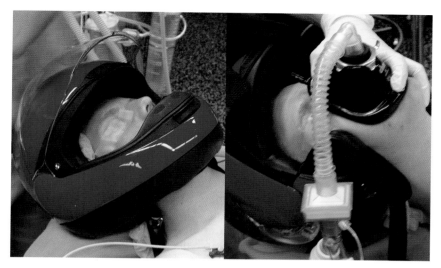

FIGURE 16-2. Modular type helmets allow more options for airway interventions (Left). Displacement of the face shield cephalad (Right) allows full access to the patient's nose, mouth, and neck as well as ventilation using a face mask.

standard prior to airway management. However, in sports medicine it is currently recommended that emergency medical personnel have the tools to remove face shields in order to provide airway management with the helmet in place.[8] Hospital-based airway practitioners should expect situations in which prehospital personnel have deferred definitive airway management until arrival at the hospital and therefore should be prepared for any scenario.

16.3.3   Describe a systematic approach to manage the airway of a patient wearing a motorcycle helmet

When a patient is wearing a motorcycle helmet, assessment of their airway should be completed in the standard fashion aiming to assess the feasibility of providing oxygenation and ventilation by (1) bag-mask, (2) extraglottic device (EGD), (3) endotracheal intubation by direct laryngoscopy, or (4) via a surgical airway. The first part of the assessment of a patient wearing a motorcycle helmet is identifying whether the helmet is open or full-face configuration.

In a patient wearing an open-face helmet, airway management can be performed with the helmet in place and the patient's head can be manually stabilized by an assistant to minimize movement of the head and neck. Bag-mask-ventilation, EGD insertion and surgical airway access are commonly straightforward in this scenario. If the open-face helmet has a visor, it should be removed to optimize line of vision during direct laryngoscopy.

In a patient wearing a full-face helmet, the practitioner must now determine whether the helmet is a modular type or not. If it is a modular type full-face helmet, the helmet may be left in place and the face shield portion should be carefully retracted superiorly to expose the face and neck. Once this is done, the airway can be managed with considerations similar to an open-face style helmet. It should be noted that a retracted face shield might obscure the line of vision during direct laryngoscopy. Alternative orotracheal intubating devices such as the Trachlight™ lighted stylet, the Glidescope™, a rigid or flexible fiberoptic intubation device are potentially useful.

In a patient wearing a full-face helmet that is not modular, several important issues must be carefully considered. Bag-mask-ventilation and EGD insertion are practically impossible because access to the mouth and face is extremely limited by the face shield. Direct laryngoscopy is practically impossible for the same reason. Access to the neck for a surgical airway is often possible, and the anatomical landmarks for cricothyrotomy should be carefully assessed. At this juncture, the practitioner should decide (1) can the helmet be removed prior to airway management and (2) should the helmet be removed prior to airway management? In many cases, it may be most appropriate to remove the helmet prior to airway interventions since this provides practitioners with the opportunity to properly assess the patient and optimally expose all relevant anatomy. Although there is no consensus on the proper technique for helmet removal, most authors advocate a two-person technique as described above. Some helmets have special mechanisms to facilitate emergency removal. Instructions can sometimes be found written on the sides of the helmet and may prove useful. Once the helmet is removed, oxygenation and ventilation can be provided in the standard fashion.

16.3.4   Should the endotracheal intubation be performed awake?

The patient wearing a motorcycle helmet, especially a full-face helmet, has significant predictors of difficult airway management. Bag-mask-ventilation is impossible in patients wearing full-face helmets and is suboptimal in patients wearing open-face helmets because of full stomach considerations. Laryngoscopy is difficult or impossible with full-face helmets, as is EGD insertion. In light of this, an awake intubation approach should be considered and is a reasonable option in cooperative patients. When possible, an "awake look" laryngoscopy can be a useful adjunct to the airway assessment as well. Unfortunately, this group of patients is challenging to intubate awake because they are often uncooperative and have significant secretions in their airway limiting the efficacy of topical anesthesia. Practitioners must consider the benefits of an awake technique and be prepared to proceed to an alternative plan.

16.4   DIFFICULT SITUATIONS: WHEN THE HELMET CANNOT BE REMOVED

16.4.1   Describe how you would provide oxygenation and ventilation in a situation where you cannot remove a nonmodular, full-face helmet

Arguably the most challenging situation for a practitioner is when a patient wearing a full-face helmet needs oxygenation and ventilation but the helmet cannot be removed easily. Many circumstances can make helmet removal difficult or impossible. Examples of such situations include patients with foreign objects penetrating the helmet and embedded in the skull and patients in whom removal of the helmet causes them extreme pain or distress, or individuals trapped in confined spaces where the helmet cannot be removed (e.g., race car). A systematic assessment of the airway management options for this patient will show that bag-mask-ventilation is impossible because the helmet's face shield obscures mouth and chin. Similarly, insertion of an EGD is practically impossible because access to the mouth is so limited. The two remaining options are (1) surgical airway using a cricothyrotomy or (2) nasotracheal intubation. Rapid assessment of the surgical landmarks relevant to cricothyrotomy, either percutaneous or open, is essential since this part of the patient's airway is usually unobstructed by the helmet or face shield. Securing the airway by a nasotracheal route is relatively simple and potentially useful and lifesaving. Airway practitioners familiar with nasotracheal intubation techniques should review the contraindications to this approach, such as evidence of basal skull fracture, prior to proceeding. Blind nasal intubation in a spontaneously breathing patient has a reasonable success rate. A recent report showed that blind nasal intubating technique has a 90% success rate for pre-hospital trauma patients requiring an endotracheal tube (ETT).[9,10] However, the success of blind nasotracheal intubation is limited by operator familiarity. A lighted stylet, such as the Trachlight™, loaded on a nasotracheal tube can be effectively used to achieve endotracheal intubation in a patient wearing a full-face helmet.[11] In this technique, transtracheal illumination using the Trachlight™ indirectly confirms proper placement of the nasotracheal tube.[12] If blood is present in the airway, the potential for a false passage in the airway makes a blind technique relatively contraindicated. Using a fiberoptic bronchoscope can be a helpful guide, especially in situations where blind techniques are contraindicated, but its efficacy may be limited by the presence of blood or secretions in the airway. Fiberoptic intubation can be performed with the patient awake and the nasopharyngeal mucosa topically anesthetized or with the patient under general anesthesia and muscle relaxed. The risks of each approach should be considered in the context of the patient's comorbidities and the operator's familiarity with the techniques.

Airway practitioners should consider a "double setup" plan that includes both a primary intubation approach (e.g., a light-guided nasotracheal intubation, fiberoptic bronchoscope, etc.) and a secondary backup surgical approach for the patient wearing a full-face helmet that cannot be removed. Since the patient's neck is almost always accessible regardless of the type of helmet worn, a "double setup" facilitates prompt airway control via a surgical access in case the primary plan is unsuccessful. Two separate equipment trays should be prepared: the first contains all the equipment needed for oral or nasotracheal access, and the second tray contains all the instruments needed for a surgical airway. Having a second skilled practitioner available who is familiar with surgical airway access is ideal. Prior to initiating the airway intervention, the patient should be optimally positioned, the neck should be prepped, and the airway management team should agree on clear end points that determine when the primary approach has failed and when to activate the secondary approach (i.e., surgical airway).

16.4.2 How do you perform a light-guided nasotracheal intubation for this patient if it becomes necessary?

An appropriate size uncut ETT should be used. While it is not possible to warm and soften the ETT in this emergency situation, generous lubrication of the ETT will facilitate nasal intubation and minimize injury. The Trachlight™ is prepared as previously described (see Section 10.3.6) with the stiff internal wire stylet removed so that the ETT/Trachlight™ (ETT/TL) unit is pliable and suitable for nasal intubation. Ideally, a vasoconstrictor, e.g., xylometazoline hydrochloride (Otrivin™) nasal spray (if available and time permits), should be administered prior to the insertion of the ETT/TL through the nostril. Following the placement of the ETT/TL tip into the nasopharynx, it is advanced gently into the glottic opening using the transillumination of the soft tissues of the anterior neck. As it is not possible to perform a jaw lift with the full-face helmet in place, a gentle jaw thrust with minimal neck movement can be performed by an assistant to elevate the tongue and epiglottis. Using the light glow, the tip of the ETT/TL is then guided to the glottic opening. When the tip of the ETT enters the glottic opening, a bright circumscribed glow can be seen readily just below the thyroid prominence and the ETT/TL unit is then advanced into the trachea.

Occasionally, the tip of the ETT/TL will repeatedly go posteriorly into the esophagus. To overcome this problem, the tip of the ETT can be easily elevated anteriorly by flexing the neck. However, movement of the neck should be avoided for this patient with a potential cervical spine injury. It is also possible to elevate the tip of the ETT anteriorly and align it with the glottis by inflating the ETT cuff of the ETT in the hypopharynx with 20 mL of air.[13] The tip of the ETT/TL can then be guided by transillumination toward the glottic opening. When the tip enters the glottic opening, a bright circumscribed glow is seen below the thyroid prominence. At this point, the ETT cuff should be deflated to allow the advancement of ETT/TL further into the trachea. Following the inflation of the cuff, ETT placement should be confirmed using auscultation and the presence of end-tidal CO_2.

16.4.3 Would your approach to airway management change for a patient who is wearing a football helmet or hockey helmet?

The approach to a patient who is wearing a different type of protective helmet is similar. Sports helmets can be open-face, full-face, and can have various styles of face shields. Of note, many of these face shields can be easily removed with simple tools, such as a screwdriver. Current recommendations suggest that injured athletes requiring emergency medical care should have their face shields removed and their helmets left in place for airway management.[14,15] This highlights the fact that sports helmets have face shields that are easily removed and takes heed of research suggesting that cervical spine motion is lessened when the helmet is left in place.

16.5 SUMMARY

Airway management in patients wearing helmets can present a major challenge to practitioners. The principles of airway management remain the same regardless of whether or not the patient is wearing a helmet; however the type of helmet can significantly impact the options available to practitioners. It is worth remembering that almost all patients wearing helmets are trauma patients, and therefore the usual considerations of full stomach, head injury, and cervical spine precautions are applicable. If a patient's airway can be managed with the helmet in place, this is often a safer option if an unstable cervical spine injury is suspected. Removing a helmet prior to airway management is often appropriate to optimize intubating conditions, but should be done carefully. Rarely, situations occur where a patient's helmet cannot be removed but oxygenation and ventilation must be provided, and practitioners must have a plan and the skills to deal with this scenario.

REFERENCES

1. American College of Surgeons: Committee on Trauma. *Advanced Trauma Life Support program for doctors: ATLS®.* 6th edn. Chicago, IL: American College of Surgeons, 1997.
2. Tintinalli JE, Kelen GD, Stapczynski JS (eds.): *Emergency Medicine, A Comprehensive Study Guide.* 6th edn. New York, NY: McGraw Hill Professional Publishing. 2003.
3. Hurt HH, Ouellet J., Thom, DR: Motorcycle Accident Cause Factors and Identification of Countermeasures, Volume 1: Technical Reports, Traffic Safety Center, University of Southern California, Los Angeles, 1981.
4. Mancino M, Cunningham MR, Davidson P, et al.: Identification of the motor vehicle accident victim who abuses alcohol: an opportunity to reduce trauma. *J Stud Alcohol.* 1996;6:652–658.
5. Kolman JM, Hung OR, Beauprie IG, et al.: Evaluation of cervical spine movement during helmet removal. *Can J Anesth.* 2003;50:A18.
6. Brimacombe J, Keller C, Kunzel KH, et al.: Cervical spine motion during airway management: A cinefluroscopic study of the posteriorly destabilized third cervical vertebrae in human cadavers. *Anesth Analg.* 2000;5:1274–1278.
7. Laun RA, Lignitz E, Haase N, et al.: Mobility of unstable fractures of the odontoid during helmet removal. A biomechanical study. *Unfallchirurg.* 2002;105(12):1092–1096.
8. Waninger KN: On-field management of potential cervical spine injury in helmeted football players: Leave the helmet on! *Clin J Sport Med.* 1998;2:124–129.
9. Dauphinee K: Nasotracheal intubation. *Emerg Med Clin North Am.* 1988;6(4):715–723.
10. Weitzel N, Kendall J, Pons P: Blind nasotracheal intubation for patients with penetrating neck trauma. *J Trauma.* 2004;56(5):1097–1101.
11. Vu M, Guzzo A, Hung OR, et al.: A novel method for endotracheal intubation in patients wearing full-face helmets. *World Cong Anesth.* 2003:CD014.
12. Hung OR, Pytka S, Morris I, et al.: Clinical trial of a new lightwand device (Trachlight) to intubate the trachea. *Anesthesiology.* 1995;83(3):509–514.
13. Gorback MS: Inflation of the endotracheal tube cuff as an aid to blind nasal endotracheal intubation (Letter). *Anesth Analg.* 1987;66:913.
14. Laprade RF, Schnetzler KA, Broxterman RJ, et al.: Cervical spine alignment in the immobilized ice hockey played. A computed tomography analysis of the effect of helmet removal. *Am J Sports Med.* 2000;23(6):800–803.
15. Swenson TM, Lauerman WC, Blanc RO, et al.: Cervical spine alignment in the immobilized football player. Radiographic analysis before and after helmet removal. *Am J Sport Med.* 1997;25(2):226–230.

SELF-EVALUATION QUESTIONS

16.1. You are about to perform a tracheal intubation in an unconscious, 29-year-old male motorcycle driver who was involved in a high-speed MVC. His open-face helmet is in place. His airway examination is favorable, and he has no predictors of difficult bag-mask-ventilation, EGD insertion, or laryngoscopy. Regarding his helmet, which of the following statements is true?

A. a skilled assistant should hold maintain inline stabilization of the patient's head and neck during the airway intervention

B. if the open-face style helmet is not obstructing the line of sight for laryngoscopy, it may remain in place during the airway intervention

C. a rapid sequence induction technique with a muscle relaxant is a reasonable choice to facilitate endotracheal intubation

D. all of the above are true

16.2. A 20-year-old motorcycle driver is involved in a high-speed MVC. He is brought to your hospital on a spine board still wearing his full-face style helmet. His vital signs are stable and he is cooperative. He complains of pain in his left leg and his neck. You should

A. remove his helmet immediately and provide supplemental oxygen

B. carefully remove the helmet by yourself and ask the patient to inform you of any discomfort

C. ask the patient to carefully remove the helmet himself while you assist him

D. complete your primary survey assessment, provide oxygen through his helmet if necessary, and complete lateral C-spine x-rays with the helmet in place prior to removing the helmet with the assistance of a skilled colleague

16.3. You assess a 50-year-old male motorcyclist who was involved in a high-speed MVC. He is wearing a modular full-face helmet with the face shield retracted. He is unconscious, breathing spontaneously, and is receiving oxygenation and ventilation via a Combitube™ placed in the field by paramedics after multiple failed attempts at laryngoscopy. He is obese and has a full beard. His SpO_2 on FiO_2 1.00 is 87%, blood pressure 110/70, heart rate 100, respiratory rate 24 assisted. You quickly review this case with a colleague and decide that your safest plan to establish a definitive airway is

A. leave the Combitube™ in place indefinitely

B. replace the Combitube™ with an LMA

C. give succinylcholine, remove the Combitube™, and replace it with an orotracheal tube under direct laryngoscopy

D. perform a cricothyrotomy with the Combitube™ in place and the patient breathing spontaneously

CHAPTER (17)

Airway Management of a Morbidly Obese Patient Suffering from a Cardiac Arrest

Saul Pytka and Idena Carroll

17.1 CASE PRESENTATION

A 67-year-old woman presented in the emergency department (ED) by ambulance with a 3-hour history of increasing dyspnea associated with chest pain. She had a history of coronary artery disease, hypertension, and hyperlipidemia, but no known allergies. Her medications included atenolol, low-dose Aspirin, atorvastatin, acetaminophen with codeine, and nitroglycerin spray as needed. Prior to notifying the emergency medical services, the patient had used three sprays of nitroglycerin every 5 to 10 minutes with no relief.

Upon arrival at the ED, she was placed on 10 L·min^{-1} oxygen by face mask. Her vital signs were heart rate 113 beats per minute and irregular, respirations 31 breaths per minute, blood pressure 85/45 mm Hg, and SaO_2 86%. On examination, she appeared to be in severe respiratory distress and was unable to speak more than three to four words in one breath. She was morbidly obese with an estimated weight of over 300 lb (137 kg) and was about 5 ft (151 cm) tall. Chest auscultation revealed faint breath sounds with crackles over the entire lung fields, a significant decrease in air entry in both bases combined with mild wheezing. Other findings included 1 + bilateral ankle edema, S_4, heart sound, and a grade III/VI systolic murmur radiating to axilla. Her jugular venous pressures (JVP) could not be assessed because of her marked obesity and short neck. Her electrocardiogram showed a pattern consistent with an acute anterolateral myocardial infarction. The chest x-ray revealed poor inflation and was consistent with pulmonary edema.

Following the initial assessment, the SaO_2 decreased to 81% with respirations increasing to 35–40 breaths per minute. Pink froth appeared from her mouth.

As you prepare for airway intervention, she loses consciousness. The monitor shows ventricular tachycardia (VT), which is pulseless. What do you do to secure the airway at this time?

17.2 INTRODUCTION

17.2.1 Define obesity

Obesity is the presence of an excess of body fat when compared to average values for age and gender. When the percentage of body fat exceeds 15–18% in men, or 20–25% in women, the individual is considered obese. Unfortunately, measuring body fat is not practical as it requires sophisticated techniques.

The ideal body weight (IBW) has been used frequently in clinical settings to define obesity:

$$IBW\ (Kg) = height\ (cm) - x,$$

where x is 100 for males and 105 for females.

Patients who weigh 20% above IBW are considered overweight, and they are considered morbid obese if they weigh 200% above the IBW.[1]

The World Health Organization (WHO), on the other hand, has utilized body mass index (BMI) as the international method of classifying obesity.[2] It is now the standard method for defining obesity.[3]

$$BMI = \frac{body\ weight\ (kg)}{height^2\ (m)},$$

Using the BMI, obesity is categorized as follows[4]:

- A person is considered overweight with a BMI of 25–29.9 $kg \cdot m^{-2}$.
- Obese individuals have a BMI > 30 $kg \cdot m^{-2}$.
- Morbidly obese individuals have a BMI > 35 $kg \cdot m^{-2}$.
- Super morbidly obese individuals have a BMI > 55 $kg \cdot m^{-2}$.

It has been well established that obesity is associated with multiple medical issues including hypertension, heart disease, congestive heart failure, diabetes mellitus, stroke, obstructive sleep apnea (OSA), an increased incidence of perioperative wound infection, and respiratory complications.

Recently, a more important predictor of long-term outcome has been shown to be the type of fat distribution, rather than BMI. "Male" or android-pattern central obesity (trunk and abdomen) has been shown to correlate more with negative outcomes and increased risk of cardiac disease and premature death than "female pattern," gynecoid obesity (peripheral).

"Metabolic syndrome" (syndrome x) describes truncal obesity as being a waist-to-hip ratio of >0.9 in men, or >0.85 in women, or a waist circumference of >40 in. (approximately 100 cm) in men and 35 in. (approximately 88 cm) in women. This syndrome is associated with glucose intolerance ("type II" diabetes), hypertension, dyslipidemia, microalbuminuria, prothrombotic states, and proinflammatory states (e.g., elevated C-reactive protein) and represents a particularly high-risk group for the development of cardiovascular and cerebrovascular diseases.[5,6]

Reducing the degree of obesity has been shown to favorably impact the progression of these disorders.[7,8]

17.2.2 What are the anatomic and physiologic factors that might contribute to the difficulty of airway management in the morbidly obese patient?

Numerous factors have been implicated as contributing to difficult bag-mask-ventilation (BMV), extraglottic device (EGD) use, laryngoscopy and intubation, and the performance of a surgical airway in this population. These include large breasts (male and female), excess adipose tissue in the face and cheeks, short neck, large tongue, redundant palatal and pharyngeal tissue, superior and anterior larynx, limited mouth opening, limited access to the anterior neck, and limited cervical spine mobility.[4]

Experience, and the literature, suggest that morbidly obese patients do not represent a "difficult airway" (see Chapter 1) based on weight alone. Even when a morbidly obese patient has favorable airway assessment parameters (i.e., Mallampati I, full range of motion of neck, adequate mouth opening, etc.), other factors can make the airway intervention more difficult.

There is a significant decrease in tolerable apnea time as compared with that of nonobese subjects. This decrease occurs in a linear fashion as obesity increases and relates to both a decreased respiratory reserve and an increase in metabolic requirement.[9] This decreased "respiratory reserve" is the result of a decrease in functional residual capacity (FRC) combined with a closing capacity that intrudes on tidal volume ventilation.[9,10] Furthermore, the high FiO_2 employed in all intubations induces absorption atelectasis, further reducing the amount of lung tissue available for gas exchange. Because of these factors, precipitous oxygen desaturation occurs rapidly should the patient be rendered apneic during airway management.[10] Data from Jense suggest that in the morbidly obese patient, apneic time before the development of hypoxemia during rapid sequence induction (RSI) permits only a single intubation attempt.[9]

The morbidly obese patient also has a restrictive lung defect resulting in a decreased vital capacity, expiratory reserve volume, and inspiratory capacity.[9,11] Auler et al. found that the morbidly obese patient under general anesthesia presents a higher resistance of the total respiratory system.[12]

The presence of morbid obesity is considered a predictor for difficult mask-ventilation by many.[4,9,13] Adequate BMV requires an open airway and a tight mask seal. Creating a patent airway in the morbidly obese and maintaining a competent mask seal in the face of elevated airway pressures sufficient to overcome the restrictive defect imparted by obesity mitigate effective BMV. Anterior translation of the mandible (jaw thrust) to effect airway opening has been shown to be more difficult and less effective in the obese.[14] In the cited study, nine nonobese and nine obese subjects were anesthetized and given neuromuscular blocking agents. Once apneic, and with steady airway pressure applied via a nasal device, the oropharynx and velopharynx (nasopharynx) were visualized with an endoscope. The cross-sectional areas were measured, both with resting state and a jaw thrust applied. In both groups of patients, the jaw thrust improved the cross-sectional area of the oropharynx. However, although an improvement with the jaw thrust maneuver occurred in the measurements of the velopharynx in the nonobese population, no improvement was noted to occur with this maneuver in the obese patients. The authors found that obstruction persisted in the lateral plane rather than that in the anteroposterior dimension, and postulated that this was due to the traction allowing the redundant soft tissue around the tonsillar pillars to close in from the sides as the tonsillar pillars were stretched anteroposteriorly. This may explain why continuous positive airway pressure (CPAP) or positive end-expiratory pressure (PEEP) augments ventilation in the obese patient, as both laterally splint the airway.[14,15] It may also explain why the LMA has been found to be an effective rescue device in the obese population (see below).

17.2.3 What are the special considerations in patients with obstructive sleep apnea?

About 5% of morbidly obese patients have OSA.[4] In studying over 6,000 subjects, Nieto[16] reported that the majority of patients with OSA are not obese. Consequently, questioning patients regarding OSA should not be reserved for only the obese. The presence of snoring may be the only indicator of OSA in the general population. Snoring and obesity are important predictors for difficult BMV.[13]

Although statistically difficult to quantify, a significant relationship exists between difficult tracheal intubation and OSA.[17] In patients with OSA, airway patency is disturbed by relaxation of pharyngeal dilator muscles during sleep. The upper airway is soft, pliable, and narrow in these patients, which makes it collapsible during sleep. Turbulent air flow through these structures produces vibrations (snoring) and collapse (apnea).[18] This obstruction continues until the level of sleep is interrupted and the individual regains pharyngeal muscle tone. This snoring/obstruction/apnea cycle is exacerbated by drugs or alcohol. Consequently, sedatives, particularly the long-acting agents, given in the perioperative period can have a pronounced deleterious effect on the ability of this patient population to maintain airway patency when asleep.[4]

The obesity hypoventilation syndrome (OHS), also known as Pickwickian Syndrome, is characterized by chronic respiratory insufficiency, with both obstructive and restrictive features on pulmonary function testing. Chronic hypoxemia and hypercarbia, polycythemia, somnolence, pulmonary hypertension, and right ventricular dysfunction (cor pulmonale) characterize this condition. These patients all exhibit a marked reduction in hypoxic and hypercarbic drives, measuring one-sixth and one-third the response to that of controls, respectively.[19] Although some similarities exist between OSA and OHS, they are not the same disease. As pointed out above, not all patients with OSA are obese, and patients with OHS do not necessarily have OSA. Due to the significant underlying pulmonary and cardiac dysfunction with the OHS population, they are at significant perioperative risk.

17.2.4 Is tracheal intubation more difficult in morbidly obese patients?

There is some disagreement as to whether morbid obesity predicts difficult intubation. The incidence of difficult intubation in the morbidly obese population has been reported to be approximately 13–20%.[20–22]

However, in a study of 100 morbidly obese patients with BMIs of >40 kg·m^{-2}, Brodsky et al.[23] concluded that obesity, per se, was not a predictive factor in determining difficulty of intubation. Of the many parameters measured in the study population, the only two that correlated with difficult laryngoscopy following RSI with cricoid pressure were large neck circumference and high Mallampati scores. A neck circumference (measured at the level of the thyroid cartilage) of 40 cm was associated with a 5% incidence of difficult intubation. In the same study, 35% of patients with a neck circumference of 60 cm were difficult intubations.[23] Of interest is that larger neck circumference has also been associated with increasing severity of OSA.[24]

In a separate study, Ezri also found that obesity, by itself, was not a predictor of difficult intubation.[25]

17.3 AIRWAY MANAGEMENT PREPARATION

17.3.1 Are obese patients at increased risk of aspiration?

Obesity has been frequently listed as a risk factor for aspiration. However, recently this belief has been challenged by a number of studies that have found no increase in gastric volumes or acidity in obese subjects.[26,27] Maltby et al.[28] demonstrated that gastric emptying was no different in obese than in nonobese patients and suggested that the same guidelines for fasting can be applied to both patient populations. Aspiration risks and prophylaxis should be applied in the obese patients using the same criterion as the nonobese. For a detailed discussion of aspiration and risks, see Chapter 5.

17.3.2 How should the morbidly obese patient be positioned for airway management?

Because of the decreased oxygen reserve in this patient population, it is crucial to position these patients carefully for tracheal intubation prior to induction of anesthesia. Appropriate positioning prior to the induction of anesthesia can significantly reduce the apnea time required for intubation as well as increase the oxygen reserve. While recent literature has questioned the advantage of the sniffing position over simple head extension,[29] these studies still advocate the sniffing position for obese patients. Proper sniffing position has been defined as head extension and a 35-degree flexion of the neck onto the chest.[30]

Achieving adequate sniffing position in a patient of IBW may mean only placement of a pillow under the neck and extending the head. However, in a morbidly obese patient, optimal position often requires building a ramp of sheets or towels under the shoulders, neck, and head (Figures 17-1 and 17-2). This is referred to as "extreme sniffing" or a "ramped" position. A comparison study of 60 morbidly obese patients by Collins et al.[31] demonstrated a significant improvement of laryngoscopic grade in patients in the "ramped" position. Determinants of proper "ramped" positioning have been described as follows: at least a 90-degree angle between the mandible and chest; the face higher than the chest; and external auditory meatus at the same horizontal level as the sternal angle.[31]

A second and important positioning principle involves the use of the reverse Trendelenberg position. Bed placement of 30-degree head up tilt increases FRC and compliance (both lung and chest wall) thereby permitting greater degrees of pulmonary oxygen reserve. Adding CPAP of 10 cm of H_2O pressure has been shown to be an effective maneuver in reducing the degree of atelectasis associated with induction. Patients receiving PEEP/CPAP prior to induction can be expected to have higher PaO_2 values than the control groups that do not.[32,33]

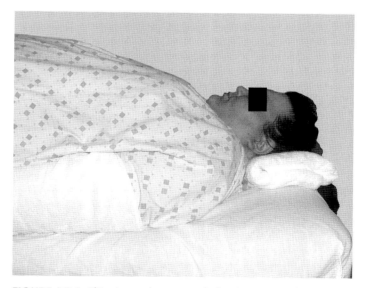

FIGURE 17-1. This picture shows a morbidly obese patient lying in a supine position with the neck and head resting on a regular pillow. It is difficult to access the mouth as well as perform direct laryngoscopy in this patient lying in this position.

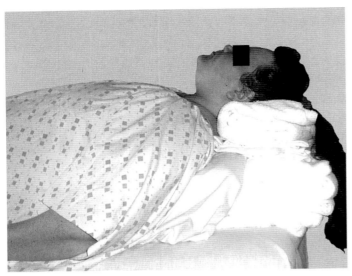

FIGURE 17-2. This picture shows a morbidly obese patient lying in a supine position with the shoulder, neck and head resting on a stacked "ramp" of hospital linen. This is an optimal position for airway management and laryngoscopic intubation for obese patients as the external auditory meatus is at the same horizontal level as the sternal angle.[31]

17.3.3 How should medications be dosed in the morbidly obese patient?

When determining the dosage of a drug, the IBW or lean body weight (LBW) are generally used. The LBW is a measured value, but can be estimated by the formula as follows:

$$LBW = (a)(weight) - b\left[\frac{weight^2}{(100 \times height)^2}\right],$$

where a and b = 1.1 and 128 for men, and 1.07 and 148 for women, respectively, weight in kg, and height in m.[34]

The IBW (as presented above) can be approximated by a simple formula.

$$IBW \ (kg) = height \ (in \ cm) - x,$$

where x is 100 for males and 105 for females.[1]

The use of total body weight (TBW) to calculate the dose is particularly problematic for lipophylic drugs. For some lipophylic agents, the use of TBW leads to an over calculation of the required dosage, and hence toxicity.

Perhaps the best way to calculate the appropriate dose of these agents is to employ the adjusted body weight (ABW):[35]

$$ABW = IBW + 0.4 \ (TBW - IBW).$$

There are a number of reasons for not using the TBW in calculating drug dosing. In the obese person, not all of the excess weight is fat. Lean mass is increased in the obese person and represents 20–40% of the increased weight, and in addition, blood supply to adipose tissues is quite low, accounting for only 5% of cardiac output. For all practical purposes, protein binding (a major influence on volume of distribution) in obese patients is essentially unaltered from their nonobese counterparts.[36]

17.4 AIRWAY MANAGEMENT

17.4.1 Discuss the appropriate methods for denitrogenation of the morbidly obese patient

While the term preinduction oxygenation or "preoxygenation" has been used by most to reflect denitrogenation of the lungs, the authors believe that the term "denitrogenation" should be used as it more accurately reflects the desired end result of nitrogen being washed out of the lungs. Two denitrogenation methods have been described and are equally effective techniques for the obese patient.[9] They included (1) four vital capacity breaths of 100% oxygen and (2) breathe 100% oxygen normally (tidal-volume breathing) through a snug-fitting face mask for 5 minutes. Denitrogenation employing CPAP with 100% oxygen showed no significant difference when compared with standard denitrogenation techniques on one study,[10] but proved beneficial in another.[32]

17.4.2 How effective is the laryngeal mask airway in the obese patient?

Numerous papers have been published recently illustrating the effectiveness of the various laryngeal mask devices available. Frappier et al.[37] studied 118 morbidly obese surgical patients with BMIs of >45 kg·m^{-2}. Following induction, all initially underwent laryngoscopy to determine the Cormack/Lehane (C/L) grade. Subsequently, they all underwent attempted tracheal intubation using the intubating laryngeal mask airway (ILMA). Tracheal intubation was successful in 114 patients (96.3%). Laryngoscopic intubation was successful for the remaining four patients with failed ILMA attempts. No correlation between laryngoscopic grade and failure with the ILMA was evident.

In a study of the efficacy of the LMA ProSeal™ laryngeal mask airway (PLMA) in the morbidly obese, Keller[38] induced anesthesia in 60 morbidly obese (BMI > 35 kg·m^{-2}) patients and inserted a PLMA. Insertion of the PLMA was successful in all patients; 90% on the first attempt and the remaining 10% on the second attempt. Following adequate oxygenation, the PLMA was removed, and laryngoscopic intubation was successful in 54 patients (90%) on the first attempt and 4 patients (7%) on the second attempt. Failure to intubate the trachea occurred in the remaining two patients (3%). These patients had the PLMA reinserted and the surgery proceeded using the extraglottic airway. No significant hypoxemia was reported in any patient during the study.

17.4.3 What are the plans to secure the airway of this patient?

Pulseless VT renders this patient a "Crash Airway" (Chapter 2). Airway management of this patient should take into account the principles discussed above.

As with any emergency intubation, every effort is made to ensure that the first attempt is the "best attempt":

• Best person,

• Best position,

• Best paralysis,

- Best BURP,
- Best length and type of laryngoscope blade.

If possible, placing the patient in a "ramped position" (see Figure 17-2) with reverse Trendelenberg immediately has the potential to improve pulmonary mechanics, improve the success of BMV, and optimize the ability to provide preintubation oxygenation saturations. Help should be summoned and adjuncts and alternative airway devices, such as the rigid fiberoptic laryngoscopes or videolaryngoscopes (Plan B and Plan C), should be immediately available. Direct laryngoscopy may not be difficult, unless there is a history of difficult intubation (OSA, previously failed intubation, etc.) or predictors of difficulty such as a thick neck or a high Mallampati score elicited precollapse.

Induction agents are not indicated in the crash airway. Neuromuscular blocking agents (e.g., succinylcholine) may be required in the event the first attempt at oral intubation fails and residual muscle tone is suspected to be a factor contributing to that failure (see Chapter 2). However, it is of questionable benefit to administer succinylcholine in the presence of a pulseless VT.

The risk of aspiration depends upon a number of factors, including the fact that it is an emergency, her stomach is likely to be full, and her history of GERD, to name a few. As failed or difficult intubation increases the risk of aspiration, cricoid pressure is employed from start to finish.

Should the decision to intubate her trachea have been made prior to her arrest, the decision to employ neuromuscular blockade to facilitate that intubation depends on the certainty that it will be able to effect gas exchange (BMV or EGD in the event that intubation fails). The selection and dosing of induction agents in the event that the decision to paralyze is taken should be based on the hemodynamic stability of the patient. In the event that effective gas exchange may not be possible, an "awake look" may be employed to further evaluate the potential for a successful intubation (see Chapter 2).

17.4.4 What are the rescue options for the failed airway in the morbidly obese patient?

The first rescue from failed BMV is improved BMV. BMV is likely to be difficult in this patient due to soft-tissue collapse of the upper airway, difficult or impossible mask seal, and noncompliant lungs due to her obesity and pulmonary edema. Having an experienced assistant to facilitate two-handed BMV technique may be crucial.

Management decisions in the face of the Failed Airway depend on whether it is a "can't intubate, can ventilate" failed airway or a "can't intubate, can't ventilate" (CICV) failed airway. In the former situation, one has time and may select an EGD or an alternative airway device or technique of greatest familiarity.

In the latter situation, there is no time and a cricothyrotomy must be performed. While preparing to perform the surgical airway, an EGD may be attempted concurrently.

In the CICV situation, it is appropriate to use alternative intubating techniques, such as the intubating LMA, the Bullard Laryngoscope, or the Glidescope® guided by the skill of the practitioner. These devices have been shown to be effective in placing tracheal tube in morbidly obese patients.

Due to the short, thick neck, performing a surgical airway in this morbidly obese patient is anticipated to be difficulty.

17.5 SUMMARY

The incidence of morbid obesity is increasing in our society, posing both long- and short-term risks to the patient requiring airway management. Associated medical conditions affecting vital organ system reserve intrude into our decision making when airway management is required. Obesity alone may not predict difficult laryngoscopy therefore highlighting the importance of thorough airway examination. However, a thick neck or high Mallampati scores do predict difficulty with laryngoscopic intubation. Difficulty with mask-ventilation is common. Preparation for failure is important. The various airway devices highlighted in this chapter have been shown to be effective in the obese patient.

Rapid desaturation and hypoxemia following induction and paralysis is to be expected. However, proper positioning to maximize FRC and recruit alveoli and proper denitrogenation practices mitigate the speed with which this desaturation occurs.

Drug dosing adjustments due to obesity remains poorly understood for many agents, but careful titration to effect with intravenous induction agents, time permitting, may prove to be effective and safer than dosing according to body weight.

Finally, the recognition of failure is crucial, as is the recognition of what type of failure has supervened. Management pathways are guided by the availability of time.

REFERENCES

1. Zeman F: *Clinical Nutrition and Dietetics*, 2nd edn. Upper Saddle River, NJ: Prentice Hall, 1991:470–516.
2. Report of WHO consultation on obesity: Preventing and managing the global epidemic, World Health Organization. Geneva, June 3–5, 1998.
3. Bray GA: Pathophysiology of obesity. *Am J Clin Nutr.* 1992;55:488S–494S.
4. Adams JP, Murphy PG: Obesity in anaesthesia and intensive care. *Br J Anaesth.* 2000;85:91–108.
5. Deen D: Metabolic syndrome: time for action. *Am Fam Physician.* 2004;69:2875–2882.
6. Mitka M: Metabolic syndrome recasts old cardiac, diabetes risk factors as a "new" entity. *JAMA.* 2004;291:2062–2063.
7. Anderson JW, Konz EC: Obesity and disease management: effects of weight loss on comorbid conditions. *Obes Res.* 2001;9:326S–334S.
8. Kenchaiah S, Evans JC, Levy D, et al.: Obesity and the risk of heart failure. *N Engl J Med.* 2002;347:305–313.
9. Jense HG, Dubin SA, Silverstein PI, O'Leary-Escolas U: Effect of obesity on safe duration of apnea in anesthetized humans. *Anesth Analg.* 1991;72:89–93.
10. Cressey DM, Berthoud MC, Reilly CS: Effectiveness of continuous positive airway pressure to enhance pre-oxygenation in morbidly obese women. *Anaesthesia.* 2001;56:680–684.
11. Doyle DJ, Arellano R: Upper airway diseases and airway management: a synopsis. *Anesthesiol Clin North America.* 2002;20:767–787.
12. Auler JO, Jr., Miyoshi E, Fernandes CR, et al.: The effects of abdominal opening on respiratory mechanics during general anesthesia in normal and morbidly obese patients: a comparative study. *Anesth Analg.* 2002;94:741–748.
13. Langeron O, Masso E, Huraux C, et al.: Prediction of difficult mask ventilation. *Anesthesiology.* 2000;92:1229–1236.
14. Isono S, Tanaka A, Tagaito Y, Sho Y, Nishino T: Pharyngeal patency in response to advancement of the mandible in obese anesthetized persons. *Anesthesiology.* 1997;87:1055–1062.
15. Rothfleisch R, Davis LL, Kuebel DA, deBoisblanc BP: Facilitation of fiberoptic nasotracheal intubation in a morbidly obese patient by simultaneous use of nasal CPAP. *Chest.* 1994;106:287–288.

16. Nieto FJ, Young TB, Lind BK, et al.: Association of sleep-disordered breathing, sleep apnea, and hypertension in a large community-based study. Sleep Heart Health Study. *JAMA*. 2000;283:1829–1836.

17. Hiremath AS, Hillman DR, James AL, et al.: Relationship between difficult tracheal intubation and obstructive sleep apnoea. *Br J Anaesth*. 1998;80:606–611.

18. Loadsman JA, Hillman DR: Anaesthesia and sleep apnoea. *Br J Anaesth*. 2001;86:254–266.

19. Zwillich CW, Sutton FD, Pierson DJ, Greagh EM, Weil JV: Decreased hypoxic ventilatory drive in the obesity-hypoventilation syndrome. *Am J Med*. 1975;59:343–348.

20. Buckley FP, Robinson NB, Simonowitz DA, Dellinger EP: Anaesthesia in the morbidly obese. A comparison of anaesthetic and analgesic regimens for upper abdominal surgery. *Anaesthesia*. 1983;38:840–851.

21. Juvin P, Lavaut E, Dupont H, et al.: Difficult tracheal intubation is more common in obese than in lean patients. *Anesth Analg*. 2003;97:595–600.

22. Voyagis GS, Kyriakis KP, Dimitriou V, Vrettou I: Value of oropharyngeal Mallampati classification in predicting difficult laryngoscopy among obese patients. *Eur J Anaesthesiol*. 1998;15:330–334.

23. Brodsky JB, Lemmens HJ, Brock-Utne JG, Vierra M, Saidman LJ: Morbid obesity and tracheal intubation. *Anesth Analg*. 2002;94:732–736.

24. Katz I, Stradling J, Slutsky AS, Zamel N, Hoffstein V: Do patients with obstructive sleep apnea have thick necks? *Am Rev Respir Dis*. 1990;141:1228–1231.

25. Ezri T, Medalion B, Weisenberg M, et al.: Increased body mass index per se is not a predictor of difficult laryngoscopy. *Can J Anaesth*. 2003;50:179–183.

26. Juvin P, Fevre G, Merouche M, Vallot T, Desmonts JM: Gastric residue is not more copious in obese patients. *Anesth Analg*. 2001;93:1621–1622.

27. Harter RL, Kelly WB, Kramer MG, Perez CE, Dzwonczyk RR: A comparison of the volume and pH of gastric contents of obese and lean surgical patients. *Anesth Analg*. 1998;86:147–152.

28. Maltby JR, Pytka S, Watson NC, Cowan RA, Fick GH: Drinking 300 mL of clear fluid two hours before surgery has no effect on gastric fluid volume and pH in fasting and non-fasting obese patients. *Can J Anaesth*. 2004;51:111–115.

29. Adnet F, Borron SW, Lapostolle F, Lapandry C: The three axis alignment theory and the "sniffing position": perpetuation of an anatomic myth? *Anesthesiology*. 1999;91:1964–1965.

30. Benumof JL: Comparison of intubating positions: the end point for position should be measured. *Anesthesiology*. 2002;97:750.

31. Collins JS, Lemmens HJ, Brodsky JB, Brock-Utne JG, Levitan RM: Laryngoscopy and morbid obesity: a comparison of the "sniff" and "ramped" positions. *Obes Surg*. 2004;14:1171–1175.

32. Coussa M, Proietti S, Schnyder P, et al.: Prevention of atelectasis formation during the induction of general anesthesia in morbidly obese patients. *Anesth Analg*. 2004;98:1491–1495.

33. Perilli V, Sollazzi L, Modesti C, et al.: Comparison of positive end-expiratory pressure with reverse Trendelenburg position in morbidly obese patients undergoing bariatric surgery: effects on hemodynamics and pulmonary gas exchange. *Obes Surg*. 2003;13:605–610.

34. Bouillon T, Shafer SL: Does size matter? *Anesthesiology*. 1998;89:557–560.

35. Erstad BL: Dosing of medications in morbidly obese patients in the intensive care unit setting. *Intensive Care Med*. 2004;30:18–32.

36. Cheymol G: Effects of obesity on pharmacokinetics implications for drug therapy. *Clin Pharmacokinet*. 2000;39:215–231.

37. Frappier J, Guenoun T, Journois D, et al.: Airway management using the intubating laryngeal mask airway for the morbidly obese patient. *Anesth Analg*. 2003;96:1510–1515.

38. Keller C, Brimacombe J, Kleinsasser A, Brimacombe L: The Laryngeal Mask Airway ProSeal(TM) as a temporary ventilatory device in grossly and morbidly obese patients before laryngoscope-guided tracheal intubation. *Anesth Analg*. 2002;94:737–740.

SELF-EVALUATION QUESTIONS

17.1. Which of the following is **NOT** true about airway management in obese patients?

A. the presence of morbid obesity is a predictor for difficult mask-ventilation

B. jaw thrust has been shown to be less effective in the obese patients

C. airway obstruction under anesthesia in obese patients is due to a decrease in the aneterioposterior dimension of the velopharynx (nasopharynx)

D. precipitous oxygenation desaturation usually occurs shortly following the induction and paralysis of obese patients

E. morbidly obese patients do not represent a risk of difficult intubation, based on weight alone

17.2. Which of the following is **NOT** true of OSA?

A. the majority of patients with OSA are obese

B. larger neck circumference has been associated with increased severity of OSA

C. the presence of snoring may be the only indicator of OSA in the general population

D. in patients with OSA, airway patency is disturbed by relaxation of pharyngeal dilator muscles during sleep

E. the snoring/obstruction/apnea cycle of OSA can be exacerbated by sedative and opioid medications including alcohol

17.3. Which of the following airway techniques is **NOT** known to be difficult in obese patients?

A. bag-mask-ventilation

B. surgical airway

C. light-guided intubation using a Trachlight™

D. laryngoscopic intubation in obese patients with thick necks

E. ventilation using a LMA

CHAPTER (18)

Airway Management with Blunt Anterior Neck Trauma

David A. Caro and Steven A. Godwin

18.1 CASE PRESENTATION

A 25-year-old male runs into an unseen wire while he is snowmobiling. The wire strikes his anterior neck and separates him from his snowmobile. Paramedics have been unsuccessful in placing a tracheal tube in the field and he arrives in the emergency department (ED) in a cervical collar, on a long spine board. He is unconscious, unresponsive to painful stimuli, and stridorous. Initial vital signs include a pulse rate of 120 bpm, a blood pressure of 160/90 mm Hg, a respiratory rate of 24 breaths per minute, and an oxygen saturation of 93% on room air. A non-rebreather mask is applied, and his oxygen saturation increases to 97%.

Palpation demonstrates no obvious subcutaneous air, but there is a large abrasion across the anterior and lateral areas of the neck (Figure 18-1). Palpation of the larynx demonstrates crepitus and some mild anatomic distortion. Airway protection is indicated and plans to secure the airway begin.

18.2 INITIAL PATIENT ASSESSMENT AND MANAGEMENT

18.2.1 What are the patient evaluation considerations I should be aware of?

Upon arrival at the ED, a protocol that is consistent with the guidelines of the Subcommittee of Advanced Trauma Life Support® of the American College of Surgeons Committee on Trauma should be followed. Aggressive initial management and a high index of suspicion for associated injuries are key steps in the successful management of patients with this type of injury.

A young patient with no significant medical history should have significant cardiorespiratory reserve. His initial oxygen saturation is concerning, but it improves with supplemental oxygen. His depressed level of consciousness could be due to a number of factors and anoxic injury to the brain or spinal cord is a consideration. His normal blood pressure, elevated pulse rate, and use of accessory muscles of respiration would suggest that his cervical cord is essentially intact. Nevertheless, his cervical spine is at significant risk and should be considered unstable until proven otherwise. Despite two small studies which suggest that laryngotracheal injury is compatible with a normal cervical spine,[1,2] the airway practitioner must assume that this patient has a cervical spine fracture until proven otherwise.[3]

Other associated injuries can occur with this type of clothesline injury. These include facial laceration, laceration of the esophagus, and of the recurrent laryngeal nerve injury.[4] It is imperative to do a thorough evaluation of the patient following the initial stabilization.

18.2.2 What are the airway evaluation considerations in this patient?

Considerations in this patient include laryngeal fracture, tracheal disruption, and a hematoma that could impinge on the airway. All of these may be difficult to detect.[5] In fact, blunt anterior neck trauma can impact all four of the dimensions of difficulty that one evaluates when contemplating airway management: bag-mask-ventilation, laryngoscopy and intubation, extraglottic device (EGD), and cricothyrotomy.

Difficulty with bag-mask-ventilation could stem from either anatomical upper airway distortion due to the trauma itself, tracheal

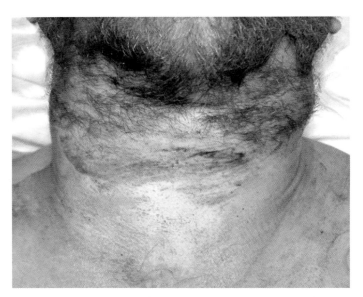

FIGURE 18-1. This picture shows that this patient has a large abrasion across the anterior and lateral areas of the neck.

disruption, or to trauma related to prior intubation attempts. Unfortunately, the use of EGDs in the setting of supraglottic or glottic disruption, or distortion, may be contraindicated.[6,7]

Difficult laryngoscopy should be anticipated. Supraglottic or glottic distortion may hinder visualization of the vocal cords. In the event one elects to pursue direct laryngoscopy, a Miller blade may be the preferable blade, as it may provide better control of the epiglottis and a more direct line of vision.[8]

One has to recognize that blunt anterior airway trauma may result in disruption of the trachea distal to the glottis. Tracheal transection may result in obstruction to tube passage or placement of the tube in a false passage through the tracheal disruption. Orotracheal laryngoscopy cannot detect this injury and may lead to a false sense of security relative to the "ease" of intubation.[9]

Cricothyrotomy may be very difficult in laryngeal trauma, as normal anatomic landmarks may be distorted, making it difficult to identify the larynx, the cricothyroid membrane, and the cricoid ring. In addition, subcutaneous air will compromise the capacity to identify the trachea with percutanous needle puncture and for this reason an open surgical technique is the preferred surgical approach.

18.3   AIRWAY MANAGEMENT

18.3.1   What are the airway management considerations in this patient?

This airway is not a crash airway, but it is a difficult one. Difficulty is expected with bag-mask-ventilation and laryngoscopy (the airway is potentially disrupted and neck mobility is limited). Difficulty can also be anticipated with EGD utilization and with cricothyrotomy (potential hematoma and laryngeal/tracheal distortion).

The mobilization of assistance is the first step in the management of this patient. There is time to formulate a plan. The patient's capacity to maintain ventilation should not be compromised by paralysis or other pharmacological respiratory depression. Conversely, coughing could further worsen the injury, or could compromise a traumatized spinal cord. Careful sedation and topical anesthesia is appropriate in this patient, and in-line stabilization of the cervical spine is an absolute requirement.

Typically, orotracheal intubation should be performed by the most experienced laryngoscopist immediately available. In addition, in-line stabilization of the cervical spine to guard against exacerbating an unstable cervical injury should be employed. Further, in a patient who has a potentially disrupted distal airway, a flexible fiberoptic bronchoscope (FFB) guided intubation is the procedure of choice.[10] This technique permits visualization as one advances into the trachea to ensure that the endotracheal tube is not advanced into a blind passage. Orotracheal laryngoscopy, following the gentle placement of an Eschmann Introducer (EI) (gum-elastic bougie), may be a distant second choice. The tactile response transmitted through the EI when it is slid against the tracheal rings may help to confirm that the EI is in the trachea and guides the endotracheal tube into place.[11] Confirmation of correct placement with an FFB is important, if feasible. A failed airway mandates an open cricothyrotomy.

18.3.2   What is the best way to intubate the trachea of this patient, step by step?

Equipment to carry out fiberoptic intubation, orotracheal intubation with an EI, and a cricothyrotomy ought to be available. Open cricothyrotomy equipment should be opened at the bedside and the patient's neck should be prepped and anesthetized. A bag-mask device, Magill forceps, functioning suction, and airway adjuncts (such as oral and nasal airway devices) should be prepared.

Denitrogenation with a bag-mask device is essential. A well-oxygenated patient gives the airway practitioner a cushion of time in the event it is needed. Steadily declining oxygen saturations may mandate assisted ventilation by a bag-mask. It is important to reiterate that EGDs are contraindicated in this scenario, as they may actually worsen the existing airway distortion. The inability to oxygenate with a bag-mask at any point mandates an immediate surgical airway. Pretreatment with intravenous medications is not indicated in this scenario, unless other conditions exist that would mandate its use. Nebulized or atomized 4% lidocaine is a consideration, provided that adequate denitrogenation can be carried out. Topical anesthesia will help to blunt the protective cough reflex that could aggravate cervical spine injury.

Numerous sedating agents may be considered, including ketamine, propofol, midazolam, or etomidate. Ketamine is a good choice for this patient as it carries the benefit of analgesia, along with sedation, with the rare complication of associated laryngospasm, or emergence reaction. Propofol and midazolam may have the advantage of operator familiarity and ease of titration, although one must recognize that both can precipitate complete obstruction through a loss of muscle tone. The advantage of etomidate is its relative cardiovascular stability. However, the potential myoclonus associated with etomidate may place the potential unstable cervical spine at risk.

Neuromuscular blocking agents ought to be avoided, as per the discussion above, although they may have a role in a Crash Airway on a risk–benefit basis. As mentioned earlier, the FFB is the intubation technique of choice for this patient. The amount of time the practitioner has to perform bronchoscopy and intubation is dependent on the maintenance of oxygen saturation. Blood and secretions may make the procedure difficult. Again, as mentioned earlier, in the event a flexible bronchoscope is not readily available, and the patient requires urgent intubation, an oral attempt, guided by an EI, is a logical alternative. The EI may be gently inserted into the larynx, with the tip of the bougie sliding across the tracheal rings to confirm intratracheal placement. However, as stated above, the trachea may not be contiguous with the larynx because of the injury. While an "awake look" may suggest that the glottis can be viewed, it gives one no confidence that the trachea is contiguous with the larynx. An inability to visualize glottic structures on the "awake look" mandates a change of plan and precludes the use of neuromuscular blockade in all but the most extreme circumstances. Further, BURP (backwards, upwards, rightwards pressure) on the larynx may be compromised due to the trauma.

Unsuccessful oral intubation after three attempts, oxygen desaturation, or failure in ventilation indicates a failed airway. In this circumstance, cricothyrotomy is in order. Open cricothyrotomy is preferable to percutaneous techniques for the reasons stated above. This method allows the practitioner to identify the trachea and intubate under direct visualization. Blind attempts at finding the distal airway are rarely successful.[12,13]

18.4 OTHER CONSIDERATIONS

18.4.1 What are the postintubation and ventilation management concerns?

Once intubated, confirmation of ventilatory exchange is the priority. The presence of end-tidal CO_2 indicates that the endotracheal tube is in the trachea and that the lower respiratory tree is being ventilated. Care must be taken to secure the endotracheal tube in place, as dislodgement would recreate the same difficult intubation scenario. Sedation is in order, as is continued protection of the cervical spine until fracture, dislocation, and ligamentous disruption of the cervical spine have been ruled out. Paralysis may also be in order if the patient is endangering his spine by excessive movement.

18.4.2 What are potential postsurgical complications associated with clothesline injuries?

If the patient survived the initial injury, and received prompt aggressive resuscitation and airway management, the outcome is generally very good.[13] However, following the repair of the laryngotracheal and cervical spine injuries, several potential, serious postoperative complications have been reported. These include mediastinal infection, tracheoesophageal fistula, and subglottic stenosis.[4] In a retrospective review of clothesline injury in children and adolescents (on all-terrain vehicles), between 1998 to 2003, Graham et al. reported that all patients ($n = 7$) had significant neck and/or facial lacerations, with long-lasting disfigurement.[14] One of the patients also had a functional impairment.

18.4.3 What other alternative should be considered if securing the airway is almost impossible for a patient with a clothesline injury?

Extracorporal circulation via a femoral–femoral cardiopulmonary bypass (CPB), placed with the use of local anesthesia and a portable unit, is a life-saving method of oxygenation and could have an important role in managing patients with a severely disrupted trachea. This can provide a safe solution for oxygenation when tracheal intubation or a surgical airway is either unsuccessful or too hazardous. However, a review of the literature did not reveal the use of CPB in airway compromise from clothesline injury. Furthermore, establishment of a femoral–femoral bypass requires at least 15–20 minutes, even in experienced hands,[15] making it impractical and impossible to apply in emergency situations.

18.5 SUMMARY

In summary, blunt anterior neck injury poses a unique and challenging obstacle to airway management. Care must be taken to protect airway reflexes whenever an inability to intubate is anticipated. The airway practitioner must recognize multiple pitfalls, including an obstructing hematoma or a transected trachea, which can prevent intubation. Intubation over an FFB is the ideal method of intubation in this scenario, as the indirect visualization provides the reassurance that the trachea is contiguous.

REFERENCES

1. Aufderheide TP, Aprahamian C, Mateer JR, et al.: Emergency airway management in hanging victims. *Ann Emerg Med.* 1994;24:879–884.
2. Penney DJ, Stewart AH, Parr MJ: Prognostic outcome indicators following hanging injuries. *Resuscitation.* 2002;54:27–29.
3. Nikolic S, Micic J, Atanasijevic T, Djokic V, Djonic D: Analysis of neck injuries in hanging. *Am J Forensic Med Pathol.* 2003;24:179–182.
4. LeJeune FE, Jr: Laryngotracheal separation. *Laryngoscope.* 1978;88:1956–1962.
5. Stassen NA, Hoth JJ, Scott MJ, et al.: Laryngotracheal injuries: does injury mechanism matter? *Am Surg.* 2004;70:522–525.
6. Pollack CV, Jr: The laryngeal mask airway: a comprehensive review for the emergency physician. *J Emerg Med.* 2001;20:53–66.
7. Wakeling HG, Nightingale J: The intubating laryngeal mask airway does not facilitate tracheal intubation in the presence of a neck collar in simulated trauma. *Br J Anaesth.* 2000;84:254–256.
8. Arino JJ, Velasco JM, Gasco C, Lopez-Timoneda F: Straight blades improve visualization of the larynx while curved blades increase ease of intubation: a comparison of the Macintosh, Miller, McCoy, Belscope and Lee-Fiberview blades. *Can J Anaesth.* 2003;50:501–506.
9. Wu MH, Tsai YF, Lin MY, Hsu IL, Fong Y: Complete laryngotracheal disruption caused by blunt injury. *Ann Thorac Surg.* 2004;77:1211–1215.
10. O'Mara W, Hebert AF: External laryngeal trauma. *J La State Med Soc.* 2000;152:218–222.
11. Steinfeldt J, Bey TA, Rich JM: Use of a gum elastic bougie (GEB) in a zone II penetrating neck trauma: a case report. *J Emerg Med.* 2003;24:267–270.
12. Shweikh AM, Nadkarni AB: Laryngotracheal separation with pneumopericardium after a blunt trauma to the neck. *Emerg Med J.* 2001;18:410–411.
13. Edwards WH, Jr, Morris JA, Jr, DeLozier JB, 3rd, Adkins RB, Jr: Airway injuries. The first priority in trauma. *Am Surg.* 1987;53:192–197.
14. Graham J, Dick R, Parnell D, Aitken ME: Clothesline injury mechanism associated with all-terrain vehicle use by children. *Pediatr Emerg Care.* 2006;22:45–47.
15. Belmont MJ, Wax MK, DeSouza FN: The difficult airway: cardiopulmonary bypass—the ultimate solution. *Head Neck.* 1998;20:266–269.

SELF-EVALUATION QUESTIONS

18.1. A patient presents with stridor and an oxygen saturation of 85%. What is the ventilation device of choice to attempt to enhance oxygenation after passive means have failed?

A. Laryngeal Mask Airway

B. Intubating Laryngeal Mask Airway

C. bag-valve-mask device

D. King LT Airway

E. Combitube™

18.2. What percentage of live patients with blunt anterior neck trauma have an associated cervical spine injury?

A. The literature is not clear

B. 5%

C. 10%

D. 15%

E. 20%

18.3. What are the limitations of percutaneous cricothyrotomy in the setting of blunt anterior neck trauma with a concomitant laryngeal fracture?

A. Subcutaneous air may mimic intratracheal air, providing false localization.

B. Airway distortion may not allow readily identifiable, percutaneous airway structures.

C. Distal tracheal disruption may not be identified.

D. Advancement of the guidewire through the needle may be difficult.

E. All of the above.

CHAPTER (19)

Airway Management in the Emergency Department

Michael F. Murphy and Ron M. Walls

19.1 CASE PRESENTATION

A 19-year-old morbidly obese male has just been brought in to the emergency department (ED) by ambulance unconscious, having been found down at a fraternity initiation party. He had been drinking heavily, though the quantity of ingested material is unknown. The patient has no identification with him and no one at the party knew his identity. The paramedics have inserted a nasal trumpet and an oral airway and are assisting his very shallow ventilations with a bag-mask. The paramedics had attempted oral and nasal intubation three times in the field but failed due to patient combativeness and obesity.

His oxygen saturation is 92%. There is no medical history, nor any other history for that matter. No Medic-Alert® bracelets are visible. He is barely breathing and responds only to painful stimuli. His blow by breath sample for ethanol reads at 220 mg/dL and his blood sugar is 90 mg/dL or 5 mmol·L^{-1}. There are no signs of trauma. In summary, we have no information as to his identity, his history of present illness, history of allergies or medications, his past medical history, his family or social history, or what or how much might be in his stomach.

19.2 INTRODUCTION

19.2.1 What is it about managing the airway in the ED that makes it "different"?

Expert management of the emergency airway is a defining skill of emergency medicine, and all necessary equipment and medications, including neuromuscular blocking agents, must be readily available in the ED. Furthermore, physicians that staff EDs must be skilled in all aspects of airway management. Patients present to the ED requiring emergency airway management, often within minutes of arrival. Many of the patients have attributes associated with difficult laryngoscopy and intubation, but the urgency of the situation usually prohibits deferral or even consultation. Frequently, others have already tried and failed to manage the airway producing an element of trauma to the airway that compounds the difficulty faced by the emergency airway practitioner. Such issues serve to highlight the importance of the verbal report given by field personnel when delivering patients to an ED.

Accordingly, the emergency physician must be both capable and constantly prepared to undertake immediate management of these airways, and to construct an approach for each one that accounts for potential difficulty, and incorporate backup plans (Plan B).

19.2.2 Who is primarily responsible for managing the airway in the ED?

Airway evaluation and management is the first priority of resuscitation and establishing a patent airway and oxygenating the brain and vital organs takes precedence over all other activities. That is not to say that concurrent evaluation and management activities should not occur, it simply says "Do this first!" In general, the emergency physician has final responsibility for definitive management of the airway for patients presenting to the ED.

19.2.3 What are the indications for tracheal intubation in the ED?

The emergency physician must be quick to recognize the presence of an inadequate airway that requires active airway intervention. The failure to maintain a patent airway and failure to effect adequate gas exchange are crucial in recognizing an impending disas-

243

ter, but equally important is the likelihood that gas exchange, airway patency, or overall patient stability might be threatened over a short period and in perhaps less-controlled environments than even the ED (e.g., in CT scan, during a transfer, etc.), or later while the patient is in the ED. Subsequent decisions with respect to *how and when* the airway will be managed will depend on the integration of numerous factors, including the skills and knowledge of the physician, the equipment available, the condition of the patient, and the anatomy of the airway.

19.2.4   Is there a conceptual framework that the emergency physician employs in approaching the airway in the ED?

It is widely recognized that a conceptual framework focusing on rapid airway evaluation, critical action analysis and performance, and facility with an array of airway management techniques minimizes the risk of failure and improves outcome.[1] Specifically, in an emergency the airway practitioner must be capable of the following:

- Rapidly assessing the urgency of the situation and the patient's need for intubation.
- Determining the best method of airway management for the particular circumstances at hand.
- Deciding which pharmacological agents to use, in what order, and in what doses.
- Managing the airway in the context of the patient's overall condition.
- Using any of a number of airway devices proficiently to achieve a definitive airway while minimizing the likelihood of hypoxemia or hypercarbia.
- Recognizing when the planned airway intervention has failed and an alternative (rescue) technique is required.
- Being able to rapidly identify when to call for help and what kind of help that might be.

19.3   HISTORY

19.3.1   How did airway management in the ED evolve to where it is today?

Emergency airway management really consisted of various forms of back-pressure/arm-lift "artificial respiration," occasional mouth-to-mouth, mouth-to-nose, and bag-mask-ventilation (BMV) until the 1960s when resuscitation research identified airway management failure as a crucial issue affecting outcome.[2–5] By the early 1970s, endotracheal intubation was recognized as an essential part of the skill set for physicians providing emergency care, many of whom had little or no formal training in emergency medicine. Intubation was generally accomplished without drugs, using either the oral or the nasal routes, and often required heavy sedation before airway management could be attempted. Later, sedation-assisted intubation without neuromuscular blockade was used, but intubation attempts not uncommonly resulted in failure and sometimes injury and other complications.

Emergency medicine practitioners began to use neuromuscular blockade to facilitate orotracheal intubation in the late 1970s. By the

late 1980s, the use of neuromuscular blockade for this purpose was well established in emergency medicine residency training programs, and had been dubbed "rapid sequence intubation" (RSI).[6] By the mid to late 1990s, neuromuscular blockade was widely used and it had become evident that neuromuscular blockade not only made the technical task of intubation easier and faster, but also resulted in lower complication rates with greater success.[6] However, a need clearly emerged to develop a consistent framework to identify patients at risk for difficult laryngoscopy (and possibly failed intubation), to develop a reliable approach to such patients, and to expand the rescue options beyond the single choice of cricothyrotomy.

The challenges facing emergency airway practitioners today include the following: How does one ensure that muscle relaxants are only employed on patients that the practitioner can confidently ventilate or perform tracheal intubation on? How to select and use an alternative approach for those with difficult or impossible tracheal intubation? How to ensure the use of the best possible rescue device or technique in the event of intubation failure?

19.4   UNIQUE FEATURES

19.4.1   How common is the difficult and failed airway in the ED?

Airways that are difficult to manage are common in emergency practice, with some estimates being as high as 20% of all emergency intubations. However, the incidence of intubation failure is quite uncommon, being in the 0.5–2.5% range. Moreover, the disastrous situation of being unable to intubate or ventilate rarely occurs (0.1–0.5%).[6]

The key difference is that in the case of a difficult airway, the same standard applies as for a routine airway: the practitioner must secure the trachea with a cuffed endotracheal tube. In the case of a failed airway, the approach is focused on rescue and in keeping the patient alive and well oxygenated until the airway can be definitively secured. Thus, the devices, techniques, and even the approach differ in the two cases. A difficult airway is managed in an anticipatory way; a failed airway is managed in a reactive way. In 2002, Walls coined the phrase "The Difficult Airway is something you anticipate; the Failed Airway is something you experience".[7]

19.4.2   What is unique about airway management in an ED?

Emergency airway management goes beyond the ED and includes the prehospital setting, the in-patient unit (when a patient abruptly deteriorates,) and other sites. Urgent and emergency airway management situations are characterized by several unique features:

- Assessment of the adequacy of ventilation and the need for intubation in an emergency is a clinical evaluation. Arterial blood gas measurement usually have no place in deciding whether or not to intubate the acutely ill patient and may, in fact, provide misleading information.
- The patient is usually at high risk for aspiration.
- The airway must be secured. That is, the patient *must have* a cuffed endotracheal tube placed in the trachea. "Canceling the case," "awakening the patient," or delaying airway management

is not an option, nor in most cases is any other form of airway management that does not protect the airway (including some extraglottic devices).

- Crucial decisions must be made on the basis of less information than in almost any other setting. This, in fact, is the essence of emergency medicine and highlights the importance of expeditious and planned strategies for airway evaluation and management (Chapters 1 and 2).

- While the need for intubation is often obvious, in other circumstances, the decision to intubate may be much more dependent on knowledge of the natural course of the disorder or injury than on the patient's precise clinical status at the time of the evaluation. There are few other situations in medicine in which judgment and knowledge of the *anticipated clinical course* of a disorder are as crucial.

- Erring on the side of caution:
  - Intubate earlier rather than later. Be especially cautious of penetrating neck wounds with evidence of injury to the airway itself (subcutaneous air) or the vascular system (hematoma—it does not have to appear to be "expanding").
  - Do not paralyze a patient (ordinarily RSI) if you are not confident that you can rapidly and successfully perform BMV, employ an EGD, or create a surgical airway. This cognitive step mandates that you have performed an evaluation for difficulty for each of these prior to embarking on Plan A (see Chapter 2).
  - Do not "sit on" patients with upper airway obstruction or insist on taking the patient out of the ED (e.g., to the CT scan or to the OR) unless it is absolutely clear that the patient's condition is stable enough and you are confident you can successfully secure the airway if needed.

19.4.3 How should one proceed in managing the airway in an emergency?

Once it has been decided that intubation is indicated, the focus must be on what kind of airway problem is present, what is the correct course of action (see Chapter 2)?

- Is this a "Crash Airway" situation in which the patient is unconscious, unresponsive, and near death?
- Is this a "Difficult Airway" in which one anticipates difficulty with bag-mask-ventilation, laryngoscopy, and intubation or cricothyrotomy?
- If neither of these exists, then an RSI is the method of choice.
- Has a "Failed Airway" supervened?

This systematic approach to airway management in the ED takes into account all possible presentations. Properly identifying the type of airway situation permits the practitioner to select an appropriate course of action. Algorithms are expeditious management strategies often used in crisis and are described in Chapter 2.

19.5 SUMMARY

Rapid Sequence Intubation by emergency practitioners is associated with high success and low complication rates. The challenge

now has become how to recognize those patients who ought to be managed in a more individualized way, given the anticipated difficulty of intubation or ventilation with bag-mask or extraglottic devices. Some patients should not be paralyzed, and require alternative procedures, such as awake fiberoptic intubation, to successfully manage the airway.

REFERENCES

1. Benumof J: The ASA difficult airway algorithm: new thoughts and considerations. 51st Annual Refresher Course Lectures and Clinical Update Program, #235. *Am Soc Anesth* 2000.
2. Daya M, Mariani R, Fernandes C: Basic life support. In: *The Airway: Emergency Management.* Dailey R, Simon B, Young G, Stewart R, eds. Philadelphia, PA: Mosby, 1992:39–61.
3. Safar P: Ventilatory efficacy of mouth-to-mouth artificial respiration; airway obstruction during manual and mouth-to-mouth artificial respiration. *J Am Med Assoc.* 1958;167:335–341.
4. Safar P, Mc MM: Mouth-to-airway emergency artificial respiration. *J Am Med Assoc.* 1958;166:1459–1460.
5. Safar P: History of cardiopulmonary resuscitation. *Acute Care.* 1986;12:61–62.
6. Walls R: *Airway, Rosen's Emergency Medicine: Concepts and Clinical Practice.* Marx J, Hockberger R, Walls R, eds. Philadelphia, PA: Mosby, 2002:2–20.
7. Murphy M, Walls RM: *Identification of the Difficult and Failed Airway, Manual of Emergency Airway Management.* 2nd edn. Walls RM, Murphy MF, Luten R, Schneider RE, eds. Philadelphia, PA: Lippincott, Williams, Wilkins, 2004:70–81.

SELF-EVALUATION QUESTIONS

19.1. All of the following are indications for emergency intubation **EXCEPT**
  A. upper airway obstruction
  B. failure to protect the airway
  C. failure to maintain reasonable oxygen saturations
  D. the need for hyperventilation
  E. cardiac arrest

19.2. Responsibility for airway management in the ED
  A. rests with the most highly trained individual in the room.
  B. rests with the anesthesia practitioner, if present.
  C. is often unclear.
  D. rests primarily with the emergency physician of record.
  E. should be negotiated at the time.

19.3. Erring on the side of caution may mean all of the following **EXCEPT**
  A. moving the patient to the OR for airway management.
  B. intubating "earlier rather than later."
  C. intubating a patient with upper airway obstruction in the ED rather than the OR.
  D. intubating awake even if you sense that you can paralyze the patient and be successful at intubation.
  E. delaying airway management at all costs until an anesthesia practitioner is present.

CHAPTER (20)

Patient with Deadly Asthma Requires Intubation

Kerry B. Broderick and Richard D. Zane

20.1 CASE PRESENTATION

This 26-year-old male has a long history of severe asthma. His trachea has been intubated multiple times in the past for his asthma, most recently 2 months ago during which he spent a week in the intensive care unit (ICU). He arrives in the emergency department (ED) after a 15 minute emergency medical service transport during which he received continuous aerosolized salbutamol (albuterol, Ventolin) via a nebulizer. He arrives with marked respiratory distress. He is awake, diaphoretic, and is speaking in two-word sentences.

He is 5' 2'' (178 cm) tall and weighs 165 lbs (75 kg). His vital signs are respiratory rate 24 breaths per minute, heart rate 134 beats per minute, and blood pressure 110/60 mm Hg. His oxygen saturation is 89% on a non-rebreather and he is becoming fatigued. As he is receiving corticosteroid chronically for his asthma, he has a steroid body habitus with an edematous face and neck.

20.2 PATIENT EVALUATION

20.2.1 What are this patient's vital organ system reserves?

Cardiovascular reserve: This is a young patient who should have adequate cardiac reserve and there should be no concerns with respect to systolic and diastolic cardiac function unless there is a significant carbon dioxide retention and respiratory acidosis. However, depending on the length of time he has been acutely ill and how adequate his oral fluid intake has been, he is likely to be relatively volume depleted. In combination with a decrease in venous return secondary air trapping and auto-PEEP (positive end-expiratory pressure) seen with acute asthma, the presence of hypovolemia can precipitate a significant hypotension, particularly if induction agents are used to facilitate intubation. The patient has been receiving a large amount of, salbutamol, a medication with significant β_1-agonist properties. In combination with stress and hypercapnia, there is a significant arrhythmia potential from large amounts of salbutamol.

CNS reserve: There is nothing to indicate that this patient will respond abnormally to standard doses of induction agents. However, one ought to be watchful for agitation, confusion, or somnolence associated with carbon dioxide retention in which case sensitivity to sedative hypnotic induction agents ought to be anticipated. Respiratory acidosis can potentiate myocardial depression associated with anesthesia induction agents.

Respiratory reserve: Severe asthmatics have prolonged expiratory phases and air trapping.[1] Tidal volume is limited with minimal or no respiratory reserve. Intubation is ordinarily indicated because these patients are exhausted and are unable to maintain gas exchange on their own. Substantial ventilation–perfusion mismatch is ordinarily present and this limits their ability to oxygenate and to denitrogenate prior to induction. Preinduction hypoxemic will rapidly deteriorate after paralytics or induction agents are administered.

20.3 AIRWAY EVALUATION AND MANAGEMENT OPTIONS

20.3.1 Employing the mnemonics suggested in Chapter 1, is this a difficult airway?

Apart from some facial and neck edema from chronic steroid dependence which may make bag-mask-ventilation (BMV) difficult, there appear to be no predictors of a difficult BMV when applying the mnemonics MOANS (see Section 1.6.1). However, acutely ill asthmatics have very high airway pressures that can be difficult or impossible to overcome with a positive pressure BMV.

Using the LEMON airway evaluation (see Section 1.6.2), the neck and face edema may make laryngoscopy difficult. As he has experienced tracheal intubation in the past, in conjunction with corticosteroids and mechanical ventilation, subglottic stenosis is a possibility that must be kept in mind. However, the geometry of his upper airway appears normal, and he has a Mallampati Class II airway. His neck appears to be freely mobile.

A recommended mnemonic to assist the assessment of the feasibility of extraglottic devices (EGDs) is RODS (see Section 1.6.3). Restricted mouth opening is not an issue in this patient and upper airway obstruction is only a possibility. However, he has severe obstructive respiratory disease and his compromised pulmonary compliance, the "stiffness of the lungs," will seriously limit usefulness of an EGD.

While there is only mild evidence that this patient has a potentially difficult airway, he is not an optimal candidate for a rapid sequence intubation (RSI). A failed intubation in a hypoxemic person with very poor lung compliance would be a very dangerous situation. On the other hand, there is no reason to believe that a surgical airway would be difficult in this patient (SHORT, see Section 1.6.4).

20.3.2 Are there any other airway concerns in a patient with status asthmaticus?

This patient has no respiratory reserves, rapid oxygen desaturation, hypotension, and possible subglottic stenosis. The insertion of a tracheal tube in a person who is already in bronchospasm will exacerbate his condition.

20.3.3 Have we medically optimized his treatment prior to tracheal intubation?

For reasons already outlined and if at all possible avoiding intubation would be the best option. β_2-agonists are the mainstay of treatment in asthma.[2] However, this patient has been on continuous bronchodilators for the 15-minute transport and had utilized his inhaler every 15 minutes at home prior to calling the paramedics. The addition of corticosteroid may be beneficial for this patient with an acute exacerbation of asthma.[3] The use of other pharmacological agents, such as methylxanthines, for acute asthmatic exacerbation remains controversial.[3]

20.3.4 What additional therapies are available to this patient?

Meta-analysis suggests that there is a modest benefit in adding this therapy to β-agonists.[4] The benefits appear to outweigh the potential risks for the patient. So anticholinergics should be considered for this patient. Two meta-analysis have been performed analyzing the effect of IV magnesium on patients with asthma.[5,6] Seven trials were identified and the investigators conclude that magnesium has no identified role in the management of mild or moderate asthma. In severe asthma, there is evidence that magnesium improves pulmonary functions and hospitalization rates, although there is no good evidence that in severe asthma magnesium decreases the need for intubation. Magnesium probably will not hurt the patient but administering it should not delay intubation.

Small studies have demonstrated both a decreased work of breathing and increased patient comfort during continuous positive airway pressure support of acute asthma exacerbations.[7,8] In one study of 17 patients with asthma and acute respiratory failure over a 3-year period, noninvasive ventilatory support (NIVS) demonstrated marked improvements in pH, $PaCO_2$, and respiratory rates. This was true even at low pressures (2.5 cm H_2O).[9] One prospective, randomized, placebo-controlled study of 30 recruited patients from a larger group of 124 asthmatics, evaluated bi-level ventilation. Fifteen patients were randomized to conventional treatment and 15 to bi-level ventilation. Using intention to treat analysis, 80% of the bi-level ventilation patients achieved the predetermined endpoints of an a forced expiratory volume$_1$ (FEV_1) of at least 50% of predicted value versus 20% in the controls and hospital admission endpoints of 17% in bi-level ventilation versus 63% in controls.[10] However, these are small studies and further studies are needed to confirm that NIVS is of clear benefit in acute asthma. It is generally felt that NIVS should be used in asthma only with extreme caution.

20.3.5 What are the possible options regarding airway management in this patient?

In this particular patient, and despite the reservations that have been articulated, RSI and a skilled practitioner is probably the best choice. Deciding ahead of time on Plans B and C in the event Plan A fails is crucial.

While recognizing the limitations of denitrogenation (described above), prior to tracheal intubation, one ought nonetheless to administer as high an oxygen concentration as possible to the patient employing a bag-mask unit if tolerated by the patient. As an added advantage, one can provide assisted ventilation to the patient, although caution to avoid inflating the stomach is crucial.

Rapid sequence induction drugs chosen should be administered to the patient in their position of comfort, often sitting upright. Once the patient loses consciousness, cricoid pressure should be applied, the patient should be placed supine, and laryngoscopy and intubation should be performed, preferably with an 8.0–9.0 mm endotracheal tube to moderate resistance and facilitate aggressive pulmonary toilette.

If time permits, patients with reactive airways disease or obstructive lung disease should be pretreated with 1.5 mg·kg^{-1} of IV lidocaine 3 minutes before tracheal intubation in order to attenuate the reflex bronchospasm in response to airway manipulation, which is thought to be mediated via the vagus nerve.[11–13] The recommendation to use IV lidocaine in RSI protocols for the severe asthmatic is extrapolated from the results of studies employing healthy volunteers with a history of bronchospastic disease.[14–16] Unfortunately, there is also evidence that IV lidocaine does not protect against intubation-induced bronchoconstriction in asthma. In a prospective, randomized, double-blind, placebo-controlled trial of 60 patients, lidocaine and placebo groups were not different in their transpulmonary pressure and airflow immediately after intubation and at 5-minute intervals.[17] Until more data are available, it seems reasonable to minimize the risk of intubation-induced bronchoconstriction by using lidocaine premedication in the asthmatic.

Ketamine is generally considered to be the induction agent of choice in the asthmatic patient because it increases circulating catecholamines and inhibits vagal outflow. In addition, it is a direct smooth muscle dilator and it does not cause histamine release.[18] While case reports of dramatic improvement in pulmonary function with ketamine have driven its popularity,[19,20] no randomized studies have been performed to demonstrate ketamine's superiority over other agents. In a case series, 19 of 22 actively wheezing asthmatics had a decrease in bronchospasm during ketamine-induced anesthesia.[21] In one prospective, placebo-controlled, double blind trial of 14 mechanically ventilated patients with bronchospasm, the 7 patients treated with 1.0 mg·kg^{-1} ketamine had a significant improvement in oxygenation but no improvement in PCO_2 or lung compliance. In addition, the outcome (discharge from the ICU) was the same in both groups. The study population was heterogeneous, making conclusions of the benefit of ketamine difficult at best.[22] A randomized, double blind, placebo-controlled trial of low-dose IV ketamine, 0.2 mg·kg^{-1} bolus followed by an infusion of 0.5 mg·kg^{-1}·hour^{-1}, in nonintubated patients with acute asthma failed to demonstrate a benefit in IV ketamine.[23]

Although evidence is limited, at the present time, based on its mechanism of action and safety profile, ketamine appears to be the best agent available for RSI in the asthmatic. Intravenous ketamine 1.5 mg·kg^{-1} should be given immediately before the administration of 1.5 mg·kg^{-1} of succinylcholine.

20.3.6   How would you conduct the tracheal intubation?

1. Preparations preprocedure:

  • The following difficult airway devices should be available and ready:

    ◦ an Eschmann Introducer (gum-elastic bougie)

    ◦ a Trachlight™

    ◦ a cricothyrotomy kit

    ◦ an intubating LMA™

  • The following drugs should be available:

    ◦ lidocaine at 1.5 mg·kg^{-1} IV in syringes

    ◦ ketamine at 1–2 mg·kg^{-1} in syringes

    ◦ succinylcholine at 1.5–2 mg·kg^{-1} in prefilled syringes

    ◦ sedation and paralytic agents for postintubation

2. The cardiac monitors are applied along with pulse oximetry. Denitrogenation is achieved with the patient sitting initially.

3. Lidocaine is administered IV at 1.5 mg·kg^{-1}. This should be given about 3–5 minutes prior to the actual laryngoscopy.

4. Ketamine is administered IV and the patient is observed until unconscious. This should take 1–2 minutes only.

5. Succinylcholine is administered. The patient is laid supine with the head and neck placed in a "sniffing" position. Cricoid pressure is applied. The patient is observed for defasiculations.

6. Laryngoscopy is performed. The cords are visualized easily and the ETT is passed and secured.

7. Capnography is used to confirmed correct tracheal placement.

8. Postintubation drugs are administered for sedation and paralysis.

20.4   ADDITIONAL CONSIDERATIONS

20.4.1   What are the appropriate ventilator settings for this patient following tracheal intubation?

All asthmatic patients have obstructed small airways and dynamic alveolar hyperinflation with varying amounts of end-expiratory residual intra-alveolar gas and pressure (auto-PEEP or intrinsic PEEP). Elevations in auto-PEEP increase the risk for baro/volutrauma. Reversal of airflow obstruction and decompression of end-expiratory filled alveoli are the primary goals of early mechanical ventilation in the asthmatic. The former requires continuous in-line nebulization with increasingly higher doses of β_2-agonists until reversal is objectively measured (decrease in peak and plateau airway pressures) or unacceptable side effects are produced. Safe, uncomplicated alveolar decompression requires a prolonged expiratory time (I:E of 1:4 to 1:5). This is achieved by using smaller tidal volumes than usual, with a high inspiratory flow (IF) rate to shorten the inspiratory cycle time, permitting a longer expiratory phase.[24]

The initial goal of ventilator therapy in the asthmatic patient is to improve arterial oxygen tension to adequate levels without inflicting barotraumas on the lungs or increasing auto-PEEP. Initial tidal volume should be reduced as necessary, to avoid barotrauma and air trapping. The speed at which a mechanical breath is delivered in liters per minute, typically 60 L·min^{-1}, is called the IF rate. In asthma, the initial IF should be increased to 80 to 100 L·min^{-1} with a decelerating flow pattern. A pressure control paradigm is preferred over volume control. If volume control is chosen, the ideal waveform is one of deceleration rather than constant (square). The ventilation rate should be relatively low in order to allow sufficient time for alveolar decompression. It is acceptable to permit the maintenance or gradual development of hypercapnia through reduced minute ventilation, as this reduces the potential for barotrauma. High intrathoracic pressure may compromise cardiac output and produce hypotension; therefore, it is to be avoided.[25,26]

The highest measured pressure at peak inspiration is the peak inspiratory pressure (PIP). The compliance of the lungs, chest wall, ventilatory circuit, and ventilator; the resistance of the endotracheal tube; and the effect of mucous plugs all contribute to the PIP. This reading has an inconsistent predictive value for baro/volutrauma but ideally should be kept under 50 cm H_2O. A sudden rise in PIP should be interpreted as indicating tube blockage, mucus plugging, or pneumothorax until proven otherwise. A sudden, dramatic fall in PIP may indicate extubation.

The measured intra-alveolar pressure during a 2–4 second end-inspiratory pause is referred to as the plateau pressure (P_{plat}). Values less than 30 cm H_2O are best and are not usually associated with baro/volutrauma. Measurement and trending of P_{plat} is an excellent objective tool to confirm optimal ventilator settings and the patient's response as well as the reversal of airflow obstruction. If initial ventilator settings disclose a P_{plat} of more than 30 cm H_2O, consider lowering minute ventilation and increasing IF, both of which will prolong expiratory time and attenuate hyperinflation. If P_{plat} is unavailable, PIP may be used as a surrogate.

Most status asthmaticus patients who require intubation are hypercapnic. The concept of controlled hypoventilation (permissive hypercapnia) promotes *gradual* development (over 3–4 hours) and maintenance of hypercapnia (PCO_2 up to 90 mm Hg) and acidemia (pH as low as 7.2). This is done primarily to decrease the risk of ventilator-related lung injury and prevent hemodynamic compromise as a result of increasing intrathoracic pressure from auto-PEEP or intrinsic PEEP ($PEEP_i$). Permissive hypercapnia is usually accomplished by reducing minute ventilation, increasing IF rate to 80–120 L·min^{-1}, and paralyzing and heavily sedating (usually paralyzing) patients who otherwise would not tolerate these settings. Permissive hypercapnia may be instrumental in promoting prolonged expiratory times and reducing auto-PEEP.[27]

20.4.2 What are the initial ventilator settings for this patient?

1. Determine the patient's ideal body weight.

2. Set a tidal volume of 6–8 mL·kg^{-1} with a F_iO_2 of 1.0 (100% oxygen).

3. Set a respiratory rate of 8–10 breaths per minute.

4. Set an inspiratory to expiratory ratio of 1:4 to 1:5. Pressure control is preferred. If using the pressure control, the I:E ratio is adjusted directly by the I:E ratio parameter, or by adjusting the inspiratory time parameter. If using volume control, the I:E ratio can be adjusted by increasing the peak flow rate, and the "ramp" inspiratory waveform should be selected. Peak IF can be as high as 80–100 L·min^{-1}.

5. Measure and maintain the plateau pressure at less than 30 cm H_2O or try to keep PIP at less than 50 cm H_2O.

6. Focus on the oxygenation and pulmonary pressures initially. If necessary, allow maintenance or gradual development of hypercapnia to avoid high plateau pressures and increasing auto-PEEP.

7. Assure continuous sedation with a benzodiazepine and paralysis with a nondepolarizing muscle relaxant.

8. Continue in-line β_2-agonist therapy and additional pharmacologic adjunctive treatment based on the severity of the patient's illness and objective response to treatment.

20.5 SUMMARY

The patient with deadly asthma constitutes a difficult airway even without features that might predict difficult laryngoscopy and intubation due to the fact that BMV and EGD rescue is likely to be difficult or impossible. A cuffed endotracheal tube in the trachea is essential to permit adequate positive pressure ventilation, and this suggests that rescue techniques, such as employing non-cuffed tracheal devices, are of no use, e.g., transtracheal jet ventilation, noncuffed Seldinger cricothyrotomy devices.

If one is contemplating using medications to facilitate intubation, careful consideration of lidocaine and ketamine ought to occur. A continuous infusion of ketamine may be of use following intubation. Postintubation hypotension ought to be expected and managed aggressively with fluids and vasopressors if indicated. Ventilation strategies ought to include low volumes and respiratory rates with long expiratory times and slow peak IF rates. Arterial carbon dioxide levels are not of immediate concern, provided the arterial pH can be maintained at a level consistent with reasonable cardiac, liver, and renal function.

REFERENCES

1. Hall J, Schmidt G, Wood L, ed. *Principles of Critical Care*, 2nd edn. New York: McGraw-Hill, 1998:1671.

2. National Heart, Lung, and Blood Institute. National Asthma Education and Prevention Program (NAEPP), Expert Panel Report 2: Practical Guide for the Diagnosis and Management of Asthma. National Institutes of Health Publication 97–4053. Bethesda, MD: US Department of Health and Human Services, 1997.

3. Levy BD, Kitch B, Fanta CH: Medical and ventilatory management of status asthmaticus. *Intensive Care Med.* 1998;24:105–117.

4. Stoodley R, Aaron S, Dales R: The role of ipatropium bromide in the emergency management of acute asthma exacerbation: A meta-analysis of randomized clinical trials. *Ann Emerg Med.* 1999;34:8–18.

5. Alter H, Koopsell T, Hilty W: Intravenous magnesium as an adjuvant in acute bronchospasm: a meta-analysis. *Ann Emerg Med.* 2000;36:191–197.

6. Rowe B, Bretzlaff J, Bourdon C, et al.: Intravenous magnesium sulfate treatment for acute asthma in the emergency department: a systemic review of the literature. *Ann Emerg Med.* 2000;36:181–190.

7. Shivaram U, Donath J, Khan FA, et al.: Effects of CPAP in acute asthma. *Respiration.* 1987;52:157.

8. Shivaram U, Miro Am, Cash ME, et al.: Cardiopulmonary responses to CPAP in acute asthma. *J Crit Care.* 1993;8:87.

9. Meduri GM: Noninvasive positive-pressure ventilation in patients with acute respiratory failure. *Clin Chest Med.* 1996;17:513.

10. Soroksky A, Stav D, Shprier I: A pilot prospective, randomized, placebo-controlled trial of Bilevel positive pressure airway in acute asthmatic attack. *Chest.* 2003;123(4):1018–1025.

11. Walls R: Lidocaine and rapid sequence intubation. *Ann Emerg Med.* 1996;27:528–529.

12. Gal T: Bronchial hyperresponsiveness and anesthesia: physiologic and therapeutic perspectives. *Anesth Analg.* 1994;78:559–573.

13. Gold M: Anesthesia, bronchospasm, and death. *Semin Anesth.* 1989;8:291–306.

14. Groeben H, Foster W, Brown R: Intravenous lidocaine and oral mexiletine block reflex bronchoconstriction in asthmatic subjects. *Am J Respir Crit Care Med.* 1997;156:1703–1704.

15. Groeben H, Silvanus M, Beste M, Peters J: Both intravenous and inhaled lidocaine attenuate reflex bronchoconstriction but at different plasma concentrations. *Am J Respir Crit Care Med.* 1999;159:530–535.

16. Downes H, Gerber N, Hirshman C: IV lignocaine in reflex and allergic bronchoconstriction. *Br J Anaesth.* 1980;52:873–880.

17. Maslow A, Regan M, Israel E, et al.: Inhaled albuterol, but not intravenous lidocaine, protects against intubation-induced bronchoconstriction in asthma. *Anesthesiology.* 2000;93:1198–1204.

18. Huber F, Reeves J, Gutierrez J, et al.: Ketamine: its effect on airway resistance in man. *South Med J.* 1972;65:1176–1180.

19. Hommedieu C, Arens J: The use of ketamine for the emergency intubation of patients with status asthmaticus. *Ann Emerg Med.* 1987;16:568–571.

20. Rock M, de la Roca S, Hommedieu C, Truemper E: Use of ketamine in asthmatic children to treat respiratory failure refractory to conventional therapy. *Crit Care Med.* 1986;14:514–516.

21. Corssen G, Gutierrez J, Reves J, et al.: Ketamine in the anesthetic management of asthmatic patients. *Anesth Analg.* 1972;51:588–596.

22. Hemmingsen C, Nielsen P, Odorica J: Ketamine in the treatment of bronchospasm during mechanical ventilation. *Am J Emerg Med.* 1994;12: 417–420.

23. Howton J, Rose J, Duffy S, et al.: Randomized, double-blind, placebo controlled trial of intravenous ketamine in acute asthma. *Ann Emerg Med.* 1996;27:170–175.

24. Corbridge TC, Hall JB: Techniques for ventilating patients with obstructive pulmonary disease. *J Crit Illness.* 1994;9:1027–1032.

25. Tuxen D: Permissive hypercapnic ventilation. *Am J Respir Crit Care Med.* 1994;150:870–874.

26. Wiener C: Ventilatory management of respiratory failure in asthma. *JAMA.* 1993;269:2128–2131.

27. Bidani A, Tzouanakis A, Cardenas V, Zwischenberger J: Permissive hypercapnia in acute respiratory failure. *JAMA.* 1994;272:957–962.

SELF-EVALUATION QUESTIONS

20.1. Hypotension following RSI facilitated tracheal intubation of the deadly asthmatic may be due to all of the following **EXCEPT**

A. increased mean intrathoracic pressure associated with positive pressure ventilation.

B. hypovolemia related to reduced oral intake pre-presentation.

C. acute respiratory acidosis.

D. reduced systemic vascular resistance due to succinylcholine.

E. an acute tension pneumothorax.

20.2. All of the following are true with respect to the pharmacologic management of asthma in the peri-intubation period **EXCEPT:**

A. IV magnesium has been shown to decrease the need for intubation.

B. antimuscarinics such as glycopyrrolate have been shown to increase the viscosity of bronchial secretions, increase the incidence of mucous plugging, and should not be used in acute severe asthma.

C. the evidence clearly supports the use of lidocaine in acute severe asthma.

D. ketamine is the induction drug of choice in acute severe asthma.

E. IV magnesium in high doses leads to skeletal muscle weakness.

20.3. Mechanical ventilation of the asthmatic ought to embrace the following parameters

A. large tidal volumes and low ventilation rates

B. small tidal volumes and low peak flow rates

C. large tidal volumes and low peak flow rates

D. small tidal volumes and high peak flow rates

E. large tidal volumes and high peak flow rates

CHAPTER (21)

Patient in Cardiogenic Shock

Kerry B. Broderick

21.1   CASE PRESENTATION

This is a 62-year-old male with a long history of hypertension and a history of an acute anterior-wall myocardial infarction (MI) 2 years ago. He presents to the emergency department by car complaining of chest pain, air hunger, and extreme weakness. His echocardiogram shows a large anterolateral MI, and his chest radiograph shows vascular redistribution and mild interstitial edema. He is on beta blockers. His last echocardiogram was done 2 months ago and showed an ejection fraction of 25%.

His respiratory rate is 40 breaths per minute, heart rate 100 beats per minute, blood pressure 68/40 mm Hg, and his oxygen saturation is at 86% with a nonrebreather mask. He is intensely diaphoretic and has two-word dyspnea. He has a beard and a normal stature.

21.2   PATIENT EVALUATION

21.2.1   What is this patient's reserve?

21.2.1.1   Cardiac Reserve

This patient is in cardiogenic shock with limited-to-no cardiac reserve. He has severe systolic dysfunction and almost certainly the same degree of diastolic dysfunction. It appears that his sympathetic nervous system is working at maximum ability just to sustain his present vital signs.

21.2.1.2   CNS Reserve

There is nothing to indicate that this patient will have any CNS problems with induction agents.

21.2.1.3   Respiratory Reserves

This patient is in pulmonary edema and will have limited respiratory reserves. Denitrogenation prior to intubation may help but is of questionable value. He is already maximizing his respiratory effort and induction may precipitate acute hypoxemia.

21.2.2   How would you evaluate the airway of this patient for difficulty?

On MOANS guided evaluation (see Section 1.6.1), you are uncertain that the patient will be a successful bag-mask-ventilation (BMV) candidate. He has a thick beard and is likely to have gastric air distention due to his increased respiratory effort and air swallowing. His lungs are likely to be stiff related to his interstitial pulmonary edema. This is of particular concern on initiating positive pressure ventilation following intubation with respect to a reduction in venous return.

On LEMON evaluation (see Section 1.6.2), *looking externally* his face and neck appear normal, although he has a beard and that may hide a small mandible. He cooperates for a *Mallampati* evaluation and appears to have a score II. He is not *obese*; his *neck* is freely mobile.

The mnemonic RODS can be used to guide the evaluation in the use of extraglottic devices (EGD) (see Section 1.6.3). His mouth opening is not *restricted*, upper-airway *obstruction* is not anticipated, and his airway does not appear *distorted or disrupted*.

However, his lungs are stiff meaning that ventilation employing an EGD may be unsuccessful.

Finally, would a cricothyrotomy be difficult (SHORT, see Section 1.6.4)? There is no history of previous neck *surgery* or evidence of anterior neck *hematoma*. He is not *obese* and there is no history of neck *radiation or tumor*.

In summary, while he may not have much cardiac or respiratory reserve, he does not appear to have any predicted difficulties in oxygenation and ventilation via a bag-mask, EGD, endotracheal tube, or a surgical airway. Therefore, he is a reasonable candidate for rapid sequence intubation should one wish to employ that technique.

21.2.3   Are there other airway management concerns in the patient with cardiogenic shock?

All medications used for induction agents have the potential for producing hypotension, less so perhaps with etomidate and ketamine than others. This patient has limited cardiac reserve, and medications that reduce cardiovascular performance are contraindicated. Induction agents, in particular, must be chosen carefully and in reduced dosages. Some would say that amnesia in situations such as this, rather than induction of anesthesia, is the goal in an effort to preserve cardiac performance as much as possible. The administration of an opioid in an individual exhibiting signs of maximal sympathetic stimulation may be contraindicated in the face of actual or incipient hypovolemia or hypotension. Finally, the onset times of medications administered intravenously may be delayed due to low cardiac output, a particular concern with the muscle relaxant in a situation where rapid intubation is desired. Under this circumstance, it is prudent to administer succinylcholine over nondepolarizing agents to achieve rapid muscle relaxation.

21.2.4   How should we medically optimize this patient prior to intubation?

21.2.4.1   Diuretics and Vasodilators

This patient is hypotensive to start with, and we are concerned that induction and intubation may acutely worsen his hypotension. The patient's hypotension makes treating the pulmonary edema with diuretics and vasodilating agents a bit of a conundrum. Small doses of nitroglycerine and furosemide may help to relieve some of the cardiac stress due to the pulmonary edema but may aggravate the hypotension.

21.2.4.2   Noninvasive Ventilatory Support

While small studies have demonstrated a beneficial effect of using noninvasive ventilatory support (NIVS) in patients with cardiac pulmonary edema (CPE), larger, prospective trials are needed before firm conclusions can be drawn. A randomized prospective study of 39 patients with pulmonary edema showed a significant decrease in need for intubation ($p = 0.005$) in patients receiving CPAP compared to patients receiving standard medical care. However, there were no significant differences in mortality and hospital length of stay between the study groups.[1] An open non-randomized study involving 29 patients with NIVS showed that oxygen saturation increased from $(73.8 \pm 11)\%$ to $(93 \pm 5)\%$, mean pH increased from 7.22 ± 0.1 to 7.31 ± 0.07 ($p < 0.01$), and $PaCO_2$ decreased from 62 ± 18.5 to 48.4 ± 11.5 mm Hg.[2] A randomized, controlled, prospective clinical trial with 27 patients comparing nasal CPAP to nasal bilevel positive airway pressure (BL-PAP) against historical controls for intubation rates and MI found that BL-PAP improved ventilation and vital signs more rapidly than CPAP. However, intubation rates, hospital stay, and overall mortality between these two modes of NIVS showed no significant differences in this study. They also reported a higher rate of MI in patients with BL-PAP (71%) as compared to CPAP (31%) and usual medical care from historical controls (38%).[3] A randomized prospective study of 40 patients comparing BL-PAP to high-dose isosorbide (HDI) reported that 80% of patients in the BL-PAP group required intubation as compared to 20% in the HDI group. In addition, there were more deaths (2 vs. 0) and a higher MI rate (55% vs. 10%) in the BL-PAP group compared to the HDI group. Unfortunately, this study was prematurely terminated.[4] One subsequent study compared the BL-PAP with mask-ventilation in patients with CPE failed to demonstrate an increase in MI or mortality in patients receiving BiPAP®.[5] A meta-analysis of NIVS studies in pulmonary edema from 1983 through 1997 found that only 3 of 497 studies were sufficiently rigorous to fulfill their study criteria. These three randomized control trials showed that NIVS patients have a decreased need for intubation (-26%, 95% CI, -13% to -38%) but the decrease in hospital mortality was not significant (-6.6%, 95% CI, $+3\%$ to -16%) as compared to standard therapy alone.[6]

In this case, one needs to carefully weigh the potential benefits of NIVS against the potential to increase mean intrathoracic pressure, which reduces venous return and cardiac output. Furthermore, it is apparent that intubation is indicated and therefore NIVS is unlikely to be a serious consideration.

21.3   AIRWAY EVALUATION AND MANAGEMENT OPTIONS

21.3.1   Which pharmacologic agents would you select for this case?

Drug selection in individuals who are moribund is particularly important, especially medications that have significant cardiopulmonary side effects.

Recalling that circulation times in cardiogenic shock are prolonged, the muscle relaxant of choice for intubation is the one with the most rapid onset, succinylcholine, unless there is a contraindication. In the face of metabolic acidosis, as is almost certainly the case in this patient, the potassium may be elevated, but this ought not deter one from choosing succinylcholine. Longer-acting neuromuscular blocking agents, such as pancuronium and vecuronium, may be employed postintubation to maintain paralysis. The relative sympathomimetic side effects of pancuronium may be of some benefit in this patient, although the degree of sympathetic activation that is evident indicates that this would be of marginal value.

The selection of an induction agent is more difficult. However, in this patient, one is more interested in amnesia than induction of anesthesia. Recognizing this as the goal, small doses of ketamine (10–20 mg) and midazolam (1–2 mg) are clearly preferable to the other induction agents. Small doses of etomidate may be used, although the amnestic effects of etomidate are less intense than with those already mentioned. Agents such as thiopental or propofol may further deteriorate this patient's hemodynamics and should not be used.

21.3.1.1   Cardiovascular Pressure Support

This patient is hypotensive, and it is likely that intubation and positive pressure ventilation may acutely worsen his hypotension. Therefore, vasopressors should be prepared and immediately available, recognizing that balanced α/β adrenergic agonists (epinephrine, norepinephrine, vasopressin) are preferable to α-agonists alone, particularly in a catecholamine-depleted heart, as in this patient.

Ionotropic support should theoretically improve outcomes in patients who present with CPE. However, they can also cause tachycardia, dysrhythmias, increase myocardial oxygen demands, and myocardial ischemia, all of which may increase mortality. These medications should be used judiciously. There are two common ionotropic classes, catecholamines and phosphodiesterase inhibitors (PDEIs). The catecholamine class includes dopamine, dobutamine, and norepinephrine. Dopamine and norepinephrine may provide blood pressure support by increasing systemic vascular resistance, which can actually worsen cardiac output. Dobutamine, while inducing some mild preload and afterload reductions, may also further lower the blood pressure. Catecholamines work through the adenoreceptors, which are often saturated with endogenous catecholamines due to the patient's condition. Therefore, higher than normal dosages may be needed in the CPE patient, and unfortunately these dosages are associated with a higher rate of adverse effects.

PDEIs work by increasing intracellular cyclic AMP, which produces a positive ionotropic effect on the heart, induces peripheral vasodilation, and reduces pulmonary vascular resistance. Together, these effects produce preload, afterload, and cardiac output improvement.[7] Studies comparing milrinone to dobutamine in patients with severe CPE did not show any improvement in hospital length of stay or mortality.[8,9]

"Calcium sensitizer" levosimendan has been suggested and studied recently as an alternative to dobutamine for CPE.[10,11] In one study comparing the two agents, levosimendan had greater improvement in their cardiac output and pulmonary pressures and also a lower 180-day mortality rate (26% vs. 38%).[12] However, its role requires further clarification.

21.3.2   So, how exactly would you handle the entire process?

1. Preprocedure preparations:

   - Get the difficult airway devices ready
     ○ Eschmann Tracheal Introducer
     ○ Trachlight™
     ○ Intubating LMA™

   - Ketamine (Ketalar®) 10–20 mg in syringes or midazolam 1–2 mg
   - Succinylcholine (Anectine®) at 1.5–2.0 mg·kg^{-1} in prefilled syringes
   - Sedation and paralytic agents for postintubation
   - Epinephrine 10 μg·mL^{-1} or vasopressin 0.4 U·mL^{-1} in 10 mL syringes

2. The patient is seated initially. The cardiac monitors are applied along with pulse oximetry. The patient is denitrogenated.

3. Ketamine or midazolam is administered IV and observe until the patient is dissociated (1–2 minutes).

4. Succinylcholine is administered and the patient is laid supine with the head and neck in a "sniffing" position and with cricoid pressure applied. The patient is observed for defasiculations.

5. Laryngoscopy is performed. The cords are visualized easily and the endotracheal tube is placed and secured.

6. Capnography and auscultation are performed to assure tracheal intubation.

7. Postintubation drugs are administered for sedation and paralysis to permit mechanical ventilation.

8. Postintubation hypotension is managed by reevaluating ventilation parameters, volume infusion, repeated small doses of epinephrine (10 μg/dose), or vasopressin (0.4 U/dose). Postintubation hypertension may be managed with small doses of propofol (10 mg/dose) or a nitroglycerine infusion.

21.4   ADDITIONAL CONSIDERATIONS

21.4.1   How should the patient be managed following tracheal intubation?

The initial goal of ventilator management in this patient is to maximize oxygenation and relieve the work of breathing while at the same time being sensitive to the adverse effects of positive pressure ventilation on venous return. It is important to realize that the air hunger exhibited by this patient is in large measure related to the metabolic acidosis associated with cardiogenic shock as he attempts to remove carbon dioxide. The ventilator should be set at tidal volumes of 8 mL·kg^{-1}. PEEP should be started at about 5 cm H_2O and then be increased depending on the cardiovascular effects and oxygenation status of the patient.

21.4.1.1   Cardiovascular Considerations

The blood pressure should be monitored immediately after intubation, expecting that the patient's hypotension may be acutely worsened. Agents that should be considered have been discussed above. If they have been started, they may need to be titrated depending on the patient's blood pressure postintubation.

21.5 SUMMARY

Patients in cardiogenic shock are desperately ill, and therefore it should come as no surprise that endotracheal intubation is often temporally associated with circulatory and cardiac arrest. Attention to detail is crucial. The maintenance of oxygenation, medication selection, dosage adjustments, and caution with respect to positive pressure ventilation are all exceedingly important in these patients.

REFERENCES

1. Bersten AD, Holt AW, Vedig AE, et al.: Treatment of severe cardiogenic pulmonary edema with continuous positive airway pressure delivered by face mask. *NEJM*. 1991;325:1825–1830.
2. Hoffman B, Welte T: The use of noninvasive pressure support ventilation for severe respiratory insufficiency due to pulmonary oedema. *Intensive Care Med*. 1999;25: 15–20.
3. Mehta S, Jay GD, Woolard RH, et al.: Randomized, prospective trial of bilevel versus continuous positive airway pressure in acute pulmonary edema. *Crit Care Med*. 1997;25:620–628.
4. Sharon A: High-Dose intravenous Isorsorbide-Dinitrate is safer and better than Bi-Pap ventilation combined with conventional treatment for severe pulmonary edema. *JACC*. 2000;36:832–836.
5. Levitt MA: A prospective, randomized trial of BiPAP in severe acute congestive heart failure. *J Emerg Med*. 2001;21:363–369.
6. Pang D, Keenan SP, Cook DJ, et al.: The effect of positive pressure airway support on mortality and the need for intubation in cardiogenic pulmonary edema: A systematic review. *Chest*. 1998;114:1185–1192.
7. Shipley JB, Tolman D, Hastillo A, et al.: Milrinone: basic and clinical pharmacology and acute and chronic management. *Am J Med Sci*. 1996;311:286–291.
8. Yamani MH, Haji SA, Starling RC, et al.: Comparison of Dobutamine-based and Milrinone-based therapy for advanced decompensated congestive heart failure: hemodynamic efficacy, clinical outcome, and economic impact. *Am Heart J*. 2001;142:998–1002
9. Cuffe MS, Califf RM, Adams KF Jr, et al.: Short term intravenous milrinone for acute exacerbation of chronic heart failure: A randomized controlled trial. *JAMA*. 2002;287:1541–1547.
10. Nieminen MS, Akkila J, Hasenfuss G, et al.: Hemodynamic and neurohumoral effects of continuous infusion of levosimendan in patients with congestive heart failure. *J Am Coll Cardiol*. 2000;36:1903–1912.
11. Slawsky MT, Colucci WS, Gottlieb SS, et al.: Acute hemodynamic and clinical effects of levosimendan in patients with severe heart failure. *Circulation*. 2000;102:2222–2227.
12. Follath F, Cleland JG, Just H, et al.: Efficacy and safety of intravenous levosimendan compared to dobtamine in sever low-output heart failure (the LIDO study): a randomized double-blind trial. *Lancet*. 2002;360:196–202.

SELF-EVALUATION QUESTIONS

21.1. Hyperventilation and air hunger in patients with cardiogenic shock is most likely related to

A. metabolic acidosis

B. anxiety

C. pulmonary edema

D. hypoxemia

E. hypotension

21.2. Hypotension following intubation in patients with cardiogenic shock is likely due to

A. the underlying disease

B. positive pressure ventilation

C. respiratory acidosis

D. the use of an induction agent

E. all of the above

21.3. With respect to the selection of induction agents for patients in cardiogenic shock

A. etomidate demonstrates remarkable cardiovascular stability

B. opioids are preferable to other induction agents as they offer impressive cardiac stability

C. no induction agent should be used because these patients have unstable hemodynamics

D. amnesia rather than induction of anesthesia is a better endpoint if one is going to use an induction agent

E. ketamine is preferable to etomidate or propofol as it maintains muscle tone

CHAPTER (22)

Airway Management of a Patient with Cardiogenic Pulmonary Edema

Kirk J. MacQuarrie

22.1 CASE PRESENTATION

You are asked by a colleague to assist with the airway management of a patient with acute cardiogenic pulmonary edema. The clinical presentation is as follows.

A 63-year-old retired fisherman presented to the emergency department complaining of severe shortness of breath which is worse lying down. His wife says that he has been getting worse over the last several days. He has a history of hypertension for which he takes diltiazem. Aside from an occasional bedtime dose of lorazepam, he takes no other medications. He has no known drug allergies. He admits to smoking a pack of cigarettes a day for many years. He had an appendectomy as a teenager but no other operations. He weighs 264 lbs (120 kg) and is 6'2"(191 cm) tall. He is agitated and confused although not combative, is diaphoretic, and obviously short of breath. His blood pressure is 180/100 mm Hg. His pulse is 100 bpm and is regular. Respiratory rate is 36 breaths per minute and oxygen saturation on 3 L·min^{-1} O_2 by nasal prongs is 83%. Auscultation of his chest reveals bilateral diffuse rales and significantly decreased breath sounds to lung bases. He displays jugular venous distention and a third heart sound is present. He has no peripheral edema and remainder of examination is unremarkable.

22.2 INTRODUCTION

22.2.1 Discuss the basic pathophysiology of acute cardiogenic pulmonary edema

Acute cardiogenic pulmonary edema is an end result of severe decompensated heart failure. Congestive heart failure (CHF) itself is actually a symptom complex rather than a discrete disease[1] and is defined as a condition in which ventricular dysfunction results in insufficient cardiac output to meet the needs of the body. There are multiple causes of CHF, but coronary artery disease (CAD) is by far the most common. CHF has been described as two types. The most common form is systolic dysfunction, which is characterized by decreased contractility and a decrease in left ventricle ejection fraction (EF). The second form is diastolic dysfunction, which is characterized by impaired filling of the left ventricle (LV). In reality, there is considerable overlap between the two forms, particularly in the extreme cases.

The body attempts to compensate for the decrease in cardiac output by three principle mechanisms: (1) retention of fluid to increase preload and improve cardiac output via the Frank–Starling mechanism; (2) left ventricular hypertrophy (LVH) to increase contractility; and (3) an increase in systemic blood pressure to increase vital organ perfusion. These changes are accomplished by a number of neuroendocrine changes: increased levels of circulating catecholamines; angiotension; aldosterone; vasopressin; B-type natriuretic peptide (BNP); prostaglandin E_2; and prostacyclin. Unfortunately, most of these compensatory mechanisms will ultimately worsen the problem of decreased ventricular efficiency.

As the LV becomes less and less efficient, filling pressures rise and this is transmitted to the pulmonary vasculature. When the pulmonary capillary wedge pressure (PCWP) rises to 18–25 mm Hg, fluid starts to accumulate in the interstitial spaces; further increases will result in alveolar edema. This leads to ventilation–perfusion (V/Q) mismatching, dead space ventilation, shunt, and increased work of breathing. The increased work of breathing results in a metabolic acidosis; initially this is accompanied by a compensatory respiratory alkalosis. As fatigue sets in, the ability to maintain PaO_2 is decreased, CO_2 rises, and plasma pH drops. With further progression, mental status is altered eventually resulting in unconsciousness, respiratory arrest, and death.

22.2.2 How do these patients typically present?

The presentation will depend on how far the disease process has progressed. The chief complaint is that of progressive shortness of breath. Typically, the patient appears anxious and is diaphoretic due to an increase in sympathetic activity. The skin may be cold and clammy due to decreased peripheral perfusion. Mental status is generally altered. Systemic hypertension is generally present due to an increase in sympathetic activity. Typically, there is a decrease in air entry with inspiratory rales and expiratory wheezes on auscultation of the chest. Meticulous cardiac auscultation may reveal a third heart sound due to decreased LV compliance. Forceful atrial contraction may give rise to a fourth heart sound, this is, of course, absent in the presence of commonly seen atrial fibrillation. Jugular venous distension may be seen. Peripheral edema may be present if there is underlying chronic heart failure. With advanced disease, there may be a decreased level of consciousness (LOC).

22.3 PATIENT ASSESSMENT

22.3.1 What are appropriate investigations for this patient?

The chest x-ray will show evidence of vascular redistribution. Acute pulmonary edema may show a classic butterfly pattern of perihilar infiltrates. Evidence of an enlarged heart is often present but may be absent in acute situations, particularly if the pulmonary edema is secondary to an acute myocardial infarction in a previously "healthy" heart.

The electrocardiogram (ECG) does not typically aid in the diagnosis of pulmonary edema but is appropriate to detect myocardial ischemia. There may be evidence of LVH. Atrial fibrillation and/or intraventricular conduction blocks are common.

Arterial blood gas analysis is generally unhelpful in terms of diagnosis and treatment. It confirms that the PaO_2 is decreased and a metabolic acidosis with a compensatory respiratory alkalosis is typical. A rising $PaCO_2$ suggests that the patient is fatiguing and will require ventilatory assistance. But the decision to intervene should be based on the clinical assessment and need not be delayed for blood gas analysis.

More recently, it has become possible to measure B-type natriuretic peptide (BNP). BNP causes venous, arterial, and coronary vasodilation. It is released from the myocardium in response to stretch (volume overload). A low BNP level makes the diagnosis of heart failure very unlikely.[2]

22.3.2 What are the clinical findings in this patient?

By the time you arrive, the patient has been treated with nitroglycerin and furosemide. He is now receiving O_2 via a non-rebreathing face mask. His SpO_2 has improved to 89%. The remainder of the clinical exam is unchanged (or better) from that given over the phone. However, the nurse says that he seems slightly more confused.

His chest x-ray is consistent with your presumptive diagnosis, showing moderate cardiomegaly, an increase in the pulmonary vasculature with perihilar infiltrates. He is in sinus rhythm with frequent premature ventricular complexes, there is evidence of left ventricular hypertrophy (LVH), and he has nonspecific sinus tachycardia changes. Blood gas analysis reveals a pH of 7.35, $PaCO_2$ of 45, PaO_2 of 50 and bicarbonate of 22 mmol·L^{-1}. A BNP was sent and came back elevated at over 500 pg·mL^{-1}.

22.4 PATIENT MANAGEMENT

22.4.1 Discuss the initial management of this patient with acute cardiogenic pulmonary edema

Basic initial management of these patients involves administration of oxygen via a tight-fitting nonrebreathing mask. Good IV access must be obtained. For patients with severe dyspnea, a head-up or sitting position will decrease anxiety and improve patient cooperation. All patients should be monitored by continuous pulse oximetry as well as ECG. A range foley catheter should be inserted to monitor urine flow and an expected diuresis.

Medical management of the patient with CHF is directed toward attenuation of the maladaptive compensatory responses. The primary goal is to decrease left ventricular filling pressures by decreasing LV preload. Secondarily, the goal is to decrease LV workload and enhance contractility by reducing afterload.

Obviously the particular management plan will depend on the patient's presentation, in particular on the blood pressure and organ perfusion. Fortunately, most patients with pulmonary edema present with elevated blood pressure. This is good because it allows for a broader choice in treatment options. Patients with pulmonary edema who are also hypotensive are difficult to manage as "most regimens" to lower LV pressures will aggravate the preexisting blood pressure problem. Predictably, it has been shown that hypotensive patients with pulmonary edema have a worsened outcome compared to patients presenting with normal or elevated blood pressure.[3]

A detailed discussion of the medical management of CHF is beyond the scope of this chapter. However, a brief overview of management options is as follows:

1. IV diuretics and nitroglycerin remain the standard treatment for pulmonary edema. In fact, most patients will improve with simple preload reduction and do not require airway intervention. Interestingly, the role of IV diuretics has recently been questioned as there is a concern that their use may be associated with a decreased long-term outcome.[2] However, for now, IV furosemide (40–80 mg) remains a common treatment.

2. Historically, morphine has been thought of as a venodilator and has been commonly used in the setting of acute pulmonary edema. The main benefit of morphine may be to relieve some of the anxiety that often accompanies the dyspnea. Its hemodynamic effects at low doses have not been firmly established. Respiratory depression is a side effect and may occur even in small doses (2–5 mg). This is a particular concern in patients who are bordering on respiratory failure. In fact, the use of morphine has been associated with an increased need for intubation and ICU admission.[4]

3. In contrast to morphine, use of the angiotension-converting enzyme (ACE) inhibitor, captopril, given sublingually has been associated with a decreased need for intubation and ICU admission.[4]

4. Severe systemic hypertension not relieved with nitroglycerin and/or an ACE inhibitor may require sodium nitroprusside (SNP), a very potent combined venous and arterial dilator. Patients receiving SNP should have continuous invasive blood pressure monitoring as profound hypotension is possible with the use of this powerful agent.

5. Tachycardia may be treated with titrated doses of selective β_1 blockers. Patients with severe chronic obstructive pulmonary disease (COPD) may require other agents to control heart rate. In addition, patients with significant bronchospasm may need inhaled bronchodilators, even though these may increase heart rate.

6. Inotropic agents such as dopamine, dobutamine, and norepinepherine should be reserved for patients with severe systemic hypotension. These agents will unfortunately increase myocardial workload and could result in ischemia, tachycardia, or both.

7. Recently a recombinant form of BNP has become available. Nesiritide is identical to the BNP that is released from the ventricles. IV nesiritide seems to hold promise, although its ultimate role in the management of acute pulmonary edema has not been established.[5,6]

22.4.2 What are the indications for airway intervention in patients with acute pulmonary edema?

Most of these patients will respond to medical management and will not require airway intervention other than oxygen administration. If the pulmonary edema does not resolve with medical management, then the ongoing increased work of breathing can eventually result in fatigue and respiratory failure. This may manifest as an increase in $PaCO_2$. However, to wait for a rise in CO_2 prior to intervention is to wait too long.

Persistent hypoxia despite appropriate medical treatment is an indication for airway intervention. There is no absolute PaO_2 or SpO_2 that should automatically trigger intervention. Airway management is a clinical decision based on how the patient is responding to the medical therapy. A worsening LOC is typically an indication for intervention as is the clinical diagnosis of respiratory failure.

22.5 AIRWAY MANAGEMENT

22.5.1 What are the potential options for airway intervention? What are the pros and cons of each?

Historically, if medical management had been ineffective, these patients would have undergone mechanical ventilation through an endotracheal tube. While this approach remains an option, there are other therapies which may be considered first.

Endotracheal intubation is indicated if there is hemodynamic instability, advanced respiratory fatigue, heavy secretions, or a significantly decreased LOC. Endotracheal intubation provides the best airway protection against aspiration and permits adequate mechanical ventilation, particularly for patients with low lung compliance or high airway pressure. In addition, endotracheal intubation permits airway suctioning to clear secretions. Patient cooperation is generally not needed, particularly for patients who are unresponsive or apneic.

Unfortunately, endotracheal intubation can be associated with serious complications. The process of intubation itself may cause airway trauma. Sedation is often required to facilitate both intubation and positive pressure ventilation (PPV). The use of sedative agents can lead to hemodynamic instability and may prolong the weaning process. Patients with an endotracheal tube cannot talk, eat, or drink and are predisposed to infections. Endotracheal intubation, when used in the management of CHF, has been associated with an increase in mortality and length of hospitalization.[7–10]

The complications associated with intubation fueled the search for alternative and less-invasive methods of respiratory support. Currently, there are two major methods of noninvasive respiratory support: (1) continuous positive airway pressure (CPAP) and (2) bilevel positive airway pressure (BLPAP).

CPAP, as the name describes, provides continuous positive pressure to the airway. Typically 5–10 cm H_2O of CPAP is delivered via either a full face mask or a nasal mask. CPAP has been shown to decrease the need for intubation and to improve patient outcome.[7–9]

However, certain prerequisites must be met for CPAP to be a reasonable option. The patients must be cooperative and hemodynamically stable with spontaneous respiration. They should be able to swallow and clear secretions. An adequate mark seal must be obtained. And last, there needs to be sufficient trained personnel available as these patients require intensive monitoring and care. Contraindications to CPAP include an untreated pneumothorax, apnea, hemodynamic instability, severe facial trauma or abnormality, heavy secretions, advanced fatigue, or impending arrest. Potential complications include patient discomfort, aerophagia, gastric aspiration, and facial skin necrosis.

BLPAP, also known as BiPAP® (Respironics Inc, Murraysville, PA), is a relatively new technique that, like CPAP, provides continuous positive pressure throughout the respiratory cycle. However, unlike CPAP, BLPAP provides increased pressure during inspiration similar to traditional pressure support ventilation. BLPAP has been shown to be beneficial in hypercapneic respiratory failure caused by COPD.[7–10] BLPAP would seem to offer a theoretical advantage over CPAP in the management of patients in acute pulmonary edema. However, concerns remain unanswered regarding potential increased risk of myocardial infarction and subsequent increased mortality.[7–10] Currently, the role of BLPAP in management of acute cardiogenic pulmonary edema has yet to be defined.

22.5.2   What are the indications for tracheal intubation in these patients?

Provided the patient meets the criteria for CPAP and has no contraindications, it is reasonable to attempt CPAP first. However, in the presence of significantly decreased LOC, advanced fatigue, and hemodynamic instability, it would be imprudent to delay tracheal intubation while trying to make CPAP work. Delayed intubation has been cited as a reason for a worse outcome in patients treated with some forms of noninvasive ventilation.[10]

22.5.3   How do you prepare the patient for tracheal intubation?

The goal of the tracheal intubation is to safely secure the airway while taking precautions to avoid aspiration and hypoxia. Maintenance of hemodynamic stability is also a priority. Many of these patients will have significant CAD, and increases in heart rate and blood pressure may worsen myocardial ischemia. Hypotension is also poorly tolerated as CAD, LVH, and acutely increased filling pressures all mandate an increased aortic root pressure to ensure adequate myocardial perfusion. Although an increase in blood pressure in a patient with acute CHF is a favorable sign, hemodynamic responses to anesthetic agents are unpredictable. The challenge is to secure the airway while maintaining hemodynamic stability with minimal myocardial depression.

As is the case with all patients requiring tracheal intubation, an airway assessment must be performed. Fortunately, most of these patients will not present a technical challenge in terms of placement of the tracheal tube. The main issue is the potential impact that intubation, PPV, and sedative/anesthetic agents will have on the patient's hemodynamics.

A thorough airway assessment can help the clinician to choose between an awake intubation versus one in which sedation is used. Predicted difficulty with two or more aspects of airway management (bag-mask-ventilation, direct laryngoscopy, extraglottic devices, and surgical airway) will lead one to choose an awake approach. It is important to note that although insertion of an extraglottic device (such as an LMA) will not generally be a problem in these patients, the poor lung compliance secondary to pulmonary edema may severely impair the ability to render effective ventilation. Furthermore, the risk of aspiration cannot be ignored when using a LMA in the presence of a full stomach.

22.5.4   What are the advantages and disadvantages of awake intubation for this patient?

Although the decision to perform an awake intubation is usually based on anatomic factors that affect the ability to visualize the vocal cords and insert the endotracheal tube, the patient's underlying disease must also be considered. In acute cardiogenic pul-

monary edema, one should anticipate hemodynamic instability and ventilation difficulties following intubation. The advantage of an awake approach is that one avoids the use of induction agents that can further depress a failing myocardium and lower blood pressure. It is important to remember that all induction agents, even etomidate,[11] ketamine,[12,13] and midazolam,[14] can adversely lower blood pressure.

Postintubation decrease in blood pressure is common[15] and a predictable consequence of PPV in CHF patients. It is imperative to avoid drugs which may further aggravate this situation. Minimizing the use of sedating medications may also help with the eventual weaning process.

Another potential advantage of an awake approach to intubation is the preservation of spontaneous ventilation. This is of benefit if one expects technical difficulties in securing the airway.

Although an awake approach may be favored in order to maintain blood pressure, there remains the risk that blood pressure and heart rate may increase and could cause myocardial ischemia. Good topical anesthesia can attenuate this risk, along with careful technique and titrated medications.

An awake approach may be technically more difficult than a rapid sequence intubation (RSI), and patient cooperation is required. Unfortunately, by the time it becomes evident that these patients require tracheal intubation, an altered consciousness is common, making cooperation less likely.

22.5.5   What are the pros and cons of tracheal intubation under RSI for this patient?

The decision to induce general anesthesia must be followed by a decision as to whether maintenance of spontaneous ventilation is desirable or even practical. Tracheal intubation for these patients is generally to manage respiratory failure, which essentially makes spontaneous ventilation under general anesthesia an impractical option. Many of these patients will become apneic with even subhypnotic doses of sedative agents. For this reason and because of extreme V/Q mismatching, inhalation induction with spontaneous ventilation is generally not a reasonable option.

Since it is not reasonable to expect spontaneous ventilation following intubation, there is no benefit in avoiding the concomitant use of muscle relaxants. When not contraindicated, the use of muscle relaxants makes intubation substantially faster, easier, and safer.

Most of these patients are not fasted and therefore must be assumed to have a "full stomach." RSI remains the standard approach to secure the airway of patients with a "full stomach" once the decision has been made to induce general anesthesia. RSI has the benefit of minimizing the time that the airway is unprotected, but the use of predetermined bolus dosing makes attenuation of the hemodynamic responses unpredictable. An alternative approach is to perform a modified RSI in order to titrate induction agents and/or vasoactive agents to minimize hemodynamic disturbance. In a "modified approach," following denitrogenation the patient is given a "sleep" dose of induction agent followed by the muscle relaxant and cricoid pressure is applied. Bag-mask-ventilation is provided with cricoid pressure continued, and additional agents are administered to achieve hemodynamic stability prior to actual tracheal intubation.

22.5.6 Which pharmacological agents can be used to attenuate the hemodynamic response to intubation?

As previously discussed, the hemodynamic goal of intubation is to avoid tachycardia and hypertension as well as hypotension. Direct laryngoscopy and intubation tend to cause an increase in heart rate and blood pressure, and a judicious amount of medication is required to attenuate these responses.

Propofol, and to a lesser extent thiopental, will attenuate the hemodynamic response to intubation,[16] although a decrease in blood pressure is not uncommon. In the setting of hypoxia and respiratory failure, anesthetic requirements are decreased, and therefore substantially smaller doses should be used (e.g., 0.25–1.0 mg·kg^{-1} of propofol). However, hypotension can occur even with small doses of propofol.

Ketamine, via sympathetic stimulation, tends to cause an increase in blood pressure and heart rate making it less attractive for patients with CAD. Although the sympathetic effects tend to predominate, ketamine is primarily a negative inotrope and in the presence of overstimulation of the sympathetic system (e.g., hypovolemic shock) administration of ketamine can result in hypotension.

While etomidate is generally considered to be hemodynamically neutral, it does not reliably block the response to intubation.[13] Adjunctive agents such as opioids and β$_1$ blockers are necessary to block the rise in heart rate and blood pressure. The clinician should be aware that etomidate can decrease blood pressure in sick patients. Since the anesthetic requirements in these patients are decreased, it is prudent to reduce the dose of etomidate if this agent is chosen (0.1–0.3 mg·kg^{-1}). Although it is controversial, clinicians must be aware of the potential adrenal suppression caused by etomidate.[17,18]

Although fentanyl has been shown to blunt the hemodynamic response to intubation, reliable attenuation of the response occurs only with large doses.[19,20] Despite this, fentanyl 1–3 μg·kg^{-1} is commonly administered as a pretreatment in RSI and does seem to be at least partially effective.[21] The problem with large doses of fentanyl is that the effect will last a long time and may contribute to postintubation hypotension.[22] As more experience is garnered with the ultrashort acting opioid, remifentanil, it may become a more attractive opioid to attenuate the response to intubation. The advantage of remifentanil is its ultrashort duration of drug effect, making management of postintubation hypotension easier. The dose of induction agent should be adjusted downward if fentanyl (or remifentanil) is employed as a pretreatment.

Lidocaine has been purported to, among other things, attenuate the hemodynamic response to intubation. Unfortunately, examination of the literature yields conflicting views on the use of lidocaine for this indication (see Section 4.2.2).[23,24] However, there does not seem to be any evidence of adverse affects when lidocaine is given for this reason.[23]

β-blocking agents have been used to control the heart rate response to intubation. The ultrashort acting agent, esmolol, is preferable to other agents in that its effect lasts only several minutes, which is particularly suitable to attenuate the brief sympathetic response associated with intubation. Esmolol 1–2 mg·kg^{-1} IV has been shown to attenuate the heart rate response to intubation.[24,25] It should be noted that these agents are also appropriate to consider for the patient undergoing an awake intubation.

Although much of the preintubation agents seek to blunt the sympathetic response to intubation, one must be prepared as well to deal with postintubation hypotension. Certainly, this can be minimized by using prudent doses of pretreatment and induction agents. As already mentioned, a modified RSI, which allows judicious titration, will also minimize postintubation hypotension. Despite these precautions, postintubation hypotension may still occur. Perhaps, prior to RSI, the ongoing vasodilator administration (e.g., nitroglycerin infusion) should be decreased. In addition, vasopressor agents must be readily available prior to initiating intubation. Aliquots of IV ephedrine (5–10 mg) or phenylepherine (50–100 μg) are generally effective. Refractory hypotension may require an infusion of a powerful inotrope such as dopamine, dobutamine, or norepinepherine.

22.5.7 How do you intubate the trachea of this patient?

In this case, despite appropriate medical management, the patient's oxygenation is not improving. Unfortunately, he does not tolerate the CPAP via a nasal mask. He remains slightly confused. His vital signs at this time are SpO$_2$ of 83%, blood pressure of 170/90 mm Hg, heart rate of 87 bpm, and respiratory rate of 36 breaths per minute. It is felt that endotracheal intubation and mechanical ventilation are necessary.

An assessment of his airway gives no reason to expect difficulty with direct laryngoscopy. As discussed earlier, bag-mask-ventilation and extraglottic devices are expected to be less effective due to decreased lung compliance. His neck is normal and in the unlikely event a surgical airway is required, technical problems are not anticipated. The last consideration is hemodynamic stability in this patient. As discussed above, maintenance of adequate hemodynamics may be a challenge. Therefore, an awake intubation is planned.

Although he is confused, he has remained mostly cooperative and generally follows commands. While an awake approach will be employed, equipment and medications for an RSI will also be prepared should the awake technique fail. Due to impending respiratory failure, minimal sedation with 0.5 mg of midazolam and 25 μg of fentanyl are administered IV. Airway anesthesia is achieved with 5% lidocaine ointment applied to the base of the tongue. This is followed by nebulized 4% lidocaine via a DeVilbiss atomizer. Prior to laryngoscopy, 100 mg of IV esmolol is administered to blunt the heart rate response to intubation. Gentle direct laryngoscopy is then performed. Unfortunately, only the tip of the epiglottis can be exposed; additional lifting gives a glimpse of the arytenoids but results in significant patient agitation. The patient now becomes completely uncooperative and attempts to push away while pulling at his lines. His SpO$_2$ decreases to the mid 70s. The laryngoscope is withdrawn and oxygen is provided via a face mask which brings his SpO$_2$ up to 85%. Unfortunately, he remains agitated and requires physical restraint to keep him from pulling out lines. Based on the degree of agitation, and the difficulties with direct laryngoscopy with the patient "awake," tracheal intubation is planned under RSI. Following the administration of propofol 50 mg and succinylcholine 140 mg IV, and with an assistant applying cricoid pressure, a direct laryngoscopy is performed. A Grade 1 laryngeal view is achieved, and tracheal intubation is easily accomplished with an 8 mm ID endotracheal tube.

22.6   OTHER CONSDIERATIONS

22.6.1   Discuss the postintubation management

Following intubation, the main focus continues to be reducing LV pressures without further reducing cardiac output. But first of all, successful endotracheal intubation must be confirmed preferably by visualization of the endotracheal tube going through the vocal cords and the presence of end-tidal CO_2. The tracheal tube should be secured properly to avoid accidental extubation. The blood pressure should be checked immediately postintubation, and frequent blood pressure checks should continue into the early postintubation period. In fact, consideration should be given to early placement of an arterial line.

It should rarely be necessary to paralyze these patients in order to facilitate PPV, and this will make the administration of sedatives more straightforward. Minimal amounts of sedative agents should be used; IV morphine in 1–2 mg increments is frequently effective.

A detailed discussion of ventilation strategies for patients with heart failure is beyond the scope of this chapter. It would be reasonable to start off using simple volume control ventilation with a rate of 12 and tidal volume set at 10 mL·kg^{-1}. Adding positive end-expiratory pressure (PEEP) of 5–10 cm H_2O is also common and helps improve oxygenation. These settings can be adjusted to maintain peak pressures less than 35 cm H_2O. Additional adjustments or "fine tuning" can be done in consultation with the receiving intensivist or cardiologist.

PPV and PEEP will generally improve oxygenation by recruitment of atelectatic lung segments. Oxygen consumption will also be decreased due to the fact that the work of breathing is reduced. The effects of PPV on hemodynamics are more variable. PPV will decrease preload by reducing venous return to the heart. In normal patients, this will typically result in a reduction of cardiac output. In hypovolemic patients, the cardiac output may be significantly reduced, resulting in profound hypotension. In CHF patients with an overloaded LV, it is possible for PPV and PEEP to actually improve cardiac output. This may not always translate into an increased blood pressure as other factors must be considered. The relief of acute dyspnea may result in a reduction of endogenous catecholamines and adversely affect blood pressure. As well, sedative agents used to facilitate both intubation and mechanical ventilation will tend to lower blood pressure.

Preintubation medical management can be continued into the postintubation period, taking into account the potential effects of PPV on hemodynamics.

22.7   SUMMARY

Successful oxygenation and ventilation of patients with cardiogenic pulmonary edema depends on several key points. Initial consideration should be given to noninvasive forms of ventilatory assistance, but endotracheal intubation should not be delayed once it is indicated. Hemodynamic responses to laryngoscopy and intubation should be carefully attenuated without impairing cardiac (and cerebral) perfusion. Regardless of whether predictors of difficult laryngoscopy are present, intubation with the patient awake is an acceptable option in order to avoid the myocardial depressant effects of the induction agents. One must be aware of the limitations of bag-mask-ventilation and extraglottic devices in these patients with a marked decrease in lung compliance. Finally, even in the hypertensive patient one must anticipate and be prepared for hypotension postintubation and initiation of PPV.

REFERENCES

1. Jessup M, Brozena S: Heart Failure. *NEJM.* 2003;348:2007–2018.
2. Peacock WF, Emerman CL: Emergency department management of patients with acute decompensated heart failure. *Heart Failure Review.* 2004;9: 187–193.
3. Goldberger JJ, Peled HB, Stroh JA, et al.: Prognostic factors in acute pulmonary edema. *Arch Intern Med.* 1986;146:489–493.
4. Sacchetti A, Ramoska E, Moakes ME, et al.: Effect of ED management on ICU use in acute pulmonary edema. *Am J Emerg Med.* 1999;17:571–574.
5. Colucci WS, Elkayam U, Horton DP, et al.: Intravenous nesiritide, a natriuretic peptide, in the treatment of decompensated congestive heart failure. Nesiritide study group. *NEJM.* 2000;343:246–253.
6. Publication Committee for the VMAC Investigators (Vasodilatation in the Management of acute CHF): Intravenous nesiritide vs nitroglycerin for treatment of decompensated congestive heart failure: a randomized controlled trial. *JAMA.* 2002;287:1531–1540.
7. Murray S: Bi-level positive airway pressure (BiPAP) and acute cardiogenic pulmonary oedema (ACPO) in the emergency department. *Aust Crit Care.* 2002;15:51–63.
8. Pang D, Keenan SP, Cook DJ, et al.: The effect of positive pressure airway support on mortality and the need for intubation in cardiogenic pulmonary edema: a systematic review. *Chest.* 1998;114:1185–1192.
9. Panacek EA, Kirk JD: Role of noninvasive ventilation in the management of acutely decompensated heart failure. *Rev Cardiovasc Med.* 2002;3:35–40.
10. Wood KA, Lewis L, Von Harz B, et al.: The use of noninvasive positive pressure ventilation in the emergency department: Results of a randomized clinical trial. *Chest.* 1998;113:1339–1346.
11. Erhan E, Ugur G, Gunusen I, et al.: Propofol—not thiopental or etomidate— with remifentanil provides adequate intubating conditions in the absence of neuromuscular blockade. *Can J Anesth.* 2003;50:108–115.
12. Cromhout A: Ketamine: its use in the emergency department. *Emerg Med.* 2003;15:155–159.
13. Bergen JM, Smith DC: A review of etomidate for rapid sequence intubation in the emergency department. *Pharm Emerg Med.* 1997;15:221–230.
14. Choi YF, Wong TW, Lau CC: Midazolam is more likely to cause hypotension than etomidate in emergency department rapid sequence intubation. *Emerg Med.* 2004;21:700–702.
15. Franklin C, Samuel J, Hu TC: Life-threatening hypotension associated with emergency intubation and the initiation of mechanical ventilation. *Am J Emerg Med.* 1994;12:425–428.
16. Barker P, Langton JA, Wilson IG, et al.: Movements of the vocal cords on induction of anaesthesia with thiopentone or propofol. *Br J Anaesth.* 1992;69:23–25.
17. Jackson WL: Should we use etomidate as an induction agent for endotracheal intubation in patients with septic shock? A critical appraisal. *Chest.* 2005;127:1031–1038.
18. Murray H, Marik PE: Etomidate for endotracheal intubation in sepsis. Acknowledging the good while accepting the bad. *Chest.* 2005;127: 707–709.
19. Kautto UM: Attenuation of the circulatory response to laryngoscopy and intubation by fentanyl. *Acta Anaesth Scand.* 1982;26:217–221.
20. Murkin JM, Moldenhauer CC, Hug CC: High-dose fentanyl for rapid sequence induction of anaesthesia in patients with coronary artery disease. *Can Anaesth Soc J.* 1985;32:320–325.
21. Adachi YU, Satomoto M, Higuchi H, et al: Fentanyl attenuates the hemodynamic response to endotracheal intubation more than the response to laryngoscopy. *Anesth Analg.* 2002;95:233–237.
22. Splinter WM, Cervenko F: Haemodynamic responses to laryngoscopy and tracheal intubation in geriatric patients: effects of fentanyl, lidocaine and thiopentone. *Can J Anaesth.* 1989;36:370–376.

23. Lev R, Rosen P: Prophylactic lidocaine use in preintubation: a review. J Emerg Med. 1994;12:499–506.
24. Kindler CH, Schumacher PG, Schneider MC, Urwyler A: Effects of intravenous lidocaine and/or esmolol on hemodynamic responses to laryngoscopy and intubation: A double-blind, controlled clinical trial. *J Clin Anesth*. 1996;8: 491–496.

SELF-EVALUATION QUESTIONS

22.1. With regards to the drugs used during airway management of patients with acute CHF, which of the following is the **CORRECT** statement?

   A. Fentanyl 1–3 $\mu g \cdot kg^{-1}$ will reliably block the hemodynamic response to intubation.

   B. The use of etomidate for an RSI will ensure no hypotension postintubation.

   C. IV lidocaine has been proven to reliably attenuate the heart rate and blood pressure response to intubation.

   D. Esmolol 1–2 $mg \cdot kg^{-1}$ IV has been shown to reliably attenuate the heart rate response to intubation.

   E. All of the induction agents, even in reduced doses, are capable of producing hypotension.

32.2. Which of the following is **CORRECT** in managing the airway of patients with acute CHF?

   A. Extraglottic devices may fail to provide adequate ventilation due to decreased lung compliance.

   B. Intubation should not be considered until either the Pa_{CO_2} is greater than 55 mm Hg or the Pa_{O_2} is less than 55 mm Hg (Rule of 55).

   C. In a patient with normal airway anatomy, RSI is always the method of first choice.

   D. The use of noninvasive ventilation (such as CPAP) will delay but not decrease the need for tracheal intubation.

   E. BLPAP (BiPAP®) should be avoided in patients with acute CHF.

32.3. Concerning airway management of patients with acute CHF, which of the following statements is **CORRECT?**

   A. Awake intubation should only be considered if intubation looks technically difficult as it is more stressful than RSI.

   B. Most patients will require paralysis postintubation in order to facilitate mechanical ventilation.

   C. A downside of RSI is that the use of predetermined bolus dosing of induction agents makes attenuation of the hemodynamic responses unpredictable.

   D. Inhalation induction is a good choice in these patients because spontaneous ventilation is preserved.

   E. In a patient with an abnormal airway anatomy, RSI is always the method of first choice.

CHAPTER (23)

Airway Management of a Patient with a Stab Wound to the Neck

Michael F. Murphy

23.1 CASE PRESENTATION

A previously healthy 36-year-old male is admitted to the emergency department (ED) with a penetrating wound to his neck. The wounding instrument is a steak knife which is sitting on the left of the neck just above the cricoid cartilage, and lateral to the anterior border of the sternomastoid muscle (see Figure 23-1). The patient's voice is normal, and there are no signs of upper-airway obstruction. The wound is 0.5 cm in length in an oblique fashion and is slightly swollen at the site of puncture. A local wound exploration reveals that the wound penetrates deep to platysma.

His vital signs upon admission are temperature 36.8°C, pulse 94 beats per minute and regular, respiratory rate 18 breaths per minute, and blood pressure 134/88 mm Hg.

Trauma surgery is consulted.

23.2 INTRODUCTION

23.2.1 How are penetrating neck wounds classified and how does this classification affect management?

Penetrating wounds to the neck may involve one of the three anatomic zones.[1] The zone of injury dictates investigation and management, particularly the urgency of management, based on the accessibility of deep structures to surgical exploration. The three zones are (Figure 23-2)[2]:

- Zone I is the horizontal area between the clavicle/suprasternal notch and the cricoid cartilage encompassing the thoracic out-

let structures. The proximal common carotid, vertebral, and subclavian arteries and the trachea, esophagus, thoracic duct, and thymus are located in zone I.

- Zone II is the area between the cricoid cartilage and the angle of the mandible. It contains the internal and external carotid arteries, jugular veins, pharynx, larynx, esophagus, recurrent laryngeal nerve, spinal cord, trachea, thyroid, and parathyroids.

- Zone III is the area that lies between the angle of the mandible and the base of the skull. It has the distal extracranial carotid and vertebral arteries and the uppermost segments of the jugular veins.

The structures at risk in penetrating neck injury are primarily the airway, vascular structures, the esophagus, spinal column including the spinal cord, the lower cranial nerves, and the brachial plexus. The thoracic duct is also at risk in wounds of the left neck.[1]

Penetrating neck injuries present a difficult challenge in management, given the unique anatomy of the neck. Immediate surgical exploration is indicated for patients who present with signs and symptoms of shock and continuous hemorrhage from the neck wound.

Zone I and III injuries are difficult to explore and manage surgically, and unless the patient is in extremis, investigation is by indirect techniques (e.g., angiography, CT scanning, etc.) and governed by symptoms and signs (e.g., dysphagia, subcutaneous emphysema, etc.).

Controversy surrounds the approach to zone II injuries; mandatory versus selective exploration. Mandatory exploration of all neck wounds found to penetrate the platysma leads to a significant number of unnecessary operations and extra cost. However the consequences of a missed injury are potentially high. To what

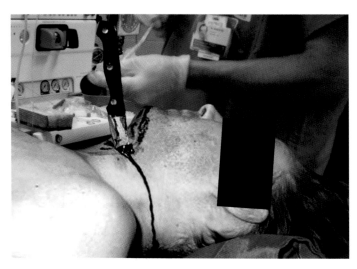

FIGURE 23-1. Neck wound with knife impaled on the left side of his neck above the cricoid ring. The knife penetrates platysma and is pulsating.

extent clinical examination can be relied upon, and which diagnostic adjuncts should be employed remain a subject of some debate. Most trauma physicians feel that patients who are not exsanguinating and do not have an evolving stroke should have a careful physical examination. If there is no expanding hematoma, no shock, and no evolving stroke, patients may be observed in a critical care area. Although angiography will exclude a significant vascular injury, physical examination has been shown to be as accurate in the assessment of zone II injuries. Soft signs such as proximity injuries, nonexpanding hematomas, and a history of hemorrhage are not indications for angiography or surgery.[1]

On the basis of an extensive literature review, Asensio et al. concluded that neither approach is obviously superior. A selective approach is safe in the asymptomatic and hemodynamically stable patient, provided that accurate invasive diagnostic means are immediately available. The mandatory approach is safe, reliable, and time tested. The greatest problem appears to be the accuracy of detection of cervical esophageal injuries: radiologic evaluation may be inaccurate, rigid esophagoscopy carries a risk of perforation, and the injury may easily be overlooked during surgical exploration.[3]

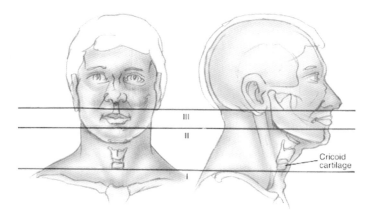

FIGURE 23-2. Zones I–III of the neck used in planning management.

Recently, Inaba et al. prospectively studied the effectiveness of the multislice helical computed tomographic angiography (MCTA) as a stand-alone screening examination for the initial evaluation of hemodynamically stable patients with penetrating neck injuries.[4] The MCTA is a minimally invasive, reproducible technique which is less expensive than conventional angiography. Their data showed that the MCTA had 100% sensitivity and 93.5% specificity in detecting all vascular and aerodigestive injuries. MCTA correctly identified two tracheal and two carotid artery injuries requiring operative or endovascular repair in stable asymptomatic patients. More importantly, no injuries requiring intervention were missed by the MCTA. Based on these findings, they concluded that in the initial evaluation of stable penetrating neck injuries, MCTA appears to be a sensitive and safe screening modality. However, further investigation with a larger number of patients is warranted to confirm these findings.

It should be emphasized that the actual management plans will depend not only on the specific patient and the injury sustained, but also on available staffing, expertise, monitoring, and available diagnostic modalities.

23.2.2 Are airway injuries common in stab wounds to the neck?

Injury to the larynx and trachea is fairly uncommon in stab wounds to the neck. Vassiliu et al. found that the aerodigestive tract is injured in only 4.9% of all blunt and penetrating neck injuries.[5]

While airway injuries in patients with penetrating neck injuries are uncommon, many of these patients may require airway management. In a retrospective review of patients ($n = 240$) admitted to the ED in Denver Health Medical Center for penetrating neck trauma, Weitzel et al. reported that 89 patients (37%) required airway management and 40 patients (17%) underwent prehospital airway management.[6]

23.3 AIRWAY ASSESSMENT AND MANAGEMENT

23.3.1 How should the airway be assessed in patients with stab wounds to the neck?

Immediate airway intervention may be indicated in the face of upper-airway obstruction suggested by a "hot potato" or muffled voice, difficulty in swallowing secretions, or stridor. This latter sign in the setting of an acute process may indicate that the upper-airway caliber is 4.0 mm or less[7] and constitutes an immediate threat to the airway. More subtle signs may include hoarseness, dysphonia, hemoptysis, and subcutaneous emphysema.

Diagnosis may be confirmed by direct or flexible laryngoscopy and tracheoscopy. Again, these maneuvers may lead to complete airway obstruction and should be performed in the appropriate environment, with personnel and equipment capable of performing an emergency intubation or a surgical airway as necessary.[8–10]

23.3.2 When should the airway be managed in this patient?

It really depends on numerous factors. The most important of which are:

- the pace of any visible expanding hematoma,
- the onset of symptoms of upper-airway obstruction, or
- whether or not the patient is to be transferred to another hospital or to diagnostic areas within the same hospital.

There is a school of thought that early or even prophylactic intubation of the trachea is indicated, particularly if the patient is to be moved to less safe environments (e.g., diagnostic imaging facilities). This belief rests on the fact that bleeding from a vascular neck structure tracks along fascial planes, particularly the precervical fascia. This may push the larynx forward rendering it anterior and if unilateral pushing its posterior aspect to the side. In both instances, the glottis may be difficult or impossible to locate during direct laryngoscopy. Furthermore, signs of airway compromise may be nonexistent or subtle right up to the point of total obstruction at which point rescue may be impossible.

23.3.3 How should this airway be managed?

Because of the propensity of penetrating neck wounds to distort the upper airway, the airway practitioner is well advised to consider this a difficult airway and help summoned. If the oxygen saturation is poor or airway obstruction is imminent, one may have to divert to a failed algorithm immediately and prepare to undertake a surgical airway.

If one has time, it is prudent to determine if the airway is in the normal midline position by employing an awake look with a flexible fiberoptic nasopharyngoscope or by oral means under topical anesthesia. If all is normal with stable hemodynamics and the airway practitioner is confident of success, a rapid-sequence technique may not be unreasonable, provided that Plans B and C are well thought out and evaluated in advance for difficulty. These include tracheal intubation using a rigid fiberoptic laryngoscope (e.g., the Bullard laryngoscope), videolaryngoscope (e.g., the GlideScope®), or a surgical airway.

Although Weitzel et al. reported no associated complications with blind nasotracheal intubation in their series of patients (n = 40) with penetrating neck trauma, blind intubating techniques, such as blind nasal intubation, light-guided intubation, or intubation through LMA Fastrach™ are ill advised.[6] Similarly, extraglottic devices, such as the LMA and Combitube™, may not circumvent an obstructing lesion or seat properly in the hypopharynx, making reliance on them for rescue undependable.

23.4 OTHER CONSIDERATIONS

23.4.1 Should the knife be removed prior to airway management?

Conventional wisdom states that impaled objects must be left in situ until removed in the controlled atmosphere of the operating room with the patient adequately anesthetized. However, if the impaled object prevents one from managing the airway of the patient, removal may be contemplated. In this case, the impaled object may hinder the insertion of a laryngoscope blade into the mouth due to the position of the handle of the laryngoscope on insertion. The use of a "stubby" handle or placement of the blade detached from the handle and subsequently attaching it will obviate the need to perform the unsafe maneuver of removing the knife before airway management.

23.4.2 What are the outcomes of a penetrating neck injury?

In a retrospective review, Nason et al. reported the outcomes of 130 patients presented to a Canadian trauma centre at a tertiary care institution with penetrating neck injuries.[11] Fifty patients were managed by a conservative approach with observation alone and 80 were managed surgically. The majority (67%) of neck explorations in asymptomatic patients were negative. Significant injuries, including major vascular (12), nerve (13), and aerodigestive tract (19) injuries were identified in 34 patients. Two of the 130 patients (1.5%) died of major vascular injuries. Seventy-six percent of significant injuries, including all zone II major vascular injuries, were symptomatic on presentation. All long-term disability (nine patients) was neurologic in nature. Nason and colleagues concluded that penetrating neck trauma, in particular stab wounds to zone II in asymptomatic patients, is associated with low morbidity and mortality.

23.5 SUMMARY

Airway involvement with penetrating neck wounds is notoriously unpredictable. Sudden, unexpected upper-airway obstruction that cannot be rescued is an ever present fear in these cases. Rapid-sequence techniques mandate a thorough evaluation assuring the airway practitioner of a high degree of certainty that this technique will be successful. Blind techniques are ill advised due to the propensity for airway distortion with these injuries. Prophylactic intubation may be advisable, particularly if transport to other facilities or remote locations is necessary.

REFERENCES

1. Kendall JL, Anglin D, Demetriades D: Penetrating neck trauma. *Emerg Med Clin North Am.* 1998;16:85–105.
2. Cheng E: Penetrating Neck Trauma. Available at: www.emedicine.com/MED/topic2802.htm, 2006.
3. Asensio JA, Valenziano CP, Falcone RE, Grosh JD: Management of penetrating neck injuries. The controversy surrounding zone II injuries. *Surg Clin North Am.* 1991;71:267–296.
4. Inaba K, Munera F, McKenney M, et al.: Prospective evaluation of screening multislice helical computed tomographic angiography in the initial evaluation of penetrating neck injuries. *J Trauma.* 2006;61:144–149.
5. Vassiliu P, Baker J, Henderson S, et al.: Aerodigestive injuries of the neck. *Am Surg.* 2001;67:75–79.
6. Weitzel N, Kendall J, Pons P: Blind nasotracheal intubation for patients with penetrating neck trauma. *J Trauma.* 2004;56:1097–1101.
7. Donlon JV, Jr: Anesthetic management of patients with compromised airways. *Anesth Rev.* 1980;7:22–31.

8. Desjardins G, Varon AJ: Airway management for penetrating neck injuries: the Miami experience. *Resuscitation.* 2001;48:71–75.
9. Grewal H, Rao PM, Mukerji S, Ivatury RR: Management of penetrating laryngotracheal injuries. *Head Neck.* 1995;17:494–502.
10. Mandavia DP, Qualls S, Rokos I: Emergency airway management in penetrating neck injury. *Ann Emerg Med.* 2000;35:221–225.
11. Nason RW, Assuras GN, Gray PR, Lipschitz J, Burns CM: Penetrating neck injuries: analysis of experience from a Canadian trauma centre. *Can J Surg.* 2001;44:122–126.

SELF-EVALUATION QUESTIONS

23.1. 22-year-old male is admitted to the ED with a stab wound to the anterior neck, and a large slash wound to the volar wrist that you feel has severed the median nerve. The neck wound is at the level of the cricoid cartilage at the anterior margin of the sternomastoid muscle. There is a small hematoma surrounding the wound. He is asymptomatic and has normal vital signs. You are about to transfer him by helicopter to a trauma center. The best way to manage his airway is

A. immediate RSI

B. administer a "sleep dose" of propofol and then have a quick look to see if the trachea can be intubated

C. send him with an ALS crew and instruct them to intubate him if he develops signs of upper-airway obstruction

D. perform an "awake look," and if all is midline intubate the trachea using an RSI technique

E. attempt a blind nasal intubation

23.2. A Trachlight™ intubation of a patient with a stab wounds to the neck is contraindicated because

A. it causes substantial elevations in blood pressure and may lead to increased bleeding

B. this technique of intubation relies on the anatomic structures being in normal position and they may not be in this situation

C. the neck hematoma obscures transillumination

D. it may stir up bleeding that will cause airway obstruction

E. the anterior position of the larynx in these patients cannot be accessed by this technique of intubation

23.3. Zone I contains

A. the superior laryngeal nerve

B. the larynx

C. the trachea

D. the pharyngeal structures

E. the cricothyroid space

CHAPTER (24)

Airway Management in the Patient with Burns to the Head, Neck, Upper Torso, and the Airway

Robert J. Vissers

24.1 CASE PRESENTATION

The emergency department receives a call from EMS about a burn victim coming to your facility in about 5 minutes. In an attempt to kill himself, a 40-year-old man set himself on fire with gasoline, while locked inside his vehicle. Because of a prolonged extrication and transport, he is about 1 hour out from the incident and has significant burns to the anterior trunk, thighs, head, and neck. The EMS personnel advise that a difficult airway ought to be anticipated.

Attempts to examine his airway, establish IV access, and oxygenate are foiled by his severely agitated and uncooperative state.

24.2 INITIAL ASSESSMENT AND MANAGEMENT

24.2.1 How can airway assessment and management, resuscitation, patient comfort, and cooperation be achieved?

The evaluation of the airway in the burn victim is critical to successful airway and patient management. Challenges to bag-mask-ventilation (BMV), the use of extraglottic devices, laryngoscopy, and surgical airways may all be present and should be anticipated.

Despite extensive burns, these patients are often awake, alert, and in severe pain. These patients are likely to face significant fluid resuscitation needs early in the course of their care. However, unless there is associated trauma, the immediate priorities for burn victims are early airway control, fluid resuscitation, and pain management. Accurate assessment of the airway and the patients'

underlying physiological status may be impossible, until control of pain and agitation is achieved. Immediate IV access is desirable to facilitate this but access may also be restricted by the location of the burns.

In this case, the patient arrived very agitated, in severe pain, and without IV access. Haloperidol and morphine were given intramuscularly to achieve cooperation. Because of the location of his burns, access was restricted to his lower extremities and groin, where skin was spared due to his seated position. While nursing staff attempted peripheral access in his feet, a right femoral venous catheter was placed under ultrasound guidance.

Limited IV access requires that everything possible be done to optimize success. Utilization of the most experienced practitioners, avoidance of burned or contaminated skin, and the use of ultrasound guidance are recommended. Attention to sterile technique is particularly important in this population, in whom delayed infections represent a significant cause of morbidity.

24.2.2 Are there difficulties with BMV that might be anticipated in this patient?

Anatomical features predictive of difficult BMV also apply to burn victims, although other barriers to effective ventilation with a bag-mask must be considered. This patient is not obese, not elderly, and there is no facial hair or edentulous state to suggest a poor seal. However, edema associated with the burn may have created anatomic changes affecting airway patency, airways resistance, and compliance that may affect the ability to deliver effective BMV or extraglottic-device-aided gas exchange.

In this case, inspection of the face and neck revealed significant deep burns in these areas (Figure 24-1). The loss of skin elasticity was impressive, restricting the mouth opening to several centimeters

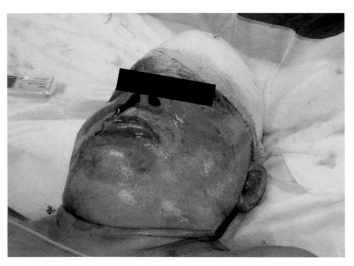

FIGURE 24-1. A photograph of the patient shortly after presentation to the emergency department.

and preventing full movement of his jaw and extension of his neck. Further inspection revealed nasal hair singing, pharyngeal erythema, and soot present in his posterior oropharynx. No obvious swelling or stridor was appreciated.

While the indirect markers above strongly suggest the presence of thermal injury, even the absence of facial burns, singed hairs, or carbonaceous sputum cannot reliably exclude the presence of supraglottic and laryngeal edema. Even if the external examination is normal, when managing a significant burn injury that took place in an enclosed space, one should assume airway swelling and inhalation injury, which cannot be excluded without direct visualization. The obstruction caused by thermal injury is related to progressive swelling and may also be complicated by skin sloughing. Early in the course of this evolving upper airway obstruction, BMV with positive pressure manual ventilation may be able to overcome it. Bronchospasm and mucosal edema of the lower airways may accompany inhalation injury, further complicating attempts at BMV. Fourth-degree burns and deep third-degree burns to the chest may cause a significant restrictive defect related to decreases chest wall compliance, particularly if it is circumferential. Eschar of the neck may prevent appropriate positioning of the patient for airway management. Emergency escharotomies of the chest or neck may be required (see below).

24.2.3 Are there issues with laryngoscopy and intubation that need to be considered in this patient?

The fundamental principle of airway management in the acute burn victim is early tracheal intubation and airway control, before conditions deteriorate. The intrinsic difficulties related to laryngoscopy uncovered with the LEMON assessment (see Section 1.6.2) remain relevant and need to be assessed. Reduced mouth opening, airway obstruction, and restricted neck mobility are the most common difficulties encountered. Edema caused by thermal injury to the perioral area, oropharynx, and glottis represents the primary difficulty in airway management. Associated swelling may

obscure visualization and the ability to identify the vocal cords. Mouth opening may be reduced further by loss of skin elasticity. Neck immobilization may be required if there is associated trauma, or may be produced by neck eschar.

This patient has a reduced mouth opening. Despite the neck burn, mobility appears reasonable and there is no suspicion of a cervical fracture. The mechanism of an enclosed space burn, associated with facial burns and carbonaceous sputum, all strongly suggest the presence of thermal injury to the glottis. There is no stridor present. However, this is considered a late finding in an adult. Only 50% of patients with airway thermal injury present with hoarseness or respiratory distress and only 20% will present with stridor.[1]

Despite the potential for difficult laryngoscopy in this patient, airway management should not be delayed and definitive airway control must be achieved urgently. The natural evolution of upper airway burn injury is progressive swelling, and airway narrowing for 12–24 hours, with resolution in 3–5 days. Although significant airway edema may be present in the first 2 hours, visualization sufficient to permit intubation is usually possible at this time, and will only deteriorate with delay. Immediate airway evaluation and consideration of early intubation is strongly recommended.

24.2.4 Are there physiologic issues that need to be considered in this patient while managing the airway?

Other issues to consider in the burn patient are fluid resuscitation, the presence of trauma, and the presence of inhalation injury. In this circumstance, there is no history to suggest associated trauma; however, when the burn is associated with a blast injury, concurrent assessment of traumatic injuries is necessary. The presence of associated injuries may enhance the need for early intubation, to facilitate therapy or operative intervention. Associated hemorrhagic shock will increase the need for aggressive volume resuscitation and the early consideration of blood replacement. In the absence of trauma, the fluid resuscitation needs can still be significant in burn patients (see discussion below).

Evidence of inhalation injury may take up to 24 hours to become evident.[2] Due to the impressive heat exchange capacity of the upper airway, thermal injury is usually most significant above the vocal cords. However, heat-induced injuries may be present in the lower airway. Smoke inhalation can cause significant, progressive, toxicity and hypoxemia by three mechanisms: the inhalation of hypoxic gas; airway inflammation from direct pulmonary toxins; and tissue hypoxia from systemic toxins such as cyanide and carbon monoxide. Any burn that takes place in an enclosed space, such as the patient described above, should raise the suspicion for inhalation and smoke injury. Chest radiography at presentation is a poor predictor of inhalation injury, since it is often normal initially. The presence of pulmonary infiltrates on initial evaluation suggests severe injury and a poor prognosis.[3]

24.2.5 How can carbon monoxide poisoning be identified?

Most pulse oximeters cannot reliably differentiate between oxygenated hemoglobin (HbO_2) and carboxyhemoglobin (COHb) and will give a spuriously high measurement of oxygen saturation. Reliance on pulse oximetry or a calculated SpO_2 (as may occur with arterial blood gas measurement) rather than a co-oximeter measured hemoglobin oxygen saturation will fail to diagnose carbon monoxide poisoning, and would provide false reassurance that adequate tissue oxygenation is occurring. An arterial blood gas specifying measured rather than calculated oxygen saturation should be obtained early in the course of management, and a COHb determination performed. High flow oxygen through a non-rebreather mask should be applied immediately, regardless of the pulse oximetry reading. Depending on the level of COHb and patient presentation, other therapies such as hyperbaric oxygen may be considered. The presence of significant carbon monoxide poisoning is another indication for early intubation to facilitate ventilation with 100% oxygen.[4]

24.3   AIRWAY MANAGEMENT CONSIDERATIONS

24.3.1   What would be the best way to manage this airway?

This patient represents potential difficulties to laryngoscopy and intubation, as well as ventilation with a bag-mask. Cricothyrotomy is possible despite the burn but the open technique is preferred. Despite the difficulties discussed above, the extent of the burns, the involvement of the face and neck, and the potential for associated inhalation injury mandate definitive airway management. As stated previously, the fundamental principle is early airway intervention. Any existing difficulties will only become worse with delay.

Anticipating these difficulties, there are a few options possible in this patient. Regardless of the strategy employed, there needs to be a bedside rescue device and surgical airway available before proceeding with any airway management technique. With limited mouth opening and restricted neck movement in the patient described above, it is advisable to have a device at the bedside that may be inserted blindly. Rescue devices such as the Trachlight™, the intubating LMA, the Combitube™, or a rigid fiberoptic laryngoscope, such as the Shikani Optical Stylet or the Bullard laryngoscope, may be used in this setting. One case report describes the successful use of a Combitube™ in a patient with facial burns, reduced oral opening, and known tracheal stenosis.[5] Because of the potential for severe delayed facial edema, the placement of an oral tube is preferred over a nasal approach. However, severe oral swelling from local chemical burns (ingestions, Freon "huffing," etc.) may prevent an oral approach and blind nasotracheal or fiberoptic-assisted nasal intubation may be the only non-surgical option. Regardless of the intubating technique chosen, an open surgical cricothyrotomy kit should be available at the bedside.

Three approaches may be considered in this patient:

1. An awake look with topicalization and sedation using a laryngoscope. This technique has been well described in other chapters. If assessment suggests that the cords are likely to be visualized, the practitoner may undertake a rapid sequence induction (RSI) technique. The urgency of the situation may preclude the use of an antisialagogue as it takes 15–20 minutes to be effective, enhancing the effectiveness of a topical application of local anesthetic agent. A combination of IV midazolam and ketamine would be a reasonable choice in this patient. The analgesic properties of ketamine are desirable and the potential for inhalation-induced bronchospasm favor the selection of this agent. Pain associated with this injury and respiratory distress may make it difficult to achieve an adequate level of cooperation unless high doses are utilized. Inability to gain cooperation without compromising ventilation may require the practitioner to move directly to RSI as outlined in option three, below.

2. Assessment of the airway with a flexible fiberoptic bronchoscope. The technique is similar to that described above, including topical anesthesia of the nares. This also requires a level of cooperation that cannot be achieved without sedation and analgesia. Utilizing the fiberoptic bronchoscope, the practitioner may consider intubation over the scope, or proceeding to RSI if assessment suggests this is likely to be successful.

3. Another option is going directly to RSI. This may be considered if:
   a. difficulty with laryngoscopy and intubation is not anticipated,
   b. the urgency or uncooperative state of the patient prevents the two options described above, or
   c. success was felt to be likely after an awake look.

The RSI procedure should not begin until Plans B and C are prepared and available at the bedside. Plan B should incorporate one of the rescue devices above. Plan C should be rapid movement to the performance of an open surgical cricothyrotomy. If difficulties are anticipated but urgency requires RSI, a double setup with the neck prepped and the surgical kit open is recommended. Attendance by another practitioner skilled in cricothyrotomies is desirable, if they are immediately available. An intubating stylet should be part of the initial laryngoscopic attempt, particularly since the glottic opening may be narrowed or difficult to visualize. Failure of laryngoscopy should be recognized early with no more than three attempts. Persistent laryngoscopic attempts are unlikely to be successful and are associated with adverse outcomes. Instead, be prepared to move rapidly to Plan B or C.

24.3.2   If the airway appears normal on presentation, should the trachea be intubated prophylactically?

As described above, not all airway injuries manifest immediately. Edema and associated obstruction will continue for at least 24 hours. Significant generalized edema may progress over several days secondary to the increased microvascular permeability of all tissues and the significant fluid requirements of burn patients (see below). Tracheal intubation and paralysis may be required to facilitate care, such as escharotomies, wound management, associated traumatic injuries, and pain control. If transportation is required, the initial presentation may present the best conditions for airway management and intubation, and is strongly encouraged before any transportation takes place. Even if the upper airway is normal, progression of inhalation injury, particularly in the face of an increased work of breathing, may require tracheal intubation and positive pressure ventilation. As a general rule, it is always better to intubate early than late in a burn patient.

24.3.3   Is cricothyrotomy contraindicated in a patient with burns involving the anterior neck?

No. In fact, there are no absolute contraindications to a surgical airway when the patient cannot be oxygenated and the trachea cannot be intubated, and the alternative is death. Many of these patients have a tracheotomy in their course of treatment (see discussion below), even when burns involve the neck. However, endotracheal intubation is the preferred method of primary airway control. In patients with burns to the anterior neck, elective tracheotomy is generally delayed until 5–7 days after skin grafting.[6]

A cricothyrotomy remains the rescue airway of choice should attempts to secure the airway fail and the lungs cannot be ventilated. In this patient, the significant anterior neck burns have created a noncompliant skin and eschar, obscuring landmarks and causing difficulty with neck extension. An open cricothyrotomy technique as opposed to a percutaneous Seldinger technique is therefore recommended in this patient, using a generous midline vertical incision. This will serve as an escharotomy to release the contracted tissue and enhance the ability to identify the cricothyroid space by palpation through the wound.

24.4   POSTINTUBATION AND VENTILATION MANAGEMENT

24.4.1   How does the presence of an inhalation injury affect ventilation?

The clinical effects of inhalation injury include upper airway edema from thermal injury, capillary leak of fluids into the airways, bronchospasm from toxins, and small airway occlusion from sloughed mucosal debris and impaired ciliary clearance. This can lead to increased dead space, intrapulmonary shunting, and decreased lung and chest wall compliance. These problems are compounded if pulmonary infection supervenes.[2]

Bronchospasm may well respond to inhaled β_2-agonists. Air trapping can occur and adequate expiratory times should be permitted. Vigorous pulmonary toilet will be required in the days following injury due to endobronchial debris, alveolar fluid, and infection. Positive end-expiratory pressure is often required to maintain small airway patency. Avoidance of excessive inflating pressures may be needed to avoid secondary lung injury. The concept of permissive hypercapnia has been associated with improved pulmonary outcomes in these patients.[7] Prophylactic steroids in the burn patient have not been associated with improved outcome, and may increase mortality.

24.4.2   Are there other concerns specific to postintubation management in the burn victim?

The role of tracheotomy in the management of inhalation injury and burns remains controversial.[8] Advantages include ease of pulmonary

toilette and the avoidance of dislodged orotracheal tubes. The potential long-term sequelae, such as tracheal stenosis and fistula formation, require careful decision making by the attending of surgeon. The two emergency indications for a surgical airway are the failure to achieve endotracheal intubation upon initial airway management, or if the endotracheal tube is inadvertently dislodged, and the subsequent edema makes replacement impossible. Anticipating that significant airway edema will evolve, cutting the endotracheal tube short is not advised. Great care should be taken to ensure tube security and prevention of accidental extubation. Exchange of a defective endotracheal tube should only be attempted by employing a tube exchanger with rescue devices immediately available.

24.5   ADDITIONAL CONSIDERATIONS

24.5.1   When should escharotomy be considered in the burn patient?

Severe third-degree and fourth-degree burns cause the collagen in skin to lose its elasticity, shorten, and become rigid. When this occurs in the chest wall, particularly in circumferential burns, significant restrictive pulmonary mechanics can occur with a reduction in pulmonary compliance. Incisional escharotomy may be needed to improve compliance of the lungs and maintain ventilation. The same can be said of circumferential burns of the extremities where circulation may be compromised.[9] Chest wall escharotomies are typically performed by a burn surgeon, although they are easily performed by any physician if required as a life-saving intervention. Vertical incisions are made bilaterally in the anterior axillary lines, from below the level of the clavicles to the lower rib margin. The top and bottom of the incisions are then joined to form a square across the chest. A tight neck eschar may draw the neck into flexion and impair ventilation. This may require a vertical incision from the sternal notch to the chin to release the constricting eschar.

Escharotomies will usually follow airway management. Significant circumferential chest burns with persistent ventilatory compromise may indicate immediate escharotomies, particularly if transport is contemplated.

24.5.2   Is succinylcholine contraindicated in acute burns?

The risk of lethal hyperkalemia following succinylcholine administration is well established in patients with >5% of body surface area burned. The greatest risk would appear to be between 18 and 66 days postburn.[10,11] However, it should be noted that one author found that the risk of hyperkalemia was present just 9 days postburn.[12] It seems reasonable to consider succinylcholine safe if used in the first week after the burn is sustained and then not used until the burn is fully healed.

24.6   SUMMARY

Unless there is associated trauma, the immediate priorities for burn victims are early airway control, fluid resuscitation, and pain management. The acutely burned patient should always be evaluated for heat-induced airway injury and inhalation injury, particularly if the injury occurred in a confined space, more so if superheated steam is involved. Signs of upper airway obstruction ought to motivate further evaluation of the upper airway to determine if endotracheal intubation is indicated. Ventilatory failure is potentially multifactorial in these patients being related to heat-induced upper airway obstruction, inhalation injury, and the acute restrictive defects related to chest wall eschar. Finally, as in all patients presenting to the ED, one must be vigilant for the "second diagnoses" such as blunt or penetrating trauma and underlying medical conditions.

REFERENCES

1. Darling G, Keresteci M, Pugash R, et al.: Pulmonary complications in inhalation injuries associated with cutaneous burn. *J Trauma*. 1996;40:83–89.
2. Miller K, Chang A: Acute inhalation injury. *Emerg Med Clin North Am*. 2003;21:533–557.
3. Masanes MJ, Legendre C, Lioret N, et al.: Using bronchoscopy and biopsy to diagnose early inhalation injury. *Chest*. 1995;107:1365.
4. Ernst A, Zibrak JD: Carbon monoxide poisoning. *N Engl J Med*. 1998;339:1603–1608.
5. Hagberg CA, Johnson S, Pillai D: Effective use of the esophageal tracheal Combitube following severe burn injury. *J Clin Anesth*. 2003;15:463–466.
6. Langford RM, Armstrong RF: Algorithm for managing injury from smoke inhalation. *BMJ*. 1989;299:902.
7. Sheridan RL, Kacmarek RM, McEttrick MM, et al.: Permissive hypercapnia as a ventilatory strategy in burned children: effect on barotrauma, pneumonia and mortality. *J Trauma*. 1995;39:854–859.
8. Jones WG, Madden M, Finkelstein J, et al.: Tracheostomies in burn patients. *Ann Surg*. 1989;209:471–474.
9. Sheridan RL: Scientific reviews: burns. *Crit Care Med*. 2002;30:S500–514.
10. Gronert GA, Dotin LN, Ritchey CR, Mason AD, Jr: Succinylcholine-induced hyperkalemia in burned patients. II. *Anesth Analg*. 1969;48: 958–962.
11. Schaner PJ, Brown RL, Kirksey TD, et al.: Succinylcholine-induced hyperkalemia in burned patients. 1. *Anesth Analg*. 1969;48:764–770.
12. Viby-Mogensen J, Hanel HK, Hansen E, Graae J: Serum cholinesterase activity in burned patients. II: anaesthesia, suxamethonium and hyperkalaemia. *Acta Anaesthesiol Scand*. 1975;19:169–179.

SELF-EVALUATION QUESTIONS

24.1. Airway burns
  A. are asymptomatic 50% of the time.
  B. are associated with stridor 20% of the time.
  C. are more common if the patient is trapped in an enclosed space at the time of the burn.
  D. may progress to upper airway obstruction over 6–12 hours.
  E. All of the above are correct.

24.2. The time course of upper airway swelling leading to total upper airway obstruction is
  A. 1–3 hours
  B. 5–8 hours
  C. 12–24 hours
  D. unpredictable
  E. seconds to minutes

24.3. The risk of succinylcholine-induced hyperkalemia
  A. is limited to patients with >20% third-degree burns.
  B. is causally related to burn-induced myoglobinuric renal failure.
  C. may be seen as early as 24 hours postburn.
  D. can be eliminated by pretreating with a nondepolarizing muscle relaxant.
  E. is a risk until the burn injury is fully healed.

CHAPTER (25)

Airway Management in a Patient with Angioedema

Michael F. Murphy and Neilson J. McLean

25.1 CASE PRESENTATION

This 25-year-old black female presents to the emergency department (ED) 2 hours after the onset of lip swelling that has progressed to difficulty in breathing. With the exception of newly diagnosed hypertension, she is otherwise well. Yesterday, her primary care physician began a course of a new antihypertensive medication, lisinopril. She has had no history of swelling and there is no family history of disorders characterized by swelling. Her vital signs are temperature 37°C, heart rate 100 bpm, respiratory rate 22 breaths per minute, blood pressure 165/90 mm Hg, and SpO_2 is 99% on 2 L·min^{-1} of O_2 by nasal prongs.

The patient is seated (Figure 25-1) with markedly edematous lips. She has a muffled voice ("hot potato voice") and is unable to swallow her own secretions due to the swelling. There is no stridor. The remainder of the physical examination is unremarkable.

25.2 DIAGNOSIS AND INVESTIGATIONS

25.2.1 What is the pathophysiology of angioedema?

Angioedema is defined as the abrupt onset of nonpitting swelling of the skin, mucous membranes, and deep subcutaneous tissues, including the linings of the upper respiratory and intestinal tracts.[1] Angioedema develops because of a local increase in permeability of the submucosal or subcutaneous capillary vessels, causing local plasma extravasation. This is exacerbated by the release of vasoactive substances such as histamines,

prostaglandins, bradykinins, and cytokines.[2] Angioedema can be divided into hereditary angioedema (HAE) and acquired angioedema.

Hereditary Angioedema is extremely rare, affecting 1 in 50,000 people.[2] It develops due to a C1 esterase inhibitor deficiency, which is inherited in an autosomal dominant pattern. This deficiency results in an abnormal increase in the activation of C1 and subsequently, excessive formation of the enzyme kallikrein. The excess kallikrein transforms kininogen into kinins, including bradykinin. Bradykinin is highly vasoactive and produces the characteristic tissue swelling.[2] HAE is commonly precipitated by trauma and stress, and can recur. If the patient has known HAE, then treatment with fresh frozen plasma (FFP) is beneficial, as it contains C1 esterase inhibitor. In some centers, vapor-heated C1 inhibitor concentrate is available and is proving beneficial in recurrent attacks of HAE.[2]

Acquired angioedema is due to faulty activation of the complement and kallikrein–kinin systems. It comprises several types, including the traditional mast-cell-mediated allergic response, precipitated by exposure to an allergen (such as peanuts and shellfish; traditional IgE-mediated responses), and those types associated with medications such as angiotensin-converting enzyme inhibitors (ACEIs) and nonsteroidal anti-inflammatory agents (NSAIDs).[3,4]

The development of angioedema secondary to ACEIs is of particular interest. In addition to inhibiting the conversion of angiotensin I to angiotensin II, the suppression of ACE results in a decrease in the breakdown of bradykinin and substance P. As outlined above, this can result in severe tissue swelling.[1] ACEI-induced angioedema has a predilection for the head and neck,[2] rendering it a particular challenge in airway management. It appears that this drug effect is associated specifically with the class

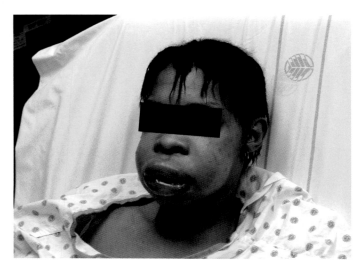

FIGURE 25-1. Patient with angioedema.

of drugs known as ACEIs.[2] Treatment with IV steroids, antihistamines, and subcutaneous epinephrine (0.3 mg) may be beneficial in allergy-induced angioedema, but has been shown to be ineffective in HAE and of limited use in ACEI-induced angioedema.[5] There is no role for FFP in ACEI-induced angioedema.

ACEI-induced angioedema affects more women than men and in the United Sates and is most common among 40–50-year-olds. Close to half of those affected with angioedema are African American.[6] According to the literature, the incidence of ACEI-induced angioedema ranges from 0.1% to 0.2% of all patients taking this class of drugs.[1,2,7] However, ACEI-induced angioedema is the most common cause of angioedema seen in US EDs, accounting for 17–38% of all angioedema cases.[8] Results of the omapatrilat cardiovascular treatment assessment versus enalapril (OCTAVE) trial investigating a new ACEI known as omapratilat suggest an increased incidence of the disorder in African American patients, those older than 65, and those with a history of drug rash or seasonal allergies.[7] Approximately 50% of all ACEI-induced angioedema cases occur within 1 week of starting the medication, with the remainder occurring anywhere from weeks to years after starting the drug.[2]

25.2.2   What is the general clinical course of the disorder?

Patients with HAE usually report trauma, often minor (e.g., dental visit), followed by tissue swelling. They can present with swelling in such widespread anatomic areas as the face, hands, arms, legs, GI tract, and genitalia but often respond to treatment. In one large series, 10% of the patients with HAE required definitive airway intervention because of upper airway edema.[2]

The clinical course of ACEI-induced angioedema is extremely unpredictable, and life-threatening presentations requiring airway interventions are reported in up to 20% of these patients.[2] According to the literature, 0–22.2% of patients with angioedema will require intubation.[6] It is extremely difficult to predict which patients who present with a stable airway will progress to a requirement for airway intervention. Researchers from Boston[6] retrospectively analyzed cases of ACEI-related angoiedema and determined that increasing age and oral cavity/oropharyneal involvement

predicted the need for airway intervention. These predictors had a sensitivity of 65.2% and specificity of 83.7%.

Since the clinical course of angioedema, especially ACEI-induced, is very unpredictable, it is recommended that these patients be admitted to an intensive care environment and closely monitored for at least 24 hours.

25.2.3   What investigations might one employ to aid in the diagnosis and evaluate the severity of the disorder?

The severity of airway compromise on presentation will determine the extent of initial investigations of these patients, and thus the workup for HAE is typically undertaken after the acute episode has resolved. The unpredictable clinical course of this disorder demands that each of these patients be triaged as "emergencies" to a resuscitation area of the ED and attended to immediately by nursing and physician staff. Evaluation and management is carried out concurrently, as is appropriate in patients with life-threatening conditions. As a result, early airway intervention is strongly advised. It is often obvious that the airway is in immediate jeopardy and this should trigger calling for assistance and implementing a strategy to secure the airway, from either above or below (surgically). The decision for airway intervention will be based largely on the clinical signs of respiratory distress: air hunger, agitation, stridor, etc.

If one has time, the most important diagnostic maneuver to undertake immediately is a flexible fiberoptic nasopharyngoscopy.[9] It is prudent to prepare for this procedure as though one was intending to perform an awake fiberoptic-guided nasal intubation. This assumes that one has anesthetized the nasal passage and inserted a nasotracheal tube through which the fiberoptic scope is passed in case the findings mandate intubation. It is preferable that the fiberoptic scope used for this procedure be of sufficient length and stiffness to guide an endotracheal tube into the trachea.[9]

A portable cross-table soft tissue x-ray of the airway may prove useful, particularly when one is questioning the diagnosis or suspecting that only the larynx is involved in the process. However, this investigation *must not* delay care if the airway is compromised and *must not* mean that the patient has to leave the resuscitation area. Patients are usually reluctant to lie flat to perform studies such as CT scanning and MRI evaluations and this hesitancy ought to alert the clinician that the degree of airway obstruction is significant, rendering such studies contraindicated. Ballooning of the hypopharynx suggests the presence of significant laryngeal involvement and may indicate an early need for upper airway endoscopy. Arterial blood gases and other blood studies are generally not helpful in the management of these patients.

25.3   AIRWAY MANAGEMENT

25.3.1   How does one make the decision that intubation is indicated?

This decision is most often made on clinical grounds and based on the degree of upper airway obstruction present and the pace at which it changes. Diagnostic studies, with the exception of flexible fiberoptic evaluation of the airway, are not usually helpful in deciding when to intubate. As mentioned above, early airway intervention is the safest course of action,[10] particularly as the clinical course may be erratic and unpredictable. In the hope perhaps to halt or reverse the progression of airway compromise, the practitioner may decide on a course of steroids and racemic epinephrine when securing the airway should have been the priority.

Any evidence of upper airway obstruction, including a muffled voice, difficulty managing secretions, or stridor, ought to trigger urgent airway intervention. Other clinical signs motivating immediate intervention include air hunger (dyspnea), confusion, agitation, or falling oxygen saturations.[11]

25.3.2   How should the airway be evaluated for difficulty?

These airways should always be considered "difficult airways" and managed according to the Difficult Airway Algorithm (see Chapter 2). Specifically, they fail the MOANS analysis (see Section 1.6.1) for difficult bag-mask-ventilation in that mask seal may be difficult. But more importantly, adequate gas exchange may be prevented by edematous upper airway tissue, occluding the airway even in the face of high pressures generated by bag-mask devices.

Based on the airway evaluation using the mnemonic RODS (see Section 1.6.3), the use of extraglottic devices (EGDs) will be difficult. Insertion of the device will be difficult if not impossible and the larynx itself may be edematous to the point of obstruction. Furthermore, the EGD may not provide an effective seal in an edematous hypopharynx.

The failure of MOANS and RODS alone would prohibit the use of paralytic agents, even if one felt that the LEMON analysis (see Section 1.6.2) might permit a successful direct laryngoscopy and intubation. In other words, rapid sequence intubation (RSI) is contraindicated. An assessment for cricothyrotomy is particularly germane in these patients, as it may emerge as the preferred and primary intervention for airway management performed awake under local anesthesia.

25.3.3   How should this patient's airway be managed?

Some patients with angioedema have had prior episodes and may be able to provide some reassurance that this episode will resolve under close observation. However, such patients are few and far between. It is much more likely that the clinical course will be unpredictable and a more aggressive approach to airway management is therefore justified.

Management is driven by the Difficult Airway Algorithm. In the event that oxygen saturations are poor and cannot be improved, one is directed to the Failed Airway Algorithm and immediate cricothyrotomy. RSI is not an option in these patients. If there is time, the next step will depend on the practitioner's access to, and ability to use, a flexible fiberoptic bronchoscope (FFB). If an experienced practitioner is available, then intubation using FFB ought to be performed with immediate cricothyrotomy as backup Plan B (double setup). The nasal route mentioned above is ordinarily much easier for those who infrequently perform fiberoptic intubations. In the event one does not have, or cannot

use, a fiberoptic bronchoscope then an "awake look" employing a conventional laryngoscope may help create a more informed decision to intubate awake or to move to cricothyrotomy.

It is often a weighty decision to use sedative hypnotic agents to facilitate airway evaluation and management in patients with upper airway obstruction in general and angioedema in particular. Patients with upper airway obstruction maintain their airways by using every airway muscle at their disposal, and even small doses of these sedative agents may precipitate total upper airway obstruction. In small titrated doses, ketamine may be preferable in that it maintains muscle tone and respiratory drive. The disadvantages of "laryngeal sensitization," salivation, and confusion must be weighed against the positive aspects of using this drug.

The use of topical local anesthetic agents in patients with upper airway obstruction is also not without risk. Several cases have been reported in the last decade of topicalization, converting partial upper airway obstruction to complete obstruction (see Section 3.3.3). However, a practitioner may have no choice but to employ topicalization in an attempt to secure the airway. Blind (nondirect vision) techniques such as blind nasal intubation and light-guided techniques are relatively contraindicated due to the potential for airway distortion and the risk of producing further trauma and bleeding.

25.4   SUMMARY

The incidence of angioedema has increased dramatically over the past two decades with the introduction of angiotensin-converting enzyme (ACE) inhibitors for the treatment of hypertension. The clinical course of an episode is unpredictable. For this reason, securing the airway early is generally a safer course than "watching and waiting." Available therapies, including intravenous steroids and nebulized alpha agonists (e.g., racemic epinephrine), are of marginal value and ought not delay airway intervention. Intubation over an FFB may be the preferred technique, the nasal route being recommended for those who perform fiberoptic intubation infrequently. Alternatively, employing sedation and topical anesthesia may enable one to intubate using direct laryngoscopy. However, the preferred Plan B may be cricothyrotomy performed under local anesthesia with the patient awake.

REFERENCES

1. Muelleman RL, Tran TP: Allergy, hypersensitivity and anaphylaxis. In: Marx JA, Hockberger R, Walls R (eds), *Rosen's Emergency Medicine: Concept and Clinical Practice,* 5th edn. St. Louis: Mosby, 2002:1619–1634.
2. Kaplan AP, Greaves MW: Angioedema. *J Am Acad Dermatol.* 2005;53: 373–392.
3. Chiu AG, Krowiak EJ, Deeb ZE: Angioedema associated with angiotensin II receptor antagonists: challenging our knowledge of angioedema and its etiology. *Laryngoscope.* 2001;111:1729–1731.
4. Gannon TH, Eby TL: Angioedema from angiotensin converting enzyme inhibitors: a cause of upper airway obstruction. *Laryngoscope.* 1990;100: 1156–1160.
5. Reid M, Euerle B: Angioedema. Available at http://www.emedicine.com/med/topic135.htm 2005.
6. Zirkle M, Bhattacharyya N: Predictors of airway intervention in angioedema of the head and neck. *Otolaryngol Head Neck Surg.* 2000;123:240–245.
7. Kostis JB, Kim HJ, Rusnak J, et al.: Incidence and characteristics of angioedema associated with enalapril. *Arch Intern Med.* 2005;165:1637–1642.

8. Roberts JR, Wuerz RC: Clinical characteristics of angiotensin-converting enzyme inhibitor-induced angioedema. *Ann Emerg Med.* 1991;20:555–558.
9. Bentsianov BL, Parhiscar A, Azer M, Har-El G: The role of fiberoptic nasopharyngoscopy in the management of the acute airway in angioneurotic edema. *Laryngoscope.* 2000;110:2016–2019.
10. Thompson T, Frable MA: Drug-induced, life-threatening angioedema revisited. *Laryngoscope.* 1993;103:10–12.
11. Bernstein S, Buckley PJ, Pollack CV, Walls R: Intubation strategies in patients with angioedema or intraoral obstruction: a multicenter study. *Acad Emerg Med* 1999;6:518.

SELF-EVALUATION QUESTIONS

25.1. ACEI-induced angioedema patients

A. usually respond to subcutaneous and aerosolized epinephrine

B. have a notoriously unpredictable clinical course with respect to the airway

C. can usually be safely observed as long as they do not have stridor

D. usually respond to high dose intravenous steroids

E. can be managed with fresh frozen plasma

25.2. All of the strategies for definitive airway management are acceptable in patients with angioedema **EXCEPT**

A. awake fiberoptic intubation

B. awake direct laryngoscopy

C. rapid sequence intubation

D. cricothyrotomy

E. tracheotomy

25.3. Which of the following symptoms would suggest an obstructed airway with a diameter of 4.0 mm or less and necessitate definitive airway management?

A. stridor

B. muffled voice

C. oxygen desaturation

D. difficulty managing secretions/drooling

E. use of accessory muscles

CHAPTER (26)

Airway Management for Blunt Facial Trauma

David A. Caro and Aaron E. Bair

26.1   CASE PRESENTATION

A 40-year-old officer was thrown from his police boat causing him to strike his face on a concrete bridge abutment. He was found lying face down and unconscious by other officers on the scene. Upon paramedic arrival, his initial Glasgow Coma Scale (GCS) score was 9, with facial bleeding and a tenuous airway. He was positioned so as to optimize airway patency and expeditiously transported to the nearest emergency department (ED).

The patient presented to the ED with sonorous respirations and an oxygen saturation of 95%, despite an inspired oxygen concentration (FIO_2) of >0.9. Vital signs included a pulse of 65 beats per minute, a blood pressure of 155/90 mm Hg, a respiratory rate of 12 breaths per minute, and a temperature of 37°C. Upon initial examination (Figure 26-1), he had ongoing oral and nasal hemorrhage; periorbital, nasal, and lip ecchymoses; mobility of his maxilla; and multiple broken teeth. The patient appeared somnolent and his GCS score was 6. In light of his injuries, and their mechanisms, cervical spine precautions were initiated in anticipation of tracheal intubation (for airway protection).

26.2   PATIENT ASSESSMENT

26.2.1   What are the airway evaluation considerations in this patient?

This patient presents with clinical issues that may influence his airway management. In addition to airway protection and maintenance, strategic adjustment of his ventilation will likely be required.

As this is not a "crash" intubation situation, an unhurried evaluation of airway difficulty is possible.

The presence of mid-face instability and orofacial disruption will likely hinder the success of bag-mask-ventilation (BMV) due to a poor mask seal. Similarly, in the presence of soft tissue edema and foreign bodies (teeth, clots, etc.), use of an extraglottic device (EGD) may be difficult. Laryngoscopy will likely be complicated by the presence of blood, tissue edema, and possible airway disruption. In addition, the use of cervical spine precautions limits the ability to position the head and neck optimally during laryngoscopic intubation.

26.2.2   What is the LeFort classification system?

Significant mid-face injuries that involve the maxilla and pterygoid plates can be categorized by the LeFort system (Figure 26-2). While fractures can be of mixed type, they are generally classified as follows: the fracture lines of a LeFort I fracture follow the course of the overlying nasolabial folds (i.e., involve the maxilla inferior to the nose only); LeFort II fractures involve a larger portion of the maxillae, triangulating from the premolar region on both sides to the nasal bones; and LeFort III fractures include the zygomatic arches, thereby allowing for total mobility of the facial structures (craniofacial disjunction).

By definition, LeFort fractures require that the maxilla be fractured in two separate places, leaving an essentially free-floating segment of bone. This alters the structural integrity of the face and potentially complicates airway visualization. LeFort II and III fractures can significantly impair the airway practitioner's ability to ventilate the patient using a bag-mask, due to poor mask fit and associated obstruction of the nares.[1–3]

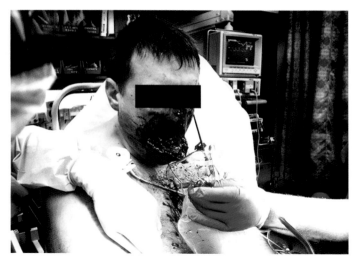

FIGURE 26-1. A photograph of the patient shortly after presentation to the emergency department.

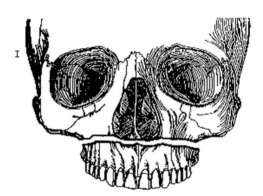

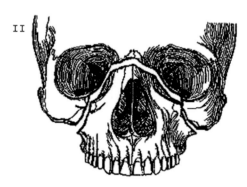

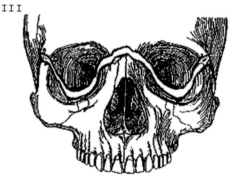

FIGURE 26-2. Diagrams of the LeFort classification of facial fractures.

26.2.3   How is a "basal skull" fracture different from a "LeFort fracture"?

Blunt facial and head trauma are often associated with other injuries, including basilar skull and cervical spine fractures. Basilar skull fractures most commonly involve the petrous portion of the temporal bone. However, the sphenoid and ethmoid bones can also be involved. The possibility of ethmoid fracture may be of particular concern, as a free passage may ensue between the nasal and intracranial cavities. Inadvertent intracranial placement of nasally introduced tubes and catheters has been reported, making the blind insertion of nasal airway devices contraindicated.[4,5]

26.2.4   How often is a major facial fracture associated with cervical spine injury?

The incidence of associated cervical spine fracture with severe blunt facial trauma ranges from 1% to 2.6% of patients.[6–9] This potential for associated cervical spine injury requires that, in the absence of the C-spine that has been fully cleared, the airway practitioner makes every effort to maintain the cervical spine in a neutral position. An assistant will be needed to maintain in-line cervical immobilization during attempts at laryngoscopy.

26.2.5   What other concerns do you have for this patient?

There are other issues for this patient. The patient has sustained a head injury that is moderately symptomatic. An increase in intracranial pressure (ICP), or even an intracranial hematoma, is possible. The principles of management for the brain-injured patient include the avoidance of hypotension and hypoxia, as both are independently associated with aggravating secondary brain injury and higher patient mortality. In addition, gratuitous intracranial engorgement due to patient coughing should be controlled. Modulation of the patient's cerebral metabolic oxygen demand is desirable to mitigate increases in cerebral blood flow to areas of normal brain with the potential to cause an increase in ICP.

Pretreatment with intravenous lidocaine, fentanyl, and a defasciculating agent (if succinylcholine is chosen as the paralytic) should be considered prior to induction and paralysis in an effort to blunt further ICP rise with laryngoscopy. For induction, a cerebroprotective sedative (e.g., barbiturates) is warranted, but care must be taken not to induce hypotension that could exacerbate the patient's brain injury. While etomidate may be attractive because of its associated "hemodynamic stability," it is not a cerebral protectant. The choice of agents is of particular importance when caring for patients with a diminished cardiac reserve, such as those with severe cardiac disease, those who are critically ill, or patients who are elderly. These patients are more prone to a hypotensive response than are healthier patients with similar injuries.

26.2.6 What investigations are warranted for this patient before proceeding to airway management?

The priority in managing patients with trauma is adequate gas exchange and oxygenation. Clearly, airway intervention takes precedence over any further investigations. Some may argue that a cross-table lateral cervical spine x-ray ought to precede airway intervention. However, since such an investigation would not alter the manner in which the airway is managed (in-line stabilization and RSI) it ought not delay airway management. Concurrent resuscitation and evaluation is the hallmark of trauma management, meaning that relevant investigations are underway at the same time intubation is undertaken and do not delay management.

26.3 AIRWAY MANAGEMENT

26.3.1 What are the airway management considerations one needs to be aware of?

The initial plan should anticipate both difficult laryngoscopy and difficult BMV. This is at least in part related to the potential for an unstable cervical spine prohibiting positioning of the airway by neck flexion or extension with the potential for spinal cord injury. An induction with full paralysis might be desirable, although it must be recognized that failure of both intubation and BMV is a significant possibility in this patient. In such a circumstance, the efficacy of many of the common alternative devices would also be compromised. Transillumination with the lightwand could be problematic. The intubating laryngeal mask airway might be difficult to place. Vision with the Bullard™ laryngoscope and GlideScope® would be clouded in the presence of blood. Basic backups, such as the Combitube™, or surgical airway, would have to be available.

26.3.2 What procedure should be used to intubate the trachea of this patient?

With a deteriorating neurological status and a possible increase in ICP, the default approach (Plan A) is a standard approach to rapid sequence intubation (RSI) with in-line cervical spine stabilization. Plan B would be an EGD and Plan C a surgical airway—in other words a "triple setup." Preparation begins by assembling standard intubating equipment, alternative airway devices, and a surgical airway kit. Denitrogenation with a non-rebreather mask should be initiated well in advance of induction. Uncontrolled epistaxis may impede this process, can lead to aspiration, and may require immediate packing, or cauterization. Adequate suctioning is essential.

Pretreatment with lidocaine, an opioid, and a defasciculating dose of a non-depolarizing paralytic agent should be given 3 minutes prior to intubation, time permitting, in order to prevent fasciculations. RSI will ordinarily include propofol or etomidate, followed by succinylcholine. Antiaspiration maneuvers such as

Sellick's maneuver ought to be employed, although cautiously to avoid internal jugular vein compression and impeded venous return from the cranial vault. Dosages of the opioids and the induction agents should be moderated to avoid hypotension, particularly in the face of substantial sympathetic nervous system activation.

A sequence of predetermined steps ought to be employed if failure with laryngoscopy or oxygenation occurs. The alternative airway device of choice should be the one with which the practitioner has the most experience. An intubating LMA has particular advantage, as it may circumvent the problem of a traditional mask seal on top of a mobile maxilla. It can also be manipulated by the guiding handle to best fit the hypopharynx. As an additional backup, the patient's neck should be prepped, and cricothyrotomy equipment should be opened and ready for use, in the event that the preceding steps fail to secure the airway.

26.4 POSTINTUBATION MANAGEMENT

26.4.1 What other issues should be considered following tracheal intubation?

Stable hemodynamics, as well as intracranial dynamics with adequate cerebral perfusion, together with adequate oxygenation and ventilation, are mandatory for this patient. Serial arterial blood gas measurements to monitor for hypo- or hyperventilation are recommended. Continuous capnography, if available, can be useful in this setting. Importantly, during the time of initial evaluation in the ED, the patient should be adequately sedated and paralyzed to limit the possibility of accidental extubation.

26.5 SUMMARY

A maxillofacial injury can significantly impair both the ability to bag-mask-ventilate a patient and perform laryngoscopy. Careful consideration must be given to the approach to this difficult airway, which is complicated further by the significant risk of cervical spine injury, as well as brain injury. The lesson from this patient is to have multiple backup devices ready to use, along with a predetermined plan on how to employ them, in the event that the trachea cannot be intubated orally.

REFERENCES

1. Manson PN: Some thoughts on the classification and treatment of LeFort fractures. *Ann Plast Surg.* 1986;17:356–363.
2. Ghysen D, Ozsarlak O, van den Hauwe L, et al.: Maxillo-facial trauma. *JBR-BTR.* 2000;83:181–192.
3. McRae M, Frodel J: Midface fractures. *Facial Plast Surg.* 2000;16:107–113.
4. Martin JE, Mehta R, Aarabi B, et al.: Intracranial insertion of a nasopharyngeal airway in a patient with craniofacial trauma. *Mil Med.* 2004;169: 496–497.
5. Schade K, Borzotta A, Michaels A: Intracranial malposition of nasopharyngeal airway. *J Trauma.* 2000;49:967–968.

6. Ardekian L, Gaspar R, Peled M, Manor R, Laufer D: Incidence and type of cervical spine injuries associated with mandibular fractures. *J Craniomaxillofac Trauma.* 1997;3:18–21.
7. Bayles SW, Abramson PJ, McMahon SJ, Reichman OS: Mandibular fracture and associated cervical spine fracture, a rare and predictable injury. Protocol for cervical spine evaluation and review of 1382 cases. *Arch Otolaryngol Head Neck Surg.* 1997;123:1304–1307.
8. Beirne JC, Butler PE, Brady FA: Cervical spine injuries in patients with facial fractures: a 1-year prospective study. *Int J Oral Maxillofac Surg* 1995;24:26–29.
9. Haug RH, Wible RT, Likavec MJ, Conforti PJ: Cervical spine fractures and maxillofacial trauma. *J Oral Maxillofac Surg.* 1991;49:725–729.

SELF-EVALUATION QUESTIONS

26.1. After denitrogenation, attempts at RSI fail. The oxygen saturation decreases into the high 80% range. What is the next step in your management?

A. attempt to intubate by using Eschmann Introducer

B. change laryngoscope blade types

C. place an LMA

D. improve attempts at BMV with improved technique

E. cricothyrotomy

26.2. After multiple attempts at intubation and recognized inability to ventilate with either bag-mask or LMA, what is your next step in management?

A. place an invasive airway (e.g., open cricothyrotomy or percutaneous cricothyrotomy)

B. call for assistance

C. attempt fiberoptic-assisted intubation

D. support with bag-mask until awakening and resumption of spontaneous respirations

E. blind nasal intubation

26.3. The incidence of associated cervical spine fracture with severe blunt facial trauma

A. is negligible

B. is not a concern provided a cervical collar that provides rigid immobilization is used

C. ranges from 1% to 2.6% of patients

D. in some studies approaches 20%

E. is unknown

CHAPTER 27

Airway Management in a Patient with Retropharyngeal Abscess

Kirk J. MacQuarrie and David Kirkpatrick

27.1 CASE PRESENTATION

A 32-year-old man (Figure 27-1) presented to the emergency department (ED) with dysphagia, dysphonia, and dyspnea. Further inquiry revealed a 1-week history of left-sided jaw pain. This was initially treated with oral antibiotics and analgesics by his family doctor while awaiting an appointment with his dentist. He saw his dentist the preceding day and had an abscessed molar tooth extracted from his left mandible. His pain unfortunately continued and he developed swelling and fever prompting him to present to the ED. His past medical history was unremarkable and aside from his remaining prescription of the penicillin and hydromorphone he was on no medications. He had no known allergies.

27.2 INTRODUCTION

27.2.1 Incidence and etiology of deep neck infections in adults

The management of the patient whose airway is compromised due to a deep neck infection is a challenge for even the most experienced practitioner. Fortunately for all, such cases are relatively rare. A typical ENT referral center may see one to three adult cases per year that require airway management. As in this case, the origin of deep neck infections is often odontogenic. Intravenous drug abuse is another important cause; however, many cases do not have an identifiable etiology.[1]

27.2.2 Do all deep neck infections require airway intervention?

The majority of cases of deep neck infections can be managed conservatively without surgical intervention and do not require intervention to maintain the patient's airway.[2,3] This conservative approach is similar to the management of adenotonsillar hypertrophy secondary to infectious mononucleosis, which will typically respond to steroids with or without antibiotics. Even epiglottitis in the adult population only rarely will require airway manipulation in the form of intubation or tracheotomy. Early deep neck infections are usually a cellulitis that can be successfully treated with antibiotics alone. Small, localized abscesses such as peritonsillar abscesses can often be treated with needle aspiration followed by antibiotics.

27.2.3 What is Ludwig's angina and how does it differ from retropharyngeal abscess?

Ludwig's angina is characterized by edema of the entire floor of the mouth and, if left untreated, may result in complete airway obstruction. The infection may cause swelling of the tongue and epiglottis that will then impair the ability to swallow and clear secretions. Total airway obstruction may result from the progressive swelling or from laryngospasm secondary to aspiration of pus secretions, or both.[4] Surgical intervention is usually required if abscess formation and airway compromise occur. While most cases of deep neck infections can be managed conservatively, true cases of Ludwig's angina typically require more aggressive intervention.

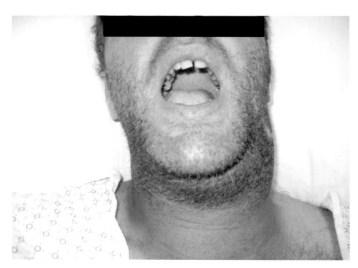

FIGURE 27-1. A 32-year-old man presented with dysphagia, dysphonia, and dyspnea. There is marked swelling on the left side of the neck. Due to marked discomfort, he was unable to protrude his tongue for proper pharyngeal evaluation.

27.3   ASSESSMENT OF THE PATIENT

27.3.1   Why might airway management be difficult in patients with a retropharyngeal abscess?

Patients with retropharyngeal abscess frequently have features that create difficulty in carrying out several airway management techniques: bag-mask-ventilation, ventilation using extraglottic devices (EGDs), direct laryngoscopy, indirect laryngoscopy, and even a surgical airway.

Bag-mask-ventilation may be challenging in these patients for a number of reasons. Patients with stridor will have significantly decreased airway caliber, necessitating high airway pressures to produce adequate gas flow. It may not be possible to generate these pressures with bag-mask-ventilation. Both the awake or obtunded patient may poorly tolerate application of the face-mask and airway opening maneuvers due to pain and anxiety. It may prove difficult (to impossible) to open the airway of the sedated or unconscious patient due to the loss of muscle tone and the resultant further narrowing of the airway decrease in airway caliber. Copious secretions may increase the risk of laryngospasm and tongue swelling may preclude use of an oral airway. A nasal airway is an option but possible bleeding could trigger laryngospasm. Although Brimacombe et al. reported the successful use of a small laryngeal mask airway (#2) as a rescue device for a hypoxic adult patient with quinsy,[5] extraglottic "rescue devices" for failed bag-mask-ventilation may be ineffective in these patients, particularly if the edema involves the glottis.

Edema (particularly tongue swelling) and secretions will make direct laryngoscopy more difficult regardless of the type of blade chosen. Nuchal rigidity, trismus, or both may be improved with sedation or muscle relaxants but there is no guarantee that these agents will be effective. Blind intubation techniques, such as the

intubating LMA (LMA Fastrach™, LMA North America Inc., San Diego, CA) and light-guided intubation (Trachlight™, Laerdal Medical Corp., Wappingers Falls, New York) would not generally be considered for first-line use in these patients as these techniques run the risk of disrupting infected tissue and potentially soiling the airway. Furthermore, these blind intubating techniques could result in laryngospasm during the intubation attempt. Alternatively, in the absence of blood and secretions in the upper airway, techniques that rely on indirect visualization of the glottis (Bullard and Wu laryngoscopes as well as Glidescope™) could be reasonably employed by experienced operators.

Unfortunately, performing a surgical airway in this patient population is generally difficult. The anatomy is often distorted due to swelling and hyperemic tissues may increase the likelihood of bleeding. In some patients, the abscess may involve the area surrounding the trachea. Supine positioning of the patient to perform a surgical airway may worsen dyspnea and reduce the patient's cooperation. Managing the airway of this patient is extremely difficult as all the possible options of ventilation and oxygenation are fraught with danger. The ultimate decision will be made based on the urgency of the clinical circumstance, the available resources, setting careful priorities, as well as the skill and experience of the airway team (anesthesia practitioner and surgeon).

27.3.2   Role of CT scan in assessing these patients

The advent of the CT scan has revolutionized the ability to accurately assess the swollen, inflamed neck. In addition to determining the severity of the infection involving different tissue planes and neck spaces, the resolution of the CT scan can help to differentiate between a cellulitis and an abscess. It can also detect the presence or absence of thrombosis of the jugular vein. Unfortunately, in the presence of a rapidly deteriorating airway, it is necessary to proceed with an emergency airway management before a CT examination of the neck becomes available.

27.3.3   Technique of nasopharyngoscopy and its role in the management of patients with deep neck Infections

Nasopharyngoscopy is a safe and simple technique that should become familiar to anesthesia practitioners, otolaryngologists, and contemporary emergency physicians. Following the application of topical vasoconstrictor and topical anesthetic (10% Xylocaine), the flexible fiberoptic scope is passed into the nasopharynx. The glottis should not be anesthetized as this could trigger laryngospasm. With the flexible fiberoptic scope, the glottis can be viewed from above without the risk of provoking laryngospasm. The technique is usually first done in the ED as part of the initial evaluation and repeated at the bedside or in the operating room (OR) as required to provide an ongoing evaluation of the airway.

27.3.4   How was this patient assessed?

On examination, he appeared anxious and in severe discomfort. He was febrile with a temperature of 38.7°C. His respiratory rate

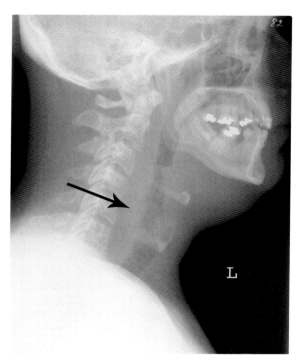

FIGURE 27-2. Although this lateral x-ray view of the head and neck did not show any obvious sign of airway obstruction, it showed an increase prevertebral soft tissue (swelling of the posterior pharyngeal wall [arrow]), an important diagnostic sign of retropharyngeal abscess.[16] There was also a loss of normal lordotic curvature of the spine.

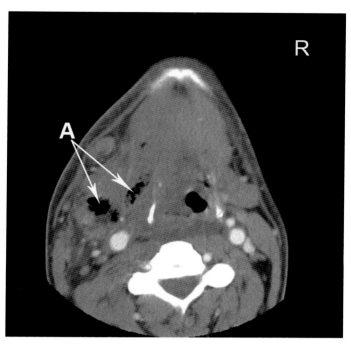

FIGURE 27-3. The axial CT image of the neck showed marked tissue swelling of the neck with air (arrows) in the soft tissue swelling on the left and deviation of the trachea to the right.

was 26 breaths per minute. His heart rate was 104 beats per minute, and his blood pressure was 132/76 mm Hg. His oxygen saturation was 91% on 40% oxygen delivered through the face mask. He was observed to have marked decrease in the range of motion of his neck. Erythema and swelling were extending from the left submandibular region down the neck to include his left upper chest. Marked submandibular swelling was seen in a lateral x-ray of the neck (Figure 27-2). Retropharyngeal swelling and a diminished airway caliber were also noted.

Nasopharyngoscopy was performed in the ED by the ENT resident and was significant for left lateral pharyngeal swelling and posterior displacement of the epiglottis making it impossible to visualize the vocal cords. A CT scan (Figure 27-3) showed that the initial odontogenic submaxillary space infection had extended to the left parapharyngeal space by a fascial connection between those spaces and had formed an abscess that was encroaching on the airway.

27.3.5 How do you assess the severity of airway obstruction?

Airway obstruction is assessed clinically by history and physical examination looking specifically at signs and symptoms, such as oxygen saturation, respiratory rate, stridor, tracheal tug, intercostal indrawing, and accessory muscle use. Lateral x-ray and CT scan of the head and neck can quantify the degree of obstruction (Figures 27-2 and 27-3). With nasopharyngoscopy, it is also possible to examine the dynamic aspect of the obstruction.

27.4 AIRWAY MANAGEMENT

27.4.1 What are the indications for establishing a definitive airway in patients with deep neck infections?

Indications for definitive airway management in these patients are either ongoing or impending airway obstruction or sepsis. The decision to secure the airway will generally be made by the ENT surgeon based on impending airway obstruction. In some instances, the ED physician may be forced into airway intervention if the patient is acutely decompensating (Crash Algorithm). Once the decision to intervene is made, anesthesia and ENT consultants (if not already involved) should be consulted immediately. These patients are ideally managed in the OR.

27.4.2 What was the plan in this case?

Given the severity of the obstruction and the patient's worsening symptoms, the decision was made to establish a definitive airway. An anesthesia practitioner was immediately consulted and the plan was made to proceed to the OR for either endotracheal intubation or tracheotomy, followed by surgical drainage of the abscess.

27.4.3 Do these patients require a primary surgical airway or can an attempt be made to intubate from above?

Once the need to secure the airway has been established, the next decision is whether to attempt intubation from above (either oral or nasal) or to go directly to a surgical airway. The choice of airway should be a joint decision between the anesthesia practitioner and the surgeon on the basis of the predicted difficulties of each of the following: face-mask ventilation, EGD ventilation, direct laryngoscopy, alternative intubation, and surgical access. The skill and experience of the airway team will also affect this decision. Potter et al.[7] reviewed the literature in 2002 and found that the background of the involved surgeon had a significant influence on preferred management. They found primary surgical airways to be favored by otolaryngologists, while oral and maxillofacial surgeons favored oral or nasal intubation.

27.4.4 "Double Setup" and Plan C

In many cases it will be reasonable to make an initial attempt at securing the airway nonsurgically. The specific route (awake, asleep, oral, and nasal) will be discussed below but the important thing is to have a well-developed Plan B (and sometimes Plan C). The "Double Setup" is the recommended approach for most of these cases, meaning that the surgical team is ready to go should attempts to secure the airway from above fail. This may involve having the surgical team gowned and gloved, and the neck prepped. Many times a formal tracheotomy can be performed but in the event of serious airway compromise consideration should be given to a cricothyrotomy.

The surgical airway typically represents Plan B and this may solve the airway problem. Surgical access could, however, prove difficult for any of the reasons discussed above. Loss of the airway during tracheotomy has been reported[8] and such an eventuality must be prepared for with Plan C. This will typically involve sedation (IV or inhalation) to facilitate patient cooperation, but in rare circumstances could require muscle relaxation and an attempt at direct laryngoscopy while attempts at obtaining surgical access continue.

27.4.5 What are the pros and cons of securing the airway with the patient awake versus under general anesthetic?

One must decide whether to intubate the patient awake or asleep. As discussed above, these patients invariably have features that pose problems in airway management. The safest initial approach with these patients is to manage the airway while they are awake. Sedation may indeed be necessary in some cases, but it is preferred to keep the patient cooperative and spontaneously breathing. Reassurance and relieving the patient's fear and anxiety is crucial; repeated reassurance and a confident demeanor on the part of the practitioner are essential. As well, the patient will often need to be maintained in a sitting or semi-sitting position in order to preserve comfort (and therefore ensure cooperation).

27.4.6 What could cause an awake intubation to be unsuccessful?

Awake intubation remains the safest initial approach to airway management but it is important to realize that sudden deterioration may occur even with the use of minimal or no sedation.[9-11] Reports of complete airway obstruction and others of failed fiberoptic intubation emphasize the importance of managing these patients under "double setup."[12] Inadequate airway anesthesia, laryngospasm, operator inexperience, oversedation, copious secretions, bleeding, or both, are all reasons that an attempted awake intubation may fail.

27.4.7 What is the plan if awake intubation fails or is not an option?

If an awake intubation is not possible, then the next safest route is to induce general anesthesia while preserving spontaneous ventilation. Inhalation induction followed by direct laryngoscopy and intubation is a common practice in children with airway obstruction since awake intubation is rarely a practical option in pediatrics. Inhalation induction of adults with airway obstruction may be more difficult in that the relatively longer excitement phase predisposes to aspiration, laryngospasm, or both. As anesthetic depth increases, complete airway obstruction can also occur due to loss of muscle tone. Inhalation induction typically requires at least some degree of patient cooperation but can be accomplished without.[13] As with awake intubation, it is critical to have a well-rehearsed backup plan (Plans B and C).

Preservation of spontaneous ventilation under anesthesia may be accomplished also with IV agents. However, preservation of spontaneous ventilation has been shown to be difficult when inhalational agents are used to achieve adequate anesthesia. Recent evidence suggests that remifentanil may be a more attractive IV sedation option. Machata et al. have demonstrated excellent intubating conditions when remifentanil was used for conscious sedation.[14] A bolus of 0.75 $\mu g \cdot kg^{-1}$ followed by an infusion of 0.075 $\mu g \cdot kg^{-1} \cdot min^{-1}$ provided good intubating conditions.

Rapid-sequence intubation is unlikely to represent a first-line management option in these patients. However, in the event that the airway is completely lost, consideration should be given to the use of muscle relaxants to facilitate intubation while attempts are made to achieve surgical airway access concurrently.

27.4.8 What are the "pros and cons" of nasal versus oral intubation?

Following the decision to attempt intubation from above, the next major choice is whether to use the nasal or oral route. Each has its advantages and drawbacks.

The nasal route bypasses the tongue (which may be swollen) and often provides a convenient passage to the glottic opening. At one time, blind nasal intubation was a common choice in these patients, but with the general availability of flexible fiberoptic bronchoscopes this technique is now seldom indicated. Furthermore, blindly advancing the endotracheal tube (ETT) into the glottic opening may rupture the abscess with resultant soiling of the trachea. Potential epistaxis is a major concern with the nasal approach. Bleeding may hamper visualization and could trigger laryngospasm.

The oral approach avoids the risks of nasal bleeding, and tube size is limited only by size of the glottic opening. For these reasons, the oral route is generally preferred, unless it appears impossible due to massive tongue swelling or inability to open the mouth.

27.4.9 How can one minimize the risk of bleeding associated with nasal intubation?

The risk of bleeding during nasal intubation can be minimized with the liberal use of topical vasoconstrictors (e.g., xylometazoline) and by using a small ETT (7 mm inner diameter, ID, or smaller). Reinforced ETTs may cause less trauma and are therefore preferable in these patients. Regular ETTs may be made less damaging to tissues by softening them in warm saline prior to use.

The practice of "dilating up the nasal passage" using different sizes of nasal trumpets may also decrease bleeding and allow for passage of a larger tube. Following application of local anesthesia and vasoconstrictors, a small soft nasal airway lubricated with 2% lidocaine jelly can be inserted into the right nasal passage (larger in most people). If resistance is encountered, the left nares can be tried. The process can then be repeated with the next larger size airway. The goal is to get easy passage of at least a size 8 nasal airway. An ETT a half size smaller can then be used for the intubation. A larger tube (7 mm ID or greater) is advantageous in that it allows for insertion of the adult flexible bronchoscope with its superior optics and suction capabilities.

27.4.10 What is the best tool to facilitate intubation?

For the most part, the tool that one chooses to facilitate intubation in these patients is less important than the approach discussed above. The technique chosen should reflect the practitioner's skill and comfort with the technique, as well as its safety and practicality. Blind techniques are discouraged due to risks of soiling the airway and of possible laryngospasm. For reasons discussed earlier, techniques that allow visualization of the airway are preferred, e.g. a direct-vision laryngoscopy. Other methods may be acceptable provided the practitioner is skilled in their use.

27.4.11 Advantages and disadvantages of fiberoptic intubation

Although advancement of the ETT through the glottis is not under vision, flexible fiberoptic bronchoscope (FFB) offers the advantage of being able to see "around the obstruction" and is usually well tolerated in the awake patient. Unfortunately, heavy secretions, bleeding, or both, may limit the usefulness of the FFB. Use of the adult FFB can lessen the effect of secretions compared to the pediatric FFB but necessitates the use of at least a size 7 mm ID ETT. FFB may be more difficult in the unconscious patient with decreased muscle tone.

27.4.12 Advantages and disadvantages of direct laryngoscopy

Direct laryngoscopy will often be advantageous in the presence of heavy secretions being present. It can be performed quickly and is generally the technique of first choice in the unconscious patient. Direct laryngoscopy is highly stimulating to reflexes and may not be tolerated in the awake patient, particularly if much force is needed to expose the glottis.

27.4.13 Description of the plan to secure the airway in this case

In the OR, the airway was reevaluated and, in consultation with the ENT surgeon, the decision was made to perform an awake orotracheal intubation under "double setup." The patient was positioned with head slightly elevated and standard monitors were applied. Supplemental oxygen was delivered with nasal prongs. A judicious dose of midazolam (0.5 mg boluses) was administered intravenously to reduce the patient's anxiety and improve cooperation. The neck was prepped and the surgical team was gowned and ready to perform an emergency surgical airway (Plan B).

27.4.14 Airway anesthesia for patients with deep neck abscess

There are multiple techniques to anesthetize the airway and these are discussed in Chapter 3. The chosen technique depends largely on the preference of the practitioner. However, care must be taken to avoid early stimulation of the airway which can result in fatal laryngospasm.[5]

Inflammation and infection can, in theory, decrease the efficacy of local anesthetics due to changes in local pH. However, this is generally not of any clinical significance. Heavy secretions, bleeding, or both, can decrease the amount of local anesthetic that actually reaches the mucosa and this should be taken into account, but there are many reports of successful airway anesthesia in the presence of infection.[15]

27.4.15 How was airway anesthesia achieved in this case?

Airway anesthesia was achieved with a combination of lidocaine ointment and inhaled tetracaine. Approximately 2 cm of 5% Lidocaine ointment was applied to the back of the tongue with a tongue depressor. The DeVilbiss atomizer was then used to deliver 15 mL of 0.45% tetracaine as an aerosol. No attempts were made to specifically block the superior laryngeal nerve due to concerns of disrupting the abscess and potentially soiling the airway.

27.4.16 How was this patient's airway secured?

Using a #3 Macintosh blade, direct laryngoscopy was attempted but no airway structures could be identified despite the patient's cooperation. A pediatric bronchoscope loaded with a 6.5 mm ID ETT was then introduced into the oral cavity. After identifying the glottic opening, which was significantly deviated to the right, the bronchoscope was directed into the trachea and the ETT was then advanced off into the airway. Following CO_2 confirmation of successful tube placement, general anesthesia was induced with 200 mg of propofol. Surgical drainage of the abscess was then accomplished without incident. Following 24 hours of ventilation in the ICU, the patient was uneventfully extubated and made a full recovery.

27.5   SUMMARY

It is clear that there is more than one approach to the management of the airway in these patients. The choice will be based on the particular patient presentation and the skills and experience of the airway team. In 2002, Jenkins et al. surveyed the management choices for the difficult airway by Canadian anesthesia practitioners.[16] Regarding the management of a patient unable to swallow, due to a retropharyngeal abscess, 70% chose an awake approach, 23% chose inhalation induction, and only 7% chose an IV induction of anesthesia. FFB was the initial technique chosen by 50%, 37% chose direct laryngoscopy, and 8% chose primary surgical airway.

Deep neck infections with abscess formation resulting in airway compromise provide a challenge for both the airway practitioner and the surgeon who are dependent upon each other for a successful outcome. The likelihood of a satisfactory result is enhanced by early involvement of both parties planning an approach to such challenges.

REFERENCES

1. Parhiscar A, Har-El G: Deep neck abscess: a retrospective review of 210 cases. *Ann Otol Rhinol Laryngol.* 2001;110:1051–1054.
2. Mayor GP, Millan JM, Vidal AM: Is conservative treatment of deep neck space infections appropriate? *Head & Neck.* 2001;23:126–133.
3. Sichel J, Dano I, Hoewald E, et al.: Nonsurgical management of parapharyngeal space infections: a prospective study. *Laryngoscope.* 2002;112:906–910.
4. Neff SPW, Merry AF, Anderson B: Airway management in Ludwig's angina. *Anaesth Intensive Care.* 1999;27:659–661.
5. Brimacombe J, Perry A, Van Duren P: Use of a size 2 LMA to relieve life-threatening hypoxia in an adult with quinsy. *Anaesth Intensive Care.* 1993;21:475–476.
6. Wholey MH, Bruwer AJ, Baker HL, Jr: The lateral roentgenogram of the neck; with comments on the atlantoodontoid-basion relationship. *Radiology.* 1958;71:350–356.
7. Potter JK, Herford AS, Ellis E: Tracheotomy versus endotracheal intubation for airway management in deep neck space infections. *J Oral Maxillofac Surg.* 2002;60:349–354.
8. McGuire G, El-Beheiry H, Brown D: Loss of the airway during tracheostomy: rescue oxygenation and re-establishment of the airway. *Can J Anaesth.* 2001; 48:697–700.
9. Ho AM, Chung DC, To EW, Karmakar MK: Total airway obstruction during local anesthesia in a non-sedated patient with a compromised airway. *Can J Anesth.* 2004;51:838–841.
10. Shaw IC, Welchew EA, Harrison BJ, Michael S: Complete airway obstruction during awake fiberoptic intubation. *Anaesthesia.* 1997;52:582–585.
11. McGuire G, El-Beheiry H: Complete upper airway obstruction during awake fiberoptic intubation in patients with unstable cervical spine fractures. *Can J Anesth.* 1999;46:176–178.
12. Pahl C, Yarrow S, Steventon N, et al.: Angina bullosa haemorrhagica presenting as acute upper airway obstruction. *BJA.* 2004;92:283–286.
13. Smith CE, Fallon WF: Sevoflurane mask anesthesia for urgent tracheostomy in an uncooperative trauma patient with a difficult airway. *Can J Anesth.* 2000;47:242–245.
14. Machata AM, Gonano C, Holzer A, et al.: Awake nasotracheal fiberoptic intubation: patient comfort, intubating conditions, and hemodynamic stability during conscious sedation with remifentanil. *Anesth Analg.* 2003;97: 904–908.
15. Ovassapian A, Tuncbilek M, Weitzel E, et al.: Airway management in adult patients with deep neck infections: a case series and review of the literature. *Anesth Analg.* 2005;100:585–589.
16. Jenkins K, Wong DT, Correa R: Management choices for the difficult airway by anesthesiologists in Canada. *Can J Anesth.* 2002;49:850–856.

SELF-EVALUATION QUESTIONS

27.1. What is Ludwig's angina?

   A. epiglottitis

   B. unstable angina

   C. deep neck infection and edema involving the entire floor of the mouth

   D. lingual tonsillitis

   E. mediastinitis

27.2. Which of the following airway management strategies may be difficult in patients with a retropharyngeal abscess?

   A. bag-mask-ventilation

   B. ventilation using extraglottic devices

   C. direct laryngoscopy

   D. surgical airway

   E. all of the above

27.3. Which of the following is **NOT** an acceptable intubating technique in managing patients with a retropharyngeal abscess?

   A. surgical airway

   B. fiberoptic intubation

   C. intubation using an intubating LMA

   D. laryngoscopic intubation

   E. intubation using a GlideScope™

CHAPTER (28)

Airway Management in the Intensive Care Unit

Stephen Beed

28.1 CASE PRESENTATION

A grossly intoxicated and obese 52-year-old female slips while leaving a restaurant, striking her head on a concrete step. She loses consciousness and while lying on her back vomits and aspirates. She is transported by ambulance to the emergency department (ED). By the time she reaches the ED, she is awake and complaining of difficulty breathing. She has a heart rate of 122 beats per minute (sinus rhythm on the cardiac monitor), respiratory rate (RR) of 28 breaths per minute (and labored), oxygen saturation (SpO_2) 90% (on a "non-rebreather"), and a blood pressure 154/88 mm Hg. Computed tomography (CT) of her head is negative and she has no other injuries. The patient is admitted to the intensive care unit (ICU) for management of her aspiration pneumonitis.

Following admission to the ICU, she becomes more distressed and her oxygen saturations fall into the low 80s despite optimal medical management and attempts at noninvasive ventilation. The decision to intubate is made. Airway evaluation reveals a thyromental distance of 4 cm; she has both upper and lower dentures. The initial attempt to intubate her trachea awake is unsuccessful and is complicated by further vomiting and aspiration. A second attempt employing a rapid sequence intubation (RSI) technique including Sellick's maneuver is successful. During the intubation, particulate matter in the pharynx is noted. The laryngeal view with laryngeal manipulation is a Cormack/Lehane Grade 2. Tracheal placement is confirmed with end-tidal carbon dioxide ($ETCO_2$) detection. Bronchial lavage with a flexible fiberoptic bronchoscope (FFB) is performed immediately after intubation.

The patient subsequently develops severe adult respiratory distress syndrome (ARDS) requiring deep sedation, with FiO_2 1.0 and pressure controlled ventilation, adjusted by using ARDSNet parameters[1-4] to the following: pressure level (PC) 20 cm H_2O, positive end-expiratory pressure (PEEP) 16 cm H_2O, FiO_2 1.0, tidal volume (TV) 500–550 mL, and RR 24 breaths per minute. She receives aggressive supportive care. On ICU day 5, corticosteroids are started and the patient subsequently improves. Her sedation is decreased and by day 7 she is switched to a PC of 18 cm H_2O, FiO_2 0.45, PEEP 12 cm H_2O, RR 24–30 breaths per minute, and TV 385–760 mL.

On day 11, the patient develops a new fever, an increased WBC, hypotension requiring inotropic support, and falling oxygen saturations requiring an increase in FiO_2 to 0.50. Bronchoscopy and CT scanning confirms a ventilator-associated pneumonia. On return from CT scan she self-extubates and within 30 minutes requires reintubation. This is accomplished with topicalization of the airway, 1 mg of midazolam, 50 μg of fentanyl, a styletted orotracheal tube (OTT), and BURP (backwards, upwards, and right-side-orientated pressure on the larynx). Broad-spectrum antibiotics are started. She undergoes a bedside percutaneous tracheotomy on day 13 and is weaned from ventilator support by day 20. She is transferred to the intermediate medical care unit on day 22.

28.2 UNIQUE AIRWAY ISSUES IN THE ICU

28.2.1 What is unique about the ICU patient?

Patients admitted to the ICU generally have limited physiologic reserve. They need minute-to-minute monitoring and treatment and usually require respiratory and/or hemodynamic support. Physicians choosing to practice in the ICU environment must possess excellent airway management skills for a variety of reasons. Some patients, initially without tracheal intubation, will decompensate while in ICU and require tracheal intubation. Others are admitted to the ICU having been intubated elsewhere and will be extubated during their ICU stay (planned or unplanned). Still others, having been extubated, will fail and require reintubation. As with any intervention, an understanding of the dynamic and often subtle interplay among commonly utilized medications, the physiologic responses associated with intubation and the physiologic reserve of the compromised patient must be understood.

In addition to limited cardiopulmonary reserve, other important concerns such as hepatic and renal dysfunction, a "full stomach," and altered neurological function are also common in this patient population. Intensive care patients are as complex as the environment in which they are cared for. The practitioner tasked with airway management in this setting must be aware of these factors and make sound decisions, often very quickly, to improve patient outcome.

28.2.2   How common is airway management in ICU patients?

It is not uncommon for airway management to be performed outside the controlled operating room (OR) environment. A recent review of cardiac arrest associated with emergency airway management outside the OR in 3,035 patients confirms that many of these occur in the ICUs.[5] Further, we know that the incidence of cardiac arrest in the ICU setting is as high as 2%, much higher than the 0.068% rate in the OR.[6] Interestingly, the authors of these two cited studies note that hypoxemia is a harbinger of cardiac arrest, and comment that improvements have been seen since the introduction of more experienced staff and the use of ancillary airway devices in ICU.

Nonintubated patients with cardiorespiratory decompensation are admitted to the ICU for monitoring. Some of these patients will deteriorate, as with the patient described above, and require tracheal intubation and mechanical ventilation.

28.2.3   Does the ICU environment influence how we manage the patient's airway in the ICU?

The American College of Critical Care Medicine describes three levels of intensive care: A level one center provides comprehensive care across all disciplines and is typically located in a large urban hospital environment affiliated with an academic medical center; a level two center provides comprehensive care, but not in all disciplines; a level three center can provide some intensive care support and stabilization of the critically ill patient.[7] Common to all such facilities is the need to manage the airway of the critically ill patient from time to time.

Perhaps more so than other environments, physical barriers may complicate the management of an airway crisis in the ICU. The presence of equipment (mechanical ventilators, monitors, infusion pumps, dialysis machines, etc.) and vascular lines can make it difficult to even get to the head of the bed. Specialized apparatus for patient care (air beds, cervical spine collars, orthopedic frames, etc.) in an already overcrowded environment also contribute to the difficulty in accessing the airway or positioning

the patient for airway management, particularly if it is an emergency. Space limitations may make it difficult for other members of the resuscitation care team to access the patient. Finally, finding room for the equipment needed for airway management such as the difficult airway cart and the bronchoscopy cart can be a challenge (see Chapter 56).

28.2.4   Does the airway management skill set of ICU medical personnel have an impact on patient outcome?

Presently, physician staffing in the ICU varies widely from low-intensity models (no intensivist or elective consultation) to high-intensity models (trained intensivists, mandatory intensivist consultations or "closed" unit).[8] The involvement of intensive care trained physicians in the care of patients in the ICU can result in as much as a 30% decrease in mortality and decreased length of stay.[8,9]

Many intensive care practitioners have significant expertise in airway management[10] and it follows that these airway skills contribute to the improved outcomes which have been documented when ICUs are staffed by trained physicians. However, not all "intensivists" are airway experts. The various entry points for critical care training (internal medicine, surgery, anesthesia, pediatrics, and emergency medicine) result in intensivists with varying skill levels and comfort with airway management, especially for this challenging patient population. Some have gone so far as to suggest that the management of these "life or death" clinical situations should be the domain of the airway expert, such as an anesthesia practitioner, or an individual with equivalent training and experience.[11] However, presently, there is no convincing evidence to support these claims. It is suggested by the Society for Critical Care Medicine Guidelines for Critical Care Medicine Training that outcomes differ as the skill set of the operator increases.[12]

Expertise comes through the acquisition of a core of clinical knowledge, the development of technical skills, a degree of familiarity with advanced approaches to the airway, and the proper use of ancillary equipment. The adoption of standardized approaches, such as the ASA Difficult Airway Algorithm, the use of specialized equipment for advanced airway management, as well as the use of appropriate monitors to confirm tracheal intubation likely improves patient outcomes. But there is still much room for improvement.[12,13]

28.2.5   How should we equip the ICU to manage the airway of critically ill patients?

The need to maintain a standard and difficult airway kit in the ICU deserves emphasis. A recent survey of ICUs revealed that most ICUs maintain an airway cart but only about 50% maintain a "difficult" airway cart, and less than 5% conform to the suggested list of equipment offered by ASA guidelines. Devices used to confirm tracheal intubation and detect esophageal intubation are present in 93% of ICUs but only routinely used in 68% of cases. Only 4% of ICUs had both a bulb syringe and $ETCO_2$ detectors, as suggested by the American Heart Association.[13]

A FFB is the most popular device selected for use in a difficult airway situation, even though it is immediately available less than one-third of the time. When surveyed, 51% of respondents thought the FFB was the primary backup when conventional intubation fails. In a "can't intubate, can't ventilate" situation, 20% thought the FFB was the method of choice, a laryngeal mask airway (which was in only 50% of the airway kits) was only chosen 36% of the time, and a cricothyrotomy was the first choice for 32% of respondents. The authors commented on the underutilization of the laryngeal mask airway (LMA) and the need for "continued efforts to educate medical personnel on airway management in the ICU setting."[13]

Respondents to this survey who were aware of an adverse outcome (morbidity 43% and mortality 20% of respondents) that occurred the previous year acknowledged that they needed to restructure their airway management strategies much more frequently than those who were unaware of such events.[13]

28.3 PHARMACOLOGY OF DRUGS USED IN THE ICU FOR AIRWAY MANAGEMENT

28.3.1 What are commonly used induction agents in the ICU?

Attention to the hemodynamic effects of commonly used induction drugs is crucial and mandates careful selection of agents and doses. The recommended induction doses are generally applicable to the healthy ambulatory population undergoing surgical procedures. These doses are excessive and dangerous in most ICU patients, especially those with limited cardiopulmonary reserve and/or hypovolemia. Coexistent hepatic or renal dysfunction may prolong the duration of pharmacological effects, depending on the metabolic and elimination pathways of the drug. Therefore, it is crucial to select the appropriate drug(s), appropriate dose, and have immediate availability of agents to support the circulation following induction.

The most commonly utilized "induction" drug is propofol. Significant hypotension (10–40% decrease in systolic blood pressure) does occur related to direct myocardial depression and altered sympathetic output with decreased arterial tone. Blood pressure is better preserved with ketamine (0–40% increase) or etomidate (0–17% increase), so that these drugs may be better choices for induction.[14]

Etomidate's favorable cardiovascular profile makes it the induction agent of choice for the patient with minimal cardiovascular reserve. However, adrenocortical suppression, even after a single dose, has been well described. Therefore, this drug has been abandoned as a long-term sedative in the ICU. The clinical significance of this adrenal suppression is unknown, but is a factor to be considered before choosing this drug as an induction agent in the critically ill patient.[14–16]

Ketamine is a direct myocardial depressant but its indirect sympathomimetic effects result in a stable hemodynamic profile when used as an induction agent in patients with resilient cardiovascular and sympathetic nervous systems.[14] The option of administering this drug intramuscularly extends its utility, particularly in patients with no vascular access. The tachycardia and hypertension sometimes seen with this drug may increase myocardial oxygen demand, a factor to be considered in the population at risk.[9] Ketamine increases the production of secretions which may precipitate laryngospasm and be bothersome during awake upper airway examination in the difficult airway patient or during procedural sedation. Ketamine produces sedation, analgesia, and amnesia in low doses. Higher doses produce the "dissociative state." Emergence dysphoria is not uncommon and its incidence and intensity may be attenuated by combining ketamine with a small dose of a benzodiazepine.[17] But its relevance following a single-dose administration for induction and airway management in ICU patients is unclear.

28.3.2 Should opioids be used to facilitate tracheal intubation in the ICU?

Opioids can be useful. Opioids attenuate the reflex sympathetic response to laryngoscopy (RSRL), and thus the hemodynamic responses to laryngoscopy.[18] Due to the array of opioids available, choices can be made with respect to potency, speed of onset, route of metabolism/excretion, and pharmacologic half-life. Although the blunting of adverse responses related to airway management may be of clinical value, it is important that the risks of attenuating existing sympathetic support of hemodynamic performance, the production of respiratory depression, and the potential for chest wall rigidity are balanced against this potential benefit.

Most opioids undergo oxidative metabolism in the liver, the capacity for which may be reduced in patients with end-stage liver disease. However, a single dose of opioid when employed in the pretreatment phase of an intubation does not require adjustment in patients with liver dysfunction. Prolonged infusions are associated with the risk of accumulation. The pharmacokinetics of some opioids, such as fentanyl and sufentanil, are unaffected in liver disease and thus are reasonable choices for intubation, if an opioid is needed.[19] This is particularly true for remifentanil, which has an alternative elimination pathway. A particularly useful property of opioids is relative hemodynamic stability.[14,19]

28.3.3 Do benzodiazepines have a role in airway management for the critically ill in the ICU?

Anxiety frequently accompanies dyspnea and respiratory distress. The anxiolytic properties of benzodiazepines, in addition to their antegrade amnestic effects and their ability to raise seizure threshold, enhance their utility for airway management in the critically ill. However, benzodiazepines, like all sedative hypnotic agents, are respiratory depressants, depressing the slope of the CO_2 response curve and shifting it to the right.[20] Opioids and benzodiazepines potentiate each other's respiratory depressant activities when administered simultaneously.[21]

28.4 AIRWAY MANAGEMENT OPTIONS

28.4.1 What is the general approach to airway management in the critically ill patient?

Several options exist to manage most situations. The route chosen is dictated by the needs of the patient and the beliefs and skills of the care team, with the caveat that practitioners responsible for these decisions possess the experience and skills to do so. This may entail a request for more experienced help as time permits. To reiterate, the skills and experience of the airway practitioner fundamentally decide who and how the airway of the critically ill patient will be managed.

The timeline of respiratory deterioration will strongly influence the approach. Acute decompensation may mandate immediate intervention (see Crash Airway Algorithm, Chapter 2). Drugs to facilitate intubation are not usually indicated in these cases but ancillary equipment may be required, particularly if intubation is anticipated to be difficult. On the other hand, clinical deterioration may be more gradual, providing time to summon help as required and an opportunity to plan for a more methodical approach.

Pharmacologic adjuncts, while affording better intubating conditions, may blunt or stop spontaneous ventilation.[21] The inability to effectively oxygenate and ventilate these critically ill patients may reasonably be expected to result in higher rates of morbidity and mortality than does the more robust population presenting for elective surgery. These factors serve to emphasize the importance of decision making with respect to the use of medications, particularly sedative hypnotics and muscle relaxants in these patients. For these reasons, most advise that these drugs should only be employed by those skilled in an array of airway rescue techniques.[22] As always, the decisions are the result of a risk/benefit analysis.

It has been shown repeatedly that in the hands of a skilled airway practitioner, the safest and most successful method is a rapid sequence intubation (RSI) technique. However, this assumes that one has taken the necessary steps to evaluate the airway for difficulty beforehand (see Chapter 1), perhaps deferring the identified difficult airway to more skilled practitioners. Likewise, in the event intubation, ventilation, or both fail, the practitioner must be capable of rescuing the airway (see Chapter 2). The ASA Difficult Airway Algorithm is specifically designed to be used in the OR environment and is of limited use in the ICU setting, though Mort recognizes that it may be of some use in this setting.[5,23]

In the event that RSI is contraindicated, the judicious use of medication may facilitate an "awake" intubation by providing better conditions for the practitioner while providing for patient comfort. As a general principle, the *minimal* amount of drug required to optimize intubating conditions and provide patient comfort during intubation should be used. The skills and experience of the practitioner and acuity of the situation will guide these decisions. These management decisions are best dictated by practitioner experience, rather than dogma.

28.4.2   How do you perform an awake tracheal intubation in the ICU?

Many patients requiring tracheal intubation in the ICU are managed with a combination of topical anesthesia and a combination of other drugs for sedation, Lidocaine is the most commonly employed local anesthetic. Systemic absorption through oral and pharyngeal mucosa is rapid and thus toxicity is a consideration.[24] A variety of approaches have been successfully employed, with

various delivery methods (see Chapter 3). In addition to local anesthetics, judicious use of benzodiazepines is common. Anxiety frequently accompanies the dyspnea seen in the hypoxemic patient and the prospect of an "awake" intubation is daunting, even for the patient in extremis. A small dose of a benzodiazepine can be helpful, as can small doses of opioids. Remifentanil has emerged as a popular adjunct to the traditional opioids in facilitating awake intubation (see Section 3.5). The availability of opioid (naloxone) and benzodiazepine (flumazenil) antagonists provides a small margin of safety if respiratory depression ensues. The opportunity to reverse the effects of administered opioids, or benzodiazepines, must not prevent the clinician from exercising good clinical judgment in the titration of dose. The ability to recognize and immediately deal with complications must be part of the armamentarium of the practitioner responsible for airway management.

28.4.3   Is RSI appropriate for tracheal intubation for critically ill patients in the ICU?

This question raises several issues related to the RSI technique that are more or less unique to the ICU environment:

- The patient is critically ill and may not tolerate predetermined bolus doses of induction agents.
- The critically ill patient typically has limited functional residual capacity (FRC) and tolerates apnea poorly.
- As discussed above, these patients are often difficult to position optimally for intubation.
- Plan B and Plan C alternatives may be also difficult (e.g., intubating laryngeal mask ventilation may not be possible in patients with adult respiratory distress syndrome (ARDS) and severely reduced pulmonary compliance: "S" of RODS (see Section 1.6.3).
- Access to the neck to perform a cricothyrotomy may be difficult or impossible.

The rapid infusion of an induction agent and a rapid acting muscle relaxant provides optimal intubating conditions and is appropriate in patients who do not have an anticipated difficult tracheal intubation. This approach has been advocated in emergency medicine where it has been associated with high success rates, low complication rates, and a low failure rate provided meticulous attention is paid to the identification of the difficult airway.[22] This approach would be expected to produce similar results if employed in the ICU as long as the airway practitioner is appropriately skilled in airway management.

Bag-mask-ventilation (BMV) is fundamental to airway management, particularly in the event RSI has failed, or the failure of any technique. It is often said that the best rescue from failed BMV is improved BMV. A variety of factors in the critically ill patient affect the ability to provide effective BMV: physical factors such as obesity; a crowded environment; illness related conditions (i.e., head and neck trauma, impaired GI motility, or gastric ileus); and pulmonary factors such as restrictive lung disease and reduced pulmonary compliance which are common in the ICU patient.

Extraglottic devices (EGDs), such as the laryngeal mask airway (LMA), intubating laryngeal mask airway (ILMA), or Combitube™ may be lifesaving in situations such as these, provided they are available and one has experience in using them.

Most ICU patients receive infusions of multiple medications concurrently. The resultant confusion of infusion pumps and lines presents an array of risks related to the bolus administration of induction agents and muscle relaxants:

- Medication compatibility
- unintended bolus of the baseline infusion medication
- interruption of essential infusions

The use of a dedicated injection port, in a dedicated intravenous line, for infusion of drugs during airway management warrants emphasis.

28.5 PREPARATION AND TRACHEAL INTUBATION FOR THIS PATIENT

28.5.1 Airway evaluation

During initial assessment, this patient was in extremis. Difficulty with BMV ought to be anticipated due to her toothlessness, obesity, and reduced pulmonary compliance (see Section 1.6.1).

Laryngoscopy and intubation were not predicted to be especially difficult. However, on the evaluation of the airway, she looked somewhat difficult due to her obesity and other factors: her thyromental distance was somewhat decreased, her decreased level of consciousness made assessment of her Mallampati score impossible, there was concern that vomitus might have partially obstructed her airway, and there was no evidence of limited neck mobility (see Section 1.6.2).

If required, an EGD was an option. However, this was somewhat problematic because of potential upper airway obstruction related to her obesity and particulate matter after vomiting. In addition, poor pulmonary compliance related to body habitus and lung volume loss, or collapse, after aspiration can make ventilation difficult with an EGD (see RODS in Section 1.6.3). Except for the access issues presented by her obesity, a surgical airway was not considered to be difficult (see SHORT in Section 1.6.4).

28.5.2 Are there any medical considerations that may impact airway management of this patient?

The urgency of the situation when this patient was first encountered was related to the marked hypoxemia that was refractory to high-inspired concentrations of oxygen and a trial of noninvasive ventilation. An initial attempt at orotracheal intubation awake was unsuccessful. Due to the risk of further vomiting and aspiration in a patient with a decrease in level of consciousness and limited ability to cooperate, further attempts at an "awake" intubation were deemed unreasonable.

Under the more controlled circumstances, in the ICU, the self-extubation situation on day 11 presents a different array of considerations:

- There was more time to review the options available including calling for airway management help if needed;
- hemodynamic instability related to sepsis and hypotension provided relative contraindications to RSI;
- she was cooperative;
- as she was stable for 30 minutes postextubation, the care team had a fairly accurate assessment of her "physiologic reserve";
- knowledge that her previous tracheal intubation was successful.

There are also some considerable challenges. She was hypoxemic due to increased dead space ventilation, reduced FRC, and increased shunt fraction related to her pneumonia. Her fever together with the increase in work of breathing associated with the resolving ARDS probably led to an increased O_2 consumption. Her trachea had been intubated for 11 days presenting the possibility of upper airway edema. She likely had a gastric ileus and full stomach related to her immobility and the fact that she had been receiving sedatives and opioids.

28.5.3 How should you have performed tracheal intubation for this patient?

More often than not, the limited skill set and the comfort level of the practitioner with RSI favors a non-RSI approach as a safer alternative. Alternatively, if the practitioner has the ability to properly assess the airway, to perform RSI and to rescue the airway should RSI fail, then RSI becomes an option. The initial attempt at an awake intubation in this patient not only failed but lead to vomiting and further aspiration. In retrospect, the decision to employ an RSI technique controlling for the risk of regurgitation and aspiration was the correct one.

Had the attempt utilizing RSI failed and gas exchange could be maintained, modifying head position, the type or length of laryngoscope blade and the use of an Eschmann Introducer may have made a subsequent attempt successful. If at any point gas exchange is not possible, the situation becomes a failed airway. An arrangement must be made for an immediate surgical airway. Recognizing the potentially limited success in the face of decreased pulmonary compliance, an EGD (e.g., LMA or a Combitube™) may be tried while these preparations are underway.

Following self-extubation in the ICU, it was reasonable to permit a brief trial of spontaneous respiration. Reintubation could be performed under controlled circumstances if it failed. At the time of reintubation, the patient was slightly confused but cooperative. Her hemodynamic instability made her particularly susceptible to bolus dose induction medications. Judicious titration of a benzodiazepine to produce anxiolysis and amnesia coupled with topical anesthesia of the airway were employed. An opioid was used to attenuate the RSRL. A difficult airway cart with airway adjuncts, EGDs, and a bronchoscope were immediately available at the bedside. Experienced help (ICU nurse, RT, and a senior resident) was present.

As recovery was expected to take some time, and as the patient had previously been on a ventilator for a significant period, an elective tracheotomy was done after the intubation. Doing this at the bedside averted the need to transfer the patient to an OR and consuming valuable OR time (see Chapter 32 for detail).

28.5.4   What are postintubation management issues?

Intubation of the trachea is confirmed by watching the ETT pass through the glottis, but confirmation of tracheal placement should be routinely done using qualitative assessment of ETCO$_2$. The chest is auscultated and the ETT secured in place by ties. If the patient is considered to be at high risk of dislodging the ETT (copious secretions, craniofacial injury or deformity, bandages, full beard, morbid obesity), an oral Endotracheal Tube Attachment Device (ETAD™, COS Medical, Inc. Atlanta, GA) should be used to secure the tube. A chest x-ray is routine to identify *where* the tip of the ETT is positioned within the trachea, not that it is *in* the trachea. Vital signs are continuously monitored throughout the procedure. A postintubation arterial blood gas is only done if the clinician feels this is clinically indicated.

Postintubation sedation, usually a combination of a continuous infusion of an opioid and a benzodiazepine, is employed to allow for patient comfort as well as to optimize the efficiency of mechanical ventilation. Increasingly, a minimal sedation approach is employed with the adoption of sedation protocols that commonly require a sedation "holiday." Improved patient outcomes have been demonstrated. More readily titratable drugs, such as propofol, are often used so that depth of sedation can be lightened quickly and reliably. The use of muscle relaxants to facilitate intubation must be viewed separately from their use to facilitate mechanical ventilation. For mechanical ventilation, paralytics should be viewed as a last resort and they are unnecessary in most cases. The use of muscle relaxants may contribute to the development of "polymyopathy of critical illness," a devastating complication with unfavorable patient outcome. Nonetheless, in isolated cases, these drugs may be necessary.

28.6   EXTUBATION CONSIDERATIONS

28.6.1   Planned extubation for ICU patients

Planning extubation is a routine part of intensive care, and has been generally considered to be effective, with reasonable reintubation rates.[25] Clinical assessment by intensivists for readiness to extubate by clinical criteria alone has been shown to be inadequate, so a myriad of parameters (i.e., negative inspiratory force, forced vital capacity maneuver, tidal volume (TV), rapid shallow breathing index (f/TV), T piece trial, arterial blood gases—66 in total) have been proposed to help predict the likelihood of successful extubation.[26]

Nonetheless, reintubation is occasionally necessary, the failure rate for patients undergoing planned extubation being in the 2–19% range.[27] The majority of reports dealing with patients requiring reintubation describe an increase in patient morbidity.[28] Chapter 2 describes an Extubation Algorithm employing an endo-

tracheal tube exchange catheter. Such devices may prove invaluable in the event that reintubation is required, particularly in patients with a difficult airway.

28.6.2   How do you manage a patient with an unplanned extubation?

Not all extubations are planned. Unplanned extubation occurs in 3–14% of ICU patients[13,29] with reintubation commonly required. When unplanned extubations occur, self-extubation by the patient accounts for 85% of the incidents and accidental extubation (often during nursing intervention or procedures) about 15%.[30] About 40% of the self-extubated patients will be stable without reintubation. Most of the patients who fail extubation will do so quickly and require reintubation within 2 hours.[28] In the self-extubated patient, factors identified predictive of the need to be reintubated included a Glasgow Coma Scale score <11, accidental extubation and a PaO$_2$/FIO$_2$ <200.[28]

Various authors have attempted to determine features of the patient at risk of self-extubation. The following have been identified: agitation, use of sedatives, use of physical restraints, older age, and oral route of intubation. Nursing workload and the inability to be constantly attentive to the patient at risk have also been suggested as factors.[22,23,25]

Complications related to airway management in this situation are much more common than in the planned extubation cohort. This translates into an increased length of stay in the ICU and higher mortality rates.[28–30] Efforts to reduce the risk of unplanned extubations must be made. These include the appropriate management of sedation, appropriate management of the delirious patient, and the appropriate use of physical measures to prevent extubation. These interventions do decrease the rate of unplanned extubation.[30]

28.6.3   When do you consider a tracheotomy for an ICU patient?

The timing of tracheotomies for patients expected to require prolonged ventilatory support has been influenced by the technology available. The more rigid endotracheal tubes in the 1960s, with their increased risk of laryngeal injury, supported early tracheotomy. With the more pliable modern polyvinyl chloride (PVC) ETTs, more prolonged translaryngeal intubation is well tolerated and elective placement of a tracheotomy is sometimes delayed until after 2 or 3 weeks of intubation.[24,31] According to recent French and American studies, practices vary widely showing great variability in indications, timing, and approach.[20,32,33] At present, the timing of tracheotomy "remains one of professional judgment,"[24] although there is some evidence that early percutaneous tracheotomy (within 48 hours) is associated with lower mortality, morbidity, decreased length of mechanical ventilation, and length of ICU stay, relative to tracheotomy at 14–16 days postintubation.[32]

The challenge is to predict early in the ICU course those patients who might require prolonged ventilatory support (and who might then definitely benefit from needed surgery) versus those who will be successfully extubated within 10–14 days.

28.7   SUMMARY

The ICU is a highly specialized environment mandated to provide intense, continuous, active monitoring and treatment for the critically ill patient. Highly trained personnel focus their skills and resources to meet the needs of these patients. A particular challenge is in the area of expert airway management.

Increasing the proportion of units staffed with practitioners with airway skills (intensivists), lobbying for compliance with the ASA recommendations regarding airway management, providing necessary equipment for the difficult airway, identifying patients at risk of self-extubation, and encouraging the application of experience and skill in the approach to the airway needs of the critically ill will improve outcomes.

REFERENCES

1. Bernard GR, Artigas A, Brigham KL, et al.: Report of the American-European consensus conference on ARDS: definitions, mechanisms, relevant outcomes and clinical trial coordination. The Consensus Committee. *Intensive Care Med.* 1994;20:225–232.
2. International consensus conferences in intensive care medicine. Ventilator-associated lung injury in ARDS. American Thoracic Society, European Society of Intensive Care Medicine, Societe de Reanimation Langue Francaise. *Intensive Care Med.* 1999;25:1444–1452.
3. Kallet RH, Jasmer RM, Pittet JF, et al.: Clinical implementation of the ARDS network protocol is associated with reduced hospital mortality compared with historical controls. *Crit Care Med.* 2005;33:925–929.
4. Artigas A, Bernard GR, Carlet J, et al.: The American-European Consensus Conference on ARDS. Part 2: Ventilatory, pharmacologic, supportive therapy, study design strategies, and issues related to recovery and remodeling. Acute respiratory distress syndrome. *Am J Respir Crit Care Med.* 1998;157:1332–1347.
5. Mort TC: The incidence and risk factors for cardiac arrest during emergency tracheal intubation: justification for incorporating the ASA guidelines in the remote location. *J Clin Anesthesia.* 2004;16:508–516.
6. Olssen GL, Hallen B: Cardiac arrest during anesthesia: A computer aided study in 250542 anesthetics. *Acta Anesthesthesiol Scand.* 1988;32:653–654.
7. Haupt MT, Bekes CE, Brilli RJ, et al.: Task force of the American College of Critical Care Medicine, Society of Critical Care Medicine Guidelines on critical care services and personnel: recommendations based on a system of categorization of three levels of care. *Crit Care Med.* 2003;31:2677–2683.
8. Pronovost PJ, Angus DC, Dorman T, et al.: Physician staffing patterns and clinical outcomes in critically ill patients a systematic review. *JAMA.* 2002;228:2151–2162.
9. Birmeyer JD, Dimick JD: The Leapfrog group's patient safety practices 2003: the potential benefits of universal adoption. Available at http://www.leapfroggroup.org/media/file/Leapfrog-Birkmeyer.pdf.
10. Dorman T, Angood PB, Angus DC, et al.: American College of Critical Care Medicine Guidelines for critical care training and continuing education. *Crit Care Med.* 2004;32:263–272.
11. Nayyar P, Lisbon A: Non operating room airway management and endotracheal intubation practices: a survey of anesthesiology program directors. *Anesth Analg.* 1997;85:62–68.
12. SCCM Guidelines for critical care medicine training and continuing education. *Crit Care Med.* 2004;32:263.
13. Oliwas N, Mort T: National ICU difficult airway survey: preliminary results. *Anesthesiology.* 2003;99:A403.
14. Reves JG, Glass PSA, Lubarsky DA, McEvoy MD: Intravenous non-opiod anesthetics. In: *Miller's Anesthesia.* New York: Elsevier, 2005:323.
15. Roberts RG, Redman JW: Etomidate adrenal dysfunction and critical care. *Anesthesia.* 2002;57:413.
16. Absalom A, Pledger D, Kong A: Adrenocortical function in critically ill patients 24 hours after a single dose of etomidate. *Anaesthesia.* 1999;54:861–867.
17. Chudnofsky C, Weber JE, Stoyanoff PJ, et al.: A combination of midazolam and ketamine for procedural sedation and analgesia in adult emergency department patients. *Acad Emerg Med.* 2000;7:228–235.
18. Jeng CS, Lin CJ, Huang CH, et al.: The optimal injection time of alfentanil for blunting circulatory response to tracheal intubation. *Acta Anaesthesiol Taiwan.* 2005;431:3–9.
19. Tegeder I, Lotsch J, Geisslinger G: Pharmacokinetics of opioids in liver disease. *Clin Pharmacokinet* 1999;37:17–40.
20. Sunzel M, Paalzow L, Breggren L, Eriksson I: Respiratory and cardiovascular effects in relation to plasma levels of midazolam and diazepam. *Br J Pharmacol.* 1988;25:561–569.
21. Bailey PL, Pace NL, Ashburn MA, et al.: Frequent hypoxemia and apnea after sedation with midazolam and fentanyl. *Anesthesiology.* 1990;73:826–830.
22. Blanda M: Emergency airway management. *Emerg Clin North Am.* 2003;21:1–26.
23. Practice guidelines for management of the difficult airway. An updated report by the American Society of Anesthesiologists Task Force on Management of the Difficult Airway. *Anesthesiology.* 2003;98:1269–1277.
24. Heffner JE: Tracheostomy application and timing. *Clin Chest Med.* 2003;24:389–398.
25. Chevron V, Manard JF, Richard JC, et al.: Unexplained extubation: risk factors of development and predictive criteria for reintubation. *Crit Care Med.* 1998;26:1049–1053.
26. Meade M, Guyatt G, Cook D, et al.: Predicting success in weaning from mechanical ventilation. *Chest.* 2001;120:400S–424S.
27. Macintyre N: Evidence based guidelines for weaning and discontinuing ventilatory support. A collective task force facilitated by the American College of Chest Physicians, American Association for Respiratory Care and the American College of Critical Care Medicine. *Chest.* 2001;120:375S–395S.
28. Mort T: Unplanned extubation outside the operating room: a quality improvement audit of hemodynamic and tracheal airway complications associated with emergency tracheal reintubation. *Anesth Analg.* 1998;86:1171–1176.
29. Boulain T: Unplanned extubations in the adult intensive care unit: a prospective multicenter study. *Am J Resp Crit Care Med.* 1998;157:1131–1137.
30. Christie JM, Dethlefson M, Cane RD: Unplanned tracheal extubation in the intensive care unit. *J Clin Anesth.* 1996;8:289–293.
31. Rumbak MJ, Newton M, Truncale T, et al.: A prospective randomized study comparing early percutaneous dilational tracheostomy to prolonged translaryngeal intubation (delayed tracheostomy) in critically ill medical patients. *Crit Care Med.* 2004;32:1689–1694.
32. Blot F: Indications timing and techniques of tracheostomy in 152 French ICU's. *Chest.* 2005;127:1347–1353.
33. Freeman BD, Borecki IB, Coopersmith CM, Buchman TG. Relationship between tracheostomy timing and duration of mechanical ventilation in critically ill patients. *Crit Care Med.* 2005;33:2513–2520.

SELF-EVALUATION QUESTIONS

28.1. Polyneuropathy is a possible side effect of prolonged use of which of the following agents

A. Propofol

B. Ketamine

C. Midazolam

D. Vecuronium

E. Etomidate

28.2. Cardiorespiratory depression is a predictable side effect of which of the following

A. Propofol

B. Etomidate

C. Ketamine

D. Fentanyl

E. Midazolam

28.3. Which of the following respiratory care statements is **NOT** true in the adult ICU patient population?

A. Tracheotomy within 14 days of prolonged intubation is desirable;

B. there is no evidence of an advantage of tracheotomy within 2–3 days;

C. tracheotomy is likely unwarranted for intubation that is less than 3 weeks duration;

D. Distinct advantages have been shown with percutaneous tracheotomy at the bedside;

E. With the more pliable modern PVC ETTs, more prolonged translaryngeal intubation is well tolerated.

CHAPTER (29)

Management of Extubation of a Patient Following a Prolonged Period of Mechanical Ventilation

Richard M. Cooper

29.1 CASE PRESENTATION

A 60-year-old male with chronic obstructive lung disease and limited exercise tolerance had tracheal intubation because of hypoxemic respiratory failure resulting from pneumonia. Direct laryngoscopy (DL) performed by an experienced practitioner using a Macintosh 3 blade yielded a Cormack/Lehane (C/L) 3 view. The first attempt at intubation using a malleable stylet was unsuccessful. The second attempt using the Macintosh 3 with an Eschmann Tracheal Tube Introducer (ETTI) was successful. After 6 days of assisted ventilation, he has now been weaned to a FiO_2 of 0.4, positive end expiratory pressure of 5 cm, and pressure support of 5 cm H_2O. The pulmonary infiltrates are much improved. His respiratory rate is 24. A cuff-leak test is performed.

29.2 EXTUBATION STRATEGIES

29.2.1 What is a high-risk extubation?

In anesthesia, and most likely in critical care and emergency departments (EDs), adverse respiratory events are more frequently associated with extubation than intubation.[1,2] Nonetheless, little attention has been paid to the management of extubation. A stratification of risk associated with extubation has been proposed,[3] and although unsupported by controlled, randomized clinical trials, the need for an extubation strategy has been advocated by expert panels.[4,5] The extubation of patients, who were easily intubated and in whom no intervening event has occurred to jeopardize their airways, can be regarded as *routine extubations*. Those

who were easily intubated but who are at greater risk of requiring reintubation (due to hypoxemia, hypercapnia, inadequate clearance of secretions, inability to protect their airway, or airway obstruction) are *intermediate-risk extubations*. Those in whom airway management is likely to be challenging or complex if reintubation was to be required represent *high-risk extubations*. The last group includes: (1) patients with a difficult tracheal intubation (failure to visualize their glottis—C/L $\geq$ 3—requiring multiple attempts or alternative techniques); (2) those with interval complications (airway edema, extrinsic compression, glottic injuries); and (3) those with clinical conditions associated with difficult ventilation and/or intubation. This latter group would include, for example, patients with paradoxical vocal cord motion, morbid obesity, obstructive sleep apnea, airway surgery, maxillofacial surgery (particularly when it involves intermaxillary fixation), deep neck infections, cervical surgery, or prolonged intubation.[6]

For most patients, there is little likelihood that reintubation will be required. The results of three studies involving nearly 50,000 patients presenting for a wide variety of surgical procedures indicated that only 0.09–0.19% required reintubation.[7–9] Certain surgical procedures such as panendoscopy and a variety of head and neck operations are associated with a risk of required reintubation approximately 10 times higher (1–3%).[10–14] Patients in critical care units often have limited physiologic reserve, altered secretions, or an impaired capacity to protect their airways. In this group of patients, required reintubation is substantially higher still.[15–17]

When patients require emergency reintubation, the practitioner may have limited clinical information, equipment, supportive personnel, and preparation time. Furthermore, the patient may be hemodynamically unstable with associated airway obstruction, hypoxemia, and acidosis. There may be a reluctance to administer paralytics when there is uncertainty about the airway. Topical anesthesia may be ineffective due to time constraints or the presence of secretions and edema. Thus a struggle could ensue between the practitioner and a confused and possibly hypoxic patient. Generally, any *urgent reintubation is likely to be more challenging than the original intubation procedure.*

29.2.2 What strategies can be used for the high-risk extubation?

In patients requiring high-risk extubation, it is especially important that every effort be taken to ensure that conditions are optimal. Optimal conditions include oxygenation, ventilation, the ability to clear secretions, and protect and maintain patency of their airway. Even when such conditions are optimal, reintubation may be required. Assessment of the airway prior to removing the endotracheal tube (ETT) might include:

- Laryngoscopy with the ETT in situ, although this is of limited value and is unlikely to reveal the extent of periglottic edema or vocal cord movement. Neither is direct visualization of the tube in situ helpful in predicting whether laryngoscopy and reintubation will be successful after the ETT has been removed.

- Laryngeal examination adjacent to the ETT using a flexible fiberoptic bronchoscope (FFB) has some of the same limitations as laryngoscopy.[18] Alternatively, an FFB can be positioned within the ETT, and as the latter is withdrawn, an effort can be made to inspect the airway below and above the vocal folds. Unfortunately, this technique often fails. As the ETT is withdrawn, the patient may cough, swallow, or secretions may obscure the view. Even if a laryngeal view is achieved, it is likely to be too hurried to be of value. This technique is further limited by the need to withdraw the FFB shortly after the examination.

- If an LMA is inserted and the ETT is withdrawn, an FFB can be passed through the LMA. This technique is compatible with either controlled or spontaneous ventilation, and it keeps extraglottic secretions from obscuring the view. It allows regulation of the FIO_2 and can facilitate reintubation should it be required. This technique does require a properly seated LMA and is hazardous if the airway is significantly compromised.

- An ETTI (Portex Limited, Hythe, UK) or METTRO Mizus obturator (Cook Critical Care, Bloomington, IN) can be introduced into the ETT. When the latter is withdrawn, the introducer can serve as a guide over which the ETT can be reintroduced if necessary. As in the case of intubating over an FFB, ETT insertion is not without challenges. Because these devices are solid, they cannot be used to insufflate oxygen or provide ventilation.

- A hollow tube exchanger can be introduced.

29.3 DEVICES TO ASSIST EXTUBATION

29.3.1 What types of hollow tube exchangers are available?

There are several commercial tube exchangers including the Cook Airway Exchange Catheter (C-AEC, Cook Critical Care), the Endotracheal Ventilation Catheter (ETVC, Cardiomed International),* and the Sheridan Tracheal Tube Exchanger (Hudson Respiratory Care). These hollow devices can be used to insufflate or ventilate. Devices with a secure proximal connection and multiple distal end holes are preferred (C-AEC and ETVC). As in the case of the ETTI or the METTRO Mizus obturator, these hollow devices are introduced through the existing ETT, and the distance markings on the tube exchanger are aligned with those on the ETT to ensure insertion to an appropriate depth within the trachea. The tube exchanger remains in the airway after the ETT is withdrawn.

29.3.2 How long a duration should a tube exchanger remain in the airway?

Most patients tolerate the tube exchanger surprisingly well. It is possible for patients to speak and cough with the device in situ.[19] Tube exchangers are more easily secured (and better tolerated) when inserted nasally. A patient with an ETT tube in place for a short time generally tolerates the tube exchanger less well than one who has had an ETT in place for a longer duration. If the patient has been intubated for several hours, coughing may indicate that the catheter is endobronchial or near the carina. The distance marking should be checked and a chest x-ray performed to confirm correct placement. If the patient remains intolerant of the exchanger despite proper placement, it may be appropriate to remove the device, although the need for reintubation may not declare itself for several hours. A more cautious approach would be to instill topical anesthesia through the tube exchanger. Rather than advocating a specific and arbitrary time period, it is this author's practice to leave the device in place until the concern for the airway is resolved. It would probably be unwise to discharge a patient from a monitored facility with a tube exchanger. Any patient requiring a tube exchanger would require the vigilance of a postanesthetic care unit (PACU), intensive care unit (ICU), or ED. Furthermore, inexperienced personnel may confuse the tube exchanger with a gastric tube with disastrous consequences.

29.3.3 How is a tube exchanger used to support oxygenation or ventilation?

A tube exchanger can serve as a conduit for oxygen by insufflation; however, if used for more than a few hours, the oxygen should be humidified. Insufflation should be at low flows of 2–4 L·min^{-1} and may be used in lieu of a face mask or nasal cannulae. Insufflation should always be attempted before considering jet ventilation.

If insufflation fails to correct hypoxemia, reintubation may be necessary and insufflation may continue even while intubation is being attempted. If reintubation is delayed or prolonged and hypoxemia is persistent or worsening in spite of oxygen insufflation, jet ventilation should be considered. To avoid the morbidity associated with jet ventilation, the following points should be addressed:

- Confirm that the tube exchanger is appropriately positioned, since jet ventilation into the bronchus or oropharynx can produce barotrauma.

---

*The author was a consultant to Cook in the development of the C-AEC and the inventor of the ETVC (Cardiomed International). He receives no royalties or consultancy fees from either of these companies.

- Delegate an assistant to hold the proximal connector to ensure that the device does not get ejected during ventilation.

- Administration of a muscle relaxant with appropriate sedation (if tolerated) will facilitate both endotracheal intubation and jet ventilation and will lessen the risks of barotrauma.

- Attach the tube exchanger to the jet ventilator by means of a Luer-Lok adapter (both C-AEC and the ETVC have these).

- Using a pressure-reducing valve, select the lowest driving pressure that results in chest expansion. "Wall pressure" of 50 psi is equivalent to 3,500 cm H_2O and can produce dramatic, life-threatening barotrauma very quickly.

- Correct hypoxemia—this should be the primary objective. One breath causing adequate chest expansion may correct hypoxemia even though it may take a short while for this to become apparent.

- To avoid "breath stacking," the chest must be carefully observed. Subsequent breaths should not be delivered until it is clear that the chest has recoiled to a "resting volume."

- Facilitate exhalation by minimizing airway obstruction (vocal cord relaxation, positioning, tongue displacement, suctioning, etc.).[19]

Jet ventilation may prove life-saving, but it requires fastidious attention to detail to ensure that life-threatening complications do not develop.[20]

29.4   AIRWAY EDEMA

29.4.1   What factors lead to airway edema?

Airway edema is not restricted to the vocal folds. In children subglottic swelling is the greatest concern, whereas in adults glottic and supraglottic edemas are the focus of concern. Patients may have airway swelling due to prone or Trendelenburg positioning, angioneurotic edema, and thermal injuries or generalized swelling as in anaphylaxis, anasarca, and massive volume overload. They may have sustained injury to their tongue, uvula, or epiglottis during tracheal intubation or as a result of subsequent trauma, such as suctioning or seizures.

Insertion of a round tube through a triangular glottis results in contact and pressure at the posteromedial aspect of the larynx. Injury can occur very early but this is usually of little consequence. Excessive or prolonged pressure can result in perichondritis or chondritis which heals poorly. Healing may result in fibrosis, producing subacute or chronic laryngeal or tracheal stenosis or an exuberant growth of granulation tissue. Early postextubation obstruction is likely to be a consequence of edema, bleeding, and occasionally granulation tissue or arytenoid dislocation.

Much has been written about the duration of intubation and resultant airway injuries. However, the association between duration and incidence of airway injuries remains controversial. Most would maintain that the longer the duration of intubation, the greater the likelihood of airway edema. Significant airway injury may, however, occur early as a result of inadequate ETT immobilization, persistent attempts to phonate or cough, gastroesophageal reflux, traumatic laryngoscopy or intubation, and vocal fold granulomas. Some authorities recommend DL at approximately day 7 under general anesthesia, using telescopes and image magnification

to assess the severity of injury. Only then can a judgment be made regarding the feasibility of extubation, prolonging translaryngeal intubation, or the need for a tracheotomy.[18]

29.4.2   What techniques are useful to assess airway edema?

We have discussed the limited value of DL with the ETT in situ in contrast to extubation under general anesthesia with DL and image magnification. An alternative approach consists of controlled visualization using a flexible FFB through an LMA. DL with image magnification provides the best anatomical evaluation; the LMA/FFB examination with spontaneous ventilation provides a good assessment of both form and function.

If tissue swelling is sufficiently severe, it may encroach on the ETT at any point along the length of the ETT. Prior to extubation, a "cuff-leak test" can be used to assess this. The oropharynx is suctioned and the cuff is slowly deflated. The patient is asked to inhale and exhale slowly as the ETT is occluded.[21] An audible leak indicates the flow of air around the ETT. This has been found to be a useful predictor of successful extubation in pediatric trauma and burn victims as well as children with croup[22] and was sensitive but not specific in predicting postextubation stridor and the need for reintubation in adults.[23] The cuff-leak test can be enhanced by quantifying the leak during controlled ventilation. Lower cuff-leak volumes are predictive of postextubation stridor, a need for reintubation, or both.[24,25] Engoren did not find this to be predictive in postoperative cardiothoracic surgical patients[26] though others have suggested that the cuff leak, expressed as a proportion of the delivered tidal volume, may be more predictive.[27–30]

29.4.3   Are there methods of reducing airway edema?

Studies involving the prophylactic benefit of *corticosteroids* to reduce postextubation stridor have yielded contradictory findings. The benefits may be restricted to high-risk patients and may require multiple doses.[31] *Elevation of the head of the bed* may be helpful. If the patient manifests signs or symptoms suggestive of airway obstruction, laryngospasm and upper-airway obstruction should be considered. If these are excluded, *racemic epinephrine* (2.25%, 0.5 mL in 2–3 mL saline) by inhalation often results in rapid improvement of airway edema by means of transient local vasoconstriction. Racemic epinephrine can be administered as tolerated, although caution must be observed in patients with hypertension, tachycardia, or conditions in which these are poorly tolerated. Rebound vasodilation can also occur. Additional management measures might include fluid restriction or diuretic therapy.

Being less dense than nitrogen, *helium* can be used as an alternative to nitrogen when turbulent airflow is present, as a transport medium for oxygen. This mixture consists of a blend of oxygen and helium, typically 30:70, although the oxygen concentration can be enriched if required. The benefits are proportional to the concentration of helium and the extent to which turbulent flow is present. Helium–oxygen (Heliox) can be used concurrently with head elevation, corticosteroids, and racemic epinephrine. The benefits from Heliox and racemic epinephrine should be apparent within minutes, whereas deteriorating conditions should prompt reintubation.

29.5   TECHNIQUE OF REINTUBATION

29.5.1   How should reintubation over a tube exchanger proceed?

If conservative measures are ineffective and reintubation over a tube exchanger is required, the exchanger can serve as a "jet stylet."[32] Supplementation of oxygenation begins with insufflation and, if necessary, progresses to jet ventilation. Depending upon the design of the device, the proximal connector can be removed to permit the loading of a replacement ETT. If the fit is tight, a water-soluble lubricant can be applied to the tube exchanger, although care must be taken to ensure that this does not interfere with secure handling. The tube exchanger must be long enough to ensure that the part protruding from the patient's mouth or nose is at least as long as the replacement ETT. If necessary, the tube can be cut. In general, the smaller the size difference between the outer diameter of the tube exchanger and the inner diameter of the replacement ETT, the easier reintubation is likely to be. The tube exchanger is held securely at the mouth or nose as well as its proximal end. After the ETT is passed over the exchanger, the connector can be reattached and insufflation or jet ventilation can resume. Throughout the procedure, the clinical condition of the patient should be monitored and any additional medications to provide sedation, hemodynamic control, or neuromuscular blockade should be administered. The team should review its plans and, if appropriate, call for additional help and equipment. If oxygenation is sufficiently maintained, there is no urgency and it is perhaps more important to ensure that the team is aware of the primary and backup strategies.

A laryngoscope can be used to elevate the tongue and epiglottis to facilitate advancement of the ETT over the tube exchanger. The ETT is passed over the tube exchanger as it might be over an FFB. If resistance is encountered, the ETT should be rotated counterclockwise, but force should never be applied. If the patient is still breathing, the operator should wait for an inspiratory effort and advance the ETT as the vocal folds abduct. Frequently, the tube exchanger is inadvertently advanced while the ETT is being introduced. If the ETT has passed easily, the tube exchanger can be removed, whereupon intratracheal placement of the ETT should be verified by capnography and auscultation.

29.5.2   What if reintubation over the tube exchanger fails?

If reintubation over the tube exchanger fails, several options exist. The adequacy of oxygenation by bag-mask or jet ventilation with the tube exchanger in situ should be assessed:

- Oxygenation is adequate. Time and expertise may permit the use of an alternative device such a flexible or rigid fiberoptic scope or a video laryngoscope. (These devices might also be considered prior to the removal of the ETT, along with the tube exchanger.) It is preferable to leave the tube exchanger in place, if possible, during the reintubation attempt.

- Oxygenation or ventilation is inadequate. If possible, confirm that the tube exchanger is still in the trachea. If jet ventilation is

available, it should be used as described above, but an assessment that the device has not become displaced should be made during the first breath. An assistant should listen over the epigastrium to ensure *the absence* of air entry during ventilation. If this is successful, jet ventilation may continue while alternative plans are being put in place.

- If intubation over the tube exchanger was not successful, prior to its removal, consider the following possibilities: (1) the use of a laryngoscope to facilitate tongue retraction; (2) the use of a smaller size ETT; and (3) the use of a fiberoptic or video laryngoscope to visualize the glottis.

- If tongue retraction, a smaller size ETT, and a fiberoptic or video laryngoscope fail to facilitate reintubation and jet ventilation is not immediately available, assess the feasibility of mask-ventilation with the tube exchanger in situ. If this cannot be accomplished, the tube exchanger may be removed and further attempts made to achieve mask-ventilation.

- If mask-ventilation still cannot be achieved, the operator should refer to the Failed Airway (can't intubate/can't ventilate) Algorithm. Time is critical and if adequate ventilation cannot be achieved quickly, a surgical airway is mandatory. An extraglottic airway may be used if immediately available while preparing for a surgical airway.

29.5.3   How should reintubation of the difficult airway without a tube exchanger proceed?

If a patient with a difficult airway requires replacement of an existing ETT and a tube exchanger is not available, an FFB loaded with an ETT can be introduced alongside the existing ETT. The pharynx should be carefully suctioned. If the existing ETT still has an intact cuff, it can be deflated to allow FFB passage alongside. Once tracheal access by the FFB has been confirmed by visualizing tracheal rings and carina, the original tube can be withdrawn and the new ETT advanced over the FFB.

For the patient requiring reintubation in whom intubation had previously been difficult, many alternatives to DL exist and have been addressed elsewhere in this text. Rigid fiberoptic or video laryngoscope equipment, for example, may produce an excellent glottic view and permit visualized tracheal reintubation.

29.6   TRACHEAL EXTUBATION

The trachea of the patient described at the beginning of this chapter was intubated using DL and an ETTI. The ETTI is placed blindly and successful placement cannot be guaranteed. A recent study found that when intubation by DL was unsuccessful, an ETTI would lead to successful intubation in 80/89 cases (10% failure rate); out of the successful intubations 50% required more than one attempt.[33]

Laryngoscopy that fails to reveal the larynx is a "failed laryngoscopy" whether intubation succeeds or fails. An extubation strategy should anticipate that reintubation might be required; reintubation may very well be more challenging than the initial intubation—the strategy should be to increase the likelihood of success and permit simultaneous intubation as well as oxygenation even if the glottis cannot be visualized. Extubation over a tube exchanger may best meet these objectives.

The patient demonstrated criteria that are associated with a successful wean from mechanical ventilation. However, such criteria are not synonymous with successful extubation. Demonstration of a large cuff leak reduces the likelihood of postextubation stridor or a need for reintubation. Examination of the vocal cords following extubation, either using an FFB through an LMA or by DL with image magnification, may provide additional certainty.

The oropharynx was suctioned, a cuff leak was demonstrated, a tube exchanger was inserted, the ETT was withdrawn, and the tube exchanger was secured to the patient's cheek and forehead. The exchanger was well tolerated and left in place for 3 hours during which time the patient continued to improve. He was able to talk and clear his secretions. The tube exchanger was then removed.

Had a cuff leak not been present, the options are less clear. A significant number of these patients would not require a tracheotomy. The patient can be taken to the operating room to have the glottis examined using DL and image magnification under general anesthesia with paralytics.[18] An alternative approach would be to use intravenous anesthesia and a short-acting muscle relaxant, followed by the insertion of an LMA and extubation. The LMA would then be inflated; its position would be optimized using an FFB. The relaxant would be allowed to wear off or be reversed, and spontaneous ventilation could resume. Flexible endoscopy would be used to assess the glottic appearance and function, while the adequacy of spontaneous ventilation would also be assessed.

Three outcomes might result:

- The assessment is unfavorable. Reintubation can be achieved over the FFB using, for example, an Aintree catheter (Cook Critical Care) or a tube exchanger.[34] If reintubation is then contemplated, a tracheotomy is probably indicated. This can be done at the bedside using one of several techniques, including percutaneous dilatational tracheotomy or translaryngeal tracheotomy ("Fantoni technique").[35,36]

- The examination is favorable. The sedation is discontinued and the LMA is removed when appropriate. There remains the possibility that reintubation will subsequently be required; however, the anatomy and glottic function have been assessed, and the patient has undergone a trial of extubation.

- The examination is indeterminate. A tube exchanger can be introduced and left in situ until the clinical status of the glottis is clarified.

29.7 SUMMARY

The risk associated with tracheal extubation (or tube exchange) may be stratified into low, intermediate, and high risk depending upon the probability of complications, including the need for reintubation. A high-risk extubation exists when a complication such as reintubation is likely to be difficult or very difficult to achieve; examples include conditions when a patient's airway access is limited by maxillomandibular or cervical fixation. It should be assumed that any emergency reintubation will be more challenging due to the patient instability or limited resources. Strategies were described to increase the probability of successful reintubation, including the substitution of a extraglottic airway and the use of a tube exchanger. Some tube exchangers have been designed to allow the administration of supplemental oxygen and ventilation. Jet ventilation through a small caliber catheter must be performed with care to avoid complications.

REFERENCES

1. Peterson GN, Domino KB, Caplan RA, et al.: Management of the difficult airway: a closed claims analysis. *Anesthesiology.* 2005;103:33–39.
2. Asai T, Koga K, Vaughan RS: Respiratory complications associated with tracheal intubation and extubation. *Br J Anaesth.* 1998;80:767–775.
3. Cooper RM: Extubation and changing endotracheal tube, In: *Airway Management Principles and Practice*, 1st edn. Benumof JL, ed. Philadelphia, PA: Mosby, 1995:864–885.
4. Crosby ET, Cooper RM, Douglas MJ, et al.: The unanticipated difficult airway with recommendations for management. *Can J Anaesth.* 1998;45:757–776.
5. Practice Guidelines for Management of the Difficult Airway: an Updated report by the American Society of Anesthesiologists Task Force on Management of the Difficult Airway. *Anesthesiology.* 2003;98:1269–1277.
6. Cooper RM: *Extubation and Changing Endotracheal Tubes, Benumof's Airway Management Principles and Practice*, 2nd edn. Hagberg CA, ed. Philadelphia, PA: Mosby, 2007:1146–1180.
7. Hill RS, Koltai PJ, Parnes SM: Airway complications from laryngoscopy and panendoscopy. *Ann Otol Rhinol Laryngol.* 1987;96:691–694.
8. Mathew JP, Rosenbaum SH, O'Connor T, Barash PG: Emergency tracheal intubation in the postanesthesia care unit: physician error or patient disease? *Anesth Analg.* 1990;71:691–697.
9. Rose DK, Cohen MM: The airway: problems and predictions in 18,500 patients. *Can J Anaesth.* 1994;41:372–383.
10. Levelle JP, Martinez OA: Airway obstruction after bilateral carotid endarterectomy. *Anesthesiology.* 1985;63:220–222.
11. Tyers MR, Cronin K: Airway obstruction following second operation for carotid endarterectomy. *Anaesth Intensive Care.* 1986;14:314–316.
12. Emery SE, Smith MD, Bohlman HH: Upper-airway obstruction after multilevel cervical corpectomy for myelopathy. *J Bone Joint Surg Am.* 1991;73:544–551.
13. Lacoste L, Gineste D, Karayan J, et al.: Airway complications in thyroid surgery. *Ann Otol Rhinol Laryngol.* 1993;102:441–446.
14. Venna RP, Rowbottom JR: A Nine year retrospective review of post operative airway related problems in patients following multilevel anterior cervical corpectomy. *Anesthesiology.* 2002;95:A1171.
15. Demling RH, Read T, Lind LJ, Flanagan HL: Incidence and morbidity of extubation failure in surgical intensive care patients. *Crit Care Med.* 1988;16:573–577.
16. Marini JJ, Wheeler AP: *Weaning from Mechanical Ventilation, Critical Care Medicine: The Essentials*, 1st edn. Marini JJ, Wheeler AP, eds. Baltimore: Williams & Wilkins, 1997:173–195.
17. Gandia F, Blanco J: Evaluation of indexes predicting the outcome of ventilator weaning and value of adding supplemental inspiratory load. *Intensive Care Med.* 1992;18:327–333.
18. Benjamin B: *Laryngeal Trauma from Intubation: Endoscopic Evaluation and Classification, Otolaryngology: Head and Neck Surgery*, 3rd edn. Cummings CW, Fredrickson JM, Harker LA, et al. eds. St. Louis, MO: Mosby-Year Book, Inc., 1998:2018–2033.
19. Cooper RM, Cohen DR: The use of an endotracheal ventilation catheter for jet ventilation during a difficult intubation. *Can J Anaesth.* 1994;41:1196–1199.
20. Benumof JL: Airway exchange catheters: simple concept, potentially great danger. *Anesthesiology.* 1999;91:342–344.
21. Adderley RJ, Mullins GC: When to extubate the croup patient: the "leak" test. *Can J Anaesth.* 1987;34:304–306.
22. Kemper KJ, Izenberg S, Marvin JA, Heimbach DM: Treatment of postextubation stridor in a pediatric patient with burns: the role of heliox. *J Burn Care Rehabil.* 1990;11:337–339.
23. Fisher MM, Raper RF: The 'cuff-leak' test for extubation. *Anaesthesia.* 1992; 47:10–12.
24. Miller RL, Cole RP: Association between reduced cuff leak volume and postextubation stridor. *Chest.* 1996;110:1035–1040.

25. Efferen LS, Elsakr A: Post-extubation stridor: risk factors and outcome. *J Assoc Acad Minor Phys*. 1998;9:65–68.

26. Engoren M: Evaluation of the cuff-leak test in a cardiac surgery population. *Chest*. 1999;116:1029–1031.

27. Sandhu RS, Pasquale MD, Miller K, Wasser TE: Measurement of endotracheal tube cuff leak to predict postextubation stridor and need for reintubation. *J Am Coll Surg*. 2000;190:682–687.

28. De Bast Y, De Backer D, Moraine JJ, et al.: The cuff leak test to predict failure of tracheal extubation for laryngeal edema. *Intensive Care Med*. 2002;28:1267–1272.

29. Jaber S, Chanques G, Matecki S, et al.: Post-extubation stridor in intensive care unit patients. Risk factors evaluation and importance of the cuff-leak test. *Intensive Care Med*. 2003;29:69–74.

30. Kharasch ED, Sivarajan M: Gastroesophageal perforation after intraoperative transesophageal echocardiography. *Anesthesiology*. 1996;85:426–428.

31. Shemie S: Steroids for anything that swells: dexamethasone and postextubation airway obstruction. *Crit Care Med*. 1996;24:1613–1614.

32. Bedger RC, Jr., Chang JL: A jet-stylet endotracheal catheter for difficult airway management. *Anesthesiology*. 1987;66:221–223.

33. Combes X, Le Roux B, Suen P, et al.: Unanticipated difficult airway in anesthetized patients: prospective validation of a management algorithm. *Anesthesiology*. 2004;100:1146–1150.

34. Bogdanov A, Kapila A: Aintree intubating bougie. *Anesth Analg*. 2004;98:1502.

35. Westphal K, Byhahn C, Wilke HJ, Lischke V: Percutaneous tracheostomy: a clinical comparison of dilatational (Ciaglia) and translaryngeal (Fantoni) techniques. *Anesth Analg*. 1999;89:938–943.

36. Byhahn C, Wilke HJ, Lischke V, Rinne T, Westphal K: Bedside percutaneous tracheostomy: clinical comparison of Griggs and Fantoni techniques. *World J Surg*. 2001;25:296–301.

SELF-EVALUATION QUESTIONS

29.1. Which of the following is a reliable method in assessing airway edema?

   A. direct laryngoscopy

   B. airway assessment using a flexible fiberoptic bronchoscope

   C. performing a "cuff-leak test"

   D. presence of facial edema

   E. none of the above

29.2. Which of the following is **NOT** a useful step to minimize the morbidity associated with jet ventilation through a hollow tube exchanger?

   A. ensure that the tip of tube exchanger is not positioned in the bronchus

   B. avoid "breath stacking"

   C. use the lowest driving pressure that results in chest expansion

   D. avoid the administration of a muscle relaxant

   E. facilitate exhalation by minimizing airway obstruction

29.3. Which of the following may be helpful to reduce airway edema?

   A. elevation of the head of the bed

   B. the use of racemic epinephrine

   C. fluid restriction

   D. the use of diuretic therapy

   E. all of the above

CHAPTER (30)

Management of an Accidental Extubation in a Patient in a Halo Jacket

Michael Frass and Michael F. Murphy

30.1 CASE PRESENTATION

A 46-year-old lady sustained a severe injury as the result of a car crash while driving on a rural Austrian road during wintertime in the middle of a snowstorm. The patient was the driver of a car that collided with a truck which sheared off the roof of her car. After ensuring that the crash scene was safe, the ambulance crew, which in this case included an emergency physician, found the patient apneic, sitting in the driver's seat (Figure 30-1). The physician and team instituted immediate airway intervention.

30.2 INITIAL PATIENT MANAGEMENT

30.2.1 What kind of airway challenge does this patient demonstrate?

This patient is in urgent need of immediate airway intervention. This patient has a "crash" airway (see Section 2.5.3) and needs to have her airway immediately managed. A "crash airway" in emergency medicine is defined as the airway of a patient that is "newly dead or nearly dead." In this situation, one anticipates little or no response to oral laryngoscopy so medications to facilitate intubation are unnecessary.

30.2.2 How was this patient's airway approached and managed?

The prevailing weather conditions, the patient's position, and the position of the vehicle combined to make bag-mask-ventilation (BMV) inadequate. With in-line stabilization of the cervical spine

(C-spine), intubation by direct laryngoscopy was attempted but failed because the physician was not able to get adequate access to the patient's head. After three unsuccessful attempts at visualization of the vocal cords, the physician decided to insert a Combitube™ (Esophageal Tracheal Combitube™ [ETC], Tyco Healthcare, Pleasanton, CA) while standing on the remnants of the hood of the car facing the patient (Figures 30-1 and 30-2).[1–3]

Ventilation via the ETC in its proper esophageal position worked well and the oxygen saturation (SpO_2) rose above 95%. A colorimetric breath indicator (EasyCap™, Tyco Healthcare, Nellcor) was attached between tube connector and ventilatory circuit. End-tidal CO_2 was identified by clear color change. The hemodynamic parameters were well within the normal range. Therefore, mechanical ventilation was continued via the longer blue tube (No. 1 of the ETC) leading to the pharyngeal lumen. With continued ventilation via the ETC, the patient was then extracted and was transferred to the ambulance. The patient was transported to the emergency department of the local trauma hospital.

X-ray examination revealed severe injury to the patient's C-spine. She suffered from a C5 on C6 subluxation with C6 pedicle fracture and a C7 crush fracture. The patient was taken to the operating room (OR) for C-spine stabilization using a Halo Jacket completely immobilizing the patient's head and neck. After deflation of the oropharyngeal balloon of the ETC, fiberoptic replacement of the ETC with a 7.5 mm inner diameter (ID) endotracheal tube (ETT) was performed successfully under sedation and topical anesthesia.

Additional procedures to address fractures of the limbs were uneventful. The patient was hemodynamically stable at the conclusion of immobilization of the C-spine in the OR and was then transferred to ICU. During transport to the ICU, the ETT was accidentally dislodged.

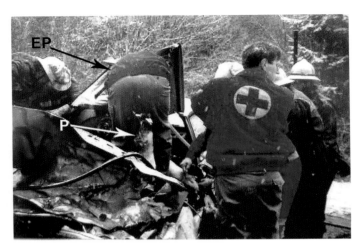

FIGURE 30-1. A scene with the emergency physician (EP) managing the airway of a patient (P) in the middle of a snowstorm.

30.3   MANAGEMENT OF AN ACCIDENTAL EXTUBATION IN A PATIENT WITH A HALO JACKET?

30.3.1   What should the immediate first steps be?

The initial response to loss of the ETT, particularly in the hallway on the way to the ICU, should be the insertion of an oral or nasal airway, and two-hand, two-person BMV. In the event such equipment is not available, a quick decision as to which is closer: ICU or OR will dictate where the patient is taken. If ventilation is inadequate, mouth-to-mouth should be instituted if no equipment is immediately available. It is not inconceivable to imagine that mouth-to-mouth ventilation may be needed since no appropriate equipment is immediately available.

The patient was returned to the OR.

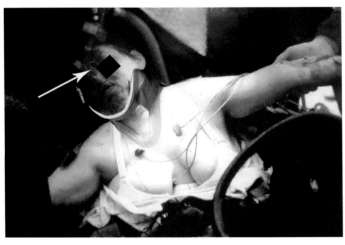

FIGURE 30-2. The patient at the scene in the driver's position with the roof of the vehicle avulsed. A Combitube™ (arrow) is in place to provide ventilation and oxygenation.

30.3.2   What should be done on arrival back in the OR?

BMV was of marginal success, with oxygen saturations hovering in the high 80s and low 90s. This is a near-failed airway. The attending anesthesia practitioner immediately attempted direct laryngoscopy. However, neck movement was impossible because of the halo jacket and had to be strictly avoided at any rate. Furthermore, blood and mucus precluded visualization of any laryngeal structures. The anesthesia practitioner now attempted the insertion of a #3 intubating LMA (ILMA; LMA Fastrach™). However, due to limited mouth opening, the ILMA could not be advanced. Since surgical airway equipment was not immediately available (though requested and en route), the anesthesia practitioner inserted an ETC 37-F Small Adult. The ETC could be inserted easily and ventilation worked well in the esophageal position. With the ETC in place, the patient was ventilated manually with 100% oxygen and emergency cricothyrotomy was not needed.[4]

30.3.3   What alternatives might be considered in a case such as this?

In the event that an extraglottic device (EGD) failed to immediately rescue the airway, cricothyrotomy should be performed. In the event cricothyrotomy is not possible, one has no choice but to release the head from the halo device while maintaining in-line stabilization manually and reattempting oral intubation.

30.3.4   How was the airway eventually managed in a definitive fashion?

Leaving the ETC in place in a patient with a potentially full stomach is not without controversy.[5–7] But this issue is not unique to the ETC among EGDs.[6,7] In our opinion, after stabilization of the patient's condition, the ETC should be replaced using the method described by Gaitini et al.[8] Gaitini described replacement of the ETC by a nasotracheal tube using a flexible fiberoptic bronchoscope (FFB) in 40 patients with Mallampati class III or IV. After partial deflation of the oropharyngeal balloon of the ETC, the FFB was introduced behind the balloon. The unique advantage of this method is that no interruption of airway control and/or ventilation occurs.

After deflation (about 50 mL) of the oropharyngeal balloon, an FFB loaded with a 7.5 mm ID ETT was passed through the right nostril into the pharynx and from there behind the partially deflated oropharyngeal balloon into the trachea. The laryngeal aperture could be identified within 2 minutes. During the procedure, ventilation was maintained without interruption via the ETC.

30.4   SUMMARY

Airway management of a patient in a halo jacket is difficult, particularly if tracheal intubation is required. The challenge of airway management is increased by the inability to position the head and neck to obtain optimal airway patency for BMV as well as laryngeal visibility for direct laryngoscopy.

If BMV is possible, then time is available to choose a definitive airway management technique. It is well known that immobilization of the head and neck will frequently result in a Grade 3 or worse Cormack/Lehane (C/L) laryngeal view.[9–11] Further, neck immobilization is associated with a reduced ability to fully open the mouth, thus hindering the utilization of an EGD.[11] While intubating stylets are most suitable for the Grade 3 C/L laryngoscopic view, orotracheal intubation can be still very difficult. In the event that the patient cannot be ventilated and the trachea cannot be intubated, a failed airway is present and immediate cricothyrotomy is indicated. As a temporizing measure, while setting up for the cricothyrotomy an EGD (e.g., ETC or LMA Fastrach™) may be attempted.

If cricothyrotomy equipment is not available, then one must release the patient's head from the halo jacket and attempt direct laryngoscopy or EGD insertion while employing in-line stabilization. With the alternative being death, oxygenation and ventilation should always have a higher priority than protecting the cervical cord.

REFERENCES

1. Davis DP, Valentine C, Ochs M, Vilke GM, Hoyt DB: The Combitube as a salvage airway device for paramedic rapid sequence intubation. *Ann Emerg Med.* 2003;42: 697–704.
2. Rabitsch W, Schellongowski P, Staudinger T, et al.: Comparison of a conventional tracheal airway with the Combitube in an urban emergency medical services system run by physicians. *Resuscitation.* 2003;57:27–32.
3. Rumball CJ, MacDonald D: The PTL, Combitube, laryngeal mask, and oral airway: a randomized prehospital comparative study of ventilatory device effectiveness and cost-effectiveness in 470 cases of cardiorespiratory arrest. *Prehosp Emerg Care.* 1997;1:1–10.
4. Deroy R, Ghoris M: The Combitube elective anesthetic airway management in a patient with cervical spine fracture. *Anesth Analg.* 1998;87:1441–1442.
5. Mercer MH: An assessment of protection of the airway from aspiration of oropharyngeal contents using the Combitube airway. *Resuscitation.* 2001;51:135–138.
6. Hagberg CA, Vartazarian TN, Chelly JE, Ovassapian A: The incidence of gastroesophageal reflux and tracheal aspiration detected with pH electrodes is similar with the Laryngeal Mask Airway and Esophageal Tracheal Combitube—a pilot study. *Can J Anaesth.* 2004;51:243–249.
7. Cook TM, Hommers C: New airways for resuscitation? *Resuscitation.* 2006;69:371–387.
8. Gaitini LA, Vaida SJ, Somri M, Fradis M, Ben-David B: Fiberoptic-guided airway exchange of the esophageal-tracheal Combitube in spontaneously breathing versus mechanically ventilated patients. *Anesth Analg.* 1999;88:193–196.
9. Gabbott DA: Laryngoscopy using the McCoy laryngoscope after application of a cervical collar. *Anaesthesia.* 1996;51:812–814.
10. Hastings RH, Wood PR: Head extension and laryngeal view during laryngoscopy with cervical spine stabilization maneuvers. *Anesthesiology.* 1994;80:825–831.
11. Heath KJ: The effect of laryngoscopy of different cervical spine immobilization techniques. *Anaesthesia.* 1994;49:843–845.

SELF-EVALUATION QUESTIONS

30.1. You are called to a ward to intubate the trachea of a 78-year-old male who has suffered a respiratory arrest but continues to have a perfusing rhythm with a BP of 180/100 mm Hg. He is in a halo jacket following a C-spine procedure for ankylosing spondylitis. Which of the following is correct?

A. Immediate RSI employing etomidate and succinylcholine is the best course of action.

B. A retrograde intubation with an FFB should be attempted.

C. A tracheotomy should be your first choice.

D. In the event laryngoscopy is unsuccessful and no other airway management devices are immediately available, one should release patient's head from the halo device with in-line stabilization and reattempt direct laryngoscopy.

E. BMV is virtually always possible in these patients.

30.2. Which of the following statements is true with regard to C-spine immobilization in a halo device?

A. It is associated with a 50% incidence of Grade 3 views on direct laryngoscopy.

B. It is associated with difficult cricothyrotomy.

C. It is not associated with a reduced mouth opening.

D. It has been shown that tracheal intubation through an ILMA is difficult in a patient in a halo jacket.

E. All of the above.

30.3. Which of the following is **NOT** true with the Combitube™?

A. It is a disposable device.

B. It provides some protection against gastric aspiration.

C. The device is designed so that regardless where the Combitube™ is placed (the esophagus or the trachea) adequate ventilation and oxygenation can be provided.

D. The Combitube™ consists of a double-lumen tube with a tracheal tube and a closed distal-end esophageal obturator tube which has perforations at the pharyngeal level.

E. There is a pediatric size Combitube™.

CHAPTER (31)

Management of a SARS Patient Admitted to the ICU with Impending Respiratory Failure and a Clinical Suspicion of Difficult Airway

David T. Wong

31.1 CASE PRESENTATION

A 47-year-old previously healthy male physician presented to hospital with the acute onset of fever, nonproductive cough, dyspnea, and malaise. As an intensive care unit (ICU) physician, he had intubated the trachea of a known Severe Acute Respiratory Syndrome (SARS) patient in the emergency department 2 weeks earlier. He began to have respiratory symptoms 1 week later. He was admitted and placed in an isolation room. Both sputum and blood cultures were negative. In spite of empiric treatment with broad-spectrum antibiotics, his respiratory status progressively worsened over the next 24 hours, necessitating ICU admission. His vitals on admission to the ICU were respiratory rate 24, breaths per min heart rate 100 bpm, blood pressure 130/90, and temperature 38.6°C. Oxygen saturation was 95% on a FiO_2 of 60%, and arterial blood gases (ABGs) revealed the following: pH 7.45, $PaCO_2$ 30, PaO_2 60. With the PaO_2 to FiO_2 ratio (PF ratio) determined to be 100, respiratory failure was diagnosed. The chest x-ray (CXR) showed progressive bilateral basal infiltrates. A complete blood count, electrolytes, creatinine, and liver function tests were all normal, but lactate dehydrogenase (LDH) was elevated. Neurological and cardiovascular systems were intact on examination.

Anesthesia was consulted regarding possible intubation for respiratory failure due to probable SARS with an acute respiratory distress syndrome (ARDS) picture. The patient was agreeable to intubation. On airway examination, the patient was noted to be of average body habitus (5 ft 10 in. [176 cm] and 154 lb [70 kg]) with no obvious dysmorphic facial features. He had no beard and no history of obstructive sleep apnea. Although he was dyspneic, there was no evidence of stridor. With full dentition, the patient was able to open his mouth 5 cm, had a 4 cm thyromental distance, and had a Mallampati Class III pharyngeal view. He exhibited good jaw protrusion, and head and neck mobility was unrestricted. The cricothyroid membrane was easily palpable in the midline.

31.2 MEDICAL CONSIDERATIONS—SARS

31.2.1 What is the epidemiology of SARS? How did SARS come out of nowhere to affect thousands of people worldwide?

SARS stands for Severe Acute Respiratory Syndrome. In November 2002, a cluster of atypical pneumonia cases of unknown etiology was discovered in Guangdong Province, China. In late February 2003, a symptomatic Chinese physician traveled to Hong Kong and transmitted the illness to others staying in the same hotel, initiating a worldwide epidemic. On March 12, 2003, the World Health Organization (WHO) issued a global alert warning of a wave of severe atypical pneumonia of unknown etiology.[1–3] On April 13, 2003, the causative agent for SARS was identified as a new coronavirus (SARS-CoV). By the end of July 2003, there were over 8,000 cases of SARS worldwide with over 700 deaths.[4] Countries and regions with the highest caseloads were China, Hong Kong, Taiwan, and Canada.

31.2.2. How is the SARS virus transmitted?

SARS is thought to be transmitted by respiratory droplets or by direct/indirect contact.[2] It is a moderately transmissible virus with a secondary infection rate of approximately 2.7 per case. The majority of SARS patients do not infect others while a small number of "super spreaders" may be highly infectious.[5,6] There is no evidence of airborne transmission.

31.2.3 What are the risk factors for SARS viral transmission?

SARS patients develop nonspecific viral symptoms in the first week of their illness and respiratory symptoms in the second week, during which they are most infectious. Fowler et al. assessed the risk factors for SARS transmission among 122 health care workers in a critical-care setting.[7] They found that performing endotracheal intubation and caring for patients receiving noninvasive positive pressure ventilation were associated with 13 and 2.3 times the risk of acquiring infection compared to those who did not. Loeb et al. studied risk factors for SARS transmission among 43 critical-care nurses.[8] They found that assisting with intubation, suctioning prior to intubation and manipulation of the oxygen mask were high-risk activities. In a third report, bag-mask-ventilation (BMV), endotracheal intubation, airway suctioning, noninvasive ventilation, and high-frequency oscillation were identified as high-risk procedures for SARS transmission in the ICU.[9]

31.2.4 What is the definition of SARS?

The WHO definition[10] of a suspect SARS patient is a person presenting after November 1, 2002, with a history of:

(a) fever >38°C;

(b) cough and respiratory difficulty; and

(c) known exposure to SARS patient or traveling in endemic area within 10 days of presenting illness.

The WHO definition *of a probable SARS patient* is a suspect person with:

(a) radiologic evidence of infiltrates consistent with pneumonia or respiratory distress syndrome;

(b) one or more assays positive for SARS coronavirus; *or*

(c) autopsy findings consistent with the pathology of respiratory distress syndrome without an identifiable cause.

31.2.5 What is the typical clinical course of a SARS patient?

The incubation period is 2–5 days but can be up to 10 days.[11] The most common symptoms at admission to hospital are fever, nonproductive cough, myalgia, dyspnea, headache, malaise, chills, and diarrhea (Table 31-1). The majority of patients have unilateral or bilateral infiltrates on the chest radiograph. The overall death rate is 10–13% but is as high as 50% in the 23–26% of patients requiring intensive care admission.[11–13] Risk factors for death include age, comorbidities, and Acute Physiology and Chronic Health Evaluation II (APACHE II) scores.[13]

TABLE 31-1

Symptoms of SARS Reported at Admission to Hospital

Fever	99.3%
Nonproductive cough	69.4%
Myalgia	49.3%
Dyspnea	41.7%
Headache	35.4%
Malaise	31.2%
Chills	27.8%
Diarrhea	23.6%
Nausea or vomiting	19.4%
Sore throat	12.5%
Arthralgia	10.4%
Chest pain	10.4%
Productive cough	4.9%
Dizziness	4.2%
Abdominal pain	3.5%
Rhinorrhea	2.1%

Adopted from Booth et al.[11]

31.3   PATIENT CONSIDERATIONS

31.3.1 What are the major considerations in this patient?

This patient fulfills the WHO definition of probable SARS and clinical criteria for ARDS (bilateral lung infiltrate with PF ratio ≤200 mm Hg). The patient has increased pulmonary shunting due to fluid-filled alveoli and atelectasis, leading to a high A-a gradient and a low PF ratio. He has little pulmonary reserve and is prone to the development of hypoxemia during intubation. He is also at risk of barotrauma (e.g., pneumothorax) with positive-pressure ventilation.

The patient is likely to have a depleted extracellular fluid volume due to his fasting status and large amounts of fluid loss from his respiratory system. This volume depletion, coupled with institution of positive-pressure ventilation and removal of sympathetic drive, puts him at risk of hypotension during and immediately following intubation.

31.3.2 What is the differential diagnosis of a patient with bilateral pulmonary infiltrates of unknown etiology?

The patient may be suffering from bacterial, viral, fungal, or parasitic pneumonia. Tuberculosis, pneumocystis carinii, and atypical pneumonia such as mycoplasma and legionella are the possibilities. In addition, bilateral lung infiltrates may be due to leaky pulmonary capillaries caused by diverse causes such as sepsis or pancreatitis. Of these causes, tuberculosis and SARS pose the highest risk of transmission to the health care workers and appropriate personal protection precautions should be exercised (see below).

31.4 AIRWAY CONSIDERATIONS

31.4.1 Is this patient predicted to have a difficult airway?

All airway examination should focus on the ability in providing ventilation and oxygenation through a bag-mask, an extraglottic device, an endotracheal tube, and a surgical airway. The mnemonics MOANS, LEMON, RODS, and SHORT described in Chapter 1 provide a useful framework to assess these aspects of patient's airway. It should be emphasized that while the ASA task force on management of the difficult airway outlined 11 criteria for preoperative airway assessment for laryngoscopy and intubation,[14] no single airway test has perfect sensitivity or specificity in predicting difficult laryngoscopic intubation. In general, all single airway predictors share a common set of characteristics: low sensitivity, high specificity, and low positive predictive value. The combination of several airway predictors tends to improve the positive predictive value for difficult laryngoscopic intubation.

With reference to the airway examination presented in the Section 31.1, it is apparent that this patient has several predictors of a difficult laryngoscopic intubation: borderline mouth opening, a reduced thyromental distance, and a Mallampati III classification. In combination, these characteristics place this patient at a *moderately* high risk for difficult laryngoscopy. However, alternative intubation devices such as the intubating LMA (ILMA) or lighted stylet should be successful, and with adequate control of secretions, and so should flexible or rigid fiberoptic devices. BMV if needed should be possible, although not optimal. Should extraglottic device placement and use be required, decreased pulmonary compliance due to ARDS may present a problem with "pop-off" leak developing at higher airway pressures: availability of a LMA ProSeal™ might be advisable. Cricothyrotomy should be possible. Note that although some of these techniques are not desirable in the patient with SARS, their predicted success must still be assessed, particularly in the patient with predictors of difficulty.

31.4.2 What do you do differently when establishing an airway in a SARS patient?

A SARS patient poses a unique risk to the health care workers due to its highly infectious nature and a high mortality rate for those infected. In developed countries such as Canada and Singapore, approximately 50% of SARS cases were health care workers involved in caring for SARS patients. The processes of tracheal intubation, BMV, and suctioning were associated with the highest risk of acquiring SARS.[7–9] A cluster of nine health care workers who cared for a single SARS patient around the time of intubation in the ICU themselves developed SARS.[15]

In order to minimize the risk of SARS cross-transmission to health care workers, guidelines have been developed to reduce the risk of aerosolization of SARS droplets during the process of intubation.[2,16,17] It is critical that the health care workers apply and remove personal protection equipment (PPE) (see Section 31.5.5) prior to and after intubation. In addition, BMV, nebulization, and application of topical airway anesthesia are to be avoided. The patient should thus be sedated and paralyzed unless contraindicated. However, with the high potential for difficult laryngoscopy, there may be a conflict of priorities.

31.4.3 How are you going to approach this patient's airway?

This patient's situation presents us with a real dilemma. On the one hand, an awake intubation following application of topical airway anesthesia is generally considered to be the safest method of securing the airway in the patient presenting with potential difficult laryngoscopic intubation. On the other hand, to minimize the risk to health care personnel of SARS transmission, avoiding BMV is preferred, as is paralysis of the patient because of the potential for coughing. Protecting the patient and the health care worker are both important priorities.

Ultimately the method chosen for intubation is determined by how likely one is to encounter a failed airway situation (see Chapter 2). The possibility for such a situation will become evident as the patient is assessed for predictors of difficulty in all aspects of airway management. If the patient presents with evidence that airway control will be difficult using various techniques of endotracheal-tube placement, BMV, an extraglottic device, or cricothyrotomy, the clinician should accept the risk of disease transmission and perform an awake intubation. However, in this case, as outlined above, the patient presents predictors of only moderate difficulty with laryngoscopy and no predictors of difficulty with alternative intubation (e.g., ILMA, lighted stylet, fiberoptic) equipment use. Bag-mask and extraglottic device ventilation, if needed, will most likely be successful in spite of reduced pulmonary compliance. Cricothyrotomy should pose few problems.

Thus, a reasonable "Plan A" approach in this patient is to attempt tracheal intubation by direct laryngoscopy after induction using short-acting anesthetic and paralytic agents. The intubation should be undertaken by an experienced airway practitioner, wearing full protection, and with a full complement of alternative intubating devices. In addition, extraglottic rescue device and cricothyrotomy equipment should be readily available in the room.

If direct laryngoscopy fails after one or two attempts, and oxygenation remains acceptable, "Plan B" calls for an alternative device to be used, in this case the flexible fiberoptic bronchoscope (FFB). If intubation is not successful after three attempts, the patient should be awakened with the intention of proceeding with an awake intubation. If at any time between attempts oxygenation cannot be maintained with BMV, "Plan C" calls for the immediate use of a LMA ProSeal™ or LMA Fastrach™, while concurrently preparing to perform a cricothyrotomy in this "can't intubate, can't ventilate" situation.

31.5   PREPARATION AND PLANNING FOR ESTABLISHMENT OF AN AIRWAY IN THE SARS PATIENT

31.5.1   Where in the ICU should the patient be placed?

In order to minimize the spread of SARS virus, the patient should be placed in an isolation room, equipped with negative-pressure ventilation.[2,16,17] The room should have a pre-entry room (anteroom) to allow application and removal of PPE.

31.5.2   Who should perform and who should assist with tracheal intubation?

Only those persons required to carry out the intubation should be permitted in the immediate vicinity of the patient. This team may consist of an experienced airway practitioner, respiratory therapist, and an ICU nurse. Students should be excluded. Additional personnel should stand by outside the room in the event that help or equipment is required during the airway management procedure. In this situation, this may include another individual with airway management expertise.

It is critically important that all team members are aware of "Plan A, Plan B, and Plan C" and have had the chance to rehearse the sequence of events prior to securing the airway.

31.5.3   What airway equipment should be available in the patient's room?

- General equipment. The room should contain a ventilator with hydrophobic filters (e.g., PALL®) on the inspiratory and expiratory limbs, suction, capnography, oximetry, ventilation bag with expiratory filter, and oropharyngeal airway.[2]
- "Plan A" equipment. A laryngoscope handle, an appropriately sized curved and straight blade, a tracheal tube introducer (e.g., Eschmann Introducer), several sizes of endotracheal tubes, and endotracheal tube stylets.
- "Plan B" rescue airway equipment. At least two alternative intubation devices such as an FFB, lighted stylet, ILMA, or Glidescope®.
- "Plan C" equipment. The equipment necessary to perform a surgical airway, as Plan C stipulates, ought to be immediately available and opened.

31.5.4   What other equipment is considered essential?

Two functioning intravenous lines should be placed. Induction and emergency drugs should be prepared. Induction drugs consist of midazolam, fentanyl, propofol, succinylcholine, and a non-depolarizing muscle relaxant. Emergency drugs consist of atropine, ephedrine, phenylephrine, and epinephrine.

31.5.5   How should health care workers dress in order to minimize SARS transmission?

All health care workers in direct contact with SARS patients should be wearing basic PPE. Enhanced PPE should be worn by all health care workers involved in high-risk procedures such as intubation.[2,17] (Table 31-2)

Basic personal protection strategy consists of airborne precautions, contact precautions, and eye protection.

TABLE 31-2

Infection Control for an ICU Patient Requiring Endotracheal Intubation[1]

DRESS PRECAUTIONS
Basic PPE
- N-95 or equivalent face mask
- Contact—gloves, gown, hat, shoe covers
- Eye protection—goggles or face shields
- Pens, pagers, or personal items should not be brought into or out of the room

Enhanced PPE for high-risk procedures
- Air-Mate® PAPR system
- Stryker T4 PAPR system

ENVIRONMENT/EQUIPMENT PRECAUTIONS
- Isolation rooms
- Negative pressure rooms preferable
- ICU rooms should be stocked with a full supply of airway and intubation equipment, induction, and emergency drugs
- Equipment and stationary (e.g., computer keyboard, pens, stethoscope) should be cleaned frequently with antiviral disinfectants
- Frequent hand washing with alcohol-based disinfectant
- No sharing of equipment

AIRWAY AND VENTILATOR MANAGEMENT
- Allow plenty of time to prepare for intubation
- The whole team to discuss and rehearse Plans A and B for intubation
- Avoid topicalization of the airway
- Avoid nebulization therapy
- Avoid suctioning of an unprotected airway
- Avoid noninvasive positive-pressure ventilation
- The most experienced physician to perform intubation
- Minimize the number of personnel in the room during intubation
- Have a second parallel team on standby outside the room
- Sedate and paralyze patient prior to intubation unless contraindicated
- Use filters for Ambu bag and ventilator
- Ensure functioning scavenging system
- Usage of closed suctioning system

31.5.4.1 Basic PPE: Airborne Precautions

An N-95 mask or equivalent is used for airborne precaution. N-95 masks offer 8 hours of protection while PCM-2000 masks provide 4 hours. Touching the mask or lifting the mask to wipe the face with gloved fingers immediately contaminates the mask and it must be replaced. It is crucial to test for proper mask fitting. An improper mask fit may not provide airborne protection. A properly fitted N-95 mask can be a very uncomfortable experience for users who may need to wear them for a prolonged period of time.

31.5.4.2 Basic PPE: Contact and Eye Precautions

Contact precautions include double gloves, double gown, disposable hats, and shoe covers.[2] Following contact with each patient and removing gloves, an alcohol-based skin disinfectant should be used to wash hands. Eyes should be protected against contamination using disposable goggles or face shields.

31.5.4.3 Enhanced PPE

Enhanced PPE consists of basic PPE plus powered air purification respirator (PAPR) systems.[17] They should be worn by all health care workers involved in high-risk procedures for these patients. One example of a commonly used PARR system is the Air-Mate® (3M, St. Paul, MN). The Air-Mate® PAPR system consists of a belt-mounted powered air purifier (Figure 31-1, right) with a HEPA filter, connected via a tube to a lightweight headpiece (Figure 31-1, left). The HEPA filter removes particles of 0.3–15 μm with an efficiency of 98–100%.[4] Experience of several years duration using the PAPR system in the bronchoscopy suite has revealed no documented disease transmission to health care workers. Chee et al. reported their experience in Singapore among health care workers caring for SARS patients undergoing 41 surgical procedures.[18] With rigid adherence to basic and enhanced PPE, none of 124 health care workers directly exposed to SARS patients was infected.

It takes time to properly setup the room and apply PPE.[17] Therefore, it is crucial to be advised well in advance of patients requiring tracheal intubation. Furthermore, staff involved in the intubation must be trained and familiar with the PPE so that it can be applied properly and expeditiously, and removed properly to avoid contamination.

31.5.6 What conditions must be satisfied before proceeding with intubation?

Just before performing intubation, a checklist should be completed and Plans A, B, and C rehearsed so that all parties involved are absolutely clear as to each person's responsibilities and course of action until the airway is secured (Table 31-2).

The ventilator, monitors, airway equipment, suction, intravenous access, induction, and emergency drugs should be in the room. An endotracheal tube with stylet, along with a second endotracheal tube loaded on an FFB, should be at the ready. The primary intubation team members apply basic and enhanced PPE including PAPR system and enter the patient's room. A second, parallel team is dressed and ready to enter the room if needed. A practitioner experienced in securing a surgical airway should be part of the second team on standby.

31.6 ACTUAL CONDUCT OF TRACHEAL INTUBATION

31.6.1 Describe the actual steps of tracheal intubation in this patient

The patient was denitrogenated while spontaneously breathing with FiO$_2$ of 1.0 for 5 minutes. At no time was positive-pressure ventilation applied prior to intubation. Topicalization of the airway and nebulization of drugs were likewise avoided. The ventilator was set on volume-control mode.

Once the patient was adequately denitrogenated, fentanyl 50 μg and midazolam 1 mg were given intravenously. A sleep dose of propofol was given followed by succinylcholine 1.5 mg·kg^{-1}.

After the patient was anesthetized and paralyzed, laryngoscopy was attempted with a Macintosh 3 blade. A Grade 3 laryngeal view was observed despite external laryngeal pressure and a head lift. The decision was made not to attempt blind intubation with direct laryngoscopy. Flexible fiberoptic guided intubation was the next option.

A propofol infusion was administered using a syringe pump at 100 μg·kg^{-1}·min^{-1}. Additional succinylcholine of 40 mg was given. The patient's vital signs were stable with a SpO$_2$ of 100%. Gentle tongue traction was performed by an ICU nurse. A 5.1 mm OD FFB was introduced orally and guided successfully through the larynx into the trachea under indirect visualization. A 7.5 mm ID endotracheal tube was advanced easily over the FFB into the trachea. The endotracheal tube was positioned 3 cm above the carina and taped at the 22 cm mark at the teeth. The endotracheal tube

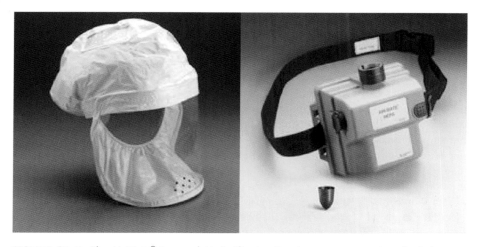

FIGURE 31-1. The Air-Mate® Powered Air Purification Respirator system consists of a belt-mounted powered air purifier (right) with a HEPA filter, connected via a tube to a lightweight headpiece (left).

pilot balloon was inflated and a ventilation bag was used to ventilate the patient. A colorimetric CO_2 indicator further confirmed endotracheal placement of endotracheal tube.

31.7   OTHER CONSIDERATIONS

31.7.1   Outline your postintubation management

The patient's endotracheal tube was connected to the ventilator, and mechanical ventilation in a volume-control mode was begun.[19] As the patient's blood pressure and heart rate remained stable, the infusion of propofol was continued for patient sedation.

The airway management team proceeded to remove their PPE. Utmost care was taken to remove the gloves, gown, PAPR head gear, goggles, cap, and shoe covers in the proper sequence so that the health care workers' bodies were not contaminated.[2] Disposable equipment was discarded while reusable equipment such as the PAPR head gear was carefully wiped down using a disinfectant agent (e.g., Virox®).

All health care workers who participated in the care of the SARS patient were advised to be on high alert for the subsequent development of any symptoms or signs of SARS.[20]

31.7.2   What other airborne pathogens may pose serious danger during airway management? Would precautions differ in any way from those presented above?

There are a number of airborne viruses or bacteria that can pose a risk to health care workers. Active pulmonary tuberculosis carries a high risk of transmission to health care workers. Similarly, active anthrax pulmonary infection may also pose a significant risk to them. Fortunately, most airborne viruses, which can potentially infect health care workers, are not associated with high morbidity or mortality. In general, health care workers at risk of coming in contact with respiratory secretions from patients with febrile respiratory illness of unknown etiology should wear PPE including gloves, goggle, gown, and N95 face mask.

Recently, the world has been on the alert for the Avian Influenza viruses (bird flu) of the H5N1 subtype. H5N1 viruses have been found in birds in many countries and normally do not cause disease in humans. However, since 1997, cases have been reported of poultry-to-human transmission resulting in very aggressive clinical courses with close to 50% mortality rate. At the time of writing, human-to-human transmission has been very rare and there has not been any spread beyond a first generation of close contacts.

With the current situation in which human-to-human transmission is generally not seen, caring for a patient with suspected H5N1 would involve PPE including gloves, goggle, gown, and N95 face mask. However, if the virus has evolved and human-to-human transmission is becoming more common, then enhanced PPE including PAPR system and isolation rooms would become necessary in caring for patients with suspected H5N1 infection.[20,21]

31.8   SUMMARY

In summary, the recent SARS epidemic illustrates the rapidity and severity with which a new virus can strike worldwide. A global surveillance system for new infections and a national coordinated response must be in place should future viral infection alerts occur. There is a need in our health care system for emphasis on and compliance with ordinary infection-control measures such as hand washing, and the use of gloves, masks, and eye protection. Health care workers should be familiar, and hospitals must be equipped, with enhanced PPE should the need arise to care for suspected SARS patients. In order to minimize the risk of contamination and SARS transmission, they should be aware of the modifications of techniques for intubation.

REFERENCES

1. Chow KY, Lee CE, Ling ML, Heng DM, Yap SG: Outbreak of severe acute respiratory syndrome in a tertiary hospital in Singapore, linked to an index patient with atypical presentation: epidemiological study. *BMJ.* 2004;328:195.
2. Peng PW, Wong DT, Bevan D, Gardam M: Infection control and anesthesia: lessons learned from the Toronto SARS outbreak. *Can J Anaesth.* 2003;50:989–997.
3. Varia M, Wilson S, Sarwal S, et al.: Investigation of a nosocomial outbreak of severe acute respiratory syndrome (SARS) in Toronto, Canada. *CMAJ.* 2003;169:285–292.
4. WHO: Summary of probable SARS cases with onset of illness from 1 November 2002 to 31 July 2003. Available at: www.who.int/csr/sars/country/table2004_04_21/en/.
5. Poutanen SM, Low DE, Henry B, et al.: Identification of severe acute respiratory syndrome in Canada. *N Engl J Med.* 2003;348:1995–2005.
6. Shen Z, Ning F, Zhou W, et al.: Superspreading SARS events, Beijing, 2003. *Emerg Infect Dis.* 2004;10:256–260.
7. Fowler RA, Guest CB, Lapinsky SE, et al.: Transmission of severe acute respiratory syndrome during intubation and mechanical ventilation. *Am J Respir Crit Care Med.* 2004;169:1198–1202.
8. Loeb M, McGeer A, Henry B, et al.: SARS among critical care nurses, Toronto. *Emerg Infect Dis.* 2004;10:251–255.
9. Scales DC, Green K, Chan AK, et al.: Illness in intensive care staff after brief exposure to severe acute respiratory syndrome. *Emerg Infect Dis.* 2003;9:1205–1210.
10. WHO: Case definition for surveillance of Severe Acute Respiratory Syndrom (SARS). Available at: www.who.int/csr/sars/casedefinition/en/.
11. Booth CM, Matukas LM, Tomlinson GA, et al.: Clinical features and short-term outcomes of 144 patients with SARS in the greater Toronto area. *JAMA.* 2003;289:2801–2809.
12. Choi KW, Chau TN, Tsang O, et al.: Outcomes and prognostic factors in 267 patients with severe acute respiratory syndrome in Hong Kong. *Ann Intern Med.* 2003;139:715–723.
13. Lew TW, Kwek TK, Tai D, et al.: Acute respiratory distress syndrome in critically ill patients with severe acute respiratory syndrome. *JAMA* 2003;290:374–380.
14. Caplan RA, Benumof JL, Berry FA, et al.: Practice Guidelines for management of the difficult airway. An updated report by the American Society of Anesthesiologists task force on management of the difficult airway. *Anesthesiology.* 2003;98:1269–1277.
15. Ofner M, Lem M, Sarwal S, Vearncombe M, Simor A: Cluster of severe acute respiratory syndrome cases among protected health care workers-Toronto, April 2003. *Can Commun Dis Rep.* 2003;29:93–97.
16. Kamming D, Gardam M, Chung F: Anaesthesia and SARS. *Br J Anaesth.* 2003;90:715–718.
17. Wong DT: Protection protocol in intubation of suspected SARS patients. *Can J Anaesth.* 2003;50:747–748.
18. Chee VW, Khoo ML, Lee SF, Lai YC, Chin NM: Infection control measures for operative procedures in severe acute respiratory syndrome-related patients. *Anesthesiology.* 2004;100:1394–1398.
19. Yam LY, Chen RC, Zhong NS: SARS: ventilatory and intensive care. *Respirology.* 2003;8(suppl):S31–S35.

20. Avian Influenza frequently asked questions. Available at: www.who.int/csr/disease/avian_influenza/avian_faqs/en/index.html.
21. Interim Recommendations for Infection Control in Health-Care Facilities Caring for Patients with Known or Suspected Avian Influenza. Available at: www.cdc.gov/flu/avian/professional/infect-control.htm.

SELF-EVALUATION QUESTIONS

31.1. Which of the following is considered the basic personal protection equipment in managing a patient with SARS?

A. N-95 or equivalent face mask

B. contact—gloves, gown, hat, shoe covers

C. eye protection—goggles or face shields

D. pens, pagers, or personal items should not be brought into or out of the room

E. all of the above

31.2. All of the following principles in managing the airway of a patient with SARS are true **EXCEPT**

A. awake fiberoptic intubation is the preferred airway technique for all SARS patients with a potential difficult laryngoscopic intubation

B. intubation should be undertaken by an experienced airway practitioner, wearing full protection

C. it is necessary to reduce the risk of aerosolization of SARS droplets during the process of intubation

D. it is critical that the health care workers apply and remove personal protection equipment prior to and after intubating the patient

E. bag-mask-ventilation, nebulization, and application of topical airway anesthesia are to be avoided

31.3. All of the following should be in the airway management team for patients with SARS **EXCEPT**

A. an experienced airway practitioner

B. an experienced surgeon for a surgical airway

C. an experienced paramedic

D. an ICU nurse

E. a respiratory therapist

CHAPTER (32)

Performing an Elective Percutaneous Dilational Tracheotomy in a Patient on Mechanical Ventilation

Angelina Guzzo, Liane B. Johnson, and Orlando R. Hung

32.1   CASE PRESENTATION

A 28-year-old, previously healthy female was thrown off an ATV and sustained blunt trauma to her chest. Her injuries included a flail chest with fractures of the right first and second ribs, a pulmonary contusion, as well as a right femur fracture and ruptured spleen. Following a splenectomy on the first night, she stabilized hemodynamically and subsequently underwent an open reduction internal fixation of the femur. On the 10th day, an extubation attempt was aborted due to hypoxemia. Currently, she is being ventilated with a pressure support of 12, positive end expiratory pressure (PEEP) of 5, and FiO_2 0.50. Her arterial blood gas shows a pH 7.47, $PaCO_2$ 37, PaO_2 60, and HCO_3 26 torr. Her respiratory rate is 20 breaths per minute. All other vital signs are stable. You have been consulted to help perform a tracheotomy.

32.2   INTRODUCTION

32.2.1   Why would you perform a tracheotomy on this patient?

Local changes occur in airway mucosal surfaces following as little as 2 hours of endotracheal intubation. These pathophysiologic changes include well-documented progression of mucosal ulceration, pressure necrosis, granulation tissue with subsequent healing, fibrosis, and occasionally stenosis.[1,2] There exists no consensus on the ideal timing of a tracheotomy performed in an attempt to minimize long-term airway complications,[3] but standard practice dictates a range of 7–10 days following the initial intubation.

However, if prolonged intubation is expected based on patient circumstances, such as a high spinal cord injury, then earlier conversion to tracheotomy may be considered.

32.2.2   What are the advantages of a tracheotomy over a prolonged translaryngeal intubation?

The potential advantages of a tracheotomy over a prolonged translaryngeal intubation include a reduced risk of direct endolaryngeal injury, a decreased risk of nosocomial pneumonia in certain patient subgroups,[3,4] more effective pulmonary toilet, and possibly decreased airway resistance and anatomical dead space to promote weaning from mechanical ventilation. Additional benefits include improved patient comfort, communication and mobility, increased airway security, decreased requirements for sedation, better nutrition, and earlier discharge from ICU.

32.3   AIRWAY CONSIDERATIONS

32.3.1   If a tracheotomy is going to be performed anyway, why is it important to know whether this patient has a difficult airway or anatomical features associated with difficult laryngoscopic intubation?

In fact, it is extremely important to assess the airway prior to performing a tracheotomy. When performing either a traditional tracheotomy (TT) or a percutaneous dilational tracheotomy (PDT), the indwelling ETT must be carefully withdrawn above the tracheotomy site during the procedure to accommodate insertion of the tracheotomy tube. This maneuver carries with it a potential risk of premature extubation and a need for ventilation and reintubation. Ultimately, preparing for a successful procedure requires a thorough chart review, patient airway assessment, proper equipment preparation (including the difficult airway cart if the patient has a history of difficult laryngoscopic intubation), and proper patient positioning. Attention to these factors and having qualified, informed assistants will minimize the need for emergency airway access should unanticipated difficulty arise.

While the importance of assessment and preparation are well accepted as basic principles of airway management, the dynamic nature of upper-airway anatomy is often overlooked. Surgical procedures or radiotherapy that alters skeletal or soft tissues of the head and neck can change the upper-airway anatomy, making laryngoscopic intubation difficult. The likelihood of deformed anatomy should be suspected in patients who have undergone recent surgery of the temporomandibular joints and mandible, reconstructive orthognathic or cosmetic surgery, fusion of the cervical spine, or patients with severe burns to the head and neck.[5,6] For example, Coonan et al.[7] reported a patient with an unanticipated difficult laryngoscopy secondary to contracture of the temporalis muscle causing ankylosis of the jaw several weeks following a temporal craniotomy. Many patients presenting for tracheotomy will have undergone recent surgery. When evaluating these patients, one must always consider the potential for such dynamic changes to what may previously have been an easily managed airway.

32.3.2   How would you assess this patient's airway?

The patient's chart should be reviewed to determine if there is a history of difficult laryngoscopic intubation or difficult bag-mask-ventilation. Chapter 1 has reviewed anatomic and physiologic factors, which may predict difficulty with each. The neck should also be assessed for cervical spine (C-spine) stability and other factors that could create difficult conditions for surgical airways such as cervical flexion deformity, previous neck surgery or radiation therapy, active neck infection, edema, or tumor.

32.4   PREPARATION AND TECHNIQUES

32.4.1   Describe the anatomy of the airway with respect to performing a PDT

Surgical access to the airway through the trachea requires a knowledge and recognition of the surface anatomy, landmarks of the larynx, as well as the important adjacent structures in the neck. Most importantly, dexterity and familiarity with flexible bronchoscopy are essential to safely carry out a PDT.

Easily palpable landmarks include the following: the hyoid bone situated high in the neck just below the submental space has a primary suspensory role for the airway; the thyroid notch is more prominent in adult males than others and identifies the superior aspect of the thyroid cartilage; and the cricoid cartilage is the only complete ring and is bridged by the cricothyroid membrane to the inferior portion of the thyroid cartilage (Figure 32-1). With the neck extended, palpation inferiorly from this point may reveal proximal tracheal rings and the thyroid gland. The vocal cords are protected by the body of the thyroid cartilage anteriorly and attach to the arytenoid cartilages, which articulate on with the posterosuperior margin of the cricoid ring.

An experienced practitioner must perform flexible fiberoptic bronchoscopy to identify the level of important internal laryngeal structures (supraglottis, glottis, and subglottis) and to transilluminate the area between the second to fourth tracheal rings. In patients with poorly palpable surface anatomy, transillumination, and visual confirmation of the guide needle will ensure proper positioning of the tracheotomy tube.

32.4.2   Compare and contrast the different sites at which surgical airway access can be performed

Surgical access to the airway can be gained at the cricothyroid space, subcricoid space, or between any of the tracheal rings. To secure an emergency airway rapidly, a cricothyrotomy is preferable because the cricothyroid membrane is superficial, easily identifiable, and thus easiest to access.[3] Controversy exists about the long-term use of cricothyrotomy due to early reports of subglottic stenosis (SGS), limiting its use to emergency airway access.[8] Re-exploration of this notion in a recent prospective study involving

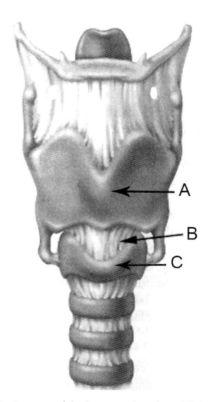

FIGURE 32-1. Anatomy of the larynx and trachea: (A) the larynx; (B) the cricothyroid membrane; and (C) the cricoid cartilage.

118 patients showed the incidence and severity of complications to be similar in both TT and cricothyrotomy techniques.[8]

The first modern-day tracheotomy performed by Chevalier Jackson in the early 1900s involved entering the trachea at the second or third tracheal rings.[9] He advocated avoiding the first and second tracheal rings due to a high incidence of subsequent SGS.[10] Current consensus dictates that in ideal circumstances, a tracheotomy is performed between tracheal rings two to four. Injury to the first ring or cricoid cartilage can increase the risk of SGS, whereas placing it too low may predispose to erosion of the anterior tracheal wall and possible creation of a tracheoinnominate fistula.[11]

The first percutaneous tracheotomy not requiring neck dissection was described in 1955 by Shelden et al.,[12] during which a slotted needle was introduced blindly into the tracheal lumen. Several deaths occurred secondary to laceration of vital structures in proximity to the airway.[13] Toye and Weinstein[14] performed the first tracheotomy using a Seldinger technique in which a single tapered dilator was introduced with a recessed cutting blade. In 1985, Ciaglia et al.[15] introduced a dilational Seldinger technique which has since been refined and has now become one of the most popular techniques for PDT.[16] Initially, PDT was performed in the immediate subcricoid space.[15] But in a follow-up publication the space between the first and second tracheal rings was advocated.[17] The more distal approach was recommended due to the risk of bleeding from the thyroid isthmus.[17]

32.4.3 Describe the different techniques used to perform an elective surgical airway*

32.4.3.1 Traditional Tracheotomy

TT is usually performed under general anesthesia in the operating room. The neck is extended to elevate the trachea into the neck. Depending on the length of the patient's neck, a horizontal incision is generally made crossing the midline approximately 2 cm above the sternal notch. The subcutaneous tissue and platysma muscle are divided transversely. The remainder of the dissection is performed longitudinally through the superficial cervical fascia and the linea alba dividing the strap muscles. Lateral retraction of the strap muscles often reveals the thyroid isthmus, which is commonly surgically divided to provide better surgical access and to minimize the risk of bleeding by manipulation of the thyroid isthmus.[11] Various types of tracheal incisions have been used. Quite frequently, a window is made by unroofing the second or third tracheal ring anteriorly.

To avoid damaging the ETT cuff during tracheotomy, it is a common practice to deflate the cuff and purposely advance the ETT distally into the right mainstem bronchus prior to making an incision in the trachea. Following tracheal access, the ETT is withdrawn under direct vision to just above the tracheotomy site by the practitioner. Superior retraction on the cephalad tracheal ring with a tracheal hook and spreading of the tracheal incision facilitates subsequent insertion of the tracheotomy tube.

Endotracheal positioning is confirmed by connecting the tracheotomy tube to the ventilatory circuit and monitoring for the presence of end-tidal CO_2 and bilateral breath sounds on auscultation. These final measures, in addition to assessing lung compliance and airway pressures, are ascertained prior to the complete removal of the ETT. The tracheotomy tube is then secured with sutures, and a tie passed around the neck.[11]

32.4.3.2 Percutaneous Dilational Tracheotomy

The PDT technique is easily performed at the bedside with two operators: one performing the tracheotomy while the second provides ventilation and oxygenation. It is essential to continuously monitor vital signs including pulse oximetry, blood pressure, heart rate, and rhythm. The patient should be ventilated with 100% oxygen throughout the procedure. The patient's current sedative regimen can be supplemented with an opioid and an intravenous sedative/hypnotic such as a benzodiazepine or propofol.[18] It is important to maintain immobility during insertion of the needle to prevent inadvertent puncture of the posterior tracheal wall or coughing during the insertion of the tracheotomy tube, e.g., the use of a nondepolarizing muscle relaxant, such as rocuronium. For continued mechanical ventilation during the procedure, the cuff of the ETT is deflated and adjustments to tidal volume, respiratory rate, and PEEP are made to compensate for the air leak. At our institution, the patient is manually ventilated with an Ambu bag with 100% oxygen throughout.

Flexible fiberoptic bronchoscopy through the ETT to facilitate PDT insertion was introduced in 1989.[19] Bronchoscopy allows indirect visualization of the needle entering the trachea by helping to confirm its location in the midline at the correct tracheal interspace, as well as ensuring that the ETT is not punctured or impaled, and minimizes the risk of damaging the posterior tracheal wall.[16] In the case of accidental premature extubation, the bronchoscope can also be used to guide ETT reinsertion. There may also be a role for videoscopic bronchoscopy during teaching as there is a "learning curve" associated with performing PDT.[13] The disadvantages of fiberoptic bronchoscopy include difficulties with ventilation and oxygenation leading to hypercarbia and hypoxia[16] and the potential for damage to the bronchoscope by the needle or guidewire.

Alternative methods have been advocated of confirming adequate ETT withdrawal prior to tracheal puncture. These include use of direct laryngoscopy with a tube exchanger, ETT cuff palpation, and premeasured blind withdrawal.[16] In 2000, our group described a technique using the Trachlight™ (Laerdal Medical Inc., Wappingers Fall, NY), a common and inexpensive intubation device, as an alternative to bronchoscopy to facilitate the PDT. In order to place the lightbulb of the Trachlight™ at the tip of the ETT, the number markings on the Trachlight™ wand shaft must be aligned with those on the ETT. Anterior neck transillumination[20] can then be used to confirm adequate withdrawal of the ETT prior to the needle puncture.

Since the original report of PDT by Ciaglia, the procedure has undergone three modifications. These include the movement of the tracheal cannulation site to one or two interspaces caudal to the cricoid cartilage; the use of fiberoptic bronchoscopy; and the use of a single, beveled dilator instead of multiple dilators.[16] While

---

*For techniques to manage an emergency surgical airway, see Chapter 12.

currently several kits are available for the Ciaglia single dilator technique, only the Ciaglia Blue Rhino™ kit (Cook Critical Care®, Bloomington, IN) will be presented.

If time permits, as in a nonurgent situation, the neck is extended and the surgical field is aseptically prepared (Figure 32-2A). The tracheotomy tube cuff must be checked for leaks and then well lubricated. The first or second tracheal interspace is located and local anesthetic injected. A vertical skin incision is made in the midline from the level of the cricoid cartilage downward 1–1.5 cm (Figure 32-2B). The wound is dissected bluntly to the subcutaneous fascia using a hemostat. The ETT should be withdrawn to 1 cm above the anticipated needle insertion site under bronchoscopic or transillumination guidance. A 17-gauge sheathed introducer needle is advanced in the midline, in a posterior and caudad direction. The tracheal air column is identified when air is aspirated into a syringe filled with fluid (e.g., lidocaine) (Figure 32-2C). The outer sheath is advanced into the trachea while the introducer needle is removed. At this time, the ETT is advanced and withdrawn 1 cm to verify that the needle does not concomitantly move, to rule out inadvertent impalement of the ETT. A syringe is then reattached to the sheath and its position in the trachea is reconfirmed by free flow of air. The syringe is removed and a 1.32 mm diameter J-wire is advanced through the sheath into the trachea caudally (Figure 32-2D). The sheath is then removed. Although not specified by the manufacturer, in our experience, it is beneficial to make a second cut around the guidewire with the scalpel to provide room for the dilator. A short 14 French introducing minidilator is advanced over the guidewire using a slight twisting motion and then removed. After soaking in water, the Ciaglia Blue Rhino Dilator™ is then advanced over the guidewire while the wire position is maintained (Figure 32-2E). The dilator and guidewire are advanced together into the trachea up to the black skin-level mark. The dilator is withdrawn and advanced several times to help create the stoma, whereupon it is removed. The lubricated tracheotomy tube with its dilator as a unit is then inserted over the guidewire and advanced until it reaches the flange (Figures 32-2F and G). The guidewire and dilator are then removed leaving the tracheotomy tube in place (Figure 32-2H). The cuff of the tracheotomy tube is inflated and connected to a ventilator or an Ambu bag device (Figure 32-2I). Once correct intratracheal placement of the tracheotomy tube has been confirmed by end-tidal CO_2, the translaryngeal ETT is removed.

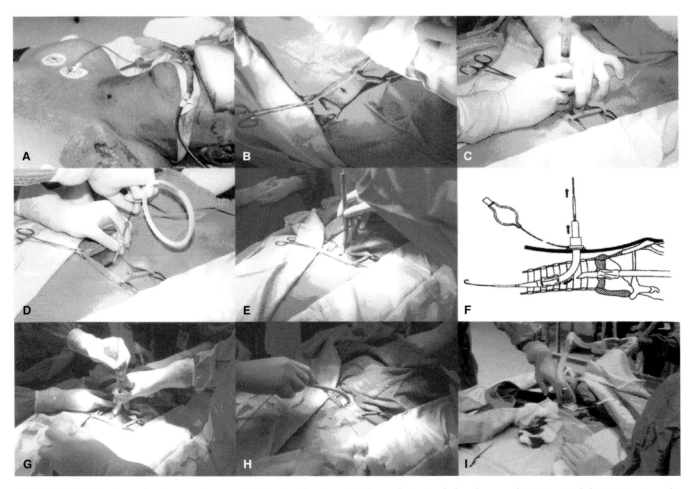

FIGURE 32-2. Steps in performing percutaneous dilational tracheotomy: (A) The neck is extended and prepped; (B) A vertical skin incision is made in the midline from the level of the cricoid cartilage downward 1–1.5 cm; (C) An introducer needle is inserted into the trachea with a syringe and aspirated until a free flow of air is obtained; (D) A J-wire is guided into the trachea caudally through the needle; (E) A dilator is advanced over the guidewire; (F, G) The tracheotomy tube and dilator are advanced as a unit over the guidewire into the trachea. (F Reproduced with permission from Cook Critical Care, Bloomington, IN); (H) The dilator is then removed leaving the tracheotomy tube in place; and (I) The cuff of the tracheotomy tube is inflated and correct intratracheal placement is confirmed by end-tidal CO_2 prior to connecting the tracheotomy tube to the ventilator.

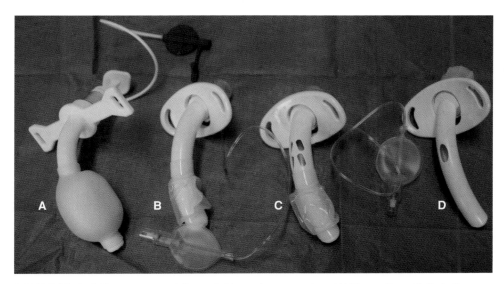

FIGURE 32-3. Different commercially available tracheotomy tubes: (A) Bivona Foam-Cuffed silicone tube (Bivona Medical Technologies, Gary, IN). (B) Shiley cuffed nonfenestrated tube (Shiley Mallinckrodt, St. Louis, MO). (C) Shiley cuffed fenestrated tube (Shiley Mallinckrodt, St. Louis, MO). (D) Shiley uncuffed fenestrated tube (Shiley Mallinckrodt, St. Louis, MO).

Three other PDT techniques have been developed.[16] The Rapitrach method had a high rate of posterior tracheal wall lacerations and balloon cuff tears and was subsequently removed from the US market.[16] It used a dilating tracheostome with blades designed to slide over the guidewire into the trachea. When squeezed, the blades opened to create a stoma.[21] The Griggs technique uses a Howard-Kelly Forceps that is introduced into the tracheal lumen using a guidewire.[22] A stoma is created when the forceps are opened, similar to the Rapitrach method, but without a cutting blade. This technique is popular in South America and Europe.[16] The third method is a translaryngeal approach developed by Fantoni and Ripamonti.[23] With this technique, a guidewire is inserted retrograde into the tracheal space and pulled out through the mouth. A trocar-tracheotomy tube with a pointed tip is then advanced over the wire and with traction applied to the guidewire; the trocar-tracheotomy tube assembly is advanced through the mouth into the trachea. A pretracheal incision is then made over the skin so that the trocar end of the tracheotomy tube can be pulled through the anterior neck. The trocar is then cut away leaving the tracheotomy tube in place. This technique avoids the downward direction of dilation and thus may minimize damage to the posterior tracheal wall.[16]

32.4.4 Describe and compare different tracheotomy tubes. Which tube should be chosen for this patient?

In selecting a tracheotomy tube, patient anatomy and ventilatory needs must be considered. These needs will influence choice of tube diameter and length, cuff design, use of an inner cannula, and presence or absence of a fenestration. Sizing usually refers to the inner diameter. The smallest outer diameter that satisfies the requirement for ventilation should be chosen.[11] Optimal sizing should aim for a tracheotomy tube approximately three-quarters of the diameter of the tracheal lumen.

In this case presentation, the indication for tracheotomy is prolonged intubation and ventilation, and therefore a cuffed tube that seals the airway and prevents loss of tidal volume represents a good selection. An example of such a cannula is a No. 6 Shiley (Mallinckrodt, St. Louis, MO) with a large-volume, low-pressure, air-filled cuff (Figure 32-3B).[11] It is important to maintain an inflated cuff pressure of less than 30 cm H_2O to prevent tracheal mucosal ischemia and minimize the risk of erosion. Once the patient is weaned from the ventilator, conversion to a fenestrated tube (Figure 32-3C) might be appropriate because it reduces resistance to the flow of air through the lumen of the tube, enabling vocalization.[11] Another option is to downsize the nonfenestrated tracheotomy tube which permits the patient to vocalize, while minimizing the risk of granulation tissue formation at the site of the fenestration. This choice often represents an individual preference based on the experience practitioner. Excessive granulation tissue can cause tracheotomy tube obstruction and may produce impressive bleeding from the airway.

The obese patient requires special consideration. Standard tracheotomy tubes are unlikely to conform to the anatomy of these patients meaning that a better choice might be a flexible tube which is extra long and adjustable.[11] The disadvantage of these tubes is that they have a single lumen without an inner cannula. They do have the advantage of minimizing risks of an inappropriately fitted tube, such as tube obstruction if the tube is too short, or necrosis of the anterior tracheal wall if too long.

32.4.5 What are the advantages of performing PDT over TT?

In general, the complications of PDT are few and are comparable to TT.[24] Theoretical advantages of PDT include a smaller skin incision, less dissection, and tissue trauma that leads to less hemorrhage, fewer infections, fewer tracheal problems, and fewer cosmetic deformities. Additionally, the procedure can be performed at the bedside, by nonsurgical personnel, decreasing the risks inherent in patient transport to the operating room. Furthermore, there is less overall cost and fewer personnel demands.[10,17,25]

The disadvantages of performing PDT in the ICU relate mainly to lack of proper facilities and equipment. Poor lighting conditions and a crowded environment can be hazardous. The risks of performing tracheotomy outside the operating room can be minimized by proper preparation of a readily available backup surgical set including drapes, tracheotomy tubes, portable electrocautery, and a surgical lamp. A difficult airway cart should be immediately available with anesthetic drugs, including muscle relaxants.

32.5   COMPLICATIONS

32.5.1   What are the contraindications from performing a PDT?

Physiologic contraindications include a patient who is hemodynamically unstable, requires an $FiO_2 > 0.60$, PEEP > 10 cm H_2O,[4] or has an uncontrolled coagulopathy.[3] Anatomic contraindications include a previously documented difficult tracheal intubation, morbid obesity, obscure cervical anatomy, goiter, short thick neck, previous tracheotomy or neck surgery, cervical infection, facial and cervical trauma and fractures, halo traction, or known presence of SGS.[3,4] Although it is controversial, PDT has been shown to be safe in the morbidly obese and in those patients who have undergone a previous tracheotomy.[26]

32.5.2   What are the complications of PDT compared to TT?

Complications common to both PDT and TT are listed in Table 32-1. Two meta-analyses have been published comparing PDT to TT.[10,25] In their comparison of TT and PDT trials from 1985 to 1996, Dulguerov et al.[10] showed that perioperative complications were more frequent with PDT (PDT 10% vs. TT 3%), whereas postoperative complications occurred more often with TT (TT 10% vs. PDT 7%). The major differences were seen in minor complications; however, perioperative death (PDT 0.44% vs. ST 0.03%) and serious cardiorespiratory events (PDT 0.33% vs. ST 0.06%) were higher in the PDT trials. Freeman et al.[25] analyzed data from five prospective trials that compared PDT performed using the Ciaglia method[15] to TT. No difference was found in the operative complication rate. However, PDT was associated with less perioperative and postoperative bleeding and stoma infection, resulting in an overall lower postoperative complication rate. Mortality rates did not differ between the two techniques. The differences in the findings of these two meta-analyses could be attributed to the fact that Dulguerov et al. included randomized studies of all PDT techniques, which may have different complication rates.[3]

32.6   POSTINTUBATION MANAGEMENT

32.6.1   What should be done immediately after the placement of a PDT?

Following insertion of the tracheotomy tube, one must ensure that the tube is properly positioned and well secured until the tract has healed, usually requiring approximately 7 days. Because PDT is a dilational technique, creation of a false passage may easily occur. Should accidental decannulation occur within the first 7 days of PDT, and if a tracheal tube is needed, an oral ETT should be immediately placed instead of attempting reinsertion of a tracheotomy tube through the stoma.[27] Chest x-ray following the procedure is somewhat controversial: studies have shown that the incidence of pneumothorax following endoscopically guided PDT is less than 3%, while when nonguided, it may range up to 12%.[28] However, because no compelling prospective data to the contrary exist at this time, postprocedure chest x-ray should be routine.

TABLE 32-1

Complications of Tracheotomy[3,4,11]

INTRAOPERATIVE	POSTOPERATIVE (<24 H)	UP TO 2 WK	WK TO MO
Damage to great vessels	Tube dislodgement with loss of airway	Peristomal cellulitis	Suprastomal or tracheal granulation tissue with airway obstruction
Injury to posterior tracheal wall	Tube occlusion by dried secretions	Stomal granulation tissue	Poor stomal healing
Injury to cupula of lung with pneumothorax	Stomal hemorrhage	Stomal hemorrhage	Subglottic or tracheal stenosis
Tracheal ring rupture	Cuff leak		Tracheomalacia
Recurrent laryngeal nerve injury			Tracheoesophageal fistula
Paratracheal insertion			Tracheoinnominate fistula
Fire in the airway			

32.6.2 Discuss the special care of a tracheotomy tube

Surgical cannulation of the trachea will cause an increase in airway secretions requiring frequent suctioning of the tracheotomy tube.[27] The suction catheter should be measured so that suctioning beyond the tip of the tracheotomy tube is not performed. If this simple measure is followed, then subsequent risks of deep suctioning will be eliminated. The risks of deep suctioning include tracheal excoriation, bleeding, ulceration and tracheitis, production of granulation tissue, and scarring of the bronchi and carina.

Creation of a tracheotomy bypasses the nose so that supplemental humidity and filtering of the air must be provided.[27] Humidity, in conjunction with tracheal irrigation, will prevent encrusting of tracheal secretions and minimize mucus plugging of the tracheotomy tube. A filter may be placed on the tracheotomy tube to remove particulate matter in the air and from the ventilator.

The first tracheotomy tube change is usually performed on approximately the seventh day postcannulation. The tract is sufficiently mature at this time to minimize the risk of creating a false passage[27] and will also allow proper examination and cleaning of the stoma. The tracheotomy tube should be changed on a routine basis thereafter, between 1 and 4 weeks, depending on patient care needs.

32.7 SPECIAL CONSIDERATIONS

32.7.1 Should PDT be performed in the pediatric population?

Traditionally, PDT is not recommended for individuals younger than 16 years of age, the main drawbacks being the small airway diameter and the pronounced pliability of the cartilaginous framework. Fantoni and Ripamonti[29] have performed trials comparing three different techniques in the pediatric population, one of which consisted of PDT guided by rigid bronchoscopy. This eliminated the main cartilaginous compliance issue seen in the pediatric population and elevated the trachea to a more superficial position, facilitating cannulation. Ideally, any surgical technique in the pediatric population should be performed in the operating room with specialized surgical staff and anesthesia support. PDT remains experimental in the pediatric patient population, but in experienced hands with the use of a rigid bronchoscope, an overall reduction in complications is noted. These include smaller operative incisions in the skin and trachea, less blood loss, and virtual elimination of pleural dome injury and posterior tracheal wall trauma.[29]

32.7.2 Can you perform a PDT in a patient with subglottic stenosis?

Subglottic stenosis (SGS) is a known late complication of prolonged intubation or any type of tracheotomy. However, little has been published on the use of PDT in a patient with SGS. SGS is a graded problem, ranging from mild asymptomatic stenosis to complete obstruction. If the stenosis exceeds 50–75% of the lumen diameter, then the patient may be quite symptomatic, possibly requiring acute airway intervention. In known cases of SGS, optimal airway control may be achieved with an extra-long, small, noncuffed pediatric ETT, or more likely a controlled tracheotomy performed on an awake patient or over a rigid bronchoscope.

It would be most imprudent to undertake PDT in the face of SGS as the vertical length, or thickness, of the stenosis may not be known even if the diameter is not significantly narrowed. To maximize patient safety and minimize otherwise preventable complications from PDT, this technique should not be used in a patient with known SGS.

32.7.3 What is the role of an extraglottic device in providing oxygenation and ventilation while performing the PDT?

To avoid the risk of an inadvertent puncture of the ETT cuff by the needle, tube transfixion, or accidental extubation, some reports suggest the use of an extraglottic airway device during the placement of the PDT. During the last decade, the laryngeal mask airway (LMA), intubating LMA (ILMA), LMA ProSeal™, Cobra PLA™, Airway Management Device (AMD™), and the Combitube™ have all been used successfully during PDT placement.[30-36]

While these extraglottic devices may have a theoretical advantage over the ETT in ventilating critically ill patients during PDT, they also have limitations. The placement of these devices may sometimes be difficult. In a prospective comparative study with patients using an ETT, Ambesh et al. showed that 33% of patients using the LMA during the PDT suffered potentially catastrophic complications.[37] These included loss of the airway, inadequate ventilation resulting in hypoxemia, gastric distension, and regurgitation. In contrast, there were substantially fewer complications in the ETT group.

Until more clinical efficacy and safety data are available concerning the use of these extraglottic devices, an in-place ETT remains the best option during PDT as it would appear to be a safer practice than removing the ETT to replace it with an extraglottic device in ventilated, critically ill patients with low lung compliance, airway edema, cervical spine instability, or a difficult airway. However, in the event that the airway is lost or in the presence of an accidental extubation, these extraglottic devices may play an important role in oxygenating these patients while continuing with the PDT.

32.8 SUMMARY

Mechanically ventilated patients in the intensive care setting frequently require a tracheotomy to minimize long-term airway complications. During the last two decades, elective PDT has been shown to be an effective and safe alternative to the TT. Theoretical advantages of PDT over the TT include less tissue trauma, fewer infections, fewer tracheal problems, and fewer cosmetic deformities. In addition, the procedure can be performed at the bedside, by nonsurgical personnel, decreasing the inherent risks of patient transport to the operating room with less overall cost and fewer demands on personnel. However, practitioners should also be aware of the disadvantages of performing PDT in the intensive care unit. These include a lack of proper facilities and equipment, poor lighting conditions, and a crowded environment.

REFERENCES

1. Sue RD, Susanto I: Long-term complications of artificial airways. *Clin Chest Med.* 2003;24:457–471.
2. Liu H, Chen JC, Holinger LD, Gonzalez-Crussi F: Histopathologic fundamentals of acquired laryngeal stenosis. *Pediatr Pathol Lab Med.* 1995;15:655–677.
3. Heffner JE: Tracheotomy application and timing. *Clin Chest Med.* 2003;24:389–98.
4. Angel LF, Simpson CB: Comparison of surgical and percutaneous dilational tracheotomy. *Clin Chest Med.* 2003;24:423–429.
5. Block C, Brechner VL: Unusual problems in airway management. II. The influence of the temporomandibular joint, the mandible, and associated structures on endotracheal intubation. *Anesth Analg.* 1971;50:114–123.
6. Boorin MR: Unanticipated difficult endotracheal intubation related to preexisting chin implant and mandibular condylar resorption. *Anesth Analg.* 1997;84:686–689.
7. Coonan TJ, Hope CE, Howes WJ, Holness RO, MacInnis EL: Ankylosis of the temporo-mandibular joint after temporal craniotomy: a cause of difficult intubation. *Can Anaesth Soc J.* 1985;32:158–160.
8. Francois B, Clavel M, Desachy A, et al.: Complications of tracheostomy performed in the ICU: subthyroid tracheostomy vs surgical cricothyroidotomy. *Chest.* 2003;123:151–158.
9. Bowen CP, Whitney LR, Truwit JD, Durbin CG, Moore MM: Comparison of safety and cost of percutaneous versus surgical tracheostomy. *Am Surg.* 2001;67:54–60.
10. Dulguerov P, Gysin C, Perneger TV, Chevrolet JC: Percutaneous or surgical tracheostomy: a meta-analysis. *Crit Care Med.* 1999;27:1617–1625.
11. Walts PA, Murthy SC, DeCamp MM: Techniques of surgical tracheostomy. *Clin Chest Med.* 2003;24:413–422.
12. Shelden CH, Pudenz RH, Freshwater DB, Crue BL: A new method for tracheotomy. *J Neurosurg.* 1955;12:428–431.
13. Powell DM, Price PD, Forrest LA: Review of percutaneous tracheostomy. *Laryngoscope.* 1998;108:170–177.
14. Toye FJ, Weinstein JD: Clinical experience with percutaneous tracheostomy and cricothyroidotomy in 100 patients. *J Trauma.* 1986;26:1034–1040.
15. Ciaglia P, Firsching R, Syniec C: Elective percutaneous dilatational tracheostomy. A new simple bedside procedure; preliminary report. *Chest.* 1985;87:715–719.
16. deBoisblanc BP: Percutaneous dilational tracheostomy techniques. *Clin Chest Med.* 2003;24:399–407.
17. Ciaglia P, Graniero KD: Percutaneous dilatational tracheostomy. Results and long-term follow-up. *Chest.* 1992;101:464–467.
18. Schwann NM: Percutaneous dilational tracheostomy: anesthetic considerations for a growing trend. *Anesth Analg.* 1997;84:907–911.
19. Paul A, Marelli D, Chiu RC, Vestweber KH, Mulder DS: Percutaneous endoscopic tracheostomy. *Ann Thorac Surg.* 1989;47:314–315.
20. Addas BM, Howes WJ, Hung OR: Light-guided tracheal puncture for percutaneous tracheostomy. *Can J Anaesth.* 2000;47:919–922.
21. Schachner A, Ovil J, Sidi J, Avram A, Levy MJ: Rapid percutaneous tracheostomy. *Chest.* 1990;98:1266–1270.
22. Griggs WM, Worthley LI, Gilligan JE, Thomas PD, Myburg JA: A simple percutaneous tracheostomy technique. *Surg Gynecol Obstet.* 1990;170:543–545.
23. Fantoni A, Ripamonti D: A non-derivative, non-surgical tracheostomy: the translaryngeal method. *Intensive Care Med.* 1997;23:386–392.
24. Feller-Kopman D: Acute complications of artificial airways. *Clin Chest Med.* 2003;24:445–455.
25. Freeman BD, Isabella K, Lin N, Buchman TG: A meta-analysis of prospective trials comparing percutaneous and surgical tracheostomy in critically ill patients. *Chest.* 2000;118:1412–1418.
26. Ernst A, Critchlow J: Percutaneous tracheostomy—special considerations. *Clin Chest Med.* 2003;24:409–412.
27. Wright SE, VanDahm K: Long-term care of the tracheostomy patient. *Clin Chest Med.* 2003;24:473–487.
28. Gonzalez I, Bonner S: Routine chest radiographs after endoscopically guided percutaneous dilatational tracheostomy. *Chest.* 2004;125:1173–1174.
29. Fantoni A, Ripamonti D: [Tracheostomy in pediatrics patients]. *Minerva Anestesiol.* 2002;68:433–442.
30. Dexter TJ: The laryngeal mask airway: a method to improve visualisation of the trachea and larynx during fibreoptic assisted percutaneous tracheostomy. *Anaesth Intensive Care.* 1994;22:35–39.
31. Lyons BJ, Flynn CG: The laryngeal mask simplifies airway management during percutaneous dilational tracheostomy. *Acta Anaesthesiol Scand.* 1995;39:414–415.
32. Verghese C, Rangasami J, Kapila A, Parke T: Airway control during percutaneous dilatational tracheostomy: pilot study with the intubating laryngeal mask airway. *Br J Anaesth.* 1998;81:608–609.
33. Craven RM, Laver SR, Cook TM, Nolan JP: Use of the Pro-Seal LMA facilitates percutaneous dilatational tracheostomy. *Can J Anaesth.* 2003;50:718–720.
34. Agro F, Carassiti M, Magnani C: Percutaneous dilatational cricothyroidotomy: airway control via CobraPLA. *Anesth Analg.* 2004;99:628.
35. Johnson R, Bailie R: Airway management device (AMD) for airway control in percutaneous dilatational tracheostomy. *Anaesthesia.* 2000;55:596–597.
36. Mallick A, Quinn AC, Bodenham AR, Vucevic M: Use of the Combitube for airway maintenance during percutaneous dilatational tracheostomy. *Anaesthesia.* 1998;53:249–255.
37. Ambesh SP, Sinha PK, Tripathi M, Matreja P: Laryngeal mask airway vs endotracheal tube to facilitate bedside percutaneous tracheostomy in critically ill patients: a prospective comparative study. *J Postgrad Med.* 2002;48:11–15.

SELF-EVALUATION QUESTIONS

32.1. You are asked to assist in a percutaneous dilational tracheotomy on the 28-year-old female in the ICU. The surgeon has just inserted the tracheotomy tube and you are ventilating the patient using an Ambu bag through the ETT that you have pulled back to 1 cm above the tracheotomy insertion site. Once the tracheotomy tube is in place, you connect the Ambu bag to the tracheotomy tube and start to ventilate the patient. However, you notice that there is a lot of resistance to ventilation, the oxygen saturation is slowly declining, and there is some subcutaneous emphysema in the neck area. What is your immediate response?

   A. remove the tracheotomy tube and the ETT and begin bag-mask-ventilation

   B. tell the surgeon to reinsert the tracheotomy tube

   C. tell the surgeon to prepare for a surgical cricothyrotomy

   D. push the ETT into the trachea 2–4 cm and ventilate through the ETT

   E. assess the location of the tracheotomy tube using a fiberoptic bronchoscope

32.2. You have secured the airway and placed the patient back on the ventilator. About 5 minutes later while you are catching up on your charting, the ventilator starts to alarm high airway pressures and the blood pressure has declined. Auscultation reveals decreased breath sounds on the right. What do you do next?

A. administer 500 mL of Ringers Lactate intravenously and vasopressor to raise the propofol-induced hypotension

B. call for a chest x-ray

C. fiberoptic bronchoscopy to remove mucus plugs

D. do a needle decompression in the midclavicular line at the right second intercostal space of the chest

E. perform CPR

32.3. Complications of percutaneous dilational tracheotomy include all of the following **EXCEPT**

A. hemorrhage

B. pneumothorax

C. tracheal rupture

D. subglottic stenosis

E. glossopharyngeal nerve injury

CHAPTER (33)

Uncooperative Down Syndrome Patient

Michael F. Murphy

33.1 CASE PRESENTATION

This 43-year-old white female patient with Down Syndrome (Figure 33-1) has had repeated episodes of aspiration pneumonia felt to be related to grossly carious teeth and is scheduled for a full mouth dental extraction. Her sister has cared for her for the past 20 years (parents are deceased). As far as her sister knows, she is perfectly healthy and has never had an anesthetic before. She is on no medication and has no allergies. She does not smoke.

On examination, she is 5′2″ (157.5 cm) tall and weighs (210 lb) (96 kg) with a moderately severe mental handicap. Vital signs are normal with a blood pressure of 120/80 mm Hg and the oxygen saturation on room air is 99%. She is not cooperative and will not permit an IV to be started. She does not answer questions. She sits with her head flexed forward and will not extend her neck when requested, nor will she permit you to. Her sister does not know if she can extend it or not. She will not open her mouth as per your request. Blood work done one week ago is normal as is the ECG. She had a normal echocardiogram, performed because you had requested it preoperatively.

She will require a general anesthetic with an endotracheal tube, preferably passed nasally.

33.2 PATIENT EVALUATION

33.2.1 What kind of vital organ system reserve does this patient have?

Cardiovascular reserve. There is nothing on history or examination to suggest any problem with the cardiovascular reserve.

Her echocardiogram does not reveal any evidence of an endocardial cushion defect.

CNS reserve. She is moderately disabled and may be anticipated to awaken slowly or combatively. Her response to sedative hypnotic agents and ketamine for sedation is unpredictable.

Respiratory system reserve. She is moderately obese and is expected to have some restrictive lung disease with predictable consequences. Postoperative mechanical ventilation is not anticipated, though postoperative supplemental oxygen should be readily available.

33.3 AIRWAY EVALUATION AND MANAGEMENT OPTIONS

33.3.1 Employing the mnemonics suggested in Chapter 1, does this patient have a difficult airway?

On MOANS guided airway evaluation (see Section 1.6.1), you gain no confidence that you will be able to ventilate this patient using a bag-mask-ventilation (BMV) when it becomes necessary. If her neck cannot be extended, a *mask* seal will be difficult. She is *obese* and the *stiffness* of her lungs (decrease in compliance) may hinder BMV.

Employing LEMON (see Section 1.6.2) to assess the difficulty of laryngoscopy and intubation reveals that the *look* of this patient suggests difficulty. When you attempt to *evaluate* the geometry of her upper airway, you are unable to assess the volume of her mandibular space. This is particularly problematic in a person with Down Syndrome where the impression is that the tongue is relatively large for the volume of the mouth to begin with. You also

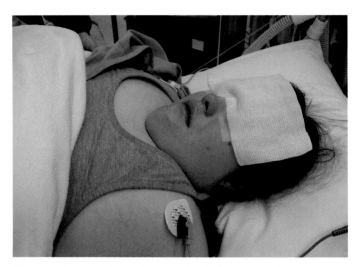

FIGURE 33-1. This figure illustrates the challenges that the airway practitioner faces in managing the airway of this moderately obese, uncooperative patient with Down Syndrome who requires a general anesthetic for dental extraction.

have no idea where her larynx is relative to the base of her tongue. You are unable to evaluate a *Mallampati* and get some idea as to airway access. Additionally, she is *obese* and you are unable to evaluate the degree of *neck* mobility.

The mnemonic for difficulties in using extraglottic devices (EGD) is RODS (see Section 1.6.3). Whether there is *restricted* mouth opening or not is unknown. There does not appear to be any upper-airway *obstruction* and the airway is neither *distorted* nor *disrupted*. As mentioned above, she is obese and the decreased compliance ("*stiff*") may mitigate against successful ventilation with an EGD.

Finally, the patient should be assessed for a potentially difficult cricothyrotomy using the mnemonic SHORT (see Section 1.6.4). There is no history of prior anterior neck *surgery, hematoma,* or other overlying process that masks the anatomy. However, she is *obese*, and in addition, one is unable to ascertain whether access to the anterior neck is possible. There is no history or evidence of *radiation* or *tumor*.

In summary, she has a potentially difficult airway and is not a candidate for a rapid sequence induction.

33.3.2 What other airway concerns do you have in patients with Down Syndrome?

An increased incidence of subglottic stenosis in Down Syndrome patients is well known.[1–4] It has been attributed, at least in part, to the increased incidence of regurgitation and aspiration in these patients during infancy and early childhood.[1] These patients may require an endotracheal tube that is one to two sizes smaller than the standard size appropriate for the patient's age.

In addition, the Down Syndrome patient is predisposed to obstructive sleep apnea due to a relatively narrow nasopharynx and large tongue.[5,6]

C-spine subluxation is also seen in these patients and may be of concern in airway management.[7] Presently there is no consensus of

opinion with respect to the need for preoperative radiological evaluation of the cervical spine for subluxation for patients with Down Syndrome.

33.3.3 What are the airway management options?

This patient gives every indication that the management of her airway will be difficult. However, the more pressing problem is deciding how to pharmacologically manage her behavior and airway in a controlled fashion without compromising her ability to maintain ventilation and oxygenation.

Ideally, one would like to identify a preferable airway technique (Plan A), and two alternative methods (Plans B and C). However, with the limited airway evaluation, the most appropriate method chosen must have the least chance of producing apnea, aspiration, or a requirement for rapid action. This really leaves two primary options for consideration:

1. Sedation and awake intubation employing an intubating device other than a laryngoscope (e.g., a flexible fiberoptic bronchoscope—FFB).
2. Tracheal intubation utilizing an intubating device other than a laryngoscope under general anesthesia, employing an inhalation induction.

No matter which route is chosen, a variety of alternative airway devices must be immediately available, particularly an intubating laryngeal mask, a Trachlight™, and a cricothyrotomy kit.

33.4 MANAGING THE AIRWAY

33.4.1 What are the "pros and cons" of each method?

As there is no IV access, Option 2 (inhalation induction) may be potentially hazardous given that many individuals may be needed to restrain the patient which constitutes a certain loss of control. In addition, an inhalation induction creates the hazard of the excitement phase and its potential to lead to deadly laryngospasm. Intramuscular (IM) or oral (PO) ketamine may be employed to facilitate mask induction in this uncooperative patient.

Option 1 is also not without hazards. The use of sedative hypnotic agents in large PO or IM dosages may provoke paradoxical excitement, or worse, lead to hypoventilation or apnea. Ketamine is an attractive option in that 7 mg·kg^{-1} (ideal body weight)[8–11] can be given orally with the expectation that the patient will be dissociated within 20 minutes, at least to the point that an IV can be started. If the degree of cooperation is not sufficient after this dose, half the original dose can be repeated at 20 minutes. The margin of safety with ketamine is greater when administered in this manner compared to sedative hypnotics such as midazolam, as it preserves ventilatory function, muscle tone, and airway protective reflexes. The disadvantages of ketamine include the risk of laryngospasm, increase in secretions, emergence reactions, and postprocedure nausea and vomiting.

33.4.2 How exactly would you manage the airway of this patient?

1. Preprocedure preparations:

   - An FFB is prepared; a 7 mm ID endotracheal tube (ETT) is placed in a bottle of warmed sterile saline to soften it; and four 5 mL syringes with 1% lidocaine are prepared to be injected as needed through the FFB. The tip of the FFB is placed in a bottle of warmed saline to prevent fogging during the procedure.

   - 0.25% phenylephrine nasal spray and 5% lidocaine ointment are immediately available, and 3 mL of Lidocaine 4% is prepared in a Mucosal Atomization Device (MAD) atomizer (Wolfe Tory Medical, Salt Lake City, UT).

   - Ketamine 1 mL (50 mg) is diluted to 5 mL with saline in a 10 mL syringe and 5 mL of propofol 10 mg·mL^{-1} is added to the same syringe. The resulting mix is 5 mg·mL^{-1} of each drug. Four of these syringes are prepared.

   - Propofol 20 mL and succinylcholine 140 mg are drawn up.

   - The following airway devices are immediately available.

     ◦ LMA Fastrach™ (Intubating LMA)
     ◦ Trachlight™ loaded onto a 7 mm ID ETT cut at 26 cm
     ◦ Cricothyrotomy kit (ready but not opened)

2. The patient is seated initially. In the operating room holding area (with the prepared equipment immediately available), the patient's sister administers ketamine 500 mg in two ounces of apple juice orally with the airway practitioner beside her. An antisialogogue is not administered due to the fact that it must be administered intramuscularly (see below). A pulse oximeter is applied when the patient permits, as is supplemental oxygen by mask or nasal prongs. Within 20 minutes, the patient ought to be sufficiently sedated, or perhaps even dissociated to permit the placement of an IV using local anesthetic, and placed supine (if she permits).

3. With the patient dissociated or near dissociated, she is moved into the operating room and onto the operating room table. Supplemental IV ketamine/propofol is titrated carefully to maintain spontaneous ventilation and continuing airway protection. Phenylephrine 0.25% is sprayed in the larger nostril. Two to three minutes later, 4% lidocaine is atomized into the nostril employing the MAD. A tongue depressor is used to access the oral cavity and 4% lidocaine atomized to the posterior pharynx. 4% lidocaine is sprayed over the back of the tongue, and atomized solution is delivered into the airway to coincide with inspiration.

4. A nasopharyngeal airway (#6 or #7) is gently and fully inserted into the selected nostril to dilate it. Immediately after the nasopharyngeal airway is withdrawn, the softened ETT is inserted to a point just beyond the posterior nasopharynx.

5. The FFB is inserted through the ETT to visualize the glottis. Supplemental topical 1% lidocaine is injected through the FFB as required to enter the trachea. The FFB is advanced to a point just above the carina and the ETT advanced over the FFB into the trachea. Propofol and succinylcholine are administered rapidly after the airway is secured and confirmed.

33.5 ADDITIONAL CONSIDERATIONS

33.5.1 Should an antisialogogue be given when ketamine is employed?

As a general comment, antisialogues are typically used whenever topical anesthesia of the oro- and hypopharynx is to be attempted because it minimizes the dilution of local anesthetic agent by saliva and improves the degree of topical anesthesia achieved. In this particular case, it was omitted because it would have required an IM injection.

Ketamine does stimulate tracheobronchial and salivary secretions, and this effect of the drug is theorized to be a precipitating factor for laryngospasm.[12] An antisialogogue such as glycopyrrolate or atropine is often given 15–20 minutes prior to the administration of ketamine to reduce these secretions. Glycopyrrolate is preferred because it produces less intense tachycardia. Unlike other tertiary substituted antimuscarinics (scopolamine and atropine), glycopyrrolate is a polar quaternary substituted ammonium compound, which does not cross the blood–brain barrier and therefore avoids the risk of producing confusion and sedation.

33.5.2 How common is laryngospasm with ketamine?

Laryngospasm is associated with all of the sedative hypnotics to some extent, including ketamine. The incidence of laryngospasm with ketamine is about 1% (ranging between 0.017% to 1.4% in various studies including studies with data from over 11,000 patients).[13–16] It manifests as transient stridor. It is likely related to ketamine-induced sensitization of laryngeal reflexes, and in some cases is thought to be related to excessive upper respiratory secretions.[12] Thus, the recommendation has been made that an antisialogogue be coadministered with ketamine. Risk factors for laryngospasm include respiratory infection (fivefold increase) and age (three times greater risk in infants aged 1–3 months than the average).[17] One study of nearly 1,200 pediatric patients with laryngospasm reported the incidence of complications as hypoxia 3.2%, aspiration 1.1%, and cardiac arrest 0.5%.[15]

33.5.3 How common are emergence reactions with ketamine?

Emergence delirium is the most common side effect of ketamine.[18] This response is thought to be caused by the drug's depression of CNS visual/auditory relay nuclei causing altered perception and interpretation of visual and auditory stimuli.[19] The occurrence of emergence reactions is associated with age (adults > children), gender (females > males), anxiety level, and psychological state prior to the procedure.[18,20,21] The incidence varies but may be as high as 10–30% in adults with a much lower occurrence in children. Severe agitation occurs in 1.6% and mild agitation in 17.6% of pediatric patients.[19] Emergence reactions are less common in older children (12.1% in those more than 5 years vs. 22.5% in children under 5 years of age).[20]

Small doses of midazolam have been used to treat severe emergence reactions. However, the prophylactic coadministration of benzodiazepines is not recommended since they have no proven benefit, delay ketamine metabolism thereby prolonging recovery, may actually increase the incidence of recovery agitation in specific patient populations, and increase the risk of respiratory depression.[17,22–29]

33.5.4 Should these patients be recovered in a dark and quiet environment to prevent emergent reactions?

Whether or not a quiet, secluded environment which limits stimuli during the postrecovery period decreases the incidence of emergent reactions is debatable.[12] Some suggest that preprocedure discussions with the patient (adult or child) have a greater impact on reducing the incidence of recovery agitation.[12,23] However, the prevailing impression is that less stimulation is advantageous.

33.5.5 How often do patients given ketamine vomit postprocedure?

Vomiting occurs in 6.7% of patients, often persists into the recovery phase, and is also age-related, being more common in younger children (12.5% incidence in children under 5 years vs. 3.5% in those more than 5 years of age).[20] There have been no documented reports of "clinically significant" aspiration with ketamine when used in patients without contraindications.[26]

33.6 SUMMARY

This case study serves as a prototype for the uncooperative, difficult airway. In this case, it is not an emergency. Therefore, one has time to methodically plan an approach. In an emergency, one does not have the luxury of time and rigid adherence to the difficult and failed algorithms is advised.

This case melds two concurrent and important issues:

- The uncooperative patient in need of airway management,
- The difficult airway.

Patient control is achieved with oral or IM ketamine. The airway is secured employing a fiberoptic technique. The difficult airway algorithm (Chapter 2) guides individuals who do not have skills or equipment to perform fiberoptic intubation to consider an awake technique.

At each step, the imperative is to ensure that adequate gas exchange occurs and one does not "burn bridges."

REFERENCES

1. Boseley ME, Link DT, Shott SR, et al.: Laryngotracheoplasty for subglottic stenosis in Down Syndrome children: the Cincinnati experience. *Int J Pediatr Otorhinolaryngol.* 2001;57:11–15.
2. Mitchell RB, Call E, Kelly J: Diagnosis and therapy for airway obstruction in children with Down syndrome. *Arch Otolaryngol Head Neck Surg.* 2003; 129:642–645.
3. Jacobs IN, Gray RF, Todd NW: Upper airway obstruction in children with Down syndrome. *Arch Otolaryngol Head Neck Surg.* 1996;122:945–950.
4. Miller R, Gray SD, Cotton RT, Myer CM, III, Netterville J: Subglottic stenosis and Down syndrome. *Am J Otolaryngol.* 1990;11:274–277.
5. Resta O, Barbaro MP, Giliberti T, et al.: Sleep related breathing disorders in adults with Down syndrome. *Downs Syndr Res Pract.* 2003;8:115–119.
6. Dahlqvist A, Rask E, Rosenqvist CJ, Sahlin C, Franklin KA: Sleep apnea and Down's syndrome. *Acta Otolaryngol.* 2003;123:1094–1097.
7. Kanamori G, Witter M, Brown J, Williams-Smith L: Otolaryngologic manifestations of Down syndrome. *Otolaryngol Clin North Am.* 2000;33: 1285–1292.
8. Rosenberg M: Oral ketamine for deep sedation of difficult-to-manage children who are mentally handicapped: case report. *Pediatr Dent.* 1991;13:221–223.
9. Younge PA, Kendall JM: Sedation for children requiring wound repair: a randomised controlled double blind comparison of oral midazolam and oral ketamine. *Emerg Med J.* 2001;18:30–33.
10. Turhanoglu S, Kararmaz A, Ozyilmaz MA, Kaya S, Tok D: Effects of different doses of oral ketamine for premedication of children. *Eur J Anaesthesiol.* 2003;20:56–60.
11. Zane R: The morbidly obese patient. In: *Manual of Emergency Airway Management*, 2nd edn. Walls R, Murphy M, Luten R, Schneider R, eds. Philadelphia, PA: Lippincott Williams and Wilkins, 2004:302–306.
12. Green S: *Dissociative Agents, Pediatric procedural sedation and analgesia.* Kraus B, Bructowicz R, eds. Philadelphia, PA: Lippincott, Williams and Wilkins, 1999:47–54.
13. Green SM, Johnson NE: Ketamine sedation for pediatric procedures: Part 2, Review and implications. *Ann Emerg Med.* 1990;19:1033–1046.
14. Green SM, Nakamura R, Johnson NE: Ketamine sedation for pediatric procedures: Part 1, A prospective series. *Ann Emerg Med.* 1990;19:1024–1032.
15. Green SM, Rothrock SG, Lynch EL, et al.: Intramuscular ketamine for pediatric sedation in the emergency department: safety profile in 1022 cases. *Ann Emerg Med.* 1998;31:688–697.
16. Green SM, Rothrock SG, Harris T, et al.: Intravenous ketamine for pediatric sedation in the emergency department: safety profile with 156 cases. *Acad Emerg Med.* 1998;5:971–976.
17. Sachetti A, Gerardi M: *Emergency department procedural sedation and analgesia, Pediatric Emergency Medicine.* Strange G, Ahrens W, Lelyveld S, et al., eds. New York, NY: McGraw Hill, 2002:185–196.
18. Muse D: *Conscious and Deep Sedation: The Clinical Practice of Emergency Medicine.* Harwood-Nuss A, Wolfson A, Linden C, et al., eds. Philadelphia, PA: Lippincott, Williams and Wilkins, 2001:1758–1762.
19. Reeves J, Glass P, Lubarsky D: *Nonbarbiturate Intravenous Anesthetics, Anesthesia.* Miller R, Cuehiara R, Miller E, et al., eds. Philadelphia, PA: Churchill Livingstone, 2000:249–256.
20. Green SM, Kuppermann N, Rothrock SG, Hummel CB, Ho M: Predictors of adverse events with intramuscular ketamine sedation in children. *Ann Emerg Med.* 2000;35:35–42.
21. Hostetler MA, Davis CO: Prospective age-based comparison of behavioral reactions occurring after ketamine sedation in the ED. *Am J Emerg Med.* 2002;20:463–468.
22. Reich DL, Silvay G: Ketamine: an update on the first twenty-five years of clinical experience. *Can J Anaesth.* 1989;36:186–197.
23. White PF, Way WL, Trevor AJ: Ketamine-its pharmacology and therapeutic uses. *Anesthesiology.* 1982;56:119–136.
24. Wathen JE, Roback MG, Mackenzie T, Bothner JP: Does midazolam alter the clinical effects of intravenous ketamine sedation in children? A double-blind, randomized, controlled, emergency department trial. *Ann Emerg Med.* 2000;36:579–588.
25. Dachs RJ, Innes GM: Intravenous ketamine sedation of pediatric patients in the emergency department. *Ann Emerg Med.* 1997;29:146–150.
26. Green SM, Krauss B: *Procedural Sedationi and Analgesia: Clinical procedures in Emergency Medicine.* Roberts J, Hedges J, eds. Philadelphia, PA: Saunders, 2004:596–620.
27. Mace SE, Barata IA, Cravero JP, et al.: Clinical policy: evidence-based approach to pharmacologic agents used in pediatric sedation and analgesia in the emergency department. *Ann Emerg Med.* 2004;44:342–377.
28. Sherwin TS, Green SM, Khan A, Chapman DS, Dannenberg B: Does adjunctive midazolam reduce recovery agitation after ketamine sedation for pediatric procedures? A randomized, double-blind, placebo-controlled trial. *Ann Emerg Med.* 2000;35:229–238.
29. Lo JN, Cumming JF: Interaction between sedative premedicants and ketamine in man in isolated perfused rat livers. *Anesthesiology.* 1975;43: 307–312.

SELF-EVALUATION QUESTIONS

33.1. Down Syndrome patients are known to have the following attributes that may lead to failed intubation

A. obstructive sleep apnea

B. large tongue

C. tendency to have subglottic stenosis

D. C-spine subluxation

E. all of the above

33.2. Ketamine used in the uncooperative patient

A. aggravates the degree of cooperation because it is a dissociative agent

B. produces such salivation that laryngospasm is a common problem

C. is contraindicated because of the high incidence of emergency delirium

D. can be administered PO or IM

E. midazolam has been proven to reduce the incidence of ketamine-induced emergency delirium in adults and children

33.3. Oral or IM ketamine is useful in the management of the uncooperative patient. Which of the following are **TRUE?**

A. the dose of oral ketamine is 7.0 mg.kg^{-1}

B. midazolam prevents emergence reactions

C. glycopyrrolate should be coadministered with ketamine to prevent laryngospasm

D. ketamine is contraindicated in mentally challenged individuals

E. all of the above

CHAPTER (34)

Airway Management in the Operating Room of a Patient with a History of Oral and Cervical Radiation Therapy

Ian R. Morris

34.1 CASE PRESENTATION

This 68-year-old male was found on CT to have a right lung nodule and paratracheal lymphadenopathy. He presents to the operating room for bronchoscopy and mediastinoscopy.

Twenty years ago, the patient was diagnosed with carcinoma of the right submandibular gland, which was treated by excision of the gland, right radical neck dissection, and a course of radiotherapy. He subsequently developed metastatic disease in both kidneys, underwent bilateral radical nephrectomies, and is currently on chronic ambulatory peritoneal dialysis (CAPD). He also underwent wedge resection of a right lung metastasis 10 years ago.

Two months prior to this admission, he experienced an episode of chest pain relieved by nitroglycerin and associated with atrial fibrillation which converted spontaneously. There was no ECG or enzyme evidence of infarction. However, subsequent cardiac catheterization revealed critical two-vessel coronary artery disease, a mildly dilated left ventricle, and inferior hypokinesis with an ejection fraction (EF) of 39%. He was managed medically and has had no further chest pain. He complains of shortness of breath on exertion but is able to walk up to one block. He quit smoking several years ago and has had hypertension for about 5 years. His medications include: ECASA, ramipril, amlodipine, transdermal nitroglycerin, and metoprolol.

On examination, he is in no distress at rest. His vital signs are blood pressure 140/90 mm Hg, heart rate 70 bpm, and respiratory rate 18 breaths per minute. His weight is 207 lbs (94 kg) and he is 5′7″ (170 cm) tall. Auscultation of the chest reveals decreased breath sounds bilaterally but no rales or rhonchi, and normal heart sounds. No carotid bruits are evident.

Airway examination reveals a Mallampati IV classification. Mouth opening is 2.5 cm and mandibular protrusion is less than 1 cm. Full upper dentition is present but the mandible is edentulous. The thyromental distance is normal. Cervical spine extension is decreased. Palpation of the submandibular tissues reveals a woody, indurated consistency. On inspection, telangiectasia and pallor of the submandibular skin are noted. The right neck has the typical appearance of a previous neck dissection.

Laboratory data reveal a serum creatinine of 1000 μmol·L^{-1}, serum potassium of 4.5 mmol·L^{-1}, normal serum bicarbonate, and hemoglobin of 95 g·L^{-1}. ECG reveals sinus rhythm, and no evidence of previous infarction.

34.2 PATIENT CONSIDERATIONS

34.2.1 Medical considerations—is this patient fit for anesthesia?

The patient has stable ischemic heart disease on a beta blocker with decreased left ventricular function and is anephric on CAPD. His hypertension is adequately controlled for his operative procedure. His anemia probably has several causes. Carcinoma of the lung is suspected on diagnostic imaging. His medical conditions are well characterized, and he appears to be medically optimized at present.

34.2.2 Surgical considerations—what anesthetic technique is required?

General anesthesia (GA) with endotracheal intubation is required for a brief but stimulating surgical procedure.

34.2.3 Airway considerations

34.2.3.1 What Anatomic and Pathophysiologic Changes Occur Following Radiotherapy to the Structures of the Oral Cavity and Neck?

Radiotherapy inflicts a radiochemical injury to both normal and malignant cells.[1] The damage is related to total radiation dose and the method of radiotherapy delivery. In order to achieve adequate tumor control, damage to normal tissues is inevitable.[1,2] Acute tissue toxicities from radiotherapy are considered to occur within 90 days of the commencement of treatment, and late effects beyond 90 days of treatment.[3] Late effects may not be manifested until years following radiotherapy.[4] In general, tissues with rapidly dividing cell populations such as mucous membranes and skin demonstrate acute effects of radiation (mucositis, desquamation), whereas those with slowly proliferating cells such as connective tissue demonstrate late effects.[5] The severity of the late effects of radiation therapy in general cannot be predicted by the severity of the acute effects.[5]

The mechanism of late tissue toxicity may be parenchymal or stromal cell death, or irradiation injury to the microvasculature.[5] Increased vascular permeability leads to deposition of fibrin and subsequent replacement by collagen in the perivascular interstitium.[6] An increase in collagen content can be seen as early as 1 week following irradiation.[6] Following radiation therapy to the oral cavity, pharynx, or larynx, the mucous membranes can become erythematous within 1 week, and develop areas with white pseudomembranes (mucositis) at about 2 weeks.[5] The patches of mucositis may coalesce by the third week.[5] This acute mucosal reaction usually heals within 2 to 4 weeks following completion of radiotherapy, although ulceration and necrosis can occur.[4] Late effects of radiation on the mucosa are characterized by thinning or atrophy of the epithelium, telangiectasia, dryness, a loss of mucosal mobility, submucosal induration, and occasional chronic ulceration and necrosis.[6] The mucosa is fragile and more susceptible than normal to mechanical injury.[5] Edema is seen in the subcutaneous or submucosal soft tissue in the early phase following radiotherapy, can persist for 6 to 12 months,[7] and can become chronic.[3,8] Fibrosis, one of the most common delayed radiation-associated manifestations, usually appears in subcutaneous tissues within 6 to 12 months of treatment,[5] although it can occur as early as 4 to 12 weeks.[6] The fibrosis tends to be slowly progressive,[5] nonhomogeneous, and variable in extent and severity from site to site.[9] The severity of the fibrosis increases when high total doses of radiation and large fraction sizes are used.[4] The risk of developing moderate to severe fibrosis has been reported to be about 40%.[3] The affected soft tissue loses elasticity and subcutaneous fat[6] and is indurated to palpation.[1,6] In the presence of moderate to severe fibrosis, contracture of the tissues also occurs.[1] In severe cases, the soft tissues develop a woody consistency and may form a hard mass fixed to skin and underlying muscle or bone (see Figure 34-1).[5] Obstructive lymphedema may also be associated with fibrosis.[5]

Radiation therapy to the neck can produce a limitation of neck extension (see Figure 34-2).[6,10] High-dose irradiation of metastatic cervical lymphadenopathy results in more subcutaneous fibrosis in the neck than does a comparable dose in the absence of palpable

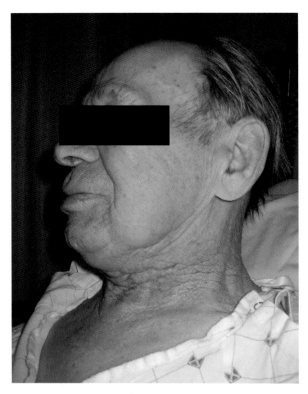

FIGURE 34-1. Appearance of the external neck following radiotherapy. The anterior neck demonstrates telangiectasia and a thickened appearance.

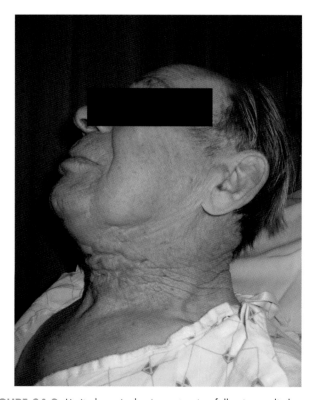

FIGURE 34-2. Limited cervical spine extension following radiotherapy.

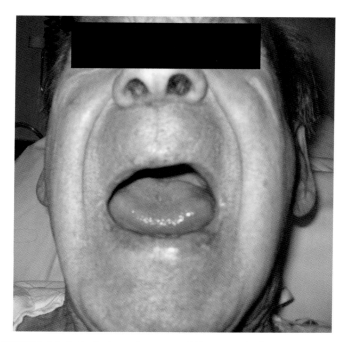

FIGURE 34-3. Limited mouth opening following radiotherapy.

lymphadenopathy.[5] Hypothyroidism occurs in 5–10% of patients who undergo irradiation of the lower neck,[4] and fibrosis of the apical segments of the lungs can also occur.[5]

Voluntary muscle exposed to high-dose irradiation can also develop fibrosis, and when the muscles of mastication (the temporalis, masseter, and pterygoid muscles) are involved, trismus can be produced (see Figure 34-3).[5] Trismus can be seen following radiotherapy for carcinoma of the nasopharynx or oropharynx. The temporomandibular joint itself is relatively resistant to ankylosis secondary to radiation injury.[5] Fibrosis of the pharyngeal musculature can produce swallowing dysfunction[11] and a predisposition to aspiration.[2] Stenosis of the pharynx or supraglottic larynx can occur and lead to airway compromise (see Figures 34-4 to 34-10).[5]

Laryngeal cartilage covered by normal mucous membrane usually tolerates conventional fractionated high-dose radiation therapy.[4,5] However, arytenoid edema, chrondritis, vocal cord palsy,[2] and rarely, chondronecrosis can occur Laryngeal edema can occur at any time following the completion of radiation therapy[12] and can produce airway compromise (see Figures 34-4(B), 34-5(B), 34-7, 34-8(B), 34-9(B), and 34-10).[8] Laryngeal chondronecrosis has been reported to occur up to 22 years following radiotherapy.[8]

Radiation therapy also can produce vascular injury which includes intimal thickening, fragmentation of the internal elastic membrane, atheroma formation, and fibrosis of the media and adventitia.[5] A reduction in the microvascular network can ultimately lead to ischemia, and narrowing or obstruction of larger arteries can occur, as can occlusive thrombosis.[9] The changes in the vessel walls are similar to those associated with artherosclerosis due to aging.[6] Symptomatic carotid atherosclerosis can be a result of cervical irradiation and may require surgical intervention.[12]

Radiation injury to the salivary glands produces a decrease in saliva production and a change in the composition of saliva.[5] Typically, about 60–65% of the total salivary volume is produced by the parotid glands, 20–30% by the submandibular glands, and 2–5% by the sublingual glands.[6] The remainder of the salivary volume is produced by anonymous minor salivary glands distributed throughout the oral cavity and pharynx, which are variable from patient to patient.[6] The degree of salivary gland dysfunction depends on the volume of the salivary glands included in the radiation field and the total dose administered.[6] It is usually not possible to irradiate the pharynx or the upper jugular nodes without irradiating the submandibular glands; however, the parotid and submandibular glands can be partially shielded during treatment.[4] A significant reduction in salivary flow occurs within 1 week of fractionated radiotherapy to the head and neck.[6] Salivary flow may become barely measurable by the end of a 6–8 week course of treatment and the xerostomia may be permanent.[6] Xerostomia causes discomfort, alters taste acuity, and contributes to a deterioration in dental hygiene because the tissues become tender.[5] The diminished salivary flow has an altered electrolyte content and reduced pH, and promotes dental decay as the normal oral microflora is altered to a highly cariogenic microbial population.[5] In the absence of stringent measures to protect the teeth, caries can develop within 3 to 6 months and lead to complete destruction of the dentition within 3 to 5 years.[5] Dental extractions from an irradiated mandible can precipitate osteoradionecrosis.[4]

34.2.3.2 What Airway Management Difficulties Can Be Anticipated Following Radiotherapy to the Oral Cavity, Pharynx, Larynx, or Neck?

Radiotherapy to the oral cavity, pharynx, larynx, or neck can produce limited mouth opening, limited cervical spine extension, and noncompliant immobile fibrotic soft tissue in the floor of the mouth and pharynx, as well as alteration of laryngeal anatomy. Airway management

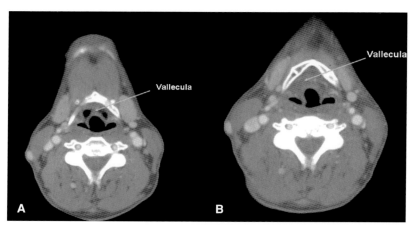

FIGURE 34-4. CT scans of the head and neck. (A) This CT scan shows normal soft tissues of the upper airway with normal vallecula. Note the bilateral air-filled depressions at this level. (B) This CT scan shows the postradiotherapy soft-tissue swelling in the vallecula.

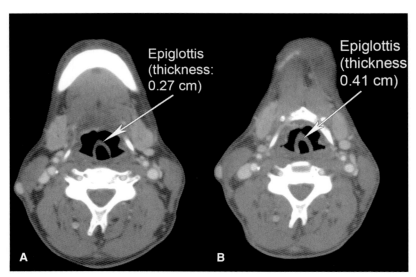

FIGURE 34-5. CT scans of the head and neck. (A) This CT scan shows normal soft tissues of the upper airway with normal vallecula. Note the bilateral air-filled depressions at this level. (B) This CT scan shows the postradiotherapy soft-tissue swelling in the vallecula.

can be difficult in the presence of these anatomic changes. The degree of difficulty is dependent on the site and extent of the altered anatomy.

34.2.3.3 Can Ventilation by Bag-Mask or Extraglottic Device Be Anticipated to Be More Difficult After Radiotherapy to the Structures of the Upper Airway?

Tomioka et al. reported ventilation by bag mask under GA to be easy in a patient who had undergone radiotherapy for a pharyngeal tumour.[13] However, intubation with a #7.0 endotracheal tube was not possible due to tracheal stenosis, which Tomioka et al. postulated, may have been produced by the radiation therapy.[13] Giraud et al. also reported bag-mask-ventilation (BMV) to be easy after induction of GA in nine patients after oral or cervical radiation.[10]

LMA placement was often difficult but was successful in all five patients who had received oral radiotherapy, and ventilation was satisfactory.[10] Two patients required lateral introduction of the LMA due to limitation of mouth opening.[10] LMA placement was easy in the four patients who had received cervical radiation, but positive-pressure ventilation was difficult.[10] On fiberoptic examination through the LMA, the vocal cords could not be visualized in any of these four patients due to vestibular-fold collapse. A large epiglottis was also seen in two of these patients. Muscle relaxation did not improve the laryngeal view. Ventilation was impossible in two of the four patients; however successful orotracheal intubation was performed. Fiberoptic intubation via the LMA was not attempted as the glottis could not be visualized. The authors theorized that the presence of the LMA in a narrowed, nondistensible hypopharynx may have compressed the larynx and thereby produced glottic collapse.[10]

Following cervical radiotherapy then, the use of an LMA for airway management may not be successful due to obstruction at the level of the larynx.[10] Laryngeal obstruction would also preclude ventilation using other extraglottic devices such as the Combitube™ or cuffed oropharyngeal airway (COPA). Furthermore, Combitube™ placement may not be possible in the presence of limited mouth opening.

Anecdotally, BMV can also be difficult in the presence of anatomic distortion of the upper airway produced by radiotherapy; however, reported experience in this clinical setting is limited.[10,13,14]

34.2.3.4 Can Endotracheal Intubation Be More Difficult Following Oral or Cervical Radiotherapy?

Reduced mouth opening due to fibrosis of the muscles of mastication, reduced cervical spine extension, and fibrosis of the structures of the floor of the mouth can make visualization of the glottis by direct laryngoscopy difficult or impossible. Fibrotic subcutaneous and submucosal soft tissues lack compliance and may constitute a

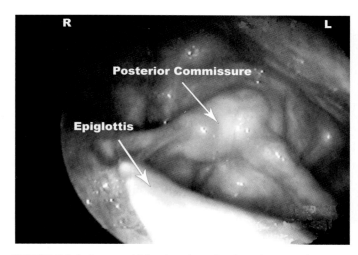

FIGURE 34-6. Laryngeal inlet view through a bronchoscope shows a normal epiglottis. Note the sharp leaflike edge along the right lateral aspect.

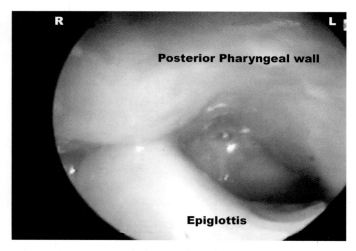

FIGURE 34-7. Laryngeal inlet view through a bronchoscope shows the appearance of the edematous epiglottis following radiotherapy.

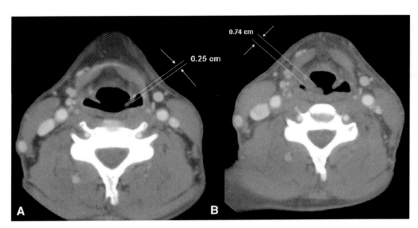

FIGURE 34-8. CT scans of the head and neck: (A) normal soft tissues of the upper airway with normal aryepiglottic folds (0.25 cm); and (B) thickening of the right aryepiglottic fold following radiotherapy (0.74 cm).

poorly mobile woody mass that cannot be elevated easily, if at all, on direct laryngoscopy. Postirradiation atrophic mucosa is also easily traumatized and bleeding can readily occur. A thickened edematous epiglottis can obscure glottic visualization, and decreased vocal cord mobility may interfere with glottic cannulation (see Figures 34-5(B), 34-7, and 34-9(B)).

Alternative intubation techniques can also be more difficult following radiation-induced changes to the upper airway. The light-guided technique using a lightwand is best avoided in the presence of anatomic distortion of the airway.[15] Retrograde intubation may be feasible although laryngotracheal abnormality has been cited as a relative contraindication to this technique as well.[16] Limited mouth opening may preclude rigid fiberoptic techniques, and flexible fiberoptic intubation under general anesthesia may be more difficult in the presence of distorted anatomy and decreased mobility of the airway structures.

34.2.3.5 Can a Surgical Airway Be More Difficult in this Group of Patients?

Subcutaneous fibrosis in the neck can obscure surface anatomical landmarks, obliterate tissue planes, and make a surgical approach

to the airway technically challenging (see Figure 34-2). Percutaneous cricothyrotomy may fail in this setting, and tracheotomy may require more time to complete and be associated with more bleeding.[14]

34.3 AIRWAY MANAGEMENT PLAN

34.3.1 What should be the approach to airway management in these patients?

Airway management of the patient following cervical or oral radiotherapy therefore requires a careful airway assessment. The assessment should focus on the four "dimensions" of airway management as outlined by Murphy et al. and be used to predict potential difficulty with (1) BMV, (2) ventilation using an extraglottic device, (3) tracheal intubation, and (4) surgical access to the airway.[17]

If BMV and intubation are both predicted to be difficult after radiotherapy, then the airway should be secured with the patient awake. Should GA be induced in this setting and BMV be inadequate, rescue ventilation by means of an LMA may also fail.[10] The use of an LMA after cervical radiotherapy may in fact be contraindicated.[10] Furthermore, rescue by means of a surgical airway may also be difficult.[14] Topical anesthesia of the upper airway has been reported to produce transient glottic obstruction resulting in a profound reduction in maximum inspiratory and expiratory flows in some normal subjects,[18] and in the presence of preexisting airway compromise an increase in resistance to gas flow may be poorly tolerated.[19] Complete obstruction has been reported during topicalization and instrumentation of the airway.[14,20,21] However, awake fiberoptic intubation, in general, maintains a wide margin of safety and has been said to be the recommended method in the patient with predicted difficult intubation postradiotherapy.[10] Nonetheless, extreme caution must be exercised in the presence of severe airway obstruction if complete obstruction is to be avoided.[22] If BMV is predicted to be easy but intubation difficult, then fiberoptic intubation under GA may be considered, although anatomic distortion and decreased tissue mobility can make fiberoptic visualization more difficult. Following radiotherapy to the floor of the mouth and/or pharynx, severe trismus may preclude oral intubation techniques, and in this setting awake nasal fiberoptic intubation may be the most reasonable alternative. Intubation via an LMA may be possible following oral radiotherapy if adequate visualization can be achieved.

Alternatively, in the presence of anatomic distortion but when intubation is predicted to be possible, inhalation induction of GA may be a reasonable option.[19,23,24] When an adequate depth of GA has been achieved, intubation can be performed during spontaneous ventilation utilizing a curved or straight blade laryngoscope, an operating laryngoscope such as the tubular Lindholm scope, or a rigid bronchoscope.[19,23] If intubation is not possible, tracheotomy can be performed under GA. Inhalation induction in the presence of airway compromise can

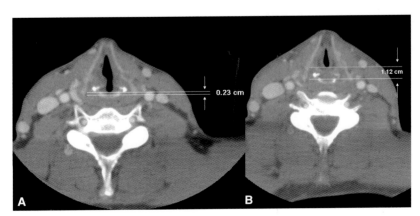

FIGURE 34-9. CT scans of the head and neck: (A) normal soft tissue thickness at the posterior commissure (0.23 cm); and (B) edema at the level of the arytenoid cartilages and the posterior commissure (1.12 cm) following radiotherapy.

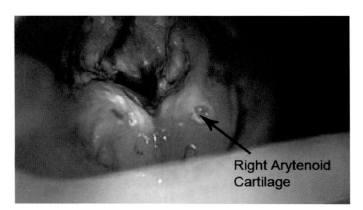

Right Arytenoid
Cartilage

FIGURE 34-10. Laryngeal inlet view through a bronchoscope shows the appearance of the arytenoid cartilages and adjacent supraglottic area following radiotherapy. Note the extensive thickening and tissue distortion.

however be difficult.[19,24] Complete airway obstruction can occur and an emergency surgical airway may be required.[19,24] Meticulous attention to detail is necessary, in particular the maintenance of spontaneous ventilation and the avoidance of airway instrumentation until an adequate depth of GA is achieved.[19] The use of a nasal airway to alleviate obstruction at the level of the soft palate during inhalation induction may be helpful.[19]

Patients who have an extremely compromised airway, severe stridor, gross anatomic distortion, or a larynx that cannot be visualized on endoscopy should undergo awake tracheotomy performed under local anesthesia.[19,23,24]

34.4   AIRWAY MANAGEMENT PROCEDURE

34.4.1   How should this patient's airway be managed?

An anesthetic record from 2 years prior to this admission was available for review. BMV had been recorded as "moderately easy" and intubation had been achieved using a lightwand on the third attempt.

Difficult direct laryngoscopy was predicted based on the examination of the airway (Mallampati IV, reduced mouth opening, limited mandibular protrusion, decreased cervical extension, woody induration involving the mandibular space). The predicted ease of BMV was also uncertain due to the presence of the submandibular induration and limited cervical extension. The recorded experience with BMV at the previous surgery is not reassuring. Ventilation by means of an LMA or other extraglottic device may be difficult as well, particularly in the presence of the existing anatomic distortion. Surgical access to the airway was not predicted to be difficult. An awake fiberoptic intubation was planned.

Routine monitors were attached and IV access established. No sedation was administered. The patient gargled and then expectorated 30 mL of 4% lidocaine. The DeVilbiss atomizer was then used to administer 12 mL of 3% lidocaine aerosolized into the right nostril and the mouth. Five percent lidocaine paste was

applied to the posterior one-third of the tongue, and an internal approach superior laryngeal nerve block was performed using Jackson forceps and cotton pledgets soaked in 4% lidocaine. The adult bronchoscope was then easily passed through the mouth into the trachea with the patient in the sitting position and using gentle tongue traction. A #8.5 endotracheal tube was then passed easily over the bronchoscope during maximum inspiration to widely abduct the vocal cords. The patient tolerated the intubation well. GA was then induced and bronchoscopy and mediastinoscopy performed uneventfully.

34.5   EXTUBATION MANAGEMENT

34.5.1   How should this patient be extubated?

Laryngeal edema was judged to be unlikely following this relatively brief surgical procedure during which the volume of IV fluid administered was small. Furthermore, no evidence of airway obstruction existed preoperatively. The patient was therefore extubated *fully awake* in the semi-sitting position in the operating room immediately following surgery. The postoperative course was uneventful.

34.6   SUMMARY

Radiotherapy to the head and neck can produce limited mouth opening, limited cervical spine extension, noncompliant fibrotic soft tissue in the floor of the mouth and pharynx, and alteration of laryngeal anatomy. Airway management of the patient following cervical or oral radiotherapy therefore requires a careful airway assessment. While complete obstruction has been reported during topicalization and instrumentation of the airway, awake fiberoptic intubation, in general, maintains a wide margin of safety and is the preferred method in the patient with predicted difficult laryngoscopic intubation postradiotherapy. Patients who have an extremely compromised airway, severe stridor, gross anatomic distortion, or a larynx that cannot be visualized on endoscopy should undergo awake tracheotomy performed under local anesthesia.

REFERENCES

1. Larson DL: Management of complications of radiotherapy of the head and neck. *Surg Clin North Am.* 1986;66:169–182.
2. Wu C-H, Ko J-Y, Hsiao T-Y, et al.: Dysphagia after radiotherapy. Endoscopic examination of swallowing in patients with nasopharyngeal carcinoma. *Ann Otol Rhinol Laryngol.* 2000;109:320–325.
3. Trotti A: Toxicity in head and neck cancer: a review of trends and issues. *Int J Radiation Oncology Biol Phys.* 2000;47:1–12.
4. Vikram B: Complications of radiation therapy. In: *Complications in Head and Neck Surgery.* Krespi YP, Ossoff RH, eds. Philadelphia, PA: WB Saunders Company, 1993:311–319.
5. Parsons JT, Mendenhall WM, Million RR: Complications of radiotherapy for head and neck neoplasms. In: *Complications of Head and Neck Surgery.* New York, NY: Thieme Medical Publishers Inc., 1995:194–229.
6. Cooper JS, Fu K, Marks J, et al.: Late effects of radiation therapy in the head and neck region. *Int J Radiation Oncology Biol Phys.* 1995;31(5):1141–1164.
7. Gaitini LA, Somri M, Fradis M, et al.: Pneumomediastinum due to ventura jet ventilation used during microlaryngeal surgery in a previously neck irradiated patient. *Ann Otol Rhinol Larynngol.* 2000;109:519–521.

8. Weissler MC: Management of complications resulting from laryngeal cancer treatment. *Otolaryngol Clin North Am.* 1997;30:269–278.
9. Fajardo LF: Morphology of radiation effects normal times. In: *Principles and Practice of Radiation Oncology,* 2nd ed. Perez CA, Brady LW, eds. Philadelphia, PA: JB Lippincott Company, 1992:114–123.
10. Giraud O, Bourgain JL, Marandas P, et al.: Limits of laryngeal mask airway in patients after cervical or oral radiotherapy. *Can J Anesth.* 1997;44:1237–1241.
11. Mittal BB, Pauloski BR, Haraf DJ, et al.: Swallowing dysfunction—preventive and rehabilitation strategies in patients with head and neck cancers treated with surgery, radiotherapy, and chemotherapy: a critical review. *Int J Radiation Oncology Biol Phys.* 2003;5:1219–1230.
12. Francfort JW, Smullens SN, Gallagher JF, et al.: Airway compromise after carotid surgery in patients with cervical irradiation. *J Cardiovasc Surg.* 1989;30:877–1981.
13. Tomioka T, Ogawa M, Sawamura S, et al.: A case of post radiation therapy patient with difficulty in intubation unexpected preoperatively. *Masui.* 2003;52:406–408.
14. Ho AMH, Chung DC, To EW, et al.: Total airway obstruction during local anesthesia in non-sedated patients with a compromised airway. *Can J Anesth.* 2004;51:838–841.
15. Hung OL, Stewart RD: Illuminating stylette (Lightwand). In: *Airway Management Principles and Practice,* Benumof JL, ed. St. Louis, MO: Mosby, Inc., 1996:342–352.
16. Sanchez AF, Morrison DE: In: *Handbook of Difficult Airway Management.* Hagberg CA, ed. Philadelphia, PA: Churchill Livingstone, 2000:115–148.
17. Murphy M, Hung O, Launcelott G, et al.: Predicting the difficult laryngoscopic intubation: are we on the right track? *Can J Anesth.* 2005;52:1–2.
18. Listro G, Stanescu DC, Veriter C, et al.: Upper airway anesthesia induces airflow limitation in awake humans. *Am Rev Repir Dis.* 1992;146:581–585.
19. Mason RA, Fielder CP: The obstructed airway in head and neck surgery (editorial). *Anaesthseia.* 1999;54:625–628.
20. McGuire G, El-Beheiry H: Complete upper airway obstruction during awake fiberoptic intubation in patients with unstable cervical spine fractures. *Can J Anesth.* 1999;42:176–178.
21. Shaw IC, Welchew EA, Harrison BJ, et al.: Complete airway obstruction during awake fiberoptic intubation. *Anesthesia.* 1997;52:576–585.
22. Ovassapian A, Wheeler M: Flexible fiberoptic tracheal intubation. In: *Handbook of Difficult Airway Management.* Philadelphia, PA: Churchill Livingstone, 2000:83–114.
23. Deam R, McCutcheon C: Management choices for the difficult airway (Letter). *Can J Anesth.* 2003;50:623–624.
24. Wong DT, McGuire GP: Management choices for the difficult airway (Author reply). *Can J Anesth.* 2003;50:624.

SELF-EVALUATION QUESTIONS

34.1. Which of the following is **NOT** true with regard to the airway management of a patient with a history of radiotherapy to the head and neck?

A. surgical airway should be uncomplicated

B. limited mouth opening may preclude rigid fiberoptic intubating techniques

C. fibrosis of the structures of the floor of the mouth can make direct laryngoscopy difficult

D. a decrease in vocal cord mobility may interfere with glottic cannulation

E. in the presence of anatomic distortion of the airway, the light-guided technique using a lightwand is best avoided

34.2. Which of the following is true with regard to the oxygenation and ventilation of a patient with a history of radiotherapy to the head and neck?

A. bag-mask-ventilation can be difficult

B. the LMA may not ensure a patent airway following cervical radiotherapy

C. Combitube™ placement can be difficult

D. glottic visualization by direct laryngoscopy may be impossible

E. all of the above

34.3. A patient with a history of radiotherapy to the head and neck arrives in the operating room with severe stridor. Which of the following is the most appropriate technique to secure the airway?

A. fiberoptic intubation under general anesthesia

B. awake retrograde intubation under local anesthesia

C. awake intubation through an intubating LMA under local anesthesia

D. awake tracheotomy performed under local anesthesia

E. awake fiberoptic intubation under local anesthesia

CHAPTER (35)

Intraoperative Accidental Dislodgement of the Endotracheal Tube in a Patient in the Prone Position

Dennis Drapeau and Orlando R. Hung

35.1   CASE PRESENTATION

A 50-year-old obese male (265 lb [120 kg], 5′8″ [173 cm]) was scheduled for lumber spine instrumentation. Preoperative airway examination revealed no obvious indicators of difficult laryngoscopic intubation apart from the fact that he had a beard. Following induction with fentanyl, propofol, and rocuronium, a Cormack/Lehane (C/L) Grade 2 laryngoscopic view was obtained with a #3 Macintosh blade. Laryngoscopic intubation was achieved easily while using backward, upward, and rightward pressure (BURP) externally on the larynx. After securing the endotracheal tube (ETT), the patient was then turned to prone position for the surgical procedure. Two hours after the start of surgery and after 1,500 mL of blood loss and the administration of 4 L of crystalloid, a leak in the ventilation system was identified.

35.2   INTRODUCTION

35.2.1   What are your concerns when a patient is placed in the prone position for a surgical procedure?

Proper patient positioning for any medical procedure is an important consideration for a safe and successful outcome. The proper position provides appropriate surgical access and guards against injury due to pressure points and strain on neurological and musculoskeletal structures. Prone positioning is required for some surgical procedures on the spine and for other neurosurgical procedures. The prone position is complicated by an increased risk of stretch and pressure injury, cardiovascular instability, difficulty with ventilation, and problems in providing cardiopulmonary resuscitation. Airway considerations for patients placed in the prone position may include difficult access to the airway, migration of ETT (tip of the ETT moving cephalad or caudad with head extension and flexion, respectively), limited ability to reposition the head and neck for bag-mask-ventilation (BMV), and airway edema.

This case represents one of the most challenging situations for airway practitioners, in that control of the airway must be regained promptly with the patient in the prone position. Limited information is available in the literature to assist critical decision making.

35.3   INITIAL PATIENT MANAGEMENT

35.3.1   What is the differential diagnosis of a ventilation system leak?

A ventilation system leak is a fairly common occurrence during surgery and is usually easy to manage. However, it is more complex and dangerous when it occurs in the prone patient. It is often challenging for the airway practitioner and is life-threatening for the patient. In diagnosing and managing this situation, the source of the leak must be determined promptly. This is usually accomplished by inspecting all portions of the anesthesia circuit in an organized and sequential manner. With the prone patient, it is usually easier to start at the anesthesia machine and work your way to the patient. This would include checking flow rates, ventilator/bag volumes valves, circuit tubing, and connections.

Leaks within the anesthesia machine or circuit may involve circuit disconnects, leaks around circuit connections or valves, and undetected holes in circuit components. Management of such leaks may include increasing the fresh gas flow, or replacing part or all, of the anesthesia circuit or machine. Potential leaks associated with an airway device include: (1) partial or complete dislodgement of the device; (2) inadequate volume in the ETT cuff; (3) disruption of the ETT cuff; and (4) a leak from the pilot cuff apparatus (pilot valve or tubing leak). These leaks may require reinsertion of a defective airway device.

35.3.2 If the ETT was found to be dislodged from the trachea, what is your initial management?

The goals of management are to regain control of the airway and to ventilate and oxygenate the patient as soon as possible. If feasible, this should be achieved by turning the patient into the supine position. Operating room personnel must be informed of the emergency and additional help should be summoned. The difficult airway cart, the patient's stretcher or bed, and the resuscitation cart should be brought into the operating theater immediately. The surgical team should close the surgical wound as soon as possible to allow transfer of the patient (in supine position) to a stretcher.

35.4   AIRWAY CONSIDERATIONS

35.4.1 If a stretcher is not immediately available, how do you provide ventilation to a patient in the prone position?

Options to regain control of the airway in a prone patient are similar to those for the supine patient. A BMV should be provided as soon as possible. However, BMV in the prone patient can be difficult due to limited access to the airway, difficult mask seal because of gravity, and lack of clinical experience performing BMV in a prone patient. It may be necessary to use a two-person BMV technique, with one person achieving a mask seal using both hands and the other person providing manual ventilation. Provided that a good mask seal can be maintained, BMV should be reasonably easy in a patient lying prone since gravity tends to move the tongue away from the posterior pharyngeal wall.

If BMV is not possible, an extraglottic device, such as the laryngeal mask airway (LMA), can be used to provide ventilation and oxygenation for a patient in the prone position. Raphael et al. and Dingeman et al. have reported successful use of the LMA in regaining the control of the airway and in providing positive-pressure ventilation following ETT dislodgement in the prone position.[1,2] Insertion of the LMA in a patient lying prone should be attempted using the classic insertion technique recommended for patients in the supine position.[3] Successful insertion of the LMA may actually be easier in the prone position because of the anterior movement of the tongue and epiglottis[4] away from the posterior pharyngeal wall and decreased down folding of the epiglottis.

Other extraglottic devices (including the Combitube™) may be used while the patient is prone, depending on the skill and experience of the practitioner as well as the available resources. However, there are currently no reports in the literature of the successful use of extraglottic devices other than the LMA for patients in the prone position.

35.4.2 Would you proceed with the surgical procedure, if adequate ventilation and oxygenation can be achieved following the successful placement of an LMA?

As mentioned, successful insertion of the LMA in patients lying prone has been reported. Ng et al. reported successful LMA insertion following induction of general anesthesia for brief surgical procedures in 73 prone adult patients.[4] However, difficulties were encountered with malposition of the LMA in four patients (5.5%), hypoventilation in two patients (2.7%), and bleeding in two patients (2.7%). Although these were considered to be minor problems, the authors stated clearly that successful insertion of an LMA in patients lying prone requires not only skill that comes from practice, but also the assurance that at any time the patient can be turned into the supine position should emergency airway management be necessary. Herrick and Kennedy[5] and Kee[6] have reported incidences of airway obstruction of 3.5% and 3%, respectively, when the LMA was used in pediatric patients placed prone for radiotherapy. It is probably reasonable to use the LMA for short surgical procedures, in the prone position as long as the patient can be positioned supine in the event that airway management becomes problematic. However, it would be unwise to use the LMA for long surgical procedures with the potential of massive bleeding and fluid shifts, such as in this case scenario. It is common to observe an increase in the airway pressure during the course of the surgery with patient lying prone, particularly when there is massive blood loss and fluid shifts. In this patient, the LMA should only be considered as a temporizing measure until a more definitive airway can be secured. Therefore, we believe that it is necessary to replace the ETT prior to resuming the surgical procedure in this case presentation.

35.4.3 How can airway edema be minimized in a patient in the prone position?

Tissue edema, particularly in dependent areas, can occur in surgical procedures involving significant blood loss and/or fluid shifts. Intraoperative dislodgement of the ETT in the prone patient with significant airway edema can be a disaster. Therefore, all attempts should be made to minimize the development of edema during procedures performed in the prone position. In lieu of large amounts of crystalloid solutions, it is perhaps prudent to administer colloid solutions, such as hydroxyethyl starch preparations. Although the efficacy of this approach has not been scientifically validated, it is our practice to use colloid solutions, after administering 2–3 L of crystalloid solutions.

Venous drainage of the head and neck can be optimized by keeping the head elevated, if possible, and avoiding compression or "kinking" of jugular veins. If the head must be turned to one side for airway or surgical access, the degree of rotation should be minimized.

35.4.4   How can airway edema be assessed and managed?

The development of edema in the hypopharynx and larynx while in the prone position can produce airway obstruction following extubation. Clinical signs, such as facial, orbital, or conjunctival edema, distended neck veins, and venous congestion of the head may indicate the presence of upper airway edema. The use of a flexible fiberoptic nasopharyngoscope to assess the extent of airway edema prior to tracheal extubation may be helpful,[7] but there have been no studies to confirm its utility.

There are no scientifically validated methods to assess the degree of postoperative airway edema or to predict postextubation airway obstruction (see Section 29.4.1). However, the performance of a leak test prior to extubation in patients with suspected airway edema has been suggested.[8] The leak test measures the decrease in exhaled volume returned to the ventilator following deflation of the ETT cuff. A positive leak test (>110 mL) has been shown to indicate that airway patency is sufficient to tolerate extubation without postextubation stridor (PES) (84% specificity, 97% negative predictive value), although a *negative* leak test is not predictive of the development of PES.[9] The leak test can also be performed by deflating the ETT cuff in a spontaneously breathing patient without ventilator support and then occluding the end of the ETT. The patient is observed for signs of an audible leak or coughing around the ETT. The absence of a leak and/or coughing are positive predictors for PES.[10] Ding et al. recently reported the results of a pilot study using a laryngeal ultrasound to predict PES in 41 patients.[11] The investigators used real-time ultrasonography to evaluate the air leak and to determine the relationship between the air column width during cuff deflation and the development of PES. The results of this study suggest that laryngeal ultrasonography could be a reliable, noninvasive method in the evaluation of laryngeal morphology and airflow through the upper airway. Other predictors of PES include length of intubation, female gender, body mass index, and ratio of ETT size to laryngeal diameter have also been reported.[9,12]

If the patient passes the leak test but still displays clinical evidence of facial and possible airway edema, we believe it would be prudent to perform extubation over an ETT exchange catheter (Cook Critical Care®, Bloomington, IN) to provide a means for ventilation should postextubation airway obstruction occur. Any patient failing the leak test should continue to be managed with an ETT in place until the airway edema resolves and a subsequent satisfactory leak test. Appropriate treatment of airway edema includes elevation of the head and the use of steroids and diuretics. The efficacy of these measures has not yet been formally validated. Steroids may reduce the amount of airway edema and decrease the risk of postextubation airway obstruction; however, evidence supporting a decreased rate of reintubation exists only in the pediatric population.[13–16]

35.4.5   How do you manage a patient with a difficult airway who requires surgery in the prone position?

Airway management of the patient with a difficult airway who requires surgery in the prone position poses unique challenges for the anesthesia practitioner. These issues can be categorized according to the etiology of the difficult airway: (1) anatomical characteristics making ventilation and/or tracheal intubation difficult; and (2) cervical spine instability. If difficult laryngoscopic intubation secondary to anatomical characteristics is predicted (LEMON, (see Section 1.6.2), the technique utilized to manage the airway is dependant on whether or not BMV, i.e., placement of an extraglottic device, and a surgical airway are also predicted to be difficult, as well as aspiration risk, the available resources, and the expertise of the practitioner. Once endotracheal intubation has been achieved, the ETT must be carefully secured.

The situation becomes more challenging when possible cervical spine instability or spinal cord damage exists. It is generally believed that awake fiberoptic intubation and positioning of the patient in prone prior to induction of anesthesia is ideal because this allows verification of neurological integrity prior to surgery. However, there is no clinical evidence to support this practice. Suderman and Crosby in a retrospective review of 150 patients found no difference in neurological outcomes in cervical spine injured adult patients intubated awake or under general anesthesia, with or without in-line cervical spine immobilization[17] (see Chapter 14).

35.5   PREPARATION AND PLANS FOR ENDOTRACHEAL INTUBATION

35.5.1   Can intubation be performed in the lateral position?

While ideal, transfer of the patient to a supine position can be extremely difficult to achieve in a timely manner and is not without considerable risk to the patient. Therefore, it is desirable to have several alternative approaches for reestablishing endotracheal intubation in this particularly difficult situation. If it is feasible to place the patient in a lateral position, the left lateral decubitus is preferred for laryngoscopy and intubation, as gravity will help to displace the tongue to the left and facilitate visualization of the glottis. However, BMV may be easier in the right lateral decubitus position. Nathanson et al. found tracheal intubation of a manikin in the lateral position to be more difficult than in the supine position.[18] The ease of intubation increased with each subsequent attempt, indicating that operator experience was a confounding factor.[18] Difficulty in intubating manikins in the lateral position may not apply to humans due to the beneficial effects of gravity, which displaces the tongue as mentioned. An assistant may be necessary to stabilize the head, neck, and body.

Blind endotracheal intubation techniques such as the intubating LMA (LMA Fastrach™, LMA North America Inc., San Diego, CA) and the lighted-stylet have also been described for use with a patient in the lateral position.[19–21] Experience with these intubation techniques will improve the operator's chance of success. Blind techniques should be attempted only after direct visualization techniques have failed, as anatomic distortion may be present.

35.5.2   What are the options for endotracheal intubation in the prone position?

Reintubation while the patient is still in the prone position would eliminate the inherent risks associated with turning the patient. In addition to direct laryngoscopic intubation, alternative intubating techniques can be considered. These include the use of a flexible fiberoptic bronchoscope (FFB), an intubating LMA (LMA Fastrach™), light-guided intubation using the Trachlight™ (Laerdal Medical Corp., Wappingers Falls, New York), and digital intubation. There is limited clinical information with regard to the effectiveness and safety of these techniques in patients lying in prone position.

Baer performed endotracheal intubation using a laryngoscope in the prone position in 200 patients undergoing lumbar surgery.[22] Two failed intubations occurred and these patients were then intubated in the lateral or supine positions, but with difficulty.[22] This experience emphasizes the importance of airway assessment and management in the supine position when difficulty is predicted. We believe that tracheal intubation of patients in the prone position should be reserved for rescue situations and that elective intubation in patients requiring prone positioning should be performed in the supine position as this is most familiar to the airway practitioner. Intubation in the prone position may be necessary if:

1. ventilation and oxygenation are ineffective using BMV, the LMA, or the Combitube™;

2. ventilation using BMV, the LMA, or the Combitube™ is adequate but a definitive airway is desired (e.g., prolonged case, risk of aspiration);

3. transfer of the patient to the supine position is impossible or is associated with extreme risk.

35.5.3   How can endotracheal intubation be performed in the prone position?

Airway control in this case scenario can be reestablished by means of several techniques. An intact ETT (unobstructed with a competent cuff) can be reinserted into the trachea by simple advancement as long as the tip of the ETT is still in the glottis. This can be facilitated if a throat pack had been placed following the initial intubation. The ability to ventilate the patient through the ETT and the presence of an end-tidal CO_2 waveform indicate that simple advancement of the tube may be all that is required. If ventilation through the ETT is difficult, it may still be possible to advance the ETT into the trachea with the aid of a lighted stylet, FFB, or a tube exchanger. When using a tube exchanger, the intratracheal location of the tube should be verified by the end-tidal CO_2 waveform or FFB.

The tracheal tube should be replaced if there is evidence of tube damage and a significant leak exists. Small air leaks may be overcome by increasing inspired gas flow, if the remaining surgical time is short. Larger leaks can be attenuated by the insertion of throat packing, if not already present. If a throat pack was in place around the original ETT, it may be possible to pass a new ETT with a deflated cuff into the trachea through the cast (or track) made by the throat pack, or it maybe possible to change the tube over an

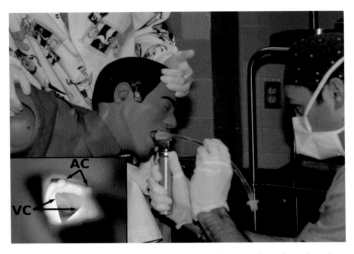

FIGURE 35-1. Laryngoscopic intubation of a manikin placed in the prone position. Laryngoscopic intubation can be performed from the front of the manikin with the right hand holding the laryngoscope. The insert shows the laryngoscopic view of this technique. The vocal cords (VC) and the arytenoid cartilages (AC) can be visualized easily.

airway exchange catheter. If these measures fail and airway control is lost, oxygenation and ventilation of the patient must be reestablished as soon as possible.

Tracheal intubation by direct laryngoscopy can be performed in a prone patient by a practitioner who is positioned at the head of the patient facing caudad and uses the right hand to insert the laryngoscope into the pharynx and expose the glottis (Figure 35-1). The practitioner then uses the left hand to insert the ETT into the trachea. Alternately, direct laryngoscopy and intubation can be performed in a more conventional manner from either side of the patient (Figure 35-2). An assistant can turn the patient's head to the side and elevate the shoulder to facilitate access to the mouth. The head and neck can also be placed in the familiar sniffing

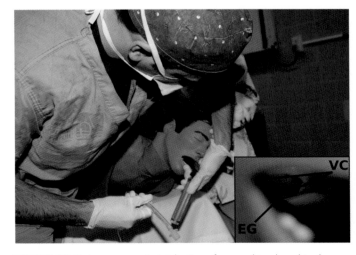

FIGURE 35-2. Laryngoscopic intubation of a manikin placed in the prone position. Laryngoscopic intubation can also be performed from the side (right) of the manikin. The insert shows the laryngoscopic view of this technique. The vocal cords (VC) and the epiglottis (EG) can be visualized easily.

position. A previous study has shown this to be an effective (99% success rate) and safe technique of laryngoscopic intubation in prone patients.[22]

The intubating LMA can also provide a conduit through which an ETT can be advanced into the trachea blindly, or with the aid of a lightwand or FFB (see Chapter 11). However, insertion of the LMA Fastrach™ (relative to the classic LMA) can be difficult in the prone position.

35.5.4 Upon turning the patient into the supine position, BMV is easy, but direct laryngoscopy reveals a grade 3 view. What is the appropriate airway management?

A previously easy intubation may be difficult upon returning the patient to the supine position. Anatomic distortion of the airway can occur due to factors inherent to the surgical procedure, to the prone position, to trauma during intubation, or to dislodgement of the ETT. Cervical vertebral fixation and surgical manipulation of oropharyngeal and neck tissues can alter airway anatomy. Bleeding into the airway and hematoma formation can be associated with neck surgery. Prolonged surgical procedures with significant blood loss may be associated with generalized edema due to fluid resuscitation. Airway edema can alter the appearance of laryngeal structures and can make visualization of the larynx difficult.[23–25] Edematous tissues may also be more easily traumatized. Direct pressure on facial and neck structures and a dependent position compromise venous drainage and contribute to edema formation.

In this case scenario, the patient was placed in the supine position and direct laryngoscopy revealed a Cormack/Lehane (C/L) grade 3 laryngoscopic view. The application of BURP[26] may improve the C/L view.[27] If BURP does not improve the view of the glottis, alternative intubating techniques can be used as long as effective ventilation and oxygenation can be provided by BMV. These techniques include the use of an Eschmann Introducer, lightwand (Trachlight™), intubating LMA, GlideScope® (Keomed, Minnetonka, MN), Bullard laryngoscope, or FFB. As each intubation attempt will likely decrease the chance of success on subsequent attempts, it is critical that the practitioner employs the technique with which he/she is most experienced. In general, in the presence of an abnormal upper airway (edema), tracheal intubation should be performed under direct or indirect vision, if at all possible. Use of the Eschmann Introducer can be considered to be a logical extension of direct laryngoscopy and has a high success rate in the presence of a C/L grade 3 view.[28] It is also helpful to use a smaller ETT to minimize the resistance to passage through the larynx.

If a visual technique is unsuccessful but BMV is adequate, blind intubation techniques may be used but great caution when preparing the patient for a surgical airway.

The lightwand is an invaluable tool. However, it is most useful in nonobese patients. Furthermore, in this scenario, the failed laryngoscopic intubation is probably secondary to airway edema and/or trauma. The use of a blind intubating technique, such as the lightwand, would likely be unsuccessful in this setting.

35.6 POSTINTUBATION AND VENTILATION MANAGEMENT

35.6.1 How can the ETT be secured following intubation in a patient with a beard?

To minimize the risk of ETT dislodgement, it is imperative to secure the ETT properly, particularly for patients in a prone position. The most common method of securing the ETT is to tape it to the face. Unfortunately, the presence of facial hair, oils on the skin, perspiration, oropharyngeal secretions, and surgical skin preparation solutions can impair the adhesiveness of the tape. Generous use of waterproof tape and the use of multiple attachment points can reinforce the bond to the face. Although adequate taping is required for the prone patient, complete sealing off of the mouth should be avoided as oropharyngeal secretions should be allowed to drain. This will minimize pooling of saliva and secretion, which may loosen the tape. The application of tincture of benzoin to the skin may improve tape adhesion. Placement of gauze packing into the airway or a gauze bite block may also limit the amount of secretions available to disrupt the bond between the tape and the skin. However, the airway practitioner must always be aware of the potential for local pressure injury associated with these packs and blocks. The use of an antisialogogue (e.g., glycopyrrolate) may be helpful in minimizing secretions.

Patients with facial hair often pose additional problems in securing the airway. For these patients, it may be best to tie the ETT around the neck with an umbilical tape. It is important not to tie the ETT too tightly and thereby obstruct venous return from the head. If the ETT cannot be tied around the neck (e.g., cervical laminectomy or post-fossa craniotomy), other options to secure the ETT can be considered. These include: (1) suturing the ETT to the lips; (2) tying the ETT to the upper incisors (if present) or nares; and (3) shaving the patient's beard prior to induction of anesthesia.

35.7 SUMMARY

Of all the potential complications associated with prone positioning for a surgical procedure, managing a failed airway is probably the most challenging. The inability to ventilate and oxygenate the patient is life-threatening for the patient and demands immediate action from the airway practitioner. The ETT must be well secured to prevent dislodgement. In the event that the ETT is dislodged from the trachea, oxygenation should be promptly provided by BMV, or through an extraglottic device such as the LMA, until endotracheal intubation is reestablished. Provided that oxygenation can be maintained, the choice of intubating technique is dependant on the available resources, the patient position, and the skills of the airway practitioner. All airway practitioners must have a strategy to manage a failed airway in a patient in the prone position. Every effort must be made to minimize airway edema while the patient is prone. This is particularly important for long surgical procedures involving significant blood loss and fluid shifts. Airway practitioners must pay special attention to the assessment of airway edema prior to tracheal extubation.

REFERENCES

1. Raphael J, Rosenthal-Ganon T, Gozal Y: Emergency airway management with a laryngeal mask airway in a patient placed in the prone position. *J Clin Anest.* 2004;16:560–561.
2. Dingeman RS, Goumnerova LC, Goobie SM: The use of a laryngeal mask airway for emergent airway management in a prone child. *Anesth Analg.* 2005;100:670–671.
3. Brain A: Proper technique for insertion of the laryngeal mask. *Anesthesiology.* 1990;73:1053–1054.
4. Ng A, Raitt D, Smith G: Induction of anesthesia and insertion of a laryngeal mask airway in the prone position for minor surgery. *Anesth Analg.* 2002;94:1194–1198.
5. Herrick MJ, Kennedy DJ: Airway obstruction and the laryngeal mask airway in paediatric radiotherapy. *Anaesthesia.* 1992;47:910.
6. Kee WD: Laryngeal mask airway for radiotherapy in the prone position. *Anaesthesia.* 1992;47:446–447.
7. Bentsianov BL, Parhiscar A, Azer M, Har-El G. The role of fiberoptic nasopharyngoscopy in the management of the acute airway in angioneurotic edema. *Laryngoscope.* 2000;110:2016–2019.
8. Miller RL, Cole RP: Association between reduced cuff leak volume and postextubation stridor. *Chest.* 1996;110:1035–1040.
9. Kriner EJ, Shafazand S, Colice GL: The endotracheal tube cuff-leak test as a predictor for postextubation stridor. *Respir Care.* 2005;50:1632–1638.
10. Maury E, Guglielminotti J, Alzieu M, et al.: How to identify patients with no risk for postextubation stridor? *J Crit Care.* 2004;19:23–28.
11. Ding DL, Wang HC, Wu HD, Chang CJ, Yang PC. Laryngeal ultrasound: a useful method in predicting post-extubation stridor. A pilot study. *Eur Respir J.* 2006;27:384–389.
12. Erginel S, Ucgun I, Yildirim H, Metintas M, Parspour S: High body mass index and long duration of intubation increase post-extubation stridor in patients with mechanical ventilation. *Tohoku J Exp Med.* 2005;207:125–132.
13. Anene O, Meert KL, Uy H, Simpson P, Sarnaik AP: Dexamethasone for the prevention of postextubation airway obstruction: a prospective, randomized, double-blind, placebo-controlled trial. *Crit Care Med.* 1996;24:1666–1669.
14. Markovitz BP, Randolph AG: Corticosteroids for the prevention of reintubation and postextubation stridor in pediatric patients: A meta-analysis. *Pediatr Crit Care Med.* 2002;3:223–226.
15. Darmon JY, Rauss A, Dreyfuss D, et al.: Evaluation of risk factors for laryngeal edema after tracheal extubation in adults and its prevention by dexamethasone. A placebo-controlled, double-blind, multicenter study. *Anesthesiology.* 1992;77:245–251.
16. Meade MO, Guyatt GH, Cook DJ, Sinuff T, Butler R: Trials of corticosteroids to prevent postextubation airway complications. *Chest.* 2001;120:464S–468S.
17. Suderman VS, Crosby ET, Lui A: Elective oral tracheal intubation in cervical spine-injured adults. *Can J Anaesth.* 1991;38:785–789.
18. Nathanson MH, Gajraj NM. Newson CD: Tracheal intubation in a manikin: comparison of supine and left lateral positions. *Br J Anaesth.* 1994;73:690–691.
19. Dimitriou V, Voyagis GS, Iatrou C, Brimacombe J: Flexible lightwand-guided intubation using the intubating laryngeal mask airway in the supine, right, and left lateral positions in healthy patients by experienced users. *Anesth Analg.* 2003;96:896–898.
20. Komatsu R, Nagata O, Sessler DI, Ozaki M: The intubating laryngeal mask airway facilitates tracheal intubation in the lateral position. *Anesth Analg.* 2004;98:858–861.
21. Cheng KI, Chu K. S, Chau SW, et al.: Lightwand-assisted intubation of patients in the lateral decubitus position. *Anesth Analg.* 2004;99:279–283.
22. Baer K: Is it much more difficult to intubate in prone position? *Lakartidningen.* 1992;89:3657–3660.
23. Farcon EL, Kim MH, Marx GF: Changing Mallampati score during labour. *Can J Anaesth.* 1994;41:50–51.
24. Samsoon GL, Young JR: Difficult tracheal intubation: a retrospective study. *Anaesthesia.* 1987; 42:487–490.
25. Mallampati SR: Clinical sign to predict difficult tracheal intubation (hypothesis). *Can Anaesth Soc J.* 1983;30:316–317.
26. Knill RL: Difficult laryngoscopy made easy with a "BURP". *Can J Anaesth.* 1993;40:279–282.
27. Cormack RS, Lehane J: Difficult tracheal intubation in obstetrics. *Anaesthesia.* 1984;39:1105–1111.
28. Kidd JF, Dyson A, Latto IP: Successful difficult intubation. Use of the gum elastic bougie. *Anaesthesia.* 1988;43:437–438.

SELF-EVALUATION QUESTIONS

35.1. Following dislodgement of the endotracheal tube (ETT) in the prone position, all of the following are acceptable initial methods to provide oxygenation and ventilation to the patient **EXCEPT**

A. advancing the ETT over a fiberoptic bronchoscope into the trachea.

B. reintubation of the trachea using a laryngoscope.

C. insertion of a laryngeal mask airway.

D. BMV.

E. establish a surgical airway.

35.2. Following orotracheal intubation, which of the following is the **LEAST** acceptable method of securing the endotracheal tube (ETT) in a patient with facial hair?

A. Tie the ETT around the neck with an umbilical tape.

B. Suture the ETT to the lip.

C. Tie the ETT to the upper incisors.

D. Secure the ETT with a waterproof tape after the appliation of tincture of benzoin to the face.

E. Shave the patient's beard prior to induction of anesthesia.

35.3. Which of the following is **MOST** reliable in assessing postoperative airway edema in a patient who was placed prone for the procedure?

A. The amount of intraoperative fluid administered to the patient.

B. The presence of facial edema.

C. The leak test.

D. Duration of placing the patient in a prone position.

E. None of the above.

CHAPTER (36)

Airway Management of Patients with a History of Difficult Intubation for a Peripheral Procedure

Lorraine J. Foley

36.1 CASE PRESENTATION

A 38-year-old obese male is scheduled for the operating room for ruptured left achilles tendon repair. The patient is 5′7″ (169 cm) tall and weighs 308 lb (140 kg). He has no known drug allergies. Past medical history is significant for obstructive sleep apnea (OSA) and he is on continuous positive airway pressure (CPAP) at home. He has no other medical problems and has no gastroesophageal reflux disease (GERD). His past surgical history is significant for laparoscopic cholecystectomy 2 years ago at which time he was told that he had a difficult intubation but he does not know the details. On examination, his Mallampati Class is III, he has a large tongue, a short thick neck, and full dentition. His mouth opening is 4.0 cm.

36.2 AIRWAY EVALUATION

36.2.1 Would this patient be difficult to ventilate using a bag-mask-ventilation or an extraglottic device?

There are five predictors of difficult mask-ventilation.[1] These predictors can be evaluated using the MOANS mnemonic (see Section 1.6.1). This patient has two of the five predictors of difficult mask-ventilation. He is obese and has OSA requiring CPAP at home.

RODS is a mnemonic that is intended to identify problem patients when using an extraglottic device (EGD) (see Section 1.6.3). Apart from potential upper airway obstruction (OSA), there are no other predicted difficulties in using an EGD.

36.2.2 Would direct laryngoscopy and intubation be difficult in this patient?

A prediction of the likelihood of a difficult direct laryngoscopy can be made using the "LEMON" mnemonic (see Section 1.6.2). The Mallampati Score and the history of OSA of this patient are positive predictors of difficult direct laryngoscopy. His short thick neck is also not reassuring.

36.2.3 Would it be difficult to perform a cricothyrotomy in this patient?

The SHORT mnemonic (see Section 1.6.4) can be used to predict difficult cricothyrotomy. Performance of a surgical airway may be difficult as the patient is morbidly obese (with a BMI > 49 kg.m^{-2}) and has a short neck.

36.3 SPECIAL ANESTHETIC CONSIDERATIONS

36.3.1 Would a regional anesthesia be acceptable for this patient?

In the revised ASA algorithm, regional anesthesia is considered to be an acceptable option if either awake intubation or intubation after induction of general anesthesia (GA) fails.[2] Rosenblatt has also described a decision-tree approach to preoperative airway assessment, the Airway Approach Algorithm.[3] The first decision point in this algorithm is in response to the question "must the airway be 'managed'?" If the answer is no, then regional/infiltrative techniques should be considered.[3] In a survey of management choices for the difficult airway by anesthesiologists in Canada, a spinal anesthetic was chosen by 16% of respondents for a case scenario of emergency cesarean section for fetal distress and "airway looks difficult" even though the survey specified that the patient required GA and endotracheal intubation.[4] Another survey of anesthesia practitioners described a patient with a known difficult airway presenting for elective caesarean section and assumed that regional anesthesia was the preferred technique.[5] For parturients, it is felt that regional anesthesia should be the technique of choice for a cesarean section if circumstances permit.[6,7] Anesthesia-related maternal mortality was reviewed by Hawkins in 2003.[8] Of pregnancy-related deaths during live birth in the United States between the period 1991–1997, 1.8% were causally linked to an anesthetic cause. Further, between 1991 and 1996, the case fatality rate for GA was estimated at 16.8 per million, whereas the case fatality for regional anesthesia was 2.5 per million.[8] Airway problems were the most common causes of anesthesia-related deaths.[8]

However, regional anesthesia in a patient with a known difficult intubation does not negate a difficult airway. The anesthesia practitioner must be prepared to manage the airway should it become necessary in the event of a failed regional technique or a complication related to the regional technique. Complications associated with regional anesthesia as documented in the ASA closed claims database have recently been reviewed.[9] Of the regional anesthesia claims resulting in death or brain damage, 51% were associated with spinal anesthesia, 41% with epidural anesthesia, 2% with interscalene block, 1% with axillary block, and 5% with miscellaneous blocks.[9] Multiple case reports of complications related to regional anesthesia have been published. According to one such report, rapid unexpected obtundation and respiratory paralysis developed after placement of a lumbosacral plexus block.[10] In another case, immediately after injection for an interscalene block the patient became unresponsive and apneic, with loss of muscle tone.[11] Twelve cases of asystole and severe bradycardia during epidural anesthesia in orthopedic patients have also been reported.[12] The ASA closed claims database has no denominator and therefore no incidence can be calculated. However, a prospective survey in France reported serous complications related to regional anesthesia and allows the incidence to be determined.[13] Of the 103,730 regional anesthetics performed, 98 severe complications were reported of which 89 were attributed either fully or partially to the regional anesthesia. Cardiac arrest occurred in 32 cases, with spinal anesthesia having the highest incidence.[13]

Many factors must be taken into account before deciding to proceed with a regional anesthetic technique in a patient with a known difficult airway. First and foremost, the expertise of the anesthesia practitioner, in both regional anesthesia and airway management, must be considered. It would be inappropriate to have a junior anesthesia trainee perform the regional anesthesia technique. Kopacz et al. looked at the learning curves for the placement of spinals and epidurals and concluded that for a 90% success rate, 45 and 60 placements of spinal and epidural anesthesia respectively may be necessary.[14]

Second, the patient must have no contraindications to the regional technique and must be cooperative and calm. Heavy sedation cannot be a supplement for an inadequate regional anesthetic in a patient with a known difficult airway, especially in the presence of obesity and OSA as in this patient. The patient must

understand the full implications of a regional technique and be prepared for an awake intubation should that become necessary.

Third, the surgeon must also understand the implications of a failed or incomplete regional block, be willing to supplement with local anesthetics if required as dose limits permit, and must be cooperative if GA is required. The anesthesia practitioner and surgeon must function as a team and have good communication.

Fourth, the type and duration of the surgery as well as the positioning of the patient must be considered. The anesthesia practitioner must have easy access to the patient's airway and the surgeon must be able to stop operating at any time during the surgery. A carotid endarterectomy is therefore not a good case for a regional technique (e.g., cervical block) in a patient with a difficult airway. The prone position should be considered risky but possible if a bed or stretcher is immediately available, the patient can easily be turned to the supine position, and airway equipment must be immediately available at all times especially while placing a regional block.

36.3.2 Would an "awake look" (awake direct laryngoscopy) be useful?

When a difficult direct laryngoscopy is predicted on preoperative assessment, the airway can be further evaluated by means of an awake direct laryngoscopy, also called the "awake look".[15] The purpose of an awake direct laryngoscopy is to examine the airway in the awake state such that a prediction of the direct laryngoscopic view following induction of GA can be made. However, how much visualization of the airway structures is sufficient to ensure that the direct laryngoscopic view under GA will be adequate for endotracheal intubation has not been clearly defined.

Careful examination is required to determine the presence of fixed or nonfixed anatomic features which may make direct laryngoscopy difficult. The upper airway consists of a bone and cartilage framework including the mandible and spine surrounded by muscle and other soft tissue.[16,17] Fixed anatomic features include decreased mouth opening and prominent front teeth. Nonfixed features include soft tissue such as muscle. Muscle tone is dynamic and typically changes as the degree of consciousness changes. These dynamic changes affecting the upper airway muscle activity depend partly on a centrally mediated drive from the brainstem and partly on local reflexes in the upper airway. The most important stimulus for these changes is negative intrapharyngeal pressure related to spontaneous respiration.[18] In an anesthetized and paralyzed patient, these dynamic anatomic changes may decrease the patency of the upper airway and obstruct a direct view of the vocal cords. It has also been shown that the larynx moves to a more anterior position under GA and paralysis,[19] such that an awake Cormack/Lehane grade 2 or 3 view becomes a grade 4 under GA.

Anesthetic agents have been shown to alter upper airway muscle activity locally at upper airway mechanoreceptors and centrally in the brain stem. Most of these agents appear to inhibit upper airway muscle activity more than the diaphragm.[20] Sedation with midazolam has been shown to decrease muscle activity and tone and may lead to airway obstruction—a fact that is crucial in patients who present with upper airway obstruction for any reason.[21] Volatile anesthetic agents such as isoflurane have also been associated with decreased muscle activity and increased collapsibility of the upper airway, particularly at the level of the soft palate.[22]

Investigations such as lateral radiographs, and more recently MRI, have been used to determine the effects of GA on airway patency in both adults and children. Nandi et al. studied 18 normal patients under GA, not paralyzed with no history of OSA.[23] They noted that radiographic occlusion of the airway occurred consistently at the level of the soft palate, and sometimes at the epiglottis, but not the base of the tongue. It was also noted that there was a caudad shift of both the epiglottis and hyoid bone under anesthesia.[23] This was also seen by Shorten et al. using MRI. They found a decrease in the anteroposterior diameter of the airway at the level of the soft palate and epiglottis in sedated patients as compared to their awake state.[24] In children, the cross-sectional area of the entire pharyngeal airway decreased with increasing depth of propofol anesthesia, with the greatest reduction occurring at the level of the epiglottis.[25] Healthy nonobese (within 20% of their ideal body weight) adult volunteers with no history of sleep disturbances or upper airway pathology were administered propofol anesthesia in a study by Mathru et al.[26] The investigators found that the anteroposterior diameter of the pharynx at the level of the soft palate was reduced, but not at the epiglottis or base of the tongue.[26]

OSA is also considered to be a risk factor for a difficult airway.[27] Several studies have looked at the relationship between OSA and difficult tracheal intubation.[27–29] Many conditions associated with difficult tracheal intubation are associated with upper airway geometric features that decrease the space available for anterior displacement of the tongue during direct laryngoscopy and decreased hypopharyngeal dimensions predisposing to OSA.[28] Isono et al. compared the mechanics of the paralyzed pharynx in normal patients and patients with OSA under GA and concluded that the passive pharynx was narrower and more collapsible in OSA patients.[17]

There are no robust studies that correlate an awake direct laryngoscopic view with that under GA in patients with possible difficult intubation. The likelihood of difficult direct laryngoscopy is usually inferred from fixed and dynamic anatomic factors known to be associated with difficulty. Fixed anatomic characteristics such as micrognathia, prominent upper incisors, or lack of neck extension cannot be expected to change under anesthesia. Therefore, if the "awake look" direct laryngoscopy in these patients is inadequate, it follows that there is a very high probability that the view under anesthesia will also be inadequate.

With respect to the dynamic anatomic characteristics, MRI and other radiographic studies of normal patients infer that a correlation may exist between the laryngoscopic view of the vocal cords and epiglottis awake versus anesthetized.[1,17,19,24–26,28,29] However, the same cannot be said of patients with OSA. In individuals without OSA, once anesthetized there is a decrease in the caliber of the entire pharyngeal airway with the greatest reduction at the level of the soft palate, being less at the level of the epiglottis.[17,23–28]

It is this author's opinion that if the awake look is to be used to predict difficult direct laryngoscopy, a Cormack/Lehane Grade 1 or 2 view should be obtained in the awake state before proceeding with GA. The laryngoscopist must always keep in mind that an awake look is *not* helpful in the detection of subglottic pathology or the determination of its extent.

36.4 ANESTHETIC AND AIRWAY MANAGEMENT

36.4.1 Is there a preferred technique (Plan A)?

The patient is having a peripheral procedure in the prone position. He may be difficult to ventilate using bag-mask-ventilation and has a history of difficult intubation. His cricothyroid membrane is easily identifiable. Regional anesthesia is a reasonable first choice in this case, although the anesthesia practitioner must be prepared to manage the airway should that become necessary. Regional anesthesia options include spinal, epidural, femoral three-in-one block combined with sciatic nerve block, and tibial, common peroneal, and saphenous nerve blocks at the knee. A description of regional techniques is beyond the scope of this chapter. In the setting of a difficult airway, the anesthesia practitioner should choose the technique with which he or she is most comfortable and experienced.

The implications and risks of the regional anesthetic must be discussed in detail with the patient and surgeon as well as the back up plans should the regional anesthetic technique (Plan A) fail. In this case, the patient must be aware that only light sedation will be administered because of his difficult airway, OSA, and the prone position. He must also be aware that if the regional technique fails, an awake intubation may be required. The surgeon must be prepared to stop surgery and turn the patient into the supine position should that be necessary in the event of inadequate anesthesia or other complications. The stretcher should be kept in the OR during the procedure for immediate availability should supine positioning become necessary. A spinal anesthetic could be placed with the patient in the sitting position; 1.3 mL of 0.75% hyperbaric bupivicaine is adequate for a 2 hour procedure. During the procedure, oxygen can be administered by facemask and end tidal CO_2 monitored. Other standard monitors should be employed.

36.4.2 What action should be taken if Plan A fails (Plan B)?

If the spinal anesthesia is unsuccessful, Plan B is an awake fiberoptic intubation. This patient has already been identified as a difficult intubation and an awake direct laryngoscopy is unlikely to be helpful. The airway can be anesthetized with 4% lidocaine aerosolized via an atomizer. The superior laryngeal nerves can be blocked via the piriform fossae, using lidocaine soaked pledgets held in Jackson forceps. The glottis can be further anesthetized using supplemental lidocaine injected through the working channel of the fiberoptic scope (see Chapter 3 for a detailed description of topical anesthesia of the airway). Awake intubation can be performed using no adjunctive sedation. Alternatively, sedation using a combination of midazolam and fentanyl can be administered and titrated to effect. The use of dexmedetomidine, an alpha-2 agonist which has analgesic and sedative properties but does not cause respiratory depression, has recently been reported in the setting of awake intubation[30] (loading dose 1 $\mu g \cdot kg^{-1}$ over 10 minutes followed by an infusion of 0.7 $\mu g \cdot kg^{-1} \cdot hr^{-1}$).

36.4.3 Is there a Plan C?

During the placement of regional anesthesia, should the patient lose consciousness due to intravascular injection or a high spinal, the first step in resuscitation is airway control. Mask-ventilation should be attempted initially. If mask-ventilation is inadequate then an EGD should be placed. Placement of the laryngeal mask airway (LMA) is part of the ASA difficult airway algorithm[2] and the European Difficult Airway Society Guidelines.[31] Parmet et al. reported the use of an LMA in 17 of 25 cases of unanticipated difficult intubation and difficult ventilation.[32] Ventilation via the LMA was successful in 16/17 cases.[32] The one case in which ventilation via the LMA failed was due to thrombus in the trachea from a traumatic cricothyroid membrane puncture.[32] The LMA ProSeal™ has a modified cuff thus providing a better seal for positive pressure ventilation as well as a drainage tube that channels fluid regurgitated from the esophagus and permits placement of a gastric tube.[33,34] Alternatively, an intubating LMA (LMA Fastrach™) could be used. A retrospective study of patients with a difficult airways in whom the LMA Fastrach™ was used electively or urgently reported successful ventilation via the device in 100% of the patients.[35] Intubation was successful in 96.5% after the fifth blind attempt and in 100% with flexible fiberoptic guidance.[35] Other EGDs such as the King LT™ and Combitube™ could also be used in the presence of difficult mask-ventilation and difficult intubation in this scenario.

If ventilation is inadequate by mask or EGD, then either endotracheal intubation or a surgical airway is urgently required. Since no attempt at tracheal intubation has yet been attempted, it would be reasonable to attempt tracheal intubation, perhaps employing devices with a track record of success in patients with difficult airways, such as a Bullard laryngoscope or the GlideScope®. If tracheal intubation using these devices is not possible or acceptable oxygen saturations cannot be maintained, a surgical airway should be performed.

36.4.4 What actually happened in this case?

The patient underwent an uneventful spinal anesthetic and tendon repair. He was admitted to a monitored setting where systemic analgesia was titrated to effect. CPAP and oxygen were administered. The remainder of his hospital stay was uneventful.

36.4.5 What postoperative airway management is required?

Following successful regional anesthesia, the patient will require postoperative analgesia. The use of systemic opioids in the presence of OSA may exacerbate pharyngeal obstruction and precipitate hypoxic episodes.[21] Supplemental oxygen should be administered. If the patient was on CPAP preoperatively, it should be continued postoperatively. A monitored setting may be required. Continuous peripheral neuroblockade can also be utilized for postoperative analgesia. Should an awake intubation have been required, then awake extubation is prudent followed by postoperative analgesia, as in a regional technique. Should emergency airway intervention have been necessary, then postoperative airway management would depend on what intervention had been performed and the presence of airway trauma, if any. Management could include awake extubation or prolonged intubation pending resolution of airway edema.

36.5 SUMMARY

If an obese patient with a history of a difficult tracheal intubation presents to the operating room for a nonurgent peripheral surgical procedure, a detailed history and airway evaluation must be obtained. In particular, potential difficulties in bag-mask-ventilation, use of an EGD, tracheal intubation, and a surgical airway must be assessed. Provided that there are no contraindications, regional anesthesia is a reasonable first choice although the anesthesia practitioner must be prepared (Plan B and Plan C) to manage the airway should that become necessary.

REFERENCES

1. Langeron O, Masso E, Huraux C, et al.: Prediction of difficult mask ventilation. *Anesthesiology.* 2000;92:1229–1236.
2. Practice guidelines for management of the difficult airway: an updated report by the American Society of Anesthesiologists Task force on management of the difficult airway. *Anesthesiology.* 2003;98:1269–1277.
3. Rosenblatt WH: The Airway Approach Algorithm: a decision tree for organizing preoperative airway information. *J Clin Anesth.* 2004;16:312–316.
4. Jenkins K, Wong DT, Correa R: Management choices for the difficult airway by anesthesiologists in Canada. *Can J Anaesth.* 2002;49:850–856.
5. Popat MT, Srivastava M, Russell R: Awake fibreoptic intubation skills in obstetric patients: a survey of anaesthetists in the Oxford region. *Int J Obstet Anesth.* 2000;9:78–82.
6. Dennehy KC, Pian-Smith MC: Airway management of the parturient. *Int Anesthesiol Clin.* 2000;38:147–159.
7. Ezri T, Szmuk P, Evron S, et al.: Difficult airway in obstetric anesthesia: a review. *Obstet Gynecol Surv.* 2001;56:631–641.
8. Hawkins JL: Anesthesia-related maternal mortality. *Clin Obstet Gynecol.* 2003;46:679–687.
9. Lee L: Complications associated with regional anesthesia. *APSF Newsletter.* 2004:5–6.
10. Muravchick S, Owens WD: An unusual complication of lumbosacral plexus block: a case report. *Anesth Analg.* 1976;55:350–352.
11. Dutton RP, Eckhardt WF, 3rd, Sunder N: Total spinal anesthesia after interscalene blockade of the brachial plexus. *Anesthesiology.* 1994;80:939–941.
12. Liguori GA, Sharrock NE: Asystole and severe bradycardia during epidural anesthesia in orthopedic patients. *Anesthesiology.* 1997;86:250–257.
13. Auroy Y, Narchi P, Messiah A, et al.: Serious complications related to regional anesthesia: results of a prospective survey in France. *Anesthesiology.* 1997;87:479–486.
14. Kopacz DJ, Neal JM, Pollock JE: The regional anesthesia "learning curve". What is the minimum number of epidural and spinal blocks to reach consistency? *Reg Anesth.* 1996;21:182–190.
15. Benumof JL: Management of the difficult adult airway. With special emphasis on awake tracheal intubation. *Anesthesiology.* 1991;75:1087–1110.
16. Goldberg AN, Schwab RJ: Identifying the patient with sleep apnea: upper airway assessment and physical examination. *Otolaryngol Clin North Am.* 1998;31:919–930.
17. Isono S, Remmers JE, Tanaka A, et al.: Anatomy of pharynx in patients with obstructive sleep apnea and in normal subjects. *J Appl Physiol.* 1997;82:1319–1326.
18. Malhotra A, Pillar G, Fogel RB, et al.: Pharyngeal pressure and flow effects on genioglossus activation in normal subjects. *Am J Respir Crit Care Med.* 2002;165:71–77.

19. Sivarajan M, Fink BR: The position and the state of the larynx during general anesthesia and muscle paralysis. *Anesthesiology*. 1990;72:439–442.
20. Brouillette RT, Thach BT: A neuromuscular mechanism maintaining extrathoracic airway patency. *J Appl Physiol*. 1979;46:772–779.
21. Drummond GB: Comparison of sedation with midazolam and ketamine: effects on airway muscle activity. *Br J Anaesth*. 1996;76:663–667.
22. Eastwood PR, Szollosi I, Platt PR, Hillman DR: Collapsibility of the upper airway during anesthesia with isoflurane. *Anesthesiology*. 2002;97:786–793.
23. Nandi PR, Charlesworth CH, Taylor SJ, Nunn JF, Dore CJ: Effect of general anaesthesia on the pharynx. *Br J Anaesth*. 1991;66:157–162.
24. Shorten GD, Opie NJ, Graziotti P, Morris I, Khangure M: Assessment of upper airway anatomy in awake, sedated and anaesthetised patients using magnetic resonance imaging. *Anaesth Intensive Care*. 1994;22:165–169.
25. Evans RG, Crawford MW, Noseworthy MD, Yoo SJ: Effect of increasing depth of propofol anesthesia on upper airway configuration in children. *Anesthesiology*. 2003;99:596–602.
26. Mathru M, Esch O, Lang J, et al.: Magnetic resonance imaging of the upper airway. Effects of propofol anesthesia and nasal continuous positive airway pressure in humans. *Anesthesiology*. 1996;84:273–279.
27. Siyam MA, Benhamou D: Difficult endotracheal intubation in patients with sleep apnea syndrome. *Anesth Analg*. 2002;95:1098–102.
28. Hiremath AS, Hillman DR, James AL, et al.: Relationship between difficult tracheal intubation and obstructive sleep apnoea. *Br J Anaesth*.1998;80:606–611.
29. Isono S, Tanaka A, Nishino T: Lateral position decreases collapsibility of the passive pharynx in patients with obstructive sleep apnea. *Anesthesiology*. 2002;97:780–785.
30. Scher CS, Gitlin MC: Dexmedetomidine and low-dose ketamine provide adequate sedation for awake fibreoptic intubation. *Can J Anaesth*. 2003;50:607–610.
31. Henderson JJ, Popat MT, Latto IP, Pearce AC: Difficult Airway Society guidelines for management of the unanticipated difficult intubation. *Anaesthesia*. 2004;59:675–694.
32. Parmet JL, Colonna-Romano P, Horrow JC, et al.: The laryngeal mask airway reliably provides rescue ventilation in cases of unanticipated difficult tracheal intubation along with difficult mask ventilation. *Anesth Analg*. 1998;87:661–665.
33. Brimacombe J, Keller C: The ProSeal laryngeal mask airway: A randomized, crossover study with the standard laryngeal mask airway in paralyzed, anesthetized patients. *Anesthesiology*. 2000;93:104–109.
34. Brimacombe J, Keller C: Airway protection with the ProSeal laryngeal mask airway. *Anaesth Intensive Care*. 2001;29:288–291.
35. Ferson DZ, Rosenblatt WH, Johansen MJ, Osborn I, Ovassapian A: Use of the intubating LMA-Fastrach in 254 patients with difficult-to-manage airways. *Anesthesiology*. 2001;95:1175–181.

SELF EVALUATION QUESTIONS

36.1. In normal patients under general anesthesia, radiographic occlusion of the airway has been found to occur consistently at

A. the level of the soft palate

B. the epiglottis

C. the base of the tongue

D. the glottic opening

E. none of the above

36.2. Correlation of the "awake look" with direct laryngoscopy under general anesthesia

A. has not been clearly defined

B. is within the same laryngoscopic grade

C. is within one laryngoscopic grade

D. is within two laryngoscopic grade

E. none of the above

36.3. From the ASA Closed Claims database, claims for death or brain damage associated with regional anesthesia occurred most often with

A. epidural anesthesia

B. interscalene block

C. spinal anesthesia

D. 3 in 1 femoral nerve block

E. axillary block

CHAPTER 37

Airway Management of a Patient with an Unanticipated Difficult Laryngoscopy

John J. Henderson

37.1 CASE PRESENTATION

A 40-year-old female is scheduled for laparoscopic cholecystectomy. She has no comorbidity. Previous anesthesia was for tonsillectomy during childhood and for hysterectomy 10 years before the current admission. Both operations were performed in other hospitals, but the patient was not aware of any problems or complications associated with anesthesia. Preoperative airway assessment showed an interincisor distance of 4 cm, a full set of healthy teeth with healthy gums, Mallampati Class II,[1] and head extension 30 degrees.[2] Thyromental distance was 6.5 cm.[3] The mandibular incisors could be protruded anterior to the maxillary incisors.[4] No difficulties with direct laryngoscopy or tracheal intubation were anticipated.

37.2 PATIENT CONSIDERATIONS

There were no special considerations for this patient.

37.3 AIRWAY CONSIDERATIONS

37.3.1 What factors influence the choice between tracheal intubation and the use of an extraglottic device for airway management of a patient scheduled for laparoscopic cholecystectomy?

The choice is controversial. Factors that should be considered include aspects of physiology, positioning, and management of surgical complications.

37.3.2 What are the most important changes in respiratory and cardiovascular physiology during uncomplicated laparoscopic cholecystectomy?

The most important respiratory and cardiovascular changes that occur during laparoscopy are a consequence of carbon dioxide pneumoperitoneum, which elevates intra-abdominal pressure (IAP) and leads to carbon dioxide absorption.[5] Elevated IAP raises the diaphragm and hence reduces lung volume and compliance and increases airway resistance. The reduced lung volume promotes uneven distribution of ventilation, leading to hypoxemia and hypercarbia. The risk of accidental endobronchial intubation is increased as the carina is pushed cephalad. An elevated IAP also increases the risk of regurgitation of gastric contents. As carbon dioxide is absorbed the blood concentration rises, leading to cardiovascular changes and the need to increase ventilation. Cardiovascular changes are produced by a combination of hypercarbia, the head-elevated position, and raised IAP. The net effect of these respiratory and cardiovascular effects is much greater in patients undergoing laparoscopic cholecystectomy than in those undergoing gynecological laparoscopy because patients in the former group are older and the duration of surgery is longer.

37.3.3 What complications of laparoscopic cholecystectomy have the greatest bearing on airway management?

Conversion to open cholecystectomy (1–7%[6] of patients) may be required if laparoscopic surgery proves to be not possible or if repair to the bile duct, blood vessels, or other structure proves necessary. Such a conversion may be urgent if there is uncontrolled bleeding. Other surgical complications include extraperitoneal gas insufflation, venous gas embolism, and pneumothorax.[7]

37.3.4   What are the claimed advantages of the LMA, LMA ProSeal™, and other extraglottic airway devices in laparoscopic surgery?

Recovery is generally smoother with the LMA; in particular there is a lower incidence of coughing.[8] Other arguments for use of the LMA are based on the limitations of tracheal intubation, such as difficulty or failure of intubation and complications such as dental damage.

37.3.5   What are the disadvantages of extraglottic airway devices in laparoscopic cholecystectomy?

In my opinion, the use of extraglottic devices (EGDs) for laparoscopic cholecystectomy has many disadvantages in comparison with tracheal intubation. The presence in the trachea of a cuffed tracheal tube provides the best protection against aspiration of regurgitated gastric contents. The cardiovascular effects induced by hypercarbia and the respiratory effects induced by raised IAP can be reversed by increasing ventilation. This is achieved most reliably by positive pressure ventilation through a cuffed tracheal tube. The incidence of dangerous intraoperative deterioration of the airway is much higher with an EGD[8] than with a tracheal tube. Although tracheal intubation can be performed during surgery, intubation in this situation is more hazardous than in ideal conditions at induction of anesthesia. Intraoperative tracheal intubation may interrupt surgery and threaten the sterility and integrity of tissues. It may be necessary to perform tracheal intubation in a suboptimal patient position so that there is an increased risk of airway trauma or failure to intubate. Furthermore intraoperative intubation will usually be performed in a situation in which the patient has not been denitrogenated optimally or is already hypoxemic so that the risk of hypoxemic damage is increased. Surgical complications of laparoscopic cholecystectomy are best managed if the surgeon has the best operating conditions, full neuromuscular blockade, and when the airway is best secured with a cuffed tracheal tube.

37.3.6   Use of the LMA ProSeal™ for airway management of nonobese patients undergoing laparoscopic cholecystectomy has been advocated.[8,9] What is the evidence that it is a good alternative to tracheal intubation for slim and obese patients undergoing laparoscopic cholecystectomy?

The LMA ProSeal™ provides a higher leak pressure and better protection against pulmonary aspiration than the standard LMA. The LMA ProSeal™ has features which might make it a more appropriate EGD for laparoscopic cholecystectomy;[8] however, it requires more attempts at insertion than the classic LMA and may fail.[10] The LMA ProSeal™ should be used only by those who have

demonstrated a high success rate with the device and have a meticulous technique.[9] Tracheal intubation should be performed if ventilation is inadequate or the LMA ProSeal™ is malpositioned.[9] In Maltby's study, 4 of 16 obese patients required conversion to tracheal intubation because of airway obstruction or leak,[8] obstruction occurring 60–90 minutes after induction of anesthesia in 2 patients. There must be serious doubt about the role of the LMA ProSeal™ in laparoscopic cholecystectomy.

37.3.7   What expert opinions have been expressed on the role of EGDs in laparoscopic cholecystectomy?

Early reviews of anesthetic management of laparoscopic cholecystectomy recommended use of controlled ventilation[6] with tracheal intubation[5,6] for airway management in order to facilitate adequate ventilation and to minimize the risk of pulmonary aspiration. Concerns about the general safety of artificial ventilation of the paralyzed patient through the LMA[11] and more specifically its use in laparoscopic surgery in the obese patient[12] are discussed in recent editorials. Some studies have come out strongly against use of the original LMA for airway management during laparoscopic cholecystectomy.[9,13]

37.3.8   What are the advantages of tracheal intubation for airway management of patients undergoing laparoscopic cholecystectomy?

First, tracheal intubation avoids all the disadvantages of EGDs discussed above. Second, regular tracheal intubation has real advantages for the anesthesia practitioner. Maintenance of expertise with more than one technique of tracheal intubation under vision should be the aim of every anesthesia practitioner.[14] The risk of complications is minimized when the anesthesia practitioner has an extended range of skills.[14]

37.4   PREINTUBATION PREPARATION AND PLANS

Standard preparations were made. Venous access and monitoring[14] were established. The pharmacology plan was denitrogenation, followed by intravenous induction of anesthesia with propofol, and neuromuscular blockade with vecuronium. Tracheal intubation under vision with the Macintosh laryngoscope was planned.

37.5   TRACHEAL INTUBATION

37.5.1   What actually happened in this case?

Bag-mask-ventilation (BMV) was effective after induction of anesthesia. Direct laryngoscopy with the Macintosh laryngoscope was performed after full neuromuscular blockade developed. It was not possible to see even the epiglottis (Cormack/Lehane (C/L) grade 4 view[15]) and a second attempt at direct laryngoscopy was performed with the McCoy laryngoscope. The best view of the larynx achieved was again C/L grade 4. Direct laryngoscopy was then attempted with a straight laryngoscope, using the paraglossal technique.[16] The epiglottis was seen to be displaced posteriorly such that it lay against the posterior pharyngeal wall. It proved very difficult to pass the tip of the straight laryngoscope posterior to the epiglottis, and further attempts at direct laryngoscopy were abandoned. BMV remained easy and effective throughout and good oxygenation was maintained. Anesthesia was continued with volatile anesthesia in 100% oxygen.

The anesthesia practitioner suspected that a lesion in the vallecula might be responsible for the posterior displacement of the epiglottis. Digital examination of the tongue revealed a firm mass in the vallecula and lingual tonsillar hypertrophy (LTH) was suspected. Blind techniques of tracheal intubation were not attempted. Surgery was postponed. Ventilation and oxygenation with bag and mask continued to be effective and anesthesia was maintained with volatile anesthesia and nitrous oxide until the first twitch of the train of four could be identified. Neuromuscular blockade was then reversed, spontaneous ventilation was established, anesthesia was stopped, and consciousness returned. Subsequent investigation with nasendoscopy, lateral radiograph of the neck, and MRI scan confirmed the diagnosis of LTH.

Laparoscopic cholecystectomy was rescheduled. On this occasion the airway was secured by tracheal intubation under topical anesthesia, using the flexible fiberoptic laryngoscope, before induction of anesthesia. Subsequent anesthesia, surgery, and recovery were uneventful.

37.5.2 What is lingual tonsil hypertrophy?

The lingual tonsil is part of a ring of tonsillar tissue that surrounds the entrance to the upper airway. Lingual tonsillar tissue is situated bilaterally on the dorsal surface of the tongue.[17] Unlike the palatine tonsil, the lingual tonsil is not encapsulated.[17,18] Pathological processes affecting the lingual tonsil are relatively uncommon, but any condition causing enlargement of the lingual tonsil can cause life-threatening airway problems, particularly in the anesthetized patient. The most frequent pathological process is hypertrophy. Hypertrophic lingual tonsils vary in size,[17,19,20] commonly filling and extending beyond the vallecula and displacing the epiglottis posteriorly. The size of the lingual tonsil may change greatly in a few weeks[20] in any individual patient.

LTH is usually asymptomatic. However, it may produce many nonspecific symptoms[21] including dysphagia,[22] globus sensation, alteration of voice, choking, and dyspnea.[21] It may cause intermittent airway obstruction.[23,24] Snoring[25–28] is a major complaint of many patients. Infection may precipitate airway obstruction or hemorrhage.[29] Most patients have a past history of palatine tonsillectomy.[17,21,30]

37.5.3 In what way does LTH (and other vallecular lesions) affect tracheal intubation?

Functionally similar lesions such as lingual thyroid[31,32] and vallecular and epiglottic cysts[25,33,34] have a similar effect on airway management and cases of these conditions will be used to illus-

trate aspects of airway management of patients with LTH. In some cases, the mass is pedunculated and intermittently obstructs the glottis. When these lesions are large enough to fill the vallecula, they make it almost impossible for Macintosh[20,35–37] (or similar such as McCoy[20,35]) laryngoscopes to be properly positioned; therefore, indirect elevation of the epiglottis is not possible. Furthermore LTH displaces the epiglottis posteriorly so that it requires some expertise to pass a flexible, straight, or Bullard-type laryngoscope behind the epiglottis and then move the tip of the device anteriorly to allow visualization of the glottis.

An example of LTH is shown in Figure 37-1. The LTH fills the vallecula and displaces the epiglottis so that it lies against the posterior pharyngeal wall. Although it is occasionally possible to push a small lesion to the side with the Macintosh[32] or straight laryngoscope[38] or the tracheal tube,[39] it is very unlikely that the Macintosh will facilitate a view of the larynx.[29,36,40] Blind intubation with the Macintosh laryngoscope may be successful,[20,34] but this is a consequence of good luck on which one should not rely. The LMA will sometimes provide a clear airway,[20,30,41,42] but neither classic LMA[20,35,36] nor intubating LMA[35] may work satisfactorily. Blind techniques such as use of a Eschmann Tracheal Tube Introducer ("bougie") may have a higher risk of failure than normal[25,43] and can easily traumatize the tonsillar tissue. The safest plan is to awaken the patient and subsequently perform elective flexible fiberoptic intubation (FFI) under topical anesthesia,[20,35,43] but the user may need a high skill level in order to negotiate a path posterior to the epiglottis and then anteriorly to pass between the vocal cords.

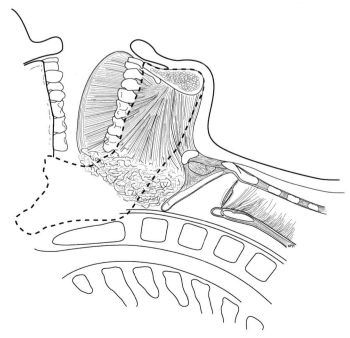

FIGURE 37-1. Hypertrophied lingual tonsillar tissue fills the vallecula and displaces the epiglottis so that it lies against the posterior pharyngeal wall.

37.5.4   How does LTH affect BMV and how should failure of BMV and tracheal intubation (the "can't intubate, can't ventilate" situation) be managed?

BMV may be difficult,[25,27,30,41] or impossible,[19,20,29,36] particularly when cricoid pressure is applied,[44] but satisfactory oxygenation can be maintained in most patients, at least initially. The first priority in management is to maintain oxygenation.[45] If the "can't intubate, can't ventilate" (CICV) situation develops and noninvasive techniques (two-person BMV with oral and nasal airway, LMA, or other EGD) do not restore oxygenation, cricothyrotomy[20,36] may be necessary (tracheotomy may take too long).[19] It is not possible to define the SpO_2 at which cricothyrotomy should be performed—it depends on the degree of hypoxemia and how rapidly it is deteriorating.[46] Cannula cricothyrotomy with high-pressure jet ventilation has long been advocated[47] as the least invasive cricothyrotomy technique for rescue oxygenation in CICV, but it may fail[20,36] in the LTH patient or cause barotrauma.[36] The airway practitioner should be prepared to perform immediate surgical cricothyrotomy[20,36] in either of these situations.

37.5.5   What is the role of blind techniques (stylet, Eschmann introducer,[48] lighted stylet[49]) of tracheal intubation when the primary technique fails to provide a view of any part of the larynx?

Most anesthesia practitioners normally resort to these blind techniques when they fail to visualize the larynx with the Macintosh laryngoscope, but caution in the use of such techniques must be exercised. If the first priority is to maintain oxygenation, the second priority is to prevent airway trauma.[45,50] Prevention of airway trauma is important in all patients, particularly in patients with conditions such as LTH. Blind techniques should be used gently, if used at all. Alternative techniques of proven value in facilitating tracheal intubation under vision may be attempted if the anesthesia practitioner has expertise with their use. If none of these techniques is successful, surgery should be postponed and the patient awakened.

The Eschmann Tracheal Tube Introducer (commonly known as the "gum-elastic bougie") is particularly important. It has a good track record (66[51]–90[52]% success rate, with the figure depending on whether data were gathered prospectively or retrospectively, the initial view, and how many attempts at laryngoscopy were made[53]), but has the disadvantages of a significant failure rate and the potential to cause trauma (mostly unreported, but present in records of the United Kingdom Medical Defense Union). Blind techniques are sometimes successful[25,54,55] in the LTH patient, although several attempts[31] may be required. However, the wisdom of making more that two blind attempts at intubation must be questioned. The disadvantage of causing serious airway trauma that could lead to CICV outweighs the diminishing possibility of achieving tracheal intubation. Trauma, usually blind, to vallecular lesions such as LTH may cause disastrous swelling and bleeding[42] with the consequence that moderate difficulty in airway management is converted to a life-threatening failure of oxygenation and ventilation,[30] when the only hope of survival for the patient is immediate creation of a surgical airway. Some guidelines for patients undergoing elective surgery have suggested a limit of four attempts at blind intubation,[45] but Combes' limit of two attempts[52] should be commended. If tracheal intubation cannot be achieved within four attempts at the primary intubation technique (Difficult Airway Society [United Kingdom DAS] Guidelines Plan A) and two attempts at the secondary technique (DAS Plan B) in the patient undergoing elective surgery, surgery should be postponed and the patient awakened (DAS Plan C).[45]

37.5.6   What investigations should be performed in patients with a history of sleep apnea?

Most cases of LTH are asymptomatic and are not diagnosed when the patient presents for surgery. However, it is desirable to detect this lesion whenever possible. Although most patients with a history of sleep apnea will not have LTH, all should be investigated[42] before elective surgery with at least a lateral neck radiograph or nasendoscopy.

37.5.7   What successful tracheal intubation techniques have been described in the presence of LTH?

Some techniques of tracheal intubation under vision may be successful when the user has a high level of skill with that technique, but success is unlikely when the user has limited skill and experience. Although not a technique under direct vision (visualizing the tracheal tube entering the glottis), the FFI has much to offer in the hands of the skilled user. Ovassapian's group achieved 100% success rate in 33 LTH patients, although passage of the flexible fiberoptic bronchoscope (FFB) was difficult in 20 (61%) and tube passage was difficult in 11 (33%).[30] Others have found FFI difficult[56] in LTH patients and it may fail as a consequence of blood in the pharynx[19,40] or difficulty in steering round the epiglottis.[20] In addition, it may prove impossible to pass a tracheal tube over a properly positioned FFB.[36,57] Techniques that involve passing a laryngoscope posterior to the epiglottis and elevating it directly may be successful. In particular, the straight anesthesia[37,38,58] or ENT[20,59] type laryngoscope, alternatively the rigid bronchoscope (passed and then exchanged for a tracheal tube[60]), and the Bullard-type[27,61] laryngoscope have been used successfully in patients with undiagnosed LTH to achieve tracheal intubation under vision. Use of the straight laryngoscope from the side of the mouth (paraglossal technique[16,37]) may succeed when a more central approach has failed.[20] Crosby suggests that the Bullard is the laryngoscope of choice in this situation.[61] The Bullard is robust, portable, and its use involves minimal distortion of tissues so that it can be used under light or topical anesthesia. These alternative techniques should be used regularly in routine practice so that the airway practitioner has the skill necessary to achieve a high success rate in the presence of undiagnosed lesions in the vallecula.

37.5.8 In what way should management of unanticipated difficult intubation due to undiagnosed LTH differ in the patient undergoing emergency surgery?

The DAS guidelines recommend that if it is not absolutely necessary to proceed with surgery the patient should be awakened and awake FFI should be used.[45] If it is absolutely essential to proceed with surgery, an EGD may be used, and the LMA ProSeal™ is probably the device of choice. However it would probably not function well in many LTH patients. The emergency patient with unanticipated difficult intubation as a consequence of undiagnosed LTH would be best managed with the straight or Bullard laryngoscope by anesthesia practitioners with sufficient expertise. The anesthesia practitioner should be prepared to perform cricothyrotomy, if necessary.[45]

37.5.9 Can LTH be diagnosed preoperatively or during laryngoscopy?

Preoperative diagnosis in the patient who does not already have a diagnosis of LTH is unlikely as most symptoms are nonspecific. Intraoperative diagnosis is not easy. In some cases it has been noted that the epiglottis is displaced posteriorly but this appearance is not diagnostic of LTH or other vallecular lesions. Intraoperative diagnosis by digital palpation may be possible in small patients.[21,35]

37.5.10 Would guidelines have helped the anesthesia practitioner in management of failed laryngoscopy in this patient?

DAS guidelines include use of an Eschmann Introducer ("bougie") in Plan A and intubating LMA as a conduit for tracheal intubation in Plan B. Both these techniques would probably fail and might cause airway trauma in many LTH patients. Guidelines are of great value for the average patient, but must be applied thoughtfully. Airway practitioners should always watch for signs of unusual anatomy. Marked posterior displacement of the epiglottis should alert one to the possibility of a lesion in the vallecula. On the other hand, application of plan D of the DAS guidelines could be lifesaving if the patient developed CICV.

37.6 POSTANESTHESIA MANAGEMENT

Postoperative discussion would take place with the patient about the consequences of her personal difficult intubation, documentation of the event, and reminder for a Medic-Alert®.

37.6.1 What responsibilities does the anesthesia practitioner have for care of the patient after recovery from anesthesia?

All patients in whom laryngoscopy proves unexpectedly difficult are entitled to a diagnosis and explanation. Such a diagnosis is impor-

tant in its own right and should lead to safer airway management during subsequent anesthesia. Fiberoptic nasendoscopy should be performed.[21,30] Soft-tissue lateral radiographs of the neck[21,40,62] may indicate posterior displacement of the epiglottis and "chicane" shape of the airway.[21,40,62]

The anesthesia practitioner has continuing responsibility for issues that may influence future care of the patient. The 1993 ASA guidelines[63] recommends documenting the presence and nature of airway difficulty, inform the patient, and evaluate and follow the patient for potential complications of difficult airway management. The latter point is reemphasized by Domino.[50] In cases such as this, there is an absolute requirement that the most effective steps are taken to inform future airway practitioners of the nature of the problem with tracheal intubation. Future airway management can then be planned in the light of this knowledge and made as safe as possible. The patient should be fully informed, a letter sent to the primary physician, and a detailed report made in the patient's record. The patient may be given a letter to carry at all times. These steps do not ensure that the patient will have the information available in the event of an accident or illness, which results in rapid reduction of consciousness. The most reliable means of communicating this information in the comatose patient is that the patient wears at all times a bracelet or necklace carrying the vital information. There is more than one such scheme, but the best established is the Medic-Alert® system.[20,64,65] It is mandatory to make strong oral and written recommendations that the patient registers with Medic-Alert® and wears the bracelet or necklace at all times.[66]

37.7 SUMMARY

Not all cases of difficult or impossible Macintosh laryngoscopy can be predicted. Although LTH is rare, all airway practitioners should be able to cope with this condition. Blind attempts at tracheal intubation can be dangerous and should be limited to a few gentle attempts. In conditions such as LTH expertise with various techniques, e.g., the straight or Bullard laryngoscope, may allow tracheal intubation under vision. All airway practitioners should be skilled in cricothyrotomy.

REFERENCES

1. Mallampati SR: Clinical signs to predict difficult tracheal intubation (hypothesis). *Can Anaesth Soc J.* 1983;30:316–317.
2. Bellhouse CP, Doré C: Criteria for estimating likelihood of difficulty of endotracheal intubation with the Macintosh laryngoscope. *Anaesth Intensive Care.* 1988;16:329–337.
3. Frerk CM, Till CB, Bradley AJ: Difficult intubation: thyromental distance and the atlanto-occipital gap. *Anaesthesia.* 1996;51:738–740.
4. Wilson ME, Spiegelhalter D, Robertson JA, et al.: Predicting difficult intubation. *Br J Anaesth.* 1988;61:211–216.
5. Chui PT, Gin T, Oh TE: Anesthesia for laparoscopic general surgery. *Anaesth Intensive Care.* 1993;21:163–171.
6. Cunningham AJ, Brull SJ: Laparoscopic cholecystectomy: anesthetic implications. *Anesth Analg.* 1993;76:1120–1133.
7. Wahba RWM, Tessler MJ, Kleinman SJ: Acute ventilatory complications during laparoscopic upper abdominal surgery. *Can J Anaesth.* 1996;43:77–83.
8. Maltby JR, Beriault MT, Watson NC, et al.: The LMA-ProSeal is an effective alternative to tracheal intubation for laparoscopic cholecystectomy. *Can J Anaesth.* 2002;49:857–862.

9. Lu PP, Brimacombe J, Yang C, et al.: ProSeal versus the Classic laryngeal mask airway for positive pressure ventilation during laparoscopic cholecystectomy. *Br J Anaesth.* 2002;88:824–827.

10. Cook TM, Nolan JP, Verghese C, et al.: Randomized crossover comparison of the proseal with the classic laryngeal mask airway in unparalysed anaesthetized patients. *Br J Anaesth.* 2002;88:527–533.

11. Sidaras G, Hunter JM: Is it safe to artificially ventilate a paralysed patient through the laryngeal mask? The jury is still out. *Br J Anaesth.* 2001;86:749–753.

12. Cooper RM: The LMA, laparoscopic surgery and the obese patient—can vs should. *Can J Anaesth.* 2003;50:5–10.

13. Asai T: Use of the laryngeal mask is contraindicated during cholecystectomy. *Anesthesia.* 2001;56:187.

14. Henderson JJ: Tracheal intubation of the adult patient. In: *Core Topics in Airway Management.* Calder IA, Pearce AC, eds. Cambridge: Cambridge University Press, 2005.

15. Cormack RS, Lehane J: Difficult tracheal intubation in obstetrics. *Anesthesia.* 1984;39:1105–1111.

16. Henderson JJ: The use of paraglossal straight blade laryngoscopy in difficult tracheal intubation. *Anesthesia.* 1997;52:552–560.

17. Puar RK, Puar HS: Lingual tonsillitis. *South Med J.* 1986;79:1126–1128.

18. Tokumine J, Sugahara K, Ura M, et al.: Lingual tonsil hypertrophy with difficult airway and uncontrollable bleeding. *Anesthesia.* 2003;58:390–391.

19. Jones DH, Cohle SD: Unanticipated difficult airway secondary to lingual tonsillar hyperplasia. *Anesth Analg.* 1993;77:1285–1288.

20. Davies S, Ananthanarayan C, Castro C: Asymptomatic lingual tonsillar hypertrophy and difficult airway management: a report of three cases. *Can J Anaesth.* 2001;48:1020–1024.

21. Golding-Wood DG, Whittet HB: The lingual tonsil. A neglected symptomatic structure? *J Laryngol Otol.* 1989;103:922–925.

22. Fitzgerald P, O'Connell D: Massive hypertrophy of the lingual tonsils: an unusual cause of dysphagia. *Br J Radiol.* 1987;60:505–506.

23. Dindzans LJ, Irvine BW, Hayden RE: An unusual case of airway obstruction. *J Otolaryngol.* 1984;13:252–254.

24. Kashyap A, Farid A, Aldridge R, King AB: Lingual tonsil causing airway obstruction. *Ear Nose Throat J.* 1994;73:830–831.

25. Mason DG, Wark KJ: Unexpected difficult intubation. Asymptomatic epiglottic cysts as a cause of upper airway obstruction during anesthesia. *Anesthesia.* 1987;42:407–410.

26. Phillips DE, Rogers JH: Down's syndrome with lingual tonsil hypertrophy producing sleep apnoea. *J Laryngol Otol.* 1988;102:1054–1055.

27. Andrews SR, Mabey MF: Tubular fiberoptic laryngoscope (WuScope) and lingual tonsil airway obstruction. *Anesthesiology.* 2000;93:904–905.

28. Dündar A, Özünlü A, Sahan M, et al.: Lingual tonsil hypertrophy producing obstructive sleep apnea. *Laryngoscope.* 1996;106:1167–9.

29. Johnson CA, Mehdiabadi RJ, Ruff T: Infection and hypertrophy of the lingual tonsil as a cause of airway obstruction. *Tex Med.* 1986;82:29–31.

30. Ovassapian A, Glassenberg R, Randel GI, et al.: The unexpected difficult airway and lingual tonsil hyperplasia: a case series and a review of the literature. *Anesthesiology.* 2002;97:124–132.

31. Fogarty D: Lingual thyroid and difficult intubation. *Anesthesia.* 1990;45:251.

32. Watt OM: Lingual thyroid, complicating general anaesthesia. *Anesthesia.* 1959;14:162–167.

33. Norris W: Epiglottic cysts complicating general anaesthesia. *Anesthesia.* 1957;12:311–316.

34. Padfield A: Epiglottic cysts. A case report and review. *Anesthesia.* 1972;27:84–88.

35. Asai T, Hirose T, Shingu K: Failed tracheal intubation using a laryngoscope and intubating laryngeal mask. *Can J Anaesth.* 2000;47:325–328.

36. Fundingsland BW, Benumof JL: Difficulty using a laryngeal mask airway in a patient with lingual tonsilar hyperplasia. *Anesthesiology.* 1996;84:1265–1266.

37. Al Shamaa M, Jefferson P, Ball DR: Lingual tonsil hypertrophy: airway management. *Anesthesia.* 2003;58:1134–1135.

38. Kamble VA, Lilly RB, Gross JB: Unanticipated difficult intubation as a result of an asymptomatic vallecular cyst. *Anesthesiology.* 1999;91:872–873.

39. Kloss J, Petty C: Obstruction of endotracheal intubation by a mobile pedunculated polyp. *Anesthesiology.* 1975;43:380.

40. Conacher ID, McMahon CC, Meikle D: 'Chicane-like' airway as a complication of lingual tonsils. *Lancet.* 1996;348:475.

41. Biro P, Shahinian H: Management of difficult intubation caused by lingual tonsillar hyperplasia. *Anesth Analg.* 1994;79:389.

42. Dell RG: Upper airway obstruction secondary to a lingual tonsil. *Anesthesia.* 2000;55:393.

43. Rivo J, Matot I: Asymptomatic vallecular cyst: airway management considerations. *J Clin Anesth.* 2001;13:383–386.

44. Georgescu A, Miller JN, Lecklitner ML: The Sellick maneuver causing complete airway obstruction. *Anesth Analg.* 1992;74:457–459.

45. Henderson JJ, Popat MT, Latto IP, et al.: Difficult Airway Society guidelines for management of the unanticipated difficult intubation. *Anesthesia.* 2004;59:675–694.

46. Henderson J, Popat M, Latto P, et al.: Difficult airway society guidelines. *Anesthesia.* 2004;59:1242–1243.

47. Benumof JL, Scheller MS: The importance of transtracheal jet ventilation in the management of the difficult airway. *Anesthesiology.* 1989;71:769–778.

48. Henderson JJ: Intubation techniques for unanticipated difficult intubation: Stylets and introducers. In: *Der schwerige Atemweg.* Dörges V, Paschen H-R, eds. Berlin: Springer-Verlag, 2004.

49. Agro F, Hung O, Cataldo R, et al.: Lightwand intubation using the Trachlight: a brief review of current knowledge. *Can J Anaesth.* 2001;48:592–599.

50. Domino KB, Posner KL, Caplan RA, et al.: Airway injury during anesthesia: a closed claims analysis. *Anesthesiology.* 1999;91:1703–1711.

51. Williamson JA, Webb RK, Szekely S, et al.: The Australian incident monitoring study. Difficult intubation: an analysis of 2000 incident reports. *Anaesth Intensive Care.* 1993;21:602–607.

52. Combes X, Le Roux B, Suen P et al.: Unanticipated difficult airway in anesthetized patients: prospective validation of a management algorithm. *Anesthesiology.* 2004;100:1146–1150.

53. Henderson JJ: The implications of different failed endotracheal intubation rates. *Anesth Analg.* 2001;93:241.

54. Kumar DS, Jones G: Is your bougie helping or hindering you? *Anesthesia.* 2001;56:1121.

55. McHugh P: Cyst of epiglottis. *Anesthesia.* 1989;44:522.

56. Nakazawa K, Ikeda D, Ishikawa S, et al.: A case of difficult airway due to lingual tonsillar hypertrophy in a patient with Down's syndrome. *Anesth Analg.* 2003;97:704–705.

57. Henderson K, Abernathy S, Bays T: Lingual tonsillar hypertrophy: the anesthesiologist's view. *Anesth Analg.* 1994;79:814–815.

58. Al SM, Jefferson P, Ball DR: Lingual tonsillar hypertrophy: airway management using straight blade direct laryngoscopy. *Anesth Analg.* 2004;98:874–875.

59. Conacher ID, Meikle D, O'Brien C: Trachesotomy, lingular tonsillectomy and sleep-related breathing disorders. *Br J Anaesth.* 2002;88:724–726.

60. Guarisco JL, Littlewood SC, Butcher RB III: Severe upper airway obstruction in children secondary to lingual tonsil hypertrophy. *Ann Otol Rhinol Laryngol.* 1990;99:621–624.

61. Crosby E, Skene D: More on lingual tonsillar hypertrophy. *Can J Anaesth.* 2002;49:758.

62. Willatt D, Youngs R: The value of soft tissue radiography in the assessment and treatment of lingual tonsillar hypertrophy. *J Laryngol Otol.* 1984;98:1217–1219.

63. American Society of Anesthesiologists Task Force on Management of the Difficult Airway. Practice guidelines for management of the difficult airway. *Anesthesiology.* 1993;78:597–602.

64. Schwartz JJ, BianRosa JJ: Medical alert—difficult intubation. *Anesthesiology.* 1985;63:343–344.

65. Liban JB: Medic Alert UK should start new section for patients with a difficult airway. *Br Med J* 1996;313:425.

66. Pasqual RT, Troianos CA, Phillips CA, III: Difficult airway warning with automated anesthesia recording. *Anesthesiology.* 1996;85:220.

SELF-EVALUATION QUESTIONS

37.1. What is the order of priorities in management of the difficult airway?

   A. prevention of airway trauma

   B. maintenance of oxygenation and prevention of airway trauma

   C. maintenance of oxygenation

   D. prevention of airway trauma and maintenance of oxygenation

   E. tracheal intubation

37.2. Which technique of laryngoscopy does Crosby et al. recommend in patients with LTH?

   A. Macintosh laryngoscope

   B. Straight laryngoscope

   C. Bullard laryngoscope

   D. flexible fiberoptic laryngoscope

   E. GlideScope®

37.3. What intubation techniques have been proven to allow tracheal intubation under direct vision in patients with undiagnosed LTH?

   A. flexible fiberoptic laryngoscope

   B. straight laryngoscope

   C. intubation using an intubating LMA

   D. Bullard laryngoscope

   E. all of above

CHAPTER (38)

Airway Management of a Patient with Superior Vena Cava Obstruction Syndrome

Gordon O. Launcelott

38.1 CASE PRESENTATION

A 55-year-old male patient with superior vena caval (SVC) obstruction secondary to a mediastinal mass is scheduled for bronchoscopy and mediastinoscopy. The patient weight 250 lbs (120 kg) and has obvious swelling of the face, neck, and upper extremities. The tongue is large (Mallampati Class IV) and the oral mucosa is bluish and plethoric. He is unable to lie flat, but is not dyspneic in the sitting position.

38.2 INTRODUCTION

38.2.1 What is the pertinent pathophysiology in SVC syndrome?

The left and right subclavian and internal jugular veins join to form the brachiocephalic (innominate) veins, which in turn join to form the SVC. Venous drainage from the head and upper extremities then finds its final conduit to the heart in this large, but easily compressible, vessel. Extensive collaterals with the SVC include the azygos, the mammary, vertebral, lateral thoracic, paraspinous, and esophageal veins. The largest of these, the azygos vein, is formed from the junction of the right subcostal and the right ascending lumbar veins. It ascends in the posterior mediastinum and then passes anteriorly over the right main stem bronchus to join the SVC as the latter enters into the right atrium. Here, the area is anatomically crowded with lymph nodes, the pulmonary artery, and the tracheobronchial structures hemmed in by the sternum anteriorly. The low pressure SVC can be obstructed, either indirectly by external compression from vascular structures, tumor, or enlarged lymph nodes or directly by primary or secondary intraluminal thrombus or tumor (Figures 38-1 and 38-2).

Obstruction of the SVC will result in upper body venous hypertension, which forces blood to seek an alternate pathway to the heart via the previously described collateral vessels and the inferior vena cava. This upper body venous hypertension results in the classic clinical signs and symptoms of the syndrome. These include facial, neck, and arm swelling and engorgement of the mucous membranes, including those of the upper airway. In some patients, it may result in laryngeal or cerebral edema and predisposes to an increased risk of surgical bleeding.

Most cases of SVC syndrome are due to extrinsic tumor compression from bronchogenic carcinoma or non-Hodgkin's lymphoma occurring in the right paratracheal space or right pulmonary hilum.[1] From even a cursory glance at the anatomy it can be clearly seen that the disease process may also compromise other major structures in the area, such as the pulmonary arteries, the right heart, and the tracheobronchial tree. With these factors in mind, the practitioner will want to determine the degree to which major structures, such as the airway, pulmonary artery, and right heart, are involved prior to embarking on anesthetic induction.

38.3 PATIENT EVALUATION

38.3.1 What evidence of airway compromise may be apparent on history and physical examination?

Airway compression may be heralded by cough, dyspnea, hemoptysis, and a history of recurrent pulmonary infection. A change in

359

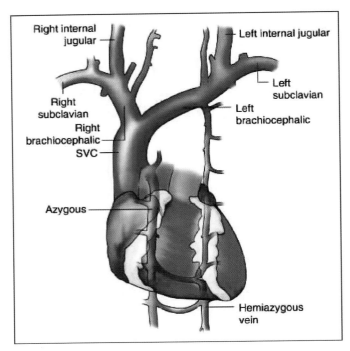

FIGURE 38-1. This diagram illustrates the venous drainage into the heart. (Reproduced with permission *from Abeloff MD: Clinical Oncology, 3rd edn.* Churchill Livingstone, Oxford, UK, 2004: 1048.)

voice may be due to recurrent laryngeal nerve involvement or vocal cord edema. Dyspnea, often with a history of syncope, may not necessarily be due to airway compromise but secondary to right ventricular outflow tract or right heart compression.[1]

In this patient, the tongue is large, perhaps as a result of upper body venous hypertension, and the mucous membranes are plethoric, suggesting that the mucous membranes of the larynx in general, and glottis in particular, may also be engorged, edematous, and friable.

38.3.2 What investigations should be done to assess the airway of the patient?

Smaller precarinal and left paratracheal tumors may not be evident but information about the size and location of the majority of mediastinal tumors can be obtained from chest radiography. Pulmonary function tests may be useful in predicting postoperative respiratory complications. In a recent prospective study, Bechard et al.[2] found a 10 fold increase in postoperative respiratory complications (pneumonia, airway edema, atelectasis) in patients with a preoperative peak expiratory flow rate (PEFR) of <40% of predicted. In the same study, however, PEFR was not predictive of airway collapse. Flow–volume loops, in the supine and upright position, have been advocated to assess the degree of airway obstruction as it relates to body position and to distinguish variable from fixed intrathoracic lesions.[3] However, Narang et al. documented that the respiratory embarrassment caused by mediastinal masses tends to be characteristic of a fixed lesion causing predominantly inspiratory impairment.[1]

Recent contrast-enhanced CT or MRI imaging is the most useful of all investigations in defining the relation of the mass to the other mediastinal structures. Viewing the CT or MRI can provide the practitioner with the necessary information with regard to the presence of pericardial effusion, the degree of anatomic compression of the airway, and the degree to which structures, such as the pulmonary arteries, right ventricular outflow tract, and the heart, may be compromised (Figures 38-3 and 38-4A). Transthoracic echocardiography (TTE) is useful in assessing the presence of pericardial effusion and the dynamic effects of tumor mass on the heart and great vessels. Significant pericardial effusion can result in cardiovascular collapse on induction of general anesthesia and positive pressure ventilation.

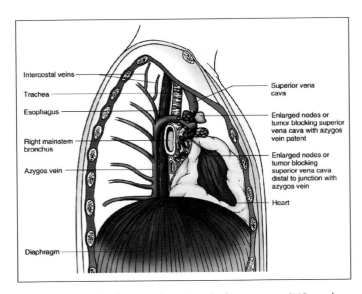

FIGURE 38-2. This diagram shows that the low pressure SVC can be obstructed, either indirectly by external compression of vascular structures, tumor, or enlarged lymph nodes, or directly by primary or secondary intraluminal thrombus or tumor. (Reproduced with permission *from Abeloff MD: Clinical Oncology, 3rd edn.* Churchill Livingstone, Oxford, UK, 2004: 1048.)

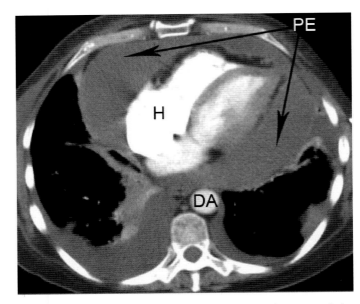

FIGURE 38-3. CT Scan of the thorax of the patient with a pericardial effusion: This CT scan of the chest shows a large pericardial effusion (PE) surrounding the heart (H), anterior to the descending aorta (DA).

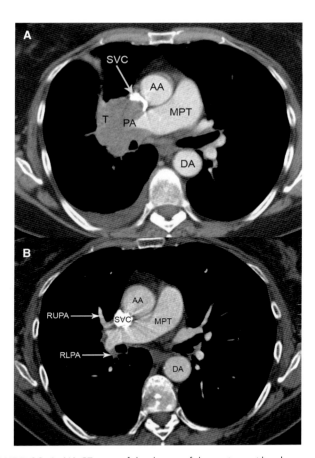

FIGURE 38-4. (A) CT scan of the thorax of the patient with a large mediastinal mass prior to chemotherapy: This CT scan of the chest shows a large right mediastinal tumor (T) encroaching the pulmonary artery (PA) and the superior vena cava (SVC). Also shown in this scan is the ascending aorta (AA), the descending aorta (DA), and the main pulmonary trunk (MPT). (B) CT scan of the thorax of the patient with a mediastinal mass after chemotherapy: This CT scan of the chest shows the normal pulmonary vasculature after chemotherapy with the disappearance of the mediastinal tumor. The superior vena cava (SVC), the anterior segmental right upper lobe pulmonary artery (RUPA), the proximal aspect of the right lower lobe pulmonary artery (RLPA), the ascending aorta (AA), the descending aorta (DA), and the main pulmonary trunk (MPT) are shown clearly without obstruction.

In this patient, chest CT findings were consistent with SVC obstruction. There was no evidence of pulmonary artery, right ventricular outflow tract, myocardial or tracheobronchial compromise and no evidence of pericardial effusion.

38.4 SPECIFIC CONCERNS FOR THIS PATIENT

38.4.1 What complications are associated with mediastinal masses and general anesthesia?

Most practitioners have a heightened sense of awareness when they are confronted with the patient with a mediastinal mass scheduled for surgery. We have all heard of the reports of airway

obstruction or cardiovascular collapse.[4,5] We may even be familiar with the anesthesia management dogmas associated with these cases. Much of the literature documenting these catastrophic scenarios, however, involves pediatric populations.[6] Furthermore, it is becoming evident that one cannot extrapolate what may happen in the adult patient from pediatric literature. The situation is further complicated by the fact that many of the sickest patients, like those with SVC syndrome, are managed with chemotherapy or radiation to shrink their tumors prior to presenting for surgery and general anesthesia (Figure 38-4A and B), or they are managed with less invasive surgical techniques not requiring general anesthesia (GA). Confusing the picture even more is the fact that some series include small or posterior mediastinal masses that are unlikely to be associated with significant cardiorespiratory compromise.[2]

The only studies that have evaluated the incidence of life-threatening cardiorespiratory compromise are those by Azarow et al.[6] and Bechard et al.[2] Azarow et al. noted that there was a significant difference in anesthetic risk between adults and children with mediastinal masses undergoing GA. The authors noted that although the mortality in both groups was similar, mortality in the pediatric group is primarily related to perioperative respiratory complications whereas that in the adult group is due to the malignancy itself.[7] Total airway obstruction in pediatric patients during GA has been associated with preoperative tracheal compression of >50%.[7] This, however, does not seem to be the case in adults. In Bechard's prospective study of 98 adult patients, there was no intraoperative airway obstruction in any of the eight patients with preoperative airway compression >50%. Further evidence for this conclusion is suggested by the fact that not a single case report could be found in the literature of an adult patient experiencing severe airway obstruction during anesthesia. Tracheal compression >50% was, however, associated with a sevenfold increase in respiratory complications, but these were related to pneumonia, airway edema, and atelectasis in the first 48 hours postoperatively.[2]

Whether the patient exhibits signs and symptoms related to the mediastinal mass effect seems to be important. A study by Hnatiuk et al.[8] suggested that symptomatic patients were more likely to experience complications, and Bechard identified stridor, orthopnea, cyanosis, jugular distension, and SVC syndrome as factors associated with perioperative complications. In Bechard's study, 3 of 105 anesthetics were complicated by severe cardiovascular compromise; two-thirds were associated with pericardial effusion. There have been reports of severe airway obstruction occurring in asymptomatic patients, but again this seems limited to the pediatric population.[2]

38.4.2 What are the airway concerns for this patient?

First of all, ventilation using a bag-mask may be difficult in this patient because he is obese, with a large tongue and edematous airway (MOANS, see Section 1.6.1). Similarly, the use of an extraglottic device may also be difficult (RODS, see Section 1.6.3).

There are several airway characteristics of this patient that would suggest a difficult laryngoscopy. He has a Mallampati Class IV pharyngeal view, in spite of the fact that he may have adequate mouth opening and thyromental distance. He is likely to have some reduction in neck mobility. In addition, he does have significant venous congestion that involves the mucous membranes of the mouth, probably the tongue and likely the larynx. Therefore, in all likelihood he will have a difficult laryngoscopy. Certainly, he is obese with swelling of his neck and evidence of upper body venous hypertension, all of which would make emergency cricothyrotomy a challenge.

38.4.3 What are the major concerns with circulation?

The major concern, from a circulatory standpoint in the patient with a mediastinal mass, is circulatory collapse on induction of anesthesia and initiation of positive pressure ventilation. This is a possibility when the mediastinal pathology results in right ventricular outflow obstruction or direct heart compression by the tumor mass, or pericardial effusion compromising cardiac output. Again, in Bechard's study, 3 of 105 patients experienced life-threatening intraoperative cardiovascular events; two-thirds had pericardial effusions.[2]

Patients with preoperative cardiovascular compromise may have symptoms such as dyspnea, orthopnea, and a history of syncope. The structural abnormalities, whether they be right ventricular outflow obstruction or direct heart compromise, can often be appreciated on chest CT scan (Figure 38-4A and B). Dynamic factors associated with these structural abnormalities can be further assessed with TTE. Significant pericardial effusions should be drained prior to presenting to the operating room for surgery. Should there be concern that there is significant right ventricular outflow obstruction, or direct heart compromise, as evidenced by clinical symptoms and/or CT and TTE findings, consideration should be given to planning for elective femoral–femoral cardiopulmonary bypass (CPB). Attempting to catheterize femoral vessels to initiate CPB following cardiovascular collapse is unlikely to be successful. Therefore, it is imperative that everything be in place prior to induction of anesthesia. A Japanese center recommended the use of a temporary extracorporeal axillofemoral venous bypass as a life-saving and auxiliary device in urgent operations for acute progressive SVC syndrome with symptoms of cerebral edema and upper airway obstruction due to intrathoracic malignancies.[9]

In patients with significant cardiovascular compromise, most surgery will be directed to obtaining a diagnosis to plan future therapy. Intrathoracic surgery under general anesthesia is a risky proposition in this group of patients. Every effort should be made to obtain a tissue sample from peripheral sites under local anesthesia. It is said that the practitioner who wishes to grow old slowly should palpate the neck and axillae of all such patients before considering GA and surgery.[1]

38.4.4 Are there any other important considerations?

In patients with SVC syndrome, there is the possibility of increased intracranial pressure due to obstructed cerebral venous drainage. Efforts to avoid the cerebral dilating effects of vapor anesthetics, such as hyperventilation and total intravenous anesthesia, may be considerations in this regard.

In the patient with SVC syndrome, large-bore IV catheters should be placed in the lower extremities as injected medications will make their way to the heart more quickly than through the obstructed route via the subclavian vein and SVC. Adequate intravascular volume is important, as is the immediate availability of inotropes and vasopressors.

38.5 AIRWAY MANAGEMENT

38.5.1 What is the most appropriate airway management option for this patient?

As a result of the factors discussed above, it is prudent to secure the airway awake using the flexible fiberoptic bronchoscope (FFB). Successful topicalization of the airway is improved by using a drying agent. This should be given subcutaneously (SC) or IV 20 minutes to 1 hour prior to bringing the patient to the induction area.[10] Following FFB intubation, the ventilation of patients with mediastinal masses can be managed in a variety of ways. In Bechard's study, only 15 out of 97 patients were induced using spontaneous ventilation and in only 3 was spontaneous ventilation used throughout.[2]

The textbook dogma of maintaining spontaneous ventilation throughout in the patients with mediastinal vascular and tracheobronchial compromise is based mostly on anecdotal information. Patients with an obstructive airway component, as may be the case in patients with mediastinal tumors, are potentially susceptible to so-called dynamic hyperinflation, or auto-PEEP, following initiation of positive pressure ventilation. This can increase global intrathoracic pressure contributing to decreased venous return and increased cardiovascular compromise.[11]

From a strictly respiratory perspective, it is a common belief that patients with airway compromise secondary to mediastinal mass effect are less subject to airflow obstruction with maintenance of spontaneous ventilation. This is based on the erroneous belief that mediastinal tumors behave more like variable rather than fixed intrathoracic lesions. Flow–volume loops in patients with variable intrathoracic lesions show a restricted expiratory flow but a largely unaffected inspiratory flow. Fixed lesions, in contrast, have an equal reduction in both inspiratory and expiratory flows compared to normal subjects.[12] Vander Els et al. studied patients with intrathoracic Hodgkin's disease. They found that these intrathoracic masses behave more like fixed than like variable lesions with equal inspiratory/expiratory flow impairment or a predominant inspiratory flow reduction. As a result, maintenance of spontaneous ventilation in these patients would appear to be of little benefit.[3]

In this patient with no evidence of tracheobronchial compression or significant cardiovascular compromise, it is unlikely that there would be any advantage in maintaining spontaneous ventilation. Following awake fiberoptic intubation, the patient can be induced while breathing spontaneously followed by neuromuscular block and controlled ventilation; or, neuromuscular block and controlled ventilation can be initiated immediately upon induction.

Spontaneous, assisted ventilation throughout may be a consideration in patients with CT or echocardiographic evidence of significant cardiovascular compromise.

38.5.2   What actually happened in this case?

The patient had no evidence of tracheobronchial, pulmonary artery, right ventricular outflow tract, or direct myocardial compromise. He received 0.4 mg glycopyrrolate subcutaneously 1 hour prior to transfer to the operating room in the sitting position. Two units of blood were immediately available. He was transferred to the operating table and was maintained in the Semi-Fowler position. Standard monitors including ECG and pulse oximetry were applied. A 14-gauge venous catheter was placed in his left greater saphenous vein at the ankle and a #20 arterial catheter placed in the left radial artery. A 1.5 L bolus of saline was given in preparation for anesthetic induction. Increased inspired oxygen via nasal cannula at the rate of 3 L·min^{-1} was applied. The airway was anesthetized with a gargle of aqueous 4% lidocaine followed by nebulized 4% lidocaine using a DeVilbiss atomizer. The trachea was intubated with an 8.5 mm ID endotracheal tube over an adult FFB. Breathing 100% oxygen, the patient received a total of 20 μg of sufentanil in divided aliquots, followed by 150 mg of propofol and 30 mg of rocuronium. Following loss of consciousness, controlled manual ventilation was initiated and sevoflurane was introduced. Cardiovascular and respiratory parameters remained stable and the patient was placed on the ventilator. The surgical procedure lasted 50 minutes and was uneventful from a surgical and anesthetic standpoint. Neuromuscular block was reversed with neostigmine and glycopyrrolate and the patient was allowed to emerge from anesthesia. He was extubated awake in the sitting position. He was then transported, in the sitting position, to the postanesthetic care unit (PACU) breathing supplemental oxygen from a Venturi mask. The immediate postoperative course was uneventful.

38.5.3   What is a reasonable approach for extubation following emergence from general anesthesia?

For all the reasons that this patient should have his airway secured awake, tracheal extubation should also be done when the patient is fully awake. In addition, worsening of airway edema can occur following endotracheal intubation and mediastinal surgery. Consideration may even be given to leaving an airway exchange catheter in the airway following extubation.[13] The catheter can be removed when the practitioner is confident that the patient has an acceptable airway, with effective gas exchange.

38.6   SUMMARY

In adult patients with SVC syndrome major considerations are with the edematous, congested mucous membranes that are prone to bleed and can make direct laryngoscopy and endotracheal intuba-

tion technically difficult and extubation potentially hazardous. It appears that life-threatening intraoperative airway obstruction in the adult is less of a problem than it is in the pediatric population. Life-threatening airway obstruction has not been reported to occur in adult patients with significantly compromised airways but pneumonia, airway edema, and atelectasis are more frequent in the first 48 hours postoperatively. The threat of postinduction cardiovascular collapse is limited to those patients with pericardial effusions, direct heart compromise by the tumor mass, and/or the potential for right ventricular outflow obstruction. These patients can be identified with careful preoperative assessment, including history, physical examination, CT scan, and echocardiography.

REFERENCES

1. Narang S, Harte BH, Body SC: Anesthesia for patients with a mediastinal mass. *Anesthesiol Clin North Am.* 2001;19:559–579.
2. Bechard P, Letourneau L, Lacasse Y, Cote D, Bussieres JS: Perioperative cardiorespiratory complications in adults with mediastinal mass: incidence and risk factors. *Anesthesiology.* 2004;100:826–834.
3. Vander Els NJ, Sorhage F, Bach AM, Straus DJ, White DA: Abnormal flow volume loops in patients with intrathoracic Hodgkin's disease. *Chest.* 2000;117:1256–1261.
4. Keon TP: Death on induction of anesthesia for cervical node biopsy. *Anesthesiology.* 1981;55:471–472.
5. Levin H, Bursztein S, Heifetz M: Cardiac arrest in a child with an anterior mediastinal mass. *Anesth Analg.* 1985;64:1129–1130.
6. Azarow KS, Pearl RH, Zurcher R, Edwards FH, Cohen AJ: Primary mediastinal masses. A comparison of adult and pediatric populations. *J Thorac Cardiovasc Surg.* 1993;106:67–72.
7. Azizkhan RG, Dudgeon DL, Buck JR, et al.: Life-threatening airway obstruction as a complication to the management of mediastinal masses in children. *J Pediatr Surg.* 1985;20:816–822.
8. Hnatiuk OW, Corcoran PC, Sierra A: Spirometry in surgery for anterior mediastinal masses. *Chest.* 2001;120:1152–1156.
9. Shimokawa S, Yamashita T, Kinjyo T, et al.: Temporary extracorporeal axillofemoral venous bypass—a beneficial device in operation for superior vena caval syndrome due to intrathoracic malignancies. *Nippon Kyobu Geka Gakkai Zasshi.* 1997;45:1827–1832.
10. Watanabe H, Lindgren L, Rosenberg P, Randell T: Glycopyrronium prolongs topical anaesthesia of oral mucosa and enhances absorption of lignocaine. *Br J Anaesth.* 1993;70:94–95.
11. Pepe PE, Marini JJ: Occult positive end-expiratory pressure in mechanically ventilated patients with airflow obstruction: the auto-PEEP effect. *Am Rev Respir Dis.* 1982;126:166–170.
12. Burrows B, Knudson RJ, Quan SF, et al.: *Respiratory Disorders: A Pathophysiologic Approach,* 2nd edn. Year Book Medical Publishers: Chicago, IL, 1983.
13. Practice guidelines for management of the difficult airway: an updated report by the American Society of Anesthesiologists Task Force on Management of the Difficult Airway. *Anesthesiology.* 2003;98:1269–1277.

SELF-EVALUATION QUESTIONS

38.1. Which of the following is **NOT** a known classic clinical sign or symptom of patients with superior vena cava obstruction syndrome?

   A. facial, neck, and arm swelling

   B. hemoptysis

   C. laryngeal edema

   D. cerebral edema

   E. engorgement of the mucous membranes

38.2. Which of the following airway management strategies may be difficult in patients with a large mediastinal mass and superior vena cava obstruction syndrome?

A. bag-mask-ventilation

B. ventilation using extraglottic devices

C. laryngoscopic intubation

D. surgical airway

E. all of the above

38.3. Which of the following is a known complication associated with mediastinal masses and general anesthesia?

A. cardiovascular collapse

B. tracheal obstruction

C. pneumonia

D. pericardial effusion

E. all of the above

CHAPTER (39)

Airway Management of a Patient with History of Difficult Airway Who Refuses to Have Awake Tracheal Intubation

Steven Abramson, Kyle Friedman, and Carin Hagberg

39.1 CASE PRESENTATION

A 50-year-old ASA II male smoker is scheduled to have a total knee replacement. His past medical history is remarkable for severe ankylosing spondylitis (AS) for which he is on a non-steroidal anti-inflammatory drug (NSAID). He has no history of gastroesophageal reflux disease (GERD). On physical examination, he weighs approximately 121 lb (55 kg) and is 5′6″ (167 cm) tall (BMI = 19.72 kg.m^{-2}). Examination of his airway reveals that he is edentulous, opens his mouth 3.5 cm, and his neck is fixed in 30 degrees of flexion. The remainder of the airway assessment is within normal limits. This same surgery was cancelled twice by the anesthesia practitioner because the patient refused to have an awake fiberoptic intubation.

39.2 PREOPERATIVE ANESTHETIC ASSESSMENT

39.2.1 What is ankylosing spondylitis? What are the anesthetic issues concerning this disease? How does ankylosing spondylitis affect the airway?

Ankylosing spondylitis is a rheumatic inflammatory disorder affecting the spine and sacroiliac joints that can also cause inflammation of the eyes, lungs, and heart valves.[1] The cause of AS is not known, but it is believed to be caused by immunogenetic mechanisms as most patients share a common genetic marker, HLA-B27.[2] AS afflicts approximately 129 out of 100,000 people in the United States and typically affects young adult males. The inflammatory process usually begins in the sacroiliac joints and spreads upward to involve the spine. The spine eventually fuses and spinal involvement may be in the cervical, thoracic, or lumbar regions.[1] When the lumbar spine is affected, this area looses its lordosis and the spine flattens. With thoracic and cervical spine involvement, patients develop increased kyphosis. Cervical spine involvement may range from limitation of neck movement to complete neck immobility. Patients with severe cervical involvement are at much greater risk for sustaining cervical injury from even minimal manipulation of the neck.[3]

In this case, in which the patient has severe cervical involvement with complete loss of cervical mobility, several anesthetic concerns must be addressed. First, any neck manipulation in order to secure the airway could result in cervical spine injury and neurologic impairment.[3] Second, involvement of one or several segments of the spine often makes lying flat difficult or impossible. Third, the inflammatory process often involves the costovertebral and costochondral joints, which may result in significant restrictive lung disease with a decrease in compliance. Thus, an assessment of pulmonary function should be performed preoperatively to determine the need for possible postoperative ventilatory support.[4] Finally, as the disease progresses, involvement may include the temporomandibular and cricoarytenoid joints.[5] With temporomandibular joint involvement, mouth opening may be significantly decreased. This patient has some decrease in mouth opening, which may present additional difficulty in airway management. Cricoarytenoid involvement may result in symptoms of airway obstruction, such as hoarseness, dyspnea, and sore throat, and may affect tracheal intubation.[6] Vocal cord fixation can occur.

The most important consideration for the airway practitioner is the degree of limitation of cervical spine mobility and possible difficulties in securing the airway. With a significant degree of fixed flexion of the cervical spine, the airway practitioner should consider the likelihood of a difficult intubation even though other commonly used predictors of difficulty may be normal (Mallampati score, mouth opening, thyromental distance, etc.).

39.2.2   What is informed consent? What are the elements of informed consent?

Consent is an expression of an individual's right to dignity and freedom, which precedes the right to health, and at the same time the condition for and a limit to medical treatment. Informed consent is the process by which a fully informed patient can participate in the decisions about their health care. Its basis, legally and ethically, is in the patient's right to direct what happens to his or her body.[7] It is generally accepted that in order to obtain proper informed consent, the following elements must be included in the discussion with the patient. First, the exact nature of the procedure must be discussed. Second, reasonable alternatives to the proposed procedure must be discussed. Third, the risks and benefits of all possibilities must be discussed. Fourth, it must be determined that the patient has a reasonable understanding of the issues being discussed. Finally, the patient must accept the proposed procedure(s) or intervention(s).[7]

In this case in which the patient refuses an awake intubation, a complete discussion and description of the process of awake intubation must take place and an assessment must be made to determine that the patient fully understands the procedure. Other alternatives to awake intubation, as well as the associated risks with these alternatives, must then be discussed with the patient. Finally, the patient and the airway practitioner need to be in agreement with the proposed airway management plan, especially as the patient's cooperation is required. It is important to remember that just as the patient can refuse to have an awake intubation, the anesthesia practitioner may also decline to provide care to a patient unless it is an emergency.

In an emergency situation in which the patient requires a life- or limb-saving procedure and no other anesthesia care provider is available, the anesthesia practitioner is obliged to proceed under emergency conditions and honor the refusal of the patient to have a particular technique. In this situation, complete documentation should be performed, including a disclosure note on the chart that all inherent risks of the treatment options were described to the patient. The anesthesia practitioner must convey to the patient what procedure(s) is in the patient's best interest. If the patient denies consent, it may be helpful for the surgeon and/or family members to become involved in the decision making. If the anesthesia practitioner ultimately fails to obtain consent for a procedure and nonetheless proceeds with that procedure he/she assumes the risk that a charge of physical assault may ensue.[7]

39.3   WHAT ARE THE ANESTHETIC MANAGEMENT OPTIONS IN THIS CASE?

39.3.1   What is the *best* technique for this patient?

When faced with either an anticipated or unanticipated difficult airway scenario, the anesthesia practitioner should consider the

ASA Difficult Airway Management Guidelines.[8] These practice guidelines and recommendations are designed to assist in decision making, which can be adopted, modified, or rejected according to clinical needs. Factors that determine these clinical needs include the patient's position during surgery, type of surgery, urgency of the situation, degree of patient cooperation, availability of equipment, and the technical skills and experience of the airway practitioner. Important take home messages from these guidelines are (1) anticipate the possibility of difficult airway management by the performance of a thorough preoperative airway assessment, (2) secure the airway awake if difficulty is anticipated, and (3) have a backup plan(s) if the initial plan to secure the airway fails (see Chapter 2).

This patient with severe AS has an anticipated difficult airway. As discussed above, these patients usually have severe fixed anterior flexion of the cervical spine, and other spinal abnormalities, making it difficult to position the patient supine, let alone in the sniffing position. Awake fiberoptic tracheal intubation is the most commonly recommended technique for securing a difficult airway and is considered the safest method in a patient with AS.[8–12] However, since this patient refuses an awake tracheal intubation, it is necessary to have alternative plan(s). Since this patient is undergoing peripheral orthopedic surgery, regional anesthesia may be considered as a safe alternative anesthetic technique. The risks and benefits of regional anesthesia will be discussed later in this chapter.

39.3.2   What are some additional preoperative considerations that may influence the choice of anesthetic management?

Positioning is an important factor for any procedure. As previously mentioned, patients with severe AS often have a fixed cervical spine and an exaggerated thoracic kyphosis. It is important to determine if this patient can lie supine in order to consider performing regional anesthesia and keeping the patient awake during surgery.

Another consideration is the ability to perform bag-mask-ventilation (BMV) either after induction of general anesthesia (GA) or following a respiratory arrest from a complication of regional anesthesia. This is extremely important to take into consideration as the inability to ventilate will have fatal consequences unless an emergency airway can be immediately established.

Difficult BMV occurs in approximately 5% of general surgical cases. In a prospective study, Langeron et al. defined five independent risk factors for difficult BMV.[13] These include the presence of a beard, a BMI > 26 kg·m^{-2}, lack of teeth, age >55 years (limited neck mobility), and a history of snoring (see Section 1.6.1). The presence of two of these factors has a sensitivity of 0.72 and specificity of 0.73 in predicting difficult BMV. This patient is edentulous and has limited neck mobility, thus he has two of the five risk factors and is considered to be at risk for difficult BMV. The significance of making this determination is that if a patient is predicted to be possibly difficult to BMV, not only must a backup plan be immediately available but a practitioner who is skilled in the performance of a surgical airway must also be immediately available.

The laryngeal mask airway (LMA) is an accepted airway management device in managing a difficult airway.[14] It is usually

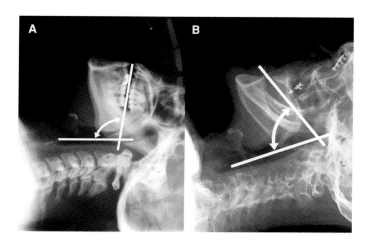

FIGURE 39-1. Lateral radiological views of the cervical spine of a normal patient (A) and a patient with a severe ankylosing spondylitis (B). With neck flexion and maximal head extension, the angle between the oral and pharyngeal axes at the base of the tongue is usually more than 90 degrees in a normal patient (A). But this angle is 70 degrees or less in this patient with ankylosing spondylitis (B).

relatively simple to insert into the pharynx and by forming a low pressure seal around the larynx permits positive pressure ventilation. However, there are instances in which the LMA may be difficult or impossible to insert and it has been suggested that AS is a contraindication to the use of an LMA.[14] Indeed, there are reports of impossible LMA insertion in patients with AS and other diseases limiting neck movement.[15-17]

One of the reasons for experiencing this difficulty is the acute angle between the oral and pharyngeal axes at the base of the tongue[15] (see Figure 39-1). Current findings suggest that if this angle is <90 degrees, LMA insertion may be impossible.[17] It is therefore suggested that a lateral neck x-ray be obtained as part of a preoperative assessment to evaluate this angle in patients with AS. This patient's neck is fixed in 30 degree flexion and he has limited mouth opening; thus, LMA insertion is very likely to be difficult. However, initial lateral insertion of the LMA may overcome this difficulty.

Lastly, although this patient does not have a history of GERD, LMA insertion may be contraindicated in AS patients with untreated GERD.[14,17] These patients should be treated preoperatively with a histamine H_2 receptor blocker, metoclopramide, and a nonparticulate antacid. Alternatively, this may motivate a decision to employ regional anesthesia. Certainly, GERD must be treated adequately prior to regional anesthesia as well, should emergency airway management be required.

39.4 GENERAL ANESTHESIA AND TRACHEAL INTUBATION

39.4.1 What anesthetic agents should be used for induction?

If there is any doubt as to the ability to perform adequate BMV or satisfactorily place an LMA, spontaneous ventilation should be maintained during induction. An inhalational induction with sevoflurane may be performed[18] to minimize the risk of sudden loss of airway control. Additionally, intravenous drugs that have mini-

mal effect on the respiratory drive, such as midazolam (low dose), ketamine, or dexmedetomidine, can be used in combination with an inhalational agent. Administration of opioids should be kept to a minimum, as they depress respiratory drive. Muscle relaxants should be avoided until BMV or LMA ventilation has been established. Although not considered as safe, there are reports of induction of anesthesia without maintaining spontaneous ventilation, followed by successful LMA placement in patients with limited neck mobility.[9,19-21] This should only be performed if there is a high level of certainty in the ability to perform adequate BMV or LMA ventilation following the induction of GA. Additionally, only short-acting drugs, such as propofol or thiopental, should be used. As with all patients undergoing a GA, a 3–5 minute period of denitrogenation with a FiO_2 of 1.0 is essential, especially in patients with diminished pulmonary reserve. Adequate denitrogenation will delay oxygen desaturation in the event the patient becomes apneic.

39.4.2 Following induction of GA, how should this patient's airway be secured?

Another principle that is ingrained in the ASA Difficult Airway Management Guidelines regarding technique choices is: Do what you do best.[8] In general, anesthesia practitioners are familiar with both the LMA and the intubating LMA (ILMA). Both can be inserted blindly into the pharynx with relative ease in most patients[14] and both of these devices can provide adequate positive pressure ventilation, without tracheal intubation. Additionally, both can serve as conduits for tracheal intubation. A 6 mm inner diameter (ID) endotracheal tube (ETT) can be passed through a #4 LMA and a 7 mm ID ETT through a #5 LMA Classic™. A special silicon-tipped ETT is designed for use with the ILMA. All silicon-tipped ETTs (up to size 8 mm ID) can be passed through the #3, #4, and #5 ILMA. Despite the suggestion that LMA insertion is contraindicated in patients with AS,[10] the literature has demonstrated that the LMA and ILMA are useful and effective devices in airway management in anesthetized patients with severe AS.[9,18-22]

The ILMA offers potential advantages over the LMA in patients with AS, since it may be easier to insert in patients with an immobile neck[18,23] and is a better conduit for intubation,[18] although LMA Classic™ or LMA Unique™ may be more advantageous in patients with limited mouth opening.[19] This patient's airway may be secured with an ILMA following an inhalational induction with sevoflurane while maintaining spontaneous ventilation. Once good positioning of the ILMA is ascertained, a muscle relaxant can be administered. If a special silicon ETT is unavailable for use with the ILMA, a flexible fiberoptic bronchoscope (FFB) can be used to guide a polyvinyl chloride ETT into the trachea. Once the scope is removed, tracheal placement should be confirmed by auscultation and capnography. The ILMA can then be removed using a special stabilizing device. If an FFB is not available, a prewarmed, softened ETT can be inserted blindly through the ILMA by feeling for a loss of resistance, with good success.[18] Additionally, a Cook airway exchange catheter (using the Rapi-fit connector, attached to the capnograph monitor to detect $EtCO_2$) or an Eschmann Introducer can be used to guide an ETT. If all these methods fail, the ILMA (or LMA) can be used alone for positive pressure ventilation throughout the case.

39.5   ALTERNATIVE AIRWAY TECHNIQUES

39.5.1   What other methods can be used to secure the airway after induction?

As previously mentioned, the prudent anesthesia practitioner should always have a backup plan(s) in case Plan A fails. If insertion of an LMA fails because of an acute oropharyngeal angle or a lack of experience or equipment, further management is dependent on the ability to perform adequate BMV.

In a nonemergency situation where the patient has received a short-acting induction agent and has not been paralyzed, he/she may be allowed to awaken and resume spontaneous ventilation if BMV is adequate. A regional anesthetic technique may also be considered appropriate and will be discussed in more detail later in the chapter. The airway can also be secured with an alternative technique. Although a complete list of all airway management devices and techniques is beyond the scope of this chapter, a few of the more commonly used devices and techniques will be discussed.

Direct laryngoscopy can be attempted in these patients. Ng and Hastings[24] reported a patient with severe AS and no neck mobility who exhibited a Cormack/Lehane Grade 4 airway on initial laryngoscopy. By placing the patient in the Trendelenburg position, it was easier to lift the laryngoscope toward the ceiling and perform tracheal intubation (Figure 39-2). If only a part of the glottis or epiglottis is visualized (Cormack/Lehane Grade 2 or 3), one of

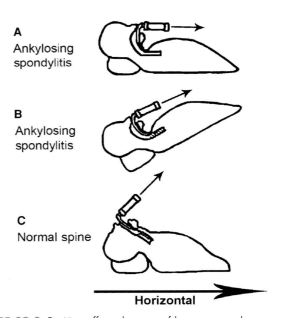

A
Ankylosing spondylitis

B
Ankylosing spondylitis

C
Normal spine

Horizontal

FIGURE 39-2. Position affects the ease of laryngoscopy because of fixed cervical flexion. (A) In the supine position, the laryngoscope had to be rotated forward and the laryngoscopist had to reach farther and toward the floor to displace the mandibular structures out of the field of view (arrow). (B) The Trendelenburg position partly compensated for the cervical flexion by facing the patient toward the ceiling. (C) The jaw could be lifted more comfortably and in a direction similar to that for a patient with a normal spine in the sniff position (Reproduced with permission from *Ng, M. and Hastings, R.: Successful direct laryngoscopy assisted by posture in a patient with ankylosing spondylitis. Anesth Analg. 1998;87:1436–1437.*)

many intubating guides, such as the Eschmann Introducer or Frova Intubating Catheter (Cook Critical Care®, Bloomington, IN), could be passed underneath the epiglottis in order to perform tracheal intubation.

A relatively new group of airway management devices, the IRM video laryngoscopes, have been shown to be very effective for intubation in patients with a difficult airway.[25] Both the Macintosh Video Laryngoscope (Karl Storz Endoscopy, Culver City, CA) and the GlideScope™ (see Chapter 9) have been shown to be useful in facilitating intubation in patients with cervical-spine immobilization.[26] As the camera is located at the distal end of the laryngoscope blade, these devices have been shown to improve the view of the larynx by one grade. The use of a styletted ETT is recommended. Either the direct view (naked eye) or the indirect view (monitor) can be used for tracheal intubation. As with traditional laryngoscopy, intubating guides can also be utilized, if necessary.

Rigid fiberoptic laryngoscopes such as the Bullard Scope (Gyrus ACMI, Norwalk, OH), the UpsherScope™ (Mercury Medical, Clear Water, FL) and the WuScope™ (Achi Corp., San Jose, CA) (see Chapter 9) have been shown to be useful in patients with limited mouth opening and neck extension,[27] but they require a measure of experience to achieve proficiency. Similarly, the lighted stylets, such as the Trachlight™ (Laerdal Medical Corp., Wappingers Falls, NY), the Bonfils Retromolar Intubation Fiberscope (Karl Storz Endoscopy, Culver City, CA), and the Shikani Optical Stylet (Clarus Medical, LLC, Minneapolis, MN), are useful in patients with limited cervical-spine mobility. Finally, retrograde intubation is a useful technique, especially when visualization of the larynx from above is impossible.[12] However, since this technique is more invasive, it should be reserved as a "Plan C" in most hands.

39.5.2   What alternative extraglottic devices can be used?

The esophageal tracheal Combitube™ is an alternative to the LMA in a difficult airway situation[28] that requires minimal mouth opening and neck mobility for its insertion. It has been shown to be useful in providing a patent airway in a patient whose neck was immobilized in the neutral position with a halo jacket.[29] Nonetheless, the ease and success of inserting a Combitube™ into a patient with severe AS is yet to be reported. Theoretically, the Combitube™ protects against aspiration since its distal cuff seals the esophagus and the tracheal lumen can be used to suction the stomach when positioned in the esophagus, yet the incidence of aspiration with the Combitube™ has been found to be similar to that with the LMA.[30]

Another new extraglottic device which could be used is the Laryngeal Tube® (VBM Medizintechnik, Sulz, Germany) (Figure 39-3 see Chapter 11). This is a single-lumen tube with a ventral ventilation aperture. The LT is designed for blind esophageal insertion. It has both esophageal and pharyngeal cuffs that are connected to the same inflation line which creates a seal above and below the ventilation aperture. Once the LT is inserted, ventilation with the cuffs inflated should be confirmed. An Aintree Extubation Catheter (Cook Critical Care®, Bloomington, IN) mounted onto a FFB can then be passed into the trachea using the

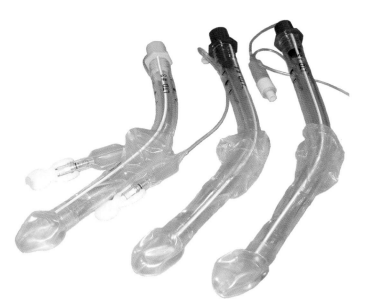

FIGURE 39-3. Laryngeal Tube®: Three different sizes of Laryngeal Tubes® are shown.

LT as a conduit. Once the FFB and the Aintree catheter are in the trachea, the FFB is removed and a 15 mm Rapi-Fit Adapter can be attached to the Aintree Catheter to aid in ventilation and to reconfirm tracheal placement by $EtCO_2$ detection. By removing the Rapi-Fit connector, the LT can then be removed and the Aintree can be used to advance an ETT into the trachea.[31] Although the LT has been shown to be an effective airway device with a high rate of successful insertion,[31] its use in patients with AS has not been sufficiently studied.

A Modified Nasal Trumpet, which is a nasal pharyngeal airway with an additional distal hole and an attached tracheal tube adaptor, has been useful in patients with difficult airways who are anesthetized and are breathing spontaneously.[32,33] It can provide supplemental oxygen and anesthetic gas delivery to facilitate a flexible fiberoptic intubation via the mouth or opposite nostril, for patients in whom LMA placement has failed or was deemed to be impossible. The patient's entire upper airway (nostrils, oral cavity, pharynx, larynx, and trachea) should be adequately anesthetized and an FFB should be available. Unfortunately, the Modified Nasal Trumpet has been shown to be ineffective as a primary airway device.[33]

39.5.3 What is your airway management plan if mask ventilation is inadequate and tracheal intubation is unsuccessful?

If both BMV and LMA ventilation are inadequate and intubation is unsuccessful, the emergency pathway of the ASA Difficult Airway Management Algorithm should be followed.[8] A call for help should be made. Appropriate responses to establish ventilation include insertion of an esophageal tracheal Combitube® (ETC), rigid bronchoscope, or transtracheal jet ventilation (TTJV).[8] If these measures fail to immediately establish ventilation, then an emergency surgical or percutaneous cricothyrotomy is indicated.[8] Alternatively, following determination of the can't

intubate can't ventilate (CICV) situation, the practitioner may proceed directly to an emergency surgical or percutaneous cricothyrotomy.[8] The elective placement of a TTJV catheter could be considered in any fasted patient considered to be difficult to BMV or for inserting an LMA. The insertion of one of these catheters can also be considered in any patient who has poor preoperative pulmonary function and is likely to rapidly desaturate after induction of GA.

39.6   REGIONAL ANESTHESIA

39.6.1 What is the possible role of regional anesthesia for this patient?

According to the ASA Difficult Airway Management Guidelines an awake intubation is the safest method to establish a secure airway in this patient. If this plan fails or the patient refuses an awake intubation, regional anesthesia is a safe alternative approach. However, it should be kept in mind that not all regional techniques are 100% effective, and regional anesthesia can lead to disastrous complications thereby requiring emergency airway management.

Although these complications are inherent for all regional anesthetic procedures, the risks vary for different procedures and are based on several factors, including the type of nerve block, needle insertion, type and concentration of drug administered, as well as the volume of injection. Therefore, risks and benefits of regional versus general anesthesia should be considered for each patient.

Chelly[34] has provided a list of important factors that should be considered in making this decision (Table 39-1). First, any contraindications to regional anesthesia should be excluded. These include infection at the site of needle insertion, systemic infection, bleeding abnormalities, and allergy to local anesthetics. In the case of neuraxial blocks, hypovolemic shock, aortic stenosis, and raised intracranial pressure should also be excluded.[36,40–44]

Additionally, possible complications of regional anesthesia should be considered. The risk of serious complications is approximately 0.1%.[36] Toxic reactions due to systemic absorption of the local anesthetic can present either with neurological or cardiovascular symptoms, such as seizures, hypotension, and cardiac arrest. The incidence of a systemic toxic reaction is approximately 1:10,000 and depends on the drug and concentration used, the volume injected, and the type of block (e.g., intercostals, interscalene, and cervical plexus blocks have a higher rate of absorption than femoral and sciatic nerve blocks).[36]

A high spinal anesthetic can result in apnea and cardiovascular collapse. The incidence of a cardiac arrest occurring from a spinal anesthetic is approximately 6:10,000, as opposed to 1:10,000 for peripheral nerve blocks.[36] Although rare, nerve injuries can occur. Complications may require emergency airway management. Furthermore, the possibility of hemodynamic instability during the case (e.g., from significant blood loss) should also be considered, as this may also require emergency airway management.

As previously mentioned, it is very important to determine if the patient can tolerate being awake during the procedure and communicate with the anesthesia practitioner. The patient's

TABLE 39-1

Factors Influencing the Choice of Regional Anesthesia Versus Control of the Airway in Patients with Established Difficult Airways[34,35]

Patient	• Informed consent
	• Cooperative and calm
	• Hemodynamically stable
	• Ability to tolerate sedation, if required
	• Ability to communicate with anesthesia practitioner throughout the procedure
	• No history of claustrophobia
	• Adequate IV access
Anesthesia practitioner	• Expertise in both RA and DA management
	• Enough preoperative time to perform RA technique
	• Appropriate RA technique for surgical procedure
	• Prepared for alternative plans for DA
Surgeon	• Dependable and reliable
	• Willing and able to supplement RA with local anesthetics, if necessary
	• Cooperative with primary and alternative plans for DA management
Types of surgery	• Nonemergency (exception c-section)
	• Short duration
	• Patient position allows easy airway access
	• Can be interrupted for DA management
	• Limited or moderate blood loss
Support	• Availability of appropriate equipment for RA and DA management
	• Staff (anesthesia practitioners/OR nurses)

RA, regional anesthesia; DA, difficult airway.

medical condition also influences this decision. For example, if the patient has severe GERD, a regional anesthetic with an awake patient may be preferable to securing the airway after induction of general anesthesia. If, however, diseases such as congestive heart failure, severe chronic obstructive pulmonary disease, or severe AS with spinal involvement prohibits the patient from lying flat comfortably, the airway should be secured.

One of the most important factors requiring consideration is the expertise of the anesthesia practitioner. This includes the appropriate experience in the chosen regional technique as well as adequate experience in managing the patient's airway in the event of a complication. The anesthesia practitioner must know which nerves to block for both the surgery and possible tourniquet pain. The approximate time that the surgical procedure will last should also be considered and the anesthesia practitioner must ensure that the regional anesthetic will last at least that long, if not longer, should delays occur. Therefore, when choosing a local anesthetic drug, consideration should be given to the safety profile of that drug, as well as its duration of action.

All of the appropriate equipment for the performance of the nerve block(s) and possible emergency airway management must be available. Additional factors to consider include the site and type of surgery. A short toe procedure requiring an ankle block will

have a lower risk of complications than a revision of total hip replacement under regional anesthesia. There must also be adequate communication and cooperation between the surgeon and the anesthesia practitioner and both must agree on the appropriateness of regional anesthesia. Expert help should be immediately available if any complications occur. If GA is necessary, a predetermined strategy to manage the airway should be in place, including the backup plans should Plan A fail. The landmarks for a surgical airway should be identified before induction of GA and the necessary personnel and equipment should be immediately available.

39.6.2 Which regional anesthetic technique would be most suitable for this patient?

If regional anesthesia is chosen for this patient, then which specific regional technique should be performed needs to be determined. When considering neuroaxial blocks in patients with AS, spinal deformity may make the technique challenging and perhaps impossible. In a retrospective study, Schelein et al.[37] demonstrated that 76% of spinals were effective whereas epidural anesthesia was generally ineffective.

This patient is also on an NSAID which, due to its antiplatelet effect, may pose a theoretical risk of spinal hematoma. However, data presented at a recent Consensus Conference on Neuraxial Anesthesia and Anticoagulation[39] concur that NSAIDs appear to represent no added significant risk for the development of spinal hematoma in patients having epidural or spinal anesthesia. The use of NSAIDs alone does not create a level of risk that will interfere with the performance of neuraxial blocks. Additionally, there should not be any specific concerns as to the timing of single-shot or catheter techniques in relationship to the dosing of NSAIDs, postoperative monitoring, or the timing of neuraxial catheter removal.[39]

A better choice for this patient may be the performance of peripheral nerve block(s), if appropriate for the surgery. Since the patient is scheduled for knee surgery, an anterior approach femoral nerve block, combined with a Labat or parasacral approach sciatic nerve block, would be most appropriate. A local anesthetic mixture of mepivicaine (1.5%) and ropivicaine (0.5%,) using a total volume of 25–30 mL for each nerve block will provide superb anesthesia for a total knee replacement and possible tourniquet pain.[38] Additional obturator and lateral femoral cutaneous nerve blocks may be required, depending on the patient's response. Although a lumbar plexus block could be considered, spinal deformities may make this approach more difficult. Additionally, this approach has a higher risk of complications.

39.7   SUMMARY

In summary, the presentation of a patient, who refuses to have an awake tracheal intubation, for surgery with a known difficult airway requires the anesthesia practitioner to consider other options. The anesthesia practitioner must be familiar with several alternative techniques to secure the patient's airway while also providing a safe anesthetic. The ASA Difficult Airway Guidelines form the basis for deciding which technique is appropriate for each individual patient. Most importantly, the anesthesia practitioner should perform the technique with which he/she is most comfortable and skilled and should always have several alternative techniques available in the event the primary technique fails to secure the patient's airway. Regional anesthesia may be an appropriate option for patients with a recognized difficult airway if certain conditions are met and the patient, surgeon, and anesthesia practitioner are prepared for the failure or complications of this technique.

REFERENCES

1. Oryzlo MA, Rosen PS: Ankylosing spondylitis. *Post Grad Med J.* 1969;45:182–185.
2. Brewerton DA, Caffrey M, Hart FD: Ankylosing spondylitis and HLA-B27. *Lancet.* 1973;1:904–907.
3. Muray GC, Persellin RH: Cervical Fracture complicating ankylosing spondylitis. *Am J Med.* 1981;70:1033–1041.
4. Kamarkar US, Chaudhari LS, Hosalkar H, et al.: Difficult intubation in a case of ankylosing spondylitits: a case report. *J Postgrad Med.* 1998;44:43–46.
5. Berendes J, Miehike A: A rare, ankylosis of the cricoarytenoid joints. *Arch Otolaryngol.* 1973;98:63–65.
6. Dave N, Sharma RK: Temporomandibular joint ankylosis in a case of ankylosing spoindylitits—anesthetic management. *Indian J Anaesth.* 2004;48: 54–56.
7. Van Norman G: Informed consent in the operating room. Ethics in Medicine. University of Washington. Available at http://eduserv.hscer.washington.edu/bioethics/topics/infc.html. Accessed February 16, 2005.
8. Practice guidelines for management of the difficult airway: an updated report by the American Society of Anesthesiologists Task Force on Management of the Difficult Airway. *Anesthesiology.* 2003;98:1269–1277.
9. Hsin S, Chen C, Juan C et al.: A modified method for intubation of a patient with ankylosing spondylitis using intubating laryngeal mask airway (LMA-Fastrach™)—A case report. *ACTA Anaesthesiol.* 2001;39:179–182.
10. Dave N, Sharma RK: Temporomandibular joint ankylosis in a case of ankylosing spondylitis—anesthetic management. *Indian J Anaesth.* 2004;48:54–56.
11. Kamarkar US, Chaudari LS, Hosalkar H, et al.: Difficult intubation in a case of ankylosng spondylitis: a case report. *J Postgrad Med.* 1998;44:43–46.
12. Lin BC, Chen IH, et al.: Anesthesia for ankylosing spondylitis patients undergoing transpedicle vertebrectomy. *ACTA Anaesthesiol.* 1999;37:73–78.
13. Langeron O, Masso E, Huraux C, et al.: Prediction of difficult mask ventilation. *Anesthesiology.* 2000;92:1229–1236.
14. Pennant T, White PF: The laryngeal mask airway—its uses in anesthesiology. *Anesthesiology.* 1993;79:144–163.
15. Ishimura H, Minami K, Sata T, et al.: Impossible insertion of the laryngeal mask airway and oropharyngeal axes. *Anesthesiology.* 1995;83:867–869.
16. Olmez G, Nazaroglu H, Arslan SG, et al.: Difficulties and failure of laryngeal mask insertion in a patient with ankylosing spondylitis. Turk. *J Med Sci.* 2004;34:369–352.
17. Takenaka I, Kadoya T, Aoyama K: Is awake intubation necessary when the laryngeal mask airway is feasible?—Letter to the editor, *Anesth Analg.* 2000;91:246–247.
18. Lu PP, Brimacombe J, Ho ACY, et al.: The intubating laryngeal mask airway in severe ankylosing spondylitis. *Can J Anesth.* 2001;48:1015–1019.
19. Pothmann W, Eckert S, Fullekrug B: Use of laryngeal mask in difficult intubation. *Anaesthesist.* 1993;42:644–647. Abstract (in German).
20. Steib A, Beller JP, Lieu JC, et al.: Difficult intubation managed by laryngeal mask and fibroscopy. *Ann Fr Anesth Reanim.* 1992;11:601–603. (in French)
21. Defalgue RS, Hyder ML: Laryngeal mask airway in severe cervical ankylosis. *Can J Anesth.* 1997;44:305–307.
22. Smigovec E, Sakic K, Tripkovic B, et al.: The laryngeal mask—news in orthopedic anesthesia. *Lijec Vjesn.* 1993;155:166–169. (in Croatian).
23. Asai T, Wagle AU, Stacey M: Placement of the intubating laryngeal mask is easier than the laryngeal mask, during manual in-line neck stabilization. *Br J Anaesth.* 1999;82:712–714.
24. Ng M, Hastings R: Successful direct laryngoscopy assisted by pressure in a patient with ankylosing spondylitis. *Anesth Analg.* 1998;87:1436–1437.
25. Cooper RM: Use of a new videolaryngoscope (Glidescope) in the management of a difficult airway. *Can J Anaesth.* 2003;50:611–613.
26. Agro F, Barzoi G, Montecchia F: Tracheal intubation using a Macintosh laryngoscope or a Glidescope in 15 patients with cervical spine immobilization. *Br J Anaesth.* 2003;90:705–706.
27. Gorback MS: Management of the challenging airway with the Bullard laryngoscope. *Clin Anesth.* 1991;3:473–477.
28. Frass M, Frenzer R, Zahler J: Ventilation via the esophageal tracheal combitube in a case of difficult intubation, *J Cardiothor Anesth.* 1987;1:565.
29. Mercer M: Respiratory failure after tracheal extubation in a patient with halo frame cervical spine immobilization—Rescue therapy using the combitube airway. *Br J Anaesth.* 2001;86:886–891.
30. Hagberg C, Vartazarian TN, Chelly JE, et al.: The incidence of gastroesophageal reflux and tracheal aspiration detected with pH electrodes is similar with the laryngeal mask airway and esophageal tracheal combitube—A pilot study. *Can J Anaesth.* 2004;51:243–249.
31. Genzwuerker HV, Vollmer T, Ellinger K: Fibreoptic tracheal intubation after placement of the laryngeal tube. *Br J Anaesth* 2002;89(5):733–738.
32. Mets S, Beattie C: A modified nasal trumpet to facilitate fiberoptic intubation. *Br J Anaesth.* 2003;90:388–391.
33. Mets S: Perioperative use of the modified nasal trumpet in 346 patients. *Br J Anaesth.* 2004;92:694–696.
34. Chelly JE: Regional anesthesia and the difficult airway. In: *Airway Management: Principles and Practice,* 2nd edn. Hagberg CA, ed. St. Louis: Mosby, 2007:1009–1015.
35. Benumof JL: Management of the difficult airway. *Ann Acad Med Singapore.* 1994;23:589–591.
36. Auroy Y, Narchi P, Messiah A, et al.: Serious complications related to regional anesthesia: results of a prospective survey in France. *Anesthesiology.* 1997;87:479–486.
37. Schelew BL, Vaghadia H: Ankylosing spondylitis and neuroaxial anaesthesia—a 10 year review. *Can J Anaesth.* 1996;43:65–68.
38. Lau HP, Yip KM, Jiang CC: Regional nerve block for total knee arthroplasty. *Formos Med Assoc.* 1998;97:428–430.
39. Horlocker TT, Wedel DJ, Benzon H, et al.: Regional anesthesia in the anticoagulated patient: defining the risks (the second ASRA Consensus Conference on Neuraxial Anesthesia and Anticoagulation). *Reg Anesth Pain Med.* 2003;28:172–197.
40. Caplan RA, Ward RJ, Posner K, Cheney FW: Unexpected cardiac arrest during spinal anesthesia: a closed claims analysis of predisposing factors. *Anesthesiology.* 1988;68:5–11.
41. Chester WL: Spinal anesthesia, complete heart block, and the precordial chest thump: an unusual complication and a unique resuscitation. *Anesthesiology.* 1988;69:600–602.
42. Frerichs RL, Campbell J, Bassell GM: Psychogenic cardiac arrest during extensive sympathetic blockade. *Anesthesiology.* 1988;68:943–944.
43. Hodgkinson R: Total spinal block after epidural injection into an interspace adjacent to an inadvertent dural perforation. *Anesthesiology.* 1981;55: 593–595.
44. Liguori GA, Sharrock NE: Asystole and severe bradycardia during epidural anesthesia in orthopedic patients. *Anesthesiology.* 1997;86:250–257.

SELF-EVALUATION QUESTIONS

39.1. Ankylosing spondylitis

  A. can cause a decreased range of movement of the cervical spine

  B. can cause restrictive lung disease

  C. can involve the temporal mandibular joints

D. can involve the cricoarytenoid joints and cause airway obstruction.

E. all of the above

39.2. Proper informed consent must include the following elements:

A. a discussion of the exact nature of the procedure with the patient

B. reasonable alternatives to the proposed procedure must be discussed with the patient

C. the risks and benefits of all alternatives must be discussed with the patient

D. it must be determined that the patient has a reasonable understanding of the issues being discussed

E. all of the above

39.3. Predictors of difficult mask ventilation include

A. absence of a beard

B. full dentition

C. age greater than 50 years

D. a history of snoring

E. BMI < 20 kg·m^{-2}

CHAPTER (40)

Airway Management in the Operating Room for a Morbidly Obese Patient in a "Can't Intubate, Can't Ventilate" Situation

David T. Wong

A diagnosis of cervical radiculopathy has been made.

40.1 CASE PRESENTATION

A 68 year old male is scheduled for an elective anterior cervical decompression and fusion due to a progressive cervical radiculopathy with numbness and pain in C6 distribution bilaterally. He has stable coronary artery disease (CAD) with class II angina and well controlled type II diabetes mellitus. He is a nonsmoker and has no history of sleep apnea. He has no allergies and is taking metoprolol, amlodipine, Nitrodur, and glyburide.

His chest is clear and heart sounds are normal. His airway examination reveals that he is edentulous with a full beard. He has a Mallampati Class II pharyngeal view, a 6 cm thyromental distance, and mouth opening of 4 cm. There is a slight reduction of neck extension (approximately 30 degrees). He is 5'7" (170 cm) tall and weighs 242 lbs (110 kg) with a BMI 38 kg·m^{-2}. His vital signs are: BP 140/95 mm Hg, HR 64 bpm, RR 20 breaths per minute, SpO$_2$ 95% on room air.

Laboratory investigations reveal normal CBC, electrolytes, and creatinine. The random blood glucose is 7.1 mmol·L^{-1}. He has a normal ECG. Magnetic Resonance Imaging (MRI) of the cervical spine (c-spine) shows disc protrusion at C4–5 and C5–6 levels causing nerve root compression at C6 level bilaterally and CSF effacement in front of C4–5 and C5–6 levels without signal changes in the spinal cord.

40.2 PATIENT CONSIDERATIONS

40.2.1 What are the anesthetic considerations for a morbidly obese patient?

Morbid obesity is associated with a number of anatomic, physiologic, and biochemical changes (see also Chapter 17).[1] The cardiovascular system of obese patients is characterized by increased cardiac output, increased circulatory blood volume, and an increased incidence of systemic hypertension and coronary artery disease. In the respiratory system, they have increased oxygen consumption, increased carbon dioxide production, reduced functional residual capacity, increased premature airway closure and shunt, decreased chest wall compliance, and increased work of breathing. There is an increased incidence of pulmonary hypertension and obstructive sleep apnea. There is also a higher incidence of hiatus hernia, gastroesophageal reflux, glucose intolerance, and diabetes mellitus. Airway considerations are detailed below.

40.2.2 Is this patient at an increased risk of having a perioperative cardiac event?

Yes. This patient has several risk factors and is at a higher risk of having a perioperative cardiac event. There are several well-established perioperative cardiac risk assessment tools. He has diabetes and stable, class II angina, which according to the 2002 American College of Cardiology/American Heart Association Guidelines[2] puts him in the "intermediate medical risk" category. Utilizing the Lee cardiac risk score,[3] he has two (CAD and diabetes) of six risk factors and is predicted to have a perioperative cardiac event rate of approximately 5%. Utilization of perioperative beta-blockade may be useful in reducing the risk of cardiac events.

40.2.3 Some patients with cervical pathology scheduled for anterior decompression and fusion undergo awake intubations. Does our patient need one?

In my opinion, three categories of patients may require awake endotracheal intubation:

- The first group has signs and symptoms of cervical myelopathy. Clinically, this may manifest itself as bilateral upper extremity numbness, pain or weakness, or long track signs such as bilateral leg symptoms. These symptoms may worsen with certain neck movements. Radiologically, cerebral spinal fluid effacement, deformation of spinal cord contour, and particularly signal changes within the spinal cord are suggestive of myelopathy. Although there are no studies showing that patients with spinal cord pathology or injury have improved outcome when intubated awake versus asleep,[4–6] I believe that patients with clinically evident myelopathy should have an awake endotracheal intubation to avoid the possibility of further spinal cord compromise with neck movement encountered during asleep intubation.

- Second, patients with cervical-spine ligamentous or bony instability constitute another potential indication for awake intubation. Examples include C1–2 subluxation from rheumatoid arthritis or traumatic cervical-spine instability.

- Third, patients with proven or suspected difficult airways should be considered for awake intubation.

40.2.4 Should this patient be admitted to the ICU postoperatively to monitor for airway swelling and compromise?

Patients undergoing anterior cervical decompression and fusion are at a slightly increased risk of postoperative airway obstruction. However, it is reasonably safe to observe these patients in the post anesthetic care unit (PACU) 4–6 hours postoperatively, and if they have an uneventful course, discharge them to the floor. We have used the above mentioned protocol for management of postoperative anterior cervical-spine fusion patients for more than 6 years and not encountered any significant airway problems in the first day postoperatively. Patients who undergo prolonged surgery, multiple segmental fusion, corpec-

tomy, difficult surgical exposure with excessive traction, massive fluid shifts, or those who have received large amounts of intravenous (IV) fluids should be admitted directly to the ICU.

Postoperatively, it is crucial that the patient be followed closely for the onset of stridor, increasing difficulty in swallowing or breathing, or signs of increasing external neck swelling. Airway obstruction can occur rapidly in the face of a neck hematoma, edema, lymphatic obstruction, or nerve palsies. Patients exhibiting any of the above mentioned signs or symptoms in the immediate postoperative period should immediately have an awake flexible fiberscope examination of the airway under topical anesthesia. Should the airway look normal and intubation is deemed to be unnecessary, close and continuous observation is indicated. If the airway is narrowed or partially obstructed, it should be secured using an awake endotracheal intubation technique. Life-threatening airway obstruction can rapidly ensue either spontaneously, with airway topicalization, or upon airway instrumentation.[7] It is imperative to have immediate availability of equipment and personnel skilled in insertion of an infraglottic airway in anticipation of complete airway obstruction.

40.3 AIRWAY CONSIDERATIONS

40.3.1 How often does difficult intubation occur in clinical practice? How is difficult intubation defined?

The incidence of difficult intubation depends on its definition. In 1993, the ASA Task Force[8] defined difficult intubation as occurring when "proper insertion of the tracheal tube with conventional laryngoscopy requires more than three attempts or more than 10 minutes." In 1998, the Canadian Airway Focus Group[9] used the following definition: "when an experienced laryngoscopist using direct laryngoscopy, requires: 1) more than two attempts with the same blade or; 2) a change in the blade or an adjunct to a direct laryngoscope or; 3) use of an alternative device or technique following failed intubation with direct laryngoscopy." The incidence of difficult intubation reported in the literature ranges from 1.15% to 3.8%.[9]

40.3.2 Is the patient predicted to have a difficult airway? How accurate are our predictions for difficult intubation?

The ASA Task Force on management of the difficult airway outlined 11 criteria for preoperative airway assessment.[10] No single airway test has perfect sensitivity or specificity in predicting difficult intubation. In general, many single airway predictors share a common set of characteristics: low sensitivity, high specificity, and low positive predictive value. Combinations of several airway predictors tend to improve the positive predictive value for difficult intubation (see Section 1.6.3).

Our patient had a Mallampati class II score, a thyromental distance of 6 cm, mouth opening of 4 cm, slightly reduced cervical extension, and a full set of dentures. In combination, these characteristics place this patient at low risk of difficult intubation.

40.3.3 Is there a concern about difficult bag-mask-ventilation in our patient? How is difficult mask ventilation defined?

The ASA Task Force on management of the difficult airway defined difficult bag-mask-ventilation (BMV) as: "it is not possible for the anesthesia practitioner to provide adequate face mask ventilation due to one or more of the following problems: inadequate mask seal, excessive gas leak, or excessive resistance to the ingress or egress of gas."[10] The incidence of difficult mask ventilation is in the range of 5%[11] while that of failed bag-mask-ventilation is in the range of 0.01–0.08%.[9]

Langeron identified five risk factors for difficult mask ventilation: beard, obesity (BMI > 26 kg·m^{-2}), age >55, lack of teeth, and history of snoring (MOANS, see Section 1.6.1).[11] Our patient has four of the five risk factors and is at a moderately increased risk of difficult mask ventilation.

40.3.4 How often does the "can't intubate, can't ventilate" situation arise in clinical practice?

Can't intubate, can't ventilate (CICV) situations are life threatening. In 1991, the incidence of CICV was estimated to be 0.01 to 2 per 10,000 patient cases.[12] The LMA has since been shown to be effective in providing rescue ventilation in the majority of CICV situations.[13] The current incidence of CICV requiring emergency infraglottic airway insertion may be lower than 2:10,000 patients. Anesthesia practitioners need to be fully prepared to insert an infraglottic airway in this rare but deadly situation.

40.4 PREPARATION AND PLANS

40.4.1 How do you plan to intubate the trachea of this patient?

The patient is undergoing an anterior cervical fusion and will require general anesthesia with endotracheal intubation. As he does not have cervical myelopathy, instability, or prediction of a difficult intubation, the plan is to proceed with endotracheal intubation after IV induction of general anesthesia.

40.4.2 Are you concerned about difficulties in BMV?

Yes. The patient is at an increased risk for difficult mask ventilation BMV but is not predicted to be a difficult intubation. Therefore, a variety of airway devices are prepared, including face masks, nasopharyngeal airways, oropharyngeal airways, laryngeal mask airways, and the Combitube™. OR personnel are alerted to the possible need to perform two person BMV.

40.4.3 What are your plans if after the induction of general anesthesia intubation with a direct laryngoscope is unsuccessful but ventilation is easy using BMV technique?

This unsuccessful intubation, but adequate ventilation clinical setting, places us in the second tier of The Failed Airway Algorithm (see Chapter 2) and in the middle of the ASA Difficult Airway Algorithm nonemergency pathway.[10] If all six factors defining an optimal laryngoscopic attempt (see Section 1.6.2) have been met, it makes no sense to persist with further attempts with direct laryngoscopy. Instead, since one has time, alternative approaches such as use of the flexible fiberoptic bronchoscope, intubating laryngeal mask, lighted stylet, or the GlideScope® may be attempted.[14,15] It is important to impose a time or number of attempts limit when using these alternative techniques such that a CICV situation following repeated airway instrumentation does not occur. In the event that intubation is unsuccessful after multiple attempts with alternative techniques in a nonemergency scenario, the patient should be awakened and an awake intubation performed.

40.4.4 Should this evolve into a CICV situation after the induction of general anesthesia, what should one do?

CICV is an absolute medical emergency. Hypoxic brain damage and death can ensue unless successful corrective measures are undertaken immediately (Table 40-1). CICV may occur immediately after induction of anesthesia or during the course of repeated airway instrumentation. The Failed Airway Algorithm directs one to immediately prepare to perform a cricothyrotomy, although while preparations are underway one may attempt an extraglottic device (EGD [LMA or Combitube™]). This differs from the ASA Difficult Airway Algorithm[10] in that these initiatives occur concurrently rather than sequentially. If ventilation and oxygenation become adequate with an EGD, there is time to attempt alternative techniques.

40.4.5 A CICV situation wherein the patient becomes progressively hypoxemic necessitates an immediate surgical airway. What is your preferred technique and instrument?

The most common techniques employed to secure an infraglottic airway include percutaneous IV catheter cricothyrotomy, percutaneous dilational cricothyrotomy, open surgical cricothyrotomy, and surgeon performed tracheotomy (Table 40-1). In a Canada-wide anesthesiologist survey,[16] respondents preferred using cricothyrotomy by IV catheter (51%), followed by percutaneous dilational cricothyrotomy (28%) and tracheotomy by surgeon (7%).

TABLE 40-1

Can't Intubate, Can't Ventilate Management Options

Optimization of lung ventilation	• Reposition the head, apply jaw lift • Optimize mask: change face mask, adjust the amount of air in the face mask • Insert oropharyngeal and two nasopharyngeal airways (appropriately sized) • Use a two-person, BMV technique: one practitioner applies a two hand mask hold and the second practitioner provides manual bag ventilation • Insert an LMA (appropriately sized) • Consider shaving the beard or applying vaseline on the beard to improve mask seal
Insertion of an infraglottic airway: options	• IV catheter: nonkinkable • Percutaneous dilational cricothyrotomy kit • Open surgical cricothyrotomy • Open surgical tracheotomy by surgeon
Adjuncts for infraglottic airway	• Handheld transtracheal jet ventilator with pressure reduction to 20 psi • Saline soaked ribbon gauze throat pack

40.4.6 What are the advantages and disadvantages of these infraglottic airway techniques?

Although cricothyrotomy by IV catheter is the simplest to perform, it is difficult to fixate the catheter, difficult to maintain patency, offers no airway protection, provides variable amounts of ventilation, lacks a conduit for suction, is associated with significant risks of barotrauma, and requires a special attachment for jet ventilation.[16] Anesthesia practitioners are generally uncomfortable performing an open cricothyrotomy. The percutaneous dilational cricothyrotomy technique incorporates many advantages of the open cricothyrotomy. It is more stable, offers airway protection, provides a conduit for suctioning, and can be readily connected to a ventilation bag with a 15 mm connector. Furthermore, the percutaneous Seldinger dilational technique is familiar to all anesthesia practitioners who perform central venous cannulation. Most anesthesiologists in the survey mentioned above were unfamiliar with the methodology and instruments involved in open tracheotomy or cricothyrotomy.[16]

40.4.7 Is there evidence in the literature to indicate which cricothyrotomy technique is superior to others in terms of speed of insertion and success rates?

Review of the literature reveals few randomized controlled trials using infraglottic airway techniques and no trials in actual patients in CICV situations.[17,18] Eisenburger et al.[19] compared the performance of percutaneous and surgical cricothyrotomy by intensive care trainees on cadavers. The cricothyrotomy times were 100 seconds

and 102 seconds, respectively. Chan et al.[20] did a similar comparative study for emergency medicine of physicians and residents. He found similar times (75 vs. 73 seconds) for the percutaneous and surgical cricothyrotomy groups. Schaumann et al. compared the performance of percutaneous and surgical cricothyrotomy on cadavers by emergency physicians.[21] The cricothyrotomy times were significantly shorter in the percutaneous compared to the surgical group (108.6 vs. 136.6 seconds). Bainton[22] assessed 23 physicians using the percutaneous cricothyrotomy technique on dogs. All completed the cricothyrotomy successfully with a mean time of 40 seconds.

40.4.8 Many anesthesia practitioners have never performed a cricothyrotomy or encountered a CICV situation. How can one acquire proficiency in the performance of infraglottic airway insertion?

To optimize the success rate of surgical cricothyrotomy, one needs to commit to memory all the sequential steps and to acquire experience in a simulated setting. Bainton reported that the time taken to perform a cricothyrotomy on dogs improved significantly after practicing on cricothyrotomy simulator models.[22] Wong et al.[23] showed that procedure times and success rates improved significantly in 102 subjects, each performing 10 consecutive cricothyrotomies on mannequins. From the first to tenth attempt, procedure times improved from 41.2 seconds to 24.4 seconds (41% change) and success rate went from 62% to 99% (37% change). Knowing the cricothyrotomy equipment, familiarity with a cricothyrotomy procedure algorithm, and practical experience with using such devices on mannequins provide the practitioner the best chance of success when called upon to perform a cricothyrotomy in an emergency such as a CICV airway.

40.4.9 How do you plan to denitrogenate this patient prior to anesthesia induction?

There are many reasons to ensure adequate oxygenation prior to induction. First, the patient is morbidly obese, which is associated with reduced functional residual capacity, increased airway closure and shunt, decreased chest wall compliance, and increased work of breathing. He will desaturate much faster than a normal individual with hypoventilation. Second, he is potentially difficult to bag-mask-ventilate. Provision of supranormal denitrogenation will provide the patient a wider margin of safety on induction. Third, he has significant coronary artery disease. With his increased cardiac oxygen requirement due to obesity and reduced coronary reserve, he may not be able to tolerate arterial hypoxemia.

Therefore, the goal should be to provide denitrogenation for at least 3 minutes and end-tidal $O_2 \geq 90\%$, similar to that in rapid sequence induction.

40.5   ACTUAL CONDUCT OF TRACHEAL INTUBATION

40.5.1   How was the induction and airway management approached?

Anesthesia equipment and drugs were fully prepared prior to induction. The patient was denitrogenated for 5 minutes, pre-treated with fentanyl, induced with propofol, and paralyzed with rocuronium. After 2 minutes, direct laryngoscopy with a MAC #3 blade was attempted. Only the epiglottis was visible. A MAC #4 blade was tried with the application of anterior laryngeal pressure with no improvement of laryngeal view. Insertion of a styletted endotracheal tube behind the epiglottis was performed, but no CO_2 waveform was detected and the endotracheal tube was removed. Bag-mask-ventilation was performed but due to a large mask leak the SpO_2 decreased to 88%.

We now have a failed intubation coupled with borderline bag-mask-ventilation. A 9 mm oral pharyngeal airway and two nasal airways were inserted. The anesthesia practitioner then performed a "two hand" mask hold while ventilation was provided by the OR an assistant.

40.5.2   Confronted with a CICV situation, what ought to happen next?

Cricothyrotomy! In the meantime as the cricothyrotomy equipment is being set up one may attempt an intubating LMA or other EGD. This should not be a *sequential* step as indicated in the ASA Difficult Airway Algorithm; it is *concurrent* with preparation to perform a surgical airway as in The Failed Airway Algorithm (Chapter 2). If the EGD rescue is successful and adequate ventilation is restored, then intubation attempts with alternative intubation equipment such as a flexible fiberoptic bronchoscope and GlideScope® are appropriate. However, in the CICV situation, attempts to intubate with alternative techniques such as the flexible fiberoptic bronchoscope and GlideScope® are not appropriate and waste valuable time.

In this case scenario, the patient was hypoxic and deteriorating in a CICV situation. A decision was made to insert an infraglottic airway immediately. The anesthesia practitioner decided to use a percutaneous dilational cricothyrotomy technique.

40.5.3   Describe the actual steps taken to insert the percutaneous dilational cricothyrotomy

The instrument used to perform cricothyrotomy was a preassembled Melker emergency percutaneous dilational Set (Cook® Critical Care, Bloomington, IN) which consisted of a needle, syringe, guide wire, scalpel, dilator, and airway, which in the newer sets is cuffed (see Chapter 12 for details). The cricothyroid

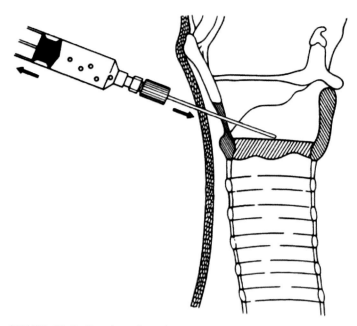

FIGURE 40-1. Cricothyroid membrane puncture: The cricothyroid membrane is punctured with an 18-gauge needle directed caudally and correct intraluminal location is confirmed by the aspiration of air. (Reproduced with permission from Cook® Critical Care, Bloomington, IN.)

membrane was located and punctured with an 18-gauge needle directed caudally. Correct intraluminal location of the needle in the airway was confirmed by the aspiration of air (Figure 40-1). The 0.038 inch guide wire was inserted via the needle into the airway (Figure 40-2) and the needle was removed over the wire. The puncture site was enlarged by a stab with a #15 scalpel blade and a cuffed tracheotomy tube or airway catheter (5 mm ID) with the dilator (18-Fr) (Figure 40-3) inserted into the trachea over the

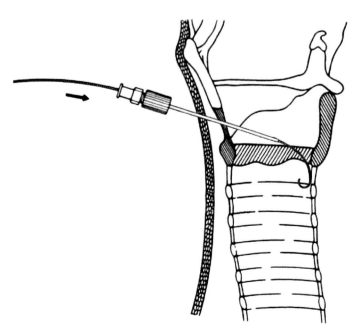

FIGURE 40-2. Insertion of the guide wire: A guide wire is inserted via the needle into the trachea. (Reproduced with permission from Cook® Critical Care, Bloomington, IN.)

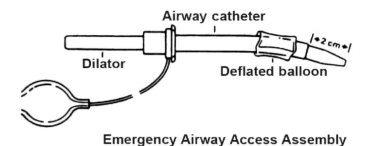

Emergency Airway Access Assembly

FIGURE 40-3. Cuffed tracheotomy tube: This figure depicts a cuffed airway catheter or tracheotomy tube with the dilator. (Reproduced with permission from Cook® Critical Care, Bloomington, IN.)

wire (Figure 40-4). The dilator and the wire were removed, ventilation was performed, and correct placement was confirmed using capnography and auscultation. A CO_2 waveform was obtained and the SpO_2 improved to >90% 2 minutes after establishment of ventilation via the cricothyrotomy.

40.5.4   Is it feasible to perform an open surgical cricothyrotomy instead of the percutaneous dilational approach?

Yes, it is a feasible option, although most anesthesia practitioners are uncomfortable with this procedure.[16] The technique consists of locating the cricothyroid membrane, making a midline longitudinal incision through skin, followed by a transverse incision through the cricothyroid membrane using a scalpel, insertion of a tracheotomy hook placed beneath the inferior border of the thyroid cartilage, applying traction in an anterior/cephalad direction to expose the airway lumen, placement of an

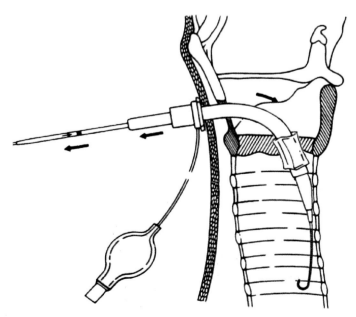

FIGURE 40-4. Insertion of tracheotomy tube: With the dilator in place, the cuffed tracheotomy tube is inserted into the trachea over the guidewire. (Reproduced with permission from Cook® Critical Care, Bloomington, IN.)

endotracheal or cricothyrotomy tube, and confirmation of positioning using capnography and auscultation (see Section 12.2.1). Open cricothyrotomy kits are commercially available. Alternatively, the necessary equipment can be assembled by the individual institution and potential practitioners can be made aware of the contents.

40.6   POSTINTUBATION MANAGEMENT

40.6.1   At present, oxygenation and ventilation are satisfactory. What is your next step?

Although there is some controversy, most consider a cricothyrotomy to be a temporary life-saving airway which should not be maintained for prolonged periods (see Chapters 12 and 32). Therefore, a surgeon was requested to perform a tracheotomy. A size 8 mm ID cuffed tracheotomy tube was inserted and the temporary cricothyrotomy was removed.

40.6.2   Now that the airway is secured, the neurosurgeon is anxious to proceed with the anterior cervical fusion. Should we go ahead?

No. The surgery is elective. The patient almost died due to a failed intubation and was subjected to repeated airway instrumentation before a surgical airway was secured. There are three reasons for not performing the surgery at this time. First, anterior cervical fusion involves traction and manipulation in the neck. Should the tracheotomy tube be dislodged, it may be very difficult to reinsert through the track of a newly created tracheotomy. Second, cervical surgery in addition to the intubation attempts will increase the risk of postoperative airway edema. Third, having a tracheotomy tube in the immediate vicinity of a fresh surgical incision increases the potential for surgical site infection.

40.6.3   As a decision has been made not to proceed with cervical surgery, what do we do next?

The patient was brought to the ICU. He was ventilated and allowed to awaken. Once awake and adequate spontaneous ventilation reestablished, he was removed from the ventilator and placed on a tracheotomy mask. The patient was discharged to the surgical floor after overnight observation.

40.6.4   When can we bring him back for his cervical fusion?

A reasonable course of action is to remove his tracheotomy tube 24 hours post ICU discharge and allow the track and skin to close. He will be brought back for his surgery in 1–2 months. An awake intubation could then be performed before induction of general anesthesia.

40.7 SUMMARY

In summary, CICV is a rare but life-threatening situation that all anesthesia practitioners should be prepared to manage. If intubation fails and oxygenation cannot be maintained by bag-mask-ventilation despite a two-person technique employing oropharyngeal and nasopharyngeal airways, an immediate decision should be made to perform a cricothyrotomy. Time and again, patients suffer hypoxic brain damage or death from a delayed decision to proceed with an infraglottic airway.

Every airway practitioner must be familiar with the cricothyrotomy equipment available locally and must acquire the necessary skills by performing cricothyrotomy on mannequins or cadavers such that emergency cricothyrotomy can be rapidly performed if required in the clinical setting. It is better to have a live patient with a neck incision than a dead patient with a nice looking neck.

REFERENCES

1. Buckley FP, Martay K: Anesthesia, obesity and gastrointestinal disorders. In: *Clinical Anesthesia*, 4th edn. Barash PG, Cullen BF, Calkins H, et al., eds. Philadelphia, PA: Lippincott Williams & Wilkins, 2001: 1035–1041.
2. Eagle KA, Berger PB, Calkins H, et al.: ACC/AHA guideline update for perioperative cardiovascular evaluation for noncardiac surgery–executive summary: a report of the American College of Cardiology/American Heart Association Task Force on Practice Guidelines (Committee to Update the 1996 Guidelines on Perioperative Cardiovascular Evaluation for Noncardiac Surgery). *J Am Coll Cardiol.* 2002;39:542–553.
3. Lee TH, Marcantonio ER, Mangione CM, et al.: Derivation and prospective validation of a simple index for prediction of cardiac risk of major noncardiac surgery. *Circulation.* 1999;100:1043–1049.
4. Criswell JC, Parr MJ, Nolan JP: Emergency airway management in patients with cervical spine injuries. *Anaesthesia.* 1994;49:900–903.
5. Meschino A, Devitt JH, Koch JP, Szalai JP, Schwartz ML: The safety of awake tracheal intubation in cervical spine injury. *Can J Anaesth.* 1992;39:114–117.
6. Suderman VS, Crosby ET, Lui A: Elective oral tracheal intubation in cervical spine-injured adults. *Can J Anaesth.* 1991;38:785–789.
7. Ho AM, Chung DC, To EW, Karmakar MK: Total airway obstruction during local anesthesia in a non-sedated patient with a compromised airway. *Can J Anaesth.* 2004;51:838–841.
8. Caplan RA, Benumof JL, Berry FA, et al.: Practice guidelines for management of the difficult airway: a report by the American Society of Anesthesiologists Task Force on Management of the Difficult Airway. *Anesthesiology.* 1993;78:597–602.
9. Crosby ET, Cooper RM, Douglas MJ, et al.: The unanticipated difficult airway with recommendations for management. *Can J Anaesth.* 1998;45:757–776.
10. Caplan RA, Benumof JL, Berry FA, et al.: Practice guidelines for management of the difficult airway: an updated report by the American Society of Anesthesiologists Task Force on Management of the Difficult Airway. *Anesthesiology.* 2003;98:1269–1277.
11. Langeron O, Masso E, Huraux C, et al.: Prediction of difficult mask ventilation. *Anesthesiology.* 2000;92:1229–1236.
12. Benumof JL: Management of the difficult adult airway. With special emphasis on awake tracheal intubation. *Anesthesiology.* 1991;75:1087–1110.
13. Parmet JL, Colonna-Romano P, Horrow JC, et al.: The laryngeal mask airway reliably provides rescue ventilation in cases of unanticipated difficult tracheal intubation along with difficult mask ventilation. *Anesth Analg.* 1998;87:661–665.
14. Jenkins K, Wong DT, Correa R: Management choices for the difficult airway by anesthesiologists in Canada. *Can J Anaesth.* 2002;49:850–856.
15. Rosenblatt WH, Wagner PJ, Ovassapian A, Kain ZN: Practice patterns in managing the difficult airway by anesthesiologists in the United States. *Anesth Analg.* 1998;87:153–157.
16. Wong DT, Lai K, Chung FF, Ho RY: Cannot intubate-cannot ventilate and difficult intubation strategies: results of a Canadian national survey. *Anesth Analg.* 2005;100:1439–1446.
17. Chang RS, Hamilton RJ, Carter WA: Declining rate of cricothyrotomy in trauma patients with an emergency medicine residency: implications for skills training. *Acad Emerg Med.* 1998;5:247–251.
18. Erlandson MJ, Clinton JE, Ruiz E, Cohen J: Cricothyrotomy in the emergency department revisited. *J Emerg Med.* 1989;7:115–118.
19. Eisenburger P, Laczika K, List M, et al.: Comparison of conventional surgical versus Seldinger technique emergency cricothyrotomy performed by inexperienced clinicians. *Anesthesiology.* 2000;92:687–690.
20. Chan TC, Vilke GM, Bramwell KJ, et al.: Comparison of wire-guided cricothyrotomy versus standard surgical cricothyrotomy technique. *J Emerg Med.* 1999;17:957–962.
21. Schaumann N, Lorenz V, Schellongowski P, et al.: Evaluation of Seldinger technique emergency cricothyroidotomy versus standard surgical cricothyroidotomy in 200 cadavers. *Anesthesiology.* 2005;102:7–11.
22. Bainton CR: Cricothyrotomy. *Int Anesthesiol Clin.* 1994;32:95–108.
23. Wong DT, Prabhu AJ, Coloma M, Imasogie N, Chung FF: What is the minimum training required for successful cricothyroidotomy? A study in mannequins. *Anesthesiology.* 2003;98:349–353.

SELF-EVALUATION QUESTIONS

40.1. The major difference between the ASA Difficult Airway Algorithm and The Failed Airway Algorithm in Chapter 2 of this book is

A. the definition of the failed airway is different.

B. the ASA algorithm recommends that LMAs and cricothyrotomy be performed sequentially; this text recommends that they be performed concurrently.

C. the ASA algorithm recommends that LMAs and cricothyrotomy be performed concurrently; this text recommends that they be performed sequentially.

D. the role of videolaryngoscopes is different.

E. the ASA algorithm recommends canceling the case; this text makes no mention of canceling the case.

40.2. The evidence with respect to cricothyrotomy suggests

A. that practice on manikins improves performance

B. that anesthesia practitioners do not like to perform it

C. that, on an average, anesthesia practitioners do not know how to perform one

D. two of a, b, c

E. all of a, b, c

40.3. Difficult bag-mask-ventilation

A. may be mitigated by the use of an oral airway and two nasal airways

B. is associated with an age >45

C. is less common with the use of transparent masks

D. is less common in the elderly with no teeth

E. is associated with difficult laryngoscopy and intubation

CHAPTER (41)

Unique Airway Issues in the Pediatric Population

Robert C. Luten, Niranjan "Tex" Kissoon,
Stephen A. Godwin and Michael F. Murphy

41.1 CASE PRESENTATION

A previously healthy 2 year old boy is brought to your emergency department (ED) having been involved in a motor vehicle crash. He was wearing a seat belt but was not in his car seat. Initial assessment by the paramedics at the scene showed that he was awake, crying, breathing spontaneously with stable hemodynamics and normal oxygen saturation. In the ED, you note that the child has a laceration on his forehead and alternates between episodes of extreme irritability and drowsiness. A CT scan is ordered. While in CT, you are summoned because the child will not lie still and requires sedation to the point that he is unable to maintain his own airway.

41.2 INTRODUCTION

41.2.1 Is the pediatric airway truly *unique*?

Somewhat. The pediatric airway possesses an array of unique features, particularly to practitioners who do not manage them every day. Unless one is a pediatric specialist, managing the pediatric airway is not a common event, therefore, it is unique. Furthermore, the *difficult* pediatric airway is decidedly rare. So not only does the pediatric airway possess unique anatomic features at different ages, the frequency with which one is confronted by a *difficult* pediatric airway is an additional unique experience.

The unique nature of the pediatric airway is most evident in the newborn to 2 year age group. Not only is the airway smaller, but the proportions of the upper airway structures are different from adult proportions. Most often, discussions of the pediatric airway really focus on the unique nature of the newborn to 2 year age

group. From the age of 2 to the age of 8, the airway gradually changes, more closely resembling the adult airway.

41.2.2 What is the clinical challenge of managing the pediatric airway?

The geometry and physical appearance of the pediatric airway, characteristics of lung anatomy and physiology and the rate at which the physiology matures, represent the elements that constitute "the pediatric airway."

The clinical challenge of pediatric airway management requires the appreciation of the continuously evolving anatomy as development proceeds from infancy to adolescence. This challenge is compounded by the fact that this evolution is accompanied by age and size related differences in drug dosing and equipment sizes, as well as the psychological stress that invariably accompanies the resuscitation of a critically ill child.[1]

Congenital anomalies notwithstanding, the pediatric airway and pediatric physiology are remarkably consistent from one patient to another. Furthermore, many of the factors that are associated with difficult airways in adults are not present in children, such as obesity, beards, edentulousness, and kyphosis, to name a few.

41.3 AIRWAY ASSESSMENT

41.3.1 What is unique about the evaluation of the pediatric patient who requires airway management?

Evidence suggests that the resuscitation of a child (including airway management) imposes an additional "mental (cognitive) burden" on the airway practitioner, compared to an adult resuscitation.[2] Age- and size-related variables in children introduce the need for more complex, nonautomatic, or knowledge-based mental activities, such as calculating drug doses and selecting equipment. Mental assets called into play to undertake these additional decisions may be thought of as "subtracting" from other important cognitive activities crucial to the task, such as assessment, evaluation, prioritization, and synthesis of information. This is referred to in the resuscitative process as "critical thinking activity." The cumulative effect of this process leads to inevitable time delays and a corresponding increase in the potential for decision-making errors in the resuscitation of the pediatric patient. It has been shown that the use of a color-coded, length-based resuscitation aid, such as the Broselow-Luten System® (Vital Signs, Inc., Totowa, NJ), in pediatric resuscitation significantly reduces the additional cognitive load associated with dosing and equipment selection, permitting more time for critical thinking and reducing performance anxiety.[3,4]

41.3.2   How do you properly assess the airway of a child?

There is sparse literature relating specifically to the systematic evaluation of the pediatric patient in difficult airway management. Most reports deal with airway management in patients with specific congenital anomalies, perhaps because in general the evaluation of the pediatric airway is no different than the evaluation of the adult airway, cooperation notwithstanding!

The strategies and mnemonics described in Chapter 1, employed in evaluating airways for difficulty in bag-mask-ventilation (BMV), laryngoscopic intubation, the use of extraglottic devices (EGDs) and the surgical airway (MOANS, LEMON, RODS, and SHORT), are useful in principle. However, it must be recognized that many of the evaluation points in these mnemonics have not been validated, and may not be applicable in the pediatric population.

The task of constructing an organized and thoughtful approach to evaluating and managing the airway can be made easier with the LEMON mnemonic. The use of MOANS may be inappropriate for the pediatric population as children do not have facial hair, are not usually edentulous, and are obviously not older than 55 years of age. Using SHORT to evaluate the airway for difficult cricothyrotomy is also less useful in children than in adults.

In infants and younger children, an assessment of the size and proportions of the jaw, the mandibular space, the face, and the tongue will suffice to uncover many difficulties. The most common congenital anomaly associated with airway management difficulty in children is micrognathia. Difficult airways in infants and young children, usually associated with a *syndrome*, are usually diagnosed in the neonatal period and may well have led to a tracheotomy. This removes establishing an airway as a consideration in resuscitation.

41.3.3   How do you evaluate vital organ system reserve as it relates to airway management in pediatric patients?

The evaluation of "vital organ system reserve" in children ought to focus on the acute disorder with which the child presents and how

this might influence the manner in which the airway is managed. Exceptions to this general rule include those children suffering from some notable disorders such as cystic fibrosis, asthma, congenital heart disease, and mental disability. Other than the disorder for which the child is being intubated, acquired conditions that specifically affect vital organ system *reserve* in children are decidedly uncommon. The same cannot be said of congenital disorders that affect the cardiovascular, respiratory, and central nervous systems. Though these are rarely encountered in adult practice, they may influence the degree of reserve, and evaluating for the extent of that reduction in reserve is important in the context of airway management.

41.4.   ANATOMICAL AND PHYSIOLOGICAL CONSIDERATIONS

41.4.1   What are the age-specific anatomic features of the upper airway and how do they change over time?

The most obvious difference between adult and pediatric airways, in addition to size, is the position of the airway in the neck relative to the cervical bodies. The pediatric airway is often described as "anterior" because at its normal position at the C2–3 level (depending on age), it is "tucked up" beneath the posterior aspect of the tongue, which is relatively larger in relation to the oral cavity and the mandibular space in children as compared to adults. So, in reality, the pediatric larynx is more superior than anterior, and the tongue may be more difficult to move out of the visual field than in adults.

The epiglottis is also proportionally larger in the child than the adult. The ligamentous connection between the base of the tongue and the epiglottis (the hypoepiglottic ligament) is not as well defined in children as it is in the adults. This fact renders less effective attempts to elevate the proportionally larger epiglottis by manipulation of the vallecular space with a curved blade. For this reason, and because the large tongue is more difficult to elevate anteriorly out of the field of vision with a curved blade, a *straight blade* inserted past the epiglottis to lift it out of the field of vision is usually preferred in the first 1–2 years of life when these differences are most pronounced.

The narrowest portion of the child's airway is at the level of the cricoid ring, as opposed to the adult where the narrowest portion is at the level of the vocal cords. An interesting observation is that while an adult may demonstrate the presence of laryngitis with changes in the voice, the small child becomes "croupy." The significance of this anatomical variation is that in the adult patient endotracheal tube (ETT) size is less critical since a low-pressure, high-volume cuff can be inflated to assure adequate fit. In children, uncuffed ETTs are preferred (see Section 41.6.7), and size becomes more important to minimize leak, particularly with positive pressure ventilation. A tube that is too small impairs one's ability to provide positive pressure ventilation and a tube that is too large can cause pressure ischemia and necrosis of the subglottic (cricoid) tracheal mucosa, with result in subglottic stenosis. By the age of 8, cuffed tubes can generally be used.

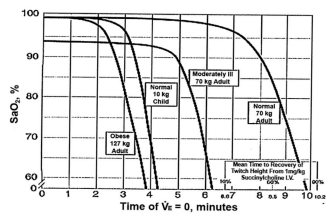

FIGURE 41-1. The time course of oxygen desaturation following apnea: Note how quickly the child desaturates compared to the adult in this desaturation curve. This speed of desaturation is related to the increased oxygen utilization and the relatively reduced FRC of the child versus the adult. (*Reproduced with permission from Benumof J, Dagg R, Benumof R: Critical hemoglobin desaturation will occur before return to an unparalyzed state following 1 mg·kg⁻¹ intravenous succinylcholine. Anesthesiology. 1997;87:979.*)

41.4.2 Is there anything unique with respect to pulmonary physiology in the child? if so, how does that influence the way one manages the airway?

Combinations of physiological factors conspire to decrease the effectiveness of denitrogenation in pediatric patients compared to adults. First, and most important, is the fact that a child metabolizes oxygen twice as fast as an adult does (6.0 mL·kg⁻¹ vs. 3.0 mL·kg⁻¹).[5] Second, a child has a proportionally smaller functional residual capacity (FRC) due to the fact that the elastic recoil of the lung is high, as is chest wall compliance. Third, the supine position may further complicate management as the abdominal contents restrict diaphragmatic movement, effectively reducing thoracic volume. For these reasons, denitrogenation[6] in the apneic child results in a significantly shorter period of acceptable oxygen saturations than that in the apneic adult (see Figure 41-1).[6] The clinical significance is that the child may be expected to desaturate more quickly during rapid sequence induction (RSI) and is more likely to require BMV while maintaining cricoid pressure.

41.5 PHARMACOLOGICAL CONSIDERATIONS

41.5.1 How do we improve the safety of drug administration in pediatric emergencies?

The timely and accurate delivery of medications to the pediatric patient is crucial, particularly in an emergency, such as an emergency intubation. The use of systems, such as the Broselow-Luten System®, can improve the safety and reduce errors in emergency situations.[2,7]

41.5.2 Is succinylcholine safe to use in children?

Perhaps the most controversial drug issue in pediatric airway management is the use of succinylcholine. The dose of succinylcholine in children is different than that in adults due to the relatively larger proportion of extracellular water in children: at birth, 45% of the weight is extracellular fluid water; at 2 months, approximately 30%; at 6 years, 20%; and at adulthood, 16–18%.[1] The recommended dose of succinylcholine therefore is higher in children.

In addition, the US Food and Drug Administration, in conjunction with pharmaceutical companies, revised the package labeling of succinylcholine in 1993 because of the reports of hyperkalemic cardiac arrests in patients with undiagnosed neuromuscular disorders who were given succinylcholine. The warning initially stated that succinylcholine was contraindicated for elective anesthesia in pediatric patients because of this concern, though the wording of the warning has since been softened. Further, both the initial advisory warning and the revised warning continue to recommend succinylcholine be used, as is current practice, in emergency or full stomach intubation of children.[8,9]

41.5.3 Should atropine be used routinely when succinylcholine is being administered?

Atropine is generally recommended during pediatric tracheal intubation to prevent bradycardia due to succinylcholine use or secondary to vagal stimulation with airway instrumentation. Younger children (less than 2 year old) are especially prone to developing bradycardia because of well-developed parasympathetic vagal responses. The optimal dose of atropine has been debated, with recommendations ranging from 0.01 to 0.02 mg·kg⁻¹. Some question the use of the higher dose as it may have deleterious side effects in the very young,[10] while others feel that the higher dose is needed to achieve consistent vagolysis if succinylcholine is to be administered.[11] Most practitioners feel that the higher (0.02 mg·kg⁻¹) dose is more reasonable, particularly if a second dose of succinylcholine is required, or if the child is less than 2 years of age.[11] It is also somewhat dependent on whether the child has intravenous (IV) access in place, which would permit the rapid administration of atropine if needed.

Although the predominance of parasympathetic tone is most evident in the very young child, the transition to the adult sympathetic/parasympathetic balance occurs gradually over time. This fact supports an empirical approach whether or not to administer atropine in conjunction with succinylcholine. Most practitioners consider the use of atropine on a case-by-case basis, taking into consideration of age, heart rate, venous access, and past experience. Some clinicians recommend a dose of 0.02 mg·kg⁻¹ of atropine IV in the pretreatment phase of RSI for *all children* under 10 years of age who will receive succinylcholine.[1]

41.5.4 Should a defasciculating agent be employed if one is using succinylcholine as part of an RSI technique?

Most experts on pediatric airway management feel that the risk of using a defasiculation agent, including the possibility of dosage errors, outweigh the marginal, if any, benefit that such use may confer to intracranial and intragastric pressures. They do not recommend its use in children less than 10 years of age.[1]

41.5.5   Can etomidate be used in children?

The package insert for etomidate in the United States makes no reference to the use of this drug in children below the age of 10 years. Despite this, there is evidence that it is safe.[12,13] There is also evidence documenting that plasma cortisol levels indicate the drug is safe in children, and a wealth of experience with the drug in this population would confirm this.[14]

41.5.6   Are there any special concerns with the use of rocuronium in children?

No. Rocuronium represents the best alternative for RSI in pediatric patients when succinylcholine is contraindicated. Although the duration of action of rocuronium far exceeds succinylcholine (45 minutes vs. 5–10 minutes), studies in children have demonstrated that the time to produce equivalent intubating conditions is similar between the two drugs at the 1.0 mg·kg^{-1} dose for rocuronium.[15–17]

41.6   AIRWAY MANAGEMENT

41.6.1   What are the unique issues with respect to specific forms of airway management in children?

The major issues with respect to specific airway management decisions in children relate to drug dosages and equipment sizes; strategies for error reduction such as the Broselow-Luten Color Coded System®.

41.6.2   How do you optimally position the head and neck for BMV and tracheal intubation in the pediatric population?

The optimal position for alignment of the tracheal, pharyngeal, and oral axes for BMV and orotracheal intubation in children is the *sniffing position*. In the adult, optimal axes alignment is accomplished by flexion of the neck on the chest (usually accomplished by placing a towel or other support beneath the occiput) and extension of the head at the atlanto-occipital joint. In most children, because of the proportionally large occiput, it is unnecessary to place a support under the occiput to flex the neck. Slight extension of the head at the atlanto-occipital joint (not extension which can actually cause obstruction) is all that is necessary (see Figure 41-2).[1] To achieve the sniffing position in small infants, it is sometimes necessary to balance the disproportionate occipital size by placing a support under the shoulders (Figure 41-2A). Older children and adolescents are positioned in a manner similar to that of

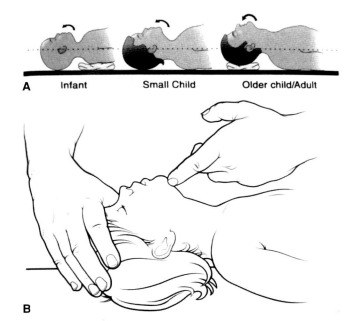

FIGURE 41-2. This figure depicts options to be considered for positioning children of various age groups for BMV and tracheal intubation. (*Reproduced with permission from Luten R, Godwin S: Pediatric airway techniques. In: Manual of Emergency Airway Management. Walls RM, Murphy MF, Luten R, Schneider R, eds. Philadelphia: Lippincott, Williams, Wilkins, 2004:228–235, Figure 20-1*)

adults. At all ages, the best position for intubation can be estimated by positioning the head in such a way that an imaginary horizontal line can be drawn through the external auditory canal just anterior to the shoulders. The anatomical features described are depicted in Figure 41-3.

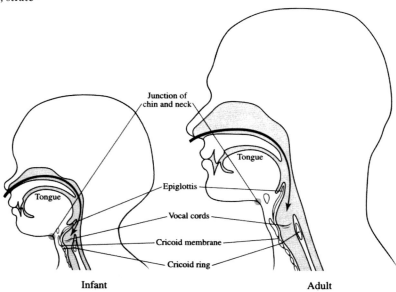

FIGURE 41-3. This figure depicts the differences in the location of the larynx in the neck of adults compared to children. Note that the larynx of the child is positioned higher in the neck rendering it more "anterior" and creating a more acute angle of approach for intubation, particularly if nasal intubation is contemplated. (*Reproduced with permission from Luten R, Kissoon N: Approach to the pediatric airway. In: Manual of Emergency Airway Management. Walls RM, Murphy MF, Luten R, Schneider R, eds. Philadelphia: Lippincott, Williams, Wilkins, 2004:212–227, Figure 19-2.*)

41.6.3 Other than position, what additional factors ought to be considered in optimizing BMV in children?

Due to the relatively large size of the infant's and the small child's tongue it is usually necessary to place an oral airway. Nasal airways in pediatric sizes are also available. Furthermore, it is often necessary to disable the positive-pressure-relief valves ("pop-off valves") that manufacturers provide with pediatric bag ventilation units. While intended to attenuate the risk of pneumothorax and other forms of barotrauma, they may hinder the delivery of sufficient positive pressure to overcome the normal anatomic airway obstruction produced by a large tongue or other forms of upper airway obstruction, such as laryngospasm, often seen in children.

41.6.4 When should you consider a surgical airway for a child?

As in the adult, a surgical airway is indicated in the face of a failed airway in a child. Any practitioner who manages pediatric airways must be familiar with needle and open cricothyrotomy, and their indications. They also must have access to the appropriate equipment. Cricothyrotomy is indicated in the failed-airway situation in patients when the obstruction is at or above the glottic opening. The classic indication is epiglottitis, in which BMV and intubation have failed. Other indications include facial trauma, angioedema, and other conditions that prevent proximal access to the glottic opening. Both forms of cricothyrotomy are rarely helpful in patients who have aspirated a foreign body that cannot be visualized by direct laryngoscope. They are also of questionable value in the patient with croup.

The type of procedure performed varies with the age of the patient. Birth to 5 years of age: needle cricothyrotomy with bag insufflation; 5–10 years of age: needle cricothyrotomy with jet ventilation; greater than 10 years of age: open cricothyrotomy.

41.6.5 What is a needle cricothyrotomy and how is it done?

In this procedure a catheter over needle (ordinarily 12–14 gauge) is passed into the trachea of a young child. No attempt is made to locate the cricothyroid space as it is generally small or nonexistent (see Figure 41-4). Various manufacturers have produced commercial devices and kits (see Chapter 56). A kit can be assembled and kept immediately available by combining a 14-gauge IV catheter over the needle, 3 mm ETT connector, and a 5.0 mL syringe in a clear bag.[1] Alternatively, a 7 mm inner diameter (ID) ETT connector inserted into the barrel of a 3 mL syringe can be prepared.

The procedure is performed by placing the child in the supine position with the head and neck extended over a towel placed at the shoulder to further exaggerate the extension. This forces the trachea anteriorly so that it becomes easily palpable and can be stabilized with two fingers of one hand. The trachea is then cannulated with a catheter over needle setup directed caudad at a 30 degree angle. After aspirating air to confirm tracheal entry, the catheter is held in place and the needle gently withdrawn. A 3 mm

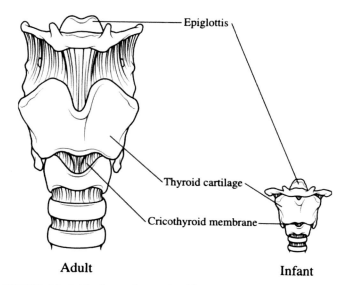

FIGURE 41-4. This figure depicts the differences in the anatomy of the upper airway. Note the very small size of the cricothyroid space in the child compared to the adult. (*Reproduced with permission from Luten R, Godwin SA: Pediatric airway techniques. In: Manual of Emergency Airway Management, Walls RM, Murphy MF, Luten R, Schinder R, eds. Philadelphia: Lippincott, Williams, Wilkins, 2004:228–235, Figure 20-2.*)

ETT connector is then attached to the hub of the catheter and ventilation is started. Bag ventilation is used in a child less than 5 years old, and jet ventilation (pressure reducing valve adjusted down to 20 psi) in the child between 5 and 10 years.[1]

41.6.6 Does a needle cricothyrotomy in a child provide sufficient oxygenation and ventilation to prevent hypoxia and hypercarbia?

Possibly. The evidence surrounding pediatric needle cricothyrotomies is based on an animal study, using a dog model, by Cote et al. Cote was able to demonstrate that dogs approximating the size of a 10 year old child (30 kg) could be oxygenated through a 12 gauge catheter and 3 mm ETT connector with a bag valve unit for a duration of at least 1 hour (the study duration). Rises in $PaCO_2$ levels were noted but were not felt to be significant as children normally tolerate mild degrees of hypercarbia well.[18]

41.6.7 When should one choose an open cricothyrotomy in a child?

Open cricothyrotomy can be performed when the child has a sufficiently large cricothyroid space to permit the insertion of a device large enough to provide adequate gas exchange. This most commonly occurs between the age of 8 and 10 years. Transtracheal jet ventilation continues to be an option, as for adults, though open cricothyrotomy is preferred by most. Cricothyrotomy using commercial kits is common, although it must be emphasized that one of the available kits on the market aimed specifically at the pediatric population (Pedia-Trake® Smiths Medical, Watford, UK) has no evidence to verify effectiveness or safety.

41.6.8   Is it possible to perform an awake tracheal intubation in children?

No. However, not all pediatric patients are *children*. The patient in the 12–18 year old age group suffering from a life-threatening airway disorder is able to appreciate the gravity of the situation and can be remarkably cooperative with efforts to secure a lifesaving airway. However, even in older pediatric patients, the use of IV sedation is crucial (e.g., ketamine or ketofol titration). Ketofol is the combination of ketamine and propofol drawn up in the same syringe. Cooperation is, of course, always a matter of degree; younger children are typically less cooperative than older children.

In large part, the ability to manage a child "awake" depends on one's ability to gain IV access in a relatively painless and non-threatening way. As a general rule, obesity notwithstanding, 5 years of age represents a threshold. Children under the age of 5 are more difficult, technically and psychologically; over the age of 5 both factors become progressively easier to manage. In reality, 'reasoning' with any young child is usually a futile exercise.

41.6.9   What EGDs are used in children?

EGDs for the most part, have been shown to be safe in children. The LMA Classic™, the King LT™ and the Combitube™ for children at least 48 inches (approximately 120 cm) tall have all been used successfully in children.

41.6.10   Is the LMA Classic™ a useful device for airway rescue in children?

The LMA Classic™ (LMA) is a safe and effective airway management device for children undergoing general anesthesia and is considered a rescue option in the event of a failed airway in children and infants. There is evidence that trainees can rapidly insert the device in children.[19,20] Case reports have demonstrated successful use of the LMA in the pediatric patient with a difficult airway, including isolated severe retrognathia, Dandy-Walker Syndrome, and Robin Sequence.[21,22] However, at least one prospective study reports that the use of the LMA is associated with a higher incidence of airway obstruction, higher ventilatory pressures, larger inspiratory leaks, and more complications in smaller children (less than 10 kg) than in the larger children.[23] To address this and similar problems in infants, Nakayama recommended a rotational placement technique in which the mask is inserted in a back-to-front manner and then rotated 180 degrees as it is advanced into the hypopharynx.[24]

As in the adult population, difficult pediatric intubations may be facilitated by the use of the LMA in combination with such devices as the bronchoscope. As in the adult, the LMA is ill-advised in the pediatric patient with intact protective airway reflexes unless the patient is adequately sedated and the airway is topically anesthetized.

41.6.11   How useful is the Combitube™ in children?

As mentioned above, use of the Combitube™ is limited to individuals taller than 48 inches (approximately 120 cm). However, it is an excellent, easily learned rescue airway device.

41.6.12   Can RSI be employed in children, and if so, how?

When emergency intubation is indicated, RSI is the technique of choice in children, as it is in adults.[25] Although there are no randomized prospective studies, large series from multiple centers support the use of RSI in children and document its safety and apparent superiority to other methods.[26,27] The sequence of events and drug selection for RSI are no different in children than it is in adults. Nor is the practice of applying Sellick's maneuver, although the pressure applied is usually reduced to avoid moving the cervical spine, and collapsing the airway.[28]

Studies in children have shown that the cricoid pressure not only prevents passive regurgitation, but also prevents gastric insufflation, even with ventilation pressures greater than 40 cm H_2O.[29–34] This is especially important in infants, in whom gastric distention may lead to decreased diaphragmatic excursion and an increased risk of aspiration.

41.6.13   Is blind nasotracheal intubation an option in children?

With respect to nasal intubation, two anatomic variations combine to *mitigate against blind nasotracheal intubation* in the child less than 8–10 years of age. The first is the presence of frequently enlarged adenoidal tissue in the nasopharynx. This tissue can easily be injured, resulting in copious bleeding, or peeled off into the tip of the advancing tube, resulting in the possibility of blowing the adenoidal tissue into the tracheobronchial tree, potentially leading to total tracheal obstruction. In addition, the angle of the nasal passages and the posterior pharynx leading to the glottic opening is much more acute in the child than the adult so that the success rate for blind nasal intubation in the child is reduced.

A direct visualization technique may be employed in small infants and children for chronic ventilator management in the intensive care unit (ICU) setting. In this technique, a nasotracheal tube is passed to the oropharynx and placed into the airway with Magill forceps under direct oral laryngoscopic vision. However, this technique is not helpful in managing the failed airway.

41.6.14   Why are noncuffed ETTs preferred over cuffed tubes in children? How are they sized?

Uncuffed ETTs are generally recommended in the younger pediatric age groups. Cuffed tubes are generally used if 5.5 mm ID or larger. The issue of cuffed versus uncuffed ETTs has been debated for years.[35] Below the age of 8–10, the subglottic area is the narrowest part of the airway and affords a degree of "seal around the ETT," making cuffed ETTs unnecessary for the most part.[35,36] Deakers and colleagues conducted a prospective but nonrandomized study involving 282 children intubated with either cuffed or uncuffed ETTs in the OR, ED, or ICU.[36] They found no difference in the incidence of postextubation stridor, the need for reintubation, or symptoms of long term upper airway disorders. Khine and colleagues studied children less than 8 years of age intubated with cuffed or uncuffed ETTs and found no difference in postextubation croup or other sequelae. Both authors stress the need to monitor intracuff inflation pressures.

The correct-sized tube for the patient can be determined by a length based system such as the Broselow-Luten System®. Beyond the age of 1 year the formula is [(age in years/4) + 4]. This is a reasonably accurate method of determining the correct tube size, provided one knows the age of the child.

In intubating the trachea of a young child, there is a tendency to insert the tube too far, usually into the right mainstem bronchus. Insertion of the tube to a predetermined distance will avoid this. Various formulas to predict the distance the tube ought to be inserted include (1) the ID of the tube times three and (2) [(age in years/2) + 12]. Perhaps the safest course is to refer to standard tables or charts such as the Broselow-Luten System®.

41.6.15   Can lightwands be used in children?

Several centers have reported the successful use of the lightwand for tracheal intubation in children with normal[37] and difficult airways.[38,39] Careful attention to the details of lightwand preparation and patient selection has been associated with high intubation success rates, particularly among novice users of the pediatric lightwand. Fisher and Tunkel identified several factors contributing to successful intubation by monitoring lightwand (Frachlight™) intubations with a flexible nasopharyngoscope.[37] These included: (1) use of a shoulder roll and slight head extension; (2) proper alignment of airway axes; (3) anterior jaw lift to elevate the epiglottis; and (4) gentle handling of the lightwand to avoid disrupting soft tissue. While these reports show promising results, usage of the lightwand for intubation among pediatric airway practitioners has not been widespread. If seems reasonable to suggest that in a difficult or failed airway situation, experienced practitioners consider employing the device only if time permits, i.e. when gas exchange and oxygen saturations can be maintained.

41.6.16   Do the various airway management algorithms work for children?

The ASA Difficult Airway Algorithm was designed for use in adults, though there is no reason to suspect that it is not applicable to the pediatric population, notwithstanding equipment options and nasotracheal intubation. The same is true of the algorithms discussed in this text. Modifying the existing algorithms to accommodate pediatric specific procedures, such as needle cricothyrotomy, is easily performed. The principles of difficult and failed airway management are no different in children than they are in adults.

41.7   SUMMARY

The principles of airway management in the pediatric and adult populations are the same. Medications used to facilitate intubation, the need for alternative airway management techniques, and many other aspects of airway management are, again, generally the same in the children and adults. There are, however, a few important differences that are most evident in the first two years of life.[5]

Some of the anxiety associated with pediatric airway management can be minimized or eliminated by employing simple clinical aids such as the Broselow-Luten Color Coded System®, coupled with planned strategies (e.g., mnemonics and algorithms) presented in this text.

REFERENCES

1. Luten R, Godwin SA: *Pediatric Airway Techniques*. Philadelphia, PA: Lippincott Williams Wilkins, 2004.
2. Luten R, Wears RL, Broselow J, et al.: Managing the unique size-related issues of pediatric resuscitation: reducing cognitive load with resuscitation aids. *Acad Emerg Med*. 2002;9:840–847.
3. Luten R: Error and time delay in pediatric trauma resuscitation: addressing the problem with color-coded resuscitation aids. *Surg Clin North Am*. 2002;82: 303–314.
4. Luten R, Broselow J: Rainbow care: the Broselow-Luten system. Implications for pediatric patient safety. *Ambul Outreach*. 1999:14–16.
5. Luten R, Kissoon N: *Approach to the Pediatric Airway*. Philadelphia, PA: Lippincott Williams Wilkins, 2004.
6. Benumof JL, Dagg R, Benumof R: Critical hemoglobin desaturation will occur before return to an unparalyzed state following 1 mg·kg^{-1} intravenous succinylcholine. *Anesthesiology*. 1997;87:979–982.
7. Shah AN, Frush K, Luo X, Wears RL: Effect of an intervention standardization system on pediatric dosing and equipment size determination: a crossover trial involving simulated resuscitation events. *Arch Pediatr Adolesc Med*. 2003; 157:229–236.
8. Robinson AL, Jerwood DC, Stokes MA: Routine suxamethonium in children. A regional survey of current usage. *Anaesthesia*. 1996;51:874–878.
9. Weir PS: Anaesthesia for appendicectomy in childhood: a survey of practice in Northern Ireland. *Ulster Med J*. 1997;66:34–37.
10. Shorten GD, Bissonnette B, Hartley E, Nelson W, Carr AS: It is not necessary to administer more than 10 micrograms kg^{-1} of atropine to older children before succinylcholine. *Can J Anaesth*. 1995;42:8–11.
11. Guyton DC, Scharf SM: Should atropine be routine in children? *Can J Anaesth*. 1996;43:754–755.
12. Guldner G, Schultz J, Sexton P, Fortner C, Richmond M: Etomidate for rapid-sequence intubation in young children: hemodynamic effects and adverse events. *Acad Emerg Med*. 2003;10:134–139.
13. Sokolove PE, Price DD, Okada P: The safety of etomidate for emergency rapid sequence intubation of pediatric patients. *Pediatr Emerg Care*. 2000;16:18–21.
14. Donmez A, Kaya H, Haberal A, Kutsal A, Arslan G: The effect of etomidate induction on plasma cortisol levels in children undergoing cardiac surgery. *J Cardiothorac Vasc Anesth*. 1998;12:182–185.
15. Cheng CA, Aun CS, Gin T: Comparison of rocuronium and suxamethonium for rapid tracheal intubation in children. *Paediatr Anaesth*. 2002;12:140–145.
16. Mazurek AJ, Rae B, Hann S, et al.: Rocuronium versus succinylcholine: are they equally effective during rapid-sequence induction of anesthesia? *Anesth Analg*. 1998;87:1259–1262.
17. Woolf RL, Crawford MW, Choo SM: Dose-response of rocuronium bromide in children anesthetized with propofol: a comparison with succinylcholine. *Anesthesiology*. 1997;87:1368–1372.
18. Cote CJ, Eavey RD, Todres ID, Jones DE: Cricothyroid membrane puncture: oxygenation and ventilation in a dog model using an intravenous catheter. *Crit Care Med*. 1988;16:615–619.
19. Lopez-Gil M, Brimacombe J, Alvarez M: Safety and efficacy of the laryngeal mask airway. A prospective survey of 1400 children. *Anaesthesia*. 1996;51: 969–972.
20. Lopez-Gil M, Brimacombe J, Cebrian J, Arranz J: Laryngeal mask airway in pediatric practice: a prospective study of skill acquisition by anesthesia residents. *Anesthesiology*. 1996;84:807–811.
21. Selim M, Mowafi H, Al-Ghamdi A, Adu-Gyamfi Y: Intubation via LMA in pediatric patients with difficult airways. *Can J Anaesth*. 1999;46:891–893.
22. Stocks RM, Egerman R, Thompson JW, Peery M: Airway management of the severely retrognathic child: use of the laryngeal mask airway. *Ear Nose Throat J*. 2002;81:223–226.
23. Park C, Bahk JH, Ahn WS, Do SH, Lee KH: The laryngeal mask airway in infants and children. *Can J Anaesth*. 2001;48:413–417.
24. Nakayama S, Osaka Y, Yamashita M: The rotational technique with a partially inflated laryngeal mask airway improves the ease of insertion in children. *Paediatr Anaesth*. 2002;12:416–419.

25. Gerardi MJ, Sacchetti AD, Cantor RM, et al.: Rapid-sequence intubation of the pediatric patient. Pediatric Emergency Medicine Committee of the American College of Emergency Physicians. *Ann Emerg Med.* 1996;28:55–74.

26. Gnauck K, Lungo JB, Scalzo A, Peter J, Nakanishi A: Emergency intubation of the pediatric medical patient: use of anesthetic agents in the emergency department. *Ann Emerg Med.* 1994;23:1242–1247.

27. Sagarin MJ, Chiang V, Sakles JC, et al.: Rapid sequence intubation for pediatric emergency airway management. *Pediatr Emerg Care.* 2002;18:417–423.

28. Stoddart PA, Brennan L, Hatch DJ, Bingham R: Postal survey of paediatric practice and training among consultant anaesthetists in the UK. *Br J Anaesth.* 1994;73:559–563.

29. Brock-Utne JG: Is cricoid pressure necessary? *Paediatr Anaesth.* 2002;12:1–4.

30. Engelhardt T, Strachan L, Johnston G: Aspiration and regurgitation prophylaxis in paediatric anaesthesia. *Paediatr Anaesth.* 2001;11:147–150.

31. Kluger MT, Willemsen G: Anti-aspiration prophylaxis in New Zealand: a national survey. *Anaesth Intensive Care.* 1998;26:70–77.

32. Moynihan RJ, Brock-Utne JG, Archer JH, Feld LH, Kreitzman TR: The effect of cricoid pressure on preventing gastric insufflation in infants and children. *Anesthesiology.* 1993;78:652–656.

33. Salem MR: Cricoid pressure for preventing gastric insufflation in infants and children. *Anesthesiology.* 1994;80:1182–1183.

34. Salem MR, Wong AY, Fizzotti GF: Efficacy of cricoid pressure in preventing aspiration of gastric contents in paediatric patients. *Br J Anaesth.* 1972;44:401–404.

35. Khine HH, Corddry DH, Kettrick RG, et al.: Comparison of cuffed and uncuffed endotracheal tubes in young children during general anesthesia. *Anesthesiology.* 1997;86:627–631.

36. Deakers TW, Reynolds G, Stretton M, Newth CJ: Cuffed endotracheal tubes in pediatric intensive care. *J Pediatr.* 1994;125:57–62.

37. Fisher QA, Tunkel DE: Lightwand intubation of infants and children. *J Clin Anesth.* 1997;9:275–279.

38. Fox DJ, Matson MD: Management of the difficult pediatric airway in an austere environment using the lightwand. *J Clin Anesth.* 1990;2:123–125.

39. Holzman RS, Nargozian CD, Florence FB: Lightwand intubation in children with abnormal upper airways. *Anesthesiology.* 1988;69:784–787.

SELF-EVALUATION QUESTIONS

41.1. Which of the following statements regarding the pediatric airway is **TRUE**?

    A. Most of the algorithms we use to guide management are not applicable to children.

    B. Extraglottic rescue devices are not useful in children.

    C. Transtracheal jet ventilation is the best rescue technique in infants when intubation has failed.

    D. Most of the medications we use in RSI are unsafe in children.

    E. The most significant difference between the adult and pediatric airway is seen in the birth to 2-year-old.

41.2. Successful BMV in children is related to all of the following **EXCEPT**

    A. positioning the head in the sniffing position is helpful

    B. oral airways are virtually always needed in infants and small children to facilitate successful BMV

    C. pediatric bag units are usually armed with a positive pressure release valve

    D. even though the positive pressure relief valve can be closed, it is unsafe to do so as pneumothorax may result

    E. nasal airways are preferable to oral airways in infants

41.3. All of the following regarding RSI in children is true **EXCEPT**

    A. Sellick's maneuver is unsafe in children and should not be preformed.

    B. The dose of succinylcholine is higher on a per kilogram basis in infants than in adolescents.

    C. Rocuronium may be used instead of succinylcholine in a dose of 1.0 mg·kg^{-1}.

    D. Defasiculation is seldom employed in children, especially the very young.

    E. Denitrogenation may provide a shorter duration of acceptable saturations in the child compared to the adult.

CHAPTER (42)

Airway Management of a Child with Epiglottitis

Christian M. Soder

42.1 CASE PRESENTATION

A previously healthy, 4 year old boy is en route to the children's hospital via helicopter. He was well until 8 hours ago when he began to complain of sore throat and pain on swallowing. His mother brought him to the local emergency department. The emergency physician on duty met a sick, flushed, aphonic, and fearful boy who sat very still and reluctantly swallowed his saliva with visible effort and discomfort. He had no visible respiratory distress or stridor. He was able to lie down on request but preferred to sit. His temperature was 39.6°C, blood pressure 142/75 mm Hg, and heart rate 145 bpm. Examination of the chest revealed no signs of distress but coarse ronchi were audible on auscultation. His throat was not examined and the remainder of the general physical examination was negative. The ER physician suspected epiglottitis and called for an emergency transfer to the nearest children's hospital. While waiting for the helicopter to arrive, was started an IV, administered 0.6 mg·kg^{-1} of dexamethasone, 25 mg·kg^{-1} ceftriaxone, and started oxygen 40% by face mask. During transport, the air medical crew administered racemic epinephrine aerosols every 20 minutes. The transport was uneventful but it was noted that the boy was developing moderate indrawing and was insisting on sitting up. His pulse oximeter read 100% on oxygen 4 L.min^{-1} flow, by non-rebreathing face mask, throughout the flight. He arrived in the ER at the children's hospital after a 25 minute flight. On examination, the physical findings were as before but the boy had now adopted the classic "tripod sniffing position." His breath sounds were muted, he was visibly drooling, and he maintained a posture of fearful rigidity. When made to speak, he had a muffled "hot potato in the mouth" voice. Chest examination revealed mild intercostal and sternal notch indrawing. Without supplementary oxygen, his oxygen saturation by pulse oximeter dropped to 89%. After preliminary assessment, he was transferred immediately to the operating room for airway management. No lateral neck airway radiographs were taken.

42.2 INTRODUCTION

42.2.1 How does epiglottitis in a child usually present and what is its pathophysiology?

Now a rarity, epiglottitis was once the most common pediatric airway emergency faced by anesthesia practitioners and ENT surgeons. Most cases were caused by infection with an invasive strain of hemophilus influenza B (HIB). The widespread introduction of conjugated HIB vaccine in the early 1990s caused a 100-fold reduction in the incidence of epiglottitis in the United States, Western Europe, Canada, and Australia.[1] However, occasional cases of epiglottitis still occur. Some represent failure of vaccination, while others are due to other bacteria known to cause the disease: hemophilus para-influenzae and other hemophilus strains; *streptococcus pneumoniae*, *staphylococcus aureus*; and beta-hemolytic *streptococcus*. Some viruses have been implicated as possible causes and fungi, or unusual bacteria, may cause epiglottitis in the immunocompromised host. Smoke inhalation and flash burns may cause a thermal epiglottitis, with many features of the infectious disease.

The pathophysiology of the non-HIB epiglottitis is similar to that of the classical form of the disease. The infection causes a local cellulitis of the epiglottis, the aryepiglottic folds (false cords), and the mucosa covering the arytenoid cartilages. In the HIB form of

389

the disease, positive blood cultures are common, while most non-HIB cases have negative blood cultures. Culture of direct swabs of the epiglottis may be positive for the responsible pathogen.

The natural history of the disease is progressive glottic inlet swelling that can progress to complete upper-airway obstruction causing death. Classic epiglottitis is most common between the ages of 2 and 5 years but cases have been reported at all ages.

Some believe that the first US president, George Washington, died of the disease at the age of 67.

Current treatment for all forms of bacterial epiglottitis consists of emergency placement of an artificial airway and a 10 day course of IV antibiotics. More recently, some centers have reported successful conservative ICU management without airway instrumentation, using humidified oxygen, inhaled racemic epinephrine, and IV steroids.[2] These measures, especially when started early, may reduce the rate of progression and prevent complete airway occlusion.

42.2.2   What is the differential diagnosis?

While epiglottitis is now rare, croup (or laryngotracheobronchitis) is still the most common cause of upper airway obstruction in preschool children. It is usually caused by a viral infection of the upper airway. Since children have small caliber tracheas, and because the cricoid ring is rigid, minor degrees of subglottic mucosal swelling produce major degrees of airway obstruction.

Despite the often dramatic symptoms, croup is normally a self-limited illness that rarely progresses to complete airway obstruction. It is almost always treated conservatively with "masterful inactivity." More severe cases are treated in hospital with humidified oxygen, steroids, and inhaled vasoconstrictors such as phenylephrine, or racemic epinephrine. Very rarely, croup may progress to severe airway obstruction and require emergency airway management.

Croup is easily differentiated from epiglottitis in most cases, but correct diagnosis is extremely important because the two illnesses run profoundly different courses. Children with croup tend to be younger, afebrile, and noisy—they have the classic "barking" cough, hoarse stridor, and vocal agitation of the unhappy toddler. Respiratory effort is often pronounced and dysphagia is not present. Occasionally, the inflammation of croup may extend to the glottic structures and present with some clinical features of epiglottitis.

Other cases suspected to be epiglottitis are actually peritonsillar and retropharyngeal abscesses. These conditions usually present with gradual onset of fever, pain, and dysphagia. Airway obstruction is a late finding in advanced severe cases. Clinical differentiation of these conditions from croup and epiglottitis is usually based on the slow rate of progression, the absence of respiratory distress, and the clinical or radiological detection of a mass.

42.3   PATIENT EVALUATION

42.3.1   How do you assess the patient's airway?

The case of the 4 year old boy presented above is a classic presentation for epiglottitis. The diagnosis is made on history and physical observation from a safe, nonthreatening distance. The patient should not be touched, or disturbed, and imaging studies should not be performed. Agitation of the patient may incite crying which is associated with increased inspiratory airflow velocity that in turn increases turbulent air flow and resistance leading to "dynamic" airway obstruction that may be fatal. Blood cultures and routine blood work can be drawn after the airway is secure. He should be moved to the operating room without delay.

The definitive diagnosis of epiglottitis is usually made in the operating room during laryngoscopy for intubation. In the current era, many patients do not present with classic features. If airway obstruction is not severe, physical examination and diagnostic imaging may be appropriate with the caveat that, as long as epiglottitis remains on the differential diagnosis, direct or optical examinations of the throat should be avoided. While some have advocated flexible endoscopy for adult patients suspected of having epiglottitis, this practice is still considered dangerous in children. The fear is that the procedure may trigger life-threatening dynamic airflow obstruction or laryngospasm.

If it is deemed appropriate to undertake investigation before intervention, the first investigation should be a lateral airway radiograph, often performed with the parent or guardian holding the child. The appearance of the classic "thumb sign," caused by the obliteration of the vallecula by the swollen epiglottis, confirms the diagnosis of epiglottitis. In contrast, if the epiglottis has its normal "pencil like" appearance and the rest of the radiographic appearance is normal, the patient probably has croup. Radiology texts[3] describe the subglottic region in croup as "blurred" on lateral view, with a "church steeple appearance" on anterior view, but these are subtle findings that may be hard to differentiate. If a peritonsillar or retropharyngeal mass is detected on clinical examination, or suspected on a plain neck radiograph, a CT scan is usually recommended to map out the location, size, and density of the lesion.[4]

42.3.2   Do you have any other medical concerns for this patient? Should you do any laboratory investigations?

Patients with epiglottitis are usually septic, toxic, dehydrated, and very afraid (high sympathetic state). In advanced states, they may be hypercarbic, hypoxemic, hypocalcemic, and hyperkalemic. Their airways are reactive, inflamed, overflowing with secretions, and obstructed. Induction of inhalational anesthesia may be complicated by complete airway obstruction, laryngospasm, hypotension, cardiac arrhythmias, and cardiac arrest.

42.4   AIRWAY MANAGEMENT

42.4.1   What are the options in airway management for this patient?

Prior to the 1980s, recommended approaches to the airway were tracheal intubations while awake, perhaps with rigid bronchoscopy, followed by general anesthesia.

In the 1980s, nasotracheal intubation under inhalational halothane anesthesia became the treatment of choice. More recently, some authors have described the use of Sevoflurane[5] or IV induction and rapid sequence intubation. The following is the airway management plan currently used by most pediatric centers:

Plan A—inhalation induction and endotracheal intubation,

Plan B—failed intubation, proceed to rigid bronchoscopy,

Plan C—failed airway, proceed to surgical airway.

Epiglottitis and croup in children represent departures from the normal algorithms for difficult airway management. There is little or no evidence or experience to support extraglottic devices, alternate intubation devices, or fiberoptic intubation, in the management of epiglottitis and croup.

Bag-mask-ventilation (BMV) and direct laryngoscopy (DL), with rigid bronchoscopy and otolaryngologist as backup, are the state of the art. Based on the skill and experience of the anesthesia practitioner and otolaryngologist, the optically enhanced telescopic rigid bronchoscope may indeed succeed when DL intubation fails. The enhancement of visualization coupled with the ability to directly advance a rigid tube through the swollen structures may help explain the long and successful history of rigid bronchoscopy in epiglottitis.

42.4.2 Discuss the preparations necessary in managing the airway of this patient?

The operating room team should include two experienced health care providers: at minimum an anesthesia practitioner and otolaryngologist (or other qualified rigid bronchoscopist). Necessary airway equipment includes a functional suction device; different size face masks; two laryngoscope handles with straight and curved blades of varying length and width; and 4, 4.5, and 5 mm ID tracheal tubes, preloaded with well-lubricated intubating stylets; two appropriate sized, lubricated, tested rigid telescope bronchoscopes connected to light source and suction; a tracheotomy tray; and a #1 Melker uncuffed cricothyrotomy set for percutaneous tracheotomy.

Succinylcholine 20 mg (for laryngospasm), atropine 0.4 mg (to treat bradycardia), and epinephrine 100 μg (1 mL of 1/10,000 solution) to respond to hypoxemia induced myocardial depression are drawn up. Other standard resuscitation drugs and equipment are at hand.

42.4.3 How do you perform tracheal intubation under inhalational anesthesia?

The child is brought into the operating room. Parental attendance is often forgone in this scenario, to minimize distraction, unless it is clear that the parents will help to calm the child (and the anesthesia practitioner!) during induction. If not already present, an IV is inserted immediately after induction of anesthesia. Atropine 0.1 mg IV may be administered to reduce secretions and mitigate vagal responses (bradycardia). Pulse oximeter, blood pressure cuff, and ECG monitors are applied.

Inhalation inductions in the presence of epiglottitis require patience, and excellent BMV technique. It is important to remember that epiglottitis produces obstruction of the glottic inlet but leaves oral, pharyngeal, glottic, and subglottic anatomy unchanged.

There is an ever-present risk of acute life-threatening events during induction. Laryngospasm, complete glottic inlet occlusion, hypoxic seizures, and obstructive pulmonary edema have all been described. Accumulated secretions above and below the vocal cords are usually present, may contribute to airway obstruction, and can trigger laryngospasm.

Induction of anesthesia starts with incremental levels of Halothane (1–4%) or Sevoflurane (5–8%) blended with 100% oxygen at 6 L·min^{-1} flow. BMV with applied mask continuous positive airway pressure (CPAP) 5–10 cm H_2O is applied to deal with increased airway obstruction during the excitement phase. While only marginally effective at overcoming anatomic glottic inlet obstruction, mask CPAP is useful in treating pharyngeal obstruction and laryngospasm. The maneuver plays a vital role in managing inhalational induction of anesthesia. There is an ever-present risk of, and need to avoid, gastric distension.

Induction is usually prolonged by the reduced alveolar ventilation and high cardiac output commonly present in epiglottitis. It is important to be patient and to persist until there is evidence of deep anesthesia, as indicated by falling heart rate and blood pressure. When the patient is judged to be deeply anesthetized, the laryngoscope blade is gently introduced. It is immediately withdrawn if the patient responds by moving, swallowing, coughing, or closing the vocal cords. In this case, anesthesia must be deepened by continuing with mask inhalation.

When laryngoscopy is fully tolerated, the blade is advanced along the lateral tongue margin until the glottic structures are identified. DL itself is not usually difficult, but visual recognition of structures at the glottic opening can be extremely difficult. Early in the course of the illness, glottic inlet structures are red and swollen, but recognizable, and the vocal cords (or at least the false cords) can be seen during DL. Such patients are easily intubated with a normal-sized endotracheal tube for age. With progression of the inflammation, the swollen tissues begin to obscure normal anatomy. The epiglottis, aryepiglottic folds, and the loose areolar tissue overlying the arytenoid cartilages become reddened and swollen. Visually, these structures merge to form the famous "red cherry" at the base of the tongue. *It is important to realize that the glottic inlet lies roughly at the center of the "cherry," not posterior to it.* In the most severe cases, all recognizable structures are effaced and the laryngoscopic appearance is that of a frightening, featureless, red mass.

Spontaneous breathing, or a stroke of chest compression, may help in identifying the glottic opening by creating bubbles of air streaming through saliva and secretions. In cases with significant distortion of normal anatomy, it is usually recommended that a tube one-half size smaller than usual (in this case a 4.5 mm ID tube), fortified by an intubating stylet, be inserted through the tiny orifice. If the appearance is that of a "cherry like" structure, the endotracheal tube is gently advanced, with the bevel aligned to the axis of the glottic opening (i.e., the tube is "sideways") toward the center of the "cherry." Often a dimple is noticed at the center of the cherry; this marks the opening, and air may be seen bubbling through it. Experienced pediatric anesthesia practitioners have often pointed out to their colleagues that the appearance of the glottis in epiglottitis is similar to that of the cervix, as visualized during gynecologic speculum exams—the os cervix represents the glottic aperture. Intubation of the trachea with epiglottitis is visually analogous to the insertion of an intrauterine device. The good news about epiglottitis intubation is that while the glottic inlet structures may be massively swollen, they are soft, not firm. Therefore, once the glottic aperture is identified, it should not be difficult to pass the endotracheal tube through the larynx.

If the diagnosis in this case unexpectedly turns out to be severe atypical croup, the glottic inlet will appear normal and airway obstruction will be isolated to the subglottic area. In this case, laryngeal visualization will be easy, but passing the endotracheal tube will be difficult. A significantly smaller than normal endotracheal tube, fortified by a straight intubating stylet, or a rigid bronchoscope, is usually required to pass through the obstruction.

In epiglottitis, repeat laryngoscopy following a failed attempt is acceptable, if the BMV airway and oxygen saturation can be restored and maintained between attempts. Second attempt laryngoscopy may include blade change, position change, and personnel change. Although it is not reported in the literature, it seems logical that external laryngeal manipulation might be helpful. There is minimal experience with the use of the intubating introducer ("bougie") or alternate intubation devices in this condition.[6] Since the problem is one of anatomic obliteration of normal structures, it is improbable that indirect intubation techniques will prove to be useful.

42.4.4   If laryngoscopic intubation is not possible, what would you do next?

If intubation fails after two or three attempts with the laryngoscope, the rigid bronchoscope should be employed. It can be inserted directly, or with the assistance of a laryngoscope. Bronchoscopy is complicated by the same factors that make intubation difficult, but the optically enhanced visualization, and rigid construction of the bronchoscope, may lead to success where laryngoscopy failed. If the bronchoscope is successfully inserted, the patient should be suctioned and ventilated through the scope and anesthesia should be deepened. A long-acting muscle relaxant may be given at this stage to facilitate intubation. An endotracheal tube can then be inserted directly, or an appropriately sized interballing introducer can be passed through the bronchoscope. The bronchoscope can then be removed, a laryngoscope positioned, and or introducer-assisted intubation completed. The process of tube change is not as intimidating as it might seem: once the airway has been opened by the passage of a bronchoscope, the glottis usually holds its shape and remains patent, and visible, for several minutes after removal of the bronchoscope. This temporary stenting effect makes reinsertion significantly less difficult than primary intubation.

42.4.5   At what stage would you consider tracheotomy appropriate for this patient?

If airway patency, oxygenation, or ventilation cannot be maintained (or recovered) by BMV at any time, or if intubation is unsuccessful after three attempts, the failed airway plan is activated. Depending on the skill and experience of the anesthesia practitioners and surgeons present, either a surgical tracheotomy is performed, or a #1 Melker percutaneous tracheotomy tube is inserted using Seldinger technique. The surgical airway is a useful option of last resort in epiglottitis, because subglottic anatomy is normal. The usual pediatric limitation applies: the cricothyroid membrane is too small to

be useful. A transtracheal approach is necessary for either surgical or percutaneous tracheotomy tube insertion.[7]

In contrast, tracheotomy is less likely to be successful in croup, because the obstruction occurs at the level of the proximal trachea. Unless the trachea is entered below the level of maximum swelling, it may be no easier to insert a tracheotomy tube than an endotracheal tube!

42.4.6   How do you manage the airway of this patient if he has a strong family history of malignant hyperthermia?

In early cases with minimal evidence of airway obstruction, denitrogenation followed by a rapid sequence induction using sodium pentothal, propofol, or midazolam, in combination with mivacurium or rocuronium, is recommended. In cases of severe airway obstruction, awake laryngoscopy, possibly facilitated by topical anesthesia, and/or anxiolytic doses of midazolam, should be attempted. If the laryngeal inlet is found to have recognizable anatomy, the awake attempt can be aborted and a rapid sequence induction performed. If the laryngeal inlet remains obscured, awake intubation, or awake rigid bronchoscopy, is recommended. Postintubation sedation with nontriggering agents should proceed, as described in the next section.

42.5   OTHER CONSIDERATIONS

42.5.1   Discuss the appropriate postintubation management

Endotracheal placement must be confirmed initially by CO_2 detection. Since inadvertent endobronchial intubation of children is common (especially under stressful circumstances), radiographic confirmation is required to confirm tube tip location. The endotracheal tube must be well secured using a commercial fixation device, or by highly adherent adhesive tape fixed to the skin of the upper lip. Tincture of benzoin (Friar's Balsam) may be used to dry and degrease the skin. The patient should be sedated and restrained in the ICU to minimize the risk of accidental extubation. Fortunately, accidental extubation is not necessarily catastrophic. Because the glottis holds its shape for some time after removal of the ETT, reintubation is usually accomplished far more easily than the original intubation. Experience has shown that extubation can be safely performed upon defervescence, as early as 6 hours after initiation of antibiotics. The average duration of intubation is approximately 24 hours.[8] Twelve hours after extubation, once it is clear that the airway will remain free from obstruction, the child may be transferred from the ICU to a regular ward (and later, home) to complete his course of antibiotics.

42.5.2   Is it necessary to have tracheal intubation for all epiglottitis?

"Conservative" management of epiglottitis has been described in adult and pediatric patients with some success, especially in early cases with mild airway obstruction. Patients are admitted to intensive care, monitored closely, and treated with IV antibiotics, dexamethasone, and inhaled catecholamines, such as racemic epinephrine or phenylephrine. This approach is still considered experimental, especially in children, and it is essential that the personnel and equipment necessary for tracheal intubation be immediately available in case of failure.

42.5.3 If orotracheal intubation is successful during laryngoscopy, is it necessary to change it to a nasal route?

The use of orotracheal versus nasotracheal tubes reflects local practice: there is no compelling evidence to favor one technique over the other. Nasotracheal intubation is considered by some to carry a lower risk of accidental extubation, but orotracheal intubation is less likely to be complicated by otitis media, or nasopharyngeal hemorrhage. The recognition that duration of intubation in epiglottitis need not be prolonged, and the observation that reintubation after accidental extubation is usually not difficult has made orotracheal intubation combined with deep sedation a popular approach in many centers.

42.6 SUMMARY

The successful treatment of epiglottitis using tracheal intubation under general anesthesia became a worldwide standard of care in the 1980s and mortality from this condition fell to near zero. The massive reduction in the incidence of this disease by widespread vaccination against HIB, while obviously a desirable outcome, has raised new concerns. Postvaccine era cases are more likely to be atypical in presentation, more delayed in recognition, and less likely to be well managed—as clinicians experienced in the diagnosis and treatment of the condition become less prevalent. As a result, it is possible that mortality in this now rare but still life-threatening condition will again rise. It is important that airway instruction continues to include epiglottitis as an area of focus.

REFERENCES

1. McEwan J, Giridharan W, Clarke R, Shears P: Paediatric acute epiglottitis: not a disappearing entity. *Int J Pediatr Otorhinolaryngology.* 2003;67:317–321.
2. Damm M, Eckel HE, Jungehulsing M, Roth B: Airway endoscopy in the interdisciplinary management of acute epiglottitis. *Int J Pediatr Otorhinolaryngol.* 1996;38:41–51.
3. Santer DM, D'Alessandro P: Acute Epiglottitis. Virtual Pediatric Hospital™. Available at//www.virtualpediatrichospital.org/providers/ElectricAirway/Text/Epiglottitis.shtml.
4. Verghese ST, Hannallah RS: Pediatric otolaryngologic emergencies. *Anesthesiol Clin North America* 2001;19:237–256.
5. Spalding MB, Ala-Kokko TI: The use of inhaled sevoflurane for endotracheal intubation in epiglottitis. *Anesthesiology.* 1998;89:1025–1029.
6. Rucklidge MW, Patel A: Failure of the single-use bougie in acute epiglottitis. *Anaesthesia.* 2004;59:925–926.
7. Navsa N, Tossel G, Boon JM: Dimensions of the neonatal cricothyroid membrane—how feasible is a surgical crycothyroidotomy? *Pediatr Anesth.* 2005;15:402–406.
8. Gerber AC, Pfenninger J: Acute epiglottitis: management by short duration of intubation and hospitalisation. *Intensive Care Med.* 1986;12:407–411.

SELF-EVALUATION QUESTIONS

42.1. Croup is distinguished from epiglottitis by all of the following **EXCEPT**

    A. age of onset

    B. rapidity of onset

    C. presence of a fever

    D. cough

    E. dysphagia

42.2. Management of significantly symptomatic pediatric epiglottitis may include all of the following **EXCEPT**

    A. airway inspection by laryngoscopy or endoscopy

    B. inhalational induction of anesthesia

    C. expedient transfer to the operating room for airway securement

    D. rigid bronchoscopy

    E. surgical airway

42.3. Intubation sequences for pediatric epiglottitis may include all of the following **EXCEPT**

    A. bag-mask-ventilation

    B. CPAP

    C. atropine

    D. extraglottic airway adjuvants

    E. tracheal tube ½ size smaller than normal, with intubating stylet

CHAPTER (43)

Management of a 12-Year-Old Child with a Foreign Body in the Bronchus

Liane B. Johnson

43.1 CASE PRESENTATION

An 80 lb (40 kg), 12 year old boy with a history of cervical spine fusion due to syringomyelia presents following the accidental inhalation of a pushpin during sneezing. There is no associated thoracic scoliosis or any neuromuscular deficits. He is otherwise healthy, takes no medications, and has no known drug allergies.

43.2 PATIENT ASSESSMENT

43.2.1 What are the initial clinical steps in patient management?

Initial management when presented with a definitive history of aspiration of a foreign body begins with the ABCs. An awake, alert patient without overt airway distress will permit a more complete workup, while a severely distressed patient with stridor and desaturation will mandate acute stabilization prior to transfer to the operating room for surgical removal. All patients should have pulse oximetry. Supplemental oxygen may be provided to maximize oxygenation.

Respiratory distress or the presence of stridor implies compromise of the airway and reduced airflow. Heliox 70/30 (70% helium/30% oxygen) will improve oxygenation by maximizing laminar airflow and reducing airflow resistance, decreasing the work of breathing, and reducing the associated anxiety and has been used as a temporizing measure in the setting of foreign body aspiration in young children.[1] Intravenous dexamethasone at a dose of 0.5 mg·kg^{-1} may be beneficial in reducing the mucosal edema which partly contributes to the airway obstruction.[2] Racemic epinephrine aerosols

may be an additional means of reducing airway edema. The use of bronchodilators is considered to be relatively contraindicated until the foreign body is removed from the airway, as its use may predispose to dislodgement and migration of the foreign body as airway caliber is increased. Bronchodilators, however, are an important adjunct to pulmonary toilet following foreign body removal.[3]

43.2.2 What are the appropriate investigations for a foreign body in the trachea?

Radiologic studies are used as an adjunct to the physical examination in diagnosing suspected aerodigestive foreign bodies. Anteroposterior and lateral chest radiographs with inspiratory and expiratory views are helpful tools if the foreign body is opaque, or if there is evidence of bronchial obstruction, though the false negative rate ranges between 24–33% when compared to bronchoscopic findings. Fluoroscopy is of little added benefit when a timely workup is of essence, especially if a radiograph has already confirmed the presence of a foreign body. Ultimately, the gold standard for diagnosing an aspirated foreign body is rigid bronchoscopy under general anesthesia.[2,4]

43.2.3 Do different types of foreign bodies (organics, metals, plastics) influence patient management and outcomes?

Organic matter (nuts, corn, seeds, etc.) and plastics are radiolucent items that are not commonly visualized on x-ray. Organics must be removed as soon as possible as the diameter of the object will increase over time due to the absorption of secretions and moisture. This may convert a stable, partial obstruction to an acute, complete obstruction, or obliterate the available space around the foreign body complicating removal with forceps. Furthermore, over time the organic matter will become more friable, potentially breaking into multiple pieces, making complete removal very difficult. This enhances the risk of obstruction and infection in the distal, smaller generation bronchi.

43.2.4 Discuss the pathophysiology of a foreign body

Determining the site of airway obstruction, the size and shape of the aspirated object, and the timeline since obstruction are crucial to patient outcomes and guide the plan for removal. Airway obstruction following foreign body aspiration may be total or partial, depending on all of the above factors. The incidence of foreign body aspiration is not dependent on socioeconomic status or geographic location. However, there is a relationship of the type of aspirated object, particularly if it is a foodstuff that is dependent on the age of the patient and the country in which the patient resides. Toddlers are at highest risk of foreign body aspiration as they explore their environment by placing encountered objects in their mouths, are more likely to talk, laugh, and run while eating, and have relatively immature laryngeal protective reflexes.[4]

A foreign body lodged in the lower airway may manifest with different pulmonary findings depending on the type of impaction. Four lower airway obstructive mechanisms have been described: check valve, ball valve, bypass valve, and stop valve.[5] Check valve implies air can be inhaled but not exhaled, creating alveolar air trapping and flattening of the ipsilateral diaphragm. This is in contrast to a ball valve which allows expiration but not inspiration of air, creating segmental bronchopulmonary collapse. A bypass valve obstruction allows partial airflow on both inspiration and expiration around the foreign body and may not exhibit specific clinical findings. A stop valve creates complete obstruction to airflow causing airway collapse and consolidation distal to the obstruction.[5]

The ability to correctly ascertain the type of obstruction and object aspirated may help determine the stability of the patient's airway and the requisite acuity of intervention. This key point is of utmost importance when the patient is not distressed, possibly lulling the physician into a false sense of (airway) security.

43.3 AIRWAY CONSIDERATIONS

43.3.1 What are the usual clinical presentations of a foreign body in the airway with or without airway obstruction and air trapping? What are the specific airway concerns in this patient?

Presenting symptoms following foreign body aspiration are related to the type of object aspirated, location of the object within the airway, and the overall duration of the obstructive event. Airway obstruction may be complete or partial. Complete obstruction of the trachea or large airway is an emergency situation usually associated with hypoxia, cardiovascular compromise, and subsequent collapse. In contrast, partial obstruction can often present with more subtle symptoms such as coughing, focal or diffuse wheezing, and decreased air entry on the affected side.[3,6] These may progress over time to drooling, dyspnea, stridor, and respiratory distress.

It is critical to appreciate that to produce symptoms a foreign body must encroach on 75% of the airway lumen to create turbulent air flow. This generally necessitates immediate intervention to avoid a disastrous outcome.[6]

In this patient, the aspirated foreign body may be found anywhere in the upper airway, down to the level of the carina and occasionally in the mainstem bronchi. Sharp objects, like pins, will generally be found with the sharp end embedded in the mucosa proximally, while the larger, blunt end is distal. It is unlikely that a pushpin, in and of itself, would cause obstruction of the larger airways. However, the associated mucosal edema, and/or displacement into the smaller generation bronchi, may create airway obstruction.

Our patient is able to provide an accurate history of aspiration and subsequent, persistent cough. His airway is currently stable. However, his previous cervical fusion may provide a challenge for both the anesthesia practitioner and endoscopist. The following sections will further delve into anesthetic management and the surgical options presented by this challenging scenario. A key principle in managing the airways of children is to ensure communication between the anesthesia practitioner and the surgeon prior to the patient's arrival in the operating suite. It is essential that the surgical setup be ready prior to the induction of anesthesia, that a backup plan has been discussed and agreed upon, and that the equipment for performing a surgical airway is available.

43.4 ANESTHESIA CONSIDERATIONS

43.4.1 What are the anesthetic options if the patient is uncooperative? How would you approach the induction of this patient?

Children with airway obstruction pose a challenge to the anesthesia practitioner. Physiologically, children have a limited functional residual capacity (FRC), reduced respiratory reserve, increased shunting, and a propensity for airway closure. In the setting of a relative increased in oxygen consumption and suboptimal ventilation, the anesthesia practitioner is faced with a patient who will likely develop hypoxemia rapidly. An inhalation induction may be prolonged if there is reduced alveolar ventilation due to airway obstruction.

Anesthetic management in the setting of foreign body aspiration is based on providing a safe anesthetic for the patient, while maintaining control of the airway and preventing the undesirable physiologic responses associated with airway manipulation. Inhalational agents are an optimal technique to maintain control of the airway.[6] Halothane and sevoflurane provide the most rapid and uneventful induction in this scenario. Sevoflurane may be the preferred inhalational agent because it allows for a smooth and rapid induction of general anesthesia. In addition, it has antitussive properties and far greater cardiorespiratory stability than halothane.[7] The other fluorinated inhalational agents, such as isoflurane, enflurane, and desflurane, are more likely to produce airway irritation on induction and are commonly avoided. However, they may be used following induction to maintain a deep plane of anesthesia.[6]

Anticholinergics (atropine and glycopyrrolate) block vagally mediated airway responses such as excessive production of airway secretions, bradycardia, and bronchoconstriction.[6] Topical lidocaine works synergistically with the inhalational agent decreasing the physiologic response to laryngoscopy and bronchoscopy. Intravenous opioids, such as $1 \ \mu g \cdot kg^{-1}$ of fentanyl, are also helpful in suppressing airway reflexes and may be used as an adjunct to the anesthetic, provided the airway is already secured, as there may be associated respiratory depression.[6] Total intravenous anesthesia with propofol infusion is also a feasible option, provided that spontaneous respiration is maintained. Similarly, small doses of short-acting muscle relaxants provide short-term neuromuscular blockade, inhibit coughing, facilitate oxygenation, and minimize atelectasis.[8] The use of muscle relaxants, once again, mandates prior stabilization and control of the airway.[8,9]

It is generally felt that positive pressure ventilation (PPV) is to be avoided as this may lead to dislodgement and distal displacement of the foreign body.[6,8] Nitrous oxide should also be avoided because it decreases the percentage of delivered oxygen, encourages atelectasis, and expands cavities containing trapped air. Indeed, augmentation of air that is trapped may be of sufficient magnitude to severely compromise pulmonary compliance and generate a pneumothorax.[6] Though some might consider awake-intubation to be an option, in this patient it is likely to be stormy with the potential to dislodge the pushpin and create a more hazardous situation.

When faced with an uncooperative patient, an intramuscular agent, such as ketamine, may provide a window of opportunity for an inhalation induction, without significant depression of respiratory drive.

Although the patient is considered at high risk for aspiration, the urgency of the airway status takes precedence. If immediate intervention is not indicated, some advocate a waiting period for the patient with a full stomach, while others believe that the stress associated with foreign body aspiration is likely to inhibit gastric emptying and advise against waiting. Likewise, some advocate a rapid sequence induction to protect the airway, though most believe that a slow inhalation induction with spontaneous ventilation is associated with minimal risk of aspiration and maximizes control. If, however, bag-mask-ventilation is required, the risks of aspiration increase mandating early control of the airway.[6–9]

In this case, the patient provides an interesting twist, as the complexity of the challenge is enhanced by limited neck extension. This case also reflects the importance of communication among the team of care givers and highlights the need for an alternate plan should the initial approach fail. The inability to predict whether the airway will be easily accessed provides a strong argument for a slow, spontaneous ventilation induction, with topicalization of the airway using lidocaine. Should the airway not be visualized on laryngoscopy, or with a rigid bronchoscope, other modalities may be attempted (lightwand, laryngeal mask airway, etc.) provided one has ascertained that blind techniques will not lead to dislodgement or impaction of the foreign body. The specifics of airway management for our patient scenario will be discussed in-depth in the next section.

43.5 AIRWAY MANAGEMENT

43.5.1 How do you perform rigid bronchoscopy for foreign body removal?

A complete airway assessment is fundamental to planning the approach to remove the foreign body and preparing for difficulties that might be encountered. Our patient has had a cervical fusion potentially limiting neck extension and making laryngoscopy and rigid bronchoscopy challenging, if not impossible. The safest means of removing a sharp foreign body requires that under direct vision it be grasped, released from its hold on the mucosa by advancing it more distally, and then sheathing it within the bronchoscope for removal when the bronchoscope is withdrawn. Removal of large tracheal foreign bodies that cannot be ensheathed within the bronchoscope are likely to become impacted at the level of the glottis during removal, potentially leading to complete airway obstruction. In situations where obstruction is, or becomes, complete, the object may need to be rapidly pushed distally, usually into the right mainstem bronchus.

It is important to note that the entire airway, trachea and first and second generation bronchi, must be visualized following removal of the foreign body to ensure the absence of a second airway foreign body, which may be present in up to 5% of foreign body aspirations.

43.5.2 How do you provide oxygenation during rigid bronchoscopy?

Provided that an appropriately sized bronchoscope is used, rigid bronchoscopy allows for oxygenation through side ports. Newer fiberoptic technology allows visualization of the airway on a monitor. The advent of fiberoptic foreign body forceps allows spontaneous ventilation through the bronchoscope, with minimal loss of anesthetic gases into the operating suite and better maintenance of the depth of anesthesia. Depending on the type and shape of the object to be retrieved, a selection of fiberoptic foreign body forceps is available.

43.5.3 What are the potential complications and limitations of rigid bronchoscopy?

Complications of rigid bronchoscopy include dental injury, cervical spine injury (due to aggressive patient positioning or underlying patient disorder) glottic or arytenoid injury, and tracheal mucosal irritation or tear occasionally leading to the formation of a tracheoesophageal fistula. Hemodynamic instability, hypercapnia, or hypoxemia may also occur in association with hypoventilation, dislodgement of the foreign body, or the use of an inappropriately large bronchoscope limiting insufflation and efflux of gases. Rigid bronchoscopes in the tracheobronchial tree cannot access secondary bronchi and smaller airways.

43.5.4   What is the role of flexible fiberoptic bronchoscopy in the management of foreign bodies in the airway?

The use of flexible fiberoptic bronchoscopy (FFB) as a primary tool for foreign body removal is not a widely practiced. Some advocate its use to evaluate the airway prior to foreign body removal by rigid bronchoscopy to allow for localization and planning.[10] It may also be used following retrieval to ensure that the foreign body has been removed in its entirety and no other foreign bodies exist. A group in Mexico is currently using FFB in approximately 40% of their pediatric airway foreign body cases, with a 93% success rate.[11]

The risks of using FFB for foreign body removal are multifaceted. The airway must be secured, usually with an endotracheal tube, prior to endoscopy, as there are no ventilation ports. There is a limited selection of grasping forceps that may be passed through the FFB. The foreign body cannot be ensheathed within the FFB to protect the airway during its removal, potentially increasing the risk of injury to the airway if the object is sharp. It also increases the risk of complete airway obstruction, if the object is dropped as it is retracted proximally.

43.5.5   What is the incidence of an open surgical procedure to remove foreign bodies from the airway?

Open surgical procedures are seldom required to remove foreign bodies from the airway. Such an approach is generally required in a setting where rigid bronchoscopy has failed or in the following situations: (1) if the foreign body is found in a small, inaccessible peripheral bronchus; (2) if the foreign body is sharp, pointed, and embedded in the tracheal or bronchial wall; (3) if it has been present for a prolonged period of time, often for several years; and (4) if there is significant difficulty in maintaining control of the airway following rigid bronchoscope insertion and manipulation. Interestingly, aspirated plastic pen caps more often require open surgical procedures, due to a high rate of bronchoscopic extraction failure secondary to their size, shape, and position in the airway.[12,13]

43.5.6   How do you remove the foreign body from this patient?

Because of the limitation of cervical spine movement and the anticipated difficulty in performing a rigid bronchoscopy in this patient, once the airway was controlled, a temporary tracheotomy was performed through which a rigid bronchoscope was passed to retrieve the pushpin.

In cases such as this, the tracheotomy may be closed primarily provided that there is minimal airway edema compromising the lumen recognizing that there is a small risk of air leak into the neck with primary closure. If the patient is expected to cough or strain, primary closure may not be the best option.

If an object still cannot be removed, an open thoracotomy is required. In such cases, a bronchotomy or partial lung

parenchymal resection may be necessary to remove the object. The latter is more commonly seen when the diagnosis of foreign body aspiration is delayed and secondary complications have occurred.[3]

43.6   POSTOPERATIVE MANAGEMENT

43.6.1   Is there a role for steroids, racemic epinephrine, bronchodilators, and antibiotics in the postoperative care of this patient?

The use of steroids in the postoperative period may be beneficial if mucosal edema and granulation tissue were present in the vicinity of the airway foreign body. Racemic epinephrine is unlikely to be needed unless faced with postoperative stridor following traumatic foreign body removal. Bronchodilators are used infrequently, but may be helpful in the presence of persistent segmental atelectasis, more commonly seen if the foreign body has been present for a prolonged period of time. Similarly, antibiotics are not used routinely, unless there is evidence of granulation tissue, or suppuration, around the foreign body, or in the distal airways.[3]

43.6.2   What investigative modalities are warranted postoperatively? What is the appropriate management of this patient if the immediate postoperative chest radiograph shows the presence of pneumomediastinum?

Postoperatively, the patient should be observed upon emergence from anesthesia to ensure that there are no sequelae following foreign body retrieval, such as airway compromise or respiratory distress. If the object was small and completely removed, with minimal underlying airway edema, the patient may be discharged following a brief period of observation. Difficult retrievals or instability in the operating or recovery rooms definitely mandate overnight-monitored observation.

If the patient exhibits pneumomediastinum on postoperative chest x-ray, clinical symptomatology must be correlated to determine whether further investigation or invasive therapies are warranted. Most commonly, there are few signs or symptoms associated with pneumomediastinum, precordial crepitus and voice change being the most common. Ideally, PPV should be avoided if possible as this may exacerbate the situation. Generally, such patients are monitored in an intensive care setting and are subject to serial chest radiographs to monitor regression or progression. Usually there is slow resolution over a few days, without significant sequelae.

43.7   SUMMARY

Airway foreign bodies in children can pose multiple challenges. The task of removing the object requires a team approach for the best possible patient outcome. Gathering as much information as possible prior to entering the operating theatre will enable better planning for foreign body retrieval, while keeping the patient's safety at the forefront. The size and nature of the aspirated object, its location in the airway, the time elapsed since aspiration, and patient factors such as age, and other associated comorbidities, all weigh into the planning of retrieval. Communication, preparation, and practice are the means by which outcomes are often successful.

REFERENCES

1. Brown L, Sherwin T, Perez JE, Perez DU: Heliox as a temporizing measure for pediatric foreign body aspiration. *Acad Emerg Med.* 2002;9:346–347.
2. Thomas GR, Dave D, Furze A, et al.: Managing common otolaryngologic emergencies. *Emerg Med.* 2005;37:18–47.
3. Rovin JD, Rogers BM: Pediatric foreign body aspiration. *Pediatr Rev.* 2000;21:86–90.
4. Gibson SE, Shot SR: Foreign bodies of the upper aerodigestive tract. In: *The Pediatric Airway—An Interdiscilinary Approach*, Chapter 12. Philadelphia, PA: JB Lippincott Co., 1995.
5. Chatterji S, Chatterji P: The Management of foreign bodies in the air passages. *Anesthesiology.* 1972;27:390–395.
6. Tan HK, Tan SS: Inhaled foreign bodies in children—anaesthetic considerations. *Singapore Med J.* 2000;41:506–510.
7. Kumra VP: Anaesthetic considerations for specialized surgeries peculiar to paediatric age group. *Indian J Anaesth.* 2004;48: 376–386.
8. Litman RS, Ponnuri J, Trogan I: Anesthesia for tracheal or bronchial foreign body removal in children: an analysis of ninety-four cases. *Anesth Analg.* 2000;91:1389–1391.
9. Holzman RS: Spontaneous for suspected airway foreign body removal. Society for pediatric anesthesia. *Summer Newsletter.* 2001.
10. Midulla F, de Blic J, Barbato A, et al.: Flexible endoscopy of paediatric airways. *Eur Respir J.* 2003;22:698–708.
11. Ramirez-Figueroa JL, Gochicoa-Rangel LG, Ramirez-San Juan DH, Vargas MH: Foreign body removal by flexible fiberoptic bronchoscopy in infants and children. *Pediatr Pulmonol.* 2005;40:392–397.
12. Ulku R, Onen A, Onat S, Ozcelik C: The value of open surgical approaches for aspirated pen caps. *J Pediatr Surg.* 2005;40:1780–1783.
13. Marks SC, Marsh BR, Dudgeon DL: Indications for open surgical removal of airway foreign body. *Ann Otol Rhinol Laryngol.* 1993;102: 690–694.

SELF-EVALUATION QUESTIONS

43.1. Which of the following is **NOT** recommended for, or to facilitate the inhalational induction of anesthesia to remove a foreign body from the trachea?

A. desflurane

B. atropine

C. midazolam

D. sevoflurane

E. halothane

43.2. All of the following aids are generally considered to be reasonable in the removal of an airway foreign body **EXCEPT**

A. LMA

B. FFB for object removal

C. avoidance of the use of nitrous oxide

D. avoidance of IPPV

E. removal of the foreign body through a rigid bronchoscope

43.3. Surgical removal of an airway foreign body is recommended under all of the following circumstances **EXCEPT**

A. if the foreign body is sharp, pointed, and embedded in the tracheal or bronchial wall

B. if the foreign body is found in a small inaccessible peripheral bronchus

C. if the foreign body has been present for a prolonged period often for several years

D. if there is significant instability in maintaining control of the airway upon insertion and manipulation with the bronchoscope

E. if the foreign body is lodged at the carnia

CHAPTER 44

Airway Management of a
Newborn with a
Tracheoesophageal Fistula

Babu V. Koka and Sabeena K. Chacko

44.1   CASE PRESENTATION

A 35 week old white male infant weighing 4.6 lbs (2.1 kg) is born by normal spontaneous vaginal delivery to a 25 year old female with a history of polyhydramnios during her pregnancy. Upon delivery, the baby is noted to be choking on his secretions and a nasogastric tube is unable to be passed into his stomach.

This is the typical presentation of a neonate with a tracheoesophageal fistula (TEF). If there is continued deterioration of respiratory status, the airway must be secured to provide adequate ventilation and to prevent further aspiration.

44.2   INTRODUCTION

44.2.1   What is the incidence of esophageal atresia and tracheoesophageal fistula?

The incidence of esophageal atresia (EA) and TEF is reported to be 1 in 3000–5000 live births.[1–3] Risk factors include maternal age, maternal race/ethnicity, and multiple gestation pregnancy, but there does not seem to be a predilection for any particular sex of the fetus.[4] Low birth weight and prematurity are common among neonates with this condition.

44.2.2   What are the common associated congenital anomalies?

During the fourth week of embryonic life, the common foregut differentiates into ventral respiratory and dorsal esophageal parts by a process of "pinching off," or apoptosis. Tracheoesophageal malformations occur when there is an incomplete separation of the trachea from the floor of the foregut. Detachment often occurs in an erratic manner causing a variety of defects of the trachea and esophagus. The most commonly cited classification system divides this anomaly into types A through F.[5] The three most common variants of this malformation are shown in Figure 44-1. Type C, which accounts for approximately 90% of the cases, is defined as EA with a distal tracheal fistula. EA and TEF may occur in isolation without any other birth defects (nonsyndromic occurrence) in about 50% of all cases. However, the treatment is more complex in children with syndromic occurrence, which is TEF in association with other congenital anomalies. The relative incidence of syndromic TEF can be as high as 30–50% and the cardiovascular system is the most commonly affected—almost 35% of the associated anomalies.

The classic cardiac lesion is a ventricular septal defect. Other cardiac defects such as patent ductus arteriosus, atrial septal defect, persistent right descending aorta, coarctation of the aorta, and tetralogy of Fallot have also been reported.

Different organ systems that may be affected include the musculoskeletal, gastrointestinal, genitourinary, and craniofacial. VATER or VACTERL (a newer, broader association) are acronyms used to describe a syndrome consisting of *V*ertebral anomalies, imperforate *A*nus, *C*ardiac defects, *T*racheo*E*sophageal fistula, *R*enal agenesis, and *L*imb abnormalities, most often radial dysplasia.[6] Many infants with TEF (15–20%) are diagnosed with VACTERL syndrome.[4] Figure 44-2 is a schematic illustration of the potential frequency of associated defects. In addition, there are several rare human single gene disorders, such as Feingold syndrome, CHARGE Syndrome, and anophthalmia-esophageal-genital syndrome, that are associated with TEF.[7,8]

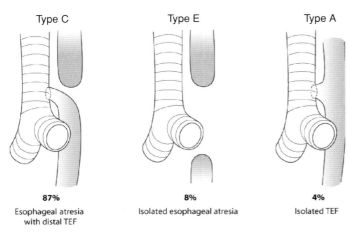

FIGURE 44-1. The three most common variants of tracheoesophageal malformations according to Gross.

44.2.3 What are the presenting signs and symptoms in neonates with TEF/EA?

The clinical signs and symptoms observed in neonates with TEF/EA include coughing, severe choking, and cyanosis, usually noted at the baby's first feeding. Abdominal distension, which often interferes with breathing, is secondary to air passing from the trachea to the esophagus. Infants present with recurrent, severe pneumonia secondary to gastric aspiration when the diagnosis is delayed.[1]

44.3   PATIENT CONSIDERATIONS

44.3.1   Discuss initial patient assessment

Initial evaluation of the neonate includes an assessment of the presence or absence of respiratory failure. Prevention of pneumonia, or other pulmonary complications prior to surgery, is essential for reducing intra- and postoperative morbidity and mortality. The neonate is kept in a semiupright, or prone, position to minimize regurgitation of gastric secretions into the trachea and all oral feeds are stopped. Suctioning of the blind esophageal pouch also helps to decrease pooling and aspiration of nasopharyngeal secretions.

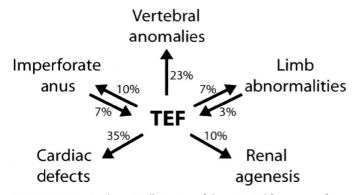

FIGURE 44-2. A schematic illustration of the potential frequency of associated defects with VACTERL syndrome.

44.3.2   What investigations are needed to make the diagnosis of TEF/EA?

The diagnosis of TEF is confirmed when a catheter passed into the esophagus stops abruptly around 10 cm from the lip. The tip of the esophagus is then determined by AP and lateral chest radiographs. In addition, a radio-opaque substance can be injected into the nasogastric tube to further delineate the proximal esophageal pouch. Complications of this procedure include gastric aspiration, leading to chemical pneumonitis, or leakage of contrast material into the mediastinum, if small esophageal perforations exist, as may occur with difficult intubations.[9] Since the contrast medium may pass into the trachea and then into the bronchi, non-ionic isotonic water-soluble contrast is suggested rather than barium, because it can be cleared from the bronchi with less irritation to the mucosa.[1]

Mediastinal sonography is a useful tool in the diagnosis of EA. Moving air bubbles ("atomizer sign") aid in the detection of an isolated TEF.[10] Abdominal radiographs will demonstrate the presence, or absence, of air in the stomach. Presence of air in the stomach with atresia of the upper esophagus is indicative of a fistula between the trachea and distal esophagus (Type C). Duodenal atresia may be ruled out by air in the small bowel and anal atresia by air in the rectum.

Reviewing the radiographs for vertebral anomalies may influence the decision to place an epidural catheter. These patients are ideal candidates for thoracic epidurals, which aid in postoperative pain control and a faster transition to spontaneous ventilation. In addition to radiographic studies, all infants with diagnosed TEF should have a renal ultrasound, echocardiogram, and cardiac catheterization, as deemed necessary prior to any surgery.[11] Echocardiography is helpful in defining intracardiac defects and aortic arch anomalies. Presence of a right-sided arch will influence the surgical approach to the lesion; however, preoperative localization of the aortic arch may be unreliable.[12] An unrecognized right aortic arch will complicate access to the fistula during surgery, as most of these fistulas are corrected via a right thoracotomy.

44.3.3   How do you assess the urgency of the airway management for this patient?

Urgent intubation and mechanical ventilation may become necessary, if the neonate is in obvious danger because of frequent cyanotic spells. Causes of respiratory failure include respiratory distress syndrome (RDS), congestive heart failure, pulmonary aspiration, and gastric distention. Neonates with TEF are often born prematurely and have low birth weights[4] and therefore are at greater risk for RDS. Cardiac failure is often due to ductal-dependent cardiac lesions requiring prostaglandin therapy. A compromise of lung compliance from any of the aforementioned causes will increase inspiratory pressures needed to maintain adequate tidal volume. A vicious cycle of higher inspiratory pressures causing even greater abdominal distention can ensue.

44.3.4   How do you assess and manage the airway of this neonate?

Airway obstruction may be present in patients with TEF who have associated anatomic defects of the upper airway. In addition, associated anomalies can cause difficulty visualizing the larynx. If a neonate is in respiratory distress, direct visualization of the vocal cords and intubation of the trachea is best accomplished with the patient spontaneously breathing. A small, straight laryngoscope blade can be used for visualization and intubation. A flexible, thin fiberoptic bronchoscope is another excellent tool to evaluate the airway. For difficult intubations in neonates, fiberoptic laryngoscopy can be used as an initial choice, or as a backup method, if direct laryngoscopy fails.

On rare occasions, TEF is associated with complete obstruction, or atresia, of the tracheal tree[13–16]; this is most often a fatal anomaly. In this situation, it might be possible to ventilate the lungs through a tube in the esophagus if a fistula exists distal to the atretic larynx. TEF may also be rarely associated with a complete laryngotracheoesophageal cleft that could be corrected.[17,18]

In a vigorous neonate, there are genuine concerns around deleterious effects of an awake intubation, such as an increase in intracranial pressure, or trauma to the vocal cords. It may be possible to place the tip of an endotracheal tube beyond the opening of a fistula in the trachea, but above the carina. This is rarely effective as the actual distances are very small in neonates and precise placement is difficult. This approach is also not possible if the fistulous connection is distal to the carina. The location of the tip of the endotracheal tube changes with movement of the baby's head and positioning of the baby, a hazardous development that can lead to severe episodes of gastric distention and hypoxemia.[19] It is best to confirm the position of the tip of the endotracheal tube with a flexible fiberoptic bronchoscope.

44.4 ANESTHETIC AND AIRWAY MANAGEMENT

44.4.1 Discuss anesthetic management of this patient

Anesthetic management in the operating room should include routine monitors (pulse oximeter, ECG, blood pressure cuff, and temperature probe) as well as an arterial line for analysis of blood gases and continuous blood pressure monitoring. A precordial stethoscope is useful in determining intraoperative airway obstruction.

In the practice of the authors, the preferred management for securing the airway in neonates with TEF is to induce general anesthesia via the intravenous or inhalational route, attempt bag-mask-ventilation (no greater than 10–15 cm water) without causing gastric distention, paralyze the patient with muscle relaxant, bag-mask-ventilate again, and then have the surgeon, or other qualified professional, perform a rigid bronchoscopy as the first attempt at airway manipulation.[20] The role of the bronchoscopy is to determine the exact location and size of the fistula and to assist in the placement of the endotracheal tube, preferably below the fistula. The rigid bronchoscope, with its side suction channel, also allows for the insertion of a Fogarty embolectomy catheter into large fistulas, especially those at the level of the carina. Inflation of the balloon on the catheter allows

occlusion of the fistula in these high-risk patients and helps prevent both inadvertent ventilation through the fistula, and gastric aspiration. Once the TEF has been corrected, the balloon is deflated and the catheter is removed.

44.4.2 Discuss different techniques in controlling air leak during the surgical procedure

If the tidal volume follows the path of lower resistance through the fistula and into the stomach, excessive positive pressure ventilation may lead to gastric distention. This, in turn, will further decrease adequate ventilation by displacing the diaphragm rostrally. However, this situation is infrequent, if lung compliance is good. A gastrostomy is not routinely performed, for though it may relieve distention, it can cause a low-resistance conduit for the loss of effective ventilation.[20,21] In addition, there is significant morbidity with gastrostomies performed in infancy.

There are reports of strategic positioning of cuffed endotracheal tubes during surgery for correction of TEF. A tracheal tube with deflated cuff can be inserted until it enters the right mainstem bronchus, as indicated by auscultation of the lung fields. The tube is then slowly withdrawn until breath sounds are heard bilaterally and air passage is heard into the stomach. The cuff is then inflated until air bubbling is no longer heard in the stomach and no air leak is present in the trachea. The cuff is deflated after ligation of the fistula.[22,23] In general, this technique has found less favor than one which employs bronchoscopy.[22]

44.4.3 What are the intraoperative problems commonly seen in these patients?

After careful tracheal intubation, the patient is turned to the left lateral decubitus position for a right thoracotomy. The fistula is ligated and the esophagus is anastomosed through a primary repair. Tracheal suctioning should be performed during the surgery to prevent the accumulation of blood, or secretions, and airway obstruction. Surgical manipulation may also contribute to airway obstruction. A clot in the tracheal tube that cannot be removed with suctioning leads to a precarious situation in which the tube must be replaced under much less than ideal conditions.

If ventilation is significantly compromised by airway leak prior to the start of surgery and an embolectomy catheter is not feasible due to patient size or condition, an emergency thoracotomy for ligation of the fistula, or a laparotomy for transabdominal occlusion of the gastroesophageal junction, should be performed until a more definitive correction can be completed.

Maintenance of adequate oxygenation can be a major intraoperative problem. In addition, positioning the baby on its side, opening its chest, collapsing the upper lung, and airway manipulation during surgery can lead to episodes of marked hypoxemia. Intravenous fluids should be administered judiciously to prevent fluid overload.

Great care should be taken during positive pressure ventilation to minimize inflation of the stomach through the fistula. Gastric perforation is a well-recognized complication of TEF when associated with extreme prematurity, hyaline membrane disease, and mechanical ventilation.[24,25] Sudden deterioration in oxygenation, increasing abdominal distention, and tension pneumoperitoneum are common warning signs of perforation.[26]

44.5   OTHER CONSIDERATIONS

44.5.1   What is the appropriate management of these patients following surgery?

The trachea is typically left intubated for an average of 3 days following thoracotomy to correct a TEF for these neonates. Nasopharyngeal and oropharyngeal suctioning is performed, as necessary, with a catheter that is carefully marked to prevent overzealous insertion into the esophagus and through an anastomosis. Excessive neck extension is also avoided to mitigate tension on an anastomotic site. Systemic opioids may be used for pain control but the immediate postoperative period is an ideal situation for a thoracic epidural, which may be beneficial in providing a quicker, less painful transition to spontaneous ventilation and extubation.

Postoperative complications of TEF repair in neonates include tracheomalacia, bronchospasm, chest-wall deformities, feeding difficulties secondary to esophageal dysmotility, gastroesophageal reflux (GERD), esophageal strictures requiring balloon dilatation, and recurrence of the fistula (in about 9% of cases).[27,28] Endoscopic followup should be continued for 3 years in all children after TEF repair and should be extended for three more years, if there is even mild esophagitis.[29] Bronchoesophageal fistulas sometimes occur after esophageal leaks and lead to recurrent lobar pneumonias.[28]

44.5.2   What are long-term outcomes of these patients?

Survival rates for neonates with TEF exceed 90%,[30] with higher mortality in those with coexisting congenital or chromosome abnormalities, such as Trisomy 13, 18, or 21.[18] Congenital heart disease, and low birth weight (<1,500 g), have been found to be independent predictors of mortality in neonates undergoing TEF repair. Ductal-dependent cardiac lesions further increase this risk and necessitate specific anesthetic considerations, in particular the use of invasive monitoring. These patients are also prone to a prolonged duration of postoperative mechanical ventilation, length of stay in the ICU, and total hospital days. TEF in association with congenital heart disease carries a 23% mortality rate. TEF, in the absence of associated heart disease, has an almost 100% chance of survival.[18,31]

Outcome in a neonate with TEF has improved significantly, in part due to advances in surgical, anesthetic, and critical-care management.[32] A decreased incidence of anastomotic leaks, in conjunction with improved nutritional and antimicrobial therapy, has had a major impact on survival. Severe tracheomalacia is now commonly treated with aortopexy and persistent GERD with a Nissen fundoplication,[33] and it is now recognized that either operation may not be successful without the other.[34] In addition, it has been possible to dramatically decrease the risk of stricture and GERD with an end-to-side repair of the EA, and ligation of the TEF, rather than the traditional end-to-end repair.[35]

Management of TEF has evolved over the past five decades.[36–40] Most neonates needing surgery are diagnosed well in advance by widespread use of prenatal ultrasound and genetic testing.[41] As the cumulative experience in treating these sick neonates accrues, certain practices that had been popular in earlier eras have been superseded. For example, staged repairs are now restricted only to the most severely ill infants, and those with long gap EA.[42] Conventional preliminary gastrostomy is no longer favored, nor is routine chest tube placement. Postoperative dilatation of a narrowed esophagus is also not commonly performed.[43] In addition, the tendency now is to attempt medical management of GERD, rather than early surgical intervention.[44]

44.5.3   Discuss newer surgical techniques and their impact on outcomes of TEF patients

Thoracoscopic repair of TEFs is possible even in the presence of severe cardiac lesions.[45] Results from thoracoscopic repair are similar to previous reports of repair through an open thoracotomy, with a shortened postoperative course.[46] Thoracotomy in infancy can lead to long-term complications such as rib deformities, winged scapula, thoracic scoliosis, and a large scar. Unilateral lung ventilation can often be associated with difficulties of oxygenation and carbon dioxide elimination with thoracotomy.[29] Congenital H-type (fistula without atresia) and recurrent TEFs are now often being treated with electrocautery and histoacryl glue through an endoscope. This technique greatly reduces traditional morbidity and mortality.[47]

44.6   SUMMARY

There are several unique issues to consider in the airway management of a neonate with TEF. These include possible difficulty in properly placing a tracheal tube because of anatomical abnormalities of the upper airway. In addition, extreme care should be taken with the use of positive pressure ventilation. Pulmonary aspiration is a significant risk and preventive measures must be undertaken. Iatrogenic inflation of the stomach, via the fistula, is a constant threat.

Innovative surgical instrumentation and operative techniques are continuing to develop. This will further serve to improve the outcome of neonates with TEF even in the face of complex associated abnormalities.

REFERENCES

1. Tarcan A, Gurakan B, Arda S, Boybat F: Congenital H-type fistula: delayed diagnosis in a preterm infant. *J Matern Fetal Neonatal Med.* 2003;13:279–280.
2. Shaw-Smith CJ: Oesophageal atresia, tracheo-oesophageal fistula and the VACTERL association: review of genetics and epidemiology. *J Med Genet.* 2005;43:545–54.
3. Depaepe A, Dolk H, Lechat MF: The epidemiology of tracheo-oesophageal fistula and oesophageal atresia in Europe. EUROCAT Working Group. *Arch Dis Child.* 1993;68:743–748.
4. Forrester MB, Merz RD: Epidemiology of oesophageal atresia and tracheo-oesophageal fistula in Hawaii, 1986–2000. *Public Health.* 2005;119:483–488.

5. Gross R: *Surgery of Infancy and Childhood*. Philadephia, PA: WB Saunders, 1953.
6. Quan L, Smith DW: The VATER association. Vertebral defects, Anal atresia, T-E fistula with esophageal atresia, Radial and Renal dysplasia: a spectrum of associated defects. *J Pediatr.* 1973;82:104–107.
7. Brunner HG, van Bokhoven H: Genetic players in esophageal atresia and tracheoesophageal fistula. *Curr Opin Genet Dev.* 2005;15:341–347.
8. Faivre L, Portnoi MF, Pals G, et al.: Should chromosome breakage studies be performed in patients with VACTERL association? *Am J Med Genet A.* 2005;137:55–58.
9. Seefelder C, Elango S, Rosbe KW, Jennings RW: Oesophageal perforation presenting as oesophageal atresia in a premature neonate following difficult intubation. *Paediatr Anaesth.* 2001;11:112–118.
10. Gassner I, Geley TE: Sonographic evaluation of oesophageal atresia and tracheo-oesophageal fistula. *Pediatr Radiol.* 2005;35:159–164.
11. Diaz LK, Akpek EA, Dinavahi R, Andropoulos DB: Tracheoesophageal fistula and associated congenital heart disease: implications for anesthetic management and survival. *Paediatr Anaesth.* 2005;15:862–869.
12. Bowkett B, Beasley SW, Myers NA: The frequency, significance, and management of a right aortic arch in association with esophageal atresia. *Pediatr Surg Int.* 1999;15:28–31.
13. Peison B, Levitzky E, Sprowls JJ: Tracheoesophageal fistula associated with tracheal atresia and malformation of the larynx. *J Pediatr Surg.* 1970;5:464–467.
14. Lander TA, Schauer G, Bendel-Stenzel E, Sidman JD: Tracheal agenesis in newborns. *Laryngoscope.* 2004;114:1633–1636.
15. Cohen MS, Rothschild MA, Moscoso J, Shlasko E: Perinatal management of unanticipated congenital laryngeal atresia. *Arch Otolaryngol Head Neck Surg.* 1998;124:1368–1371.
16. Wei JL, Rodeberg D, Thompson DM: Tracheal agenesis with anomalies found in both VACTERL and TACRD associations. *Int J Pediatr Otorhinolaryngol.* 2003;67:1013–1017.
17. Burroughs N, Leape LL: Laryngotracheoesophageal cleft: report of a case successfully treated and review of the literature. *Pediatrics.* 1974;53:516–522.
18. Kingston HG, Harrison MW, Smith JD: Laryngotracheoesophageal cleft—a problem of airway management. *Anesth Analg.* 1983;62:1041–1043.
19. Buchino JJ, Keenan WJ, Pietsch JB, Danis R, Schweiss JF: Malpositioning of the endotracheal tube in infants with tracheoesophageal fistula. *J Pediatr.* 1986;109:524–525.
20. Andropoulos DB, Rowe RW, Betts JM: Anaesthetic and surgical airway management during tracheo-oesophageal fistula repair. *Paediatr Anaesth.* 1998;8:313–319.
21. Ehlen M, Bachour H, Wiebe B, Bartmann P, Birkhold H: Esophageal atresia and severe respiratory failure—cuffed pediatric tracheal tubes as an additional therapeutic option? *J Pediatr Surg.* 2005;40:e25–e27.
22. Greemberg L, Fisher A, Katz A: Novel use of neonatal cuffed tracheal tube to occlude tracheo-oesophageal fistula. *Paediatr Anaesth.* 1999;9:339–341.
23. Lucking-Famira KM, Schulzke S, Hammer J: Cuffed endotracheal tube for occlusion of a tracheo-oesophageal fistula in an extremely low birth-weight infant. *Intensive Care Med.* 2004;30:1249.
24. Salem MR, Wong AY, Lin YH, Firor HV, Bennett EJ: Prevention of gastric distention during anesthesia for newborns with tracheoesophageal fistulas. *Anesthesiology.* 1973;38:82–83.
25. Jones TB, Kirchner SG, Lee FA, Heller RM: Stomach rupture associated with esophageal atresia, tracheoesophageal fistula, and ventilatory assistance. *Am J Roentgenol.* 1980;134:675–677.
26. Maoate K, Myers NA, Beasley SW: Gastric perforation in infants with oesophageal atresia and distal tracheo-oesophageal fistula. *Pediatr Surg Int.* 1999;15:24–27.
27. Kovesi T, Rubin S: Long-term complications of congenital esophageal atresia and/or tracheoesophageal fistula. *Chest.* 2004;126:915–925.
28. Krosnar S, Baxter A: Thoracoscopic repair of esophageal atresia with tracheoesophageal fistula: anesthetic and intensive care management of a series of eight neonates. *Paediatr Anaesth.* 2005;15:541–546.
29. Schalamon J, Lindahl H, Saarikoski H, Rintala RJ: Endoscopic follow-up in esophageal atresia-for how long is it necessary? *J Pediatr Surg.* 2003;38:702–704.
30. Seguier-Lipszyc E, Bonnard A, Aizenfisz S, et al.: The management of long gap esophageal atresia. *J Pediatr Surg.* 2005;40:1542–1546.
31. Spitz L, Kiely EM, Morecroft JA, Drake DP: Oesophageal atresia: at-risk groups for the 1990s. *J Pediatr Surg.* 1994;29:723–725.
32. Kalish RB, Chasen ST, Rosenzweig L, Chervenak FA: Esophageal atresia and tracheoesophageal fistula: the impact of prenatal suspicion on neonatal outcome in a tertiary care center. *J Perinat Med.* 2003;31:111–114.
33. Orford J, Cass DT, Glasson MJ: Advances in the treatment of oesophageal atresia over three decades: the 1970s and the 1990s. *Pediatr Surg Int.* 2004;20:402–407.
34. Nasr A, Ein SH, Gerstle JT: Infants with repaired esophageal atresia and distal tracheoesophageal fistula with severe respiratory distress: is it tracheomalacia, reflux, or both? *J Pediatr Surg.* 2005;40:901–903.
35. Touloukian RJ, Seashore JH: Thirty-five-year institutional experience with end-to-side repair for esophageal atresia. *Arch Surg.* 2004;139:371–374.
36. Poenaru D, Laberge JM, Neilson IR, Guttman FM: A new prognostic classification for esophageal atresia. *Surgery.* 1993;113:426–432.
37. Choudhury SR, Ashcraft KW, Sharp RJ, et al.: Survival of patients with esophageal atresia: influence of birth weight, cardiac anomaly, and late respiratory complications. *J Pediatr Surg.* 1999;34:70–73; discussion 74.
38. Engum SA, Grosfeld JL, West KW, Rescorla FJ, Scherer LR, 3rd: Analysis of morbidity and mortality in 227 cases of esophageal atresia and/or tracheoesophageal fistula over two decades. *Arch Surg.* 1995;130:502–508; discussion 508–509.
39. Louhimo I, Lindahl H: Esophageal atresia: primary results of 500 consecutively treated patients. *J Pediatr Surg.* 1983;18:217–229.
40. Sharma AK, Shekhawat NS, Agrawal LD, et al.: Esophageal atresia and tracheoesophageal fistula: a review of 25 years' experience. *Pediatr Surg Int.* 2000;16:478–482.
41. Skarsgard ED, Blair GK, Lee SK: Toward evidence-based best practices in neonatal surgical care-I: The Canadian NICU Network. *J Pediatr Surg.* 2003;38:672–677.
42. Healey PJ, Sawin RS, Hall DG, Schaller RT, Tapper D: Delayed primary repair of esophageal atresia with tracheoesophageal fistula: is it worth the wait? *Arch Surg.* 1998;133:552–556.
43. Yanchar NL, Gordon R, Cooper M, Dunlap H, Soucy P: Significance of the clinical course and early upper gastrointestinal studies in predicting complications associated with repair of esophageal atresia. *J Pediatr Surg.* 2001;36:815–822.
44. Konkin DE, O'Hali WA, Webber EM, Blair GK: Outcomes in esophageal atresia and tracheoesophageal fistula. *J Pediatr Surg.* 2003;38:1726–1729.
45. Mariano ER, Chu LF, Albanese CT, Ramamoorthy C: Successful thoracoscopic repair of esophageal atresia with tracheoesophageal fistula in a newborn with single ventricle physiology. *Anesth Analg.* 2005;101:1000–1002.
46. Holcomb GW, 3rd, Rothenberg SS, Bax KM, et al.: Thoracoscopic repair of esophageal atresia and tracheoesophageal fistula: a multi-institutional analysis. *Ann Surg.* 2005;242:422–428; discussion 428–430.
47. Tzifa KT, Maxwell EL, Chait P, et al.: Endoscopic treatment of congenital H-Type and recurrent tracheoesophageal fistula with electrocautery and histoacryl glue. *Int J Pediatr Otorhinolaryngol.* 2005;70:925–30.

SELF-EVALUATION QUESTIONS

44.1. Which of the following is **NOT** a true statement about the associated congenital anomalies with esophageal atresia and tracheoesophageal fistula?

   A. Other birth defects are always associated with esophageal atresia and tracheoesophageal fistula.

   B. Cardiac defects account for almost 35% of the associated anomalies.

   C. Radial dysplasia is often associated with esophageal atresia and tracheoesophageal fistula.

   D. TEF is associated with complete obstruction or atresia of the tracheal tree.

   E. VACTERL is a syndrome consisting of *V*ertebral anomalies, imperforate *A*nus, *C*ardiac defects, *T*racheo *E*sophageal fistula, *R*enal agenesis, and *L*imb abnormalities.

44.2. Which of the following is the best to confirm the proper positioning of the tip of the endotracheal tube following tracheal intubation?

A. auscultation of the chest bilaterally

B. auscultation of the abdomen

C. chest x-ray

D. flexible fiberoptic bronchoscope

E. mediastinal sonography

44.3. Which of the following is **NOT** a known postoperative complication of TEF repair?

A. tracheomalacia

B. gastric perforation

C. chest-wall deformities

D. gastroesophageal reflux

E. bronchoesophageal fistulas

CHAPTER (45)

Airway Management in a 1-Year-Old with Pierre Robin Syndrome for Myringotomy and Tubes

Christian M. Soder

45.1   CASE PRESENTATION

A 1 year old boy known to have Robin Sequence (Pierre Robin syndrome or Pierre Robin sequence) presents with chronic otitis media and significant conductive hearing loss. The pediatric otolaryngologist has booked him for bilateral myringotomy and tube insertion. Twenty minutes of operating room time has been scheduled. The patient has been evaluated in the outpatient clinic by an anesthesia colleague. The consultation report states that the infant was hospitalized for the first 3 months of his life for severe airway obstruction and feeding difficulties. The patient has never required tracheotomy, but his airway was managed by glossopexy (tongue sutured to lip) during the first month of life. The anesthesia record for this procedure indicates that the infant was intubated awake with great difficulty by a team of pediatric anesthesia practitioners employing an unorthodox combination of the infant size Trachlight™ and direct straight-blade laryngoscopy. It is noted that the infant currently still sleeps on his stomach without apparent apnea or airway obstruction, but develops stridor and apnea if placed on his back.

45.2   INTRODUCTION

45.2.1   What is Robin Sequence (RS)?

Robin Sequence (named for the eminent French dentist, Pierre Robin, who first described it) has become synonymous with the pediatric anesthesia practitioner's worst airway nightmare. The condition is believed to be the result of primary failure in fetal mandibular development. The resulting micrognathia leads to rostral displacement of the tongue termed "glossoptosis." In 50% of cases, the displacement of the normal-sized tongue into the roof of the mouth leads to failure of fusion of the maxillary arches and a resultant cleft palate. The combination of cleft palate and malposition of the tongue leads to airway obstruction, recurrent episodes of hypoxemia and hypercapnia, pulmonary hypertension, sleep apnea, swallowing difficulties, failure to thrive, and chronic ear disease.[1] Although Robin Sequence is an isolated anomaly in 2/3 of the cases, similar features are found in multiple malformation patterns including Treacher Collins syndrome, Stickler syndrome, and velocardial syndrome. Accurate diagnosis of multiple anomaly syndromes is important in formulating the airway plan because of the possible presence of associated major malformations, such as congenital heart disease.

Older texts quote a mortality of 50% for this anomaly. Good positioning (nursing in prone position), tube feeding, glossopexy (suturing the tongue to the lip to pull it forward), mandibular advancement surgery, prevention or treatment of aspiration pneumonia, and reduced incidence of pulmonary hypertension (less exposure to hypoxemia and hypercarbia) have combined to reduce mortality below 5%. After birth, growth of the mandible proceeds normally and surgical closure of the cleft palate eventually allows for the development of near normal airway anatomy, normal swallowing, normal growth, and full physical and intellectual development.

The anesthesia practitioner respects this malformation because the trachea of these patients is notoriously difficult to intubate and bag-mask-ventilation (BMV) is often difficult, which is unfortunate because they frequently need surgery. Compounding the matter, the currently recommended long-term management plan is a conservative one that does not usually include tracheotomy. The good news is that the long-term prognosis for the syndrome is excellent, if they survive repeated general anesthetics.

45.3   PATIENT CONSIDERATION

45.3.1   How do you assess the airway of this patient?

RS poses the classic "small chin conundrum": difficult BMV and difficult direct laryngoscopy (DL).[2,3] The lack of a well-developed mentum creates significant problems with mask fit (no seal below the lower lip) making BMV difficult or impossible. The glossoptosis places the tongue posteriorly and superiorly into apposition with the roof of the mouth. If Mallampati classes could be performed on these infants, they would score a IV! With the loss of consciousness, airway obstruction often becomes complete and its correction by an oropharyngeal airway (OPA) is difficult unless a perfect fit is achieved. These patients are usually at their best in the prone position because gravity helps keep the tongue off the roof of the mouth. They may develop varying degrees of obstruction when placed supine.

On the positive side, extraglottic devices, such as the Laryngeal Mask Airway (LMA), have been reported to be effective in providing ventilation and oxygenation.[4–6] An appropriately sized OPA, nasopharyngeal airway (NPA), or LMA can often be placed easily and will usually maintain the airway. The LMA may well prove to be the airway of choice for some surgical procedures in RS, particularly for minor procedures not involving or near the airway.

Glossoptosis and mandibular hypoplasia compound the difficulty in securing an airway. The glottic opening is angled away from the oral axis more than the usual 90 degrees, and the virtual absence of a submental space means that the laryngoscope blade cannot displace the tongue into this area. Fortunately, the cleft palate in RS is not accompanied by a cleft lip and therefore does not interfere with laryngoscopy. In extreme cases, mandibular hypoplasia is so severe that the tongue completely obstructs direct visualization of the larynx despite optimal direct laryngoscopic technique, delivering a Cormack/Lehane (C/L) grade 4 view of the larynx.

Although experience with alternate intubation techniques is limited, the author has successfully used blind right angle techniques (the infant-size Trachlight™), while others have reported successful use of right angle visualization techniques (Bullard™ laryngoscope)[7] and fiberoptic intubation.[8]

Subglottic anatomy is normal, but these patients are usually too young to have a useful cricothyroid membrane, making surgical or percutaneous cricothyrotomy impractical. However, open or percutaneous tracheotomy is possible and increased familiarity and experience with percutaneous tracheal access may bring this approach within the skill set of most pediatric anesthesia practitioners. Surgical backup and even a full double setup are advisable for severe cases.

How does one recognize such a "severe case"? Risk factors include hyomental distance less than 1 cm (i.e., severe mandibular

hypoplasia), inability to maintain the airway when awake and supine (severe glossoptosis), oxygen dependence, history of significant pulmonary disease, and prior episodes of failed airway in competent hands.

45.3.2   Do you have any medical concerns for this patient?

Isolated RS is not associated with major cardiac or other malformations. However, these patients usually require anesthetics during their first year of life, a time when their anatomic challenges are compounded by the normal physiologic limitations of infancy such as a reduced effectiveness of denitrogenation, increasing the risk of desaturation. In addition, some of these infants have problems with recurrent aspiration and pulmonary hypertension, further reducing cardiopulmonary reserve. In Robin Sequence infants, airway obstruction is followed almost immediately by desaturation and bradycardia. Planning for options A, B, and C is vital as there is precious little time to think once the airway is lost.

45.4   AIRWAY MANAGEMENT

45.4.1   What are the alternatives in managing the airway of this patient under general anesthesia?

At age 1, this patient is no longer at maximum risk. He has survived the neonatal period to be discharged from hospital, has continued to thrive at home without home oxygen, and has no history of serious pulmonary disease. However, the history of a previously failed airway with the need for glossopexy in the newborn period, and persistent airway obstruction when supine, are evidence of significant ongoing glossoptosis. These issues indicate an increased risk for difficult DL and BMV. The airway management plan for a RS patient must reflect these risks.

45.4.1.1   Plan A: Attempt to Maintain an Extraglottic Airway

After the placement of an IV catheter, and the application of appropriate monitors, anesthesia is induced with oxygen–sevoflurane or oxygen–halothane inhalation. Under deep anesthesia, an extraglottic device is placed. This is to be followed by myringotomy and tube insertion surgery.

45.4.1.2   Plan B: Failed Extraglottic Airway

Should an extraglottic airway fail, additional assistance should immediately be summoned. It is reasonable to attempt paraglossal DL with a straight blade. Should this maneuver fail, it may be possible to effect gas exchange by maintaining an open airway with the laryngoscope in position either, maintaining saturations and anesthesia, employing the patient's own spontaneous respiratory efforts. This is followed by the implementation of a planned sequence of alternate intubating techniques. A digital intubation is an option in these patients.

45.4.1.3 Plan C: Failed Ventilation and Intubation

After ventilation and intubation fail (can't intubate, can't ventilate or CICV), one should proceed immediately to either percutaneous tracheotomy or surgical tracheotomy depending on the available resources. Concurrent or nearly concurrent actions may be indicated depending on the ability to maintain reasonable oxygen saturations.

The airway management plan for the patient with an inadequate mandibular space presents some unusual features. The airway of choice for bilateral myringotomy and tubes in RS patient is the OPA or LMA (Plan A).

The anatomy is suitable for extraglottic device placement, and experience has shown that it usually works. The anatomy is unfavorable for laryngoscopy and an endotracheal tube (ETT) is not necessary for the surgery. However, if an extraglottic airway does fail and cannot be restored promptly, the next maneuver should be the insertion of a laryngoscope blade (Plan B). Many pediatric anesthesia practitioners have observed that displacing the glossoptotic tongue with a laryngoscope can open the obstructed RS airway, permitting spontaneous ventilation to continue. This technique can buy time while one attempts to optimize laryngoscopy, manipulate the airway, deploy airway adjuncts, and attempt alternate intubation techniques. If the airway cannot be maintained by extraglottic device and cannot be obtained by laryngoscopy, and the patient cannot be awakened, a failed airway procedure becomes necessary (Plan C).

45.4.2 How do you prepare to manage the anesthesia and airway of this patient?

Even though the procedure is scheduled for less than 1 hour and is a "minor case," it is a "major anesthetic" and this paradox must be discussed with the surgeon, the staff, and the family. In addition to the usual preanesthetic routine, airway equipment preparations ought to include assembling several potentially useful face masks and OPAs, and two laryngoscope handles with straight blades of varying lengths and widths. The Flagg or Wisconsin designs have the advantage of being completely straight (maximum optical path efficiency) and having circular cross sections (more room to see, and pass the tube). Multiple 3.0, 3.5, and 4.0 mm ID ETT with well-lubricated hockey stick shaped intubating stylets preloaded are prepared, as are number 1–2 LMAs, tested and lubricated.

A lubricated, pediatric size Eschmann Tracheal Tube Introducer ought to be considered a standard piece of airway management equipment and should be immediately available. The anesthesia practitioner, based on familiarity with the techniques, should set up appropriate alternate intubating devices such as an infant Trachlight™ with 3.5 mm ID ETT preloaded, tested, and lubricated; a pediatric Bullard™ laryngoscope tested and loaded; a Glidescope™; or an infant fiberoptic intubation scope, connected to light source, loaded, lubricated, and tested.

Surgical equipment available should include the surgical tracheotomy tray and a #1 Melker™ uncuffed cricothyrotomy set for percutaneous tracheotomy. If this patient presented with more threatening risk factors (e.g., severe pulmonary disease), the surgeon would be gloved and gowned, the tray would be opened, the tracheotomy tube selected, and the skin prepared prior to induc-

tion of anesthesia. In this case, a second anesthesia practitioner should be on stand by in the room.

Succinylcholine 20 mg (for laryngospasm on BMV or LMA), atropine 0.4 mg (to mitigate bradycardia), and epinephrine 1 mL of 1/10,000 solution (to respond to hypoxemia-induced myocardial depression) are drawn up. Other standard resuscitation drugs should be available on the cart.

45.4.3 Discuss the conduct of anesthesia for this patient

The child is brought into the operating room. Parental attendance is usually forgone in this scenario to minimize distraction. An IV is inserted prior to the induction of anesthesia. Atropine 0.1 mg IV is administered to reduce secretions and mitigate vagal responses (bradycardia). Pulse oximeter, blood pressure cuff, and ECG monitors are applied. Mask fitting and denitrogenation proceed for 2 to 3 minutes. Induction starts with 8% sevoflurane in 100% oxygen at 2 L·min^{-1} flow. The OPA or LMA is inserted after the sevoflurane excitement phase passes.

Position is confirmed by the CO_2 detection, and anesthetic depth is optimized. When sustained regular spontaneous respirations, normal pulse oximetry readings, and appropriate heart rate and blood pressure for age are achieved, the surgical procedure may begin. If the airway is lost and cannot be regained at any time, a laryngoscope (# 2 straight blade) is inserted using a paraglossal approach to displace the tongue laterally. If the airway is opened by this maneuver, and if spontaneous breathing continues, endotracheal intubation is attempted when the anesthetic depth is adequate. Laryngoscopy can be optimized by external laryngeal manipulation, and placement of the ETT can be facilitated by the traditional hockey stick shaped intubating stylette or the infant Eschmann Tracheal Tube Introducer. The ETT can also be mounted on a hockey stick shaped Trachlight™ to improve visualization and confirm location.

If a Cormack/Lehane (C/L) grade 3 laryngoscopic view can be obtained, intubation is almost always possible employing an intubating stylette. If the laryngeal view grade is 4 and/or intubation is unsuccessful, alternate intubation techniques may be helpful. With the laryngoscope blade left in situ for tongue control, oxygen and anesthetic agent are blown toward the airway, ordinarily employing sevoflurane. To effect this, a 3 mm ID ETT may be inserted into the oropharynx or nostril and connected to the anesthesia circuit. Usually, 6–10 L·min^{-1} flows permit insufflation of sufficient oxygen and agent to maintain normoxemia and anesthesia. The following maneuvers are then considered in the order most familiar to the anesthesia practitioner: repeat laryngoscopy with blade or technique change; tongue traction using a forcep or gauze to pull the tongue out of the mouth toward the left; alternate intubation technique using Glidescope™, Trachlight™, or Bullard™ laryngoscope; or attempt fiberoptic intubation with or without an LMA.

If at any time the airway or spontaneous respirations are lost and cannot be recovered by the laryngoscopy or extraglottic techniques, the failed airway Plan C is activated. Depending on the skill and experience of the anesthesia practitioners and surgeons, either a surgical tracheotomy is performed or the #1 Melker™ percutaneous tracheotomy is inserted.

45.5   OTHER CONSIDERATIONS

45.5.1   Discuss postintubation management of this patient

Endotracheal placement must be confirmed by CO_2 detection. Inadvertent endobronchial intubation of infants is common in stressful circumstances, and radiographic confirmation may be required if there is any doubt about tube tip location. It is obvious that following a difficult intubation, the ETT must be well secured using a commercial fixation device or by highly adherent adhesive tape fixed to the skin of the upper lip. Tincture of benzoin (Friar's Balsam) is recommended to dry and degrease the skin. At the end of the procedure, awake extubation is mandatory. Extubation in the prone position may be helpful. Complications of traumatic intubation, including subglottic edema, bleeding, and laryngeal injury, should be anticipated and planned for.

45.5.2   What is the extubation plan if the tracheal intubation was traumatic with significant airway edema?

Patients who have been intubated with difficulty are at risk for the development of postextubation stridor, usually caused by traumatic laryngeal inlet hemorrhage or edema. The symptoms usually appear within 2–4 hours of extubation and may persist for several days. Following a difficult intubation, there may well be a reluctance to remove the ETT because of the potential need for reintubation. In cases where trauma to the airway appears to have been minimal and a leak around the tube is present at the end of the case, awake extubation in the recovery room can be performed. If stridor develops, it is treated with nebulized or atomized racemic epinephrine or phenylephrine, and IV dexamethasone $0.5–1.0$ mg·kg^{-1}. If available, heliox (80% helium/20% oxygen) may permit adequate gas exchange, although the reduction in work of breathing must be weighed against the reduction in FIO_2. Pulse oximetry is essential. In cases where the intubation was obviously traumatic or where there is no audible leak around the tube, the patient should be transferred to ICU for delayed extubation. ICU management should include sedation, ventilation, and IV dexamethasone for 12–48 hours. When an audible leak around the tube is present, extubation should be considered. Flexible fiberoptic laryngoscopy should be considered to assess the state of the laryngeal inlet prior to extubation.

45.6   SUMMARY

RS is the pediatric prototype of the difficult airway. It is the ultimate "anterior larynx." Many congenital anomalies include RS or some of its features. There is no doubt that the severe glossoptosis in Robin sequence is intimidating, but the basic airway management should be familiar to all anesthesia practitioners.

The approach is very similar to that used for the adult case that presents a C/L grade 3 or 4 view on laryngoscopy.

Face or laryngeal mask fit is an essential prerequisite to basic airway management (and to reduce operator stress!). The first attempts at intubation usually include maneuvers such as blade change (e.g., straight blade), approach change (e.g., paraglossal), position change (e.g., flexion, head elevation), external laryngeal and/or tongue manipulation, and use of a Tracheal Tube Introducer.

Failing successful DL, indirect visualization devices (e.g., SOS™, Glidescope™, Bullard™, or fiberoptic laryngoscope) may be useful, as may blind right-angle techniques (e.g., Trachlight™). Digital intubation may also be considered.

Rescue can be accomplished with an LMA, and tracheotomy offers a final option. With anticipation and a good airway management plan, most patients with RS can be successfully intubated and tracheotomy is rarely required.

REFERENCES

1. van den Elzen AP, Semmekrot BA, Bongers EM, et al.: Diagnosis and treatment of the Pierre Robin sequence: results of a retrospective clinical study and review of the literature. *Eur J Pediatr.* 2001;160:47–53.
2. Nargozian C: The airway in patients with craniofacial abnormalities. *Paediatr Anaesth.* 2004;14:53–59.
3. Schaefer RB, Gosain AK: Airway management in patients with isolated Pierre Robin sequence during the first year of life. *J Craniofac Surg.* 2003;14:462–467.
4. Baraka A: Laryngeal mask airway for resuscitation of a newborn with Pierre-Robin Syndrome. *Anesthesiology.* 1996;83:645–646.
5. Selim M, Mowafi H, Al-Ghamdi A, Adu-Gyamfi Y: Intubation via LMA in pediatric patients with difficult airways. *Can J Anaesth.* 1999;46:891–893.
6. Ofer R, Dworzak H: The laryngeal mask—a valuable instrument for cases of difficult intubation in children. Anesthesiologic management in the presence of Pierre-Robin syndrome. *Anaesthesist.* 1996;45:268–270.
7. Baraka A, Muallem M: Bullard laryngoscopy for tracheal intubation in a neonate with Pierre-Robin Syndrome. *Paediatr Anaesth.* 1994;4:111–113.
8. Scheller JG, Schulman SR: Fiberoptic bronchoscopic guidance for intubation of a neonate with Pierre Robin Syndrome. *J Can Anaesth.* 1991;3:45–47.

SELF-ASSESSMENT QUESTIONS

45.1.   Difficult intubation correlates with all of the following signs **EXCEPT**

   A.   hyomental distance <1 cm

   B.   airway obstruction when supine

   C.   airway obstruction when prone

   D.   oxygen dependence

   E.   prior history

45.2.   Recommended airway maneuvers for a child with Robin Sequence could include all **EXCEPT**

   A.   LMA

   B.   direct laryngoscopy

   C.   oxygen/vapor insufflation

D. percutaneous tracheotomy

E. intravenous induction

45.3. Recommended extubation maneuvers after traumatic intubation include all the following **EXCEPT**

A. leak test around the tube

B. racemic epinephrine

C. dexamethasone

D. mandatory transfer to an ICU

E. heliox

Airway Management of a 6-Year-Old with a History of Difficult Airway for Bilateral Inguinal Hernia Repair

David C. Abramson

46.1 CASE PRESENTATION

A 6 year old child with Crouzon syndrome (CS) presents with bilateral inguinal hernia for repair. His parents report that a previous craniosynostosis repair, at the age of 9 months, and a LeFort III osteotomy, at the age of 4 years, were both associated with a difficult airway and that the anesthesia practitioners had told them to pass this information onto the next practitioner. The child is otherwise well and of normal intelligence.

46.2 INTRODUCTION

46.2.1 What is Crouzon syndrome?

Crouzon and Apert syndromes are the most common of the craniosynostosis syndromes. In addition to craniosynostosis, these children also have fusion of the sutures or bones in the cranial base and midface, and shallow eye sockets. This gives the appearance of a flat midface and eyes which protrude. Children with Apert syndrome (AS) also have syndactaly (webbing) of the hands and feet. The infant's shallow midface and/or small or partially obstructed nasal passages can cause airway problems, as in this case presentation. Evaluations by ENT specialists are important and a tracheotomy may be necessary to relieve the airway problems.[1]

CS occurs in approximately one in 25,000 births. It may be transmitted as an autosomal dominant genetic condition or appear as a fresh mutation (no affected parents). The appearance of an infant with CS can vary in severity from a mild presentation with subtle midface characteristics to severe forms with multiple cranial sutures fused and marked midface and eye problems. The incidence of AS is approximately one in 100,000 births and most cases are fresh mutations. The general features of a child with AS are similar to those in CS. However, there is not as much variability between cases and the degree of presentation is more severe.

46.2.2 Why is the team approach so important in cases like this?

Essential to the handling of this patient is communication and preparation. The surgeon, on scheduling the case, should contact the anesthesia practitioner to advise them of the potential of difficult airway management to prevent surprises and case cancellation. Had prior notification not occurred, it is perfectly reasonable to delay this elective surgical procedure until as much information as possible regarding the patient's past medical history is obtained. Every effort should be made to contact the previous anesthesia practitioners to discuss their past management issues and obtain previous anesthesia records to determine anesthetic and airway difficulties.

46.3 AIRWAY ASSESSMENT AND PREPARATIONS

46.3.1 How do you assess the airway of this child? What if he is uncooperative?

As 2 years have passed since the last surgery, one can expect some growth changes in the airway (see Chapter 41). Essentially, this is a "new" difficult airway and it is incumbent upon the anesthesia practitioner to take a good history, paying particular attention as to whether this child has difficulty in breathing with different body positions, and whether there are symptoms of *upper-airway resistance syndrome*[2–8] or *sleep apnea* and, if present, whether these conditions have been formally tested. Typically, CS (proptosis, craniosynostosis, and maxillary hypoplasia) patients do not present with obstructive airway symptoms.

Examination of the airway should pay particular attention to the ability to flex and extend the neck, ability to open the mouth, and, most important, the capacity of the submandibular space to accommodate the tongue on direct laryngoscopy. Even if all these measurements are "normal," a difficult airway under anesthesia should be anticipated and prepared for. Additionally, an accurate weight and height should be recorded, as well as a hematocrit.

46.3.2   What are the airway management options for this patient?

There are several options for anesthesia in this case and all have been used in children younger than 6 years:

1. local/regional anesthesia without airway intervention
2. general and local/regional anesthesia with airway intervention
3. general anesthesia with intubation
    a. direct laryngoscopy and intubation
    b. fiberoptic intubation
        • directly
        • with the use of a guide
4. awake Intubation prior to induction of general anesthesia

Practically, we are faced with a bilateral inguinal hernia repair, which does not require muscle relaxation. We also have a 6 year old child probably unlikely to cooperate with a procedure under local anesthesia for any length of time.

46.3.3   What general preparations for airway management are required?

If airway intervention is contemplated, IV access is mandatory and can be achieved either under sedation or awake. If awake, this may be facilitated by the use of either EMLA® (AstraZeneca) or LMX4® (ELA-Max) (Ferndale Laboratories, Inc., MI) applied topically to the skin 60–90 minutes, respectively, prior to the IV start.[9] Similarly, if one is considering regional anesthesia (caudal or spinal) without airway intervention, application of these agents to the relevant anatomical area can easily be achieved. Relatively painless regional anesthesia can be accomplished.

All anesthetic and emergency drugs should be prepared and drawn. In addition, a difficult airway cart with appropriate equipment should be available in the operating room and checked (see Chapter 56). Experienced airway assistants should also be available, including a surgical staff who can perform a surgical airway, should it become necessary.

46.4   ANESTHESIA AND AIRWAY MANAGEMENT

46.4.1   How exactly should the airway of this patient be managed?

Most children will require some form of sedation prior to a procedure, particularly children with multiple prior contacts with health care providers because they have a healthy suspicion of them. Midazolam is a reasonable anxiolytic in either the commercially available syrup or the concentrated IV form suspended in flavored syrup which is usually unpleasantly bitter. A dose of 0.5 mg.kg^{-1} (maximum 10 mg) is administered orally at least 15 minutes before attempting any separation from caretakers.[10] At this dose, respiratory depression has not been reported. Once IV access is obtained, further small incremental doses of midazolam can be titrated to effect, should a sedation technique be used.

Most anesthesia practitioners would employ a combined general and regional anesthesia technique using a Laryngeal Mask Airway (LMA). The anesthetic is characterized by an inhalational induction that maintains spontaneous ventilation and has the advantage to reverse the anesthetic at any point when maintenance becomes questionable. This technique is generally considered to be safe, particularly since paralytic agents are not being employed.

While many consider sevoflurane to be the preferred anesthetic agent for induction and maintenance of pediatric anesthesia, it does have several limitations:

1. much higher incidence of emergency delirium[11],
2. marked depression of respiration in high concentration,
3. too rapid a change in the level of consciousness.

If an IV is in place, some practitioners would administer glycopyrrolate, 5–10 μg.kg^{-1}, as an antisialagogue. Atropine is less desirable as it has less drying action and more tachycardia associated with its use.

IV induction may be easily achieved with a number of agents, but, in the case of potential airway manipulation, propofol is often the drug of choice as it blunts airway responses to manipulation and is easily titratable.

Once anesthetized, an LMA should be attempted. The insertion method for the LMA is described in Chapter 41.[12] Correct placement is confirmed by hearing breath sounds and can be further validated by successful ventilation with positive pressure.

46.4.2   If one wanted to perform a caudal block, how might that be done, especially if an LMA is in place?

Once the LMA is placed and secured, the child is turned into the left lateral decubitus position (for right-handed practitioner) to perform the caudal block and then returned to the supine position for surgery. Attention to securing the LMA during any positioning procedure is vital as the seal is easily lost. This is particularly important in the smaller child (less than 10 kg), where initial placement tends to be more difficult.[13]

A detailed discussion of caudal block technique is beyond the scope of this chapter. Briefly, an agent with a rapid onset is preferred to avoid potential laryngospasm with surgical incision. An equal mixture of 2% lidocaine and 0.25% levobupivacaine (or 0.2% ropivacaine) 1 mL·kg^{-1} will achieve this goal and produce a block of long duration as well. The addition of clonidine 1–2 μg·kg^{-1} has been suggested to prolong the duration of the block.[14] The caudal block can reduce the requirement of the anesthetic vapor and avoid respiratory depression associated with the use of opioid. If airway difficulty is encountered at any stage during the induction, simply turning off the inhalational agent and administering 100% oxygen will result in rapid awakening and recovery of airway reflexes.

46.4.3 How would one perform a fiberoptic intubation in this child?

If Plan A is unsuccessful or not practically feasible, Plans B and C should be designed and prepared before bringing the patient to the operating room.

Fiberoptic intubation is one of those plans. This can be done awake or asleep in this age group with patience and careful planning. These children can be very challenging, particularly if they have had previous negative interactions with health care personnel. It is difficult to employ logic and reasoning with a 6 year old child. For this reason, moderate to heavy sedation is required. Oral midazolam 0.5 mg·kg^{-1} (maximum 10 mg) is often effective as an initial sedating agent as one begins the process of preparing for the fiberoptic intubation.

Initially, both nasal passages are anesthetized with 4% aqueous lidocaine and vasoconstriction achieved with topical oxymetazoline. Nebulization of lidocaine is an effective airway anesthetic. The 4% solution commonly available can be diluted (with water, not saline, saline changes its pH) to 2% to give greater volume. Not more than 5 mg·kg^{-1} should be placed in the nebulizing chamber and allowed to be slowly inhaled either in the holding area or on the way to the operating room. The finely nebulized particles will anesthetize the glottis and trachea to varying degrees.

Once in the operating room, IV access is mandatory before proceeding further, and, once secured, 5 μg·kg^{-1} glycopyrrolate should immediately be given. Monitoring should be instituted (pulse oximetry, noninvasive blood pressure, and ECG at a minimum); suction, oxygen, emergency drugs, and airway equipment should be checked as discussed above. An experienced assistant will be required to help. If there is a failed airway and ventilation is not possible at any point during the intubating attempt, a surgeon should be immediately available to perform a rigid bronchoscopy or a surgical technique.

It is prudent to avoid the use of bolus doses of sedatives. For sedation, incremental doses of IV midazolam and propofol administered via an infusion pump should be done slowly, to allow time for the onset of drug effect after changing or increasing dosages. Haste is strongly discouraged. It is less likely to lose the airway of a spontaneously breathing patient who is awake. If the patient becomes unconscious and apneic with the propofol infusion, it can be turned off and return of spontaneous ventilation should occur rapidly. It is a matter of personal preference to employ drug infusions instead of volatile agents for sedation or anesthesia for this procedure. Generally, infusions are easier to control than volatile agents, which can pollute the operating room environment. Additionally, it may be difficult to achieve a constant anesthetic concentration during the intubation procedure.

Fiberoptic intubation through the mouth without a guide to maintain the pediatric flexible fiberoptic bronchoscope (FFB) in the midline is difficult to achieve without practice. Some practitioners use an LMA to keep the FFB in the midline position. However, most find the nasal route much easier, since the tip of the bronchoscope usually emerges in the pharynx in the midline just above the glottis. The nasal passages are dilated by passing increasingly larger diameter nasal trumpets, well lubricated with lidocaine jelly, every few minutes. The aim is to pass a trumpet slightly bigger than the proposed nasotracheal tube. As there is no contraindication to use cuffed tubes in pediatric patients, a smaller, cuffed tube is used to secure the airway of this patient.[15] Gentleness cannot be over emphasized; bleeding from the nasal passages can turn an elective controlled procedure very rapidly into an emergency disaster. In the presence of blood in the airway, the FFB becomes virtually useless.

Some manufacturers (e.g., Karl Storz Endoscopy, CA) stiffen neonatal & pediatric bronchoscopes intended for intubation. Although bronchoscopes as small as 2.3 mm in diameter are available, the procedure is usually performed with a 3.0–3.5 mm tip diameter. The major disadvantage of pediatric and neonatal bronchoscopes is the small ineffective working channel for suctioning. Generally, the insufflation of oxygen is strongly discouraged due to the risk of gastric insufflation, perforation, and death.[16,17] However, some practitioners like to insufflate oxygen down the side port, at about half a liter a minute to blow secretions out of the way being extremely careful to regulate the flow of oxygen and never advance the bronchoscope unless under direct vision.

Before using the bronchoscope, it is important to confirm the correct functioning of the light source and the controls and to ensure that it is in focus. In the event one plans to inject local anesthetic through the working channel, 2–3 mL air flush is needed to flush the drug out of the distal lumen.

Once the nasal passages are dilated and anesthetized and the patient adequately sedated, a longitudinally split trumpet is placed in the naris of choice (the larger of the two). The bronchoscope is inserted through the split trumpet into the nasopharynx during the intubation. Once the bronchoscope is placed into the trachea, the trumpet can be "peeled" off the bronchoscope so that the endotracheal tube (ETT) can be advanced over the bronchoscope. The process of repeated nasal trumpet insertion can be quite stimulating, and therefore, once the final, split trumpet has been passed and the patient is comfortable with it in place, the need for deeper sedation ought to be minimal.

An appropriately sized nasotracheal tube should be selected and loaded onto the FFB. The lumen of the ETT is lubricated with a silicon-based solution, rather than lubricating the FFB, as it becomes very difficult to manipulate once the FFB is lubricated.

Once the FFB is passed through the split nasal trumpet, the epiglottis and then the cords can be visualized in the midline. Secretions can sometimes obscure the view. Manipulation of the FFB or the trumpet can be employed to position the tip of the FFB over the glottis. With a spontaneously breathing patient, regular movement of the airway may help to guide one in the right direction. If the patient is cooperative, one can ask the patient to stick out their tongue, or ask an assistant to gently pull the tongue forward with a gauze. This serves to open the hypopharynx, which often will help expose the cords. Alternatively, a gentle jaw thrust in a drowsy patient will also help to elevate the tongue and epiglottis.[18–23]

At this point, 0.5–1.0 mL of 1% or 2% lidocaine can be instilled through the working channel onto the cords to allow easy passage of the FFB between the cords, followed by the nasotracheal tube. In some situations, particularly if violent coughing occurs, a small bolus of propofol can be administered rapidly by an assistant to facilitate the advancement of the ETT. The FFB is then removed and general anesthesia is induced. The FFB can also be used to confirm placement of the tube above the carina.

The nasal route is not always available, either due to anatomical difficulties or surgical considerations. In this case, the oral route may be used. While the nebulized lidocaine often adequately anesthetizes the nasal passages of children, oral topical anesthesia is often inadequate using this technique. Persuading a 6 year old child to gargle lidocaine may work in selected patients. Attention to the cumulative dose of local anesthetic used is important. Applying lidocaine jelly to the tongue slowly and progressively with a tongue depressor may also be effective. In an awake child, eliminating the gag reflex may be achieved by one quick squirt of local anesthetic on the uvula, which can be achieved with patience.

Passing an appropriately sized LMA has been shown to facilitate oral fiberoptic intubation.[24–30] Prior to starting the procedure, the following needs to take place.

Lubricate the inside of the LMA shaft with a silicon spray. Find an ETT that fits the lumen of the LMA. Because there are a number of manufacturers, it is difficult in a chapter such as this to publish size guidelines since outer diameters of ETTs vary from manufacturer to manufacturer. A standard ETT may be of insufficient length. In this event, the following "work around" is advised. Obtain a second, identical tube. Take the tube connector of one of the tubes and cut the shaft off the connector as close as possible to the hub. This short (about 1–2 cm) connector can be used to join the two ETTs together back to back, giving you one long ETT (Figure 46-1).[31] Since it is very slightly thickened at the joint,

make sure that this new tube will fit through the LMA/FFB combination. Alternatively, a long Microlaryngeal Tube (Rusch Inc., Duluth, GA) can be used for fiberoptic intubation through an LMA. It is reasonable to advance the ETT blindly into the trachea through the LMA and then use the FFB to confirm placement. Once the ETT is in place, the LMA may be withdrawn over the elongated tube without extubating the patient. This works for both regular tubes and RAE (Ring, Aldair & Elwyn) preformed tubes and can even be done with a cuffed tube, provided that you "load" the LMA from the distal end with the balloon and pilot tube of the cuff protruding from the distal end of the LMA.

Cobra manufactures a disposable perilaryngeal airway that comes in pediatric sizes. It operates and is placed in a similar fashion to the LMA Classic™. Its major advantage as a guide for oral fiberoptic intubation is that the bore of the shaft is wider than that of the LMA, thus allowing the easier passage of the fiberscope and accompanying ETT.

46.4.4 What if a fiberoptic intubation cannot be accomplished?

In the event that the fiberoptic intubation cannot be achieved in a child with a difficult airway, a tracheotomy in a spontaneously breathing anesthetized patient may be the best course of action, and is quite commonly done.[32]

SUMMARY

Congenital anomalies associated with CS often present a difficult airway for anesthesia practitioners. In cases that are known to be difficult airways, the relationship between surgeon and anesthesia practitioner is important from the communication and patient-management perspective. In this particular case, the patient was known to have a difficult intubation and the practitioner is prepared to manage the airway with sedation, topical anesthesia, and fiberoptic intubation through the nose. Reassurance, adequate sedation, adequate topical anesthesia, and a gentle technique are crucial attributes to success. The use of an extraglottic device, such as LMA, as a conduit to fiberoptic intubation is an important adjunct as oral fiberoptic intubation guides used in adults may not be suitable for children.

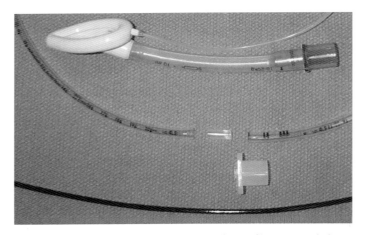

FIGURE 46-1. The equipment needed to perform a fiberoptic-guided intubation through an LMA. A tube connector is created by cutting the shaft off the connector from a similar size ETT. This short connector can then be used to join the two endotracheal tubes together back to back, thus providing a sufficiently long endotracheal tube to pass through the LMA. *(Reproduced permission, from Muraika L, Heyman JS, Shevchenko Y: Fiberoptic tracheal intubation through a laryngeal mask airway in a child with Treacher Collins syndrome. Anesth Analg. 2003;97:1298–1299)*

REFERENCES

1. Crouzon and Aprert Syndrome. Available at: www.kidsplastsurg.com/crouzon.html.
2. Exar EN, Collop NA: The upper airway resistance syndrome. *Chest.* 1999;115:1127–1139.
3. Guilleminault C, Khramtsov A: Upper airway resistance syndrome in children: a clinical review. *Semin Pediatr Neurol.* 2001;8:207–215.
4. Guilleminault C, Pelayo R: Sleep-disordered breathing in children. *Ann Med.* 1998;30:350–356.
5. Guilleminault C, Pelayo R, Leger D, Clerk A, Bocian RC: Recognition of sleep-disordered breathing in children. *Pediatrics.* 1996;98:871–882.
6. Guilleminault C, Stoohs R, Skrobal A, Labanowski M, Simmons J: Upper airway resistance in infants at risk for sudden infant death syndrome. *J Pediatr.* 1993;122:881–886.
7. Hasan N, Fletcher EC: Upper airway resistance syndrome. *J Ky Med Assoc.* 1998;96:261–263.

8. Marcus CL, Katz ES, Lutz J, et al.: Upper airway dynamic responses in children with the obstructive sleep apnea syndrome. *Pediatr Res*. 2005;57:99–107.

9. Koh JL, Harrison D, Myers R, et al.: A randomized, double-blind comparison study of EMLA and ELA-Max for topical anesthesia in children undergoing intravenous insertion. *Paediatr Anaesth*. 2004;14:977–982.

10. Khalil SN, Vije HN, Kee SS, et al.: A paediatric trial comparing midazolam(Syrpalta mixture with premixed midazolam syrup (Roche). *Paediatr Anaesth*. 2003;13:205–209.

11. Cravero JP, Beach M, Dodge CP, Whalen K: Emergence characteristics of sevoflurane compared to halothane in pediatric patients undergoing bilateral pressure equalization tube insertion. *J Clin Anesth*. 2000;12:397–401.

12. Soh CR, Ng AS: Laryngeal mask airway insertion in paediatric anaesthesia: comparison between the reverse and standard techniques. *Anaesth Intensive Care*. 2001;29:515–519.

13. Bagshaw O: The size 1.5 laryngeal mask airway (LMA) in paediatric anaesthetic practice. *Paediatr Anaesth*. 2002;12:420–423.

14. Klimscha W, Chiari A, Michalek-Sauberer A, et al.: The efficacy and safety of a clonidine/bupivacaine combination in caudal blockade for pediatric hernia repair. *Anesth Analg*. 1998;86:54–61.

15. Newth CJ, Rachman B, Patel N, Hammer J: The use of cuffed versus uncuffed endotracheal tubes in pediatric intensive care. *J Pediatr*. 2004;144:333–337.

16. Hershey MD, Hannenberg AA: Gastric distention and rupture from oxygen insufflation during fiberoptic intubation. *Anesthesiology*. 1996;85:1479–1480.

17. Ovassapian A, Mesnick PS: Oxygen insufflation through the fiberscope to assist intubation is not recommended. *Anesthesiology*. 1997;87:183–184.

18. Aoyama K, Takenaka I, Nagaoka E, Kadoya T: Jaw thrust maneuver for endotracheal intubation using a fiberoptic stylet. *Anesth Analg*. 2000;90:1457–1458.

19. Durga VK, Millns JP, Smith JE: Manoeuvres used to clear the airway during fibreoptic intubation. *Br J Anaesth*. 2001;87:207–211.

20. Schwartz D, Johnson C, Roberts J: A maneuver to facilitate flexible fiberoptic intubation. *Anesthesiology*. 1989;71:470–471.

21. Stacey MR, Rassam S, Sivasankar R, Hall JE, Latto IP: A comparison of direct laryngoscopy and jaw thrust to aid fibreoptic intubation. *Anaesthesia*. 2005;60:445–448.

22. Stella JP, Kageler WV, Epker BN: Fiberoptic endotracheal intubation in oral and maxillofacial surgery. *J Oral Maxillofac Surg*. 1986;44:923–925.

23. Uzun L, Ugur MB, Altunkaya H, et al.: Effectiveness of the jaw-thrust maneuver in opening the airway: a flexible fiberoptic endoscopic study. *ORL J Otorhinolaryngol Relat Spec*. 2005;67:39–44.

24. Benumof JL: A new technique of fiberoptic intubation through a standard LMA. *Anesthesiology*. 2001;95:1541.

25. Choi JE, Leal YR, Johnson MD: Fiberoptic intubation through the laryngeal mask airway. *J Clin Anesth*. 1996;8:687–688.

26. Ianchulev SA: Through-the-LMA fiberoptic intubation of the trachea in a patient with an unexpected difficult airway. *Anesth Analg*. 2005;101:1882–1883.

27. Johr M, Berger TM: Fiberoptic intubation through the laryngeal mask airway (LMA) as a standardized procedure. *Paediatr Anaesth*. 2004;14:614.

28. Talke PO, Nguyen H: Concept for easy fiberoptic intubation via a laryngeal airway mask. *Anesth Analg*. 1999;88:228–229.

29. Weiss M, Gerber AC, Schmitz A: Continuous ventilation technique for laryngeal mask airway (LMA) removal after fiberoptic intubation in children. *Paediatr Anaesth*. 2004;14:936–940.

30. Yilmaz AS, Gurkan Y, Toker K, Solak M: Laryngeal mask airway-guided fiberoptic tracheal intubation in a 1,200-gm infant with difficult airway. *Paediatr Anaesth*. 2005;15:1147–1148.

31. Muraika L, Heyman JS, Shevchenko Y: Fiberoptic tracheal intubation through a laryngeal mask airway in a child with Treacher Collins syndrome. *Anesth Analg*. 2003;97:1298–1299.

32. Sculerati N, Gottlieb MD, Zimbler MS, Chibbaro PD, McCarthy JG: Airway management in children with major craniofacial anomalies. *Laryngoscope*. 1998;108:1806–1812.

SELF-EVALUATION QUESTIONS

46.1. All of the following statements regarding fiberoptic intubation of the child are true **EXCEPT:**

A. The nasal route is usually easier than the oral route.

B. General anesthesia is not usually successful.

C. Inhaled anesthetic agents for sedation are preferred over IV agents in a child because starting an IV is so difficult.

D. An LMA may be used as a conduit for intubation.

E. Extreme caution needs to be taken if oxygen is to be insufflated down the scope to blow secretions away.

46.2. Pediatric fiberoptic bronchoscopes—all of the following are true **EXCEPT:**

A. are generally between 2.3 and 3.5 mm tip diameter

B. are often stiffened to permit intubation

C. have working channels that are very effective

D. are generally 500–600 mm in length

E. are more easily damaged than adult scopes because they are so small

46.3. When using an LMA as a guide to fiberoptic intubation the most significant problem one encounters in a child is

A. it is difficult to seal LMAs in children

B. the upper airway is too difficult to anesthetize to accept an LMA

C. the LMA flips the epiglottis down, and therefore you cannot get "under" it with a fiberscope

D. the lumen of the LMA is too small to pass a cuffed ETT through

E. standard ETTs are too short for this technique

CHAPTER 47

Pediatric Patient with a Closed Head Injury

Robert C. Luten, Niranjan "Tex" Kissoon, and Michael F. Murphy

47.1 CASE PRESENTATION

A 6 year old boy is brought to the emergency department (ED) by Emergency Medical Services (EMS) following an automobile crash with blunt trauma to the head, chest, and possible cervical-spine (C-spine) injury. The paramedic team reports that the child was an unrestrained front-seat passenger and was retained inside the vehicle. The driver was killed in the accident. No other information is available.

Upon arriving at the ED his vital signs were temperature 36°C, heart rate 96 beats per minute, noisy breathing with a respiration rate of 22 breaths per minute, and blood pressure of 106/86 mm Hg. His oxygen saturation is 89% on a non-rebreathing oxygen face mask. The Glasgow Coma Score (GCS) is 6. The C-spine is immobilized in a collar and paramedics are assisting the patient's respirations. The patient is estimated to be 3' 6" (100 cm) tall and weighs approximately 66 lb (30 kg).

47.2 INITIAL MANAGEMENT

47.2.1 How should the airway of this child be managed in the field?

Airway management in the field is discussed in detail in Chapter 13 and the reader is referred to that discussion. Although this is a child, the general principles in managing the airway of this patient in the field remain unchanged. After scene safety, airway is the most important initial factor to be considered and managed.

47.2.2 What are the evaluation and management priorities in this patient and where does "airway" fit?

For the most part, pediatric trauma victims do not present primarily with injuries to the airway itself, as in this case. This child has serious injuries, although airway management is particularly urgent due to head trauma.

The most important management priorities in patients with severe head injury are hypotension and hypoxia. Several issues emerge as concurrent and perhaps complicating priorities:

- The risk of C-spine injury. However, it is known that maintenance of in-line stabilization before, during, and after airway management in the C-spine injured patient prevents neurologic injury.[1–4]

- The potential for hemodynamic instability in the face of other multisystem injuries.[5–8] The resilience of the pediatric cardiovascular system may conceal substantial hypovolemia, although tachycardia may herald it and modify later decisions regarding the use and dosing of pretreatment (e.g., fentanyl) and induction agents (e.g., propofol).

- A full stomach and, in particular, acute gastric dilation, a condition that is a significant risk factor for regurgitation and aspiration. Furthermore, gastric dilation can reduce lung compliance (a restrictive lung defect).[8,9]

- The ability to rapidly gain vascular access. This is not so much a problem beyond the age of 5 as it is in younger infants and children. Lack of access constrains the options available for the airway practitioner if intravenous medications are required.

- The issue of "cognitive load" (mental burden experienced by the airway practitioner) consistent with pediatric resuscitations where drug dosing and equipment selection are not as "automatic" as in the adult.[10]
- The "angst in the room" factor that attends all pediatric resuscitations and has the potential to lead to performance deterioration.[11]

Because of their size, unique anatomy, and resilient physiology, pediatric trauma patients present special challenges that require unique solutions. As with adults, airway evaluation and management are often done concurrently with other activities that are directed toward other life and death priorities.

47.3   AIRWAY MANAGEMENT

47.3.1   Is active airway intervention required in this case?

The first question to be answered is whether or not this patient requires intubation. For the following reasons, the answer is "yes":

- Hypoxemia, as demonstrated by low oxygen saturation in spite of supplemental oxygen.
- The GCS of 6 implies the need for airway protection, and the possible management of hypercarbia.
- This patient will require multisystem evaluation, including CT diagnostic imaging, potential transfer depending on local policies, and airway patency and protection must be assured throughout.

The priority of airway in the Airway, Breathing, and Circulation (ABC) schema means that the airway must be immediately managed. In practice, this means that the airway practitioner physically positions themselves at the head of the patient and begin the process of denitrogenation, ordinarily with a bag-mask unit. In the event that this unconscious child is breathing spontaneously, the airway practitioner should coordinate ventilatory support with the child's respiratory efforts, being careful not to inflate the stomach. A methodical evaluation of the airway, including the potential for "difficult airway" may now be carried out.

The airway of a 6 year old child is anatomically in transition to the adult form. Fortunately, being well beyond the age of 2, most of the structures will be similar to those at the adult by this age.

47.3.2   What challenges do we face in managing this child's airway?

This patient does not have a "crash airway" (see Chapter 2, Figure 2-3) so immediate intubation is not indicated. The next priority is evaluating the patient for a potential difficulty airway and the suitability of rapid sequence induction (RSI) for this patient. The mnemonics introduced in Chapter 1 are designed to guide the evaluation of the airway in such a way that important features indicating potential difficulty are not missed. Though specific elements of the mnemonics may be less valid in children, the principles are the same. Employing the strategies for evaluating the airway for difficulty presented in Chapter 1:

- Will bag-mask-ventilation (BMV) of this patient be difficult (MOANS, see Section 1.6.1)? The potential for C-spine injury hinders ones ability to place the head in the sniffing position, the best position for BMV in a child. However, at the age of 6 this is unlikely to be crucial. Mask-seal ought not to be difficult and obstruction of the upper airway is not anticipated. The degree of obstruction offered by the relatively large tongue of the infant is not an issue in a 6 year old, and even so a large or obstructing tongue can be overcome by oral or nasal airways. Obviously, this patient is not aged (older than 55), is not edentulous, and is not stiff (increased resistance or reduced pulmonary compliance), though the potential for acute gastric dilation influencing thoracic compliance must be evaluated. So, evaluation using MOANS does not indicate any difficulties with BMV.

- Will the insertion of an extraglottic device (EGD) be difficult (RODS, see Section 1.6.3)? Mouth opening is not anticipated to be restricted, although head and neck immobilization, particularly with the patient in a cervical collar, is known to hinder mouth opening. Airway obstruction at or above the glottis is not suspected. There is no airway distortion to prevent a seal with the SGD, though the inability to move the neck may hinder seal characteristics of an LMA. Stiffness was evaluated with MOANS.

- Will a surgical airway be difficult (SHORT, see Section 1.6.4)? A 6 year old has such a small cricothyroid space that the surgical procedure of choice will be a transtracheal cannulation rather than an open cricothyrotomy as in the adult. The transtracheal catheter may be ventilated with a bag-mask unit (usually recommended in those less than age 5 or with a jet ventilation device attached to a wall outlet with the initial pressure reduced to 20 pounds per square inch). Alternatively, an ENK Flow Modulator (Cook Critical Care®, see Chapter 55 for contact information) attached to a wall flowmeter at 15 L·min^{-1} may be employed. This particular patient does not appear to have any potential problems with a surgical airway as he has not had prior neck surgery, has no hematoma or infection over the anterior neck, is not obese or otherwise structured to hinder access to the anterior neck, obstructed at or below the glottis, has never had radiation therapy, and has no tumor in the airway.

- Will it be difficult to perform laryngoscopy or intubation in this patient (LEMON, see Section 1.6.2)? Examination of the patient ('looking') reveals no gross features that might predict a difficult laryngoscopy or intubation. The evaluation (3-3-2) of the geometry of his airway and the position of his larynx is normal. Mouth opening is adequate, though one is unable to evaluate a Mallampati score. There is no upper airway obstruction. The neck (C-spine) is of concern, though not of sufficient concern that an awake intubation is indicated. Thus, in the absence of a difficult airway, the decision is made to proceed with an RSI as per Figure 2-3 in Chapter 2 with Plan A being RSI, Plan B is an EGD such as an LMA. The use of the Combitube™ for this patient would not be appropriate as the patient has yet to reach 48 inches (approximately 120 cm) in height. Plan C is a transtracheal approach.

47.3.3 How exactly does one proceed with an RSI in this patient?

Reflecting the previous discussion, several factors will influence how an RSI is accomplished:

- This patient has an acute severe head injury with the potential for elevated intracranial pressure (ICP).
- Prior to "clearing" the C-spine for instability by appropriate radiologic procedures, in-line stabilization is provided by a trained individual dedicated to this task and this task alone.
- A full stomach is suspected, as is the possibility of acute gastric dilation.
- Hemodynamic instability is suspected due to findings as stated.

Preparation

Equipment for Plans A, B, and C are assembled and tested. Drugs are drawn up as per the Broselow-Luten System® (Vital Signs, Inc., Totowa, NJ). A functional suction is critically important in this case and should be ready at hand.

Denitrogenation

Bag-mask assisted ventilation on high flow oxygen is already underway.

Pretreatment

Three minutes before the expected time of succinylcholine injection, 1.5 mg·kg^{-1} or 45 mg of lidocaine is injected to attenuate the rise of ICP, although its use is controversial.[12–15] Fentanyl is specifically omitted as hemodynamic instability is suspected. Defasiculation with a nondepolarizing neuromuscular blocking (NMB) agent is omitted as the child is less than 10 years of age. Although atropine may be considered in order to attenuate bradycardia associated with the use of succinylcholine, it is held since venous access is established and allows for rapid administration if needed; furthermore, the use of atropine may confound the heart rate as an indicator of hemodynamic instability. In-line stabilization is maintained.

Induction and Paralysis

Because of the suspicion of hemodynamic instability, a reduced dose of etomidate from 0.3 mg·kg^{-1} to 0.2 mg·kg^{-1} or 6 mg is selected as the induction agent and is administered rapidly as a bolus dose. Ketamine 1 mg·kg^{-1} could be employed so long as ventilation is assisted and PaCO$_2$ controlled. Succinylcholine 1.5 mg·kg^{-1} or 50 mg is administered rapidly after the induction agent is injected. Unlike the induction agent, the dose of the NMB agent is never tailored to the hemodynamic status.

Protection Against Aspiration

Cricoid pressure is applied[16] once the child is anesthetized with care taken to:

- avoid stimulation of gag during induction,
- avoid cervical spinal motion,
- not obstruct or deform the relatively compliant airway of the child.

Although BMV in this child is risky due to the potential for gastric insufflation and regurgitation, there is little choice but to perform careful bag-mask breathing in order to maintain normal oxigen saturation as well as arterial carbon dioxide levels and not to compromise ICP.

Placement of the Endotracheal Tube

With in-line stabilization of the C-spine, the placement of the endotracheal tube (ETT) is performed under direct laryngoscopy as delicately and atraumatically as possible to attenuate rises in blood pressure, heart rate, and ICP. Tracheal tube placement is confirmed with end-tidal carbon dioxide detection and a complete clinical evaluation, including auscultation. Immediately after intubation, the blood pressure is taken and if it is elevated beyond 140/90 mm Hg, managed with small bolus doses of propofol (5 mg) or midazolam (1 mg). Hypotension is managed with rapid volume infusion, up to 20 mL·kg^{-1} of balanced salt solution.

It is the practice of the authors that if the endotracheal tube is inadvertently placed in the esophagus, one of the following two maneuvers is indicated depending on the oxygen saturation:

- Oxygen saturation greater than 90—move the esophageal ETT to the left corner of the mouth and attempt reintubation.
- Oxygen saturation less than 90—quickly inflate the balloon of the ETT with as much air as it will take without breaking (ordinarily 5–15 mL depending on the size of the ETT). Compress the epigastrium to empty as much air and liquid stomach contents as possible. Deflate the balloon and remove the ETT while suctioning the hypopharynx. Perform BMV to recover the saturations and attempt orotracheal intubation.

If at any point oxygen saturation becomes unacceptable and cannot be corrected, by definition a failed airway has occurred and the appropriate algorithm should be applied.

Postintubation Management

Maintaining hemodynamic stability with acceptable blood gases (PaCO$_2$ 35–40 mm Hg) should now become a priority in this patient. Neuromuscular blockade ought to be continued using longer acting nondepolarizing agents such as rocuromium (0.6 mg·kg^{-1}), vecuronium (0.1 mg·kg^{-1}), or pancuronium (0.1 mg·kg^{-1}). Sedation with bolus doses of midazolam 0.5–1 mg/dose will be required from time to time and the need for this is ordinarily indicated by rising heart rate and blood pressure. Opioids such as fentanyl 1 μg·kg^{-1} may be necessary if pain is suspected. In either case, one must pay particular attention to the effect of small doses of sedative hypnotics and opioids on the hemodynamic stability of the patient. Gastric decompression using an orogastric or nasogastric tube is indicated.

47.3.4 What if the trachea cannot be intubated after three attempts?

This situation constitutes a failed airway. There are two types of failed airways:

- A situation in which three attempts at conventional intubation have failed but gas exchange is possible and saturations acceptable (e.g., BMV or EGD such as an LMA). This is a "can't-intubate, can-ventilate-have-time" situation. In this situation, there is time to use alternative nonsurgical techniques, such as the light-wand and flexible fiberoptic bronchoscope, despite the risk of regurgitation and aspiration.

- A situation in which neither intubation nor ventilation is possible. This is a "can't-intubate, can't-ventilate-have-no-time" situation in which a surgical airway must be performed. In this case, an LMA may be attempted as preparations are made to insert a transtracheal catheter, but not *instead of preparing* to insert one, i.e., these activities are concurrent not sequential.

47.4 SUMMARY

A child with an acute, severe head injury is a common indication for emergency tracheal intubation. While airway protection and blood gas management are the top priorities, many other factors impact decisions about airway management. These include the stability of the C-spine, elevated intracranial pressure, hemodynamic stability, and the presence of an acute gastric dilation. Because there is often a need to manage multiple problems in these patients, attention to detail is be crucial.

Given the emotional atmosphere that can surround the resuscitation of a child, there is a risk of practitioners getting sidetracked by concurrent confounding issues. Therefore, a planned, methodical, and disciplined approach to airway evaluation and management in the injured child is important.

REFERENCES

1. Holley J, Jorden R: Airway management in patients with unstable cervical spine fractures. *Ann Emerg Med.* 1989;18:1237–1239.
2. Ghafoor AU, Martin TW, Gopalakrishnan S, Viswamitra S: Caring for the patients with cervical spine injuries: what have we learned? *J Clin Anesth.* 2005;17:640–649.
3. Ollerton JE, Parr MJ, Harrison K, Hanrahan B, Sugrue M: Potential cervical spine injury and difficult airway management for emergency intubation of trauma adults in the emergency department—a systematic review. *Emerg Med J.* 2006;23:3–11.
4. Crosby E: Airway management after upper cervical spine injury: what have we learned? *Can J Anaesth.* 2002;49:733–744.
5. Schiff JS, Moore B, Louie J: Pediatric trauma—unique considerations in evaluating and treating children. *Minn Med.* 2005;88:46–51.
6. Morgan WM, 3rd, O'Neill JA, Jr: Hemorrhagic and obstructive shock in pediatric patients. *New Horiz* 1998;6:150–154.
7. Kirk JA: Pediatric trauma. *CRNA* 1997;8:135–143.
8. Jambor CR, Steedman DJ: Acute gastric dilation after trauma. *J R Coll Surg Edinb.* 1991;36:29–31.
9. Cogbill TH, Bintz M, Johnson JA, Strutt PJ: Acute gastric dilatation after trauma. *J Trauma* 1987;27:1113–1117.
10. Luten R, Wears RL, Broselow J, et al.: Managing the unique size-related issues of pediatric resuscitation: reducing cognitive load with resuscitation aids. *Acad Emerg Med.* 2002;9:840–847.
11. Lawton L: Paediatric trauma—the care of Anthony. *Accid Emerg Nurs.* 1995;3: 172–176.
12. Nakayama DK, Waggoner T, Venkataraman ST, et al.: The use of drugs in emergency airway management in pediatric trauma. *Ann Surg.* 1992;216: 205–211.
13. Bozeman WP, Idris AH: Intracranial pressure changes during rapid sequence intubation: a swine model. *J Trauma.* 2005;58:278–283.
14. Yano M, Nishiyama H, Yokota H, et al.: Effect of lidocaine on ICP response to endotracheal suctioning. *Anesthesiology.* 1986;64:651–653.
15. Robinson N, Clancy M: In patients with head injury undergoing rapid sequence intubation, does pretreatment with intravenous lignocaine/lidocaine lead to an improved neurological outcome? A review of the literature. *Emerg Med J.* 2001;18:453–457.
16. Stoddart PA, Brennan L, Hatch DJ, Bingham R: Postal survey of paediatric practice and training among consultant anaesthetists in the UK. *Br J Anaesth.* 1994;73:559–563.

SELF-EVALUATION QUESTIONS

47.1. Airway management in a child with acute severe head injury needs to respect all of the following **EXCEPT**

   A. the potential for raised ICP

   B. the potential for unrecognized hemodynamic instability exists

   C. that managing hypotension takes precedence over intubation

   D. in-line stabilization of the C-spine before, during, and after intubation is crucial

   E. acute gastric dilation is common in injured children

47.2. Rapid Sequence Intubation in a 6 year old with an acute severe head injury should include all of the following **EXCEPT**

   A. pretreatment with lidocaine

   B. pretreatment with fentanyl

   C. cricoid pressure

   D. augmented ventilation through the process

   E. succinylcholine 1.5 mg·kg^{-1}

47.3. You have attempted an RSI on a 6 year old with an acute severe head injury and have failed to intubate on the first attempt. The oxygen saturations have fallen to the mid-80s and BMV is not helping. What is the next most appropriate thing to do?

   A. attempt intubation two more times

   B. quickly attempt a nasal fiberoptic intubation

   C. attempt to insert a Combitube™

   D. move directly to a transtracheal approach

   E. try an LMA, and if that is not successful move to a Trachlight™

CHAPTER (48)

What Is Unique About the Obstetrical Airway?

Brian K. Ross

48.1 INTRODUCTION

The ability to maintain a patient's airway, provide adequate ventilation, and place an endotracheal tube remains a major concern for airway practitioners. There is no location that produces more anxiety in this regard than labor and delivery. Obstetrical anesthesia is a high-risk practice that is replete with medicolegal liability and laden with clinical challenges. On the obstetric service, the practitioner is required to provide safe anesthesia care to two patients, mother and baby, both of whom have unique and demanding anatomical and physiological requirements. The purpose of this chapter is to briefly review the status of maternal morbidity/mortality, highlight the principal reasons that airways of parturients might be difficult to manage, and propose an algorithm for the management of the obstetrical airway.

Underpinning all discussion is the critical importance of being prepared cognitively for the unexpected occurrence and being facile with appropriate emergency airway equipment. Of equal importance is teamwork between the anesthesia practitioner, the labor and delivery nurses, and the obstetrician. Practicing difficult airway scenarios is invaluable. Being unprepared will certainly guarantee failure.

48.2 MATERNAL MORBIDITY AND MORTALITY

48.2.1 Discuss anesthetic-related morbidity and mortality of parturients

Women continue to experience preventable pregnancy-related deaths. Death due to anesthesia is the seventh leading cause of pregnancy-related mortality in the United States.[1] These anesthesia-related deaths are particularly catastrophic because many of these anesthetics are elective and are provided to young, otherwise well, mothers.

Hawkins and her colleagues characterized obstetrical anesthesia deaths in the United States by specific cause, relationship to the type of anesthetic and to the type of obstetrical procedure.[2] Most women who died from anesthesia complications were undergoing cesarean section delivery (82%), whereas only about 5% of the deaths were associated with vaginal deliveries. Women who died of complications of general anesthesia (52% of all maternal deaths) primarily died as a result of airway management problems, which included aspiration, intubation difficulties, and inadequate ventilation.

In 1985, a unique perspective on anesthesia morbidity and morality was unveiled by the institution of the American Society of Anesthesiologists Committee on Professional Liability Closed Claims Project. The data from this project are an accumulation of personal damage insurance claims filed against anesthesiologists and subsequently settled.[3] Of the nearly 6,500 cases in the database, 12% have been associated with obstetrical anesthesia care and nearly three fourths of these claims have been associated with cesarean section. Critical events involving the respiratory system were the most common precipitating events in the obstetrical files. Trauma from repeated attempts at intubation was recognized as an issue of particular hazard.

Obstetrical airway catastrophes occur most frequently during emergency cesarean sections. It is in these settings that regional anesthesia may not be possible because of either maternal condition or severe fetal distress. It is also in this setting that airway evaluation may be particularly hurried and harassed. Overall incidences of difficult obstetrical airway are low (7.9%)[4] but still greater than those in the non-obstetric patients (2.5%).[5] Bag-mask-ventilation (BMV) can be difficult or impossible in approximately 0.02% of parturients, an incidence not dissimilar to other surgical patients.[6]

The literature is unclear as to the actual incidence of failed intubation under general anesthesia in obstetrical patients. Ranges have been given from 1 in 283 to 1 in 2,130; however, a composite incidence of about 0.2%[7] to 0.4%[8] is a reasonable estimate. This is ten times more frequent than in the general surgical population and these numbers have not decreased over the last 10 years.

48.3   PARTURIENT AIRWAY

48.3.1   Why do parturients have more airway complications compared to the general population?

The parturient is at significantly greater risk for airway complications and difficult intubations than her nonpregnant counterpart.[9] A wide range of both anatomical and physiological changes occur during pregnancy and many of these can impact the airway directly or indirectly (Table 48-1). Many of the changes are hormonally driven and the gravid uterus has a significant impact on the respiratory, cardiovascular, and gastrointestinal systems. Finally, there are a number of abnormal pregnancy related processes that impact heavily on the parturient airway.

48.3.2   How do the physiological changes associated with pregnancy impact the airway of parturients?

The difficulties in airway management for obstetrical patients may be related to a number of factors.

48.3.2.1   Weight Gain

During pregnancy, average weight gain can be 12–20 kg over the parturient pre-pregnant weight. This weight gain is related to increases in total body water, interstitial fluid (generalized body edema), blood volume, deposition of new fat and protein, uterine size and contents, and enlargement of the breasts.

Over the past decade, obesity (BMI > 30 kg·m^{-2}) has been encountered much more frequently in the general population. BMV is often difficult in obese patients because of reduced chest compliance and increased intra-abdominal pressure. The incidence of partially obliterated oropharyngeal structures in obese parturients is double that of nonobese parturients.[4] In addition, weight gain may create a "short neck," a large tongue, and large breasts, all of which contribute to difficult laryngoscopy. In the morbidly obese parturient (greater than 140 kg or ~300 lbs, BMI ≥ 40 kg·m^{-2}), the risks for diabetes, hypertension, preeclampsia, and primary cesarean delivery are all increased. There is also a higher incidence of difficult labor resulting in instrumental deliveries, postpartum hemorrhage, or other conditions that require anesthetic intervention.[10]

TABLE 48-1

Factors Affecting Management of the Parturient Airway

Weight gain (12–20 kg)	• Enlarging gravid uterus • Increasing total body water and interstitial fluid • Increasing blood volume • Deposition of new fat • Enlargement of the breasts
Respiratory system	• Decrease in respiratory reserve volume • Decrease in functional residual capacity (20–30%) • Increased oxygen consumption • More rapid desaturation
Airway	• Increased oral, nasal, pharyngeal, and tracheal mucosal edema • Vascular engorgement of oral, pharyngeal, and nasal capillaries • Edema of face and neck • Advancement of Mallampati classification with pregnancy • Advancement of Mallampati classification with bearing down during labor
Cardiovascular system	• Inferior caval syndrome (supine hypotensive syndrome) requiring left uterine tilt
Gastrointestinal system	• Steadily increasing intragastric pressure as pregnancy progresses • Decreased lower esophageal sphincter tone due to increasing progesterone • Symptomatic gastroesophageal reflux • Distortion of gastric anatomy • Increased gastric acidity

Morbidly obese parturients are at increased risks for anesthesia-related complications during cesarean delivery and increased risks for failed intubation and gastric aspiration if general anesthesia is required.[11] The cesarean section rate in these patients can exceed 50% with one-third of attempted tracheal intubations being difficult and 6% being failures.[12] On reviewing the ASA closed claims obstetrical files, it was found that damaging events related to the respiratory system were significantly more common among obese (32%) than among nonobese (7%) parturients.[13]

48.3.2.2 Respiratory Changes

Respiratory changes during pregnancy are of special significance to the anesthesia practitioner. Over the course of a normal gestation, the parturient experiences a 30–60% increase in oxygen consumption because of the metabolic demands of the growing fetus, uterus, and placenta. This, in combination with a reduction in functional residual capacity (FRC) which begins to decline as early as the fifth month and is reduced to 80% of nonpregnant values by term, invites exceedingly rapid desaturation with apnea. The tendency toward rapid desaturation is further aggravated by the supine position.

Displacement of abdominal contents toward the chest as a result of the enlarged uterus causes a reduction in FRC and premature airway closure with widening of the alveolar–arterial oxygen gradient. As a result of these changes, oxygenation of the mother and fetus are compromised if difficult BMV is encountered or attempts at intubation are prolonged or failed.[14]

48.3.2.3 Airway Changes

As mentioned, generalized edema seen in pregnancy may affect the oropharynx, nasopharynx, and trachea. These changes are aggravated by elevated estrogen levels that stimulate the development of mucosal edema and hypervascularity in the upper airways. Capillary engorgement of the nasal and oropharyngeal mucosa begins early in the first trimester and increases progressively throughout pregnancy. Because of this capillary engorgement, the parturient frequently appears to have symptoms of upper respiratory infection and laryngitis, with nasal congestion and voice changes due to swelling of the false vocal cords and arytenoids. Nasal breathing often becomes difficult, potentially affecting the efficacy of BMV.

Edema of the pharyngeal and laryngeal structures, and vocal cords, can hinder visualization of the cords and passage of an endotracheal tube. Tongue edema may make retraction of the tongue into the mandibular space during laryngoscopy quite difficult. Hypervascularity dictates that manipulation of the upper airway be undertaken with extreme care. An endotracheal tube one size smaller than might be usual (i.e., 6–7 mm ID) should be routinely used. The increased engorgement and vascularity also demands cautious approach when manipulating the nasopharynx (nasal trumpets, nasogastric tubes) or when considering repeated attempts at intubation. Epistaxis, excessive bleeding and swelling of the upper airway, can quickly exacerbate a crisis when a difficult intubation is encountered.

Excessive weight gain and even mild upper respiratory tract infections, preeclampsia, fluid overload, and bearing down can all exacerbate airway edema leading to a severely compromised airway. The classical Mallampati classification (Samsoon and Young modification) of mouth opening has been reported to advance by one or two classes during pregnancy.[15] The Mallampati classification of a parturient has also been reported to change even further as a consequence of bearing down, due to progression of edema of the lower pharynx, not returning to the prelabor state for a further 12 hours postpartum.[16]

48.3.2.4 Cardiovascular Changes

The supine position in these patients may result in compression of the aorta, the inferior vena cava, or both by the enlarged pregnant uterus. Compression of the aorta decreases uterine blood flow, impairing fetal oxygenation. Vena caval compression decreases venous return, cardiac output, and ultimately uterine blood flow. A combination of respiratory desaturation and compromised cardiac output is particularly lethal for the pregnant mother. It is therefore imperative that the parturient be positioned with a wedge under the right hip, creating left lateral displacement of the uterus away from the great vessels. Unfortunately, such displacement may hinder the creation of an optimum position for intubation.

48.3.2.5 Gastrointestinal Changes

The risk of aspiration in the parturient impacts how the anesthesia practitioner approaches and manages the parturient's airway. Several factors increase the risk of aspiration in these patients. While intragastric pressure increases steadily during pregnancy, as the gravid uterus enlarges, a concomitant decrease in lower esophageal tone occurs as circulating levels of progesterone increase.

The enlarging uterus distorts esophageal and gastric anatomy. The cephalad pressure of the abdominal uterus decreases the obliquity with which the esophagus contacts the stomach, permitting reflux of gastric contents at lower than usual trans-sphincter pressures. Gastric emptying appears to be unaffected by pregnancy, though intestinal transit time and gastric acidity are increased. With the onset of labor, gastric emptying slows and may be further aggravated by the administration of opioids for labor pain management. Taken together, these gastrointestinal changes mandate that precautions be taken when a parturient undergoes general anesthesia. Such precautions pay dividends in the event that attempts to intubate are not immediately successful.

48.3.2.6 Obstetrical Factors

There are a number of comorbid obstetrical factors that put the parturient at risk for airway management difficulties and related complications. Most notable of these are hypertensive diseases of pregnancy that place the parturient at higher risk for difficult intubation. Pregnancy induced hypertension as well as its more serious partners, eclampsia and preeclampsia, aggravate mucosal and interstitial edema leading to difficult intubation.[17] Concomitant proteinuria with reduced intravascular plasma protein levels in preeclamptic patients leads to increased edema of the upper airway, an enlarged and less mobile tongue, and soft tissue deposition in the neck.

Preeclampsia is frequently accompanied by coagulopathy and edema, both of which may complicate repeated attempts at direct laryngoscopy because of increased tissue friability and upper airway bleeding. Airway and laryngeal edema can develop exceedingly rapidly in preeclamptic patients. Certainly, neck and face edema and dysphonia from uvular edema should alert the practitioner to the possibility of difficult intubation.[18] In these patients, extreme caution should be exercised not only on intubation but at the time of extubation as well.

Massive peripartum hemorrhage (e.g., placenta previa, accreta, abruption) and acute fetal distress (i.e., abruption, cord prolapse) are frequently encountered obstetrical emergencies occurring acutely and unannounced. The visual impact of profuse vaginal bleeding, or the slow ominous sound of the tocodynamometer with fetal distress, frequently pushes obstetricians and anesthesia practitioners to urgently proceed to general anesthesia, without taking the time to adequately assess the patient's airway. Most airway catastrophes occur when the difficult airway is not recognized before the induction of anesthesia. Endler et al. found that emergency surgery was implicated in up to 80% of maternal deaths with general anesthesia, and difficult or failed intubation was associated with 4 of 15 deaths.[11]

48.4　AIRWAY EVALUATION

48.4.1　Why is it important to assess the airway of each parturient?

Every pregnant patient admitted to the labor and delivery service must have a thorough preanesthetic evaluation. With the always-present risk of acute onset fetal distress, an essential and critical part of airway management is an accurate assessment of the patient's airway. Even in the most urgent situations, it is critical to take the time to go through a regimented process of airway assessment.

A detailed discussion of the airway examination and those predictors associated with management difficulties can be found in Chapter 1. Most predictive studies have been conducted on general surgical populations, not parturients. Some 20 factors predicting difficult laryngoscopic intubation have been identified. The obstetrical patient presents unique assessment challenges, often the most important being a pressure of time.

48.4.2　How do you assess the airway of a parturient? What are the predictors or risk factors of a difficult airway for a parturient?

The increasing use of regional anesthetic techniques for delivery has significantly decreased opportunity for research in patients undergoing general anesthesia. While parturients pose different airway challenges to anesthesia practitioners, assessment of the difficulties in using the four basic methods (BMV, the use of extraglottic devices (EGDs), tracheal intubation, and performing a surgical airway) to provide ventilation and oxygenation should not differ from that done for the nonobstetrical population.

48.4.2.1　Difficult Bag-Mask-Ventilation

As indicated above, BMV can be difficult to impossible in approximately 0.02% of parturients. However, this incidence is comparable to the general surgical patient.[6] While the mnemonic MOANS (see Section 1.6.1) is a helpful reminder of the five patient characteristics associated with difficult BMV,[19] many of these characteristics do not apply to the obstetrical population. For example, young and healthy pregnant women are typically not older than 55 years of age or edentulous, and they do not generally have facial hair.

48.4.2.2　Difficult Laryngoscopy and Tracheal Intubation

Although "Predictions of Difficult and Failed Airway" section in Chapter 1 discusses in detail the current evidence in assessing the predictors of difficult laryngoscopy and intubation (LEMON), it is appropriate to review these assessment tools in the obstetrical population. Dupont and colleagues conducted one of the early studies in the obstetrical population[20] in which they reported that the risk of difficult laryngoscopic intubation was eight times greater than that in the general surgical population. The literature suggests a variety of clinical signs that can be employed to help determine the degree of difficult laryngoscopic intubation (Table 48-2). However, none of these has a high positive predictive value as a single tool, particularly in the obstetrical patient. A number of studies suggest that although the presence of risk factors was useful, they were not as reliable as the Mallampati classification. Benumof has frequently suggested that a patient's relative tongue/pharyngeal size (Mallampati), degree of atlanto-occipital joint extension, and adequacy of the mandibular space provide the clinician with three easy-to-perform and accurate predictors of difficulty in laryngoscopic intubation.[21]

Rocke et al. conducted one of the sentinel studies specifically looking at the obstetrical population and difficult airway predictors.[4] They prospectively evaluated the airways of 1,500 parturients presenting for elective and emergency intubations. They found that a highly predictive sign for a difficult airway was a "neutral" to "extension" sternomental distance variation of less than 5 cm. In addition, the authors built a scale of predictive factors showing clearly that the greater the number of abnormal findings, the higher the prediction accuracy for a difficult intubation (Figure 48-1). The associated risk factors included short neck (SN), protruding maxillary incisors (PMI), receding mandible (RM), and Mallampati Class III and IV airways. The relative risk of experiencing a difficult intubation in comparison to an uncomplicated Class I airway assessment was as follows: Class II, 3.23; Class III, 7.58; Class IV, 11.3; SN, 5.01; RM, 9.71; and PMI, 8.0. Using the probability index, or combination of risk factors, Roche et al. showed that a combination of either Class III or IV, plus PMI, SN, and RM, correlated with a probability of difficult

TABLE 48-2

Features of the Airway Exam Useful in Predicting Difficult Laryngoscopy

In the parturient	• Mallampati Class III or IV • Limited thyromental distance • Short, thick neck • Limited mouth opening • Prominent incisors

Risk Factors

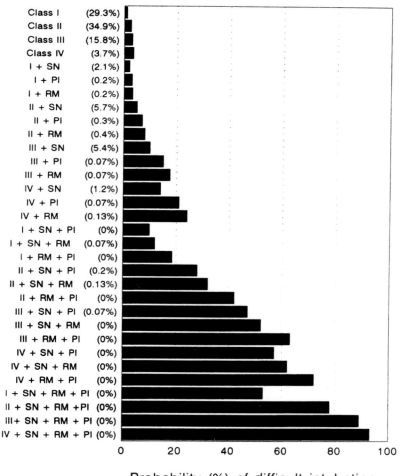

Risk factor	Incidence
Class I	(29.3%)
Class II	(34.9%)
Class III	(15.8%)
Class IV	(3.7%)
I + SN	(2.1%)
I + PI	(0.2%)
I + RM	(0.2%)
II + SN	(5.7%)
II + PI	(0.3%)
II + RM	(0.4%)
III + SN	(5.4%)
III + PI	(0.07%)
III + RM	(0.07%)
IV + SN	(1.2%)
IV + PI	(0.07%)
IV + RM	(0.13%)
I + SN + PI	(0%)
I + SN + RM	(0.07%)
I + RM + PI	(0%)
II + SN + PI	(0.2%)
II + SN + RM	(0.13%)
II + RM + PI	(0%)
III + SN + PI	(0.07%)
III + SN + RM	(0%)
III + RM + PI	(0%)
IV + SN + PI	(0%)
IV + SN + RM	(0%)
IV + RM + PI	(0%)
I + SN + RM + PI	(0%)
II + SN + RM + PI	(0%)
III + SN + RM + PI	(0%)
IV + SN + RM + PI	(0%)

Probability (%) of difficult intubation

FIGURE 48-1. The probability of experiencing a difficult laryngoscopic intubation for the varying combinations of risk factors and the observed incidence of these combinations. (*Reproduced with permission from Rocke D, Murray W, Rout C, et al.: Relative risk factors associated with difficult intubation in obstetric anesthesia.* Anesthesiology. 1992;77:67–73.)

laryngoscopy of >90%. It was interesting that neither facial edema nor swollen tongue was associated with difficult laryngoscopic intubation.

Overall, the mnemonic LEMON (see Section 1.6.2) examines almost all of the difficult laryngoscopic intubation characteristics discussed above (with the exception of the PMI) and remains a useful guide for the obstetrical population. It behooves all practitioners working on labor and delivery services to take the time necessary to evaluate for all of the predictors of difficult airway in parturients in every case.

In the obstetrical patient, features associated with airway management, obesity, and large pendulous breasts often compound problems. It is important that the parturient be assessed in the recumbent position with left uterine displacement. This is frequently omitted from the examination and this position can have considerable impact on the ease or difficulty of airway management. Adjustments in the patient's position can and should be made before induction of anesthesia to make intubating conditions easier, but there are limits to the extent that these

adjustments can be employed because of the positioning required to reduce aortocaval compression. In the morbidly obese parturient, elevations (i.e., ramping, see Figure 48-2 and Chapter 17) of the thorax, shoulders, and head may be necessary to bring the anatomical axes of the oral, pharyngeal, and laryngeal structures into alignment. Positioning on a ramp may also mitigate the problem of the laryngoscope handle abutting on the patient's chest.

48.4.2.3 Difficult Use of Extraglottic Devices

The use of an EGD is an important backup maneuver (Plan B) and it serves as a bridging attempt to reestablish gas exchange in a "can't intubate, can't ventilate" (CICV) setting while one prepares to perform a cricothyrotomy in parturients. One ought to have performed an evaluation for difficult EGD placement in all parturients. RODS (see Section 1.6.3) is a mnemonic that is intended to identify patients where the use of an EGD may be difficult.

48.4.2.4 Difficult Surgical Airway

While performing a surgical airway or cricothyrotomy in an obstetrical population is exceedingly rare, all parturients requiring a general anesthetic ought to have an assessment of the possibility of a difficult surgical airway. The mnemonic SHORT (see Section 1.6.4) can be used to quickly assess the patient for features that may indicate a difficult cricothyrotomy. Most obstetricians do not have experience in performing a surgical airway, nor do most anesthesia practitioners, although all must be competent in the performance of a surgical airway if indicated. Having said that, it may be prudent to consult with an experienced surgical colleague for assistance when a difficult airway is identified and a surgical airway is a possibility.

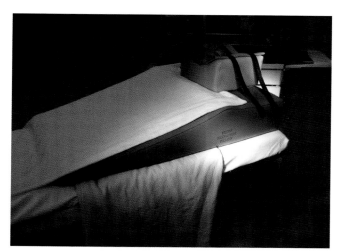

FIGURE 48-2. The Troop Elevation Pillow®: The pillow can help to raise the head and neck above the patient's chest and abdomen. The goal is to position the earlobes at the level of the angle of Louis. (*Reproduced with permission from Mercury Medical.*)

48.4.3 When a difficult laryngoscopy is anticipated in a parturient, is it useful to perform an awake direct laryngoscopy (an "awake look")?

Awake direct laryngoscopy with a topically anesthetized airway (i.e., "awake look") has been suggested as a useful assessment tool of the potentially difficult airway prior to induction of anesthesia. However, one must recognize that the airway as it appears with the patient awake and unparalyzed might look quite different with the patient under general anesthesia and with muscle paralysis (see Section 36.3.2).[22]

48.5 CONDUCT OF ANESTHESIA AND TRACHEAL INTUBATION

48.5.1 What are necessary preparations for general anesthesia for a parturient?

There are several preparations that must be made on the labor and delivery suite to ensure safe and expeditious care of the parturient should general anesthesia be required. The operating room bed should have a ramp on it at all times (see Figure 48-2 and Chapter 17). This will prove to be an invaluable aid in optimizing the head position and help align the oral, pharyngeal, and laryngeal axes in the obese parturient, and will not be problematic in the patient with easy tracheal intubation. It is important to have all difficult airway equipment in the operating room. It is also important to recognize the importance of having well-trained assistants to help with all aspects of airway management, including rescue devices as well as application of cricoid pressure. Because time is often of the essence and resources often limited, the practitioners must carefully choose devices with which they are familiar and comfortable and techniques that can be practiced regularly. Table 48-3 details some of the suggested equipment necessary to manage the difficult airway on the labor floor. A short laryngoscope handle ("stubby") can be particularly helpful.

All obstetrical patients requiring general anesthesia must receive aspiration prophylaxis (nonparticulate antacid, H_2 blocker). Induction must be in rapid sequence fashion, including the application of cricoid pressure. Recent work has shown that, even when correctly applied, cricoid pressure may not always be completely effective.[23] Nevertheless, it has the potential to convert a flood into a trickle.

Because the pregnant patient is at increased risk for hypoxemia even during short periods of apnea, it is especially important that adequate denitrogenation with 100% oxygen prior to the induction of general anesthesia is performed. Various techniques for denitrogenation have been advocated. Norris and Dewan observed that 3 minutes of denitrogenation and the four-breath denitrogenation technique resulted in similar measurements of PaO_2 in pregnant women undergoing rapid sequence induction of general anesthesia for cesarean section.[14] If the tidal volume is large and the respiratory rate is high, the duration of denitrogenation may need to be only 1 minute in duration. However, this 1 minute can be one of the most important minutes of the induction and should not be cut short.

48.5.2 Describe an appropriate algorithm for a difficult/failed intubation in a parturient

The Difficult Airway Algorithm in the parturient is significantly different from that used in the operating room for nonobstetrical surgical patients. In general, the differences focus on the presence or absence of fetal distress.

TABLE 48-3

Equipment Required for Management of Difficult OB Airway

Bed ramp	Troop pillow (see Figure 48–2)
Oral airway	3 sizes
Intubation guides	• Eschmann Tracheal Tube Introducer (Portex Limited, Hythe, U.K.); • Frova Intubation Introducer (Cook® Critical Care, Inc.,Bloomington, IN); • Lightwand
Endotracheal tubes	at least 3 different sizes (6.0, 6.5, 7.0 mm ID)
Laryngoscope	• MAC #3, #4; • Miller #2, #3, "stubby" short handle
LMA	• LMA Classic™ #3, #4; • LMA ProSeal™ #3, #4; • LMA Fastrach™ #3 ILA (intubating laryngeal airway)
Flexible fiberoptic bronchoscope	
Percutaneous cricothyrotomy kit	

TABLE 48-4

Important Points for Managing the Anticipated Difficult Obstetrical Airway

- Detailed discussions with the obstetrician concerning delivery plan
- "crash" induction is not an option
- speak to patient and family early in labor
- persist with regional techniques
- awake intubation if necessary—using a flexible fiberoptic bronchoscope
- "wishful thinking" is a poor anesthetic plan—*know* that your regional technique is working

Frequently, general anesthetics on the labor and delivery service are required in patients with whom the anesthesia practitioner has little or no foreknowledge. In addition, the environment is often chaotic with considerable pressure to proceed with an emergency induction because fetal viability is in question and fetal rescue is required. In such an event, it is imperative that the practitioner has a simple, clear algorithm to follow when a difficult airway is encountered. Equally important is that the practitioner regularly practices this algorithm with the labor and delivery personnel and that they are familiar with the airway devices that might be employed in an emergency.

48.5.2.1 Anticipated Difficult Airway

When the anesthesia practitioner anticipates a difficult airway, a regional anesthetic technique may be preferable (Table 48-4). However, there are numerous conditions that may preclude the use of regional anesthesia. When regional anesthesia is not possible, one of the first things that must occur is a thorough discussion with the obstetrician, the patient, the patient's family, and nurses, pointing out any airway management concerns that the anesthesia practitioner has. In some circumstances, the anesthesia practitioner ought to make it clear that the patient's airway management cannot be hurried, implying that a decision to go to surgery may need to be made earlier rather than later. The hope is that one is not pushed into a general anesthetic when more deliberate planning may have permitted a regional technique.

In those instances when regional anesthesia is contraindicated, an anticipated difficult airway is recognized, and if time permits, an awake intubation technique should be employed. Flexible fiberoptic bronchoscopy has become the method most frequently used. The specifics of this technique can be found in Chapter 8. However, there are several points that should be reiterated for the obstetrical patient. Because the parturient airway is often edematous, and engorged, topicalization of the upper airway can frequently be difficult and requires considerable patience. A drying agent is necessary. Aspiration prophylaxis must be initiated before topical anesthesia begins. One should not hesitate to sedate the mother as needed.

Blind nasal intubation is an option that must be approached with caution. Any attempt at nasal instrumentation incurs the risk of nasal and pharyngeal bleeding that can compromise subsequent efforts at direct or fiberoptic laryngoscopy. Retrograde intubation techniques have been shown to be valuable in the management of the difficult airway in the past but have little, if any, value today in the care of the obstetrical patient.

There are a host of specialized fiberoptic or video laryngoscope blades and handles (e.g., Bullard, GlideScope®, UpsherScope™, Storz Videoscope) each with individualized bulbs, light sources, or fiberoptic bundles ending at various distances into the oral pharynx (see Chapter 9). Considerable effort is needed to maintain them and considerable practice is necessary to become skilled in their use. Certainly, for the anticipated difficult airway in which time and technical assistance will be available, these devices may be useful. However, according to my observation, time and assistance are perpetually in short supply on labor and delivery services.

48.5.2.2 Unanticipated Difficult Airway

Table 48-5 lists several important points to remember in managing an unanticipated difficult obstetrical airway. Figures 48-3 and 48-4 are algorithms one might choose to use in the event of an unanticipated failed tracheal intubation in the obstetrical patient. Figure 48-3 outlines the critical breakpoints in the management of an obstetrical patient requiring general anesthesia: anticipated versus not anticipated, adequate ventilation versus inadequate ventilation, fetal distress versus no fetal distress.

If ventilation is possible, the decision to continue hinges on the presence or absence of fetal distress. If there is no fetal distress, the

TABLE 48-5

Important Points for Managing the Unanticipated Difficult Obstetrical Airway

Thorough and careful airway evaluations	• know your predictors—which ones work for you
Strategy for intubating the difficult airway	• pick your algorithm ahead of time
Make basic preparations for the difficult airway	• pick you equipment ahead of time (LMA ProSeal™, LMA Fastrach™, Eschmann Introducer, Combitube™, jet ventilator, cricothyrotomy kit)
	• keep it simple—get "real" with your gadgets
	• practice, practice, practice

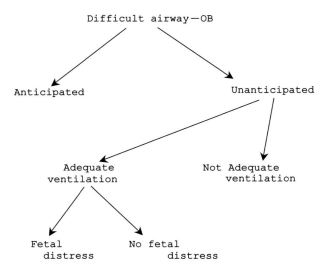

FIGURES 48-3. Basic decision points for the Difficult Airway Algorithm in the obstetrical patient.

patient should be awakened and an alternative anesthetic technique chosen. If, on the other hand, fetal distress is present, one may elect to continue with the case using BMV or an EGD. The patient continues to be at risk of aspiration and cricoid pressure should be continued.

If ventilation is impossible, the patient should be allowed to wake up regardless of the presence of fetal distress. In the interim, rescue techniques may be necessary. Placing the classic laryngeal mask airway (LMA), LMA Fastrach™ or LMA ProSeal™, could be life saving in this instance. If, during the awakening process, ventilation is reestablished, one may then elect to continue with the case if fetal distress is present. A more critical situation is one where, in addition to fetal distress, obstetrical hemorrhage or some other life-threatening condition for the mother exists. Most situations of antepartum hemorrhage do not improve until delivery of the fetus and placenta. The LMA Fastrach™ may be an excellent choice in this setting.

Several alternative methods to BMV have been described, which, of necessity, can be instituted quickly: insertion of the esophageal–tracheal Combitube™ or insertion of an LMA (LMA Classic™, LMA ProSeal™, and intubating LMA Fastrach™). If these fail, one may institute transtracheal jet ventilation (TTJV) or perform an emergency cricothyrotomy, or tracheotomy.

The Combitube™ is a plastic twin-lumen tube that can be placed blindly and when properly positioned serves to seal the esophagus and ventilate the trachea. The Combitube™ has been employed in diverse clinical circumstances to provide adequate ventilation and oxygenation. There is only one report of its use in the parturient.[24] A major drawback of the Combitube™ is that it is a disposable device that one would not use electively and, therefore, not something one can easily practice with in nonemergency situations.

LMA is a recognized device in the ASA Difficult Airway Algorithm and must be part of every difficult airway cart on the labor and delivery floor. The LMA has rapidly become a mainstay in difficult airway management because it is used on a daily basis and practitioners are comfortable with its use. The LMA has been used effectively and safely in selected healthy nonobese parturients, though this is not a practice that I would support other than as a rescue maneuver.[25] When the LMA is placed in the failed intubation/failed ventilation scenario, cricoid pressure should be continued.

The LMA ProSeal™ is a redesigned LMA that may offer a degree of safety to the parturient, in comparison with the LMA Classic™. The LMA ProSeal™, designed to facilitate controlled ventilation and to mitigate the potential for reflux, has been used successfully in failed intubation emergency cesarean section.[26] Finally, the LMA Fastrach™ may have a significant advantage over the LMA Classic™ or the LMA ProSeal™ in the obstetrical patient. Following placement of the LMA Fastrach™, an endotracheal tube can be placed through the LMA Fastrach™ device to secure the airway.

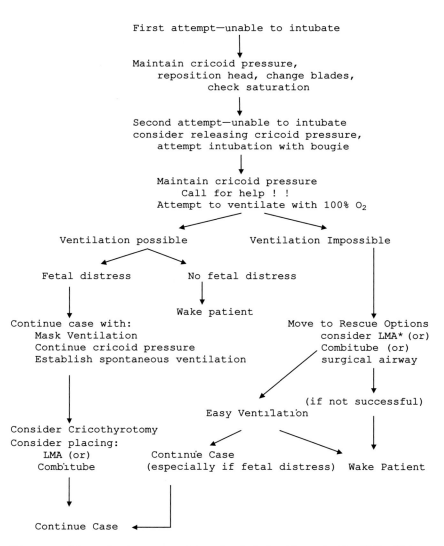

FIGURE 48-4. Difficult Airway Algorithm in the obstetrical patient.

While TTJV is said to be simple, quick, and relatively safe, it is technically difficult to perform in obstetrical patients. As reports of catastrophes have surfaced with TTJV during emergency situations, this technique has slowly lost favor and is seldom used while using the LMA or during a surgical cricothyrotomy. A surgical airway is indicated when one is confronted with a failed airway. Percutaneous surgical cricothyrotomy is a viable alternative to open surgical cricothyrotomy. Several kits have become commercially available. These kits appear to be simple, rapid, and safe to use. There is increasing enthusiasm that anesthesia practitioners learn this technique, instead of TTJV.

48.6 SUMMARY

Difficult or failed intubation is a major contributor to maternal morbidity and mortality during obstetrical emergencies. Careful preanesthetic evaluation focusing on the parturients' airway should identify patients at risk for difficult airway management. Early communication with the obstetricians, regular review, practice of a formal Difficult Airway Algorithm, and facility with current difficult airway devices should mitigate some of the risk of injuries to parturients when a failed intubation does occur.

REFERENCES

1. Berg CJ, Chang J, Callaghan WM, Whitehead SJ: Pregnancy-related mortality in the United States, 1991–1997. *Obstet Gynecol.* 2003;101:289–296.
2. Hawkins JL, Koonin LM, Palmer SK, Gibbs CP: Anesthesia-related deaths during obstetric delivery in the United States, 1979–1990. *Anesthesiology.* 1997;86:277–284.
3. Ross BK: ASA closed claims in obstetrics: lessons learned. *Anesthesiol Clin North America.* 2003;21:183–197.
4. Rocke DA, Murray WB, Rout CC, Gouws E: Relative risk analysis of factors associated with difficult intubation in obstetric anesthesia. *Anesthesiology.* 1992;77:67–73.
5. Rose DK, Cohen MM: The airway: problems and predictions in 18,5000 patients. *Can J Anaesth.* 1994;41:372–383.
6. Benumof JL: Difficult laryngoscopy: obtaining the best view. *Can J Anaesth.* 1994;41:361–365.
7. Davies JM, Weeks S, Crone LA, Pavlin E: Difficult intubation in the parturient. *Can J Anaesth.* 1989;36:668–674.
8. Hawthorne L, Wilson R, Lyons G, Dresner M: Failed intubation revisited: 17-year experience in a teaching maternity unit. *Br J Anaesth.* 1996;76:680–684.
9. Munnur U, Suresh MS: Airway problems in pregnancy. *Crit Care Clin.* 2004;20:617–642.
10. Cedergren MI: Maternal morbid obesity and the risk of adverse pregnancy outcome. *Obstet Gynecol.* 2004;103:219–224.
11. Endler GC, Mariona FG, Sokol RJ, Stevenson LB: Anesthesia-related maternal mortality in Michigan, 1972 to 1984. *Am J Obstet Gynecol.* 1988;159:187–193.
12. Hood DD, Dewan DW: Anesthesia obstetric outcome in the morbidly obese parturient. *Anesthesiology.* 1993;79:1210–1218.
13. Chadwick HS: Obstetric anesthesia closed claims update II. *Anesthesiology Newsletter.* 1999;63:1–6.
14. Norris MC, Dewan DM: Preoxygenation for cesarean section: a comparison of two techniques. *Anesthesiology.* 1985;62:827–829.
15. Pilkington S, Carli F, Dakin MJ, et al.: Increase in Mallampati score during pregnancy. *Br J Anaesth.* 1995;74:638–642.
16. Farcon El, Kim MH, Marx GF: Changing Mallampati score during labour. *Can J Anaesth.* 1994;41:50–51.
17. Izci B, Riha RL, Martin SE, et al.: The upper airway in pregnancy and pre-eclampsia. *Am J Respir Crit Care Med.* 2003;167:137–140.
18. Perlow JH, Kirz DS: Severe peeclampsia presenting as dysphonia secondary to uvular edema: a case report. *J Reprod Med.* 1990;35:1059–1062.
19. Langeron O, Masso E, Huraux C, et al.: Prediction of difficult mask ventilation. *Anesthesiology.* 2000;92:1229–1236.
20. Dupont X, Hamza J, Jullien P, Narchi P: Risk factors associated with difficult airway in normotensive parturients (abstract). *Anesthesiology.* 1990;73:A999.
21. Benumof JL: Management of the difficult adult airway. *Anesthesiology.* 1991;75:1087–1110.
22. Sivarajan M, Fink BR: The position and the state of the larynx during general anesthesia and muscle paralysis. *Anesthesiology.* 1999;72:439–442.
23. Brimacombe JR, Berry AM: Cricoid pressure. *Can J Anaesth.* 1997;44:414–425.
24. Wissler RN: The esophargeal-tracheal Combitude. *Anesth Rev.* 1993;20:147–152.
25. Han TH, Brimacombe J, Lee EJ, Yan HS: The laryngeal mask airway is effective (and probably safe) in selected healthy parturients for elective cesarean section: a prospective study of 1067 cases. *Can J Anaesth.* 2001;48:1117–1121.
26. Awan R, Nolan JP, Cook TM: Use of a ProSeal laryngeal mask airway for airway maintenance during emergency caesarean section after failed tracheal intubation. *Br J Anaesth.* 2004;92:144–146.

SELF-EVALUATION QUESTIONS

48.1. Which of the following combination of patient characteristics have been shown to have a high prediction accuracy for a difficult laryngoscopy and intubation in obstetrical population?

A. high Mallampati grade plus short neck (SN), plus protruding maxillary incisors (PMI), plus receding mandible (RM)

B. SN, plus PMI, plus RM

C. PMI plus RM

D. high Mallampati grade alone

E. none of the above

48.2. Which of the following gastrointestinal changes associated with pregnancy is **NOT** true?

A. a decrease in lower esophageal tone

B. an intragastric pressure increases steadily during pregnancy, as the gravid uterus enlarges

C. gastric emptying appears to be delayed during pregnancy

D. there is an increased risk of gastric aspiration

E. gastric acidity is increased during pregnancy

48.3. All of the following are known airway changes associated with pregnancy **EXCEPT**

A. generalized edema of the oropharynx, nasopharynx, and trachea

B. voice changes are common due to swelling of the false vocal cords and arytenoids

C. capillary engorgement of the nasal increases progressively throughout pregnancy

D. Mallampati classification of the oropharyngeal space has been reported to advance by one or two classes during labor

E. all the airway changes return to prelabor state within 12 hours postpartum

CHAPTER (49)

Airway Management of the Obstetrical Patient with an Anticipated Difficult Airway

Brian K. Ross

49.1 CASE PRESENTATION

The patient is a 32 year old black female G_1P_0 at 31 week gestation. Her medical history is notable for mild obesity (224 lbs [102 kg]; BMI 39 kg·m^{-2}), a suggestion of sleep apnea (a report of significant snoring and periods of apnea while she sleeps), and treatment for chronic hypertension for the past 6 years.

Five days prior to admission, the patient's hypertension and peripheral edema worsened and she developed new onset of proteinuria. A 6 lbs (~3 kg) weight gain during the 7 days prior to admission was also noted. At the time of admission, the patient had a blood pressure of 168/102 mm Hg, a heart rate of 85 beats per minute, a short neck, large breasts, an airway classified as Malampatti class IV, a 3 cm mouth opening with prominent incisor teeth, a thyromental distance of 2 cm, and a limited range of motion of her neck. She was placed on strict bed rest and treated aggressively with atenolol and furosemide.

Twenty-four hours prior to delivery, a nonstress test demonstrated little or no reactivity and late decelerations with the few contractions she was having. The decision was made to induce labor and deliver the fetus. In the 8 hours preceding her induction, her hematocrit rose from 32% to 41% and her platelet count fell from 178,000 × 10^9/L to 75,000 × 10^9/L. The patient was placed on a magnesium sulfate intravenous infusion. She was noted to become increasingly edematous and somnolent.

With induction of labor, the patient has developed regular contractions of appropriate strength for some 12 hours. She has progressed to 10 cm cervical dilation and has been pushing for 3 hours. The baby has remained at -1 station and does not appear to be descending. Because of the risk of inadequate coagulation the patient has been managed throughout labor with a systemic opioid. A decision has been made to perform a cesarean section. The fetus is stable at the present time.

49.2 PATIENT CONSIDERATIONS

49.2.1 What are the physiological changes of pregnancy that impact on the airway management of this patient?

This patient is at considerable risk of rapid desaturation because of her pregnancy-associated increase in oxygen consumption, decrease in functional residual capacity (FRC), increase in closing volume, and increase in alveolar–arterial oxygen gradient. She is also at risk for aspiration because of pregnancy-related decreased gastroesophageal sphincter tone, increased gastric acid production, and decreased gastrointestinal motility. Therefore, this patient must be pretreated with a nonparticulate antacid and perhaps an H2 receptor blocker. If the patient is rendered unconscious before her airway is secured, a rapid sequence induction must be employed to minimize the risk of aspiration. Most would also recommend a cricoid pressure to mitigate the likelihood of gastric content reflux.

49.2.2 What is the most likely diagnosis for this patient?

This patient has chronic hypertension, as well as superimposed severe preeclampsia, i.e., severe hypertension, edema, and proteinuria. She has been given magnesium sulfate for both seizure prophylaxis and blood pressure control. In addition, she has developed thrombocytopenia and a likely associated platelet dysfunction. Regional anesthesia, while preferred, is considered contraindicated under these circumstances.

49.2.3 What is preeclampsia?

Preeclampsia is a term that describes a subset of pregnancy-induced hypertension accompanied by proteinuria, low plasma oncotic pressure, generalized capillary leakage and edema, including the airway, after the twentieth week of gestation. Preeclampsia is more dangerous if onset is prior to 34 weeks.

Preeclampsia can be mild or severe. Severe preeclampsia is defined by the presence of at least one of the following: blood pressures ≥160 mm Hg systolic or 110 mm Hg diastolic, proteinuria ≥5 g/24 h, headache, blurred vision, epigastric or right upper quadrant pain, and pulmonary edema. Because thrombocytopenic coagulopathy frequently complicates preeclampsia, general anesthesia is usually employed, if an operative delivery is required.

49.2.4 What are the consequences of preeclampsia on the parturient airway?

The possibility of severe upper airway edema constitutes a major concern with preeclampsia.[1] Any suggestion of stridor or dyspnea should particularly alert the practitioner to the possible hazards of a difficult airway. However, extreme difficulty may be encountered in preeclamptic patients who are asymptomatic. The airway of a preeclamptic patient will be edematous and friable and thus very unforgiving if multiple attempts at intubation are required. In addition, there have been observations of pharyngeal narrowing that could contribute to difficulty in blind intubating procedures.

49.2.5 What is the impact of weight gain and obesity on the parturient?

Weight gain is a natural consequence of pregnancy. This patient has experienced a rapid weight gain of greater than 6 lbs (~3 kg) in the week prior to intervention, primarily as a result of generalized edema. This patient is of particular concern because her preeclampsia was preceded by significant obesity.

Obesity places the parturient at risk for hypertension, diabetes, preeclampsia, increased incidence of difficult labor, increased likelihood of instrumental delivery, and postpartum hemorrhage. All of these conditions frequently require surgical intervention. Difficult mask ventilation and difficult tracheal intubation, as well as increased volume and acidity of gastric contents, are also associated with obesity. Indeed, there is a documented association of obesity with airway difficulty and maternal mortality.[2,3]

49.2.6 Does labor have any effect on the parturient airway?

The incidence of Mallampati class IV airways increases by as much as 34% as pregnancy progresses from 12–34 week gestation.[4] In addition, airway status can deteriorate significantly as labor proceeds.[5] This suggests that the dynamic airway status should be examined repeatedly throughout labor, particularly in those patients where initial concerns of a possible difficult airway exist.[6]

49.2.7 Does this patient have a worrisome airway?

The patient, as described, is likely to be difficult at laryngoscopy and intubation. While no single measurement is sufficient to predict a difficult laryngoscopy, this patient certainly has more than two of the usual predictors. The Mallampati class IV assessment indicates that oral structures are large in relation to mandibular size. The small thyromental distance and prominent incisors correlate with difficulty in placing a laryngoscope blade. All of these, in association with a short thick neck, limited range of motion of the neck, and large pendulous breasts, suggest that laryngoscopic intubation would be very difficult.

In addition to an unfavorable anatomical presentation, the patient's obesity and potential sleep apnea would suggest potential difficulties with bag-mask-ventilation. The combination of potential difficult BMV and difficult laryngoscopic intubation drastically limit the options available for oxygenating this patient. If this patient's fetus was experiencing a significant distress, management of her airway would be even more problematic.

49.3 AIRWAY MANAGEMENT FOR A PARTURIENT WITH AN ANTICIPATED DIFFICULT AIRWAY

49.3.1 What initial preparations should be made with the obstetricians as induction of labor is undertaken?

One of the first things that an anesthesia practitioner must do is to communicate with the obstetricians, the nurses, the patient, and the patient's family. The health care team, and patient/family, must understand that every effort would be made to avoid the necessity for an urgent induction of general anesthesia. Nevertheless, all equipment must be readied for urgent induction and obstetrically relevant protocols should be reviewed by all caregivers. Algorithms used on the obstetrical floor are quite different from the ones used in the general operating room (see Chapter 48).

49.3.2 What anesthetic technique would be most appropriate for a surgical delivery in a parturient with in anticipated difficult airway?

Some form of regional anesthesia (epidural, spinal, continuous spinal, or combined spinal epidural) would certainly be the preferred management technique for a parturient with an anticipated difficult airway. It is very unusual for a successful regional technique to require conversion to general anesthesia. However, in this patient, her developing coagulopathy precludes the use of a regional technique.

49.3.3 What specific equipment should be available in caring for this patient—a parturient with an anticipated difficult airway, short thick neck with anatomy distorted by edema and obesity, and at considerable risk for bleeding and excessive secretions?

The operating theater should be readied, the OR bed should be "ramped" (see Section 17.5.2), the difficult airway equipment or cart (see Chapter 56) should be immediately available at the induction site.

While there are a number of alternative intubating techniques under general anesthesia, the author believes they all have limitations. Rapid sequence induction with direct laryngoscopy, under any circumstance, is dangerous. Techniques requiring transillumination are technically very difficult in obese patients with a short neck or excessive neck tissue and edema. Poor neck anatomy greatly hinders rescue techniques such as transtracheal jet ventilation, cricothyrotomy, or tracheotomy. Blind nasotracheal tube placement will inevitably lead to considerable bleeding in a pregnant preeclamptic patient; and blind placement of the endotracheal tube using an Eschmann Introducer, or its equivalent, requires at least some visualization of the epiglottis. There is some enthusiasm for the elective utilization of an LMA in a pregnant patient at term,[7] but such advocacy is usually limited to healthy nonobese patients and is rarely used in North America. The newly introduced LMA ProSeal™ (PLMA), with its incorporated esophageal vent, has the potential advantage over the LMA Classic™ of providing some protection against the aspiration of gastric contents. Unfortunately, there are also case reports of gastric aspiration during its use,[8,9] particularly if the LMA ProSeal™ is not properly placed in the hypopharynx. An intubating LMA (ILMA or LMA FastTrach™) might also be considered; however, failure with these devices is not unknown.

An awake technique is probably most appropriate for this patient. A number of practitioners employ an "awake look" technique. That is, the airway is topicalized, or anesthetized, using laryngeal nerve blocks, and then examined under direct vision using a laryngoscope. However, evidence exists of poor correlation between airway visualization in an awake patient and patients who are subsequently anesthetized and paralyzed.[10]

I would choose awake fiberoptic intubation. Sedatives and hypnotics will be required to facilitate an awake intubation, and potential impact on the newborn will require consideration. Consideration will be required in regard to unusual sensitivity in pregnant patients and patients with sleep apnea. Pharyngeal and laryngeal structures must be anesthetized adequately for awake fiberoptic intubation to be successful, and topicalization of the airway in edematous airways is usually difficult and requires patience. Some practitioners advocate laryngeal nerve blocks in this instance. However, in the edematous obese neck, nerve blocks are both difficult and frequently not successful.

49.4 POSTINTUBATION CARE OF THE PARTURIENT WITH A DIFFICULT AIRWAY

49.4.1 What precautions must be taken when the case ends?

The difficult airway case does not end with intubation. One must be equally cautious with the extubation. There are certainly many times one might consider leaving the obese preeclamptic patient intubated for several hours after her surgery to allow her time to remobilize some of the edema fluid and improve her airway conditions. The preeclamptic patient is invariably on magnesium for seizure prophylaxis and if nondepolarizing neuromuscular blocking agents have been used, complete reversal of these agents must be ensured. At extubation, the patient must be fully awake and capable of protecting her airway from aspiration. In many instances, one might consider checking for an air leak (a leak test) around the deflated cuff of the endotracheal tube to further ensure that the patient's airway will be protected after extubation.

49.5 SUMMARY

The obese preeclamptic patients with an anticipated difficult airway can be exceedingly challenging to manage and are best cared for by a thorough team effort. Thorough understanding of the pathophysiology of preeclampsia is critical in providing the optimal anesthetic care for these patients. Their care cannot be rushed and decisions must be made in a logical and methodical manner. In addition, the practitioner must continue to review the difficult airway algorithm and make a concerted effort to remain facile with those devices that may be needed in difficult airway scenarios.

REFERENCES

1. Izci B, Riha RL, Martin SE, et al.: The upper airway in pregnancy and preeclampsia. *Am J Respir Crit Care*. 2003;67:137–140.
2. Endler GC, Mariona FG, Sokol RJ, Stevenson LB: Anesthesia-related maternal mortality in Michigan, 1972 to 1984. *Am J Obstet Gynecol*. 1988;159: 187–193.
3. Ross BK: ASA closed claims in obstetrics: lessons learned. *Anesthesiol Clin North America*. 2003;21:183–197.
4. Pilkington S, Carli F, Dakin M, et al.: Increase Mallampati score during pregnancy. *Br J Anaesth*. 1995;74:638–642.
5. Farcon El, Kim MH, Marx GF: Changing Mallampati score during labour. *Can J Anaesth*. 1992;41:50–51.
6. Lewin SB, Cheek TG, Deutschman CS: Airway management in the obstetric patient. *Crit Care Clin*. 2000;16:505–513.
7. Han TH, Brimacombe J, Lee EJ, Yang HS: The laryngeal mask airway is effective and probably safe in selected healthy parturiets for elective Cesarean section: a prospective study of 1967 cases. *Can J Anaesth*. 2001;48:1117–1121.
8. Koay CK: A case of aspiration using the proseal LMA. *Anaesth Intensive Care*. 2003;31:123.
9. Brimacombe J, Keller C: Aspiration of gastric contents during use of a ProSeal laryngeal mask airway secondary to unidentified foldover malposition. *Anesth Analg*. 2003;97:1192–1194.
10. Sivarajan M, Fink BR: The position and the state of the larynx during general anesthesia and muscle paralysis. *Anesthesiology*. 1990;72:439–442.

SELF-EVALUATION QUESTIONS

49.1. Which of the following is **NOT** a physiological change of pregnancy that would impact on the airway management of the patient?

A. increase in oxygen consumption

B. decrease in FRC

C. increase in risk of aspiration

D. decrease in alveolar–arterial oxygen gradient

E. increase in closing volume.

49.2. All of the following are potential problems of preeclampsia on the parturient airway **EXCEPT**

A. severe upper airway edema

B. friable airway which can be very unforgiving if multiple attempts at intubation are required

C. pharyngeal narrowing that could contribute to difficulty in blind intubating techniques

D. fiberoptic intubation under indirect vision is contraindicated because of the potential airway bleeding

E. blind nasotracheal intubation will inevitably lead to considerable bleeding

49.3. Which of the following is a reasonable intubating technique for an obese parturient with severe preeclampsia and a history of difficult laryngoscopic intubation?

A. awake fiberoptic intubation

B. laryngoscopic intubation following a rapid sequence induction

C. awake intubation using a lightwand

D. awake blind nasal intubation

E. intubation through an intubating LMA under general anesthesia

CHAPTER (50)

Unanticipated Difficult Airway in an Obstetrical Patient Requiring an Emergency Cesarean Section

Adeyemi J. Olufolabi and Holly A. Muir

50.1 CASE PRESENTATION

A 25 year old primigravida at 39 week gestational age presents to the case room with ruptured membranes and frequent uterine contractions. She does not want to have epidural analgesia because of a serious epidural complication suffered by one of her close relatives. After 14 hours of labor, augmented with oxytocin, she is urgently taken to the operating room for emergency cesarean section, for prolonged late decelerations. She weighs 253 lbs (~115 kg) and is 5'3" (~160 cm) tall. Airway examination reveals a Mallampati III and a thyromental distance of 5 cm. She has a full neck extension with normal dentition and a normal mouth opening. She has large gravid breasts. Her blood pressure is 128/68 mmHg, heart rate 100 beats per minute (bpm), respiration rate 20 breaths per minute, and SaO_2 of 99% on a 100% O_2 rebreathing face mask. On arrival in the operating room, the fetal heart rate is 80 bpm.

50.2 ANESTHETIC CONSIDERATIONS

50.2.1 What are the anesthetic options for cesarean section in this patient?

An emergency cesarean section is mandated to deliver the fetus with persistent bradycardia (late deceleration), while minimizing potential/preventable risk to the mother. Anesthesia risk factors for airway management in this patient include her BMI (60.1 kg·m^{-2}) and enlarged breasts. Although regional anesthetic techniques have become the standard of anesthetic care for operative delivery in obstetrics,[1] this patient has refused the regional approach.

The concerns for emergency cesarean section under general anesthesia include securing the airway, reducing the sympathetic response to laryngoscopy and intubation, adequate fluid resuscitation, and the potential of blood loss due to volatile-agent-induced uterine atony. With respect to the first of these concerns, all labor and delivery facilities must have a difficult airway cart and contingency plans for failed laryngoscopic intubation.[1]

50.3 AIRWAY CONSIDERATIONS

50.3.1 What are the airway considerations in pregnant women?

Pregnancy is associated with fluid retention and weight gain. Increased tissue perfusion secondary to a markedly increased cardiac output leads to mucous membrane engorgement. These changes may be aggravated by a prolonged labor and by pushing (valsalva) during delivery. Prolonged bed confinement and the use of oxytocin further contribute to this. The result may be the deterioration of the Mallampati class a factor that is known to occur during pregnancy.[2]

The assessment of the pregnant patient must specifically address features that increase the risk of difficult laryngoscopic intubation, including receding mandible, limited mouth opening, short neck, limited neck movement, and Mallampati IV. Taken together, these features are known to increase the likelihood of a difficult laryngoscopic intubation.[3] Using the airway assessment strategies as described in Chapter 1 (MOANS, LEMON, RODS, and SHORT), her airway assessment suggests possible difficult bag-mask-ventilation (BMV), possible difficult use of extraglottic device (EGD), and possible difficult surgical airway. But there are no other predictors of a difficult laryngoscopy and intubation.[4,5]

The standard of care in obstetrical anesthesia demands that the airway of this patient be secured in such a manner that the risk of aspiration is minimized, leaving the airway practitioner with two choices in this case, rapid sequence induction (RSI) or an awake technique. An awake technique reduces the risk of a failed airway in an anesthetized and paralyzed patient. The decision to perform an awake intubation technique rather than an RSI should be based on clinical findings and the experience of the practitioner. In either case, contingency plans (Plans B and C) must be in place in the event that these techniques fail. One of the contingency plans must be a cricothyrotomy or a surgical airway.

50.4   CONDUCT OF ANESTHESIA

50.4.1   How should the anesthetic be conducted in this patient?

Reflux/aspiration prophylaxis using oral 0.3 M sodium citrate (30 mL) and intravenous ranitidine 50 mg ± metoclopramide 10 mg should be given, following the placement of an intravenous catheter. Appropriate intravenous anesthesia induction agents (propofol 2 mg·kg^{-1} or thiopentone 3–4 mg·kg^{-1}) and succinylcholine 1.5 mg·kg^{-1} are prepared. A designated assistant with experience in applying cricoid pressure during the RSI must be available.

The patient is placed in a 15 degree left tilt to minimize the threat of aortocaval compression syndrome (or supine hypotensive syndrome). In addition, the thorax, shoulders, neck, and head of this morbidly obese parturient should be elevated (ramping) to bring the anatomical axes of the oral, pharyngeal, and laryngeal structures into alignment (see Figures 17-2 and 48-2). A polio handle (short handle) laryngoscope (see Figure 7-3) may be required during intubation to facilitate laryngoscope blade insertion in the face of large breasts. Alternatively, someone may be designated to retract the breasts caudally during laryngoscopy. An airway cart with appropriate difficult airway devices must be immediately available. Denitrogenation is achieved. It should be noted that modified shorter-duration denitrogenation techniques may suffice and have been shown to be effective.[6,7]

Following an RSI with cricoid pressure, direct laryngoscopy, using a #3 Macintosh blade, reveals a Cormack/Lehane (C/L) Grade 4 view (only the hard palate is visible). A second attempt at laryngoscopy using a #3 Miller blade also fails to reveal any identifiable glottic structures despite laryngeal manipulation. Following the second attempt at laryngoscopic intubation, the patient's O$_2$ saturation falls to 85%, her heart rate is 120 bpm, and her BP is 180/120 mm Hg.

50.4.2   What does one do if one cannot visualize the cords on second attempt of laryngoscopy?

There should be no delay in summoning additional assistance and informing all team members of the gravity of the situation. It is necessary to analyze why the attempts were unsuccessful by recalling the six factors that affect the success of the attempt: the

practitioner, optimum head and neck position, optimum paralysis, best external laryngeal manipulation, type of blade, and length of blade (see Chapter 1).

Various laryngoscope blades, rigid fiberoptic laryngoscopes, and video laryngoscopes, with modified curved and straight blades, can be considered if the practitioner possesses a degree of expertise in their use. These include the McCoy, Shikani, Bullard, and GlideScope® laryngoscopes. Improperly applied cricoid pressure can make visualization of the glottic opening more difficult, necessitating guidance by the practitioner. Backward, upward, and right side pressure (BURP) on the thyroid cartilage can also be guided by the practitioner and may help to improve the laryngeal view. An Eschmann Introducer is useful if the epiglottis can be visualized, otherwise it has a limited role. In the environment of a rapidly developing crisis and a glottis that is difficult to visualize, a fiberoptic intubation would likely be inappropriate.

50.4.3   How does one apply the failed airway algorithm in this situation?

The rapid desaturation after the second intubation attempt is likely related to the decrease in functional residual capacity (FRC) and increase in O$_2$ consumption (basal metabolic rate) seen in the gravid state.[8] This patient's respiratory reserve is further compromised by her obesity and by being placed in the supine position. In addition, repeated attempts at intubation are likely to lead to upper airway trauma, particularly in the parturient, where the airway is edematous and the submucosal capillaries are fragile.

Because of these factors, and in the face of unacceptable oxygen saturations after the second attempt, it is imprudent to proceed to a third laryngoscopic attempt without first attempting BMV while maintaining cricoid pressure. Adopting a Failed Airway Algorithm approach at this point must be considered. If BMV is successful, provided the fetal distress has resolved, awakening the patient ought to be considered followed by an awake technique to secure the airway (see Chapter 48, Figure 48-4).

Providing general anesthesia via a face mask to an obese parturient is not generally considered to be safe. However, in the presence of a failed laryngoscopy and ongoing fetal distress, a mask anesthetic is acceptable, provided that oxygenation is adequate while maintaining cricoid pressure. If BMV is unsuccessful, even by easing the cricoid pressure, a rescue device should be inserted.

The ASA Difficult Airway Algorithm recommends that a laryngeal mask airway (LMA) should be inserted as a rescue device for ventilation and oxygenation in a "can't ventilate, can't intubate" (CICV) situation.[9] Failing that, the ASA algorithm recommends a surgical approach. It is the opinion of the editors that this sequential approach in an airway emergency is imprudent and a concurrent approach should be advocated (see Failed Airway Algorithm, Chapter 2).

As the parturient has an increased aspiration risk, an LMA ProSeal™ with an esophageal vent may be a more appropriate rescue device, as long as the practitioner is familiar with its placement. Anecdotal reports have demonstrated success with its use in similar circumstances, with better seating and ventilation and a reduced risk of aspiration related to the venting of contents through the gastric port.[10,11] The intubating LMA (ILMA) has the advantages of rescuing oxygen saturations, as well as serving as a conduit to secure the airway with an endotracheal tube. Placement of the tracheal tube can be achieved blindly through the ILMA device[12] or can be facilitated using a flexible fiberoptic broncho-scope (FFB). The use of an FFB allows visualization of the cords, facilitating the placement of the endotracheal tube under indirect vision and avoiding potential trauma from a blind technique.

Placement of the LMA, LMA ProSeal™, or ILMA may be hindered by cricoid pressure. It has been suggested that relaxing cricoid pressure briefly may allow higher placement success rates.[13,14] Cricoid pressure has also been shown to reduce tidal volumes and increase airway pressures.[15] These difficulties have served to highlight recent studies, questioning the efficacy of cricoid pressure in the prevention aspiration and its hindrance in airway management.[16,17] Others, however, have not demonstrated such disadvantages.[18]

50.4.4 If one is successful in providing ventilation and oxygenation with an LMA, should one proceed with the cesarean section?

When an airway cannot be secured with an endotracheal tube, devices such as the LMA are effective rescue aids. Following the insertion of the LMA, proper placement should be confirmed by end-tidal CO_2 ($ETCO_2$) detection, an unobstructed $ETCO_2$ trace pattern if capnography is employed, and adequate chest and abdominal excursion during ventilation.

While the LMA has been shown to be effective and safe in providing ventilation and oxygenation to healthy, nonobese, fasted parturients for elective cesarean section,[19] it is generally accepted that the LMA should be used only as an emergency device for airway management in the parturient when tracheal intubation is unexpectedly difficult.[20] The decision to proceed with cesarean section with an LMA in place should be based on the risk–benefit assessment on the effectiveness of oxygenation with the LMA, the condition of the fetus, the ability to expedite the delivery of the fetus, and ultimately, the safety of the parturient.

Actions that may lead to regurgitation and aspiration must be minimized if one proceeds with an LMA as the airway. Coughing related to light anesthesia may lead to regurgitation and must be avoided. High intragastric pressure, and incompetence of the lower esophageal sphincter, likewise predispose to regurgitation. There is evidence that gastric insufflation leading to elevated intragastric pressure is reduced by the application of cricoid pressure[21,22] and permits ventilation of the patient at a lower peak airway pressure.[23] Finally, the obstetrician should be advised to minimize fundal pressure, if possible, during delivery of the baby.[24]

Should there be a serious doubt with regards to the safety of the mother in the event an LMA anesthetic is contemplated, the parturient should be awakened despite the presence of fetal distress. An alternative means of intubation (such as a fiberoptic technique), or of anesthesia (regional or local anesthesia), should then be undertaken.

50.4.5 If a Combitube™ is used to secure the airway, what other management issues should be considered?

The Combitube™ is an alternative, two lumen airway device that is designed to be inserted blindly into the esophagus with over

80% success on the first attempt. It is commonly utilized among emergency medical services personnel with limited intubation experience.[25] It may also be employed as a rescue airway device. If placed properly, it permits gas exchange and probably provides a measure of protection against aspiration (see "The Combitube™" Section 11.5 for a detailed description of the device and how it is used). Little information on the use of this device in the obstetric population exists. A theoretical disadvantage may be the potential for trauma (bleeding) in an already engorged airway during its insertion.

50.4.6 When should one proceed with a surgical airway? Who should do it? What equipment should be immediately available on the labor unit?

A surgical airway in a parturient is performed when the patient's airway can neither be intubated nor ventilated (CICV airway). Clinically, the oxygen saturation declines rapidly due to increased metabolic rate and diminished FRC in the pregnant woman. Delay in recognizing a CICV failed airway contributes to adverse outcomes and increased maternal mortality.[26] Surgical and nursing support must be immediately available to assist as necessary.

Commercially available cricothyrotomy kits are standard tools that must be available in all maternal suites and its use should be regularly reviewed. A kit that provides a cuffed tracheal device is mandatory in the labor and delivery suite. Chapter 12 provides a detailed description of the commercial kit recommended and the techniques of surgical airway management.

It should be emphasized that the recognition of the potential difficult airway, avoiding delay in recognizing the CICV situation, and regular practice of a failed intubation drill all contribute toward improving the outcome. Although both surgical and anesthesia practitioners should be conversant with this procedure, the onus is on the anesthesia practitioner to perform the procedure if indicated. With the risk of the failed airway being 10 times more common in the parturient than in the general surgical population, it is mandatory that those who provide anesthesia care in the labor ward be trained in the use of these devices and techniques.[27]

50.5 POSTOPERATIVE CONSIDERATIONS

50.5.1 Having secured the airway, how does one manage this patient postoperatively?

The likelihood of successful extubation is based on several factors and guided by the condition of the patient's airway, but must err on the side of caution. In situations in which airway edema is anticipated to increase, such as significant fluid resuscitation, or an already edematous airway having suffered trauma during intubation attempts, the prudent course is to ventilate the patient for 12–24 hours postoperatively in a 15–30 degree head up position.

A trial of extubation may only be attempted if the patient is fully awake, muscle relaxation fully reversed, and preparations are in place for immediate reintubation. The Frova Introducer, or other tracheal tube exchanger (see Section 10.2.2), may be placed through the tracheal tube prior to its removal to serve as a reintubation guide should it be required. The patient usually tolerates this small diameter device reasonably well if local anesthetic is instilled down the endotracheal tube prior to placement. These devices have a hollow lumen providing limited gas exchange capacity if reintubation over the guide proves difficult or impossible. Employing a laryngoscope to straighten the angle of approach aids tracheal placement over a guide. Smaller tracheal tubes may also enhance the success rates of reintubation over a guide. Increasing obstruction, significant respiratory effort, or increasing acidosis are early indications of extubation failure.

50.6   SUMMARY

The incidence of the CICV failed airway is more than 10 fold in the parturient at term compared to a general surgical population. The obstetrical anesthesia practitioner must be prepared to manage the difficult and failed airway. Regular rehearsal of a failed airway plan of action along with the obstetric team, maintaining skills in the use of a rescue device (e.g., the intubating LMA), and ensuring that surgical airway devices are immediately available are essential components of that preparation.

REFERENCES

1. Kuczkowski KM, Reisner LS, Benumof JL: Airway problems and new solutions for the obstetric patient. *J Clin Anesth.* 2003;15:552–563.
2. Pilkington S, Carli F, Dakin MJ, et al.: Increase in Mallampati score during pregnancy. *Br J Anaesth.* 1995;74:638–642.
3. Rocke DA, Murray WB, Rout CC, Gouws E: Relative risk analysis of factors associated with difficult intubation in obstetric anesthesia. *Anesthesiology.* 1992;77:67–73.
4. Mallampati SR, Gatt SP, Gugino LD, et al.: A clinical sign to predict difficult tracheal intubation: a prospective study. *Can Anaesth Soc J.* 1985;32:429–434.
5. Rose DK, Cohen MM: The airway: problems and predictions in 18,500 patients. *Can J Anaesth.* 1994;41:372–383.
6. Baraka A, Haroun-Bizri S, Khoury S, Chehab IR: Single vital capacity breath for preoxygenation. *Can J Anaesth.* 2000;47:1144–1146.
7. Nimmagadda U, Chiravuri SD, Salem MR, et al.: Preoxygenation with tidal volume and deep breathing techniques: the impact of duration of breathing and fresh gas flow. *Anesth Analg.* 2001;92:1337–1341.
8. Russell IF, Chambers WA: Closing volume in normal pregnancy. *Br J Anaesth.* 1981;53:1043–1047.
9. American Society of Anesthesiologists Task Force on Management of the Difficult Airway: Practice guidelines for the difficult airway: an updated report by the American Society of Anesthesiologists Task Force on Management of the Difficult Airway. *Anesthesiology.* 2003;98:1269–1277.
10. Keller C, Brimacombe J, Lirk P, Puhringer F: Failed obstetric tracheal intubation and postoperative respiratory support with the ProSeal laryngeal mask airway. *Anesth Analg.* 2004;98:1467–1470.
11. Awan R, Nolan JP, Cook TM: Use of a ProSeal laryngeal mask airway for airway maintenance during emergency Caesarean section after failed tracheal intubation. *Br J Anaesth.* 2004;92:144–146.
12. Minville V, N'Guyen L, Coustet B, Fourcade O, Samii K: Difficult airway in obstetric using Ilma-Fastrach. *Anesth Analg.* 2004;99:1873.
13. Aoyama K, Takenaka I, Sata T, Shigematsu A: Cricoid pressure impedes positioning and ventilation through the laryngeal mask airway. *Can J Anaesth.* 1996;43:1035–1040.
14. Harry RM, Nolan JP: The use of cricoid pressure with the intubating laryngeal mask. *Anaesthesia.* 1999;54:656–659.
15. Hocking G, Roberts FL, Thew ME: Airway obstruction with cricoid pressure and lateral tilt. *Anaesthesia.* 2001;56:825–828.
16. Jackson SH: Efficacy and safety of cricoid pressure needs scientific validation. *Anesthesiology.* 1996;84:751–752.
17. Janda M, Vagts DA, Noldge-Schomburg GF: Cricoid pressure—safety necessity or unnecessary risk? *Anaesthesiol Reanim.* 2004;29:4–7.
18. Brimacombe JR, Berry AM: Cricoid pressure. *Can J Anaesth.* 1997;44:414–425.
19. Han TH, Brimacombe J, Lee EJ, Yang HS: The laryngeal mask airway is effective (and probably safe) in selected healthy parturients for elective Cesarean section: a prospective study of 1067 cases. *Can J Anaesth.* 2001;48:1117–1121.
20. Preston R: The evolving role of the laryngeal mask airway in obstetrics. *Can J Anaesth.* 2001;48:1061–1065.
21. Asai T, Barclay K, McBeth C, Vaughan RS: Cricoid pressure applied after placement of the laryngeal mask prevents gastric insufflation but inhibits ventilation. *Br J Anaesth.* 1996;76:772–776.
22. Lawes EG, Campbell I, Mercer D: Inflation pressure, gastric insufflation and rapid sequence induction. *Br J Anaesth.* 1987;59:315–318.
23. Moynihan RJ, Brock-Utne JG, Archer JH, Feld LH, Kreitzman TR: The effect of cricoid pressure on preventing gastric insufflation in infants and children. *Anesthesiology.* 1993;78:652–656.
24. Hartsilver EL, Vanner RG, Bewley J, Clayton T: Gastric pressure during emergency caesarean section under general anaesthesia. *Br J Anaesth.* 1999;82:752–754.
25. Davis DP, Valentine C, Ochs M, Vilke GM, Hoyt DB: The Combitube as a salvage airway device for paramedic rapid sequence intubation. *Ann Emerg Med.* 2003;42:697–704.
26. Walls RM: Management of the difficult airway in the trauma patient. *Emerg Med Clin North Am.* 1998;16:45–61.
27. Samsoon GL, Young JR: Difficult tracheal intubation: a retrospective study. *Anaesthesia.* 1987;42:487–490.

SELF-EVALUATION QUESTIONS

50.1. Which of the following is true with regard to the use of an LMA for the parturient undergoing the cesarean section under general anesthesia?

   A. LMA can be used as a rescue device in a parturient with a failed airway undergoing emergency cesarean section.

   B. LMA has been shown to be effective and safe in providing ventilation for all parturients undergoing cesarean section.

   C. There are no data to support the use of LMA for any parturient undergoing cesarean section.

   D. The LMA has been shown to be effective and safe in providing ventilation for obese parturients undergoing cesarean section.

   E. Use of LMA is associated with a reduced risk of aspiration for parturients undergoing cesarean section.

50.2. What should the anesthesia practitioner do if the vocal cords cannot be seen after three attempts at laryngoscopy in a parturient requiring an emergency cesarean section for placenta previa associated with exsanguinating hemorrhage?

   A. Awaken the patient and perform an awake fiberoptic intubation.

   B. Awaken the patient and perform the cesarean section under regional anesthesia.

   C. Immediate cricothyrotomy.

D. Ventilation using BMV or an EGD while maintaining cricoid pressure and if oxygenation is unsatisfactory proceed with the emergency surgery.

E. Reposition the head and neck of the parturient to facilitate further attempts of laryngoscopy.

50.3. Which of the following is a reasonable approach to minimize the risk of regurgitation and aspiration in a healthy parturient undergoing emergency cesarean section?

A. preoperative oral administration of 0.3 M sodium citrate (30 mL)

B. preoperative IV administration of ranitidine

C. preoperative IV administration of metoclopramide

D. a designated assistant with experience in applying cricoid pressure during the rapid sequence intubation.

E. all of the above

CHAPTER (51)

Airway Management in the Pregnant Trauma Victim

Adeyemi J. Olufolabi and Holly A. Muir

51.1 CASE PRESENTATION

A 35 year old pregnant woman approximately 36 weeks gestation is admitted to the emergency department (ED) following a motor vehicle crash. She has a closed head injury, bilateral femoral fractures, and possible abdominal trauma. Her Glasgow coma score (GCS) is 5: she does not open her eyes (1); there is no audible vocalization (1); and she is showing decorticate rigidity (3). Her heart rate is 135 beats per minute, blood pressure 85/40 mm Hg, and respiratory rate is 40 breaths per minute and shallow. Fetal heart rate (FHR) is 110 beats per minute. The oxygen saturation (SaO_2) is 90%, on a non-rebreathing oxygen mask. A cervical collar is in place and Thomas splints are being applied to the legs.

51.2 INITIAL ASSESSMENT OF THE PATIENT

51.2.1 What are the immediate evaluation and management priorities in this patient?

Initial evaluation and management priorities for the near term parturient are no different than any trauma victim—assessment of airway, breathing and circulation (ABCs), followed by a secondary survey, including assessment of the abdomen and fetus.

Unique considerations related to the pregnancy such as supine hypotensive syndrome and the significant capillary engorgement of the nasal and oropharyngeal mucosa may impact positioning, hemodynamic, and airway management.[1]

Immediate attention is directed toward the airway. Her GCS and oxygen saturations mandate endotracheal intubation and

ventilation. She is not a crash airway, and therefore an evaluation for difficulty is performed employing the MOANS, LEMON, RODS, and SHORT mnemonics (see Sections 1.6.1, 1.6.2, 1.6.3, and 1.6.4). In this particular case, difficulty should be anticipated and an approach as suggested in the Difficult Airway Algorithm (Chapter 2) adopted recognizing that parturients at term have a substantially elevated risk of aspiration, particularly in this case where protective airway reflexes are compromised.

Following airway management, attention is directed to an assessment of breathing. Her lung fields must be evaluated for presence, equality, and quality of breath sounds. This evaluation, coupled with a stat portable chest x-ray, may uncover a pneumothorax and/or hemothorax that may require treatment.

In pregnancy, minute ventilation is normally increased by approximately 45%, largely through an increase in tidal volume. This increased minute ventilation results in a fall in $PaCO_2$ to approximately 30 mm Hg. Therefore, one should initially moderately hyperventilate this patient empirically. Ventilation may be guided by arterial blood gases once resuscitation has been established.

During pregnancy, an increase in gastric acid production results not only in an increased volume but a decrease in the pH. Coupled with a decrease in the competency of the lower esophageal sphincter, a greatly enhanced risk of reflux is present. The most effective protection against aspiration in this situation is the presence of a cuffed endotracheal tube in the trachea.

The final step of the primary survey is directed to the evaluation and management of the circulation. This patient is hypotensive. Positioning to minimize supine hypotensive syndrome (or aortocaval compression syndrome) and volume resuscitation should be undertaken. A wedge should be placed under the right hip to create 30 degrees of left uterine displacement. This will reduce aortocaval compression and improve systemic and placental perfusion.[2] Large bore IV cannula and fluids must be initiated as the parturient can lose 30% blood volume before demonstrating cardiovascular changes.[3]

There is a strong correlation between hypotension and negative outcome for both an injured brain, and a fetus in utero.

Relative anemia (approximately 11 g/dL or 6.9 mmol·L^{-1}), related to an enhanced blood volume, is a physiologic response to pregnancy. In a healthy near term parturient, blood pressure may remain at near normal values until greater than 1000 mL of blood loss occurs. In addition to the usual sources of blood loss in a trauma victim, the uterus can be a source of significant hemorrhage, e.g., both placental and uterine abruption may be associated with blunt abdominal trauma (e.g., lap belt injury).

Now the attention can be turned to the secondary survey focusing on her head injury, the abdomen, and the stabilization of her fractures.

Her GCS of less than 7 indicates a significant head injury at risk of further decompensation at any time. Securing an airway in a timely fashion may be critical in limiting hypoxic brain injury and avoiding surges in intracranial pressure (ICP) related to elevations of PaCO$_2$.[4]

51.3   AIRWAY CONSIDERATIONS

51.3.1   What is unique about managing the airway urgently in the traumatic brain-injured patient who also happens to be a near term parturient?

As discussed above, the practitioner must deal with competing priorities: the patient has features suggestive of difficult intubation, specifically, difficult bag-mask-ventilation (BMV) and difficult extraglottic device (EGD) use. Additionally, she needs to have her airway managed atraumatically and quickly in the presence of traumatic brain injury and a greatly increased aspiration risk. Following the Difficult Airway Algorithm (Chapter 2) will take time; resorting to rapid sequence induction (RSI) immediately runs the risk of inducing and paralyzing a patient at high risk for aspiration and difficult airway.

The practitioner has time to call for help and a Difficult Airway Cart as the SaO$_2$ is acceptable, while borderline, and the FHR is normal. The airway practitioner should begin denitrogenation quickly using a mask with a rebreathing bag with 15 L·min^{-1} of oxygen.

Assisted ventilation may be required, taking care to avoid inflating the stomach. Her rapid respiratory rate makes this a challenge. If the practitioner is not confident of tracheal intubation or provide gas exchange using BMV or EGD, then an "awake look" with a laryngoscope may help to make the decision to move to a surgical airway or embark on an RSI pathway. As the status of the cervical spine stability is unclear, the collar is gently removed and airway evaluation and management is performed while maintaining in-line stabilization.

Should RSI be selected in the setting of a patient with acute severe head injury, the patient ought to be pretreated with an opioid, lidocaine, and defasciculating agent. The selection of an induction agent and the dose employed will be guided by the degree of hemodynamic stability, and in this case is likely to be etomidate at a reduced dose (e.g., 0.2 mg·kg^{-1}). The dose of the neuromuscular blocker, such as succinylcholine, is never modified and is 1.5 mg·kg^{-1}.

Alternatively, an "awake look" to determine "intubatability" may be performed. This patient has a GCS of 5 and may not require sedation (e.g., etomidate titration). However, patients with acute severe head injury may present with a clenched jaw, prohibiting an awake look. If this occurs, the only options are RSI and cricothyrotomy.

Induction and neuromuscular blocking agents must be prepared prior to securing the airway. A selection of intubation and rescue airway devices familiar to the airway practitioner must also be prepared. In this case, laryngoscopic intubation is judged to be highly likely (Plan A). Plan B is to use an Intubating LMA (ILMA), and Plan C is a surgical airway should both fail. Following denitrogenation with 100% oxygen, pretreatment, induction, paralysis, and the application of cricoid pressure by an experienced assistant are undertaken. A third person maintains manual in-line stabilization of the neck, and the trachea is successfully intubated. After carbon dioxide detection confirms tracheal placement, the endotracheal tube is secured. An orogastric tube may be placed to reduce the risk of aspiration.

51.3.2   How would you secure the airway if three attempts at laryngoscopic intubation failed despite laryngeal manipulation?

While maintaining cricoid pressure, ventilation should be provided by BMV with 100% oxygen. Gradual relaxation of cricoid pressure may be indicated if it is felt to hinder the ability to ventilate. If at any point the ability to maintain saturations is lost, an immediate surgical airway is indicated. As preparations for the surgical airway are underway, an ILMA can be inserted. Should this reestablish adequate ventilation, tracheal intubation through the ILMA can be considered.

Oxygen desaturation and hypotension are associated with poor outcomes in patients with acute severe head injury.

51.3.3   What specific concerns related to the airway do you have if this patient needs to be transported to the radiology suite for diagnostic imaging?

This patient will require ongoing sedation, paralysis and mechanical ventilation during transport, and diagnostic imaging to maintain oxygenation and to keep her PaCO$_2$ within her physiologic range (between 30–32 mm Hg). Although hypocapnia has traditionally been considered an important part of the management of head injury, even moderate hypocapnia can be associated with a harmful reduction in cerebral and uterine blood flow.[5] Following the acute resuscitation phase, PaCO$_2$ levels should be monitored continuously by capnometry/capnography or periodically by arterial blood gas sampling.

The endotracheal tube should be properly secured as movement from stretchers to radiology tables and back increases the risk of accidental extubation. In addition, appropriate equipment and personnel to manage reintubation should be immediately available, including drugs (both induction agents and neuromuscular blocking drugs), laryngoscopes, endotracheal tubes, and rescue devices (including a tracheal tube introducer and an LMA).

51.3.4   Are sedating drugs and muscle relaxants safe in pregnancy?

The duration of action of agents such as vecuronium and rocuronium may be prolonged in the pregnant state, and therefore, in non-resuscitation situations, dosing should be titrated using a neuromuscular block monitor.[6] Although small amounts of non-depolarizing muscle relaxants are known to cross the placenta to the fetus when administered as a bolus, there are no reports of adverse fetal effects. The effects of prolonged (greater than 24 hours) neuromuscular blocking drug administration on a fetus are unknown. It has been shown, however, that the fetal/maternal ratio of vecuronium increases significantly with prolonged induction to delivery times.[7] In a scenario such as this, personnel should be available to ventilate or intubate the trachea of a neonate should the need arise.

All patients intubated as part of an emergency resuscitation effort ought to receive sufficient sedation and muscle relaxation to facilitate mechanical ventilation and attenuate the stress responses (increased airways resistance, ICP, blood pressure, and heart rate). This is particularly important in patients with poorly controlled elevated ICP, such as in this patient. Drug selection in pregnancy is somewhat problematic as few of the available drugs are approved for use in parturients. The US Federal Drug Administration has created a classification structure for drugs administered to females during pregnancy.[8] This five-level system of classification categorizes agents from safe to use with well-controlled studies (category "A"—no risk to the fetus) to those who are clearly contraindicated (category "X").

Most anesthetic and sedating agents fall into the category "C" group in which risks cannot be ruled out (often due to the lack of controlled studies). It is recommended that category C agents be used only if the potential benefit to the mother justifies the potential risk to the fetus. Although the key teratogenic period is from 31 to 71 days postconception, fetal brain and organ development continues throughout gestation rendering them susceptible to the adverse affects of agents administered to the mother.

The prevailing wisdom in the decision-making process is to bear in mind that the general health and well-being of the fetus is *entirely* dependent on the survival and well-being of the mother. As a general principle, drugs with a known "safe" history of use in pregnancy, such as thiopental and fentanyl, can be used. There is a growing body of evidence that propofol is also safe, although the experience is substantially less than those for thiopental and fentanyl. The fact that propofol is commonly used in the care of adult patients with neurotrauma would suggest its favorable application in this case. Despite traditional cautions in regard to possible teratogenic effects of benzodiazepines, recent evidence indicates that these agents are not proven human teratogens.[9] The safety of etomidate in pregnancy has not been established. The drug crosses the placenta and has been shown to produce a fall in serum cortisol in the fetus lasting for about 6 hours. The significance of this finding

is unclear. The selection of etomidate in this case was driven by the considerable hemodynamic instability noted in the mother.

By and large, there is little evidence that a single dose of any currently available IV induction agents is harmful to the fetus.

51.4   OTHER CONSIDERATIONS

51.4.1   What fetal monitoring is required in this situation?

Fetal monitoring during trauma resuscitation is often challenging because of limited access to the abdomen. Continuous fetal monitoring is possible from about 18 weeks gestational age, although it is technically difficult to perform transabdominally early in gestation. FHR variability as an indicator of fetal well-being is usually not established until 25–27 weeks of gestation. Additionally, sedating agents affect FHR variability further limiting its usefulness.[10] Therefore, persistent and marked fetal bradycardia may be the only true indicator of fetal distress in early pregnancy or in pregnant patients receiving sedating medications.

Blunt and abdominal trauma place the fetus directly at risk, and also indirectly at risk due to the potential for placental abruption or uterine hypoperfusion related to maternal hemodynamic instability.

It is reasonable to use continuous fetal monitoring in a pregnant trauma victim if it is physically possible. This assumes that personnel skilled in fetal heart trace reading are available and a plan to deliver the fetus if there is evidence of fetal compromise. The American College of Obstetricians and Gynecologists supports a position of individualizing the use of monitoring in these situations as a team approach so as to optimize the safety of both the mother and the fetus.[11]

After 35 week gestation, delivery results in minimal morbidity to the fetus.

51.4.2   What findings would lead to a decision to expedite the delivery of the fetus?

Evaluation of the pregnant trauma victim involves the evaluation of two patients, the mother and the fetus. Assessment and stabilization of the mother is always the first priority. Occasionally, the resuscitation of the mother requires the delivery of the fetus. The classic example is during maternal cardiac arrest, if the fetus is older than 24 weeks, and if it has not been possible to resuscitate the mother after 4 minutes of cardiopulmonary resuscitation (CPR), the fetus should be delivered by emergency cesarean section. This is done to improve both fetal outcome and the effectiveness of maternal CPR, by removing any aortocaval obstruction.

In cases where the mother is hemodynamically unstable secondary to hemorrhage and placental abruption, delivery of the fetus may be necessary as part of maternal resuscitation. Immediate induction of anesthesia with airway management is mandated.

A more common scenario is that of a hemodynamically stable mother with a fetus demonstrating signs of terminal fetal distress (severe fetal bradycardia). This situation parallels any other emergency cesarean section for fetal distress. As in all situations where anesthesia induction agents and muscle relaxants are used, a strategic plan (Plans A, B, and C) must be in place for management of the failed intubation.

51.5 SUMMARY

The management of trauma in a parturient often provides significant challenges to caregivers. The physiologic changes of pregnancy must be considered when one interprets vital signs, response to resuscitative maneuvers, and laboratory investigations in these trauma victims. The fetus adds a second dimension to the resuscitation, although maternal well-being and safety should remain the primary concern.

The benefit of left uterine displacement as part of the resuscitation must be recognized. Airway protection is a critical part of management as these patients are at higher risk of aspiration due to the physiologic and mechanical changes of pregnancy. The value of airway management algorithms in crisis situations such as the resuscitation of the parturient cannot be overemphasized.

REFERENCES

1. Leontic EA: Respiratory disease in pregnancy. *Med Clin North Am*. 1977;61:111–128.
2. Camann WR, Ostheimer GW: Physiological adaptations during pregnancy. *Int Anesthesiol Clin*. 1990;28:2–10.
3. ACOG Educational Bulletin. Obstetric aspects of trauma management. Number 251, September 1998. American College of Obstetricians and Gynecologists. *Int J Gynaecol Obstet*. 1999;64:87–94.
4. Gelb AW, Manninen PH, Mezon BJ, Lee RJ, Durward OJ: The anaesthetist and the head-injured patient. *Can Anaesth Soc J*. 1984;31:98–108.
5. Morishima HO, Daniel SS, Adamsons K, Jr, James LS: Effects of positive pressure ventilation of the mother upon the acid-base state of the fetus. *Am J Obstet Gynecol*. 1965;93:269–273.
6. Khuenl-Brady KS, Koller J, Mair P, Puhringer F, Mitterschiffthaler G: Comparison of vecuronium- and atracurium-induced neuromuscular blockade in postpartum and nonpregnant patients. *Anesth Analg*. 1991;72:110–113.
7. Iwama H, Kaneko T, Tobishima S, et al.: Time dependency of the ratio of umbilical vein/maternal artery concentrations of vecuronium in caesarean section. *Acta Anaesthesiol Scand*. 1999;43:9–12.
8. FDA classification of drugs for teratogenic risk. Teratology Society Public Affairs Committee. *Teratology*. 1994;49:446–447.
9. Sheppard T: *Catalog of Teratogenic Agents*, 7th edn. Baltimore, MD: John Hopkins University Press, 1992.
10. Immer-Bansi A, Immer FF, Henle S, Sporri S, Petersen-Felix S: Unnecessary emergency caesarean section due to silent CTG during anaesthesia? *Br J Anaesth*. 2001;87:791–793.
11. ACOG Committee on Obstetrical Practice. ACOG committee opinion. Number 284, August 2003. Nonobstetric surgery in pregnancy. *Obstet Gynecol*. 2003;102:431.

SELF-EVALUATION QUESTIONS

51.1. Which of the following anesthetic induction agents has been shown in clinical trials to be safe for a pregnant patient?

A. etomidate

B. propofol

C. thiopental

D. ketamine

E. none of the above

51.2. During a rapid sequence induction for an emergency caesarean section, you are neither able to intubate nor ventilate the patient. Which of the following is **NOT** an appropriate course of action?

A. repeat laryngoscopy and intubation

B. ventilation using Combitube™

C. immediate preparations for cricothyrotomy

D. ventilation using an LMA

E. relaxing cricoid pressure to determine if BMV can be improved

51.3. Which of the following is **NOT** an indication to deliver the fetus in a trauma victim who is 37 weeks pregnant?

A. to aid in the resuscitation of the mother, the fetus must be delivered in an expeditious fashion

B. maternal cardiac arrest

C. hemodynamically stable mother and the fetus is showing signs of terminal fetal distress with severe fetal bradycardia

D. the mother is hemodynamically unstable secondary to hemorrhage and placental abruption

E. maternal respiratory arrest

CHAPTER (52)

Unique Challenges of Ectopic Airway Management

Michael F. Murphy

52.1 CASE PRESENTATION

A 42 year old obese male is undergoing renal dialysis in a hospital dialysis unit when he suddenly suffers a cardiac arrest. He is diabetic with a history of cerebrovascular disease, peripheral vascular disease and angina. He is a nonsmoker. He had no premonitory symptoms.

You are called to manage his airway. When you arrive on the scene from your unit, you see a cyanotic male looking older than his stated age, reclining at 45 degrees in a dialysis chair. He is still connected to a dialysis machine via a vascular shunt in his left arm. The head of the chair, which is not on wheels, is against the wall. A dialysis technician is straddling the patient performing cardiopulmonary resuscitation and a nurse is delivering ineffective bag-mask-ventilation (BMV) from the right side of the patient. You are informed that he receives dialysis three times a week. His "dry weight" is 414 lbs (188 kg).

The crash cart has arrived containing both oral and nasal airways, endotracheal tubes, a laryngoscope handle, and #3 and #4 Macintosh blades. There is an intubating stylet as well. This is the third time this year you have been called to this unit. Unfortunately, the equipment you prefer to use for airway management is *never* available in the dialysis unit, despite continuous reminders that you prefer a Miller blade.

52.2 INTRODUCTION

52.2.1 What is meant by the term "ectopic airway management"?

Anesthesia practitioners, emergency physicians, intensivists, hospitalists, and other health care providers with airway management expertise often become involved in emergency and urgent airway management outside of their usual operating milieu. This is referred to as *ectopic* airway management.

52.2.2 What are the common examples of ectopic venues?

There are several areas of a hospital where it should be *anticipated* that emergency airway management will be required occasionally, or even perhaps regularly. These include but are not exclusive to:

- postanesthetic care unit (PACU)
- diagnostic imaging locations where emergency and intensive care unit (ICU) patients are taken; particularly CT, MRI, ultrasound, and angiography units
- units where procedural sedation is undertaken:
  - endoscopy
  - invasive cardiology
  - interventional imaging
  - pediatric clinics such as dentistry, ophthalmology, EEG, ENT, and others
  - lithotripsy
- cardiac stress testing facilities
- medical and surgical inpatient units
- obstetrical delivery suites

Outpatient clinics, medical offices, and non-patient care areas (e.g., cafeterias, residences, waiting rooms, administrative offices, and the areas immediately external to the healthcare facility) are occasionally the site of an airway emergency.

52.3   AIRWAY MANAGEMENT CHALLENGES

52.3.1   What issues are the unique challenges of ectopic airway management?

Managing a difficult airway is always anxiety provoking and somewhat dysphoric. Most ectopic airway management is difficult for a variety of reasons; some are related to the airway anatomy, others to the patient's condition, and some are unique to the situation. The result is performance anxiety and potentially less than optimal performance. Consider the following unique challenges inherent in managing the ectopic airway:

1. medico-legal risk
2. consistency of airway kits/carts
3. unfamiliar environment
4. unknown patient medical conditions
5. assistants unfamiliar with airway management
6. emotionally charged environment; stressed response
7. postintubation management

52.3.2   What are the medical–legal risks associated with ectopic airway management?

Participating in ectopic airway management is associated with an element of medico-legal risk in the event of a poor outcome. Peterson et al. published an update of the *Management of the Difficult Airway: A Closed Claims Analysis* in 2005. Out of 179 claims for difficult airway management, 86 (48%) were from events occurring from 1985–1992 and 93 (52%) were from events occurring from 1993–1999. The majority of claims for difficult airway management (156 out of 179 or 87%) involved perioperative care and 23 claims (13%) involved ectopic locations. Out of these 23 cases of airway management "misadventures" outside the operating room environment, 25% involved endotracheal tube change, and nearly half were not related to surgical procedures. Reintubation on the ward or ICU some time after a surgical procedure was related to neck swelling with respiratory distress. The procedures included cervical fusion ($n = 3$), total thyroidectomy ($n = 1$), intraoral/pharyngeal procedures ($n = 2$), and fluid extravasation from a central catheter ($n = 1$).[1]

The typical scenario coming to litigation has the following features:

- the patient is unknown to the airway practitioner
- it is an emergency situation:
  - which is emotionally charged and chaotic
  - in which events preceding the airway emergency are unclear
  - in which the amount of information about the patient is sketchy
  - in which action is needed immediately
- it is a difficult airway (e.g., post-thyroidectomy in PACU; patient in a halo jacket)
- it is in a location that is less than familiar to the airway practitioner

- evaluation of the airway for difficulty is inadequate
- paralytic agents are inappropriately given
- the management strategy is poorly thought out and executed leading to a failed airway

The fact that the airway practitioner is thrust into an emotionally charged and unfamiliar environment provides little if any legal protection or indemnification. Furthermore, the defense of "lack of familiar or desired equipment" may be discredited. This is particularly so if it can be established that emergency airway management is *expected* to occur from time to time on that unit *and* that the individual charged with airway management in such situations (i.e., you) *knew or ought to have known* that they might be summoned to do so.

Part of the solution to this problem is to *prevent* failure by establishing policies and procedures with respect to airway management equipment and its maintenance in areas where it is predictable that emergency or urgent airway intervention will occasionally be required. This requires that the disciplines involved take ownership of this issue and communicate with each other, and among themselves, about the specifics of such policies that will insure safe, and hopefully litigation free, ectopic airway management.

52.3.3   What airway equipment or carts should be available in these ectopic facilities?

Airways are managed virtually every day in the operating rooms, emergency departments, and ICUs of most hospitals. These units ordinarily assemble routine and rescue airway management equipment into varying configurations of storage units where they are checked regularly (e.g., daily or with shift change) for availability and function, and are easily accessed in an emergency. Routine and difficult/failed airway equipment may be arranged on top of, and/or in the storage areas of the same cart (e.g., emergency departments and ICUs); or sometimes in different carts (e.g., the operating room's difficult airway cart, see Chapter 56 for details). The literature, albeit limited, provides little guidance as to what ought to be stocked in these "carts," or alternatively in a "carry out" kit that the practitioner takes along to an airway management event.[2–6]

The equipment on the carts is typically determined by the consensus among the specialists or staff who respond to manage an airway emergency in these units. The equipment should be arranged in a consistent fashion such that the drawers always contain the same airway equipment. This site-to-site consistency is particularly important when large specialty groups cover several facilities. Such consistency will likely avoid wasting valuable time to find the proper airway equipment in an emergency situation. Chapter 56 addresses the policy and content aspects of difficult airway carts in operating suites, emergency departments, and ICUs. It also serves as a resource for contacting equipment manufacturers and suppliers.

In areas of the hospital where airway management may be required on a regular basis, or patients are placed at risk for respiratory failure (see above), it is recommended that routine and rescue airway management equipment be immediately available. Furthermore, the storage of this equipment should be consistent from area to area, and the equipment should be checked for inventory and function daily.

"Carry out" emergency airway satchels that can be quickly retrieved and carried to the site of an airway emergency are used by some individuals and departments. The same issues arise with these kits as with permanent on-site carts such as:

- consistent location of kits to permit rapid retrieval
- contain both routine and rescue devices
- organized consistently to permit rapid access to the desired equipment
- regular inspections to ensure that the kits are complete and replenished after each use
- daily inspections of each kit to ensure proper function of all devices

Some areas may have unique needs that require special equipment. The most common example is areas serving pediatric patients. Some areas of a health care facility may see this population from time to time, while others may not.

52.3.4 What are the challenges associated with managing the airway in the ectopic environment?

Leaving the comfort of one's usual environment and venturing into unfamiliar territory ought not hinder appropriate airway management. Individuals who may be summoned to ectopic areas to manage airways should familiarize themselves with the staff, the equipment, and the storage systems *before* the emergency arises. Participating in the decisions as to what is stored, where it is stored, and how it is maintained (i.e., policy) is only reasonable.

The scene on arrival is generally chaotic, emotionally charged, and boisterous. As there are substantial expectations placed on the responding airway practitioner, it is critical that the airway practitioner does not participate in or inflame the chaos, which fosters the avoidance of a bad airway management decision.

52.3.5 Why is airway management in an ectopic location more challenging?

Patients requiring airway management in these ectopic locations are generally not known to the airway practitioners. Most of these patients are not prepared for airway management. For example, unprepared patients often have a full stomach and therefore a higher risk of gastric regurgitation and aspiration. Furthermore, airway assessment is not available or incomplete. Because of these poorly prepared patients, it is difficult for airway practitioners to formulate strategies to manage the airway. As indicated previously, the single most important factor leading to a failed airway is failure to properly assess a patient and predict a difficult airway.[1,7,8] Consequently, it is more common to encounter difficulties in airway management in an ectopic environment.

52.3.6 What are the challenges faced by the personnel managing these patients' airways in ectopic locations?

Airway management urgencies/emergencies presenting in PACU (e.g., post-thyroidectomy bleed) may be quite different from those occurring in the CT scanner (e.g., pediatric patients). Airway practitioners have varying skills and not many are expert at managing all different types of situations.

In addition, unlike the situation in the operating room, PACU, ICU, or emergency department, airway management assistants in these ectopic locations may be unfamiliar with subtleties. Maneuvers such as cricoid pressure, external laryngeal manipulation, head lift, or even passing the endotracheal tube in the correct orientation to the airway practitioner may not be properly handled.

To minimize these difficulties, institutions should provide basic training to both airway practitioners and assistants to manage patients in varying ectopic areas.

52.3.7 How should the airway be managed in ectopic locations?

The following simple rules of engagement may be helpful:

- Remain calm and take control of the scene.
- Speak firmly and give clear instructions to assistants without shouting.
- Consider titration of intravenous haloperidol and/or ketamine (*not* succinylcholine) if the patient's behavior hinders adequate management of ventilation and oxygenation.
- If patient behavior management is not an issue, managing oxygenation and ventilation or gas exchange must be achieved quickly:
  - Move to the head of the patient and establish ventilation and oxygenation.
- Establish airway patency.
- Take over BMV and avoid aggressive ventilation (i.e., avoid high-frequency, large tidal volume, and high airway pressure).
- Insert an oral airway and two nasal trumpets if needed.
- If this fails, inserting an LMA is reasonable.
  - Gather your wits and composure as you establish adequate gas exchange.
- While maintaining gas exchange, it is important to evaluate the airway and formulate a plan.
  - Formally evaluate the airway using the mnemonics described in Chapter 1 (e.g., with MOANS, LEMON, RODS, SHORT).
  - Identify Plans A, B, and C; assemble the required equipment and drugs.
  - Avoid muscle paralysis if the ability to maintain ventilation or gas exchange is uncertain.
  - Optimize conditions—invest time to properly position the patient at the head of the bed, elevate the bed to the proper height, and place the patient's head and neck in the appropriate (e.g., "sniffing") position.
- Execute your plan in a deliberate and a controlled manner.
- When faced with inadequate equipment (or skills) in an ectopic location, it is important to think of alternatives:
  - Call for assistance if available. A colleague or an assistant can contribute with suggestions, expertise, and more importantly, moral support.

- Does the patient really need tracheal intubation *right now* or will BMV or an extraglottic device (e.g., LMA) suffice until additional equipment or expertise arrives?
- Are there any other options (e.g., blind nasal intubation)?

52.4 POSTINTUBATION CONSIDERATION

52.4.1 What should be done following tracheal intubation in these ectopic locations?

While confirmation of tracheal intubation is critical following intubation, proper equipment (capnography and self-inflating bulb) may not be available. This important equipment, together with hemodynamic monitors and pulse oximetry, should be called for if they are not available. Ensure that the airway device (e.g., ETT, LMA) is secured properly. Long-term neuromuscular blockade may be necessary to facilitate mechanical ventilation and ensure that the patient does not self extubate. Ensure that appropriate mechanical ventilation parameters are established if indicated.

Following the airway management in these unusual environments, it is essential to document the following elements:

- any evaluation that indicated that the airway might be difficult
- ensure that the resuscitation record or nurses' notes accurately record the time you were summoned, arrived, completed key interventions, etc.
- ensure that drug doses are accurately recorded
- document the airway management, and the intratracheal verification methods employed (end-tidal carbon dioxide detection is the standard of care)

52.5 SUMMARY

To minimize the risk, adverse outcome, and the anxiety associated in airway management of patients in an ectopic environment, it is important to:

1. participate in crafting hospital and departmental policies regarding airway management equipment in areas where you are called to manage them (see Chapter 56),
2. familiarize yourself with different hospital units and their staff,
3. minimize the chaos,
4. assess the airway and formulate airway strategies quickly,
5. call for assistance early,
6. avoid paralyzing the patient if ventilation is uncertain,
7. document the airway management episode.

REFERENCES

1. Peterson GN, Domino KB, Caplan RA, et al.: Management of the difficult airway: a closed claims analysis. *Anesthesiology.* 2005;103:33–39.
2. Murphy MF: The difficult airway cart. In: *Manual of Emergency Airway Management*, 2nd edn, for PDA. Walls RM, Murphy MF, Luten RC, Schneider R, eds. Philadelphia, PA: Lippincott Williams and Wilkins, 2004.
3. McGuire GP, Wong DT: Airway management: contents of a difficult intubation cart. *Can J Anesth.* 1999;46:190–191.
4. Practice Guidelines for the Management of the Difficult Airway. A report by the ASA task force on management of the difficult airway. *Anesthesiology.* 1993;78:597–602.
5. Practice guidelines for management of the difficult airway: an updated report by the American Society of Anesthesiologists Task Force on Management of the Difficult Airway. *Anesthesiology.* 2003;98:1269–1277.
6. Crosby ET, Cooper RM, Douglas MJ, et al.: The unanticipated difficult airway with recommendations for management. *Can J Anaesth.* 1998;45:757–776.
7. Mort TC: Emergency tracheal intubation: complications associated with repeated laryngoscopic attempts. *Anesth Analg.* 2004;99:607–613.
8. Cheney FW, Posner KL, Caplan RA: Adverse respiratory events infrequently leading to malpractice suits. A closed claims analysis. *Anesthesiology.* 1991;75:932–939.

SELF-EVALUATION QUESTIONS

52.1. Ectopic airway management is associated with measurable medico-legal risk. Of the closed claims related to difficult airway management in the ASA Closed Claims Database between 1985 and 1999, the approximate percentage of those occurring at an ectopic location is

    A. 2%

    B. 5%

    C. 15%

    D. 25%

    E. 43%

52.2. The most important factor related to successfully managing an airway in an ectopic location is

    A. getting there quickly

    B. making it clear that you are the most skilled airway practitioner at the scene

    C. you have familiarized yourself with the equipment that will be available to you beforehand

    D. that you speak in a low voice to avoid fanning the flames of anxiety

    E. that you paralyze the patient quickly to enhance your success rate

52.3. All of the following are associated with ectopic airway management **EXCEPT**

    A. Chaos is the norm.

    B. Failure rates are higher than in locations where you usually work.

    C. Policies with respect to airway management equipment maintenance are the norm.

    D. Good help is usually present at the scene.

    E. The person who performs the intubation is responsible to see that it is secured in place.

CHAPTER (53)

Management of the Patient with a Neck Hematoma

J. Adam Law

53.1 CASE PRESENTATION

A 54 year old male has been in the post-anesthetic care unit (PACU) for 6 hours with a slowly expanding neck hematoma, following an uneventful anterior cervical discectomy and fusion (C5–6) under general anesthesia. Over the last 45 minutes, he has become symptomatically short of breath. Neurosurgery has booked him to return to the operating room (OR) for wound exploration and evacuation of hematoma. Preoperatively, he was otherwise healthy, taking no medications, and was noted to have normal-looking airway anatomy. Postinduction at the original surgery, he was documented to have been easy to bag-mask ventilate, presented a Cormack/Lehane (C/L)[1] Grade 1 view at direct laryngoscopy using a Macintosh #3 blade, and the trachea was easily intubated with an 8.5 mm ID endotracheal tube.

In the PACU, he is sitting upright, breathing oxygen at 10 L·min^{-1} via a non-rebreathing face mask. Although restless, he is rational and complaining of dyspnea and dysphagia. Blood pressure is 180/95 mm Hg, heart rate 100 beats per minute, respiratory rate 30 breaths per minute, and his SpO$_2$ is 95%. He is audibly stridorous. Under the dressing, the right side of his neck looks slightly enlarged. The patient is 5'10"(~178 cm) in height and weighs 176 lbs (80 kg). He has vascular access. An OR is being prepared for his return.

53.2 PATIENT EVALUATION AND MANAGEMENT OPTIONS

53.2.1 In what ways might this patient present with difficulty with airway management? What are the key aspects of the airway examination in this situation?

This is potentially an emergency situation. The patient must be quickly assessed and decisions made. While historically some patients with neck hematomas have been treated expectantly, case reports attest to the difficulty in predicting if or when these individuals will go on to sudden and catastrophic airway obstruction.[2–4] As part of the patient's evaluation, a formal airway examination must quickly be performed, seeking predictors of difficulty in all aspects of airway management.[5] Even though the patient had anatomy which earlier that day presented no difficulty with airway management, the presence of a neck hematoma changes everything. With evidence of an obstructing lesion in the airway—as manifested by stridor, neck swelling, and the patient's dyspnea and agitation—difficulty can now be anticipated with both bag-mask-ventilation (BMV) and use of an extraglottic device (EGD). Similarly, direct laryngoscopy in the presence of pathological obstruction may also be difficult, as anatomic landmarks are distorted, displaced, or obscured. Finally, transtracheal access by percutaneous or open surgical routes may also be difficult as landmarks are shifted or become indistinct.

53.2.2 What other patient factors may be relevant in this situation?

With predicted difficulty in all aspects of airway management limiting options in this patient, an awake approach at securing the airway may be judged preferable. However, for most awake airway interventions, substantial patient *cooperation* is necessary. Patient cooperation may be lost (a) as hypoxia occurs and/or (b) the patient panics as dyspnea worsens with progressive airway lumen narrowing. Both factors speak to the importance of early identification of the need for securing the airway, while cooperation can still be counted upon. Although sedative medications may help to render a patient more cooperative, sedating a patient with a tenuous airway is hazardous and may itself precipitate complete airway obstruction.[6–8] Other patient comorbidities will assume secondary importance compared to the gravity of threatened loss of the airway.

53.2.3 What are the mechanisms (anatomic and physiologic) of airway obstruction in a patient with a postsurgical neck hematoma?

Neck hematomas originate from capillary oozing or arterial bleeding. Arterial hematomas may present earlier[9]; however most post-surgical airway hematomas originate from capillary or venous sources.[9–11] Although slower in evolution, these latter hematomas can be insidious, and devastating in their ability to cause obstruction. The following mechanisms may contribute to the development of symptomatic airway obstruction in the patient with a neck hematoma:

1. *Physical pressure effect.* The presence of a hematoma in the neck can mechanically *displace* the laryngeal inlet dramatically away from the midline position,[4,9,12–14] in addition to physically *compressing* the lumen of the pharynx, laryngeal inlet or tracheal airway. While some authors consider significant compromise of the larynx and trachea unlikely due to their rigid cartilaginous structures,[15] others point out that the posterior, membranous portion of the trachea may still be compressed.[16] Indeed, some published case reports show CT scan images of impressive tracheal[17–19] compression by hematomas. Bukht described a case[20] in which a patient with a neck hematoma was intubated with difficulty with a 5 mm ETT. No leak was apparent even with the cuff deflated; however upon subsequent release of the hematoma, a large leak immediately developed.

2. *The development of perilaryngeal edema.* This is a consistent feature in case reports of patients with neck hematomas[2–4,9,13,14,17,20–22] and is often out of proportion to any degree of externally visible neck swelling. Most authors agree that this is due to interference with normal lymphatic[23] and/or venous drainage by the neck hematoma itself, as well as blood tracking into tissue planes away from the hematoma.[4,15,17,21,22] Edema may also have been exacerbated by released tissue inflammatory mediators.[21,24] At direct laryngoscopy, the resulting edema is variously described as "swollen supraglottic mucosal folds,"[4,9] or as a "watery, pale swelling of the mucosa"[15,22] which in many cases completely obscures the glottic opening. Interestingly, some case reports document the development of such perilaryngeal edema after neck surgery even in the absence of an obvious hematoma.[9,25]

3. Blood *dissection along tissue planes* in the neck. Blood from a neck hematoma can spread to further compromise the airway. Due to the contiguous nature of the parapharyngeal and retropharyngeal spaces,[16] neck hematomas can dissect into this latter space. Retropharyngeal collections of blood are often manifested symptomatically with dysphagia or odynophagia, in addition to hoarseness and dyspnea. They can also cause airway obstruction by compressing the arytenoid cartilages, which may in turn adduct the vocal cords.[26] In addition, retropharyngeal swelling can render direct laryngoscopy more difficult by: (a) shifting the laryngeal inlet anteriorly[27]; (b) apposing the posterior pharyngeal wall to the epiglottis; and (c) as it is a large dark mass,[27] a retropharyngeal hematoma can absorb light from the laryngoscope, worsening visibility.

Note that the second and third causes of airway compromise will not remit immediately upon evacuation of a hematoma, accounting for the variable success of urgently opening the surgical incision in alleviating respiratory extremis in these patients.

Two additional factors could potentially contribute to airway compromise postoperatively in patients undergoing routine head and neck surgery:

1. Simply undergoing certain operations in the head and neck region may transiently cause narrowing of the upper airway, even in the absence of a neck hematoma: Carmichael and colleagues[28,29] demonstrated a significant loss (up to 32%) of airway volume after routine carotid endarterectomy, greatest at the level of the hyoid but also present at the level of the arytenoids and cricoid ring.

2. Neck surgery can result in transient palsies to cranial nerves (IX–XII)[30] due to direct injury during dissection, retractor pressure, or other[31] causes. If unilateral, such palsies may be asymptomatic; however, particularly in patients presenting for staged bilateral procedures (e.g., carotid endarterectomies), bilateral nerve damage can result in complete airway obstruction. Vocal cord palsy can result from damage to the vagal trunk, or its recurrent laryngeal or superior laryngeal branches, while bilateral hypoglossal nerve palsies can result in airway obstruction due to loss of innervation to the intrinsic muscles of the tongue and pharyngeal musculature.[30] One final point to note in the patient undergoing staged bilateral carotid endarterectomies, is that ablation of the carotid bodies bilaterally will result in loss of the ventilatory response to hypoxia.[32]

53.3 MANAGING THE AIRWAY

53.3.1 Pending the decision of whether and where to reintubate, how can the patient be symptomatically temporized?

It should be reiterated that patients with partial airway obstruction are unpredictable in when, where, and if they will go on to complete airway obstruction. Indeed, case reports[3,4] document decisions to conservatively manage neck hematoma patients by observation, only to be confronted with sudden and catastrophic complete airway obstruction some hours later. Note that some patients going on to complete airway obstruction in this setting, have done so without first developing the physical sign of stridor.[2,3,9] It follows that nursing staff and airway practitioners must be educated to recognize the early signs of impending obstruction from a possible neck hematoma (i.e., subtle voice changes, progressing to hoarseness, dyspnea, and eventually stridor).

Dyspnea and stridor are late signs of airway compromise: the presence of inspiratory stridor is variously considered to be a symptom of an extrathoracic airway narrowed by 50%,[33] or to a diameter of 4.0 mm or less.[34] The patient in the presented case should be assumed to be in respiratory extremis. Once a compromising neck hematoma is suspected, plans should be undertaken for immediate definitive care: release and reexploration of the neck wound, and securing of the airway.

To temporize a case such as this on the short term (e.g., while organizing a return to the OR, or while obtaining equipment for reintubation), a number of maneuvers can be undertaken:

1. Elevation of the head of the bed, from 30 degrees to fully sitting, to promote venous drainage. The patient with significant airway compromise will most likely naturally wish to assume the sitting position.

2. Heliox can be administered. Heliox, a mixture of helium gas with oxygen, is less dense than air or pure oxygen. Gas flow through a stenotic area results in turbulent flow downstream from the stenosis and varies directly with density of the gas.[35] With its lower density, a helium–oxygen mixture minimizes the work of breathing by converting some or all of the turbulent flow through a critically narrowed airway to laminar flow.[36,37] Heliox is available in different oxygen/helium dilutions from 20/80 to 40/60: to maximize its clinical effect, the mixture with the highest concentration of helium should be used that is consistent with adequate oxygenation. Improved flow with heliox can lead to larger tidal volumes and less alveolar shunting, sometimes with improved oxygenation.[35,36,38] In addition, as a patient experiences alleviation of dyspnea-associated anxiety, less negative inspiratory pressure applied to the obstructed area may result in less airway collapse, thus actually improving the degree of obstruction.[36] Heliox use in the patient with a critically narrowed airway will often provide dramatic symptomatic relief, in turn potentially improving patient cooperation. In the setting of a neck hematoma, however, it should be assumed that heliox has no definitive therapeutic effect and is strictly a temporizing agent.

3. Racemic epinephrine (e.g., Vaponephrine®) given by aerosol may help temporarily shrink upper-airway edema.[39] In the adult population, it is most often used in the setting of transient post-extubation stridor and, in the setting of a neck hematoma, it would also have to be used with the understanding that it is only a temporizing measure.

4. Steroid administration can be considered, but the onset of drug effect is generally slow. Furthermore, evidence of clinical efficacy (in the short term) in the setting of pathologic airway obstruction is lacking.

5. Early consideration should be given to *opening the neck wound* in all postoperative neck hematoma cases. Some,[20,40] although certainly not all,[9,22,41] case reports document rapid clinical improvement following this maneuver. While a significant hematoma mass may be decompressed immediately, associated laryngeal edema and/or blood tracking remotely from the hematoma site will resolve more slowly. Clinical judgment dictates where and when to open the neck wound; the patient in respiratory extremis should have it opened immediately, while others may be safely managed upon returning to the more sterile conditions of the OR. However, any attempt at intubation should generally be preceded by release of the neck wound, whether in or out of the OR. It should be noted that this directive contrasts with the management of the patient with penetrating neck trauma, or likely bleeding from the carotid artery, where the possible presence of damaged major vascular structures mandates securing the airway by intubation prior to neck exploration.

53.3.2 Should tracheal intubation be performed in the PACU or in the operating room for this patient? What factors go into the decision?

The short answer is that the patient with a neck hematoma is ideally reintubated in the controlled conditions of the OR. The OR has the advantage of a more sterile environment, with availability of surgical equipment and staff should a double setup be elected, together with easier access to difficult airway equipment and expert help. In addition, the OR offers the option of an inhalational induction if desired. Ultimately, the decision about on-the-spot versus return to the OR intubation will be tempered by the following factors:

1. Is the patient *in extremis*? If so, the airway should be secured on the spot.

2. If the patient is becoming increasingly dyspneic, is the rate of decline such that a return to the OR may be safely undertaken?

3. How far is the OR from the patient's present location and is the OR located on the same floor as the PACU?

4. If the patient obstructs during transport to the OR, will one be able to bag-mask ventilate the patient? Fixed lesions (such as tumors, hematomas, or foreign bodies) that cause near-complete airway obstruction will often render the patient impossible to BMV. In contrast, more compressible pathology, such as epiglottitis, might be more amenable to BMV.

53.3.3 How should such an airway be approached, and why?

Patients with significant narrowing of the airway due to evolving pathological processes are in a dangerous situation. Onset of dyspnea, and then stridor, suggests critical airway narrowing, and in the setting of a neck hematoma should generally be regarded as signs of impending complete obstruction. Our airway assessment has suggested the potential for difficulty with BMV, laryngoscopic intubation, EGD rescue ventilation, and surgical airway. Careful consideration must therefore be given as to how best to proceed. A number of options exist:

1. *Local or regional anesthesia.* One published case series in the surgical literature[11] documents hematoma evacuation in eight patients under local anesthesia with no morbidity, which contrasted significantly from the 57% complication rate in the seven patients done under general anesthesia. Hematoma evacuation and exploration using local or regional anesthesia may be feasible before the patient is significantly short of breath, and is still able to cooperate. Regional anesthesia (e.g., superficial cervical blockade) may be difficult to perform as an enlarging hematoma obscures landmarks.[9]

2. *Awake tracheotomy under local anesthesia.* Some authorities suggest that patients with advanced degrees of airway pathology, particularly those with obstructing lesions of sufficient size to preclude passage of even a small tube, should have their airways secured with an awake tracheotomy under local anesthesia.[33,42] With patient cooperation, this is a procedure that can be done relatively quickly and painlessly. Technical difficulty can be

encountered if midline landmarks are shifted or obscured by an expanding hematoma. In addition, airway edema can also occur internally at the level of the cricoid ring, potentially impacting ease of cricothyrotomy.[24]

3. *Awake translaryngeal intubation.* Awake intubation confers the advantage of a breathing patient who is maintaining and protecting the airway, and would be judged the method of choice by many experts in this situation. In the setting of a neck hematoma, grossly distorted anatomy can be anticipated (see Section 53.2.3), yet, in the awake patient, movement of swollen mucosal folds (and bubbles) may help locate the laryngeal inlet. An attempted awake intubation must, however, confer a high probability of success in order to outweigh the risk of loss of the airway during the attempt (which can happen even in expert hands[6]). Attention to topical airway anesthesia (see Section 3.3.4 as well as Section 53.3.10 below), good fiberoptic or video bronchoscopic equipment, and the expertise to use it[9,43] will be necessary.

4. *Inhalational induction.* An inhalational induction has been espoused in a number of reports as an option for the patient with a neck hematoma.[9,23,33] However, during an inhalational induction, while spontaneous ventilatory efforts are generally maintained, it must be appreciated that volatile anesthetics have deleterious effects on upper airway tone and patency similar to those of intravenously administered sedatives.[44] While the inhalational induction may be considered for the patient unable to cooperate with an awake intubation, a double setup should be arranged, the neck wound should be opened before beginning, and close attention should be paid to maximizing airway patency as the patient loses consciousness. The latter includes: (1) maintaining the patient in a sitting or semi-sitting position; (2) keeping the head and upper C-spine extended and lower C-spine flexed (to maintain longitudinal traction on the upper airway, thus decreasing its collapsibility)[44]; (3) applying a jaw thrust to increase retropalatal and retrolingual airway caliber[44]; and (4) use of a nasopharyngeal airway to help overcome approximation of the soft palate to the posterior pharyngeal wall, while the patient is still too light to tolerate an oropharyngeal airway.[33] In addition, applying PEEP during gentle assisted BMV may help to splint open collapsible supraglottic structures. Inhalational inductions in the setting of neck hematomas in published case reports have been generally successful,[4,9,20] although in some cases prolonged or difficult.

5. *Rapid-sequence induction.* This route *cannot be recommended* for the patient with pathologic airway obstruction due to a neck hematoma. IV induction of anesthesia, with muscle relaxant administration is fraught with hazard in this setting, with case reports attesting to the lack of any identifiable landmarks at direct laryngoscopy,[4] *often in conjunction with the inability to bag-mask ventilate* the patient.[9]

53.3.4 How should we proceed in this case?

Our Plan A here is for an awake intubation under topical airway anesthesia, a viable option if good equipment and expertise is available with the flexible fiberoptic bronchoscope, and if patient

cooperation can be enlisted. In the event of an uncooperative patient, an inhalational induction can be considered. Plan B, in the event of loss of the airway during the awake intubation or inhalational induction, would be rapid conversion to transtracheal airway access (cricothyrotomy or tracheotomy).

53.3.5 How will you actually perform the awake intubation?

In the OR, a double setup should be readied, with scrubbed surgical staff and equipment for emergent cricothyrotomy or tracheotomy. The difficult airway cart should be in the room. The cricothyroid membrane should be identified and marked. If not already done, the neck wound should be opened, any easily accessible clot removed, and covered with a sterile dressing. IV access should be assured, monitors applied, and the patient placed in his position of comfort (often sitting). A drying agent such as glycopyrrolate 0.2–0.4 mg IM/IV can be given. Psychological preparation should be undertaken with confident reassurance that successful intubation will totally alleviate the patient's dyspnea, while at the same time explaining the gravity of the situation, and emphasizing the need for cooperation. If heliox had been applied, it should be interrupted for only brief periods during application of topical airway anesthesia. Topical airway anesthetic agents and techniques have been addressed elsewhere (see Chapter 3). Ideally, sedation should be omitted or minimized. An adult flexible fiberoptic bronchoscope (e.g., 5.5 mm) should be loaded with a small tube (e.g., 7 mm ID) and awake fiberoptic intubation performed, aided by gentle tongue traction. Substantial edema of perilaryngeal tissues should be expected. The patient should be encouraged to continue to protrude his tongue, while taking slow deep breaths to help elevate the epiglottis. The laryngeal inlet is located by observing movement of the cords (or overlying edematous tissue). Occasionally, looking for bubbles on expiration has been helpful.

53.3.6 During application of topical airway anesthesia, the patient's airway obstructs. What should you do now?

If the patient's airway obstructs, common sense should prevail. You should do what you would always do to ventilate the apneic patient: attempt an airway-opening maneuver, and perform BMV, using a two-person technique. An oropharyngeal, or nasopharyngeal airway, may be used, depending on the level of consciousness of the patient. Note that PEEP should be applied during BMV[44,45] to help splint open collapsed tissues and ease laryngospasm.

58.3.7 What if the BMV fails? Should a surgical airway be performed?

A failed airway situation can be defined as the inability to maintain adequate O_2 saturation with BMV *and* failure to intubate on at least one occasion (see Section 2.5.5). This is a serious situation and immediate preparations should be underway to proceed with an emergency cricothyrotomy. However, while preparing for the cricothyrotomy, it is reasonable to perform at least one direct laryngoscopy. To this point, after all, we do not know for sure that the trachea of the patient cannot be intubated using direct laryngoscopy, and emergency surgical airway is not without morbidity.

53.3.8   At direct laryngoscopy, nothing is identifiable other than the epiglottis. What are your options?

If direct laryngoscopy itself is easy, with midline structures and a visible, mobile epiglottis, but only amorphous edematous tissue beneath, it is possible that extensive supraglottic edema is the problem. If the patient is already unconscious, it may be worth performing a single chest compression to see if a bubble is produced, indicating the entrance to the airway. With or without a bubble, a tracheal tube introducer, and/or small tube, can be placed where the glottic opening would be expected to be. Alternatively, if the anatomy is even more distorted, with minimal or no exposure of an abnormally located epiglottis (e.g., with left or right deviation), time does not permit other options. In a "can't ventilate/can't intubate" failed airway situation, the default maneuver is to proceed to emergency percutaneous or open surgical cricothyrotomy, particularly as EGDs may not work well in this situation. To maximize the chances of salvaging a bad situation, it is important to proceed quickly with the surgical airway. Historically, the decision to proceed with transtracheal access is made too late to salvage the patient.

53.3.9   What is the role, if any, for an EGD such as a laryngeal mask airway?

Strictly speaking, use of a laryngeal mask airway (LMA) in this patient would be difficult: as (a) there may be problems with its seating due to a displaced laryngeal inlet; and (b) extensive edema at, or above the level of the cords may preclude effective ventilation. However, several centers have reported successful oxygenation of patients with LMAs in failed airway situations due to neck hematomas[41,46] or other obstructing pathology.[47,48] This may occur as the LMA bypasses more proximal obstruction due to tongue and soft palate, while delivering positive-pressure ventilation immediately in front of the laryngeal inlet, possibly with local delivery of PEEP. While the correct response in the failed airway (can't intubate/can't ventilate) situation is a surgical airway, if delay was encountered in obtaining the requisite equipment and an EGD was immediately available, it may be worth a quick try.

53.3.10   I thought that awake fiberoptic intubation was the foolproof gold standard for difficult airway. Why did the patient's airway obstruct during application of topical airway anesthesia?

Loss of the airway during application of topical airway anesthesia[45,48–50] or awake fiberoptic intubation[6,41,51] in the patient with a neck hematoma or other obstructing pathology is well described. Apart from the natural progression of the disease process, this may occur for a number of reasons:

1. The adverse effects of systemically administered sedative agents on the airway.[6,44]

2. *Laryngospasm* during the airway topicalization process,[33,48,49] particularly in the patient with heavier degrees of sedation.

3. *Patient panic.* As the dyspneic patient desperately tries to inspire, the high negative inspiratory pressure applied to an already narrowed, collapsible upper airway may contribute to complete collapse.[18,49]

4. *Direct effect of local anesthetic agents on upper airway mechanoreceptors.* The existence of laryngeal and supralaryngeal pressure and stretch receptors has been hypothesized, to maintain airway patency by responding to negative intraluminal airway pressure via increasing neural and muscular activity.[52,53] The activity of such receptors can be affected or abolished by application of topical airway anesthesia.[52,53] This in turn can significantly affect inspiratory flow, even in normal individuals. Pulmonary function studies have demonstrated a significant reduction in maximal,[54] peak, and forced[55] inspiratory flow rates following topical airway anesthesia. Studies of the sleep apnea population in whom topical airway anesthesia has been applied have also shown worsening of obstructive parameters. This is an underappreciated side effect of topical airway anesthesia and in the patient with a tenuous airway may be an important phenomenon to consider (see Section 3.3.4). It does not preclude choosing awake intubation with topical airway anesthesia, but does underscore the need for planning and a double setup. It may also imply that, in the patient with pathological upper airway compromise, a nasal approach may be preferable, with its lessened need for extensive pharyngeal topicalization.

53.4   OTHER CONSIDERATIONS

53.4.1   What should be the postoperative disposition of a patient reintubated for a neck hematoma?

Although the immediate mechanical compression of the airway caused by the hematoma may be relieved, other mechanisms of airway compromise, e.g., laryngeal inlet edema and blood dissection along tissue planes, may take longer to resolve. Caution must prevail and strong consideration should be given to keeping the patient intubated and ventilated for a period of time (e.g., 24 hours) in an intensive care setting. The patient should be nursed head-up to promote venous drainage and consideration can be given to administering steroids. Admittedly, many randomized controlled trials looking at the effect of steroid administration on upper airway[29] and laryngeal edema,[56] or postextubation stridor[57] in adults have failed to demonstrate a beneficial effect. Results of studies in the pediatric setting have been mixed.[58,59] Future studies looking at alternative doses, dosing intervals, or specific subpopulations may yet identify a beneficial effect of steroid administration.

53.4.2   What criteria should be met prior to extubation?

In addition to usual extubation criteria, prior to extubation of the patient intubated for airway pathology, such as a neck hematoma, an attempt should be made to evaluate both the caliber of the sub-glottic airway and the condition of the laryngeal inlet. Traditionally, presence of a "cuff leak" has been sought as a reassuring sign of an airway patent enough to withstand extubation. Clinically testing for a cuff leak has been described in a number of ways (see Section 29.4.2):

1. In the spontaneously breathing patient, simply deflating the ETT cuff, briefly manually occluding the end of the ETT, and evaluating the patient's ability to breath around the tube.[60–63]

2. With the cuff deflated, delivering a positive pressure volume with a satisfactory result being the presence of a leak at a delivered peak pressure of 15 cm H_2O or less.[4,9]

3. A more objective evaluation has been described which involves having a ventilator deliver a set volume (e.g., 10 mL·kg^{-1}) with the ETT cuff deflated, then measuring the expired volume in milliliters[64,65] and/or as a percentage of the delivered inspiratory volume.[66–68]

Most,[60–64,67,68] but not all[65] studies agree that the presence of a leak (present qualitatively or measured quantitatively)[66] is predictive of successful extubation (i.e., absence of stridor postextubation and/or no need for reintubation). Conversely, many studies also showed that the absence of a leak did not necessarily preclude successful extubation.[61–63,66–68]

This latter group of patients, however, would be particularly good candidates for further evaluation of the upper airway prior to extubation, e.g., through direct laryngoscopic or indirect fiberoptic (e.g., with a nasopharyngoscope) assessment. One would look for three features:

1. an appropriate midline location of the laryngeal inlet

2. the lack of significant perilaryngeal edema

3. appropriate bilateral vocal cord movement[31]

If extubation is elected in this group, consideration should be given to extubating over an airway exchange catheter. In worrisome cases, extubation can be done in the OR, as this may facilitate inspection of the laryngeal inlet with direct or indirect laryngoscopy, in addition to permitting easier access to equipment for a difficult reintubation.

53.4.3   What other situations or types of surgery incur the risk of neck hematomas? Are there any preventive measures which can be undertaken?

Any surgery of the head, neck, and thorax can lead to airway-compromising hematomas. Common examples include carotid endarterectomies,[9,10] parathyroid and thyroid surgery,[15,22] and anterior discectomy/fusion.[40] Central line insertion attempts are also strongly represented in the literature in the development of life-threatening and fatal neck hematomas.[2,3,12–14,17] At least for carotid artery surgery, risk factors for the development of postoperative hematomas include antiplatelet agents,[4,9] the nonreversal of intraoperatively administered heparin,[10,21] use of a vein graft,[69] and

experiencing significant hypertension (e.g., systolic blood pressure of >200 mm Hg)[4,9,10,21] in the PACU. This latter underscores the importance of aggressive control of hemodynamics in a high-dependency care environment postoperatively.

53.5   SUMMARY

Clearly, with awake intubation, or an inhalational induction in the patient with a postsurgical neck hematoma, the risk of complete loss of the airway is always present. Primary awake tracheotomy will avoid this eventuality in the patient with severe airway compromise, or, if intubation from above *is* attempted, it should be with prior release of the neck hematoma, and must always be with "double setup" availability of equipment and personnel to allow an emergency cricothyrotomy, should it become necessary.

REFERENCES

1. Cormack RS, Lehane J: Difficult tracheal intubation in obstetrics. *Anaesthesia.* 1984;39:1105–1111.
2. Randalls B, Toomey PJ: Laryngeal oedema from a neck haematoma. A complication of internal jugular vein cannulation. *Anaesthesia.* 1990;45:850–852.
3. Digby S: Fatal respiratory obstruction following insertion of a central venous line. *Anaesthesia.* 1994;49:1013–1014.
4. Munro FJ, Makin AP, Reid J: Airway problems after carotid endarterectomy. *Br J Anaesth.* 1996;76:156–159.
5. Murphy M, Hung O, Launcelott G, Law JA, Morris I: Predicting the difficult laryngoscopic intubation: are we on the right track? *Can J Anaesth.* 2005;52:231–235.
6. McGuire G, el-Beheiry H: Complete upper airway obstruction during awake fibreoptic intubation in patients with unstable cervical spine fractures. *Can J Anaesth.* 1999;46:176–178.
7. Crosby ET: Complete airway obstruction. *Can J Anaesth.* 1999;46:99–104.
8. Byard RW, Gilbert JD: Narcotic administration and stenosing lesions of the upper airway—a potentially lethal combination. *J Clin Forensic Med.* 2005;12:29–31.
9. O'Sullivan JC, Wells DG, Wells GR: Difficult airway management with neck swelling after carotid endarterectomy. *Anaesth Intensive Care.* 1986;14:460–464.
10. Nunn DB: Carotid endarterectomy: an analysis of 234 operative cases. *Ann Surg.* 1975;182:733–738.
11. Kunkel JM, Gomez ER, Spebar MJ, et al.: Wound hematomas after carotid endarterectomy. *Am J Surg.* 1984;148:844–847.
12. Smurthwaite GJ, Letheren MJ: Airway obstruction after trans-jugular liver biopsy: anaesthetic management. *Br J Anaesth.* 1995;75:102–104.
13. Knoblanche GE: Respiratory obstruction due to haematoma following internal jugular vein cannulation. *Anaesth Intensive Care.* 1979;7:286.
14. Lo WK, Chong JL: Neck haematoma and airway obstruction in a pre-eclamptic patient: a complication of internal jugular vein cannulation. *Anaesth Intensive Care.* 1997;25:423–425.
15. Hare R: Respiratory obstruction after thyroidectomy. *Anaesthesia.* 1982;37:1136.
16. Paleri V, Maroju RS, Ali MS, Ruckley RW: Spontaneous retro- and parapharyngeal haematoma caused by intrathyroid bleed. *J Laryngol Otol.* 2002;116:854–858.
17. Kua JS, Tan IK: Airway obstruction following internal jugular vein cannulation. *Anaesthesia.* 1997;52:776–780.
18. Shiratori T, Hara K, Ando N: Acute airway obstruction secondary to retropharyngeal hematoma. *J Anesth.* 2003;17:46–48.
19. Thomas MD, Torres A, Garcia-Polo J, Gavilan C: Life-threatening cervico-mediastinal haematoma after carotid sinus massage. *J Laryngol Otol.* 1991;105:381–383.
20. Bukht D, Langford RM: Airway obstruction after surgery in the neck. *Anaesthesia.* 1983;38:389–390.
21. Holdsworth RJ, McCollum PT: Acute laryngeal oedema following carotid endarterectomy. *J Cardiovasc Surg (Torino).* 1994;35:249–251.

22. Bexton MD, Radford R: An unusual cause of respiratory obstruction after thyroidectomy. *Anaesthesia.* 1982;37:596.

23. Wells DG, Zelcer J, Wells GR, Sherman GP: A theoretical mechanism for massive supraglottic swelling following carotid endarterectomy. *Aust NZJ Surg.* 1988;58:979–981.

24. Carmichael FJ, McGuire GP, Wong DT, et al.: Computed tomographic analysis of airway dimensions after carotid endarterectomy. *Anesth Analg.* 1996;83: 12–17.

25. Wade JS: Cecil Joll lecture, 1979. Respiratory obstruction in thyroid surgery. *Ann R Coll Surg Engl.* 1980;62:15–24.

26. Field JR, DeSaussure RL: Retropharyngeal hemorrhage with respiratory obstruction following angiography. *J Neurosurg.* 1965;22:610–611.

27. Myssiorek D, Shalmi C: Traumatic retropharyngeal hematoma. *Arch Otolaryngol Head Neck Surg.* 1989;115:1130–1132.

28. Carmichael F, McGuire G, Wong D, et al.: Computed tomographic analysis of airway dimensions after carotid endarterectomy. *Anesth Analg.* 1996; 83:12–17.

29. Hughes R, McGuire G, Montanera W, Wong D, Carmichael FJ: Upper airway edema after carotid endarterectomy: the effect of steroid administration. *Anesth Analg.* 1997;84:475–478.

30. Spiekermann BF, Stone DJ, Bogdonoff DL, Yemen TA: Airway management in neuroanaesthesia. *Can J Anaesth.* 1996;43:820–834.

31. Tyers MR, Cronin K: Airway obstruction following second operation for carotid endarterectomy. *Anaesth Intensive Care.* 1986;14:314–316.

32. Wade JG, Larson CP, Jr, Hickey RF, Ehrenfeld WK, Severinghaus JW: Effect of carotid endarterectomy on carotid chemoreceptor and baroreceptor function in man. *N Engl J Med.* 1970;282:823–829.

33. Mason RA, Fielder CP: The obstructed airway in head and neck surgery. *Anaesthesia.* 1999;54:625–628.

34. Donlon J, Jr: *Anesthetic and Airway Management of Laryngoscopy and Bronchoscopy.* St. Louis, MO: Mosby, 1996.

35. Khanlou H, Eiger G: Safety and efficacy of heliox as a treatment for upper airway obstruction due to radiation-induced laryngeal dysfunction. *Heart Lung.* 2001;30:146–147.

36. Ho AM, Dion PW, Karmakar MK, Chung DC, Tay BA: Use of heliox in critical upper airway obstruction. Physical and physiologic considerations in choosing the optimal helium:oxygen mix. *Resuscitation.* 2002;52:297–300.

37. Hessan H, Houck J, Harvey H: Airway obstruction due to lymphoma of the larynx and trachea. *Laryngoscope.* 1988;98:176–180.

38. Riley RH, Raper GD, Newman MA: Helium-oxygen and cardiopulmonary bypass standby in anaesthesia for tracheal stenosis. *Anaesth Intensive Care.* 1994;22:710–713.

39. MacDonnell SP, Timmins AC, Watson JD: Adrenaline administered via a nebulizer in adult patients with upper airway obstruction. *Anaesthesia.* 1995;50: 35–36.

40. Roy SP: Acute postoperative neck hematoma. *Am J Emerg Med.* 1999;17: 308–309.

41. Martin R, Girouard Y, Cote DJ: Use of a laryngeal mask in acute airway obstruction after carotid endarterectomy. *Can J Anaesth.* 2002;49:890.

42. Goldberg D, Bhatti N: Management of the impaired airway in the adult. Chapter 106. In: Cummings Otolaryngology Head and Neck Surgery, 4th edn. Cummings CW, ed. Philadelphia, PA: Elsevier, Mosby, 2005: 2441–2453.

43. Ovassapian A, Tuncbilek M, Weitzel EK, Joshi CW: Airway management in adult patients with deep neck infections: a case series and review of the literature. *Anesth Analg.* 2005;100:585–589.

44. Hillman DR, Platt PR, Eastwood PR: The upper airway during anaesthesia. *Br J Anaesth.* 2003;91:31–39.

45. Calder I, Koh K: Cervical haematoma and airway obstruction. *Br J Anaesth.* 1996;76:888–889.

46. Jones DA, Geraghty IF: Emergency management of upper airway obstruction due to a rapidly expanding haematoma in the neck. *Br J Hosp Med.* 1995;53: 589–590.

47. King CJ, Davey AJ, Chandradeva K: Emergency use of the laryngeal mask airway in severe upper airway obstruction caused by supraglottic oedema. *Br J Anaesth.* 1995;75:785–786.

48. Shaw IC, Welchew EA, Harrison BJ, Michael S: Complete airway obstruction during awake fibreoptic intubation. *Anaesthesia.* 1997;52:582–585.

49. Ho AM, Chung DC, To EW, Karmakar MK: Total airway obstruction during local anaesthesia in a non-sedated patient with a compromised airway. *Can J Anaesth.* 2004;51:838–841.

50. White MC, Reynolds F: Sudden airway obstruction following inhalation drug abuse. *Br J Anaesth.* 1999;82:808.

51. Wulf H, Brinkmann G, Rautenberg M: Management of the difficult airway. A case of failed fiberoptic intubation. *Acta Anaesthesiol Scand.* 1997;41: 1080–1082.

52. Horner RL, Innes JA, Holden HB, Guz A: Afferent pathway(s) for pharyngeal dilator reflex to negative pressure in man: a study using upper airway anaesthesia. *J Physiol.* 1991;436:31–44.

53. Berry RB, McNellis MI, Kouchi K, Light RW: Upper airway anesthesia reduces phasic genioglossus activity during sleep apnea. *Am J Respir Crit Care Med.* 1997;156:127–132.

54. Liistro G, Stanescu DC, Veriter C, Rodenstein DO, D'Odemont JP: Upper airway anesthesia induces airflow limitation in awake humans. *Am Rev Respir Dis.* 1992;146:581–585.

55. Kuna ST, Woodson GE, Sant'Ambrogio G: Effect of laryngeal anesthesia on pulmonary function testing in normal subjects. *Am Rev Respir Dis.* 1988;137: 656–661.

56. Darmon JY, Rauss A, Dreyfuss D, et al.: Evaluation of risk factors for laryngeal edema after tracheal extubation in adults and its prevention by dexamethasone. A placebo-controlled, double-blind, multicenter study. *Anesthesiology.* 1992; 77:245–251.

57. Ho LI, Harn HJ, Lien TC, Hu PY, Wang JH: Postextubation laryngeal edema in adults. Risk factor evaluation and prevention by hydrocortisone. *Intensive Care Med.* 1996;22:933–936.

58. Anene O, Meert KL, Uy H, Simpson P, Sarnaik AP: Dexamethasone for the prevention of postextubation airway obstruction: a prospective, randomized, double-blind, placebo-controlled trial. *Crit Care Med.* 1996;24: 1666–1669.

59. Tellez DW, Galvis AG, Storgion SA, et al.: Dexamethasone in the prevention of postextubation stridor in children. *J Pediatr.* 1991;118:289–294.

60. Potgieter PD, Hammond JM: "Cuff" test for safe extubation following laryngeal edema. *Crit Care Med.* 1988;16:818.

61. Fisher MM, Raper RF: The 'cuff-leak' test for extubation. *Anaesthesia.* 1992; 47:10–12.

62. Maury E, Guglielminotti J, Alzieu M, et al.: How to identify patients with no risk for postextubation stridor? *J Crit Care.* 2004;19:23–28.

63. Marik PE: The cuff-leak test as a predictor of postextubation stridor: a prospective study. *Respiratory Care.* 1996;41:509–511.

64. Miller RL, Cole RP: Association between reduced cuff leak volume and postextubation stridor. *Chest.* 1996;110:1035–1040.

65. Engoren M: Evaluation of the cuff-leak test in a cardiac surgery population. *Chest.* 1999;116:1029–1031.

66. Sandhu RS, Pasquale MD, Miller K, Wasser TE: Measurement of endotracheal tube cuff leak to predict postextubation stridor and need for reintubation. *J Am Coll Surg.* 2000;190:682–687.

67. De Bast Y, De Backer D, Moraine JJ, et al.: The cuff leak test to predict failure of tracheal extubation for laryngeal edema. *Intensive Care Med.* 2002;28: 1267–1272.

68. Jaber S, Chanques G, Matecki S, et al.: Post-extubation stridor in intensive care unit patients. Risk factors evaluation and importance of the cuff-leak test. *Intensive Care Med.* 2003;29:69–74.

69. Tawes RL, Jr, Treiman RL: Vein patch rupture after carotid endarterectomy: a survey of the Western Vascular Society members. *Ann Vasc Surg.* 1991;5: 71–73.

SELF-EVALUATION QUESTIONS

53.1. Recognizing that no method of intubation can be guaranteed 100% complication free, which of the following approaches to securing the airway is **LEAST** safe in the patient with a neck hematoma?

A. awake intubation with topical airway anesthesia

B. rapid-sequence intubation with induction agent and muscle relaxant

C. local or regional anesthesia for evacuation of hematoma and no intubation

D. inhalational induction

E. awake tracheotomy under local anesthesia

53.2. In the patient with obstructing airway pathology such as a neck hematoma, which of the following is the **LEAST** safe option to help symptomatically temporize the patient while preparing for intubation?

A. use sedative agents to alleviate patient anxiety

B. if patient oxygenation permits, use Heliox to help reducing the work of breathing

C. have the patient in the sitting or semi-sitting position

D. administer racemic epinephrine via aerosol

E. give IV steroids to help counteract any inflammatory component.

53.3. In the patient with obstructing airway pathology such as a neck hematoma, which of the following airway management techniques would be (at least relatively) contraindicated?

A. direct laryngoscopy and intubation

B. placement of a laryngeal mask airway

C. blind tube passage through an intubating (Fastrach®) laryngeal mask airway

D. awake intubation with a flexible fiberoptic bronchoscope

E. BMV with an oropharyngeal airway.

CHAPTER (54)

Respiratory Arrest in the Magnetic Resonance Imaging Suite

D. John Doyle

54.1 CASE PRESENTATION: PART I

Mr. S is a 52 year old entrepreneur in the waste management industry. He weighs 262 lbs (~119 kg), is 5'9" (~175 cm) tall, and is being investigated for "dizzy spells" that appear to be panic attacks. His medical problem list includes obesity, untreated hypertension, and possible obstructive sleep apnea (OSA) (based on his wife's nocturnal observation that "sometimes he just stops breathing"). When questioned, he admits to extreme claustrophobia, possibly the result of a protracted period of time spent in a car trunk as a child. A previous attempt at a magnetic resonance imaging (MRI) scan was unsuccessful because Mr. S, startled by the onset of the loud noises made by the MRI machine, panicked and tried to get out of the MRI scanner, pulling out his IV in the process.

On this occasion, the MRI team decides that Mr. S might be more cooperative with pharmacologic assistance and to this end has given him 5 mg of IV midazolam (Versed®). Unknown to the clinical team, just before entering the MRI suite, Mr. S had also taken 6 mg of sublingual lorazepam (Ativan®) to help reduce his considerable anxiety. For the scan, a pulse oximeter and nasal capnograph are used to monitor respiration. Oxygen is administered by nasal prongs at 3 L per minute.

About 10 minutes into the scan, the pulse oximeter alarm activates, drawing attention to an oxygen saturation reading of 83%. The pulse oximeter waveform quality appears to be good. However, no waveform can be obtained from the capnograph. Since Mr. S is deep inside the MRI machine, it is hard to see how well he is actually breathing. You are summoned to the MRI suite to help manage this patient.

54.2 THE MAGNETIC RESONANCE IMAGING (MRI) SUITE

54.2.1 What is MRI and why is it done?

MRI has steadily increased in popularity as a noninvasive, painless diagnostic imaging procedure. MRI images are produced using a strong (typically, 1.5 tesla [15,000 gauss]) magnetic field into which radiofrequency (RF) pulses are injected. MRI is the imaging method of choice for examinations in which water content differences make it possible to differentiate tissue types.[1] It offers distinct advantages over computed tomography, both in terms of the quality of the obtained images for certain types of tissue (like brain) and in the lack of exposure to ionizing radiation. MRI scans are frequently ordered by neurologists and neurosurgeons for patients of all ages with neurological disorders. In addition to intra-axial pathology, orthopedic problems such as osteomyelitis, soft tissue muscle tumors, and damaged knee menisci can be assessed using MRI techniques.[1]

54.2.2 What is unique about the MRI suite?

The extreme strength of the magnetic field in an MRI scanner can be hazardous. For example, patients with implanted ferromagnetic objects like aneurysm clips have had these fatally pulled out of position by the magnetic field.[2] Similarly, some authorities have expressed concerns about carrying out MRI scans in patients with pacemakers.[3] Likewise, ferromagnetic objects like wrenches, scissors, IV poles, pens, stethoscopes, and even hair barrettes can become accidental projectiles. In one case, a pillow containing metal springs, not detectable using a handheld magnet, flew into the magnet during positioning of a patient, fortunately without causing injury.[4] Sometimes death has been the result, as in the case of a 6 year old boy killed when a loose oxygen tank became a projectile and crushed his skull.[5–7]

Zimmer et al.[8] relate the following interesting cautionary tale. A 2 year old boy underwent abdominal MRI scanning under general anesthesia. During the case, an anesthesia practitioner carried a portable sevoflurane vaporizer into the MRI suite. When the vaporizer was placed on an examination table, it was vigorously attracted toward the scanner, and it was only by the strength of two people that the vaporizer was directed to strike against the gantry, instead of flying directly into the magnet where it might have hit the child. Quenching the magnet, i.e., emergency release of liquid helium from the scanner to collapse the magnetic field, was initially considered, but the vaporizer could be removed with the help of a third individual. Of interest, immediately after the mishap the portable vaporizer was tested for magnetism with a strong handheld magnet, and no attraction was apparent. A review of the event revealed that the vaporizer contained ferromagnetic material in the temperature compensation module.

In addition to the attractive forces of the magnetic field on ferromagnetic objects, the strong magnetic field and associated RF pulses can interfere with the operation of ordinary anesthesia machines, as well as with patient monitoring equipment, sometimes resulting in patient injury.[9]

It should be emphasized that some anesthesia machines and patient monitors that are alleged to be MRI compatible may still contain ferromagnetic components and may pose risks when safety precautions (often described in fine print in the user's manual) are violated.

54.2.3 Why might MRI require moderate or deep sedation, or general anesthesia?

Patients must remain motionless during MRI scans. However, the long duration (up to 20 minutes or more) of some MRI scans may eventually lead to significant discomfort for many patients. In addition to fidgeting, many MRI patients are fearful or claustrophobic. Moderate to deep sedation, or general anesthesia, may be required to immobilize these patients sufficiently to obtain good quality scan images, particularly in children and the mentally challenged patients.

54.2.4 What special precautions must clinicians take when responding to or working in the MRI suite?

Clinicians caring for patients in MRI suites must be careful to rid themselves of all objects with possible ferromagnetic components, such as pagers, mobile phones, keys, pens, and stethoscopes. In addition, credit cards and ID badges may be erased by the magnetic field.

There are serious concerns regarding the clinical monitoring modalities available in an MRI unit. In order to monitor the patients undergoing general anesthesia properly, it is necessary to have MRI compatible systems that support automatic noninvasive blood pressure monitoring, electrocardiography, pulse oximetry,

capnography, and even multichannel invasive pressure monitoring. Electrocardiogram electrodes must be applied at a distance from the imaging area, or (in special cases) should be replaced with special carbon MRI compatible electrodes.

54.2.5 Where can one obtain MRI-compatible anesthesia equipment?

The list of MRI compatible anesthesia equipment needed in an MRI suite can be extensive and includes, but is not limited to, anesthesia machines, patient monitors, oxygen cylinders, and laryngoscopes. Hospital purchasing departments should be able to provide useful information on the availability of this equipment. The author recommends getting information from the web site www.magmedix.com. Additional resources appear in Appendix 1 later in this chapter.

54.3 AIRWAY MANAGEMENT CONSIDERATIONS IN AN MRI UNIT

54.3.1 What airway equipment may or may not be used in an MRI unit?

The answer to the question regarding which airway management devices are safe to use in an MRI unit can be both simple and complex. The simple answer is that devices, such as conventional laryngoscopes that contain substantial amounts of ferromagnetic materials, can easily become dangerous projectiles, while items completely free of ferromagnetic materials are completely safe. The complex answer is that most airway instruments and devices that have not been specifically designed for use in an MRI environment are likely to have at least some ferromagnetic components. Even apparently benign products, like endotracheal tubes and laryngeal mask airways (LMAs), may have small amounts of ferromagnetic materials, such as metallic springs in the cuff inflation valve. While such small ferromagnetic objects do not generally present a projectile safety hazard, they can interfere with the image quality, possibly introducing an "information hole" if located near the imaging area.

54.3.2 What are some other airway management issues in the MRI environment?

Since most airway devices are not specifically designed for the MRI environment, equipments like flexible fiberoptic bronchoscopes, rigid fiberoptic laryngoscopes (such as the Bullard laryngoscope), or video laryngoscopes (such as the GlideScope®) must be specifically tested for suitability in the MRI environment, by experienced MRI personnel. In addition, there is a theoretical concern that armored endotracheal tubes and other airway devices with wire-reinforced elements may either interfere with image quality, or undergo self-heating from absorbed electromagnetic radiation. The same applies to the LMA Fastrach and CTrach™ Intubating LMA, though the newly introduced disposable Intubating LMA device is metal free.

It should also be pointed out that airway equipment containing electronic circuits could possibly be affected by strong magnetic fields, for example by the mechanism of closing a normally open switch containing ferromagnetic elements. This has been alleged to sometimes occur with the Trachlight™ intubating lightwand.

54.4   MANAGEMENT OF THIS PATIENT

54.4.1   What are immediate management options for this patient?

Let us get back to Mr. S, who is now turning blue. It is likely that he has been overly sedated and has an obstructed airway. Based on the history from his wife that he sometimes "just stops breathing" while asleep, it is likely that OSA is involved. The management options available include the following:

1. If the patient is accessible, a simple jaw thrust or head tilt often suffices to restore respiration. Most of the time, however, the scan will have to be temporarily suspended to permit this to occur. (This does not, however, mean that the magnet needs to be turned off). Some practitioners have tried taping the patient's jaw to the MRI head frame to keep the airway open.

2. The patient may also benefit from a nasopharyngeal airway. An oropharyngeal airway may also be considered but these tend to be less well tolerated.

3. If a simple jaw thrust, head tilt, or artificial airway does not promptly restore effective ventilation and oxygenation, positive pressure ventilation with 100% oxygen, using BMV, will be needed to restore oxygenation. Certainly, when the patient is severely hypoxemic, this should be the first step undertaken.

4. Pharmacologic reversal of the lorazepam/midazolam may be helpful to reduce the level of sedation and restore the airway. Intravenous flumazenil, administered in 100 μg increments (in adults), is a benzodiazepine antagonist that antagonizes the sedation produced by all benzodiazepines. In the case of opioids, pharmacologic reversal can be achieved using intravenous naloxone (Narcan®), also using 100 μg increments. It should be emphasized that since both naloxone and flumazenil have relatively short durations of action, resedation can occur. As Mr. S is a chronic user of benzodiazepines, he may be physically dependent on benzodiazepine. It is possible that flumazenil, administered in traditionally recommended doses, may induce seizures.[10]

5. Insertion of an LMA, or even tracheal intubation, may be necessary in the absence of ventilation. Although LMAs may compromise the MRI image, this is not a constant finding. As mentioned, ferromagnetic laryngoscope cannot be used. Commercially available MRI compatible laryngoscopes along with MRI compatible batteries should be readily available in the vicinity of the MRI unit.

54.5   CASE PRESENTATION: PART II

Given that Mr. S has developed respiratory difficulties, it is decided to remove him from the scanner to allow for positive pressure ventilation, or other intervention. With the commotion of being moved about, Mr. S becomes aroused, and spontaneous respirations resume. Instead of positive pressure ventilation with a bag-mask-ventilation (BMV) unit, a non-rebreathing face mask is used and the pulse oximeter is soon providing reassuring tones and numbers. Mr. S remains drowsy when left undisturbed and he continues to have intermittent obstruction of his airway. The radiologist is eager to have the scan completed, emphasizing first that Mr. S's neurologist has called repeatedly about the results (being concerned about ruling out a brain tumor) and also emphasizing that this is the second time an MRI has been attempted on Mr. S.

Your examination shows that Mr. S. has a Mallampati class III view. In addition, his considerable obesity and his apparent history of OSA raise concerns regarding possible difficult BMV, laryngoscopy, intubation, and emergency surgical airway. In addition, there are patient issues regarding cooperation, possible substance abuse, and an increased potential for rapid desaturation (because of a small functional residual capacity).

54.5.1   How should we proceed (if we did proceed) with managing the airway?

With the concerns listed above, and the urgency to proceed, a variety of means to secure the airway can be considered. Provided that BMV is not anticipated to be difficult, the first option, "Plan A," is to induce anesthesia using propofol and achieve muscle relaxation using succinylcholine. Assuming that the patient is not prone to aspiration, and expert help is readily available, induction of anesthesia could either be done in the induction area some distance from the MRI scanner or in a regular operating room. An appropriate variety of airway devices and adjuncts, like an intubating stylet and an LMA, must be immediately available.

If the view at laryngoscopy proves to be unsatisfactory, even with the external laryngeal manipulation, and the use of the intubation stylet is unlikely to be successful (Grade 3B, or Grade 4 airway [see Figure 7.1]), this author's recommended "Plan B" would be to use a GlideScope®. This instrument has proven to be especially valuable.[11,12] Failing that, "Plan C" would be to use fiberoptic intubation, either awake or under general anesthesia.

There are several possible options in the use of the flexible fiberoptic bronchoscope. These include tracheal intubation using the fiberoptic bronchoscope through the LMA Classic™ with the aid of an Aintree catheter[13] or using the GlideScope® to facilitate fiberoptic intubation.[14]

If one's overall clinical impression is that inducing general anesthesia is not a prudent course, a more cautious approach would likely be awake intubation under topical anesthesia, using a flexible fiberoptic bronchoscope or using the GlideScope®.[14]

54.5.2   Discuss postintubation management

At the end of the MRI scanning procedure, a decision should be made whether it is safe to perform tracheal extubation in the MRI suite or in the post-anesthetic care unit after a period of elective ventilation (as might be appropriate if intubation was difficult and it is suspected that the airway structures are edematous). Consideration will, at times, be given to extubation over a tube exchanger (see Chapter 29).

54.6   OTHER CONSIDERATIONS

54.6.1   How do you manage a patient with a history of difficult airway in the MRI suite?

A review of the patient's previous medical records (especially anesthesia records) can be valuable to determine why previous intubation attempts may have been difficult. Depending on what information is found in the medical records, and the results of the airway examination, options will range from maintaining spontaneous ventilation in the patient in a setting of minimal sedation to full general anesthesia preceded by awake endotracheal intubation. In particular, patients with severe reflux may require rapid sequence intubation, or awake intubation methods, to prevent aspiration from occurring. As most of the airway devices and intubating equipment may not be compatible in the MRI unit, if the patient requires tracheal intubation for the MRI scanning, it is perhaps wise to secure the airway in the operating room, prior to going to the MRI suite.

54.7   SUMMARY

The key message to be taken from this chapter is that the MRI suite is a potentially hostile environment for the patient with a difficult airway and numerous special precautions must be taken to prevent airway related problems in such patients. Such precautions include having an additional airway practitioner readily available, as well as having primary and secondary backup plans for airway management. It is also essential to consider in advance what equipment can or cannot be used near the MRI scanner. The unique role of the recently introduced disposable, metal free LMA Fastrach™ is yet to be determined, though it seems uniquely suited to the MRI environment.

Because it can be difficult to directly observe whether a patient is breathing adequately when they are deep inside the MRI scanner, other means of respiratory monitoring (such as capnography) are especially important. In some situations, tracheal intubation is necessary because of the high likelihood of airway obstruction with sedation; in such cases, consideration must be given to the possibility that tracheal intubation may be difficult, without special equipment and/or special techniques.

REFERENCES

1. Vlaardingerbroek MT, den Boer JA: *Magnetic Resonance Imaging: Theory and Practice*, 2nd edn. New York, NY: Springer-Verlag Telos, 1999.
2. Klucznik RP, Carrier DA, Pyka R, Haid RW: Placement of a ferromagnetic intracerebral aneurysm clip in a magnetic field with a fatal outcome. *Radiology*. 1993;187:855–856.
3. Pinski SL, Trohman RG: Interference in implanted cardiac devices, part II. *Pacing Clin Electrophysiol*. 2002;25:1496–1509.
4. Condon B, Hadley DM, Hodgson R: The ferromagnetic pillow: a potential MR hazard not detectable by hand-held magnet. *Br J Radiol*. 2001;74:847–851.
5. Chen DW: Boy, 6, dies of skull injury during MRI *The New York Times*. July 31, 2001; section B:1, 5.
6. Mitka M: Safety improvements urged for MRI facilities. *JAMA*. 2005;294:2145–2148.
7. Chaljub G, Kramer LA, Johnson RF, 3rd, et al.: Projectile cylinder accidents resulting from the presence of ferromagnetic nitrous oxide or oxygen tanks in the MR suite. *AJR Am J Roentgenol*. 2001;177:27–30.
8. Zimmer C, Janssen MN, Treschan TA, Peters J: Near-miss accident during magnetic resonance imaging by a "flying sevoflurane vaporizer" due to ferromagnetism undetectable by handheld magnet. *Anesthesiology*. 2004;100:1329–1330.
9. Shellock FG, Slimp GL: Severe burn of the finger caused by using a pulse oximeter during MR imaging. *AJR Am J Roentgenol*. 1989;153:1105.
10. Spivey WH: Flumazenil and seizures: analysis of 43 cases. *Clin Ther*. 1992;14:292–305.
11. Zura A, Doyle DJ, Orlandi M: Use of the Aintree intubation catheter in a patient with an unexpected difficult airway. *Can J Anaesth*. 2005;52:646–649.
12. Doyle DJ: GlideScope-assisted fiberoptic intubation: a new airway teaching method. *Anesthesiology*. 2004;101:1252.
13. Cooper RM, Pacey JA, Bishop MJ, McCluskey SA: Early clinical experience with a new videolaryngoscope (GlideScope) in 728 patients. *Can J Anaesth*. 2005;52:191–198.
14. Doyle DJ: Awake intubation using the GlideScope video laryngoscope: initial experience in four cases. *Can J Anaesth*. 2004;51:520–521.

SELF-EVALUATION QUESTIONS

54.1. Practitioners must take all of the following precautions when managing the airway of a patient in the MRI suite **EXCEPT**

   A. remove objects with possible ferromagnetic components before entering the MRI suite

   B. remove credit cards and ID badges before entering the MRI suite

   C. use special asbestos MRI compatible ECG electrodes

   D. ECG electrodes should be placed away from the imaging area

   E. use MRI compatible oxygen cylinders

54.2. What airway equipment may be used safely in an MRI unit?

   A. Laryngeal Mask Airway

   B. video laryngoscopes (GlideScope®)

   C. flexible fiberoptic bronchoscope

   D. Macintosh laryngoscope

   E. Bullard laryngoscope

54.3. Which of the following is **NOT** a known hazard in the MRI suite?

   A. patients with implanted ferromagnetic objects like aneurysm clips have had these objects fatally pulled out of position by the magnetic field

   B. patients with pacemakers

   C. the endotracheal tube

   D. stethoscopes

   E. portable sevoflurane vaporizer

APPENDIX 54.1

Where can I get more information on MRI safety issues?

A good place to start is on the web at www.mrisafety.com. Unfortunately, one must register to use this site. Another valuable resource is from the American College of Radiology Blue Ribbon Panel on MR Safety. This site offers a number of useful safety guidelines and clinical protocols and can be accessed at www.acr.org/dyna/?doc=committees/mr_safety/safe_mri.html.

An interesting report from the Institute for Safe Medication Practices (www.ismp.org/msaarticles/burnsprint.htm) explains that patient burns can occur when medication patches employing an aluminized backing are used (like many of those in common use containing nicotine, nitroglycerine, scopolamine, etc.). (What happens is that the RF pulses heat up the metal involved, even if the metal is not ferromagnetic.) Of interest, this problem can also occur when patients have tattoos using metal pigments.

A comprehensive list of MRI-forbidden objects is available at www.newmri.com/html/mr_safety.asp.

CHAPTER (55)

Postobstructive Pulmonary Edema (POPE)

Matthew G. Simms and J. Adam Law

55.1 CASE PRESENTATION

A 43 year old morbidly obese woman presented for gastroplasty. Her past medical history included treated hypothyroidism, and her past surgical history was unremarkable. She reported functional class II–III dyspnea on exertion. Her medications consisted of L-thyroxine, amitriptyline, codeine, and furosemide. Laboratory investigations and ECG were normal. She weighed 337 lbs (153 kg) and was 5'6" (168 cm) tall. Preoperative airway examination revealed normal mouth opening with full teeth, a thyromental span of 7 cm, and good jaw protrusion. She demonstrated a modified Mallampati score of III and had slightly restricted head extension. The rest of her physical examination was unremarkable.

Following appropriate positioning and denitrogenation, a rapid sequence induction (RSI) was performed using fentanyl, midazolam, propofol, and succinylcholine. Direct laryngoscopy using a Macintosh #3 blade revealed a Cormack/Lehane (C/L)[1] Grade 2 view, and although some difficulty with tube passage was encountered, successful intubation using a styletted 7 mm ID endotracheal tube (ETT) occurred on the first attempt. General anesthesia was maintained with nitrous oxide in oxygen, sevoflurane, and further doses of fentanyl, while vecuronium was used for muscle relaxation. Two liters of Ringer's lactate were given during the 2 hour case. On emergence, residual neuromuscular blockade was fully reversed, and she demonstrated a regular pattern of spontaneous respiration, with good tidal volumes.

At this time, she vigorously bit down on the ETT. For a period of approximately 90 seconds, no gas exchange occurred, even with attempted assisted manual ventilation via the anesthetic circuit. Although respiratory efforts continued, no CO_2 trace was apparent during the episode. Oxygen saturation was 80% before she relaxed slightly, allowing assisted, then spontaneous ventila-

tion to resume. She was subsequently placed in the lateral position until her eyes opened and she was able to obey commands. At this point she was extubated. Approximately 5 minutes after extubation, she began to cough up frothy, pink fluid in the absence of either retching or vomiting. Her oxygen saturation, which had been 97% on a simple oxygen face-mask immediately postextubation, dropped to 85%.

55.2 INTRODUCTION

55.2.1 What is postobstructive pulmonary edema (POPE)?

Postobstructive pulmonary edema (POPE) is characterized by the sudden onset of pulmonary edema of varying severity following vigorous inspiratory efforts against an obstructed upper airway, most often in a patient with no intrinsic cardiac, neurologic, or pulmonary disease. Patients generally present with dyspnea, tachypnea, hypoxemia, and a cough productive of pink, frothy sputum. After confirming that the obstruction has been relieved, the treatment of POPE is usually symptomatic, and varies from simple application of supplemental oxygen to intubation with mechanical ventilation and application of positive end-expiratory pressure (PEEP). The condition usually resolves within 24–48 hours and most patients suffer no long-term sequelae.

Pulmonary edema following acute upper airway obstruction was first described in children in 1973.[2] Later, Oswalt in 1977 described a number of cases of respiratory distress and pulmonary congestion following episodes of severe acute upper airway obstruction in otherwise healthy patients.[3] Since then, numerous case reports and case series have been published on this phenomenon.

55.2.2 What synonyms have been used to refer to POPE?

Many synonyms appear in the literature to describe this process. These include the following:

- Negative pressure pulmonary edema[4–12]
- postlaryngospasm pulmonary edema[13]
- laryngospasm induced pulmonary edema[7,14,15]
- postextubation pulmonary edema[16]
- noncardiogenic pulmonary edema[4]
- athletic pulmonary edema.[7]

55.2.3 What are the two types of POPE?

Two types of POPE have been described.[17] They present with similar clinical pictures, and most likely have similar pathophysiologies:

- *POPE type I:* This typically occurs shortly after relief of an episode of acute upper airway obstruction from any cause, e.g., laryngospasm.
- *POPE type II:* POPE type II occurs after relief of a chronic upper airway obstruction, caused by conditions such as chronic tonsillar hypertrophy, laryngeal tumor, goiter, or bilateral vocal cord paralysis.[4]

This chapter refers mainly to POPE type I, as this is most commonly encountered in anesthetic and airway management practice.

55.3 INCIDENCE, ETIOLOGY, AND PATHOPHYSIOLOGY

55.3.1 What is the incidence of POPE?

POPE has been estimated to occur in approximately 0.5–1 per thousand surgical patients.[6,18] Of those patients who have experienced, or required intervention for an episode of acute upper airway obstruction, published figures suggest a 5–10% incidence of progression to POPE.[8,18,19] POPE occurs most often in younger adults and children, most with ASA 1 and 2 status.[5,6] Young, athletic males are strongly represented in case series,[20] possibly because well-developed musculature enables them to develop stronger inspiratory efforts against the upper airway obstruction, with resultant highly negative intrathoracic pressures. Most cases occur following tracheal extubation.[6]

55.3.2 What predisposes adults to the occurrence of POPE?

In the adult population, the most common cause of POPE is post-extubation laryngospasm,[21] while in children younger than 10 years, most cases follow upper airway obstruction from croup, epiglottitis,[5,19] and to a lesser extent, laryngospasm. However, POPE following vigorous attempts to inspire against upper airway obstruction has been reported from many other causes, including biting down and occluding the lumen of ETTs[9,22] and laryngeal mask airways (LMAs).[11,12] POPE has also been reported following

upper airway obstruction from hanging, strangulation,[3,9] foreign body aspiration,[23,24] laryngeal tumor,[5] hematoma, goiter,[9] obstructive sleep apnea,[25] bilateral vocal cord paralysis,[26] direct suctioning on an ETT adapter during thoracotomy,[27] and anatomic variations predisposing to functional airway obstruction.[16]

55.3.3 What is the pathophysiology of POPE?

POPE occurs as a consequence of the highly negative intrathoracic pressure generated during an episode of airway obstruction, and the hyperadrenergic response to hypoxia, anxiety, and hypercarbia occurring secondary to the obstruction[5,16,17] (Figure 55-1). Variable clinical and laboratory manifestations probably reflect the multifactorial pathophysiology and various degrees of severity.

55.3.3.1 Hemodynamic Consequences of Negative Intrathoracic Pressures

Attempted forced inspiration against a glottis occluded by laryngospasm or other obstruction (the Mueller procedure) can generate markedly negative intrapleural and intratracheal pressures.[19,21,24] This negative pressure is transferred to the pulmonary interstitium, affecting Starling forces and creating a gradient favoring transudation of fluid out of the pulmonary capillaries.[4,23] Negative intrathoracic pressure also enhances venous return to the right heart. This increase in right ventricular preload increases pulmonary capillary bed blood volumes and hydrostatic pressures.[4–6,21,23] At the same time, outflow from the pulmonary capillary bed is impeded by increased left-sided pressures from decreased left ventricular compliance (due to RV distension decreasing LV diastolic compliance) and stroke volume (from increased afterload).[6,23,28,29] The resultant increase in pulmonary capillary hydrostatic pressures, coupled with a decrease in surrounding pericapillary pressures, further increases the transvascular gradient and results in transudation of fluid from capillary to interstitium.[4,5,8]

Increased pulmonary capillary volume and pressure causes increased wall stress and may cause capillary endothelium damage, with eventual disruption of the alveolar–capillary membrane and subsequent impairment of the barrier function, a process called "stress failure."[30]

55.3.3.2 Consequences of a Hyperadrenergic State

During an episode of airway obstruction, a hyperadrenergic reaction occurs as a response to significant hypoxia, anxiety, hypercarbia,[28] or cerebral anoxia. This response has been theorized to contribute further to alveolar–capillary membrane disruption,[4,6] particularly when hypoxia is prolonged.[23] In addition, systemic vasoconstriction occurring during a hyperadrenergeic state redistributes blood centrally, further increasing pulmonary blood volumes and pressures.[5,9,16,21,23,28,29] Hypoxia and acidosis cause depression of myocardial contractility,[9] further contributing to increased left atrial pressure and interference with venous outflow from the lungs. As well, hypoxic pulmonary vasoconstriction directly contributes to increases in pulmonary capillary pressures.[5,16]

POPE has a spectrum of presentations, from a transudative edema through pulmonary hemorrhage. It is likely that in milder

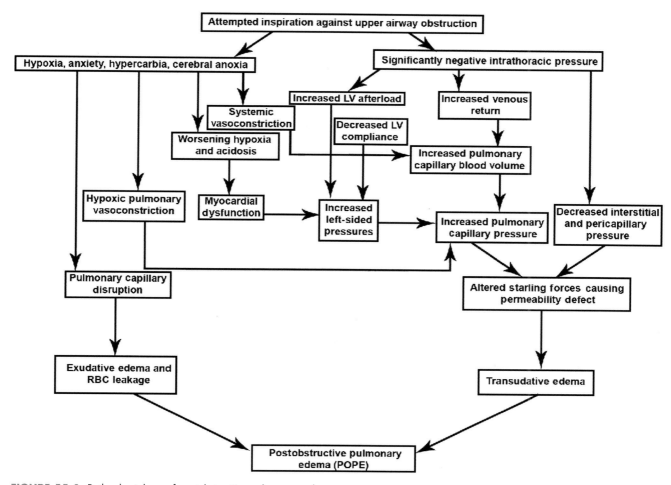

FIGURE 55-1. Pathophysiology of postobstructive pulmonary edema.

cases, with intact pulmonary capillary, integrity, simple alteration in Starling forces results in the transudative production of low-protein edema.[28] Chest radiographs in this situation would be predicted to show a primarily interstitial pattern of edema.[7] However, higher negative intrathoracic pressures, coupled with a hyperadrenergic response result in ultrastructural changes in the capillary endothelial barrier, allowing the escape of exudative edema, which is higher in protein content. Extreme cases result in breaks in the alveolar–capillary membrane, allowing red blood cell leakage and possibly frank hemorrhage. Chest radiographs in these latter situations may show more of an alveolar pattern.[7] That case reports differ in their reporting of transudative and exudative edema, or primarily interstitial or alveolar patterns of chest radiography, probably reflects the spectrum of severity of the obstructive episode causing the POPE. Once POPE becomes symptomatic, it is likely that the normal ability of lymphatic drainage to maintain fluid homeostasis in the interstitium has been impeded or overwhelmed.[16,29]

55.3.4 Why does POPE appear only after the relief of upper airway obstruction?

Type I POPE generally appears shortly after the relief of an acute upper airway obstruction. In many cases, this is a fixed obstruction

such as laryngospasm or an occluded ETT. Profoundly negative intrathoracic pressures generated during attempted inspiration (Mueller maneuvers) may be balanced during attempted expiration against the same fixed obstruction (i.e., a Valsalva maneuver), akin to an "auto PEEP" phenomenon. Although the mean intratracheal pressure is still negative in this situation, it may be that this PEEP like effect during attempted expiration is somewhat protective by limiting the transcapillary pressure gradient. Only upon relief of the obstruction does pulmonary edema become manifest[5,6,23] with the sudden increase in venous return[7] and pulmonary hydrostatic pressure.[29]

In type II POPE, chronic, usually variable, obstruction favors the Mueller maneuver in that more obstruction occurs during attempted inspiration than expiration. In this situation, the generated negative intrathoracic pressure is counteracted by more modest levels of PEEP. Although still somewhat protective against the development of pulmonary edema,[31] published reports document abnormal A-a gradients and radiographic evidence of pulmonary edema *before* relief of chronic upper airway obstructions.[5,6,23] Following the relief of both type I and type II obstructions, it is likely that altered capillary permeability, previously occult interstitial edema,[31] and LV dysfunction[23] contribute to the development of POPE in spite of now-normal lung volumes and pressures.

55.4   DIAGNOSIS AND INVESTIGATIONS

55.4.1   What are the presenting symptoms and signs of POPE?

The patient with POPE often presents within minutes[5,21] after the relief of an episode of upper airway obstruction characterized by vigorous inspiratory efforts without significant air movement.[16,28] The initial presentation is often with dyspnea,[8] tachypnea,[23,32,33] agitation,[8,20,28] and cough[11,20,21] producing pink, frothy fluid.[3,4,8,9,21,28,34] In addition to hypoxemia,[7,32] the patient is also often tachycardic[14,28] and hypertensive.[28] Other patients have presented with frank hemoptysis,[9,12,18,22] although this is less frequent. Residual partial obstruction may be present in this population, manifested by stridor[8,11,16,20,35] or intercostal and subcostal retractions.[20,23,36] On auscultation, most patients have rales,[12,16,21,23,33,34] sometimes with associated rhonchi.[3,14,21,24,28,33] Rash or jugular venous distention are absent.[21]

55.4.2   What are the results of investigations typically performed on the patient with POPE?

- *Invasive monitoring* of central venous pressure (CVP) or pulmonary artery pressure (PAP) is rarely undertaken in the patient recognized to have POPE. However, when reported, pressures, including CVP[3,21] and pulmonary capillary wedge pressures,[5,21,37,38] have generally been normal, while PAPs have been normal or only slightly elevated.[21]

- *Chest radiographs* of the patient with POPE often show signs of edema with either an alveolar (airspace consolidation)[9,16,18,36] or interstitial (perihilar haze, perivascular or peribronchial cuffing, and Kerley lines)[3,4,6,24] pattern, or both.[7,23,32] Most often the edema distribution is predominantly central and bilateral, although asymmetrical[28] or even unilateral distributions have been reported.[7,11,18] Heart size is generally normal.[7,18,23] Vascular pedicle width in one series was found to be above normal, suggesting an increase in central blood volume.[7]

- *High resolution CT scans* of the chest have shown findings of ground-glass opacities, peribronchial cuffing, and interlobular septal thickening, typical of interstitial pulmonary edema.[24] Others have shown diffuse patchy lobular airspace disease.[23]

- *Bronchoscopy* performed on patients with POPE have shown punctate bleeding lesions in both trachea and mainstem bronchi[35] or more generalized blood staining of the tracheobronchial tree.[22,28] Bronchial alveolar lavage (BAL) in one report revealed a progressively bloody return, consistent with alveolar hemorrhage,[28] while in a second report, BAL produced clear returns.[22]

- No specific *electrocardiogram (ECG) pattern* has been reported in the POPE patient population. Where comments have been made on ECG findings, they have been uniformly normal.

- *Edema fluid analysis*, on the few occasions it has been reported, has shown results consistent with an exudate (i.e., with a high protein content).[26,39] This is consistent with capillary basement membrane and alveolar–capillary membrane disruption, as opposed to a simple permeability defect, where a transudate (with a lower protein content) would be expected.

55.4.3   Should the patient presenting with POPE be referred for echocardiography?

Most case reports and case series of patients experiencing POPE have documented rapid resolution of the episode with no long-term sequelae and no special cardiac work-up performed. Echocardiograms have generally been normal.[9,16,18,24,28] One exception was a case series of six patients who had experienced POPE, all of whom had echocardiograms. In this small retrospective series, abnormalities were detected in 50% of the cases: one patient with hypertrophic cardiomyopathy and two with pulmonary and tricuspid valvular insufficiency.[4] However, in the absence of other recognized indications, the dearth of current evidence does not support a recommendation for routine echocardiographic testing of all POPE patients.

55.5   CLINICAL MANAGEMENT

55.5.1   What is the usual clinical course of POPE?

Following relief of the acute upper airway obstruction, the onset of POPE is generally rapid, i.e., within minutes, though a minority of case reports document delayed onset of up to 4–6 hours.[5,31] Therefore, some authors recommend the admission of patients to a monitored setting for 6–12 hours following an episode of acute, severe upper airway obstruction.[17] The same recommendation has been made for patients who have had surgical relief of chronic upper airway obstruction.[17] In most cases, POPE runs a benign course, with symptoms and clinical and radiologic signs clearing within 24–48 hours.[4–6,21,31,36]

55.5.2   How is POPE managed?

As the name implies, most cases of POPE present *after* the upper airway obstruction has been alleviated. After confirming airway patency, supplemental oxygen should be administered, and may be all that is required.[3,6,16,21] Continuous positive airway pressure (CPAP) by face mask has also been shown to be an effective intervention.[14,18] Hypoxemia, or patient fatigue that is unresponsive to noninvasive methods may require reintubation and positive pressure ventilation. The larger case series report reintubation rates of between 66.5%[8] and 85%.[5,6,21] Of those patients reintubated, about half require mechanical ventilation[5] with[3,4,28] or without PEEP, usually for less than 24 hours.[6]

Although diuretics are often used in the setting of POPE,[3,5,6,14,22,23,28,36] this practice has been questioned[5,23] based on the finding of normal central filling pressures and the equally rapid resolution of symptoms when they are not used.[9,36] Theoretically, diuretics may reduce pulmonary edema by decreasing intravascular volume and ventricular preload even before the onset of diuresis.[36] The use of steroids has been reported sporadically[3,14,36] to help dampen any inflammatory component to the condition, although as with the use of diuretics, their use is controversial[17] and without proven benefit. Other case reports make mention of fluid restriction[3,17] and the administration of conventional congestive cardiac failure (CCF) medications such as morphine or digoxin.[21]

The available evidence would suggest that if the diagnosis of POPE is correct, drug therapy is unlikely to be of benefit, particularly in view of the self limited and rapidly resolving course of the condition. The same can be said for invasive hemodynamic monitoring,[16] with rare exceptions.[4,10]

55.5.3 What is the differential diagnosis of POPE?

The primary alternate diagnosis to POPE is aspiration pneumonitis, which may lead to pulmonary edema even when frank regurgitation has not been noted.[5] The initial management of this condition is identical to that of POPE, unless of course the aspirate is suspected to be particulate or contaminated by bacteria. It is more important to rule out causes of pulmonary edema with management differs from that of POPE, including iatrogenic volume overload, primary cardiogenic causes, or drug reactions.

55.5.4 What are the risk factors and preventive strategies for the development of POPE?

A number of factors place the patient at higher risk for the development of POPE. Some are unavoidable, while some can be minimized by employing the principles of good airway management. The early recognition and management of acute, severe upper airway obstruction, and the conditions leading to it, are critical to the prevention of POPE:

- *Laryngospasm*: Most cases of POPE in adults, and many in children, occur following an episode of laryngospasm. Many case reports of POPE document laryngospasm following extubation during emergence from anesthesia, before the patient is fully awake.[36,40] Therefore, it is recommended that extubation be performed in patients who are either deeply anesthetized or fully awake. The prevention of intraoperative laryngospasm under mask or extraglottic device (EGD) anesthesia requires appropriately deep general anesthesia, particularly for highly stimulating surgical procedures. Prior to removing an ETT, suctioning of blood or secretions that may trigger laryngospasm is essential, particularly following upper airway surgery. Should laryngospasm occur, the initial treatment is to relieve any soft tissue obstruction together with general application of CPAP by mask. However, the administration of succinylcholine 0.2 mg·kg^{-1} (or other appropriate neuromuscular blocking agent) may be indicated in patients making vigorous inspiratory efforts against a closed glottis, particularly if it persists for more than 30 seconds.[40]

- *Tube occlusion by biting down*: POPE has been described in patients who have "bitten down" to occlude ETTs[34,36] and EGDs (e.g., LMA).[11,12,41] Most reports have documented that this occurs on emergence from anesthesia, although it has also been described during the positioning process.[11] Use of a rolled gauze bite block alongside the lumen of an ETT[9,34] or LMA (as recommended by its inventor[41]) ought to minimize this risk. As

with laryngospasm, the administration of a neuromuscular blocking agent may be indicated. Alternatively, the deflation of the cuff of the ETT or EGD may permit sufficient alleviation of obstruction to prevent marked negative intrathoracic pressure and the development of POPE.

- *Other soft tissue obstruction*: POPE has been described as a complication of obstructive sleep apnea, in patients with obesity and vocal cord paralysis, and other risk factors for upper airway obstruction.[16,33] The preoperative identification of patients at risk for these conditions mandates full recovery of neuromuscular function, and that they be fully awake prior to extubation.

- *Type of surgery*: A retrospective study by Deepika et al. showed that the majority of POPE cases (63%) occurred following surgery to the upper aerodigestive tract,[6] suggesting that vigilance be exercised in patients suffering from chronic tonsillar hypertrophy, goiter, and other conditions leading to chronic upper airway obstruction.

- *Patient*: POPE occurs about twice as often in male patients,[5,6,8] and in those with an average age of 35–45 years.[5,6,8] The male preponderance may be related to well-developed musculature and their ability to generate high negative intrathoracic pressures.[20] Early and aggressive treatment of airway obstruction in this population may be indicated.

55.6 PROGNOSIS

POPE is an important cause of morbidity in otherwise young, healthy patients that may lead to an unplanned hospital or ICU admission. However, with prompt recognition and appropriate therapy, the condition generally resolves within 24–48 hours with no long-term sequelae.[6,18] A recent review of published adult case series of POPE (excluding hanging, goiter, epiglottitis and ETT biting) reported three deaths in 146 patients a mortality rate of 2%.[8]

55.7 PATIENT MANAGEMENT

Following extubation in the operating room, the patient exhibited clinical evidence of developing pulmonary edema and increasing respiratory distress. She was placed in a semi-sitting position. Her oropharynx was suctioned. Oxygen (100%) was administered via a face mask through the anesthetic circuit and CPAP was applied. This failed to improve the SpO_2 to above 90%, so assisted bag-mask-ventilation (BMV) was attempted. However, agitation and reduced lung compliance made assisted ventilation increasingly difficult, and the SpO_2 could not be maintained above 90%. Therefore, the trachea of the patient was reintubated using a rapid sequence technique. She was ventilated with an FiO_2 of 1.0 and her SpO_2 returned to 97% within 2 minutes following intubation; suctioning revealed copious quantities of pink, frothy fluid. Midazolam for sedation and furosemide 40 mg were administered. An arterial line was placed and she was admitted to the ICU. A chest x-ray showed signs of pulmonary edema. A 12-lead ECG was normal and troponins were negative. The patient remained sedated, intubated, and ventilated overnight. By the following day, her radiographic findings and arterial blood gases had improved, and she was extubated that evening. There were no further complications.

55.8   SUMMARY

Postobstructive pulmonary edema is an uncommon, yet potentially life-threatening condition. Occurring shortly after the relief of an acute episode of upper airway obstruction of varying cause, POPE presents with dyspnea, cough, progressive oxygen desaturation, tachypnea, and agitation. In most cases, POPE resolves within 24–36 hours. In some instances, nothing more than supportive care consisting of oxygen administration is required. Mask-delivered CPAP may also be effective. However, some patients with POPE may require tracheal intubation, followed by mechanical ventilation and PEEP to maintain adequate oxygenation. Although often used, the benefits of diuretics and steroids in managing POPE remain unproven.

Practitioners must be aware of the disorder, be able to identify and avoid the predisposing risk factors, and be able to manage it if it occurs. Furthermore, the prompt management of upper airway obstruction is crucial in reducing the incidence of POPE and improving outcome, particularly in view of the fact that deaths have been reported.

REFERENCES

1. Cormack RS, Lehane J: Difficult tracheal intubation in obstetrics. *Anaesthesia.* 1984;39:1105–1111.
2. Capitanio MA, Kirkpatrick JA: Obstructions of the upper airway in children as reflected on the chest radiograph. *Radiology.* 1973;107:159–161.
3. Oswalt CE, Gates GA, Holmstrom MG: Pulmonary edema as a complication of acute airway obstruction. *JAMA.* 1977;238:1833–1835.
4. Goldenberg JD, Portugal LG, Wenig BL, Weingarten RT: Negative-pressure pulmonary edema in the otolaryngology patient. *Otolaryngol Head Neck Surg.* 1997;117:62–66.
5. Lang SA, Duncan PG, Shephard DA, Ha HC: Pulmonary oedema associated with airway obstruction. *Can J Anaesth.* 1990;37:210–218.
6. Deepika K, Kenaan CA, Barrocas AM, Fonseca JJ, Bikazi GB: Negative pressure pulmonary edema after acute upper airway obstruction. *J Clin Anesth.* 1997;9:403–408.
7. Cascade PN, Alexander GD, Mackie DS: Negative-pressure pulmonary edema after endotracheal intubation. *Radiology.* 1993;186:671–675.
8. Westreich R, Sampson I, Shaari CM, Lawson W: Negative-pressure pulmonary edema after routine septorhinoplasty: discussion of pathophysiology, treatment, and prevention. *Arch Facial Plast Surg.* 2006;8:8–15.
9. Koh MS, Hsu AA, Eng P: Negative pressure pulmonary oedema in the medical intensive care unit. *Intensive Care Med.* 2003;29:1601–1604.
10. Louis PJ, Fernandes R: Negative pressure pulmonary edema. *Oral Surg Oral Med Oral Pathol Oral Radiol Endod.* 2002;93:4–6.
11. Sullivan M: Unilateral negative pressure pulmonary edema during anesthesia with a laryngeal mask airway. *Can J Anaesth.* 1999;46:1053–1056.
12. Devys JM, Balleau C, Jayr C, Bourgain JL: Biting the laryngeal mask: an unusual cause of negative pressure pulmonary edema. *Can J Anaesth.* 2000;47:176–178.
13. Baltimore JJ: Postlaryngospasm pulmonary edema in adults. *AORN J.* 1999;70:468–479.
14. Jackson FN, Rowland V, Corssen G: Laryngospasm-induced pulmonary edema. *Chest.* 1980;78:819–821.
15. McConkey P: Airway bleeding in negative-pressure pulmonary edema. *Anesthesiology.* 2001;95:272.
16. Lorch DG, Sahn SA: Post-extubation pulmonary edema following anesthesia induced by upper airway obstruction. Are certain patients at increased risk? *Chest.* 1986;90:802–805.
17. Guffin TN, Har-el G, Sanders A, Lucente FE, Nash M: Acute postobstructive pulmonary edema. *Otolaryngol Head Neck Surg.* 1995;112:235–237.
18. McConkey PP: Postobstructive pulmonary oedema—a case series and review. *Anaesth Intensive Care.* 2000;28:72–76.
19. Galvis AG: Pulmonary edema complicating relief of upper airway obstruction. *Am J Emerg Med.* 1987;5:294–297.
20. Holmes JR, Hensinger RN, Wojtys EW: Postoperative pulmonary edema in young, athletic adults. *Am J Sports Med.* 1991;19:365–371.
21. Willms D, Shure D: Pulmonary edema due to upper airway obstruction in adults. *Chest.* 1988;94:1090–1092.
22. Sow Nam Y, Garewal D: Pulmonary hemorrhage in association with negative pressure edema in an intubated patient. *Acta Anaesthesiol Scand.* 2001;45:911–913.
23. Ringold S, Klein EJ, Del Beccaro MA: Postobstructive pulmonary edema in children. *Pediatr Emerg Care.* 2004;20:391–395.
24. Maniwa K, Tanaka E, Inoue T, et al.: Interstitial pulmonary edema revealed by high-resolution CT after relief of acute upper airway obstruction. *Radiat Med.* 2005;23:139–141.
25. Chaudhary BA, Nadimi M, Chaudhary TK, Speir WA: Pulmonary edema due to obstructive sleep apnea. *South Med J.* 1984;77:499–501.
26. Dohi S, Okubo N, Kondo Y: Pulmonary oedema after airway obstruction due to bilateral vocal cord paralysis. *Can J Anaesth.* 1991;38:492–495.
27. Pang WW, Chang DP, Lin CH, Huang MH: Negative pressure pulmonary oedema induced by direct suctioning of endotracheal tube adapter. *Can J Anaesth.* 1998;45:785–788.
28. Schwartz DR, Maroo A, Malhotra A, Kesselman H: Negative pressure pulmonary hemorrhage. *Chest.* 1999;115:1194–1197.
29. Ciavarro C, Kelly JP: Postobstructive pulmonary edema in an obese child after an oral surgery procedure under general anesthesia: a case report. *J Oral Maxillofac Surg.* 2002;60:1503–1505.
30. West JB, Tsukimoto K, Mathieu-Costello O, Prediletto R: Stress failure in pulmonary capillaries. *J Appl Physiol.* 1991;70:1731–1742.
31. Van Kooy MA, Gargiulo RF: Postobstructive pulmonary edema. *Am Fam Physician.* 2000;62:401–404.
32. Sofer S, Bar-Ziv J, Scharf SM: Pulmonary edema following relief of upper airway obstruction. *Chest.* 1984;86:401–403.
33. Brandom BW: Pulmonary edema after airway obstruction. *Int Anesthesiol Clin.* 1997;35:75–84.
34. Liu EH, Yih PS: Negative pressure pulmonary oedema caused by biting and endotracheal tube occlusion—a case for oropharyngeal airways. *Singapore Med J.* 1999;40:174–175.
35. Koch SM, Abramson DC, Ford M, Peterson D, Katz J: Bronchoscopic findings in post-obstructive pulmonary oedema. *Can J Anaesth.* 1996;43:73–76.
36. Herrick IA, Mahendran B, Penny FJ: Postobstructive pulmonary edema following anesthesia. *J Clin Anesth.* 1990;2:116–120.
37. Weissman C, Damask MC, Yang J: Noncardiogenic pulmonary edema following laryngeal obstruction. *Anesthesiology.* 1984;60:163–165.
38. Stradling JR, Bolton P: Upper airways obstruction as cause of pulmonary oedema. *Lancet.* 1982;1:1353–1354.
39. Kollef MH, Pluss J: Noncardiogenic pulmonary edema following upper airway obstruction. 7 cases and a review of the literature. *Medicine (Baltimore)* 1991;70:91–98.
40. Lee KW, Downes JJ: Pulmonary edema secondary to laryngospasm in children. *Anesthesiology.* 1983;59:347–349.
41. Brain AI: The laryngeal mask—a new concept in airway management. *Br J Anaesth.* 1983;55:801–805.

SELF-EVALUATION QUESTIONS

55.1. Which of the following situations would be **LEAST** likely to result in an episode of postobstructive pulmonary edema?

   A. 25 year old male bites and occludes the endotracheal tube for a period of less than 60 seconds on emergence from a desflurane based anesthetic. He never desaturates below a SpO_2 of 85%.

   B. 25 year old male was scheduled for appendectomy. During RSI using fentanyl, propofol, and rocuronium, tracheal intubation was achieved with a Trachlight™

following three failed intubation attempts using a Macintosh blade; difficulty with BMV was experienced between intubation attempts.

C. A 25 year old male has been extubated "deep" following surgery for a deviated nasal septum. At the time of extubation, end-tidal desflurane was 2%.

D. A 6 year old child has presented to the ED with acute epiglottitis, is "tripoding" with stridor, drooling, and respiratory distress. Intubation using an inhalational induction in the operating room is planned.

E. A 25 year old male weighing 120 kg is having banding of hemorrhoids under general anesthesia with a laryngeal mask airway. Following a propofol induction, he has been given a total of 100 μg of fentanyl and is breathing a mixture of air and sevoflurane, with an end tidal sevoflurane concentration of 1.7%.

55.2. Emerging from general anesthesia for shoulder acromioplasty and shortly after extubation, a 25 year old man experiences an episode of laryngospasm and makes vigorous, yet futile inspiratory attempts against his closed glottis. Which of the following responses would be appropriate?

A. Suction the back of the throat with rigid tonsil suction, insert an oral airway, and "ride it out."

B. Immediately give succinylcholine 100 mg.

C. As the laryngospasm is probably related to pain, give a dose of parenteral narcotic such as sufentanil 5 mg.

D. Give lidocaine 100 mg intravenously.

E. Perform an airway opening maneuver and apply gentle CPAP by mask; if this does not break the laryngospasm within 30 seconds, give succinylcholine.

55.3. Which of the following patient conditions is considered a risk factor for the development of postoperative pulmonary edema?

A. The patient with an ASA of 3 or 4.

B. The patient emerging from surgery of the aerodigestive tract.

C. The patient with a history of ischemic heart disease.

D. The patient with a history of severe gastroesophageal reflux.

E. The patient with a history of asthma.

SECTION (4) Practical Considerations in Difficult and Failed Airway Management

CHAPTER (56)

Difficult Airway Carts

Saul Pytka and Michael F. Murphy

56.1 INTRODUCTION

56.1.1 Why are difficult airway carts necessary?

The concept of emergency difficult airway carts is not a novel one. It has long been acknowledged that having emergency equipment readily available in a reliable location is the standard of care. The "cardiac crash cart," for example, is a mandatory addition to operating rooms (OR), emergency departments (ED), and other patient care areas where they may be required. Many labor and delivery rooms have an "emergency cart" ready for unanticipated "crash" cesarean sections, while trauma units have an emergency surgical setup for occasions when a chest or abdomen must be rapidly opened.

Although the literature is silent on the actual benefits of having emergency airway carts available, there is strong consensus among experts that the ready access to alternative devices for airway management has the potential for reducing risks and complications in the management of the unanticipated difficult airway.[1–3] In 1993, the American Society of Anesthesiologists Task Force on Management of the Difficult Airway published their Practice Guidelines for Management of the Difficult Airway.[1] This document, subsequently updated in 2003, contained a clear statement that "at least one portable storage unit that contains specialized equipment for difficult airway management should be readily available".[2] They followed with a suggested list of specialized equipment that this "storage unit," or cart, should contain.

Beyond the scope of the original ASA guidelines, Crosby and a group of consultants reviewed the pertinent literature on airway management in Canada and published recommendations for the management of the unanticipated difficult airway.[3] In the publication, they recommended that a "difficult airway cart" be available for emergency airway interventions in addition to the standard airway equipment available in every OR. They also suggested a minimum equipment list for such a cart.

56.1.2 Is there any evidence that airway carts are beneficial in the setting of difficult or failed airway management?

The literature is replete with the advantages of using alternative airway devices in situations where a difficult airway is encountered, both expected and unanticipated. Just as emergency drugs and the presence of a defibrillator on the "crash cart" are indispensable in the management of a cardiac emergency, the readily available rescue airway devices in an airway emergency clearly represent an improvement in patient care.

There are multiple studies describing the morbidity and mortality associated with difficulties in airway management.[4,5] Both the ASA and Canadian groups recommend limiting the number of attempts at direct laryngoscopy to three and two, respectively.[1–3] Mort has shown that the increasing numbers of attempts at intubation by direct laryngoscopy correlates with an increased incidence of respiratory and hemodynamic complications.[6] In this study, a database was created to record complications following emergency airway interventions outside the OR. When three or more attempts were made to secure an airway by direct laryngoscopy, the incidence of hypoxemia increased from 11% to 70%, regurgitation from 2% to 22%, aspiration from 0.8% to 13%, and cardiac arrest from 0.7% to 11% (Table 56-1). One could speculate that the presence of alternate airway devices would have prevented the need for repeated attempts at direct laryngoscopy.

In a separate study, Mort reviewed the incidence and etiology of out-of-OR cardiac arrests occurring during emergency intubation before and after the introduction of emergency airway carts.[7] In 1995, the institution, a level-one trauma center, studied newly introduced airway carts or kits containing "advanced" airway

TABLE 56-1

Complications by Intubation Attempts[6]

COMPLICATION	2 OR FEWER ATTEMPTS (90%)	>2 ATTEMPTS (10%)*	RELATIVE RISK FOR >2 ATTEMPTS	95% CI FOR RISK RATIO
Hypoxemia	10.5%	70%	9X	4.20–15.92
Severe hypoxemia	1.9%	28%	14X	7.36–24.34
Esophageal intubation	4.8%	51.4%	6X	3.71–8.72
Regurgitation	1.9%	22%	7X	2.82–10.14
Aspiration	0.8%	13%	4X	1.89–7.18
Bradycardia	1.6%	18.5%	4X	1.71–6.74
Cardiac arrest	0.7%	11%	7X	2.39–9.87

*All categories $P < 0.001$ when comparing 2 or fewer attempts to >2 attempts. Hypoxemia—SpO_2 <90%; Severe Hypoxemia—SpO_2 <70%. (Reproduced with permission from Mort TC: Emergency tracheal intubation: complications associated with repeated laryngoscopic attempts. *Anesth Analg.* 2004;99:607–613.)

equipment and tracheal tube verifying devices. The time periods 1990–1995 and 1995–2002 were compared retrospectively for a number of variables, the primary comparator being cardiac arrest. There was an overall reduction of 50% in airway-related cardiac arrests between the two time periods, attributable to the presence of the carts (Figure 56-1).[7]

Although the data compiled from these papers were gathered outside the OR locations, the principles that lead to the conclusion are equally applicable to other locations, including the OR. The ready accessibility of difficult airway carts is indispensable in reducing airway-related morbidity and mortality.

56.1.3   What steps should be taken to ensure that the carts remain well stocked and contain equipment in good working order?

It is important that when an airway practitioner arrives at the scene of an airway emergency, or when the "Difficult Airway Cart" is summoned, all of the equipment that is needed must be there and all of the stipulated equipment must be functional. To achieve this, departmental and hospital policies or processes must be crafted, which should identify:

- the numbers and locations of such carts;
- a process of annual review of the cart locations and how they are equipped and updated;
- a staff member (a clinician, a nurse, or a respiratory therapist), must be responsible for the cart in each assigned area as the "keeper of the cart";
- how equipment is added to and deleted from the standard list of contents, and how such changes are suggested, vetted, implemented, and communicated to the relevant staff;
- how the drawers will be labeled;
- how equipment with maintenance schedules are to be maintained (e.g., bronchoscopes);

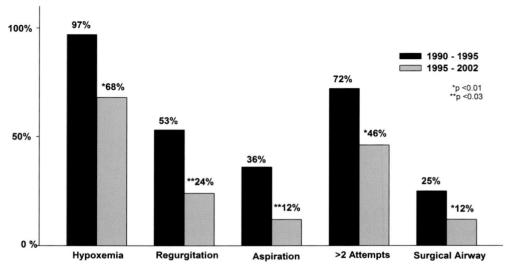

FIGURE 56-1. Complications associated with repeated attempts at laryngoscopic intubation. (Reproduced with permission from Mort TC: The incidence and risk factors for cardiac arrest during emergency tracheal intubation: a justification for incorporating the ASA Guidelines in the remote location. *J Clin Anesth.* 2004;16:508–516.)

- time frames and responsibilities regarding replenishment after equipment is used;
- who will check the inventory and how often it will be checked (e.g., every shift, every day, etc. including a checklist as part of the process. The checklist includes functions of essential equipment such as bulbs and batteries, and perishable supplies such as local anesthetic agents and vasoconstrictors;
- if cleaning is to be done, who will do it, how it will be done (e.g., bronchoscopes), and how long the "out of service for cleaning" interval will be;
- an inventory of replenishment supplies to be kept immediately on hand, particularly disposables (e.g., Combitube™, Melker Cricothyrotomy kit, etc.);
- where equipment manufacturers' literature will be kept.

Routine airway management equipment that one expects to use in most if not all airway management emergencies such as laryngoscopes, airways, endotracheal tubes (ETTs), intubating stylets (e.g., Eschmann Introducer or Frova), tonsil and catheter suction devices, etc., should be immediately available and not clutter the drawers of the cart. These equipment need not be on an OR cart as each anesthetizing location ought to have them available. Carts should be located in each area of the hospital where airway management might reasonably be expected to occur such as ED, ICU, Cardiac Cath Units, labor and delivery suites, endoscopy suites, diagnostic imaging unit, and other locations where sedatives will be administered. In locations where both children and adults are cared for, the pediatric cart should be distinctly separate from the adult cart (different style, and perhaps different color). An array of ETT sizes, masks, oral and nasal airways, etc., must be easily accessible in the event pediatric patients are cared for. Perhaps the best system currently available to meet this need is the Broselow-Luten System®.[8] Alternatively, canvaspocketed systems that are rolled up for storage can easily and quickly be unrolled to access the equipment.

If at all possible, airway carts should be in a consistent location (e.g., with the cardiac crash cart). The cart should be secured with a plastic twist removable lock. The cart is secured after each use, signaling that the cart has been replenished and is ready for use. Thus, the absence of the lock identifies that the cart needs immediate inspection. A keyed lock may be required for drawers that contain medications. The locking mechanism for this drawer must be limited to this drawer only and should not impede access to the other drawers with airway devices.

56.2   DIFFICULT AIRWAY CART IN THE OR

56.2.1   What are the guiding principles for establishing a difficult airway cart for the OR area?

Historically, the contents of the "difficult airway cart" in most anesthesia locations varied widely, as various practitioners demanded the addition of newer or their preferred devices. Unfortunately, items that nobody had ever used or would ever use were included. The contents would often be forgotten, and little or no maintenance would occur. Basically, they were difficult airway carts in name only.

Although a number of publications describe difficult airway cart setup, most are simply a description of the author's departmental cart.[9] However, such a list can be a good starting point for creating a useful cart, with the end users customizing the contents according to departmental needs, preferences, and available resources. A designated individual or committee should be responsible for soliciting input from users in determining what should be on the cart. The decision about the contents ought to be reviewed quarterly or semiannually to ensure that carts have the most up-to-date and effective equipment. Deletions and additions need to be communicated to all users in a timely manner. Surprises in the midst of a failed airway are most unwelcome!!

In principle, the cart should be one that is easily accessible and has equipment familiar to the users and other unit personnel. An assortment of well-arranged and quickly accessible devices should be available to handle most needs. Decisions about disposable versus reusable equipment should be made consistent with hospital policies and published evidence of equipment effectiveness (discussed later in this chapter).

In this all-inclusive difficult airway cart, all equipment needed for difficult airway situations (so-called Plan B and Plan C) should be present. Equipment on the cart need not duplicate routine airway equipment otherwise available on anesthetic carts in the ORs. This may be where an OR difficult airway cart differs from airway carts in other locations: in ICU or ED settings, airway kits or carts may contain both routine and alternative airway equipment.

Familiarity with the difficult airway cart and its contents is crucial. Using "difficult airway" equipment for routine intubations will add to the skills in using alternative devices and will also help the anesthesia practitioner and support personnel gain needed familiarity with cart contents and location. This in turn will lead to more effective management of an emergency unanticipated difficult and failed airway, minimizing stress for all concerned. However, with regular use of the difficult airway cart, there must be a routine to ensure that it is properly maintained: disposables must be replenished and reusable equipment disinfected and replaced as quickly as possible (see Section 56.4 below). This in turn implies that designated personnel familiar with the cart routinely check and replenish it. This is the same principle that applies to maintenance of the cardiac arrest "crash cart."

56.2.2   What equipment should be available on a difficult airway cart for the OR?

The cart containing the equipment should be mobile, small enough to be safely and easily moved by one person, and should fit into the ORs through the doorways. It should be located in a central location that is familiar and visible to all. Smooth castors on the cart and the drawers are important to ensure that the cart does not become an obstacle in itself, and is safe from being overturned. Cables and cords should be neatly attached so that nothing can be snagged while the cart is being moved or people are working around it. Failure to pay attention to this could lead to damage to equipment or injury to staff. The drawers should be clearly labeled as per their contents.

The equipment included on the cart should cover the range of options that might be needed in a difficult airway scenario. This will include categories such as:

- equipment to facilitate mechanical (bag-mask or EGD) ventilation;
- adjuncts to direct laryngoscopy;
- alternatives to direct laryngoscopy;
- equipment to facilitate transtracheal access;
- light sources, cameras, and monitors for techniques requiring, or facilitated by, this equipment;
- equipment and drugs for application of topical airway anesthesia or airway blocks;
- miscellaneous equipment as determined by each facility.

56.2.3 What equipment to facilitate mechanical (bag-mask or EGD) ventilation should be included in difficult airway cart for the OR?

At least one bag-mask device should be available for delivery of positive pressure ventilation. Nonstandard mask sizes may belong on the cart. The group or individual responsible for the airway cart should decide which extraglottic devices to stock. If classic or disposable laryngeal mask airways (LMA Unique™) are routinely stocked in the OR, then the cart may contain, for example, the LMA ProSeal™ and intubating LMA (LMA Fastrach™). Other EGDs such as the Combitube™ or King LT™ Airway can be considered, but the devices should be the ones with which the department members have experience and have found useful.

56.2.4 What adjuncts to direct laryngoscopy should be included in a difficult airway cart for the OR?

An assortment of alternate blades designed to fit standard laryngoscope handles used in the OR should be available. For example, Miller (straight) and Macintosh (curved) blades of various sizes, as well as levering tip (McCoy/CLM) laryngoscope blades, might be kept in this section. The presence of a variety of ETTs (e.g., Endotrol®) not routinely stocked in the OR, including a range of smaller sizes, is important.

The presence of a flexible, Coudé-tipped (distal 2.5 cm and angled approximately 35 degrees) Eschmann Tracheal Tube Introducer (the "gum-elastic bougie") is an essential addition to an emergency cart. It can be guided below the epiglottis when a Mallampati class II or III view of the larynx is encountered, whereupon the ETT can be advanced over it (see Section 10.2.1). Because they should be kept straight, rather than bent to fit into a drawer, some tracheal tube introducers (e.g., Portex) may be stored in their original shipping case, secured to the side of the cart (Figure 56-2). As a simple, yet useful device, most would suggest that these introducers be an integral part of standard equipment found in every room or location where anesthetics are administered.

56.2.5 What alternatives to direct laryngoscopy should be included in a difficult airway cart for the OR?

Here is where the list of objects becomes potentially extensive. Again, the principles are to not duplicate what already exists as routine airway management equipment in the OR are readily

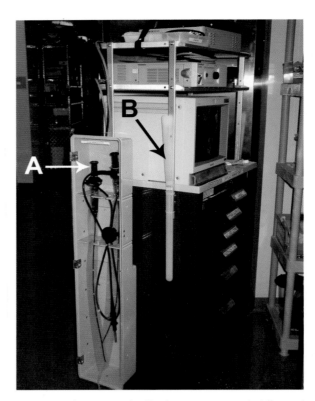

FIGURE 56-2. The proposed Difficult Airway Cart with different drawers for different airway equipment, video monitor, flexible fiberoptic bronchoscope in a secure compartment (A), and Eschmann Tracheal Introducer stored in its original shipping case (B).

available, but to stock only those devices familiar to the anesthesia practitioner and support staff. Options for inclusion in this section are as follows:

- Intubating LMA (LMA Fastrach™) in a variety of sizes (#3 - #5), their dedicated silicone-ETTs (7-8 mm ID), and the tube stabilizer to aid with subsequent LMA Fastrach™ removal.
- Intubating lighted stylet (e.g., Trachlight™). There should be at least one handle, which is tested daily to ensure that the batteries are functional, as well as two or three wands. Some institutions stock the cart with one Trachlight™ loaded with a precut (26 cm) 7.5 mm ID ETT (see Chapter 10) in the cart as well.
- Flexible fiberoptic devices. The flexible fiberoptic bronchoscope (FFB) should be kept in a secure compartment, where it can be stored so that it is not tightly curled (Figure 56-2). This ensures maximum protection of the fragile fibers and the motion cable that controls of the scope tip. FFBs ought to be handled with great care as they are fragile devices and repairs may be expensive. Discussion often arises regarding the use of pediatric versus adult scopes. In a difficult intubation, particularly where failed attempts at direct laryngoscopy have traumatized the airway, the adult scope has the advantage of having a more functional suction lumen in addition to being a more rigid (and sturdy) scope. Ideally, a scope that will allow intubation with a 6 mm ID or larger ETT should be sought. Pediatric scopes are fragile and may not have the rigidity to facilitate the insertion of a large-diameter ETT tube around tight corners, and have smaller working channels compromising their suction capacity. They are, however, indispensable in confirming the position of devices when lung isolation is required. Included in the drawer

where the FFB equipment is kept should be devices to protect the scope from being bitten, such as a bite block Tudor Williams (Figure 8-23), Ovassapian (Figure 8-24), or Berman Intubating Pharyngeal airways (Figure 8-22) in an assortment of sizes.

- Rigid fiberoptic and video laryngoscopic devices. These devices provide indirect visualization of the larynx via fiberoptics or video monitor. Some devices such as the Bullard Laryngoscope, UpsherScope™, and GlideScope® have a blade to aid with tongue control, while others, such as the Shikani SOS™, Bonfils, and Levitan FPS, are simply fiberoptic optical stylets, enabling visualization through an ensleeved ETT. Further details on these devices appear in Chapter 9. Many of these devices can be operated with batteries, making them portable.

50.2.6 What equipment to facilitate transtracheal access should be available in the difficult airway cart for the OR?

In a failed airway situation, particularly when ventilation and intubation are not possible, quick direct transtracheal access to the airway must occur (see Chapter 12 for details). For those trained in transtracheal-jet-ventilation, a nonkinking catheter should be available, together with a regulated oxygen source. The latter can be affixed directly to the cart. Recognizing the dangers of barotrauma inherent in this technique, many practitioners elect to proceed directly to open surgical or percutaneous cricothyrotomy. Commercial kits are available with equipment for one or both techniques. The percutaneous Melker cricothyrotomy kits are now available with a cuffed cannula, making this a particularly useful device. For those departments with members familiar with the technique, equipment for retrograde intubation can be considered an option in less urgent situations. Again, this is available commercially in a kit.

50.6.7 What video accessory equipment should be available in the difficult airway cart for the OR?

Many of the newer flexible fiberoptic scopes can run on a battery-powered light source, while visualization occurs through a traditional eyepiece. Other FFBs and the newer video bronchoscopes require a separate light source that attaches to the scope via a cable. This light source is generally brighter than the battery-powered light sources. A particularly useful device is a camera with an appropriate adaptor that attaches to a fiberoptic scope's eyepiece to give a video feed to a monitor (see Figure 56-2). This allows much better viewing of the airway, as the image is magnified and is brighter than that viewed through the eyepiece. It allows an assistant to visualize what is happening and in a teaching institution, it can be invaluable when explaining or directing a trainee what to do next. Still or video images can be recorded for documentation of the procedure as well as any pathology encountered.

56.2.8 What other miscellaneous equipment should be available in a difficult airway cart?

Ancillary equipment, such as medication cups for holding and mixing solutions, tongue depressors, tonsil forceps (e.g., the Kraus or Jackson forceps) for applying gauze balls for superior laryngeal nerve blocks, as well as antifog agents for the fiberoptic scopes, are a few other additions to the cart. The need for awake intubation is always a possibility, so appropriate types and volumes of local anesthetic agents should also be kept on the cart. These agents can be injected (e.g., with transtracheal injection and/or percutaneous superior laryngeal nerve blocks) or applied topically, e.g., by gargling, dripping onto the extended or tractioned tongue, or with a nebulizer or DeVilbiss atomizer. For a more detailed description of airway anesthesia techniques, see Chapter 3. Water-soluble lubricants, silicone liquid, or other antifog agents should also be available.

An array of airway exchange catheters is almost always appropriate, for use in changing tubes in difficult situations or for the extubation of the patient whose trachea was difficult to intubate. Availability of pediatric equipment will be dictated to an extent by the practice pattern of the hospital, although very small-for-age adults, disaster preparedness, and airway pathology situations make it advisable for adult hospitals to carry some pediatric equipment. Other equipment for inclusion on the difficult airway cart will be dictated by the department's practice environment. For instance, some institutions include rigid bronchoscopes and anterior commissure scopes on their cart.

56.3 DIFFICULT AIRWAY CART OUTSIDE THE OR

56.3.1 How might equipment requirements differ for out-of-OR locations such as the ICU or ED and why?

The processes governing airway carts in non-OR areas are no different than those described above. A variety of policies and practices are essential in ensuring that vital life-saving equipment is available and in working order when required, including the following:

- Who should be involved to decide what the cart contains?
- How are suggestions as to contents made and how are those decisions made?
- How are cart modifications communicated effectively to all staff that may be affected?
- How often is the cart checked for contents and equipment function and by whom?
- Who is responsible to ensure that the carts are re-stocked routinely after use?
- How is this process documented?

Some areas are more "airway intervention prone" than others. EDs, ICUs, free-standing day-surgery operations, postanesthesia care units, pediatric dental clinics, and pediatric cancer care units are obvious examples. It is reasonable to expect that airway intervention may occur with some regularity in these units and that routine and difficult airway management equipment ought to be immediately available.

Others are less obvious. These include units where procedural sedation is undertaken, such as endoscopy suites, angiography and cardiac catheterization units, and others. While routine airway management equipment ought to be immediately available on these units, it may be financially prohibitive to create potentially expensive, fully equipped carts as described above. However, it is not unreasonable to expect that such units have relatively inexpensive, proven adjuncts such as oral and nasal airways and rescue devices such as disposable LMA (LMA Unique™), LMA Fastrach™, Combitube™, and intubating stylets.

Some institutions designate that anesthesia be a part of the team that responds to declared intra-institutional airway emergencies. In response, some of these anesthesia departments have created portable airway management bags to be taken to the site of the airway emergency. Policy considerations as to contents and their working order are no different for these kits than for the cart described above.

Furthermore, and crucially important from a medico-legal perspective is the involvement of anesthesia in the design and maintenance of unit resident carts (e.g., ICU, ED) if they are responsible for responding to those units (or elect to do so) to support airway management activities. It is the duty of the hospitals and unit management *and* anesthesia practitioners to understand and embrace this accountability.

56.4   DISPOSABLE VERSUS REUSABLE DEVICES CONSIDERATIONS FOR DIFFICULT AIRWAY CARTS

56.4.1   What is transmissible spongiform encephalitis? Should airway practitioners be concerned about it?

The widespread awareness of the possibility of transmission of infectious processes via the use of reusable medical equipment has led to adherence to standards for sterilization as a routine practice. Until recently, it was assumed that the adherence to these measures would assure that equipment was sterile and the prevention of iatrogenic disease transmission by this route.

Creutzfeldt-Jakob disease (CJD), bovine spongiform encephalitis (BSE or mad cow disease), as well as variant CJD (vCJD) are examples of the transmissible spongiform encephalopathies (TSE). All these diseases are transmitted by malformed protein particles, referred to as prions. These infectious prion proteins attach themselves to native prion proteins in the recipients' brain, resulting in production of more of the distorted, abnormal prions, and the clinical specter of progressive neurological symptoms leading to death. Almost any symptom can present, from motor, to sensory, to cognitive dysfunction. This often makes the diagnosis difficult as the symptoms can be confused with other neurological conditions. Definitive diagnosis is made hisologically by biopsy or at autopsy. the term "Spongiform" refers to the spongy gross appearance of the brain caused by TSE.

The incidence of TSE in humans is extremely low. Sporadic (90% of CJD) and familial (10% of all CJD) forms of CJD occur at a frequency of 1:1,000,000 in the general population. Iatrogenic forms of CJD have occurred from transfer of infected neural tissues (pituitary extract, cornea, or dura mater) and represent <1% of all cases of CJD. In 1986, the first case of BSE was reported in

Britain. By 2001, it was estimated that 180,000 cattle were infected. One recalls the widespread control measures taken at that time, with the mass destruction of herds throughout the United Kingdom. There appears to be a link between BSE and vCJD. This variant has some significant differences from the sporadic form of CJD. Among the differences between the two disease entities is the notable discovery of a prion specific to vCJD in lymphoid tissues (tonsil, spleen, appendix, and lymph nodes). Prior to this, the only location of the agents responsible for BSE was felt to be neural tissue involving brain, spinal cord, dura mater, or eye. The discovery of prions in lymphoid tissue occurs very early in the disease process, before the onset of clinical symptoms. Furthermore, the tissues are very highly infectious. A mass of 1 µg of infected lymphoid tissue has the same risk of infectivity as 1 g of neural tissue from BSE-infected tissues.[10,11] This makes the tissue infected with the vCJD prion particle 1000 times more infectious than the neural tissue from sporadic CJD-infected subjects.

By the year 2002, a total of 134 cases of human TSE felt secondary to BSE had been reported worldwide.[10] The vast majority (126) were in the United Kingdom and Ireland, 6 in France, 1 in Italy, and 1 in the United States. The US (FL) resident, however, was from the United Kingdom and it was felt the disease had been acquired there. Clearly, the transmission of TSE has been documented through the use of neural tissues, both dural grafts and pituitary growth hormone. It has also been reported to have passed from patient to patient via reusable neurosurgical instruments, despite employing standard cleaning and disinfection methods. While it is difficult to assess the risk of transmission via reusable airway instruments, either surgical or anesthetic, that have come in contact with lymphoid tissue in an infected patient, the infectivity of the vCJD prion from such tissue as mentioned above, is approximately 1000 times that of the material from neural tissue.

56.4.2   How effective is sterilization in destroying the prion particle?

Discovery of prion transmission through the use of infected surgical instruments created an alarming realization that the usual methods of sterilization were not reliable in disinfecting medical equipment.[12,13] It has been shown that the prion particles associated with TSE are extremely resistant to accepted standard sterilization procedures; particles withstanding autoclaving (120°C), ultraviolet radiation, as well as ionizing radiation.[13] The discovery that protein residue is present in medical instruments used for airway manipulation after routine cleaning procedures creates even more concern. This is particularly worrisome in light of the presence of prions in lymphoid tissues in patients later diagnosed with vCJD. Miller showed in the assessment of 20 *cleaned* reusable LMAs that all had residual protein deposits on them, ranging from mild (55%) to heavy staining (20%). Similarly, of 61 used laryngoscope blades that had been cleaned and returned for use, 50 were contaminated.[14] This finding was confirmed by Clery and others.[15]

The recognition that: (1) prions related to vCJD were present in tonsil tissue; (2) the specific prion was much more virulent than the agent for vCJD; and (3) material from patients was present on airway instruments in spite of adequate techniques of sterilization has led to the suggestion that single-use instruments be used in place of reusable varieties where the risk of cross contamination with tonsil tissue can occur. Indeed, in 2001, the Department of Health in the United Kingdom mandated the use of disposable surgical and anesthetic instruments for use in tonsil surgery. However, within a year, the high incidence of surgical complications deemed to be secondary to the introduction of these disposable instruments led to the reversal of the directive. It was decided that the risk of complications from the disposable instruments outweighed the risk of transmission of vCJD from cross contamination of inadequately cleaned multiple use instruments. Although the ban on reusable anesthetic equipment was initially lifted, it was reimposed in 2002.

56.4.3 How well do single-use (disposable) airway devices work when compared to the reusable instruments?

Following the concern that reusable airway equipment could cause the transmission of vCJD, a large number of single-use instruments were introduced into the market. These included, but were not limited to, laryngoscope blades, tracheal tube introducers (e.g., Eschmann Introducer), LMA and other extraglottic devices, as well as disposable covers for laryngoscope blades. However, there are no strict testing or standards that must be met by any of these devices. Consequently, a great deal of controversy has arisen as to their effectiveness, when compared to the traditional equipment.

Twiggs et al.[16] compared six single-use laryngoscope blades with the "standard" Macintosh blade in a simulator model. Twenty experienced anesthesiologists used each device, both in an "easy" scenario and a simulated difficult airway. Time to intubate, need for the use of an Eschmann Introducer, Cormack/Lehane (C/L) grading, and percentage of glottic opening visible (POGO) scores were recorded. Although considerable variability existed between the disposable devices, the best performer in both "normal" and "difficult" scenarios was the Macintosh blade. Not surprisingly, it was the difficult airway that brought out the greatest differences between the best and the worst performers. Some of the single-use blades performed reasonably well, the best being the Europa, which is a metal. The results were so troubling that the investigators concluded, "We believe that intubation equipment that fails to match standard equipment should be avoided and is clinically unsafe. The unregulated use of single-use laryngoscopes must be questioned."[16]

Annamaneni et al.[17] demonstrated a difference between single-use and disposable tracheal introducers ("bougies") in simulated difficult intubations. Twenty anesthesiologists attempted intubation twice with both a reusable introducer and a single-use introducer, with success measured by tracheal as opposed to esophageal insertion. The success with first attempts was 85% versus 15% for the multiple use and disposable devices, respectively. The results were similar for the second attempt.

Evans et al.[18] compared disposable and nondisposable laryngoscopes by studying the time to intubate as well as measuring the force used to obtain an adequate laryngoscopic view, for both routine and difficult intubation in a manikin. They had 60 anesthesiologists performing intubations with five different laryngoscope blades, both routinely and with a cervical collar on the manikin. The blades included the standard Macintosh #3, a disposable metal, and three plastic blades. The time was significantly greater with the plastic blades when compared to the metal, for both the routine and "difficult" intubations. The increase ranged from 33–85%. Forces generated were statistically greater for the plastic blades when compared to those for the metal blades, by as much as 35%. The forces generated, even though they were not out of the range used clinically, were sufficient to cause three of the plastic blades to fracture during the study.

Anderson and Bhadal measured the effect on the illumination by placing a protective cover over a reusable Macintosh blade.[19] They showed that a predictable reduction in illumination occurred, with a mean reduction of 19%. Others have commented on their findings that disposable laryngoscope blades are inferior to reusable devices.[20,21]

One of the authors of this chapter (SP) had the experience of having been provided with a disposable plastic blade in the ICU when called to assist with a failed intubation. The blade fractured during the intubation attempt, causing a laceration on the patient's tongue and adding to an already stressful situation. Intubation was successful following the use of a reusable metal Macintosh blade.

56.4.4 Should reusable or disposable equipment be kept in the difficult airway carts?

The only reliable ways to avoid the transmission of vCJD is to either use disposable instruments or not perform airway manipulation on patients infected with prion agent, and thus avoid contamination of reusable equipment. Clearly, the risk of contaminating equipment depends upon the probability of caring for an infected individual. The data from the World Health Organization (WHO) show that the incidence varies worldwide and is very low, even in countries at highest risk (i.e., the United Kingdom). Indeed, the risk of transmission through the use of contaminated instruments was felt to be less than the risk of complications posed by disposable surgical instruments used for tonsillectomy in 2001. Fortunately, the risks of anesthetic-related airway mishaps are lower than the risks posed by complications from our surgical colleagues. The numbers of failed intubations are too low to have adequate power to reveal what are the increased risks posed to patients by using disposable devices. Certainly, the risk posed by cross contamination of vCJD is unknown. In their editorial, Blunt and Burchett[10] discuss the hypothetical relative risks and come to the conclusion that the risk to the patient with poorly functioning airway equipment is likely greater than that of acquiring TSE through contaminated airway instruments.

The cost and reliability must be taken into account for all single-use instruments. Although Galinski et al.[22] felt that the disposable instruments were acceptable, they also state that, "it may be advisable to maintain conventional laryngoscopes in reserve for difficult intubations." More effective cleansing methods would also reduce risk, albeit not eliminate it. In the final analysis, it is important to weigh the relative risks of possible contamination with vCJD prions, negligible in most areas of the world, to those of risks created during airway management with what could, and has been shown to be, less than optimal equipment. The decision to keep reusable or disposable equipment in the difficult airway carts should be based on sound scientific evidence, relative risk, and cost–benefit assessments.

56.5 SUMMARY

The use of alternative airway devices has clearly improved patient care. The ready availability of these devices is markedly facilitated by the creation of an airway cart. This cart should be easy to use, well laid out, and maintained to ensure optimal use. The contents should encompass a range of devices as described in various publications, and should be customized to the needs of a given department and its members. Although the decision to keep reusable or disposable equipment in these airway carts is not an easy one, it should be based on relative risk, scientific evidence, and the cost–benefit assessments.

The appendix itemizes how a difficult airway cart might be structured.[9]

REFERENCES

1. American Society of Anesthesiologists Task Force on Management of the Difficult Airway: Practice guidelines for the difficult airway. *Anesthesiology.* 1993;78:597–602.
2. American Society of Anesthesiologists Task Force on Management of the Difficult Airway: Practice guidelines for management of the difficult airway: an updated report by the American Society of Anesthesiologists Task Force on Management of the Difficult Airway. *Anesthesiology.* 2003;98:1269–1277.
3. Crosby ET, Cooper RM, Douglas MJ, et al.: The unanticipated difficult airway with recommendations for management. *Can J Anaesth.* 1998;45:757–776.
4. Rose DK, Cohen MM: The airway: problems and predictions in 18500 patients. *Can J Anaesth.* 1994;39:1105–1111.
5. Schwartz DE, Matthay MA, Cohen NH: Death and other complications of emergency airway management in critically ill patients: a prospective investigation of 297 tracheal intubations. *Anesthesiology.* 1995;82:367–376.
6. Mort TC: Emergency tracheal intubation: complications associated with repeated laryngoscopic attempts. *Anesth Analg.* 2004;99:607–613.
7. Mort TC: The incidence and risk factors for cardiac arrest during emergency tracheal intubation: a justification for incorporating the ASA Guidelines in the remote location. *J Clin Anesth.* 2004;16:508–516.
8. Luten R, Broselow J: Rainbow care: the Broselow-Luten system. Implications for pediatric patient safety. *Ambul Outreach.* 1999;14–16.
9. McGuire GP, Wong DT: Airway management: contents of a difficult intubation cart. *Can J Anaesth.* 1999;46:190–191.
10. Blunt MC, Burchett KR: Variant Creutzfeldt-Jacob disease and disposable anesthetic equipment—balancing the risks. *Br J Anaesth.* 2003;90:1–3.
11. Bruce ME, McConnell I, Will RG, et al.: Detection of variant Creutzfeldt-Jacob disease infectivity in extraneural tissue. *Lancet.* 2001;358:208–209.
12. Brown P, Preece M, Brandel JP, et al.: Iatrogenic Creutzfeldt-Jacob disease at the millennium. *Neurology.* 2000;55:1075–1081.
13. Zobeley E, Flechsig E, Corizio A, et al.: Infectivity of scrapie prions bound to a stainless steel surface. *Mol Med.* 1999;5:240–243.
14. Miller DM, Youkhana I, Karaunaratne WU, Pearce A: Presence of protein deposits on "cleaned" re-usable anesthetic equipment. *Anaesthesia.* 2001;56:1069–1072.
15. Clery G, Brimacombe J, Stone T, Keller C, Curtis S: Routine cleaning and autoclaving does not remove protein deposits from reusable laryngeal mask devices. *Anesth Analg.* 2003;97:1189–1191.
16. Twiggs SJ, McCormick B, Cook TM: Randomized evaluation of the performance of single-use laryngoscopes in simulated easy and difficult intubation. *Br J Anaesth.* 2003;90:8–13.
17. Annamaneni R, Hodzovic I, Wilkes AR, Latto IP: A comparison of simulated difficult intubation with multiple-use and single-use bougies in a manikin. *Anaesthesia.* 2003;58:45–49.
18. Evans A, Vaughan RS, Hall JE, et al.: A comparison of forces exerted during laryngoscopy using disposable and non-disposable laryngoscope blades. *Anaesthesia.* 2003;58:869–873.
19. Anderson KJ, Bhadal N: The effect of single use laryngoscopy equipment on the illumination for tracheal intubation. *Anaesthesia.* 2002;57:773–777.
20. Babb S, Mann S: Disposable laryngoscope blades. *Anaesthesia.* 2002;57:286–287.
21. Jefferson P, Perkins V, Edwards VA, Ball DR: Problems with disposable laryngoscope blades. *Anaesthesia.* 2003;58:385–386.
22. Galinski M, Adnet F, Tran D, et al.: Disposable laryngoscope blades do not interfere with ease of intubation in scheduled general anaesthesia patients. *Eur J Anaesthesiol.* 2003;20:731–735.

SELF-EVALUATION QUESTIONS

56.1. Which of the following is a known effective method of sterilization in destroying the prion particle?

  A. autoclaving (120°C)

  B. ultraviolet radiation

  C. ionizing radiation

  D. sterilization with ethylene oxide

  E. none of the above

56.2. All of the following policy issues regarding a difficult airway cart are crucial **EXCEPT**

  A. cart location

  B. who is the cart "policy" manager

  C. communications regarding contents

  D. maintenance and replacement of contents

  E. who is permitted to use the cart

56.3. Since anesthesia practitioners are called to out-of-OR locations to manage airways

  A. they are liable for negative outcomes if the equipment they need is not available.

  B. they must have input regarding contents of difficult airway carts in locations where they may be called to intervene.

  C. they must ensure that policies regarding airway equipment maintenance in out-of-OR locations are in force and followed.

  D. noncompliance in any of the scenarios listed above (including the availability of essential equipment) would be grounds to refuse to participate in airway management in those locations.

  E. all of the above.

APPENDIX 56.1

Sample contents of an OR difficult airway cart

DRAWER #1:
Topical anesthesia

- William's® Airways (9 cm × 2; 10 cm × 1)
- Berman Intubating Pharyngeal or Breakaway® Airways (sm, med, lg)—Vital Signs
- Mucosal Atomization Device (MAD®) (3)—Wolf Tory Medical
- Mucosal Atomization Device gic (MADgic®) (3)—Wolf Tory Medical
- Antifog (3); Goggles (1); Bite Blocks (2); Med Cups (4)
- Jackson Crossover Forceps (1)
- DeVilbiss Atomizer® with O_2 Tubing
- Phenylephrine 0.5% (Neosynephrine®) nasal spray 15 mL (1)
- 20% Hurricaine Gel 6.25 g (4)
- Lidocaine 4% aqueous 50 mL bottles (1)
- Tetracaine 0.45% with epinephrine 1:25,000 (40 µg·mL^{-1}) (3 × 15 mL bottles)
- Olympus light source replacement bulb (1)
- Portex fiberoptic bronchoscope swivel adapter (4)
- Adult and pediatric Magill Forceps

DRAWER #2:
Jet ventilator

- Metered dose inhaler in-line administration adapters (2)
- Jet ventilator
- Intravenous needle/catheters for transcricoid insertion (14 and 16 gauge × 2 of each) must be aspiration capable with 3 mL syringe with 7 mm ID ETT connector
- ENK Oxygen Flow Modulator®—Cook
- 6, 7, and 8 mm ID Endotrol® tubes—Mallinckrodt

DRAWER #3:
Combitube™ and Trachlight™

- Small Adult (1) and Regular Adult (1) Combitube™—Mallinckrodt
- Trachlight™ handles (2) and adult wands (10)

DRAWER #4:
LMAs

- LMA Fastrach™: #5 × 2; #4 × 1; #3 × 1
- LMA Classic™: #1; #1.5; #2, #2.5; #3; #4; #5

DRAWER #5:
Surgical airway

- Melker Cricothyrotomy Kit®—Cook
- Retrograde Intubation Kit

DRAWER #6:
Fiberoptics

- Bullard Laryngoscope
- Cook Airway Exchange Catheters® (14 F × 2; 19 F × 2)

Top of Cart

- Bronchoscope light source
- Spare Eschmann Tracheal Tube Introducer

Side Cabinet

- 3.5 "Pediatric" and 5.1 Fiberoptic Bronchoscopes

EQUIPMENT SUPPLIER CONTACT INFORMATION

The following list of the manufacturers of airway equipment is not intended to be exhaustive, nor should it be construed to represent any sort of endorsement by the authors.

Airway Management Device (AMD™); Nagor Limited, PO Box 21 Global House, Isle of Man Business Park, Cooil Road Douglas, Isle of Man IM99 1AX, British Isles, Tel.: +44 (0) 1624 625556; Fax: +44 (0) 1624 661656

Ambu Laryngeal Mask; Ambu, Inc., 6740 Baymeadow Drive, Glen Burnie, MD 21060 USA, Tel.: 1 800 262 8462 or 410 768 6464; Fax: 1 800 262 8673 or 410 768 3993; www.ambu.com

Angulated video-intubation laryngoscope (AVIL); Acutronic Medical Systems AG, Fabrik im Schiffli CH-8816 Hirzel, Schweiz/Switzerland, Tel.: ++41 44 729 70 80; Fax ++41 44 729 70 81

Beck Airway Airflow Monitor (BAAM); Alliance Medical, 8624 Rte C, PO Box 147, Russelville, MO 65074 USA, Tel.: (888) 633 6908; Fax: (800) 425 5633; www.allmed.net

Berman Intubating Pharyngeal Airway ("Berman Breakaway Airway"); Vital Signs, Inc., 20 Campus Road, Totowa, NJ 07512 USA, Tel.: (800) 932 0760; Fax: (973) 790 3307; http://www.vital-signs.com/

Bonfils Retromolar Intubation Fiberscope; Karl Storz Endoscopy-America, Inc., Attn: Human Resources, 600 Corporate Pointe, Culver City, CA 90230-7600 USA, Fax: 310 410 5520

Bullard Laryngoscope; ACMI Corporation, 93 North Pleasant St., Norwalk, OH 44857 USA, Tel.: 508 804 2600; http://www.acmicorp.com/

CobraPLA™ (Perilaryngeal Airway); Engineered Medical Systems, Inc., 2055 Executive Drive, Indianapolis, IN 46241 USA, Tel.: 317 246 5500; Fax: 317 246 5501

Combitube™; Kendall Healthcare, 15 Hampshire St. Mansfield, MA 02048 USA, Tel.: (508) 261 8000; Fax: (508) 261 8062

Cook Airway Exchange Catheter; Mercury Medical, 11300 A-49th Street North, Clearwater, FL 34622-4800 USA, Tel.: (800) 237 6418; Fax: (800) 990 6375; http://www.mercurymed.com/

Cook ILA intubating LMA; Mercury Medical, 11300 A-49th Street North, Clearwater, FL 34622-4800 USA, Tel.: (800) 237 6418; Fax: (800) 990 6375; http://www.mercurymed.com/

Cuffed Oropharyngeal Airway (COPA); Mallinckrodt, 675 McDonnell Blvd, Hazelwood, MO 63042 USA, Tel.: (800) 635 5267; http://www.mallinckrodt.com/contact/contact.html

Cricoid pressure simulators; Nasco, 901 Janesville Avenue, PO Box 901, Fort Atkinson, WI 53538-0901 USA, Tel.: 1 800 558 9595; Fax: 920 563 8296; http://www.enasco.com/Static.do?page = contact

Cricothyrotomy (open) kits and needle cricothyrotomy devices; Cook® Critical Care, PO Box 489, 750 Daniel's Way, Bloomington, IN 47402-0489 USA, Tel.: (800) 457 4500; Fax: (800) 554 8335; http://cookcriticalcare.com/

Cricothyrotomy instruments; Allegiance Healthcare, V. Meuller Division, 1435 Lake Cook Road, Deerfield, IL 60015, Tel.: (800) 964 5227; http://www.allegiance.net/products/vmueller/vmuelle1.asp

DeVilbiss atomizers; Anthony Products, Inc., 7740 Records St. Indianapolis, IN 46226, Tel.: (877) 428 1610; Fax: (317) 543 3289; http://www.anthonyproducts.com/contact/contact.htm

Endotracheal Tube Attachment Device (ETAD™); COS Medical, Inc., 3213 Post Woods Drive, Suite B, Atlanta, GA 30339 USA, http://www.continentostomystore.com/

Endotracheal tube exchangers (airway exchange catheters); Cook® Critical Care, PO Box 489, 750 Daniel's Way, Bloomington, IN 47402-0489 USA, Tel.: (800) 457 4500; Fax: (800) 554 8335; http://cookcriticalcare.com/

Endotrol® endotracheal tubes; Mallinckrodt, 675 McDonnell Blvd, Hazelwood, MO 63042 USA, Tel.: (800) 635 5267; http://www.mallinckrodt.com/contact/contact.html

ENK Oxygen Flow Modulator; Cook Critical Care, PO Box 489, 750 Daniel's Way, Bloomington, IN 47402-0489 USA, Tel.: (800) 457 4500; Fax: (800) 554 8335; http://cookcriticalcare.com/

Eschmann Tracheal Tube Introducer (Blue Line® tracheal tube introducer); SIMS Portex, Inc., 10 Bowman Drive, PO Box 0724, Keene, NH 03431 USA, Tel.: (800) 258 5361; http://www.portex.com/airway/products/dcategory = General%20Anesthesia

Fiberoptic bronchoscopes and nasopharyngoscopes; Karl Storz Endoscopy-America, Inc., Attn: Human Resources, 600 Corporate Pointe, Culver City, CA 90230-7600 USA; Fax: 310 410 5520; Pentax Precision Instrument Corporation, 30 Ramland Road, Orangeburg, NY 10962-2699 USA, Tel.: (800) 431 5880; Fax: (845) 365 0822; http://www.pentaxmedical.com/Products/Bronchoscopy.asp; Olympus America, Inc., 3500 Corporate Parkway, PO Box 610, Center Valley, PA 18034-0610 USA, Tel.: 800 645 8160; http://www.olympusamerica.com/

Flex-tip (McCoy type) laryngoscope blades; Heine USA Ltd., One Washington Street, Unit 555, Dover, NH 03820 USA, Tel.:

(800) 367 4872; Fax: 603 742 7217; http://www.heine.com/; Mercury Medical, 11300 A-49th Street North, Clearwater, FL 34622-4800 USA, Tel.: (800) 237 6418; Fax: (800) 990 6375; http://www.mercurymed.com/; Rusch, Inc., 2450 Meadowbrook Parkway, Duluth, GA 30096 USA, Tel.: (800) 553 5214; Fax: (770) 623 1829; http://www.rusch.com/; Flex-Guide endotracheal tube introducer (Green Field Medical Sourcing, Inc., 14141 Highway 290 West Suite 710, Austin, TX 78737 USA, Tel.: 512 894 3002; Fax: 512 858 1515

Frova intubating stylet; Cook® Critical Care, PO Box 489, 750 Daniel's Way, Bloomington, IN 47402-0489 USA, Tel.: (800) 457 4500; Fax: (800) 554 8335; http://cookcriticalcare.com/

GlideScope® Video Laryngoscope; Saturn Biomedical Systems, Inc., 4224 Manor Street, Burnaby, BC V5G 1B2, Canada, Tel.: 604.439.3009; Fax: 604.439.3039; email: info@saturnbiomedical.com (To purchase: Diagnostic Ultrasound Customer Care Department, Tel.: 1 800 331 2313; Fax: 1 425 883 2896; email: sales@dxu.com)

Grandview laryngoscope blade; Hartwell Medical, 6352 Corte del Abeto, Suite J, Carlsbad, CA 92009-1408 USA, Tel.: (800) 633 5900; Fax: (760) 438 2783; http://www.hartwellmedical.com/grand.html

Human Patient Simulators (Air Man, Sim Man); Laerdal Medical Corporation, 167 Myers Corners Road, PO Box 1840, Wappingers Falls, NY 12590-8840 USA, Tel.: (800) 648 1851; Fax: (800) 227 1143; http://www.laerdal.com/

Jackson Crossover or Jackson Laryngeal Forceps; Surgical Tools, 2 C Greenmanville Ave, Mystic, CT 06355 USA, Tel.: (800) 774 2040; Fax: (860) 536 8532; http://www.surgicaltools.com/

Jet ventilator; Life-Assist, Inc., 11277 Sunrise Park Dr, Rancho Cordova, CA 95742 USA; Tel.: (800) 824 6016; Fax: (800) 290 9794; http://www.life-assist.com/jetvent.html

King LT™ Airway (Laryngeal Tube Airway); King Systems Corporation, 15011 Herriman Blvd, Noblesville, IN 46060 USA, Tel.: 1 800 642 5464; http://www.kingsystems.com/Main.htm

Laryngeal Mask Airway, LMA ProSeal™, LMA Fastrach™, and LMA Unique™; LMA North America, 9360 Towne Centre Drive, Suite 200, San Diego, CA 92121-3030 USA, Tel.: (800) 788 7999; Fax: (858) 622 4130; http://www.lmana.com/prod/components/contact_us.html

LaryVent™; B + P Beatmungs-Produkte GmbH, Willy-Brandt-Allee 300, Gelsenkirchen, 45891, DEU, Tel.: +49 209 970770; http://www.masterflex.de

Levitan FPS Scope; Clarus Medical, LLC, 1000 Boone Avenue North, Minneapolis, MN 55427 USA, Tel.: 763 525 8403; Fax: 763 525 8656; http://www.clarus-medical.com/airway-management/airway_levitan.htm

MAD (Mucosal Atomization Device) and MADgic; Wolf Tory Medical, Inc., 79 W 4500 South, Suite 16, Salt Lake City, UT 84107 USA, Tel.: (888) 380 9808; Fax: (801) 281 0708; www.wolfetory.com

Melker Cricothyrotomy kit; Cook® Critical Care, PO Box 489, 750 Daniel's Way, Bloomington, IN 47402-0489 USA, Tel.: (800) 457 4500; Fax: (800) 554 8335; http://cookcriticalcare.com/

Metered dose inhaler inline adapter; DHD Healthcare, 1 Madison St, Wampsville, NY 13163 USA, Tel.: (800) 847 8000; Fax: (315) 363 9462; http://www.dhd.com/html/catalog.html

Pharyngeal Airway Express (PAxpress™); Vital Signs, Inc., 20 Campus Road, Totowa, NJ 07512 USA, Tel.: (800) 932 0760; Fax: (973) 790 3307; http://www.vital-signs.com/

Retrograde Intubation kit; Cook® Critical Care, PO Box 489, 750 Daniel's Way, Bloomington, IN 47402-0489 USA, Tel.: (800) 457 4500; Fax: (800) 554 8335; http://cookcriticalcare.com/

The Schroeder (Parker Flex-It™ Directional Stylet); Parker Medical, 7275 S. Revere Pkwy, Suite 804, Englewood, CO 80112 USA, Tel.: 303 799 1990; Fax: 303 799 1996

Sheridan Tube Exchanger; Sheridan Catheter Corp., Route 40, Argyle, NY 12809 USA, Tel.: 518 638 6101; Fax: 518 638 8493

Shikani Optical Stylet (SOS™); Clarus Medical, LLC, 1000 Boone Avenue North, Minneapolis, MN 55427 USA, Tel.: 763 525 8403; Fax: 763 525 8656; http://www.clarus-medical.com/airwaycontact.htm

Silicone fluid (Endoscopic Instrument Fluid); ACMI Corporation, 93 North Pleasant St., Norwalk, OH 44857 USA, Tel.: 508 804 2600; http://www.acmicorp.com/

Streamlined Pharynx Airway Liner (SLIPA™); ARC Medical, Inc., 322 Patterson Ave., Scottdale, GA 30079 USA, Tel.: 404 373 8300 ext. 210

StyletScope™; Nihon Kohden America, Inc., 90 Icon St., Foothill Ranch, CA 92610 USA, Tel.: 800 325 0283

Sun Med Intubating Stylet; Mercury Medical, 11300 A-49th Street North, Clearwater, FL 34622-4800 USA, Tel.: (800) 237 6418; Fax: (800) 990 6375; http://www.mercurymed.com/

Trachlight™; Rusch, Inc., 2450 Meadowbrook Parkway, Duluth, GA 30096 USA, Tel.: (800) 553 5214; Fax: (770) 623 1829; http://www.rusch.com/; Laerdal Medical Corporation, 167 Myers Corners Road, PO Box 1840, Wappingers Falls, NY 12590-8840 USA, Tel.: (800) 648 1851; Fax: (800) 227 1143; http://www.laerdal.com/

Trans tracheal jet ventilation sets, catheters, and equipment; Cook® Critical Care, PO Box 489, 750 Daniel's Way, Bloomington, IN 47402-0489 USA, Tel.: (800) 457 4500; Fax: (800) 554 8335; http://cookcriticalcare.com/

Universal Cricothyrotomy Kit (both open and Seldinger apparatus); Cook® Critical Care, PO Box 489, 750 Daniel's Way, Bloomington, IN 47402-0489 USA, Tel.: (800) 457 4500; Fax: (800) 554 8335; http://cookcriticalcare.com/

UpsherScope™; Mercury Medical, 11300 A-49th Street North, Clearwater, FL 34622-4800 USA, Tel.: (800) 237 6418; Fax: (800) 990 6375; http://www.mercurymed.com/

Videolaryngoscope; Karl Storz Endovision, Inc., 91 Carpenter Hill Road, Charlton, MA 01507 USA, http://www.karlstorz.com/

Video Macintosh Storz (VMS); Karl Storz Endovision, Inc., 91 Carpenter Hill Road, Charlton, MA 01507 USA, http://www.karlstorz.com/

Video-Optical Intubation Stylet (VOIS); Acutronic Medical Systems AG, Fabrik im Schiffli, CH-8816 Hirzel, Schweiz / Switzerland, Tel.: ++41 44 729 70 80; Fax: ++41 44 729 70 81

Viewmax® laryngoscope blade; Rusch, Inc., 2450 Meadowbrook Parkway, Duluth, GA 30096 USA, Tel.: (800) 553 5214; Fax: (770) 623 1829; http://www.rusch.com/

WuScope System™; Achi Corporation, 2168 Ringwood Avenue, San Jose, CA 95131-1720 USA, Tel.: 408 321 9581; Fax: 408 321 9587; www.achi.com

MEDICATION CONTACT SUPPLIER INFORMATION

Tetracaine 1% aqueous; Abbott Pharmaceuticals, 100 Abbott Pk Rd, Abbott Park, IL 60064 USA, Tel.: (800) 633 9110; http://www.abbott.com/

Lidocaine 4% aqueous and viscous; Lidocaine 5% ointment; AstraZeneca Pharmaceuticals LP, 1800 Concord Pike, PO Box 15437, Wilmington, DE 19850-5437 USA, Tel.: (800) 456 3669; http://www.astrazeneca-us.com/products/list.asp

Lidocaine nonaerosol tracheal spray; Odan Laboratories Ltd., 325 Stillview Ave, Point Claire, QC H9R 2Y6, Canada, Tel.: (514) 428 1628; Fax: (514) 428 9783; http://www.odanlab.com/; email: info@odanlab.com

Benzocaine 20% ointment; Beutlich LP Pharmaceuticals, 1541 Shields Dr, Waukegan, IL 60085-8304 USA, Tel.: (800) 238 8542; Fax: (847) 473 1122; http://www.beutlich.com/

CART SUPPLIER CONTACT INFORMATION

Armstrong Medical; 575 Kinghtsbridge Pkwy, Lincolnshire, IL 60069-0700 USA, Tel.: (800) 323 4220; Fax: (847) 913 0138; http://www.armstrongmedical.com/

Blue Bell Bio-Medical; 550 Bonneweitz Ave, Van Wert, OH 45891 USA, Tel.: (800) 258 3235; Fax: (419) 238 0226; http://www.bluebellcarts.com/

CHAPTER (57)

Documentation of Difficult Airway

Lorraine J. Foley

57.1 CASE PRESENTATION

A 39 year old female was scheduled for a laparoscopic cholecystectomy under general anesthesia. She was 5 ft 4 in (163 cm) tall and weighed 220 lb (100 kg). She denied a history of gastric reflux. Past surgical history was limited to a caesarean section performed under epidural anesthesia. Preanesthetic airway assessment showed that she had a Mallampati class II airway with good head and neck extension. On the 3-3-2 examination (LEMON, see Section 1.6.2), she demonstrated just less than 5 cm mouth opening, less than 5 cm mentohyoid distance, and 3.5 cm distance from the hyoid to the thyroid notch. Standard monitors were placed on the patient. With the head and neck placed in a "sniffing position," denitrogenation was achieved. Following induction of anesthesia with Propofol (200 mg), bag-mask-ventilation (BMV) was checked and easily performed. Rocuronium (50 mg) was given for muscle relaxation. After all four twitches were ablated; direct laryngoscopy was attempted with a Macintosh #3 blade. Only a large epiglottis could be seen. The Macintosh #3 was removed and a Miller #3 blade was used to lift the epiglottis. On this second attempt at laryngoscopy, the Grade III view persisted, with no aspect of the glottis visible. An Eschmann Introducer (the "gum elastic bougie") was employed without success. Following this second attempt, the patient remained easy to ventilate using BMV and oxygen saturation was maintained. Help was summoned and the difficult airway cart obtained. A #3 Intubating Laryngeal Mask Airway (ILMA) (Fastrach™) was placed easily and permitted satisfactory ventilation. An attempt at blind intubation through the ILMA was unsuccessful. A 7 mm ID endotracheal tube (ETT) was then loaded onto a flexible Foley fiberoptic Airway STylet (FAST) and introduced through the ILMA. The ILMA was manipulated until the vocal cords were seen through the FAST and the ETT

was advanced into trachea under indirect vision without further difficulty.

57.2 INTRODUCTION

57.2.1 What airway information should be documented following a routine tracheal intubation and airway management?

The short answer to this question is "whatever information *you* would like to see when seeking information from old records about a difficult airway." For example, in assessing the patient described above with predictors of possible difficult laryngoscopy, availability of an anesthetic record from 6 months previously which clearly documented, "easy BMV; easy laryngoscopy with Macintosh 3 blade, Cormack/Lehane (C/L) grade 2 view; optimal external laryngeal manipulation (OELM) improved view to C/L grade 1 with 75% of cords visible, easy tube passage with a 7.5 mm ID ETT" would be immensely reassuring, and adds objective information to the airway examination. In some patients with a questionable difficult airway, the availability of such information may spare the patient an uncomfortable awake tracheal intubation.

57.2.2 Why should we document the management of a difficult or failed airway?

The difficult or failed airway is an ongoing threat to patient safety in anesthetic practice. Careful examination of the patient seeking anatomic predictors of not only difficult laryngoscopic intubation but also difficult BMV, difficult extraglottic device use and difficult transtracheal access is advisable, as outlined in Chapter 1. However, the fact remains that these predictors, while being sensitive, are not specific, and generally have a low positive predictive value.[1] The result is that unanticipated difficult airways continue to occur. Indeed, 1–2% of patients undergoing general anesthesia present unanticipated difficult airways and intubations with conventional laryngoscopy.[2,3]

In the aftermath of the unanticipated difficult airway, every effort must be made to ensure that future anesthesia practitioners are informed of such a history. Written documentation and verbal communication providing the details of the difficulty encountered, the adequacy of BMV, and the remedy employed to manage the airway must occur.

The American Society of Anesthesiologists (ASA) Closed Claims Analysis[4] points to the importance of being able to predict difficulty with airway management. The analysis demonstrates that adverse outcomes associated with respiratory events constitute the single largest class of injury. Seventeen percent of these claims were related to difficult intubation. Cheney et al. compared the closed claims cases from the 1970s, 1980s, and 1990s.[5] Inadequate ventilation, difficult intubation, and unrecognized esophageal intubation were the three most common respiratory system related events leading to brain damage or death in all three of these time periods. Some favorable trends were noted in the study: inadequate ventilation dropped from 22% of respiratory related claims in 1970, to 15% in 1980s, and only 7% in 1990s; and the incidence of death or brain damage also decreased. However, though not statistically significant due to the small numbers of claims in the 1990s, the proportion of difficult intubation contributing to death or brain damage increased from 5% in 1970s to 12% in the 1990s.[5] It is generally felt that the introduction of pulse oximetry, end-tidal CO_2 detection, and esophageal detection devices helped to decrease the number of inadequate ventilation and esophageal intubation cases. It is also felt that the increasing incidence of difficult intubation cases is related to the increasing incidence of morbid obesity.

As a result of Caplan's closed claims analysis from the 1970s and 1980s, the ASA Task Force on Management of the Difficult Airway published guidelines for management of the difficult airway in 1993 with an update in 2003.[6] These guidelines were published in an effort to reduce the likelihood that an unanticipated difficult or failed airway will be encountered. These guidelines recommend that the preoperative evaluation include an "airway" history and physical examination.

57.3 DIFFICULT AIRWAY DATABASE AND REGISTRY

57.3.1 When was the first difficult airway registry established?

Coincident with the development of these guidelines, an advisory group with representation from anesthesia, otolaryngology, and experts in risk management was formed to work with the nonprofit MedicAlert® Foundation in the United States to establish a "National Difficult Airway/Intubation" registry. A fundamental

objective of this registry was to develop criteria for uniform documentation of difficult airway management events and mechanisms to make such information available to future airway practitioners. In 1991, the ASA Anesthesia Advisory Council ratified the nomenclature "Difficult Airway/Intubation" as a standardized nomenclature for use within the MedicAlert® identification system. Thereafter, in 1992, The World Federation of Societies of Anesthesia and the American Academy of Otolaryngology—Head and Neck surgeons officially endorsed the MedicAlert® Foundation nomenclature and documentation system.

Several years later, the MedicAlert® Foundation introduced a unique patient enrollment form and established a uniform database for difficult airway/intubation events and patients. However, due to the labor demands related to data entry, the unique patient-enrollment form is no longer employed by MedicAlert®. Presently, a physician can download a generic MedicAlert® form from the website www.medicalert.org.

At the time of writing, no difficult airway registry exists. The Difficult Airway Registry Committee of the Society of Airway Management (SAM) is presently developing a computerized database to include specific aspects of airway management and complications in an effort to ensure that pertinent patient care information is available to other airway practitioners.

57.3.2 Is there any evidence to support the use of centralized difficult airway database?

Two preliminary studies have shown a reduced incidence of adverse outcomes when prior difficult intubation information was available to the practitioner. The first publication included 111 patients enrolled in the MedicAlert® Registry database. The authors found that anticipation of a difficult airway led to fewer airway management techniques being employed, a lower incidence of adverse outcomes, and that practitioners educated about the registry would voluntarily enroll selected patients.[7] Further, despite a high frequency of negative outcomes or adverse events (e.g., tracheotomy), 100% of the patients surveyed in the study reported an element of perceived "future safety" and were satisfied that the MedicAlert® Registry fostered that notion.

A second study reported on a computerized in-hospital Difficult Airway Registry, which had been developed at the Beth Israel Deaconess Medical Center in Boston, MA.[8] From April 1995 to April 1997, 129 patients were entered into the registry. Out of these patients, 31 returned to the operating room at least once. Information regarding the patient's previous airway management episode was available from the database eliminating the need to rely on the patient's memory or paper medical records. There were no adverse airway outcomes in patients returning to the operating room. Others institutions have used their automated anesthesia recording systems as a warning system by flagging patients in whom difficult airway situations have been encountered.[9,10] The interest in having a centralized difficult airway registry has also spread to the United Kingdom.[11]

Practice guidelines published in the ASA, United Kingdom, and Canada vary with respect to the specific information that ought to be recorded in the event a difficult airway and/or intubation is encountered, where it should be documented, and to whom the information should be communicated.[12–14] Common sense suggests that greater the number of people who know about a difficult intubation in a specific patient, the more places the information is documented, it is less likely the patient will be placed at risk when that patient returns for general anesthesia.[13]

57.3.3 Who should be informed about the difficult airway?

The patient should be told about the difficulty with airway management upon regaining full alertness and orientation, and advised to acquire a Medic-Alert® bracelet. Written documentation, (see Appendix 57.1) explaining the difficulty should be given to the patient. In addition to the patient, the following individuals should also be notified of the difficult airway:

- a family member who is the caregiver of the patient
- the primary care provider
- the attending surgeon—it may be helpful for the surgeon to reiterate information regarding the airway management difficulty if the patient is seen in a followup visit.

57.3.4 Where should the information be documented?

Information about an encountered difficult airway should be entered in the following locations:

- the patient's anesthetic record—documentation of the difficult airway encountered will then become part of the patient's permanent medical records
- in-hospital Difficult Airway Registry, if available
- in a letter to the patient, as described in the next section and in Appendix 57.1
- in computerized medical records
- through MedicAlert® Foundation, as describe above
- while patient remains hospitalized, a bracelet should be worn to indicate the difficult airway status.

57.3.5 What information should be documented following the management of a difficult or failed airway?

The following information should appear on medical records and the MedicAlert® application form:

Date of operation

Type of operation

Hospital and medical record number

Anatomic features on airway examination which may have contributed to the problem, e.g., height, weight, Mallampati classification, mouth opening, thyromental span, limitations to head and neck mobility, etc.

Relevant medical conditions that may have contributed to the difficult airway, e.g., rheumatoid arthritis, diabetes, obesity, obstructive sleep apnea, etc.

Mask ventilation—easy, difficult, or impossible

Oral or nasal airway size, if used

If direct laryngoscopy attempted, blade used, view obtained, number of attempts, use of adjuncts such as OELM or tracheal tube introducer, and whether or not successful

Ultimate disposition—whether the airway was secured awake or asleep and with which technique/instrument

Use of an extraglottic device as a rescue device

Any other comments

As an example, airway documentation for the patient presented in the chapter would be as follows:

Date of operation: 4/12/05

Type of operation: laparoscopic cholecystectomy

Winchester Hospital, Winchester MA Medical Record # 333–42-35

PE 5 ft 4 in. (163 cm) 220 lb (100 kg), otherwise healthy, normal airway anatomy

Easy bag-mask-ventilation with #7 OPA throughout

Attempt 1—Macintosh 3; C/L Grade 3 laryngoscopy, long floppy epiglottis, no improvement with OELM or head lift, unsuccessful

Attempt 2—Miller 3; C/L Grade 3 laryngoscopy, bougie passed, esophageal intubation, removed

Attempt 3—ILMA #3; good ventilation, blind # 7.0 ETT passed, unsuccessful

Attempt 4—ILMA #3; ETT with FAST, successful

57.3.6 What are the problems with a difficult airway database or registry?

In principle, the difficult airway database has the potential to improve patient care and outcome. However, to establish a valid regional, national, or international difficult airway registry requires more than individual curiosity and enthusiasm. It needs dedication, time, and resources. For example, establishing and maintaining the national MedicAlert® Registry for Difficult Airway was prohibitively expensive.

Indeed, some have questioned the wisdom of setting up a MedicAlert® Registry in the United Kingdom.[15] Even though this study established that most anesthesia practitioners were willing to provide written details of a difficult airway to patients and their family physicians postoperatively, the authors argued that the time and effort entailed in a registration process may encourage non-compliance.

The dynamic nature of airway anatomy may also discourage some anesthesia practitioners from using a difficult airway registry. Hung and Morris pointed out that the anatomy of the upper airway changes with physiological conditions (e.g. pregnancy) or disease states.[16] In some cases, the changes can temporarily make laryngoscopic intubation more difficult. For example, it is well known that pregnancy, particularly if the parturient suffers from PIH (pregnancy induced hypertension; new name for preeclampsia), has a significant impact on the upper-airway edema, making laryngoscopy more difficult.[3] One would then logically question the usefulness of registering a patient in the difficult airway database after encountering an unanticipated difficult airway in an obstetrical patient as the etiology of the difficulty may disappear in the postpartum period. Similarly, one would question the usefulness of the Difficult Airway MedicAlert® bracelet in a morbidly obese patient who had a difficult airway and now, having lost more than 80% of the previous body weight, returns to have a general anesthetic for a pannectomy. Another example is a patient with a difficult airway secondary to lingual tonsillar hypertrophy, which was subsequently resected. And there are others.

While these issues ought to be addressed, they should not trivialize the critical importance of thorough documentation and dissemination of information that may prevent a lethal outcome. Furthermore, regardless of the history of a difficult airway, or the pathological airway conditions or surgeries of the head and neck that may have an impact on the airway anatomy, relevant-interval history, airway assessment (see Sections 1.6.1–1.6.4), and relevant documentation since the last airway intervention must be sought.

57.4   CASE REVISITED

The patient presented in the beginning of this chapter returned to the operating room 6 months later for a laparoscopic tubal ligation. Upon arrival at the same hospital, she was wearing a MedicAlert® stating "easy bag-mask-ventilation, difficult intubation." This was noted in the preoperative nursing assessment. In the preoperative holding area, the patient was interviewed by the anesthesia practitioner. The old medical record was obtained and the relevant anesthesia record was reviewed. The anesthesia practitioner noted on interview that the patient now weighed 90 kg and still denied reflux. Airway examination did not reveal any changes from her previous record. Prior to induction, the anesthesia practitioner had the difficult airway cart in the operating room and ensured that a colleague would be immediately available if needed. The anesthesia practitioner induced the patient and provided adequate ventilation using a BMV. Possessing the skill to use a Trachlight™, the anesthesia practitioner intubated the trachea of the patient without difficulty.

57.5   SUMMARY

Documentation is a critical part of airway management, particularly if it is a difficult or a failed airway. For every airway management event, the following should be recorded: (a) ease of BMV (if performed); (b) ease of ventilation with an extraglottic device (if used); (c) ease of laryngoscopy and intubation, including blade used, view obtained (Cormack/Lehane and/or the percentage of Glottic Opening), any adjunctive maneuvers used to obtain this view (e.g., head lift or external laryngeal manipulation); and (d) ease of the tube passage and size of ETT. If an alternative intubating technique was used (e.g., LMA Fastrach™), it should be documented with the reason why (e.g., "for skills maintenance purposes").

While some may question the cost-benefit of establishing difficult airway registries, it is the opinion of the author that thorough documentation and the dissemination of important information about a difficult airway will likely improve patient safety.

At any rate, regardless of the history of a difficult airway, the importance of careful airway assessment on each occasion in which airway management is required cannot be overemphasized.

REFERENCES

1. Yentis SM: Predicting difficult intubation—worthwhile exercise or pointless ritual? *Anaesthesia.* 2002;57:105–109.
2. Rose DK, Cohen MM: The airway: problems and predictions in 18500 patients. *Can J Anaesth.* 1994;41:372–383.
3. Samsoon GL, Young JR: Difficult tracheal intubation: a retrospective study. *Anaesthesia.* 1987;42:487–490.
4. Caplan RA, Posner KL, Ward RJ, Cheney FW: Adverse respiratory events in anesthesia: a closed claims analysis. *Anesthesiology.* 1990;72:828–833.
5. Cheney FW: Anesthesia patient safety and professional liability continue to improve. *ASA Newsletter.* 1997;61. Available at: www.asahq.org/newsletters/1997/06_97/Safety_Liability.html.
6. Practice guidelines for management of the difficult airway. A report by the American Society of Anesthesiologists Task Force on Management of the Difficult Airway. *Anesthesiology.* 1993;78:597–602.
7. Mark L, Gibby G, Fleisher L, et al.: Practice guidelines to clinical practices: medic alert difficult airway/intubation registry. *Anesthesiology.* 1994;81:A1222.
8. Foley L, Sands D, Feinstein D, Park KW: Effect of difficult airway registry on subsequent airway management: experience in the first two years of difficult airway registry. *Anesthesiology.* 1998;89:A1220.
9. Atkins RF: Simple method of tracking patients with difficult or failed tracheal intubation. *Anesthesiology.* 1995;83:1373–1374.
10. Pasqual RT, Troianos CA, Phillips CA, 3rd: Difficult airway warning with automated anesthesia recording. *Anesthesiology.* 1996;85:220.
11. Liban JB: Medic Alert UK should start new section for patients with a difficult airway. *BMJ.* 1996;313:425.
12. Practice guidelines for management of the difficult airway: an updated report by the American Society of Anesthesiologists Task Force on Management of the Difficult Airway. *Anesthesiology.* 2003;98:1269–1277.
13. Barron FA, Ball DR, Jefferson P, Norrie J: 'Airway Alerts'. How UK anaesthetists organise, document and communicate difficult airway management. *Anaesthesia.* 2003;58:73–77.
14. Crosby ET, Cooper RM, Douglas MJ, et al.: The unanticipated difficult airway with recommendations for management. *Can J Anaesth.* 1998;45:757–776.
15. Morris E, Osborne A, Jewkes C: Costs that would be incurred in establishing "difficult airway register" could be better spent. *BMJ.* 1996;313:1399.
16. Hung OR, Morris I: Dynamic anatomy of upper airway: an essential paradigm. *Can J Anaesth.* 2000;47:295–298.

SELF-EVALUATION QUESTIONS

57.1. Which of the following about the MedicAlert® bracelet for difficult airway is **NOT** true?

   A. The World Federation of Societies of Anesthesia and the American Academy of Otolaryngology—Head and Neck surgeons officially endorsed the MedicAlert® Foundation for difficult airway.

   B. The MedicAlert® Foundation developed a uniform database and specialized patient enrollment form for the Difficult Airway/Intubation category.

   C. The major objective of the MedicAlert® Registry was to develop mechanisms for a uniform documentation and dissemination of critical information to maximally protect patients.

   D. The MedicAlert® Registry is currently used worldwide.

   E. The "Difficult Airway/Intubation" has been used as a standardized nomenclature within the MedicAlert® identification since 1992.

57.2. Which of the following information should be documented following the management of an unanticipated difficult or failed airway?

A. date and type of operation

B. anatomic features of the patient on airway examination

C. ability to ventilate using a face mask or an extraglottic device

D. laryngoscopic view and the effectiveness of alternative intubating techniques

E. all of the above

57.3. Following the management of an unanticipated difficult airway, the anesthesia practitioner should inform about the difficult airway to all of the following **EXCEPT**

A. the patient

B. the primary care physician

C. the attending surgeon should be informed immediately following the difficult airway encounter

D. the MedicAlert® Difficult Airway Registry

E. a family member who is the caregiver of the patient

APPENDIX 57.1

Dear _____,

As we discussed during our postoperative visit, you did well under anesthesia. However, it was difficult to place a breathing tube into your windpipe. This is known as a difficult intubation. In addition, it was difficult to provide you ventilation through a face mask (or difficult mask ventilation). We wish to emphasize that at no time during this operation was your life at risk.

It will be important for you to inform future anesthesia practitioners of the difficulty placing a breathing tube. We also strongly advise you to enroll in the Medic Alert® Registry for difficult airway/intubations. This involves registering and paying a fee of $35. You will be issued an ID number, a wallet card, and one bracelet which will alert your medical personnel that you have a potentially difficult airway. You should also inform your relatives or close friends in the event that they need to provide this information on your behalf.

Please retain this letter in a safe place for future reference. Registering for the Medic-Alert® bracelet would be well advised. Please contact me for any further information or questions.

Sincerely,

Dr. _____

On the other side of this letter, the following relevant information ought to be recorded:

Date of operation

Type of operation

Hospital and medical record number

Anatomic features on airway examination which may have contributed to the problem, e.g., height, weight, Mallampati classification, mouth opening, thyromental span, limitations to head and neck mobility, etc.

Relevant medical conditions that may have contributed to the difficult airway, e.g., rheumatoid arthritis, diabetes, obesity, obstructive sleep apnea, etc.

Mask ventilation—easy, difficult, or impossible

Oral or nasal airway size if used

If direct laryngoscopy attempted, blade used, view obtained, number of attempts, use of adjuncts such as OELM or tracheal tube introducer, and whether or not successful

Ultimate disposition—whether the airway was secured awake or asleep and with which technique/instrument

Use of an extraglottic device as a rescue device

Any other comments

ANSWERS

CHAPTER 1
1.1.   D
1.2.   C
1.3.   B

CHAPTER 2
2.1.   A
2.2.   C
2.3.   E

CHAPTER 3
3.1.   B
3.2.   C
3.3.   E

CHAPTER 4
4.1.   C
4.2.   E
4.3.   C

CHAPTER 5
5.1.   C
5.2.   D
5.3.   E

CHAPTER 6
6.1.   E
6.2.   C
6.3.   C

CHAPTER 7
7.1.   D
7.2.   B
7.3.   C

CHAPTER 8
8.1.   E
8.2.   E
8.3.   E

CHAPTER 9
9.1.   A
9.2.   D
9.3.   A

CHAPTER 10
10.1.   D
10.2.   D
10.3.   C

CHAPTER 11
11.1.   A
11.2.   E
11.3.   C

CHAPTER 12
12.1.   D
12.2.   E
12.3.   D

CHAPTER 13
13.1. D
13.2. B
13.3. C

CHAPTER 14
14.1. E
14.2. E
14.3. B

CHAPTER 15
15.1. D
15.2. E
15.3. E

CHAPTER 16
16.1. D
16.2. D
16.3. D

CHAPTER 17
17.1. C
17.2. A
17.3. E

CHAPTER 18
18.1. C
18.2. A
18.3. E

CHAPTER 19
19.1. A
19.2. D
19.3. E

CHAPTER 20
20.1. D
21.2. C
22.3. D

CHAPTER 21
21.1. A
21.2. E
21.3. D

CHAPTER 22
22.1. E
22.2. A
22.3. C

CHAPTER 23
23.1. D
23.2. B
23.3. C

CHAPTER 24
24.1. E
24.2. C
24.3. E

CHAPTER 25
25.1. B
25.2. C
25.3. A

CHAPTER 26
26.1. D
26.2. A
26.3. C

CHAPTER 27
27.1. C
27.2. E
27.3. C

CHAPTER 28
28.1. D
28.2. A
28.3. C

CHAPTER 29
29.1. E
29.2. D
29.3. E

CHAPTER 30
30.1. D
30.2. E
30.3. E

CHAPTER 31
31.1. E
31.2. A
31.3. C

CHAPTER 32
32.1. D
32.2. D
32.3. E

CHAPTER 33
33.1. E
33.2. D
33.3. A

CHAPTER 34
34.1. A
34.2. E
34.3. D

CHAPTER 35
35.1. E
35.2. E
35.3. E

CHAPTER 36
36.1. A
36.2. A
36.3. C

CHAPTER 37
37.1. B
37.2. C
37.3. B

CHAPTER 38
38.1. B
38.2. E
38.3. E

CHAPTER 39
39.1. E
39.2. E
39.3. D

CHAPTER 40
40.1. B
40.2. D
40.3. A

CHAPTER 41
41.1. E
41.2. D
41.3. A

CHAPTER 42
42.1. C
42.2. E
42.3. D

CHAPTER 43
43.1. A
43.2. B
43.3. E

CHAPTER 44
44.1. A
44.2. D
44.3. B

CHAPTER 45
45.1. C
45.2. E
45.3. E

CHAPTER 46
46.1. C
46.2. C
46.3. E

CHAPTER 47
47.1. C
47.2. B
47.3. D

CHAPTER 48
48.1. A
48.2. C
48.3. E

CHAPTER 49
49.1. D
49.2. D
49.3. A

CHAPTER 50
50.1. A
50.2. D
50.3. E

CHAPTER 51
51.1. E
51.2. A
51.3. E

CHAPTER 52
52.1. C
52.2. C
52.3. C

CHAPTER 53
53.1. B
53.2. A
53.3. C

CHAPTER 54
54.1. C
54.2. A
54.3. C

CHAPTER 55
55.1. B
55.2. E
55.3. B

CHAPTER 56
56.1. E
56.2. E
56.3. E

CHAPTER 57
57.1. D
57.2. E
57.3. D

INDEX

Note: Page numbers followed by *f* indicate figures; those followed by *t* indicate tables.